1 MONTH OF FREE READING

at

www.ForgottenBooks.com

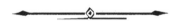

By purchasing this book you are eligible for one month membership to ForgottenBooks.com, giving you unlimited access to our entire collection of over 1,000,000 titles via our web site and mobile apps.

To claim your free month visit:

www.forgottenbooks.com/free660711

ISBN 978-0-428-93018-9
PIBN 10660711

THE

EDICAL NEWS.

A Weekly Medical Journal

EDITED BY

SMITH ELY JELLIFFE, AM., M.D., PH.D.

VOLUME 86.

MARCH
JANUARY—JUNE. 1905.

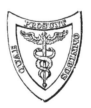

NEW YORK:
LEA BROTHERS & CO.
1905.

THE MEANY PRINTING CO.
NEW YORK

CONTRIBUTORS

TO

VOLUME EIGHTY-SIX

WILLIAM ACKERMANN, M.D., Milwaukee, Wis.
LOUIS C. AGER, M.D., Brooklyn, N. Y.
H. A. ALDERTON, M.D., Brooklyn, N. Y.
ELLICE M. ALGER, M.D., New York.
J. M. ANDERS, M.D., LL.D., Philadelphia.
E. ANDRADE, M.D., Jacksonville, Fla.
CHAMPE S. ANDREWS. Esq., New York.
EDWARD B. ANGELL. M.D., Rochester, N. Y.
JOHN P. ARNOLD, M.D., Philadelphia.
F. W. BAESLACK, B.A., Buffalo, N. Y.
L. BOLTON BANGS, M.D., New York.
W. A. BASTEDO, Ph.G., M.D., New York.
WILLIAM M. BEACH. A.M., M.D., Pittsburg, Pa.
A. L. BENEDICT, A.M., M.D., Buffalo, N. Y.
WM. N. BERKELEY, A.B., M.D., New York.
A. C. BERNAYS, M.D., St. Louis, Mo.
EUGENE P. BERNSTEIN, M.D., New York.
RUSSELL H. BOGGS, M.D., Pittsburg, Pa.
S. G. BONNEY, A.M., M.D., Denver, Col.
JOHN H. BORDEN, A.M., M.D., New York.
GEORGE EMERSON BREWER, M.D., New York.
F. TILDEN BROWN, M.D., New York.
W. SOHIER BRYANT, M.D., New York.
WILLIAM J. BUTLER. M.D., Chicago.
HIRAM BYRD, M.D., Jacksonville, Fla.
FOLLEN CABOT. M.D., New York.
C. N. B. CAMAC, A.B., M.D., New York.
R. BISHOP CANFIELD, M.D., Ann Arbor, Mich.
WALTER B. CANNON, M.D., Boston, Mass.
WILLIAM FITCH CHENEY, M.D., San Francisco, Cal.
JAMES S. CHENOWETH, M.D., Louisville, Ky.
RUSSELL H. CHITTENDEN, Ph.D., LL.D., New Haven, Conn.
MARGARET A. CLEAVES. M.D., New York.
J. R. CLEMENS. M.D., St. Louis, Mo.
G. H. A. CLOWES, Ph.D., Buffalo, N. Y.
C. G. COAKLEY, M.D., New York.
LEWIS GREGORY COLE, M.D., New York.
CHAS. F. CRAIG, M.D., San Francisco, Cal.
WILLIAM J. CRUIKSHANK, M.D., Brooklyn, N. Y.
COLMAN W. CUTLER. M.D., New York.
CHARLES L. DANA, M.D., New York.
THOMAS DARLINGTON. M.D., New York.
C. F. DAVIDSON, M.D., Baltimore, Md.
A. EDWARD DAVIS, A.M., M.D., New York.
CHARLES DENISON, A.M., M.D., Denver, Col.
GEORGE C. DIEKMAN. M.D., Ph.G., New York.
FRANK DONALDSON, M.D., San Francisco, Cal.
JULIUS DONATH, M.D., Budapest, Hungary.
ALVAH H. DOTY, M.D., New York.
CHARLES W. EDMUNDS, A.B., M.D., Ann Arbor, Mich.
GEORGE ELLIOTT, M.D., Toronto, Can.
A. G. ELLIS, M.D., Philadelphia.

CHARLES A. ELSBERG. M.D., New York.
HENRY L. ELSNER, M.D., Syracuse, N. Y.
LEONARD W. ELY, M.D., New York.
JOHN F. ERDMANN, M.D., New York.
L. A. EWALD, M.D., New York.
SIMON FLEXNER. M.D., New York.
SAMUEL FLOERSHEIM, M.D., New York. ,
W. W. FORD, M.D., Baltimore, Md.
GEORGE RYERSON FOWLER. M.D., Brooklyn, N. Y.
J. M. FRANKENBURGER, M.D., Kansas City., Mo.
MILTON FRANKLIN, M.D., New York.
HENRY W. FRAUENTHAL. M.D., New York.
ROWLAND GODFREY FREEMAN, M.D., New York.
JOHN FUNKE. M.D., Philadelphia.
HARVEY R. GAYLORD, M.D., Buffalo, N. Y.
C. L. GIBSON. M.D., New York.
E. W. GOULD. M.D., New York.
CHARLES R. GRANDY, M.D., Norfolk, Va.
FRANK C. HAMMOND, M.D., Philadelphia.
T. W. HASTINGS, M.D., New York.
J. B. HAWES, M.D., Boston, Mass.
O. HENSEL, M.D., New York.
C. D. HILL, A.B.. M.D., Jersey City, N. J.
EDWARD C. HILL. M.D., Denver, Col.
L. EMMETT HOLT, M.D., New York.
FRANCIS HUBER, M.D., New York.
R. R. HUGGINS, M.D., Pittsburg, Pa.
WILLIAM E. HUGHES, M.D., Philadelphia.
J. RAMSAY HUNT, M.D., New York.
J. M. INGE, M.D., Denton, Texas.
NATHAN JACOBSON. M.D., Syracuse, N. Y.
HERMAN JARECKY, M.D., New York.
NEWTON JAMES. M.D., New York.
SMITH ELY JELLIFFE. M.D., New York.
RICHARD H. JOHNSTON, M.D., Baltimore, Md.
DAVID M. KAPLAN, M.D., New York.
HOWARD A. KELLY, M.D., Baltimore, Md.
J. A. KELLY, M.D., New York.
E. L. KEYES, JR., M.D., New York.
HERMANN G. KLOTZ, M.D., New York.
WALTER C. KLOTZ, M.D., New York.
MARK I. KNAPP, M.D., New York.
GEORGE W. KOSMAK, M.D., New York.
CHARLES KNAPP LAW, M.D., Jersey City, N. J.
JAMES A. LE ROY, ESQ., Durango, Mexico.
HOWARD LILIENTHAL, M.D., New York.
LEO LOEB, M.D., Philadelphia.
FRANK B. LORING, M.D., Washington, D. C.
W. P. MacCALLUM. M.D., Baltimore, Md.
FRANK MARTIN, M.D., Baltimore, Md.
J. W. D. MAURY, M.D., New York.
T. M. T. McKENNAN, M.D., Pittsburg. Pa.
J. W. McLAUGHLIN, M.D., Galveston, Texas.

H. D. MEEKER, M.D., New York.
LAFAYETTE MENDEL, Ph.D., New Haven, Conn.
ALFRED MEYER. M.D., New York.
JAMES ALEXANDER MILLER. A.M., M.D., New York.
A. C. MORGAN. M.D., Philadelphia.
ROGER S. MORRIS. A.B., M.D., Ann Arbor, Mich.
PRINCE A. MORROW, A.M., M.D., New York.
WILLIAM JAMES MORTON, M.D., New York.
JOHN C. MUNRO, M.D., Boston. Mass.
HIDEYO NOGUCHI, M.D., New York.
W. P. NORTHRUP, M.D., New York.
W. B. NOYES. M.D., New York.
MAURICE PACKARD, A.M., M.D., New York.
RALPH WAIT PARSONS, M.D., Ossining, N. Y.
GEORGE L. PEABODY. M.D., New York.
FREDERICK PETERSON, M.D., New York.
R. E. PICK, M. D., New York.
HENRY G. PIFFARD, M.D., New York.
J. L. POMEROY, M.D., New York.
A. M. POND, M.D., Webster City, Iowa.
JACOB B. PRAGER, M.D., New York.
CHARLES C. RANSOM, M.D., New York.
A. ROVINSKY, M.D., New York.
ALBERT E. SELLENINGS, M.D., New York.
J. GARLAND SHERRILL, A.M., M.D., Louisville, Ky.
E. MATHER SILL. M.D., New York.
CHARLES E. SIMON, M.D., Baltimore, Md.
JUSTUS SINEXON, M.D., Philadelphia.
ANDREW H. SMITH, M.D., New York.
JACOB SOBEL. M.D., New York.
FREDERIC E. SONDERN, M.D., New York.
GEORGE A. SOPER, Ph.D., New York.
ALEXANDER SPINGARN, A.M., M.D., New York.
J. BENTLEY SQUIER, M.D., New York.
GEORGE W. STONER, M.D., New York.

ARNOLD STURMDORF, M.D., New York.
D. F. TALLEY, M.D., Birmingham, Ala. ·
ALFRED S. TAYLOR. M.D., New York.
J. MADISON TAYLOR. A.B., M.D., Philadelphia.
W, GILMAN THOMPSON, M.D., New York.
WILLIAM HANNA THOMSON, M.D., LL.D., New York.
S. W. S. TOMS, M.D., Nyack-on-Hudson, N. Y.
FRANCIS VALK, M.D., New York.
FRANK VAN FLEET, M.D., New York.
ROY M. VAN WART, B.A., M.D., C.M., New Orleans, La.
KARL M. VOGEL, M.D., New York.
JOHANNES H. M. A. VON TILING, M.D., Poughkeepsie, N. Y.
I. W. VOORHEES, M.D., New York.
JAMES D. VOORHEES, M.D., New York.
JONATHAN M. WAINWRIGHT, M.D., Scranton, Pa.
W. K. WALKER, M.D., Dixmont, Pa.
GROESBECK WALSH, M.D., Chicago.
JAMES J. WALSH, M.D., Ph.D., New York.
GEORGE GRAY WARD, Jr., M.D., New York.
NATHAN G. WARD, M.D., Philadelphia.
HARRY T. WEIL, M.D., Baltimore, Md.
RICHARD WEIL, M.D., New York.
EDWARD F. WELLS. M.D., Chicago.
J. SHERMAN WIGHT, B.S., M.D., Broklyn, N. Y.
ENNION G. WILLIAMS, M.D., Richmond, Va.
LINSLY R. WILLIAMS, M.D., New York.
ROBERT N. WILLSON, M.D., Philadelphia.
J. T. WILSON. M.D., Sherman, Texas.
RANDOLPH WINSLOW, M.D., Baltimore, Md.
CLARENCE A. WRIGHT, F.R.C.S., F.F.P.S.G., Leydenstone, England.
JONATHAN WRIGHT, M.D., New York.
WALTER WYMAN, M.D., Washington, D. C.

THE MEDICAL NEWS.

A WEEKLY JOURNAL OF MEDICAL SCIENCE.

VOL. 86.　　　NEW YORK, SATURDAY, JANUARY 7, 1905.　　　NO. 1.

ORIGINAL ARTICLES.

DISTURBANCES OF DIGESTION IN INFANTS RESULTING FROM THE USE OF TOO HIGH FAT PERCENTAGES.

BY L. EMMETT HOLT, M.D.,

OF NEW YORK;

PROFESSOR OF PEDIATRICS IN THE COLLEGE OF PHYSICIANS AND SURGEONS (COLUMBIA UNIVERSITY), NEW YORK.

THAT serious disturbances of digestion in infants may be due to an excess of any of the milk constituents in the food employed, is a trite remark, and is the daily experience of all who see much of the results of infant feeding. The practitioners and the skilled nurses who direct the feeding of infants have come pretty generally to appreciate the symptoms which usually follow too high proteids, to understand what percentages of proteids an average infant may be expected to digest under given conditions, and how these percentages may be secured in the various milk formulas used. With the methods of home modifications of milk now in vogue, it is probably true that the proteid percentages of our formulas have been rather lower than higher than we have calculated, but often to the decided advantage of the patient.

But how is it with the fat? Personally I have reached the conclusion that disturbances of digestion resulting from an excess of fat are quite as serious, if no quite so obvious, as those which follow the use of too high proteids, and that they need to be studied just as carefully. Even those who give special attention to infant feeding have been slow to learn the infant's capacity with respect to the digestion of fat, both in health and in the ever varying conditions of disease. Others who have given the question less attention have fallen into error in one of two ways: In following the formulas of the books, instead of using an ordinary milk, with a fat content of 4 per cent., they have substituted a rich Jersey milk containing from 5 to 5.5 per cent. fat. Thus unwittingly they have given from 5 to 7 per cent. fat when they have supposed they were giving a food containing 3.5 or 4 per cent. Or, they have made another mistake of intentionally increasing the fat, almost without limit, for the purpose of overcoming that most troublesome symptom in artificial feeding—chronic constipation.

Errors like these are exceedingly common and their consequences may be very serious. It is the purpose of the present paper to record some of the results seen with such feeding, all of the cases cited having come under observation in private practice in the course of a few months.

Case I.—Overfeeding with high fats, rapid increase in weight and progress in development till eight months; then general convulsions followed later by tetany, laryngismus stridulus, fatty liver (?). Recovery after three months illness. —In February, 1904, I was asked by a physician to see a baby of a medical friend whose feeding he had directed. The child had been considered a magnificent specimen of physical development, and a great triumph of the feeding art, until one week before my visit, at which time his weight, at eight months old, was twenty-one pounds. In the previous 3½ months he had gained ten pounds. The child had bright rosy cheeks; was strong in his muscles, already pulling himself up by the side of his crib and bearing his weight on his feet; and was, for his age, well advanced mentally. He seldom vomited; had a good appetite, and was taking until a few weeks before I saw him, seven feedings of six ounces each, but lately only six feedings, of a mixture made up as follows:

The upper sixteen ounces were taken from each of two quarts of a rich Jersey milk (Briarcliff Dairy) : twenty-four ounces of this top milk were used in a forty-ounce mixture. Examination of the top milk used showed it to contain 10 per cent. fat ; so that the baby was receiving in his food not less than 6 per cent. fat. With this food the bowels usually moved twice a day, the passages being smooth, large and yellow. An occasional restless night and some transient urticaria were the only clouds in the otherwise clear sky until February 16, when a stool not well digested was reported, with loss of appetite. These were not enough to make necessary any change in food.

The following morning, one hour after feeding, the child had a severe general convulsion which lasted from six to eight minutes, followed by a second one three hours later. The stomach was promptly washed out and all food stopped; calomel given and later castor oil, then bromide of soda. Five loose stools following this treatment, none of them especially foul. There was no rise of temperature and no signs of serious illness. The following day, as no unfavorable symptoms had occurred, the previous food was begun, but much diluted, the proportions being one part of the food to five parts of water. The strength of the food was gradually increased, so that at the end of four days the baby was taking five ounces of his original food diluted with only one ounce of water. During the next night some severe pain occurred, ascribed to colic: the next morning the temperature was 104.5° F. I saw him first early in the afternoon. He was, as he had been described, a splendid-looking child. The fat lay in great folds over his body and extremities. Fontanel large, but no other evidences of rickets; no teeth. Liver much enlarged, the lower border being nearly two inches below the costal margin. Hands and feet in typical position of tetany, considerable muscular rigidity, movements painful, temperature 103.5° F.

A second clearing out of the intestinal tract was advised, and the first stool passed was examined chemically and found to consist of almost pure fat. All food was omitted for one day, all milk for a week, and then very low fat percentages given. The tetany gradually passed away, but was followed three weeks later by laryngismus stridulus which continued for nearly three weeks. There was much trouble with the digestion for the next two months and the child lost five pounds in weight. When last seen, 3½ months after his severe attacks, he was digesting well and thriving, but his weight was only nineteen pounds.

Several points of interest in this case deserve attention: (1) the long period during which the child bore the high percentage of fat without any apparent disturbance; (2) the severity of the nervous symptoms, the suddenness with which they came on and their long duration; (3) the prolonged disturbance of the digestion and general nutrition; (4) the large liver (paté de foie gras?) and stools consisting of almost pure fat.

Case II.—Prolonged feeding with high fat, notwithstanding which constipation and the development of moderate rickets, followed by acute disturbances of digestion with repeated convulsions.

This patient was also seen in consultation within a few days of Case I, and the symptoms presented many points of similarity. The milk used was from the same dairy; it was prepared after almost the same formula, except that the percentage of fat in the food as given was only 5 per cent. The patient was the first child of healthy parents, nursed for three months, had suffered somewhat from facial eczema at six months, after which barley water had been substituted for plain water as a diluent. For the past month the child had been taking the following formula:

℞ Top milk .... 19 oz.
  Barley water 21
  Sugar of milk........ 4 even tablespoonfuls
  Milk of magnesia ..... 1 teaspoonful

The top milk was the upper sixteen ounces from one quart of rich Jersey milk and had been estimated by the physician to contain 7 per cent. fat. The child was taking six ounces every three hours. With the addition of the magnesia the bowels moved regularly but the stools were pale yellow. The formula begun after weaning had been a similar one with a little lower proportion of milk. The baby was gaining from six to eight ounces a week and his weight at the time of my visit, when he was eight month old, was 18¾ pounds. There had been no vomiting, the child

had a good appetite, slept well, and was considered to be in the best of health.

One week before my examination, without any change in the food or other assignable cause, the child had a slight convulsion in the evening. The following morning a second and more severe one. The temperature was elevated up to 103° F., and the child gave the appearance of being seriously ill. Food was stopped, the bowels cleared with calomel followed by magnesia, and the temperature quickly fell to normal. The child improved rapidly, and he was put back on his previous food, at first diluted, but strengthened daily until at the end of three or four days it was two-thirds the original strength. One week after the first convulsions, he had a third, and later in the day two more. I saw him in the evening. He presented all the appearance of a splendid, healthy, well-developed child with bright red cheeks, plenty of fat and muscles well developed. The head was well-shaped but craniotabes was present; no teeth. Physical examination otherwise negative. All food was stopped for twenty-four hours and a second clearing with calomel ordered. All milk was stopped for a week and then a mixture containing a low fat substituted. Three months later I saw the child again. He had one convulsion six weeks after the first group, apparently from a slight attack of indigestion. At the last visit he was in excellent condition, still no teeth at eleven months, with moderate head sweats, but general condition otherwise excellent. The craniotabes had disappeared.

It was interesting to note the development of rickets and the presence of constipation, in spite of the excessive amount of fat which his food had contained ever since he had been weaned at three months.

Case III.—Overfeeding with high fat—Convulsions.—This was an office patient, six months old, the second child of healthy parents, whose weight at birth was reported as 8¾ pounds. The mother had nursed for a few weeks then discontinued on account of illness. The child had been fed upon a milk modified at home, the proportions of which were stated to be as follows:

Milk 12   ounces
Cream .... 4½ ounces
Lime water .... 1½ ounces
Water 14   ounces

The child was given 5½ ounces every three hours. The cream used was examined and found to contain 35 per cent. fat. The proportion of fat in the food was thus about 6.75 per cent. Upon this mixture the child had gained very rapidly in weight, had had from three to four yellowish stools daily, occasionally containing masses called curds, and its progress had been considered most satisfactory until the age of four months. There had been some vomiting, but this had never been very troublesome. At four months old a severe general convulsion occurred lasting twenty minutes; a second convulsion, two hours later. The food was reduced to a mixture of equal parts of milk and water, which was continued for a few days; but as the child did not gain as rapidly as before the mother, on her own responsibility, had returned to the original formula. The father, a dentist, being convinced that the convulsions were from dentition, ascribed great benefit to gum-lancing which was practised. After the first convulsion the general condition was not so good, slight symptoms of indigestion were present—regurgitation of food many times a day, much flatulence and stools usually yellow but occasionally green. Examination showed a moderately fat infant, pale, flabby without signs of rickets.

The cream was omitted from the formula and milk substituted, reducing the proportion of fat to about 2 per cent. The child made satisfactory progress from this time, had no further convulsions and its symptoms of indigestion rapidly disappeared.

Case IV.—Habitual vomiting aggravated by high fat; serious gastric catarrh produced; finally cured by stomach washing.—This was an infant, ten months old, also seen in consultation. The chief symptoms in this case were continued wasting with persistent vomiting. The vomiting had begun almost from birth and had been a most troublesome symptom up to the time of my visit. A great variety of infant foods and milk formulas had been employed, none with any very great success. Up to the eighth month the food had been, for the greater part of the time, barley water and condensed milk. For the past two months the child had been in the care of a physician who is enthusiastic in the feeding of high fats. The formula used had been:

Top milk	17 ounces
Water	13 ounces
Lime water	2 ounces

The child was given four feedings, seven ounces each; the interval between feedings, four hours. Occasionally an extra feeding was given during the night. The top milk was the upper seventeen ounces from one quart of the Briarcliff milk. According to two analyses of similar samples, the food contained as given about 5.30 per cent. fat. During the two months that the child had been on this diet, his weight had fallen from 9 pounds 8 ounces, to 8 pounds 4 ounces. His vomiting had not improved, in fact had grown steadily worse. Now not only was food rejected, but frequently mucus in large amounts at some time almost every day. The child had never had any acute disturbance of digestion; the bowels were constipated.

Examination showed a typical marasmus child. Head 16 inches, chest 14¼ inches, length 23½, and weight 8 pounds 4 ounces; at ten months his weight being only 2¾ pounds more than at birth. After one or two minor changes the child was put upon the following:

Plain milk	18 ounces
Water	7 ounces
Lime water	5 ounces

This was peptonized. He was given 5 ounces every four hours; five feedings daily. Stomach washing was begun, at first daily and then every other day. Large amounts of mucus, often as much as two ounces at a time were removed. With the stomach washing the mucus rapidly disappeared and the quantity and strength of the food were increased. The stomach washing was continued at longer intervals for a period of nearly two months during which time the weight steadily increased. At the end of four months he had gained 6¼ pounds. The progress from this time was rapid and uneventful and one year afterward the child was reported by the attending physician to be in robust health.

The condition had been in this case persistent gastric indigestion with excessive fermentation continuing until a gastric catarrh of serious proportion had developed. The high fat mixture which had been ordered had greatly aggravated this condition, and the state of the child at my first visit was really an alarming one.

Case V.—Feeding with high fat; eczema, habitual constipation, and finally habitual vomiting.—This case is an illustration of a very rapid gain in weight and subsequent development of serious digestive disturbance from very high fat. The child at birth was very large and robust, his weight being 11½ pounds. He had increased rapidly and at eight weeks old his weight was 15 pounds, at three months it was 17 pounds 10 ounces. The weekly gain during the greater part of the time was from 12 to 15 ounces. The formula used had been:

Top milk	24 ounces
Lime water	2 ounces
Water	22 ounces
Mellin's food	3 tablespoonfuls

The Mellin's food had been added to overcome the chronic constipation. The top milk consisted of 12 ounces removed from each of two quarts of the Briarcliff milk, the same dairy as that which supplied the milk in three of the preceding cases. The proportion of fat in the food given was approximately 7 per cent. The mother reported that the child had always been constipated, and that he had had no natural movement for three weeks, enemas or glycerin suppositories being usually required to induce one. The stools passed were large, dry, and a light yellow color. There had been a good deal of straining and finally a rectal prolapse had developed. The vomiting at first had been slight but recently had greatly increased until it had become very troublesome and was repeated several times each day. He had an excellent appetite and seemed never quite satisfied with the food given. A troublesome eczema of the face had appeared about the third month.

It was interesting in this case to see that the

constipation greatly improved when the fat in the food was reduced to 4 per cent.; but it was not entirely overcome until the fat was reduced to 3 per cent. The symptoms of indigestion and eczema continued to be troublesome for the next two to three months but no serious symptoms occurred, and the progress on the whole was satisfactory.

It would be easy from my records of private patients to multiply almost indefinitely examples of acute and chronic disturbances of digestion in infants from the use of too high fat. Those cited, however, illustrate the most frequent and the most serious types. Often the very rapid and unusual gain in weight goes on steadily until the acute upset comes. In other cases the results of such feeding are shown in a gradual loss of appetite, sometimes so complete that for weeks a child will hardly take one-third of his former food. The increase in weight now ceases and there may even be a steady but a slow loss. In such cases the infant seems to take into his own hands the matter of cutting down his food and thus prevents serious acute disturbances of digestion.

That gastric disturbances—habitual vomiting or regurgitation of food, continued fermentation and finally the production of a gastric catarrh—may follow the use of very high fat has often been emphasized; but it is not so generally appreciated that disturbances of intestinal digestion may also occur, and that even chronic constipation may be greatly aggravated by such feeding. The hard, dry, gray stools passed under these conditions frequently consist almost entirely of undigested fat. Steadily raising the proportion of fat because of the constipation is the plan often followed, and this makes matters worse.

Severe nervous symptoms such as occurred in several of the cases have not in my experience been very frequently seen from this cause, and I do not feel convinced that the form of auto-intoxication present was entirely due to the fats, although this is possible. The symptoms were not very different from those which accompany other forms of acute digestive disturbance.

There are some practical conclusions to be drawn from these cases. It is evident that the errors into which both physicians and patients have usually fallen have resulted from their fondness for rich Jersey milk and cream. Although there is pretty general agreement among those who have given special study to the question of infant feeding that milk from other herds, containing from 4 to 4¼ per cent. fat, is better, still a great majority of the profession and the public will turn from such milk as being thin and blue to the rich yellow product of the Jersey or Alderney herd. I believe that one of the chief causes of failure in feeding from the milk laboratory has been the use of too high fat, it being so easy for a physician under these circumstances to increase the fat percentage, particularly if his mind has been filled with the idea that thereby chronic constipation is likely to be overcome.

Mistakes like those above described may be avoided if the physician knows approximately the fat content of the milk, cream or top milk which he is using. Too often he falls into error by disregarding this entirely and treating all specimens of milk and cream alike, using them in the formulas which he may have obtained from some book. More definite results may be obtained in several ways. In the first place, the physician may obtain from the milk laboratory a cream or milk of a definite fat percentage and thus be able to calculate closely the amount of fat which his patient is taking in the formula given. Or he may himself examine the milk, top milk or cream which his patients are using. His advice is generally asked in the choice of the milk supply and if he habitually uses milk from the same dairy he can be fairly certain of his results. Such examinations with the Babcock tester or some of its modifications can be made in a few minutes, or a specimen may be sent to a laboratory and the fat determination had for one dollar.

In order to interpret correctly the result of these milk examinations he must learn to think in percentages. In no other way can one form any idea of how much fat he is giving. Although a little difficult at first it soon becomes easy. To a student of medicine there does not seem to be very much difference between a temperature of 103° F. and one of 106° F., yet how different is the meaning they convey to the practitioner. In the same way milk percentages at first signify little to one unaccustomed to using them, and where the increase is made by percentages at the milk laboratory often the most injurious combinations are ordered. A friend told me of a physician who was feeding his own child on milk from the laboratory. The formula used was one containing 3 per cent. fat. As the child was not gaining very well he decided that an increase was needed and ordered milk containing 6 per cent. fat. He then abused the laboratory because his baby's digestion had been upset by the milk.

As to how much fat may be wisely given to infants in health, opinions may perhaps differ somewhat. I am not sure that any arbitrary standard can be fixed. Children differ very much in their capacity to digest fats as in other respects; but there is a limit with each child beyond which he may not safely go. If the percentage is raised very much above this for any length of time, disturbances are almost certain to follow. Personally I have never seen any advantage, but often much harm, from raising the fat above 4 per cent., and in my own practice I have fixed upon this as about the limit for the average child.

The physician who assumes to direct the feeding of infants must have some notion of what is proper; must know what he is giving and must appreciate the difference between giving a food which contains 3 or 4 per cent. fat and one containing 6 or 7 per cent. Although the bad results of the higher percentages may not be at once apparent they are almost certain to come later. Furthermore, simply to raise the percentage of fat seldom relieves chronic constipation; and, finally, whenever there are marked symptoms of either gastric or intestinal indigestion, the fat should be reduced much below the normal 3 or 4 per cent.

14 West Fifty-fifth Street.

MEDICAL QUACKS, THEIR METHODS AND DANGERS.

BY CHAMPE S. ANDREWS, ESQ.,

OF NEW YORK;

COUNSEL MEDICAL SOCIETY COUNTY OF NEW YORK.

"Where I killed one, a fair square death
By loss o' blood, or want o' breath,
This night I'm free to take my oath
　　That Hornbook's skill
Has clad a score i' their last cloth
　　By drop and pill."

"That's just a swatch o' Hornbook's way,
Thus goes he on from day to day,
Thus does he poison, kill and slay,
　　An's weel paid for't;
Yet stops me o' my lawful prey,
　　Wi' pills and dirt."

WHEN Burns, in his inimitable satire, selected Death as the one to expose the dangers of "Dr. Hornbook's" ignorant methods, he chose the one who had the best opportunities for accurate observation. The crimes laid by Death at the door of Doctor Hornbook, were terrible indeed, but it is not difficult to duplicate them over and over in the official records of actual crime as found in the proceedings of our Criminal Courts.

In November, 1808, one Samuel Thompson came into Beverly, Mass., and, proclaiming his ability to heal the sick without fail, declared that the country was being ruined by the regular physician. As his experience with the credulous warranted him in believing, there were those, even in enlightened Massachusetts, who took him at his word. Patients flocked to him by the score. Ezra Lovett, Jr., finding himself confined to bed by a cold, sent for the now celebrated Thompson. He came, and, I have no doubt, received his pay in advance. "Dr." Thompson had the patient's room heated as hot as the stove could make it. And the report of the case, found in 6 Mass. 134 *et seq.*, tells us in great detail of the healer's methods:

"He then placed the feet of the deceased, with his shoes off, on a stove of hot coals, and wrapped him in a thick blanket covering his head. In this situation he gave him a powder in water, which immediately puked him. Three minutes after he repeated the dose, which in about two minutes operated violently. He again repeated the dose, which in a short time operated with more violence. These powders were all given within the space of half an hour, the patient in the meantime drinking copiously of a warm decoction which the 'Dr.' called 'coffee.'

"The 'coffee' administered was a decoction of marsh-rosemary, mixed with the bark of bayberry bush. The powders called by the 'Dr.' 'well-my-gristle' and 'ram-cats,' which the prisoner said he chiefly relied upon in his practice, and which was the emetic so often administered by him to the patient was the pulverized plant trivially called 'Indian tobacco,' four grains of which was a powerful puke and cathartic."

The report goes on to relate that the learned physician ordered his patient to sleep in a warm bed, "where he lay in a profuse sweat all night." The next (Tuesday) afternoon more powders of "well-my-gristle" and "ram-cats" were administered in quick succession, washed down by "coffee." On Wednesday the patient's face and hands were rubbed with rum and he was given fifteen minutes of nature cure by exposure to the January winds in the open air. As a reward more ram-cats were washed down by more coffee. With variations this heroic treatment continued until the following Monday, when the "Dr." was specially summoned as the patient insisted he was dying.

Pearlash, "coffee" and "well-my-gristle" were administered in quick succession and the patient was asked how far the medicine had gotten down. "The patient, laying his hand on his heart, answered "here," when the "doctor" observed that the "medicine would soon get down and unscrew his vitals." It did. Between nine and ten o'clock convulsions set in, the patient lost his reason, and on the next day, after one week's treatment, Ezra Lovett, Jr., died.

The object of this article is not to point out the history and present status of the law governing illegal practice or the rules governing the trial of a quack charged with manslaughter or murder. Its object is to point out, by concrete example the great dangers resulting from the practice of the quack, and the crying necessity for the enforcement of the laws designed to protect the public against these dangers.

The law books are full of instructive cases, illustrating, among other things, how slowly the courts have progressed in a realization of the fraud and danger always present in the practice of the unlicensed practitioners.

The methods of the old time charlatan can be studied in such cases as Rice *vs.* The State (8 Mo. 561), State *vs.* Schulz (55 Ia. 628), Commonwealth *vs.* Pierce (138 Mass. 165), and many other cases both in this country and in England, too numerous to mention. But the methods of criminal practitioners of this modern day are far more interesting, and show invention and creative genius worthy of a good cause. "Doctor Thompson" and his methods would be scorned by the astute and polished medical fakir of to-day.

THE MODERN CHARLATAN.

As education has become more generally diffused and science more advanced, the medical charlatan has changed his methods to correspond with the new order of things. The modern endeavor is to imitate the true scientific methods, and, with "a little learning" to make louder claims to specialized knowledge and advanced methods than does the regular practitioner. Strange as it may seem to know that "Dr." Thompson could have deceived anybody even a hundred years ago, the helpless and afflicted in these opening years of the Twentieth Century are victimizd more completely and more artistically than was Ezra Lovett, Jr. Indeed the modern methods of advertising, the rapidity with which the false claims of the charlatan can be disseminated, and the ease with which the post-office and newspaper penetrate every section of the country have given the fakir of to-day a field of operation that "Doctor Thompson" never dared to contemplate.

THE HELPLESSNESS OF THE CHARLATANS' VICTIMS.

As one learns in detail of the methods and dangers of the modern quack, there is at first a tendency to believe that the credulity of mankind is growing alarmingly greater, but a deeper study of the subject shows that the credulity upon which the charlatan relies, is the credulity that arises from weakened powers of resistance, from disordered minds, and from the mirage that such minds see mirrored in the clear sky of hope. The victim of the medical mountebank, by reason of his susceptibilities and infirmities, is in a class to himself and should have the especial care and protection of the State.

The gambler for the most part takes away from his victims only that which the victim can again recover by prudence and industry. The political mountebank may lead the people away from the honest path for a time, but the wandering in time generally proves self-corrective. The religious frauds exist for a season with fashionable following, but in the end he talks to empty benches. The victims of the medical charlatan, however, have nothing like the same chance to retrieve their false steps as the victims of the other fakirs mentioned. The patients of the quack are either hypochondriacs, who remain eternally ill in their own diseased imaginations and furnish a never-failing harvest for the scythe of the charlatan, or else by reason of genuine maladies their power of resistance has gone and the illusions of hope created by marvelous claims and extravagant promises cause them to grasp at every cure-all just as the drowning man grasps at a straw.

In the City of New York, the danger of the charlatan is seen at its worst. The thickly settled neighborhoods where the ignorant foreigner resides are hot-beds of unlicensed and illegal practitioners, while the advertisements unblushingly accepted by a majority of New York newspapers, with their enormous circulation both in and out of the city, furnish the widest possible field for the modern quack, whose very life lies in newspaper publicity.

MEDICAL SOCIETY OF THE COUNTY OF NEW YORK.

The State of New York, in 1806, perceived the necessity of protecting the public against empirical methods in medicine, and organized in that year, by a special charter which continues to this day, the Medical Society of the State of New York with its branch society in each county of the State. The act was entitled "An Act to Regulate the Practice of Physic and Surgery."

In later years these various county societies have, to a greater or less extent, been the only organized bodies standing between the charlatan and his victim. Theoretically, the Police Department and the District Attorney's Office are charged with the prosecution of all offenses, but where life is as complex as in the City of New York, and where the regular departments of the government charged with the suppression of crime are busy with crimes of murder, arson, larceny and the more heinous crimes generally, it is found impossible in practice for these departments to suppress the unlicensed practitioners of medicine. The presence of a body composed of the organized medical profession engaged, with the sanction of the State, in suppressing not only the criminal practitioner who is licensed, but also the practitioner without a license, is a salutary force in the community and commands, I believe, the respect and confidence of the public and acts as a constant deterrent to the wrong-doer.

The Medical Society of the County of New York for a great many years has maintained a separate legal bureau for the suppression of the unlicensed and criminal practitioner. A staff of well-trained detectives and agents are constantly investigating complaints and procuring evidence where the law is being violated. The method of procuring evidence by detectives is unavoidable because the victims of the charlatan are most reluctant to appear in court as complaining witnesses. It generally brings humiliation and disgrace upon them, exposes their maladies, real and imaginary, to the public, and is in itself a confession that they have been the willing dupes of preposterous frauds.

By means of the efforts of the Medical Society of the County of New York hundreds of cases involving a violation of the Public Health Law have been presented to the criminal courts in New York City. Since 1900, the legal department of that Society has been in charge of the writer, and it has been his duty to institute these prosecutions, and by the courtesy of the District Attorney of New York County, to present the evidence to the various City Magistrates and to the Court of Special Sessions.

The charlatans operating in New York City may be divided into the following classes: (1) Those who prey upon the consumptive poor; (2) Advertising "Specialists for men only;" (3) Occultists; (4) Nature Cure and Water Cure doctors; (5) Midwives; (6) "Osteopaths," "Osteotherapists," "Somatopathists," "Mechano-Neural-Therapists," " Vitopaths," and scores of others of similar ilk, whose chief object seems to be to seek refuge in an imposing title. To these classes must be added the men and women who assume the names of deceased physicians and who practise under their diplomas. Others still boldly use their own names and falsely claim to be members of the medical profession, in the hope that in a city of four millions of people and many thousands of doctors, they may be overlooked and left unmolested.

The cases now to be mentioned, as illustrating the actual methods of each of the classes mentioned, were all presented to the courts in New York City by the Medical Society of the County of New York.

" OCCULTISTS."

The fakir who poses as a master of occult mysticism and esoteric philosophy finds a great many lovers of the mysterious willing to listen to his blandishments. In May, 1901, a complaint was received against " Doctor A. de Sarak," of 413 West Fifty-seventh Street. An agent of the Society called upon the " doctor " and was received with oriental salaams and greetings. The agent and the learned occultist soon got down to business and the doctor's inevitable card was presented to his supposed patient. It read as follows:

"Doctor A. de Sarak, Oriental Scientist, General Delegate of the Scientific Academy of ' Sauveteur' of Paris, Member of the Oriental Society of Thibet and Calcutta, etc."

"Consultations of Oriental Sciences, on Magnetism, Double Vision, Concentration, Telepathy and Palmistry. Every day, except Sundays, bet. 3 and 5 P.M. 413 West Fifty-seventh Street, New York. Consultations by correspondence. English, French, Italian, Spanish, Portuguese and Russian Spoken."

This wonderful assortment of methods and languages, together with the impressive display of decorations, medals and ribbons, soon led to a contract. The patient complained of headache, chills and sleeplessness. The doctor produced an ophthalmoscope and thermometer, and after making a few mysterious gestures and uttering weird incantations, pronounced the trouble as "nervous neurasthenia." He recommended a drug of unpronounceable name, and suffered the patient to depart after extracting $3 for the treatment. The " doctor " tried his case most vigorously—in the newspapers—but in the Court of Special Sessions pleaded guilty and without a murmur pain a fine of $50. A year or two afterward, clad in the same gorgeous attire, the " doctor " appeared for a brief season at one of the fashionable hotels in the city, where many respectable people accepted him at his own valuation. But his former experience served him in good stead, and he soon folded his tents and silently stole away.

The feminine variety of this interesting form of fakir is illustrated in "Madame Marcella Bryan," convicted on January 16, 1903. I shall let her tell her own story. Scorning the services of a lawyer, she addressed the learned judge as follows:

"I am a maker and seller of magic potions. My chief production of mysterious alchemy is ' Sympathy Water.' This one washes with and immediately does it take the devil out of one. That is why I have the great reputation and why Madame Bryan is known the world over. Shall I tell you more? Yes? I am also a clairvoyant, and I know magic and am of the mysterious spirit. I help people in business trouble. I help the maiden, the wife, the husband, the lover in the troubles of the heart. I can do anything; but practice medicine —never."

But alas for this wonderful healer, Mr. Justice Olmstead, speaking for the Court, pronounced her guilty, and forthwith she took her place along the great multitude of persecuted scientists.

MIDWIVES.

The midwife has no recognized status in the laws of the State of New York. As long as she confines her activities to the sphere that custom for generations has allotted to her, it has not been the policy of the medical profession to disturb her. But as a matter of fact, there are no bolder criminal practitioners in New York City than are to be found among the midwives. It is safe to say that a large majority of them will undertake, without hesitation, to perform criminal operations or prescribe drugs for a criminal purpose. Over fifty convictions for such offenses have been secured recently by the Medical Society. Many deaths occur every year as a result of the ignorance and criminal practice of the midwives of New York.

In the last ten days, we brought to the attention of the Courts, Yetta Prince, an East Side midwife. She undertook to relieve a poor woman of sterility. Sixteen treatments resulted in a double pyosalpinx, followed by an operation and the removal of both ovaries and the tubes. She was sentenced to a term of imprisonment.

UNWARRANTED USE OF TITLE " DOCTOR."—" DIPLOMA MILLS."

A most interesting fraud is the man who boldly assumes the title of doctor without any claims whatever to a medical education. The most brazen and successful practitioner of this kind that the Society has ever dealt with is " Dr." Charles Conrad, convicted April 21, 1904.

On April 7 he wrote to Dr. J. McPherson Scott, Secretary of Board of Medical Examiners for the State of Maryland, asking permission to register as a physician in that State. In his letter he said: ' I am not licensed in any State, but I hold a diploma from the ' Vetus Academia Physio Medica.' " He asked to be permitted to register in Maryland without going to the trouble of appearing there in person.

This letter was sent to the Regents of the University of the State of New York, who in turn forwarded it to the Medical Society of the County of New York. Upon investigation we ascertained that the defendant was formerly a Norwegian sailor with no pretense to medical knowledge. The "Vetus Academia Physio Medica" was a college of which he was the president and faculty. He printed elaborate diplomas on parchment, couched in wonderful Latin, but he was willing to sell one to every applicant for $500.

At 56 West Sixty-fifth Street, he was conducting the Platen Institute, with two branches in Harlem, each branch being in charge of a "graduate" of his celebrated school, and supplied with a staff of nurses. Almost any form of treatment desired was administered. This man went so far as to have a bill introduced into the last Senate of New York State (Bill No. 983, March 21, 1904) entitled "To define and regulate the practice of Osteotherapy." Of course, "Dr." Conrad was the founder of the great healing science osteotherapy.

His card surpasses criticism and description.

"Dr. C. Conrad, Founder, President and Medical Director of Vetus Academia Physio Medica (Inc.), Founder, President and Director in Chief of the Platen Institute (Inc.), Lecturer on Psychology and Physiology in the Old Physio Medical College; Founder of Osteotheraphy, Demonstrator and Lecturer on Osteotherapy at Platen Institute; Founder and President of New York Society of Ostheotherapeutic physicians; Founder and Editor-in-Chief of the Twentieth Century Journal in Osteotherapy. Vice-President of the American Association of Physicians and Surgeons. Telephone, 2204 Columbus. By Appointment Only. Office, 56 West Sixty-fifth Street, New York, N. Y."

None of these institutions existed save in his own vivid imagination. A similar case is that of Joseph Rohrer, convicted February 17, 1902, for practising without registration and on May 19, 1904, for using the title "M.D." as President of "International Massage and Movement Cure Institute," which he advertised in over fifty papers and described in an elaborate book of 61 pages, containing many reproductions of the learned doctor in various professional poses.

Closely akin to this form of fraud is the man who assumes the name of some licensed physician who has recently died or removed from the community. The most recent conviction of this sort was a Russian who was a former valet to a London physician, and who, at the latter's death, stole his diploma and attempted to practise in this country.

In the East Side district of New York, there have been several instances of the diploma of a deceased physician bringing at auction more than all the other assets of the estate. An advertisement recently appeared in a New York newspaper offering $1,000 for the diploma of a registered physician in this State who had not been dead over five years.

PRACTITIONERS OF OSTEOPATHY AND THE ART OF MANIPULATION.

The "Osteopath," the "Mechano-Neural Therapist," the "Somatopath," and other practitioners who attempt to cure disease by manipulation stand in a class by themselves. The cult of osteopathy has made considerable progress in this country within the past ten years in States where the standard of medical education is low. Many of the States of the Union have legalized the practice, but in New York and New Jersey and the Eastern States generally, where a high standard of medical education is maintained, the legislatures have persistently refused to grant them any recognition.

The osteopath claims that disease results from a disarrangement of the anatomy, and he includes in this disarrangement of the organs and circulation of the body, particularly nervous circulation as a result of local disturbances and influences. He insists that the proper method for cure is to remove the inflammation or dislocation by manipulation, massage, and kindred methods without the use of drugs.

A small percentage of these practitioners are, no doubt, sincere in their claims, but a great herd of them throughout the United States take up this system of healing because of the ease with which it may be mastered and the short course of study necessary to obtain a diploma. A four years' course in a medical college is now requisite in the State of New York, whereas an osteopathic degree in other States may be secured in from one to two years, or less, according to the character of the institution.

WHAT IS THE "PRACTICE OF MEDICINE?"

This cult is responsible for the prevalent belief that to practise medicine is to give drugs. The courts of original jurisdiction in New York State have uniformly held that the practice of medicine is the practice of the healing art generally, and anyone who undertakes to diagnose and cure disease is practising medicine within the meaning of the statute. None of the higher courts have yet passed upon this question, and until such a decision is obtained, the law on this point will be in confusion. One of the resulting harms from the presence of this system of healing in a community is the encouragement it gives to unlicensed practice of all sorts where drugs are not administered. The practitioner who administers only electrical treatment or baths or massage or magnetic healing is as much entitled as the osteopath to claim that he is not practising medicine because he gives no drugs. All of these practitioners unhesitatingly undertake to cure the most serious forms of diseases, and hope to escape the penalty of the law because they avoid the use of medicine. If such a decision ever comes, the most appropriate comment on it that could be made is the comment made in 1806 in the report of the Thompson case previously referred to and found in 6 Mass. 134.

"It is to be exceedingly lamented that people are so easily persuaded to put confidence in these itinerant quacks, and to trust their lives to strangers without knowledge or experience. If this astonishing infatuation should continue, and men are found to yield to the imprudent pretensions of ignorant empiricism, there seems to be no adequate remedy by a criminal prosecution, without the interference of the legislature."

The enlightened medical profession to-day makes use of all rational methods of healing, including suggestion, manipulation, massage, and electricity. It is the height of injustice in view of this fact to say to the regular physician that he must acquire a knowledge of the healing art by a four years' course of study and at the same time permit the osteopath and all of his ilk who follow a short cut to the healing art to practise their cults without molestation or conditions as long as they do not administer drugs. As was said in a recent editorial in the New York *Times* " A course in medicine and surgery is expensive, and it takes a lot of time, while a varied assortment of pseudo-religious and pseudo-philosophic phrases can be learned in a few days by any man or woman with a disinclination for honest work."

WATER CURE.

The " practitioner " who pins his faith to water, styles himself by various titles ranging from Nature Cure to Balneotechnic. The latest specimen of this variety is " Dr." Charles F. Starken. who carried on a thriving business at Fifty-second Street and Broadway before his career was cut short by the unsympathetic agents of the Society. His card read as follows:

"C. F. Starken, Physician of Natural Cure and Balneothechnic, cures all kinds of Diseases without Medicine or instrument. Gives all kinds of massage and Heat Gymnastics, Magno-Electro and Hydropathic Treatments, Also all kinds of Cure-Baths, Herbs, Mineral, Sulphur, Iron, Lithion, Pine-needles, Aromatic and all Medicated baths. Specially for Blood purifying and good Complexion. Moussir, Steam, Hot Air, Vapor and Astringent Baths, For Males, Females, and Children. Prices Liberal. Dr. C. F. Starken, Consultation: 9-10 A.M.; 2-3 P.M., 6-7 P.M. Fifty-second Street and Broadway, New York."

After the " Doctor's " methods had been called to the attention of the Medical Society by the New York Society for the Prevention of Cruelty to Children, two agents of the Society, both women, sought the professional services of the celebrated water-cure specialist. They described a variety of symptoms and pains, but the doctor was equal to the emergency and his diagnosis showed several serious complications. He scorned to cure them with drugs, but proceeded to administer a variety of baths, followed by massage. One of the agents in Court described her experience as follows:

"I told him I was troubled with fainting spells and pains in my arms and shoulders. He asked me to remove my clothes, which I refused to do. He examined my chest. He took hold of both of my arms. I do not know what he did, but I screamed, it hurt me so. I said, what do you think is the matter with me? He said I had stagnation of the lungs; perhaps he meant congestion of the lungs. He said I was troubled with neuritis."

In some unimportant particulars, the learned gentleman's testimony contradicts the testimony of the People, but I am sure his own story is more interesting than any that could be framed for him. This is his story as taken from the minutes of his trial, March 31, 1904:

" I said, what can I do for you? She said she would like a treatment. I said what is the matter with you? I said I do not want to give any treatment until I know what is the matter with you. I said this is not a Turkish bath. I said you might drop down here dead. She said she had a pain here and a pain there, and much pain all over. I said, is there a name for that and a that for that; I said there is a name for every kind of disease; if an organ is affected we call it that name, and if this organ is affected we call it that name. She said she would like to take a treatment and asked how much it was. I said $3. She left. She said she would come again. My nurse let her in again. She said she wanted to take my treatment. I said, wait a moment, and a woman will come and help you along. My nurse came along and brought her into the steam bath. I said, are you hot here? She said, yet it is quite hot. I felt of her temples, how her temperature was. Then the nurse took her to a bath and there was pine needles in it to clean the skin. Then I gave her a douche. My nurse brought her back to the table and wiped her off. When I was through with the other people I went back to the room where she was. I started to massage her. I must test the muscles—."

The Court. "Don't give us a lecture on that."

The witness continued. "I gave her a rub. She asked, What is the matter with me? I said there is a lot of uric acid in you. She said, Can you give me any medicine? I said no, I give no medicines at all. I said I did not think the treatment would do her much good, because she was too timid."

Q. "Was anything said about cirrhosis of the liver?" A. "No, sir. She said she had pains. And I said if she had a pain there it could not be cirrhosis of the liver."

His discourse did not have the desired effect, for Mr. Justice Wyatt, speaking for the Court, said:

"The sentence of the Court is that the defendant shall pay a fine of $100, and in default of payment that he shall stand committed to the City Prison for a term of thirty days. You will have to stop this business."

FRAUDS, WHO PRACTISE ON THE CONSUMPTIVE POOR.

Of all invalids the consumptive seems to believe more firmly than all others in his ultimate success in combating disease. The unscrupulous quack takes pitiless advantage of this weakness of the consumptive, and in his advertisements makes greater claims and pretensions perhaps than any other medical fraud.

In support of this assertion, I quote from a statement from S. A. Knopf, M.D., of New York City, to whom the " International Congress to Combat Tuberculosis as a Disease of the Masses," at Berlin, awarded the international prize for the best essay, on July 31, 1900. In a statement to the Charity Organization Society of New York, Dr. Knopf says:

"How many poor consumptives have lost their last little reserve fund by giving everything they had for a dozen bottles of the "sure and quick cure" only those who come in contact with them know. How unscrupulous some of these charlatans are in their method of procuring certificates of cure, which they then publish as bait to the unfortunate help-seeking sufferer, is something which can hardly be believed. Let me tell you of one instance: A poor woman in the last stages of consumption came to me seeking advice. When asked for the name of her former medical attendant, she confessed that she had been treated for a number of weeks by a quack concern, and now, her means being exhausted, she was made to understand that they would not continue to treat her unless she would give them a certified testimonial that she had been thoroughly cured of her disease, which had been pronounced an advanced case of consumption by prominent physicians. This poor sufferer had not derived any benefit whatsoever from the treatment, and as a result her conscience would not permit her to become a partner to such a fraudulent procedure.

"Some of these unscrupulous concerns resort to absolute fraud to beguile the public by using the name of the great scientist and benefactor, Prof. Robert Koch, of Berlin, as though he were associated with them in their business and treatment. They advertise his picture beside that of an individual with a similar name, and are heading their advertisements as 'Professor Robert Koch's Cure.'"

One of the advertisements referred to by Dr. Knopf reads as follows:

"*A Statement of Dr. Edward Koch.*—This is a picture of Dr. Edward Koch, the inventor of the Koch Inhalation Apparatus. He can be seen at his office, at 48 West Twenty-second Street, New York, where his diplomas are on exhibition; also his membership to the Tuberculosis Congress, which he attended in London last July. He has also as further evidence of his identity one of the group photographs taken in London, showing the two hundred physicians who were members and delegates at this Congress; of all the pictures the most prominent is that of Dr. Edward Koch.

"In the official catalogue of this Congress, on page 41, the names of Drs. Edward and Robert Koch can be seen in the order in which they were registered, Dr. Robert Koch coming first and Dr. Edward P. Koch next."

During the past year the fraud referred to by Dr. Knopf as Professor Robert Koch's Cure has been fully exposed in the New York *Herald* on evidence submitted by the Medical Society of the County of New York. From their own advertisement, it will be seen that everywhere the impression is given that Dr. Edward Phillip Koch and Dr. Robert Koch are in professional relations with each other. Their so-called cure has offices in Buffalo, Chicago, Boston, Pittsburg, Altoona, Philadelphia, Cincinnati, Baltimore, Washington, Rochester, St. Louis, Newark and other cities. Dr. Koch is advertised in connection with the various establishments. In the New York establishment the Society has never yet been able to capture Dr. Edward Phillip Koch, but he was recently brought to justice in the

District of Columbia. He was, in May, 1904, convicted of practising medicine without registration.

Dr. Robert Koch, of Germany, has written to Dr. S. A. Knopf protesting most bitterly against the use of his name by quacks and charlatans, and denying, of course, the slightest connection with any so-called cure or with any physician of a similar name anywhere in the world. As long as registered physicians can be induced to take part in such deception it will be difficult to close this establishment by law, but the conviction of Dr. Edward Phillip Koch and the wide publicity given to his methods will greatly lessen the dangers of such establishments.

SO-CALLED SPECIALIST IN "DISEASES OF MEN."

Almost as dangerous is the so-called specialist in diseases of men. Certain newspapers in New York print columns of their advertisements without apology to the public for intruding such filthy printed matter. The methods of these quacks are various. Most of them advertise in the name of a registered physician and then employ green youths and unlicensed practitioners to meet the patient after he calls. As the law as present constituted does not require a physician employed in an advertising institution to make known his identity, it is difficult to trace out the identity of the practitioner in any of these concerns. The employer generally keeps them moving and does not permit a practitioner to remain in any one office long enough for very much information to be found out about him. Other offices advertise in the name of men not licensed to practice, but put in charge of their office in New York a licensed practitioner.

The writer is reliably informed that one institution of this character in New York City made over $200,000 last year. I know of several instances where, by making a false diagnosis and frightening the patient into the belief that he had a loathsome disease, the patient has been induced to pay over as high as $2,000 for a few treatments. The law must be amended so as to compel every practitioner in an advertising institution to make known his identity just as every dentist in any advertising dental parlor is required by law to post his name above the chair where he operates.

In brief, such is the work of the Medical Society of the County of New York. With its professed antagonism to so many powerful yet corrupt influences, it has an abundance of enemies, many of them occupying the seats of the mighty. In these enemies it finds the highest testimonial to the efficiency of its work and the greatest incentive to a continuance of its labors.

In 1893, when the law regulating the practice of medicine assumed its present form, the work of the various County Medical Societies in New York State received its most complete recognition by the State, when a provision was inserted in that law authorizing the return of fines to the County Societies as follows:

"When any prosecution under this article is made on the complaint of any incorporated medical society of the State, or any county medical society of such county entitled to representation in a State society, the fines when collected, shall be paid to the society making the complaint, and any excess of the amount of fines so paid over the expense incurred by the said society in enforcing the medical laws of this State, shall be paid at the end of the year to the county treasurer."

As a matter of fact, however, the return of fines resulting from prosecutions instituted by a medical society is inadequate to meet more than a small part of that society's expenditures in this work. Again the whole principle of returning fines to societies engaged in the prosecution of crime, however well meant in theory, is vicious in practice and should not be continued by the legislature. Neither should the great State of New York put upon the shoulders of the medical profession the burden of supplying the funds with which to carry on a work to protect the citizens of the State. The treasury of the Medical Society of the County of New York, the income of which consists entirely of the dues of its two thousand members, is continually being depleted by the demands made upon it by the prosecutions it institutes. It is doubtful if, with the increasing demands made upon its legal department, the work can be continued as at present. Realizing this, the Medical Society of the County of New York and the Medical Society of the County of Kings have instituted a movement that seems certain to result in the repeal of the laws giving the fines to the Society and substituting in lieu therof a direct appropriation from the public treasury of an amount sufficient to pay the actual expenses of the Society in suppressing and punishing the charlatan. This movement has the unqualified approval of the public authorities and the sympathetic endorsement of the magistrates and judges in the City of New York, who are more familiar than anyone else with the necessity of continuing and improving the facilities for the detection of such crimes as have been described in this article.

ADDENDA.

To the Editor of the MEDICAL NEWS.

DEAR SIR: The counsel of the Medical Society of the County of New York, recently read a paper before the Society of Medical Jurisprudence entitled "Medical Quacks, Their Methods and Dangers." The newspapers have given wide publicity to the crying evils of the medical fakir pointed out on that occasion.

On one point alone does there seem to be any misapprehension. Several papers have asked why, with many thousand charlatans now practising in this city, the society has succeeded in convicting in five years only about 500 of them.

At a meeting of the Comitia Minora of the Medical Society, recently held, it was resolved that an official statement be made to the press of New York City giving the reasons why the percentage of cases taken up by us is so small.

We beg to present these reasons as follows:

1. Lack of funds. There are 2,000 members of the medical profession in the New York County Society. In order to make our work as effective as possible, the scientific features of our society have been curtailed in order to devote our funds to the suppression of the dangerous quack. For the past five years we have expended every available dollar for this purpose.

2. Inherent difficulties in the nature of prosecutions. In rarely one case out of a hundred will the real victims of the charlatan consent to give evidence. They report their cases to the society on condition that they are not called as witnesses. This is to avoid the exposure, humiliation, and disgrace which in many instances would follow publicity. This necessitates the society procuring its own evidence at great expense against every charlatan it prosecutes.

3. Radical defects in the medical law. We have no definition in this State as to what constitutes the practice of medicine. Until the legislature gives us a satisfactory definition great uncertainty will exist. We have repeatedly asked the legislature for such a definition, and have been as often refused.

4. Failure of the newspapers to cooperate. The modern charlatan could not exist without publicity given his advertisements by the press. If our New York papers would refuse advertisements for the sale of drugs for a criminal purpose, illegal lying-in establishments, and the distressing advertisements of the so-called specialists for diseases of men only, and the "consumption cure" frauds, it would not be difficult for the Medical Society, even with its present lack of funds, to rid the community of the chief offenders. These vicious advertising charlatans draw their recruits from innocent victims attracted by the advertisements unblushingly received by many New York newspapers.

COMITIA MINORA MEDICAL SOCIETY OF THE COUNTY OF NEW YORK.

New York. October 16, 1904.

ANAL FISSURE.[1]

BY WILLIAM M. BEACH, A.M., M.D.,

OF PITTSBURG, PA.

THE object of this short paper is to consider etiological factors, some of the reflexes, and finally the treatment of irritable ulcer of the rectum.

The nomenclature may be disposed of as that of anal fissure, painful, irritable or concealed ulcer of the rectum. The shape of the sore is usually long and narrow, lying between two folds; it is frequently club-shaped, sometimes round, a shape which is usually the signal of a submucous blind fistula or the concealed type.

The location is in one of three planes in the anal rectum. the special point affected bearing an important relation to the symptoms produced, especially that of pain. The lesion may be over the site of the internal sphincter, between the sphincters, or over the external sphincter extending into the skin. The stool passing over a solution of continuity at the internal sphincter will not cause any particular discomfort during the act. but in a few minutes is followed by a

---

[1] Read before Pennsylvania State Medical Society, September 28, 1904, at Pittsburg, Pa.

dull aching reflected in the back, lasting two or three hours. An ulcer located between the sphincters, that is disturbed, evinces severe smarting and burning, continuing most of the day. The victim becomes nervous, irritable and irascible. If the wound presents within and below the grasp of the external sphincter, the pain will be severe, of a tearing nature and excruciating, and may completely disable the patient. The hypertrophied muscle spasmodically contracts, adding to the suffering. On account of these trying seances, the victim becomes constipated by deferring the call of nature from time to time.

Again, the location of a fissure may be in any quadrant and plane of the anal circle; and this leads us to consider the first object of our paper, viz.: Some of the etiologic factors determining the location as well as the disease itself.

If we were to consider causes for all ulcers to be found in the anal rectum, it would be necessary to review gonorrhea, syphilis, chancroid, tuberculosis, etc., but our purpose is to discuss the simple traumatic type.

The mucous membrane in the anal region is very delicate and consequently easily wounded by the passage of hardened feces, the introduction of a syringe tip or unskilful use of specula. Fissures may follow operations for removal of hemorrhoids, fistula and adenoids. Some authors state that painful ulcer is more frequent in women on account of parturition; the fetus presses the rectal walls against the bony background and lacerates the mucosa. This may account for the fact that a greater number of fissures in women occur in the anterior quadrant. It is my observation that ulceration there is preceded by severe perineal laceration, the repair of which is neglected by the obstetrician. Nature's attempt at repair gives evidence of an unusual amount of inflammatory discharge conducing to keeping alive the rent in the rectal mucosa and producing sphincteralgia. Fissure in the anterior quadrant is less frequent in the male, but when it does occur is most intractable, owing to the mobility of the area during locomotion.

Proctitis is generally a concomitant symptom of fissure in which we find the presence of feces that finds lodgment in one of the anal pockets. The pockets are effaced during the act of defecation, as the levator muscles lift the anal canal over the protruding column. A foreign body already lodged behind the crypt, and causing the valve to swell, prevents the normal effacement and invites further damage by a fecolith or by pressure from the column itself. By a further study of the mechanics of defecation, we may determine causal factors of fissure. The line of axis changes in various planes of the rectal cavity. In the ampulla, the axis directs postero-anteriorly, to change analward to anteroposteriorly just at the site of the anal pockets, which form with the papillæ the floor of the rectal pouch. By virtue of the angle of the two

axes at this place, the object to be expelled would most likely be caught in the pocket in whatever quadrant it might happen to be located. The chief point of predilection is in the right or left posterior quadrant. Various theories are given to account for this phenomenon. A member of the American Proctologic Society advanced the idea that in the posterior and anterior commissures the fibers of the sphincter muscle decussate in a most delicate manner and approach very closely the mucosa, which fibers rupture and hold apart the torn mucosa, made so by the expulsion of hard objects in the fecal column. This idea seems to me rather tenable, but we must consider in connection with it Mr. Ball's theory that tears are most likely in the commissures owing to the fact that the anal pockets or crypts of Morgagni are most highly developed there. Fecal matter lodges in these pockets, and, being pressed upon by subsequent discharges, tears the edges of the valve,—the beginning of a painful history. Further observation by Tuttle has shown a well-developed crypt on each side of the rectum, occasionally the site of fissure.

In a certain umber of cases the foreign substance will infect a pocket and burrow its way under the mucosa, a condition commonly known as a blind fistula, but which I call a concealed ulcer. Sometimes they will kindle a suppurative process between the planes of anal fascia, and open in the skin about one-half inch from the anal orifice. In this connection I must emphasize the importance of fissure as a causal factor in the development of peri-rectal abscess. While I agree with the Ball theory, I must confess to the belief that most fissures are due to direct injury, both from within and without, and that the origin may be found in internal hemorrhoids, a pathologic condition that further predisposes to rupture of the mucosa.

In order to note some of the reflexes, we should observe the symptoms objectively and subjectively—moreover, the primary and secondary stages of the disease or, as Gant puts it, "The fresh wound ending with the inauguration of the second stage, sphincteralgia, which is the pathognomic symptom of this disease." The schedule of symptoms, as given by the same author, includes: Pain and sphincteralgia, constipation, flatulence, hemorrhages, discharges, pruritis, reflex disturbances, change in the character of feces, proctitis, melancholia and nervousness.

It is not my purpose to discuss the entire list, but to call especial attention to pain and the reflexes. A newly made fissure is comparatively free from pain. The category of subjective symptoms may be limited by a sense of fulness and slight burning. But when the stage of sphincteralgia is reached and the so-called "sentinel" pile is formed, severe pain of a tearing nature follows a stool, only to subside in two or three hours, when the paroxysms of contractions cease. If the ulcer be irregular and located between the sphincters, the nagging and sense of weight may continue the entire day. The pain is usually reflected to the sacrococcygeal region. These symptoms appear in less degree, as evidence of the high location, and in concealed ulcers.

This type of ulcer is easily overlooked; in fact, it is difficult to locate, except by the most approved method of anoscopy. I have a case on record, a male, who had an anterior fissure of this kind, forming a complete fistula without a history of abscess. Patients suffering from fissure are usually very restless, high-strung and melancholic. The severe pain, though not commensurate with the pathologic condition, renders the belief that they are suffering from cancer or incurable disease.

The reflex phenomena become quite interesting when we consider the anatomic distribution of nerves of the parts: the anal branch of the internal pudic nerve gives off numerous end organs in the anal pilasters and Hilton's line, forming the rectal sense of Stroud. These nerves are exceeding sensitive and, when exposed by a laceration, become congested and swollen. By their intimate relationship to the spinal plexus and sympathetic systems, both local and remote reflexes are easily understood. The bladder, prostate, urethra and testicles, ovaries, tubes and uterus are apt to bear the onus of direct disease, when, in fact, the pain of fissure is reflected to these organs. Again, we may mention such remote reflexes as pain in thighs, legs and heel, back of neck, and flatulent dyspepsia. I recall a young man whom I cured of this form of dyspepsia by removing an irritable ulcer of the rectum. He had been limited to a milk diet for a year, and was receiving special treatment of the stomach when referred to me.

To locate an ulcer rarely requires the use of a speculum, except in very obscure cases, where the lesion is behind one of the crypts. The trained digit, inserted to the white line, will suffice in the majority of instances. If the classical " sentinel " pile is present, as it is not in all cases, by separating the anal folds there will open to view the grayish granulations and indurated margins of an ulcer. I must herewith urge the importance of a direct examination, since the patient is liable to mislead the doctor in diagnosis. Again, the mistake is made by many in digital examination of inserting the finger too far. Most diseases of the anal rectum are found between the ental and ectal sphincters.

The problem of treatment and cure of anal fissure will depend upon the stage of the disease, —whether we shall invoke medical or surgical measures. In the first stage, a laxative and topical use of ichthyol will generally suffice to cure. But if the sphincteralgic stage has been inaugurated, nothing short of surgical procedure will avail. Since the introduction of local anesthesia, the danger of general anesthesia can be dispensed with and the associated terrors eliminated. The operation may be done in the office, and the patients lose no time. To overcome the paroxysmal contractions is the secret. It is entirely unnecessary to " stretch the sphincter " in order to put the muscle at rest. No matter how much you divulse, short of tearing, retraction will occur in twenty-four hours. The safest and most rational procedure is to cut a few fibers directly back of and beneath the ulcer, then cut through the base of the lesion; the second incision should extend above and below the margin of the sore, then the indurated margins should be trimmed and all the granulations curetted. By the use of a one-tenth per cent. solution of beta eucoine, about 100 drops injected beneath the ulcer, or by sterile water anesthesia, This operation is painless, and results are speedy and certain. Before doing this operation care must be taken to determine the presence of sinuses, so often found. These should be opened first and the technic executed as described. The subsequent care consists chiefly in keeping the margins of the wound apart, by daily inserting the finger and the application of ichthyol or silver nitrate, gr. xx to the ounce to a healthy granulation.

In 1896 I advocated the use of the electrocautery knife as a safe and painless practice, a method which has been used quite extensively since among proctologists.

THE PHYSICS AND CHEMISTRY OF DRUG ACTION.[1]

BY EDWARD C. HILL, M.D.,

OF DENVER, COL.;

PROFESSOR OF CHEMISTRY IN THE MEDICAL AND DENTAL DEPARTMENT OF THE UNIVERSITY OF DENVER.

DRUGS in general act, first, as mechanical protectives; second, as modifiers of osmosis ("salt action "); third, by combining with compounds in the blood and secretions (acids, bases, antitoxins) ; fourth, by direct combination with or catalytic action on protoplasm; fifth, by reflex influence (bitters, stimulants, antispasmodics). The action of medicines is primary (unaltered drug) and secondary (compounds formed in body), direct (local) and indirect (remote). The effect of drugs is qualitative, not quantitative (Cushny), increasing or depressing activity, but not altering its form. No new function can be created by any substance (Sollmann). Most drugs have an elective affinity for certain types of cells, comparable to the selective tendency shown by toxins and the products of digestion. Thus strychnine and the toxins of tetanus affect chiefly the motor nerve cells; morphine depresses the brain and stimulates the spinal cord; coniine, gelsemine and sparteine paralyze the endings of motor nerves; strophanthus acts primarily upon muscle tissue (Potter) by direct contact through the blood. Prussic acid is a general protoplasm poison. The thyroid attracts arsenic and iodine; the liver, iron.

[1] Read before the Rocky Mountain Interstate Medical Association, September 7, 1904.

Each cell is supposed to possess many and varied receptors, which, by appropriate combination with haptophores adapted to their metabolic requirements, maintain nutrition and function. (McFarland). Foreign haptophores, as of drugs and poisons, are more or less isomerically identical with some normal nutrient haptophores. Ehrlich holds that alkaloids, antiseptics and antipyretics do not enter into the composition of protoplasm, and so fail to call forth a specific antigenetic action (antibodies). Gowers is a believer in dynamic therapy, *i.e.*, increase or decrease of metabolic processes by catalytic " contact of molecules of allied constitution with latent energy on the point of release, so held as to blend with that which is being set free in the living tissues." The action of large doses is generally the reverse of small or moderate ones. Strychnine first stimulates and finally paralyzes by overstimulation the large multipolar ganglia in the anterior columns of the spinal cord (Potter). Hydrocyanic acid first stimulates, then paralyzes the central nervous system (Cushny). Bromides may produce transient excitement and intoxication (Bartholow). Belladonna in small doses increases intestinal peristaltic movements (paralysis of inhibitory fibers of splanchnics), whereas moderate doses completely arrest these movements (White). Small quantities of opiates make the sleep lighter than usual. General anesthetics excite the brain and heart at first. Very minute quantities of antiseptics may stimulate the development of germs (Roger). Aconitine in contact with some nerve structures induces the production of excess of energy; on others arrests all action (Gowers). Naturalistic medication furnishes us with means capable of intensifying or attenuating reactionary phenomena, when these are insufficient or excessive (Roger). The tendency of modern therapeutics is toward smaller and more frequently repeated doses (White).

The effects desired for medicines may be obtained at the area of contact with the skin or mucous membrane, or in the blood, affecting also the nerves and muscles, or on the organ which excretes them (concentration here)—one or two or all. The law of dissolution is that when a drug affects functions progressively, those first affected are the highest in development; that is, the last acquired by the individual and the last to appear in the species. Thus chloral is a general protoplasm poison, but affects the brain first, hence is used as a hypnotic.

The period during which a medicine stays in the system varies greatly. Many volatile remedies, such as ether, pass out of the body within an hour after taking, whereas a single dose of arsenic may not be entirely eliminated for several months. It appears to the writer that the alterative effect of mercury and other heavy metals may be due to their long-continued presence in the body, augmenting retrograde metabolism in virtue of their foreign nature. The accumulative action of drugs is shown when administered for some time when absorption is more rapid than excretion. It is probable that when digitalis or strychnine accumulates in the tissues to a certain amount, the renal vessels contract and excretion is arrested (White). The action of drugs and the doses required are greatly modified by the presence of disease. Enormous doses of opium are well borne in peritonitis. The conformation of the drug molecule has as much to do with the action of the remedy as has its elemental composition. In general, drugs that are closely allied chemically have a similar effect on the organism. The methane derivatives, as a class, are cerebral depressants, their toxic effects increasing with the homologous series, except as modified by insolubility; the presence of hydroxyl and acid-forming groups lessens their toxicity (Cushny). The alkaloids show many therapeutic peculiarities. Thus, jaborine is isomeric with pilocarpine, but exactly opposite in action, and a specimen of the latter drug adulterated with the former may have no therapeutic effect. Hyoscyamine differs from atropine only in the arrangement of the atoms of the molecules, but the two remedies have a slightly different action. Strychnine changed to methyl-strychnine becomes a paralyzant (White). By dehydration of morphine into apomorphine the cerebral depressant action is much reduced, while the stimulating effect (particularly on the vomiting center) is retained. Differences in pharmacologic effects may depend on physical characters (volatility, solubility) rather than chemical combinations. Most volatile substances are more or less irritant, and are used for their local or reflex effects.

Ions.—In the fluids of the body inorganic compounds in general break up largely into electrically charged parts, namely, anions and cations. In a one-per-cent. solution of NaCl only about one-fifth of the salt is present as molecules (Cushny). These ions serve as conductors of electricity and so are absolutely essential to protoplasmic activity. The function of the ions (Ott) is by their presence in definite proportions in each tissue to preserve the labile equilibrium of the colloid material of the protoplasm on which its activities depend. The positive and negative particles must be potentially equivalent (Mathews) in this electric substratum, hence there must be a mixture of salts in proper proportions. Predominance of anions increases motor activity, and *vice versa*.

The excised frog's heart does not continue beating when supplied with a solution of any non-electrolyte. The contractions are maintained longer in sodium chloride of a certain strength than in the solution of any other single salt (Ringer). Calcium antagonizes the slightly poisonous effect of sodium ions (Loeb), and the addition of a trace (1 : 1,000) of a calcium salt to a NaCl (and KCl) solution maintains cardiac contractions much longer than with the sodium salt alone. Bivalent and trivalent cations commonly antagonize univalent cations, the neutralizing effect being proportional to their valency. Univalent cations tend to keep colloid proteins in solution, while bivalent and trivalent cations precipitate them, thus counterbalancing each other and so preventing excessive or deficient fluidity in the tissues (Hardy).

The animal cell may be regarded as a semi-permeable membrane enclosing protoplasm. Unless both ions of a salt can enter a cell, neither does so (Cushny). The rate and degree of dissociation of different compounds are of great importance in their effects upon the cells of the body. The stronger acids and bases dissociate more readily than the weaker ones. Bivalent and trivalent ions resist dissociation and absorption much more than do the weaker ones. The organic compounds of arsenic (cacodylates) and bromine (monobromated camphor) dissociate with difficulty; hence they are less irritant and likewise less effective than the inorganic ones. Many non-electrolytes (urea, for example) permeate cells readily. Muscle immersed in equimolecular salt solution of Na or Li gains but little in weight; in K, gains a great deal; in Ca, loses water. Oils increase exosmosis, so there is a valid reason for greasing the nose and the chest for a cold. Glycerin is hygroscopic, and thus allays thirst and depletes inflamed tissues when applied on tampons.

Absorption.—Aqueous solutions are absorbed best from mucous membranes and subcutaneous tissues; oily or alcoholic (mix with sebum), by the skin-glands. The gums, sugars, starches, waxes and proteins of plant juices delay absorption of the active constituent. Hence laudanum or extract of nux vomica is prescribed when local action on the stomach or bowel is desired; morphine or strychnine for effects after absorption (Cushny). Acetate of lead with opium should be given in pill form, as otherwise it acts on the stomach. Nitrite of amyl by the mouth has but little effect, since the nitrous acid freed by the gastric juice is decomposed at once. It acts within a minute when inhaled. Shoemaker recommends absorption from the mouth by sucking tablet triturates, to get quick effects from aconite, belladonna or pilocarpine. Oleates of alkaloids and metallic oxides penetrate the skin more readily than solutions in fats and oils. Intramuscular injections of mercury are well given as calomel in liquid petrolatum (slow absorption—less painful). The addition of NaCl (10 parts) to $HgCl_2$ (one ion in common) lessens dissociation of the latter salt, and so renders it less germicidal but less irritant, hence more suitable for hypodermic injection in syphilis. Hypodermic medication is almost useless in marked dropsical conditions. So-called idiosyncrasies sometimes depend, no doubt, on abnormally rapid or retarded absorption or excretion. It is a general rule that medicines are to be taken after, rather than before meals (Hare), unless a local gastric effect or very rapid absorption is desired.

Acids.—Mineral acids owe their activities almost entirely to the hydrogen ion, which is stronger than potassium. Salicylic, benzoic and hydrocyanic acids have effect chiefly through their negative ions, the first two having a nearly identical action. Acids abstract water (astringent), neutralize bases and precipitate proteins, particularly globulins. They coagulate the superficial layer of proteids in the skin, mouth and throat, and so give rise to stiffness and numbness, or a puckery feeling. By reflex action they excite the flow of saliva (vinegar test in mumps) and other alkaline fluids, and so diminish febrile thirst (refrigerant). Acids are protoplasm poisons (antiseptic). When they are administered in large doses, animals die before their blood becomes even neutral (Cushny). Ammonia is liberated by the tissues for self-protection and to save the fixed alkalies from combining with the acids, mineral acids being excreted chiefly as ammonium salts. Organic acids are absorbed mostly as salts of the alkaline metals, and are oxidized to carbonates in the tissues, rendering the blood more alkaline and the urine less acid. Vegetable acids stimulate the alimentary secretions, causing flatulence and diarrhea. Benzoic acid, changed to hippuric acid in the kidneys, is the only drug that can effectually render the urine acid (White). Large doses of boric acid or of acid sodium phosphate are said to intensify urinary acidity, which is likewise augmented by the free use of carbonated waters (Ultzmann). Nitric acid by the mouth is said to increase the amount of ammonia in the urine, and thus render it slightly alkaline.

Bases.—Hydrates of the alkali metals owe nearly all their action to the relatively powerful anion hydroxyl. Carbonates and bicarbonates of these metals, by dissociation and combination with water (liberating HO), have properties similar to hydrates, though weaker. All these alkalies neutralize acids $(HO + O = H_2O)$, dissolve proteins (including mucus) and saponify fat. They soften the skin and remove horny layers of epithelium. A dilute alkaline solution checks the discharge (same reaction) of acute eczema and allays the itching, smarting and burning (Shoemaker). Alkaline medication internally is of special use in arthritic dermatoses (Huchard).

Hydrates are probably absorbed as carbonates or in combination with proteins. Alkaline hydrates and carbonates render the blood and tissues more alkaline, aiding oxidation, but have less effect on tissue change than was formerly believed (Cushny). Through a saving of tissue antacid reaction, the ammonia of the urine is often decreased and the urea correspondingly increased. The local effect on the bowels may sometimes cause an increased formation and destruction of leucocytes, and thus give rise to the appearance of more uric acid in the urine (Cushny). The organism quickly frees itself from excess of alkali by excretion of alkaline salts, with accompanying diuresis, so that the alkalinity of urine induced by sodium salts ceases on the day following their administration, and urinary acidity is then intensified (Bartholow). The alkalies in moderate doses are useful in irritable conditions of the bladder and urethra, but they are not lithontriptics (may cause a stone to fall apart by dissolving cementing mucus), and when given for some time in sufficient quantity to keep the urine alkaline are very liable to increase the size of a stone by secondary deposition of phosphates. Alkalies are of unquestioned benefit in late diabetes to neutralize oxybutyric acid and so economize the alkalies of the blood and fixed tissues. For producing effects after absorption, potassium bicarbonate is the alkali of choice, preferably administered on an empty stomach as an effervescing drink with lemonade. Ammonium hydrate has practically the same effect as ammonium carbonate, since the latter gives off ammonia freely. Owing to its volatility, ammonia is more penetrating than the fixed alkalies, but is less caustic. Alcohols are not dissociated in the body, as are the mineral hydroxides. Wood spirit is not so toxic as grain spirit, but is longer retained in the system; hence its deleterious effects on the optic nerve.

Salts.—The therapeutic effects of salts of the alkali metals depend chiefly on their relation to osmosis. Sodium chloride having a low molecular weight, and being readily dissociated, induces greater osmotic changes than most other salts. It penetrates the red blood cells with difficulty, if at all, and differs from most other binary salts in disturbing equilibrium toward the negative side (stimulating). Concentrated solutions act as counter-irritants (saline baths), while the imbibition of large amounts of a weak solution cause a mild stimulation of the gastric mucous membrane. Hypoisotonic solutions are absorbed rapidly, though not so quickly as water or alcohol; hyperisotonic solutions draw water from the blood (hydragog action) until they become isotonic. when the greater part remaining is absorbed. Salt is not necessary for the absorption of enemas (Cushny). The physiologic action of inorganic salts is an electric action, due to the changes in their ions (Mathews). Salt ions in the blood change the distribution of fluids in the tissues and exert besides a stimulating effect (diuresis) upon the kidneys. They "flush" the system by increasing the excretion osmotically of the diffusible constituents of cells (Sollmann). Slowly dissociated salts are comparatively free from local irritative effect. Ion action varies inversely as salt action. Osmotic nutritive changes produced by drugs are most pronounced in cells of the lowest vitality, hence salt action in general (iodides particularly) tends to break down pathologic formations (Sollmann).

Potassium salts are distinctly depressant to the heart and nervous system, whereas sodium has almost no effect; possibly the greater atomic weight of the former metal has to do with this difference. Lithium salts diminish the alkalinity of the blood (by reacting with Na_2HPO_4) and so lessen the elimination of uric acid. Ammonium salts are excreted as urea; hence (except the benzoate) they do not affect the reaction of the urine. The salts of strontium and calcium, being bivalent, are more slowly dissociated and absorbed than those of the alkali metals; they are less irritant locally and less effective in the blood than the latter. They are excreted chiefly through the large intestine; to a less extent by the kidneys (lime as calcium carbamate, which breaks up into the carbonate and ammonia, rendering the urine alkaline). Calcium salts lessen the phosphates in the urine (reducing its acidity) by forming insoluble phosphates in the bowel. The heavy metals have no chemical action on or in the body until changed by air to an oxide (mercury), or by secretions to chlorides, carbonates and other salts. These cations (and aluminum) combine with proteins (irritant or corrosive action), and are absorbed to a slight degree from the small intestine in such combinations and by the leucocytes. They are excreted mostly by the large bowel (causing irritation and ulceration) and to a less degree through the kidneys and in the secretions (mercury in the saliva). Double salts and organic compounds do not combine with proteins (non-irritating) until decomposed, as by acids. Inorganic iron may be more readily absorbed than food-iron enveloped in colloid matter (Cushny), aside from the much greater amount given as medicine. Hemoglobin (blood) is changed by the acid contents of the stomach to hematin ("coffee grounds"). which passes through the bowel unabsorbed (Cloetta). The soluble salts of mercury are more irritant and corrosive than those of other metals, since the protein ppt. is looser and so does not protect the deeper layers, and is further soluble in excess of proteins or in solutions of neutral salts. The chloride and nitrate (univalent anions) are particularly penetrating and corrosive. The least corrosive salts of mercury and other metals are those with the slowly dissociated organic acids. The aluminate of lead is soluble in potassium iodide, which is given to hasten the elimination of poisonous metals. Mercury is more quickly absorbed than other metals. Antimony enters the blood more slowly than arsenic, hence its effects are more localized. The effects of tartar emetic are due to antimony. It increases the sweat, saliva and bronchial mucus through reflex action in vomiting (Cushny). The colloidal salts of the metals have a distinct catalytic or oxidizing power. The halogen salts of the alkali metals owe their salty taste and medicinal properties chiefly to the negative element. Aside from their general salt action, they exert a selective influence on different tissues. Chlorine and bromine replace hydrogen in its combinations with proteids. All bromides are changed to NaBr in the stomach. They may cause considerable diminution of the urinary phosphates, by depressing mental activity. The various salts of the body are probably in definite ionic combination (not reacting to ordinary tests) with proteids, and it is possible to substitute one class of ions for another in the molecule, as when common salt in the food of epileptics is replaced with bromides and the body becomes saturated with bromine. The skin eruptions from bromides and other salts probably depend on the irritation accompanying their excretion through the cutaneous glands. Some iodides undergo decomposition—perhaps by interaction with nascent O and CO_2 (Binz)—and the free iodide thus formed is thought to cause the symptoms of iodism. Iodides in syphilis may act as a specific poison to the unknown cause of this disease. Arsenical preparations owe their therapeutic efficiency to the AsO_3 ion. The chlorate ion is a specific poison to hemoglobin. Whatever local usefulness chlorates may have is probably due, in part at least, to simple salt action (Cushny). The nitrate ion produces local irritation of mucous membrane. Sulphur is changed (by Na_2CO_3) in the bowel to H_2S and sulphides, which cause increased peristalsis, reduce oxyhemoglobin and depress the central nervous system. Sulphites and hyposulphites are absorbed and eliminated as sulphates, having a salt action only in the tissues. Hypophosphites are excreted unchanged in the urine, and there is no reason to suppose that they have any further action than other indifferent salts, such as chlorides of the same metals (Cushny). Citrates and acetates (and tartrates more slowly) are oxidized to carbonates in the tissues. They have the advantage over carbonates of not neutralizing the gastric juice. The ferrocyanids do not dissociate iron in the body.

Antiseptics, Anthelmintics, Parasiticides.—Solutions of antiseptics in oil have little or no antiseptic effect—may not diffuse into microbes. Equimolecular solutions of mercurial salts are bactericidal in the direct of their capacity for dissociation of the metal, $HgCl_2$ ranking first. A solution of this salt in ether or absolute alcohol does not affect anthrax spores, since it does not dissociate. Mercury albuminate dissolved in sodium thiosulphate forms a complex, non-dissociable, non-antiseptic salt (Dreser). A trace of mercury is sufficient to kill a cell by combining with its protoplasm, and water distilled from copper vessels is also destructive to algæ and infusoria. The antiseptic effect of silver nitrate is limited by its reactions with chlorides and proteins. Owing to the absence of the astringent NO_3 ion, the colloidal salts of silver are less irritating than the nitrate. Permanganate solution oxidizes and destroys bacteria, but does not penetrate deeply. It is of special service as an antidote for snake-bite (Brunton) and in alkaloidal poisoning. Hydrogen dioxide is catalyzed by all

forms of living (and dead) organic matter, liberating nascent oxygen. The deodorizing power of charcoal may be due partly to the absorbed oxygen. Sodium sulphite gives off the strong reducing agent, sulphur dioxide gas, in the stomach. Phenol and the aromatic acids are general protoplasm poisons, producing gangrene at times. The lower members of the aromatic series are generally more poisonous to higher animals than the more complex ones, while the latter are equally or more efficient in the destruction of the lowest living forms (Cushny). Formaldehyde renders proteins insoluble. Quinine and aromatic acids prevent the movements of protozoa and leucocytes. Acids are generally antiseptic (protoplasm poisons), hydrochloric being the most efficient for internal use. In the normal strength of gastric juice it destroys the great majority of the less resistant micro-organisms. Salol is dissolved and rendered active by the steapsin of the pancreatic juice. It has but little effect on the amount of indican in the urine (Kumagawa). Calomel, strontium salicylate (Wood) and the sulphocarbolates are among the best intestinal antiseptics, and all purgatives have an antiseptic effect by removing the culture media on which the bacteria flourish. Yeasts and microbes are precipitated by tannin (antifermentative). The use of creosote, guaiacol, etc., by the mouth for pulmonary disease gives favorable results in some cases by their disinfectant action on the stomach and bowels. The traces of volatile oils excreted by the lungs are quite incapable of any noticeable effect on microbial growth (Cushny). The inhalation of turpentine or terebene sprayed into the air lessens the foul odor of pulmonary tuberculosis or gangrene.

Volatile oils are closely related to phenols and aromatic acids. They are all antiseptic and some are germicidal, readily penetrating protoplasm and lessening its vitality by acting as foreign bodies (Cushny). They are of special service (particularly terebene) as stimulating antiseptics in the subacute and chronic stages of inflammation of the urethra or bladder. Santal oil, balsam of copaiba and oleoresin of cubeb are common examples. The benzol derivatives are excreted by the kidneys in forms much less irritant and antiseptic than that in which they are administered (Cushny). Hexamethylenetetramin passes into the urine unchanged or as formaldehyde. Its value as a genito-urinary antiseptic has been somewhat overrated. Chloroform, one minim to the ounce, is the best preservative of urine or of solutions of alkaloidal salts.

Most so-called antiseptic dressing powders act in the main merely as drying and protecting agents, although those containing iodine liberate this element slowly in the presence of moisture. Boric acid is no disinfectant, but is a useful antiseptic dusting powder in the impalpable form. Baking soda is an excellent application to moderate burns and slight wounds. Pyrogallol is said to owe its value in skin diseases to its reducing action, depriving the superficial tissues of oxygen. Balsam of Peru has largely taken the place of sulphur (SO_2) in the treatment of scabies. Ozone is antiseptic only when the air contains 13.5 mg. or more per liter, which is never attained in practice (Cushny). Pelletierine comes nearest to being a specific anthelmintic. A dilution of 1:10,000 kills tapeworms in ten minutes (Schröder), while a strong solution has practically no effect on other worms. The therapeutic action of male fern is due to the neutral bodies aspidin and aspidinin and to filicic acid. Oily substances should be avoided in conjunction with male fern, since they dissolve the filicic acid and promote its absorption, causing toxic symptoms (Poulsson). The bowels should be well cleared out with oil some hours before. Santonin (with calomel), spigelia and chenopodium are effective vermifuges against the round worm; and repeated injections of brine (dissolves mucus) or infusion of quassia will rid the rectum of thread-worms. Certain drugs may set up in the human body a reaction destructive to parasites, the dead parasites inducing the formation of immune bodies, as in the use of trypan red by Ehrlich and Shiga in cases of trypanosomiasis.

Protectives.—Emollients, to the skin, and demulcents applied to its involution, the mucous membrane, afford much relief locally and have also a reflex action. Inert oils and fine, insoluble powders (rice, starch, talc, fuller's earth, lycopodium) are used to protect an abraded surface from the air and other irritants, and to soak up secretions. Flexible collodion is a useful application for skin-cracks. Petrolatum is the usual basis for ointments, and is preferred to lard, since it does not become rancid. Liquid petrolatum, instilled into the nostrils, after cleansing with a physiological salt solution, frequently checks the night coughs of children. When glycerin is used as a protective, it should be diluted (4 parts water) to the sp. gr. of blood serum.

Demulcents consist largely of colloid and mucilaginous substances. They are slowly absorbed, and so may decompose and irritate the alimentary tract. They increase secretion, particularly when used as lozenges. Licorice is an excellent demulcent for sore throat and tickling cough. Sassafras is a mucilaginous demulcent. Bismuth salts are about the best gastric sedatives in sufficient doses (up to ½ ounce daily), soon becoming evenly distributed over the whole inner surface of the stomach. They also allay intestinal irritation with diarrhea, and serve to prevent autointoxication (hydrothionemia) by combining with the hydrogen sulphide of intestinal putrefaction (Fuller). The undoubted good effect of olive oil in some cases of biliary colic is due probably to its demulcent action on the duodenum, with consequent lessening of gall-duct irritation. Demulcent mixtures (starch,

slippery elm) are of service as soothing enemas, and do not provoke peristalsis as crystalloids would. Demulcents have a local effect only, giving "body" and agreeable taste to a draught and assuaging thirst. Triticum (a starch and sugars) increases the quantity of urine simply by the water given with it (Cushny).

Counter-Irritants and Stimulants.—It has been shown by experiments on animals that when the vessels of the skin are dilated by the application of an irritant, those of the subjacent viscera are often reflexly contracted (White). If one hand is placed in cold water, a positive fall of temperature takes place in the other. The irritation of a surface involving the end-organs of the nervous system modifies the functions of the trophic nerves (Bartholow). There is a definite reflex relation between the internal organs and that part of the skin supplied by the same nervous segment (Head). The improvement of circulation produced by slight irritation may also be of benefit in chronic inflammatory conditions in the subcutaneous tissues (Cushny). Counter-irritation applied to a considerable surface increases the action of the heart, raises body temperature, and exalts the irritability of the nervous system.

The active principle of counter-irritants and stimulants is generally a volatile substance; hence, penetrating. Ethereal oils with low boiling points and comparatively little oxygen are very penetrating; thus, turpentine is more penetrating than mustard or cantharides. The sulphur-containing volatile oil of mustard is produced from a glucosid (sinigrin or sinalbin) by the action of a ferment (myrosin) in the presence of moisture. This ferment is destroyed by heating above 60° C., hence boiling water should not be used in making mustard plasters.

Alcohol is a local irritant and, properly diluted, may quicken the healing of sluggish sores. Tincture of arnica and the distilled extract of hamamelis owe what good effects they may have simply to the contained alcohol. Ammonia is quite penetrating but is not so corrosive as the fixed alkalies, since its action is of short duration. Most liniments are composed of volatile oils or stearoptenes, alcohol and ammonia. Iodine excites a mild but steady cutaneous irritation, and induces some congestion in the underlying tissues, thus aiding the absorption of exudates in them (Cushny). It destroys epithelium and causes it to peel off. Sulphur produces mild and prolonged irritation, since it acts only as gradually converted into sulphides. The much-vaunted ichthyol is a weak counter-irritant, depending for its action on the contained sulphur. Cantharidin vesication is less painful than when produced by mustard or turpentine, because the Spanish-fly is non-volatile and therefore less penetrating. Pustulants (croton oil) act as severe irritants in contact with living tissues, as at the orifices of the cutaneous glands (Cushny). The double salt, tartar emetic, is perhaps broken up and made active by the acid in the decomposing secretions of the skin. Carbon dioxide has a weak irritant effect; hence its use in baths and as carbonated drinks (increase stomach blood-flow and appetite).

Ammonia and ether are very powerful stimulants to the cardiac and respiratory centers, whether taken by the mouth or inhaled. The aromatic spirit of ammonia is one of the best all around cardiac stimulants for tiding a patient over a short period of danger. Volatile oils and their essences stimulate the heart reflexly, in addition to their local carminative influence. The virtue of asafetida is in its volatile oil. The nitro-compounds owe their vasodilator activity to the NO_2 ion. The nitrites of sodium and potassium act more slowly than the very volatile amyl nitrite (by inhalation), but their effects are more durable (four to six hours). Nitroglycerin is absorbed unchanged, and is broken up by the alkaline ingredients of the blood into a mixture of glycerin, nitrites and nitrates; the last named salts in the small quantity given have practically no action (Cushny). Strychnine greatly increases muscular activity (may cause fever) and exalts spinal irritability (reflex tone). Caffeine stimulates the cerebrum directly. Atropine enhances the motor power of the heart and diminishes inhibitory control. Small doses of quinine have a vasoconstrictor; large doses, a vasodilator action (Butler).

Caustics, Astringents, Styptics.—A caustic action indicates affinity for water and for the proteins in the secretions and tissues. Astringents coagulate the semifluid cement substance of the endothelial cells, and so prevent filtration of fluids and emigration of cells (Sollmann). Caustic alkalies are deeper in their action than the mineral acids, which tend to form a hard, insoluble, self-limiting eschar. Lunar caustic owes its escharotic action to the nitrate ion, metallic silver being deposited in the epithelium. Dilute solutions of caustic serve as astringents, contracting vessels and diminishing exudation and secretion.

The sulphates of aluminum and the heavy metals act as caustics and astringents—metasulphuric acid has a great avidity for water. Burnt alum is a good local application to granulations and condylomata. The sulphocarbolate of zinc is an effective antiseptic astringent. Zinc chloride and chromic oxide are very hygroscopic and equally caustic. Arsenous oxide is said to destroy diseased surfaces, leaving the healthy skin unaffected. Lead preparations are usually astringent, but rarely the irritant properties of the metal may set up diarrhea. Hydrochloric acid is of considerable value in fermentive diarrhea, the double sulphates of the urine diminishing under its use. The oxide and carbonate of zinc are much used for their astringent effect in acute skin diseases. Dilute acids applied to the skin are antihydrotic. Sweating feet are well treated by sponging with formalin (hardens

epithelium) or a 1:20 solution of chromic oxide. The astringent action of lime water is probably due to the formation of insoluble compounds with surface proteids (Cushny). Carbonate of calcium (chalk mixture or aromatic powder) is a useful antacid astringent in hyperacidity with diarrhea.

Vegetable astringents owe their properties as such chiefly to some form of tannin, which precipitates proteins (not peptones in an acid medium) as digestible tannates. For intestinal effect it is better to give the colloid U. S. P. preparations (kino, catechu, krameria, hamamelis), or, still better, insoluble combinations with proteins (digested by pancreatic juice), so as to avoid the local action on the stomach. These render the stools harder and firmer, and check diarrhea. An excess, by irritating the bowels, may lead to loose stools. Tannic and gallic acids given by the mouth are absorbed to a slight extent as tannate or gallate of sodium, which has no astringent effect; hence these remedies are useless for remote hemorrhages (Cushny).

Locally applied, tannin stops bleeding by coagulating the proteins of the blood, but only when brought into immediate contact with the bleeding point. Gallic acid and tannates do not coagulate albumin. Ergot acts directly (tetanic contraction) on the blood-vessels and unstriped muscle tissue. The convulsive alkaloid cornutine is the chief factor in the action of ergot on the uterus (Kobert). Gangrene may be brought about by the prolonged contraction of the arterioles, leading to a hyaline formation (by sphacelotoxin) in the lumen and walls (Cushny). Hydrastine is also a vasoconstrictor of the peripheral vessels, and is useful in menorrhagia. Acetanilid and antipyrin act on the muscular coat of small vessels as powerfully as ergot (White). The suprarenal derivatives have a marked vasoconstrictor and styptic effect when locally applied (nose, stomach, bowels), and have been much employed for internal hemorrhages, though with somewhat indefinite result. Turpentine contracts the arterioles, and is an effective hemostatic. Opiates (except codeine) lessen the secretions and diminish normal peristalsis. The salts of lead and iron are of no value in visceral bleeding, since they are absorbed only in minute quantities and in a non-astringent form. Ferric chloride is perhaps the best of the mineral styptics in capillary and recurrent hemorrhages (Cushny). It precipitates the proteins of the plasma, and so stops the flow when brought into actual contact (styptic cotton) with the bleeding point, as in the nose or gums. It may cause a fatal embolus when injected into the uterus, a nevus or an aneurism.

Eliminants.—Intestinal evacuants act by increasing osmotic pressure (hydragogues) and by exciting peristalsis. They should not be absorbed from the stomach, and those that act chemically are generally insoluble. The colloid character of impure sugars (honey, molasses, manna) causes delay of absorption and softer evacuations. Constipation is due chiefly to a sluggish colon, and most purgatives act principally on this portion of the intestine; calomel affects the small intestine particularly, and so is properly followed by salts (affect large bowel). Purgative salts have a greater tendency to precipitate proteins and less tendency to permeate into unorganized colloids than most non-purgative salts (Hofmeister). Very dilute solutions act as diuretics, but more slowly than non-laxative salts. The greater the purgative the less the diuretic effect. The stool is softer after purgation, from increased secretion and unabsorbed water. If the muscular coat is affected there is griping, which may be prevented to some degree by combining with carminatives or an alkali.

Sulphates, phosphates, tartrates and citrates are less readily absorbed than the univalent salts of the same metals (Cushny); hence they exert osmotic pressure in the bowel. Magnesium, being bivalent, is more slowly absorbed than univalent sodium. $MgSO_4$ is more purgative than Na_2SO_4, since in the former both ions are difficult of absorption. The sodium salt (c. p.) is, however, generally preferable (Wetherill); in fact $MgSO_4$ is largely changed to the acid carbonate and Na_2SO_4 in the bowel. The fluid, drawn by osmosis chiefly from the blood-vessels, by its weight, and the distention of the large bowel, causes increased peristalsis and evacuations that are much more prompt than those from vegetable purgatives, most of the salt appearing in the feces. The more concentrated the solution of salts administered and the more fluid in the tissues, the more profuse the evacuations will be. The oxide and carbonate of magnesium are insoluble (may form concretions)' and alkaline (counteract acidity). Calcium salts would probably be aperient were they not so readily precipitated. A small amount of $CaCl_2$ added to a saline enema prevents its premature expulsion (MacCallum).

None of the so-called cholagogues have any appreciable effect on the secretion of bile (calomel decreases it; bile salts augment it), but any of them may increase its excretion by hurrying it through the bowel. Calomel preserves the bile (and food) from putrefaction, and so gives a green color to the stool. It relieves " biliousness " due to disorders of the alimentary tract. Bile acids (fel bovis) irritate the mucous membrane of the large bowel, and so induce purgation (Stadelmann). There is no condition known in which increase of biliary secretion is indicated, since when the pressure is augmented in the gall-duct the secretion is automatically arrested (Cushny).

Vegetable purgatives serve as local irritants to the muscular layer of the bowel, especially in the presence of bile, which aids in their solution or suspension, thus bringing them into intimate contact with the mucous membrane. Soaps have a similar adjuvant action (Stadelmann). Many of these purgatives act specifically on the bowel (perhaps by excretion here) when injected subcutaneously (croton oil enepidermically). Cascara, frangula, senna, aloes and rhubarb owe their activity to anthracene or anthraquinone bodies, which are commonly attached to a sugar molecule, forming a glucoside (Cushny). Some of these principles are much less active than the crude drugs, since impurities may alter solubility; thus, aloin is less certain than aloes. On account of their taste, vegetable purgatives are usually prescribed in pill or tablet form. Rhubarb contains considerable tannin, and its use is often followed by constipation. The bitter stomachic by-action is in its favor. Aloin acts largely on the lower bowel and may cause piles. Its purgative effect is increased by the addition of a little iron and alkaline salts (Cushny). The cathartic acid of senna and cascara stimulates the colon especially. Convolvulin (jalap), jalapin (scammony), elaterin, bryonin, leptandrin, euonymin and the active principles of podophyllum are irritant resinous glucosides (anhydrids). Colchicum, guaiac, sanguinaria, xanthoxylum and stillingia owe their medicinal value mainly to their selective eliminant action on the mucous membrane of the intestine. Caffeine increases secretions, and so is slightly laxative.

Castor oil on saponification by pancreatic steapsin, yields irritant ricinoleic acid, which differs from the free acids of ordinary fixed oils in being unsaturated and containing an OH group. Croton oil is likewise changed to glycerin, and the very irritant crotonoleic acid; there is some free acid (much in old specimens) in the oil. The irritant effect of glycerin injected into the rectum causes prompt evacuation. Bile is no more effective than soap in enemas.

Diuresis by means of drugs depends on vasodilation (alcohol, nitrites), increase of arterial blood-pressure (digitalis), and direct stimulation of renal cells (salts of univalent metals). Salines are diuretic, since they accumulate fluid in the blood (capillary engorgement) at the expense of the tissues. Potassium salts are more diuretic than those of sodium, as the former react with other salts, producing an excess in the blood of certain salines, which are quickly excreted by the kidneys. When sweet spirit of niter is prescribed with water, the ethyl nitrite rapidly escapes, and the effect is merely that of alcohol and ether. Calomel is an effective diuretic in cardiac dropsy, probably by a direct action on the renal epithelium. Theobromine is preferable to caffeine as a diuretic, since the first alkaloid has no vasoconstrictor action (Cushny). Uva ursi is slightly antiseptic (arbutin and methyl-arbutin), and buchu also (volatile oil.) Zea maize owes its diuretic effect to a resinous acid.

Volatile oils are excreted chiefly by the lungs and kidneys, and are used as stimulating expectorants (terpene, terebene, balsams, squill). Alkalies also increase the secretions in bronchitis and render them more fluid. Pilocarpine acts on the nerve-endings in the gland cells; it augments the proportion of urea in the sweat. Emetics act locally (emetine, antimony) and centrally (apomorphine). In the latter event they are best given hypodermically.

Digestants.—Hydrochloric acid is of the greatest value in conditions accompanied by hypo- or achlorhydria, being requisite to the action of pepsinogen, a stimulant of pancreatic secretion and an effective antiseptic. It should be given in full doses—10 drops of the strong acid just after eating, to be repeated in one-half hour and again in an hour if need be, always well diluted (Hershey). This quantity at the most is about half what nature should furnish. As an aid to peptic action HCl is exceeded only by HF and $H_2C_2O_4$, both poisonous. Alkalies give quick relief in hyperchlorhydria, and render mucus less tenacious. Alkaline salts have no action on the bile, but may be of benefit in hepatic diseases through their sedative effect on the duodenum (Stadelmann). Milk treated with lime water curdles in finer flakes and so is more easily digested.

Pepsin is not needed in the great majority of cases of dyspepsia, since the zymogen is present in quantity even when the acid secretion is insufficient. Moreover, as Cushny remarks, the doses usually given are amusingly small (nature furnishes about three ounces daily). Practical uses for the essence of pepsin are the preparation of junket and whey, and coadministration with iodides and salicylates to prevent irritation of the stomach. Pancreatic ferments are destroyed by the acid gastric juice (in about $\frac{1}{2}$ hour after food is taken), hence if diastatic mixtures are thought to be needed they should be given at the beginning of a meal or three or four hours later. It is a question whether the ordinary digestive juices are ever unable to digest the starch of food (Cushny). "Amylaceous dyspepsia" is usually a fermentive condition due to lack of HCl.

All bitter (taraxacum, quassia, calumba, hydrastis) and aromatic substances given by the mouth, reflexly increase the flow of saliva and gastric juice, and excite the appetite psychically. Nux vomica or strychnine is also a direct stimulant to the muscular coat of the stomach, rarely producing painful spasm of this organ. Bitters are best administered shortly before meals. They are of value in convalescence and sedentary habits and occasionally in chronic dyspeptic conditions (Cushny). Their long-continued use produces gastric catarrh, decrease of normal gastric juice and impaired digestion (Bartholow).

Carminatives (chiefly volatile oils) cause a sensation of warmth and comfort in the stomach and a marked increase in the gastric juice (by reflex from the mouth and nose). They accelerate the movements of the stomach, promote absorption and relieve flatulence and distention (Cushny). They are most useful in sedentary subjects with no marked gastro-intestinal irrita-

tion. Their effects in the large bowel are best obtained by giving full doses (of asafetida and turpentine, for example) in enemas of hot water and soap. For administration by the mouth cardamom is both pleasant and effective. Capsicum is much used for the dyspepsia of drunkards. Aromatic ammonia is a mild gastric stimulant in debility and alcoholism. It appears to act reflexly as a general stimulant in collapse or heart failure (Cushny). The action of viburnum and other uterine sedatives is probably of a similar nature to that of peppermint and ginger. The volatile oil in myrrh renders it a healing agent for sore gums. Spirits are all carminative and stimulant.

Restoratives.—Among nutrient medicines cod-liver oil ranks first. It is in fact little else than an easily emulsified fat, and is especially valuable to increase weight in delicate children. It is perhaps more readily oxidized in the body than other oils (Heyerdahl). Eructations result when the free acids contained in the oil are air-changed to oxyacids. The traces of halogens and alkaloids contained in the oil, and supposed to be present in wines of cod-liver oil, can hardly have any medicinal effect. Phosphorus exists in the elemental state in the blood, and its effects on the tissues are unquestionably due to the element itself and to none of its compounds (Cushny). It has a specific stimulating action on the formation of bone from cartilage, being much more effective in rickets when given in cod-liver oil (Rey). An excess causes deficient oxidation and fatty degeneration. Phosphoric acid and its salts have never been shown to be of any benefit in any cachectic conditions. Calcium salts are not likely to be of service in human rickets, since in these cases there is plenty of calcium phosphate in the blood, but the bones cannot take it up. Calcium chloride is claimed to be of service in hemophilia; its presence is necessary to the formation of fibrin ferment. Bitter tonics stimulate the production of appetite juice through psychic contrast (Pawlow). They have little or no effect in this direction when introduced directly into the stomach. Tonics favor decomposition of waste products and stimulate tissue formation by catalysis (Benedikt).

Arsenic increases appetite and promotes digestion, growth and nutrition, perhaps by selective action on epithelium (Cushny). It seems to act only on living cells. It is beneficial in many forms of chronic skin diseases (deleterious in acute stages), and temporarily in pernicious anemia. Cumulative excess lessens oxidation (H_3AsO_3 takes O from living cells) and causes fatty degeneration of the viscera. According to Bertrand, arsenic is a fundamental constituent of the human body. Iron is the hematinic par excellence, particularly in chlorosis, and is best given probably in some organic combination. The anemia of plethora requires agents to overcome suboxidation, rather than hematinics (Shoemaker). Very small doses of mercury, given for some time, increase weight, nutrition and the number and quality of the blood cells (Cushny) by stimulating metabolism (alterative). Gold is of no value in therapeutics, except possibly by suggestion. Quinine differs from most other alkaloids in acting on the general nutrition of protoplasm. It lessens the number of leucocytes, which may be one factor in reducing the size of the spleen (Cushny). It lessens the destruction of nitrogenous bodies and the formation of uric acid, thus sometimes relieving non-malarial headache and neuralgia. Sarsaparilla is not a bloodbuilder, but the reverse. Owing to its saponincontent, it induces hemolysis (Kobert) if absorbed.

The members of the digitalis series consist of glucosides or indifferent compounds of C, H and O, probably with a common nucleus belonging to the picrotoxine series (Cushny). The active principle of the adrenals (adrenalin, epinephrin) contains a pyridin nucleus. It raises the blood pressure more than any other remedy, partly by direct action on the arteriolar muscular coats, partly by enhanced cardiac contraction of vasomotor origin. Thyroid extract causes rapid loss of weight (I have noted 11 pounds loss in a month), with increase of urinary nitrogen and phosphates, in goiter, cretinism, myxedema and soft anemic obesity. This reduction is due to augmented waste of body proteids, rapid oxidation of fats, and diuresis. Part of the constituent iodine of the extract is taken up by the patient's thyroid, and part is excreted in the urine as iodides. Much more iodine is required to act in goiter when taken as the element than when ingested as thyroid extract or iodothyrin (Cushny). Thyroid extract is injurious in Graves's disease, which thymus extract is said to relieve sometimes.

Hypnotics, Antipyretics, Anodynes, Analgesics, Anesthetics.—The narcotic effect of certain drugs may depend on a reducing action, drawing oxygen out of the biogen molecules of the nerve centers. The solvent power on the fats (of neurones) of the methane derivatives may also have something to do with their general anesthetic effect. Hypnotics probably induce changes in the brain similar to those of natural sleep. Chloral does not break up into chloroform in the blood, as Liebreich thought, but is excreted in the urine in combination with glycuronic acid (urochloralic acid). Its continued use leads to imperfect oxidation (fatty degeneration) and augmented destruction of body proteids. Sulphonal and trional are almost insoluble in water, hence their action is slow and uncertain, though comparatively safe. Sulphonal is excreted as ethyl-sulphonic acid, but the narcosis produced is due to the unchanged molecule (Cushny). The resinous red oil (cannabinol) of cannabis indica seems to be the active principle. Morphine is excreted mainly by the digestive tract, only traces being found in the urine; therefore it is not contraindicated in uremic convulsions. The benefit derived

from valerian in hysteric affections is probably due to the strong mental impression produced by its odor and taste. Valerianates act only as do the salts of other organic acids.

Chemical antithermics act by diminishing exalted cellular protoplasmic activity, by modifying the function of the red blood cells and by a direct sedative action on the nervous system. Antipyrin is useful in lingering pyrexia after infection is ended, to control excessive oxidation by reducing metabolism to the needs of the economy (Roger). Except antipyrin, all modern antipyretics (phenetidine compounds) owe their activity to the formation of simple derivatives of paramidophenol in the tissues. This decomposition should be gradual, for if too rapid there result collapse and destructive blood changes (methemoglobinemia, cyanosis). The cyanosis is due to vasoconstriction and consequent engorgement of capillaries and slowing of the current therein, whereby oxyhemoglobin is unduly reduced (Sajous). Acetanilid in large doses increases tissue waste about one-third. Antipyretics affect chiefly the thermotactic nervous mechanism, thus lowering the point (as in a thermostat) at which the temperature is maintained (Cushny). They cause dilation of the cutaneous vessels, with sweating and increased thermolysis. True thermolytic drugs (alcohol, spirit of nitrous ether, ipecac, antimony) were more used formerly than at present. Sudorifics (pilocarpine, salicylates) lower febrile temperature by increased dissipation of heat. Purgatives sometimes act as febrifuges by removal of reflex irritation and of sources of intoxication. Quinine retards metabolism. Aconite, pulsatilla, gelsemium, grindelia and quebracho are motor depressants. All antipyretic phenetidine compounds have likewise an anodyne effect.

Cocaine is a general protoplasm poison (causes scars aside from infection), with some selective affinity for certain nerve-endings, and it causes transient local contraction of the blood-vessels. Its anesthesiophore function is due to the benzoyl group. Cocaine and HCN check vomiting by their local anesthetic effect. Menthol makes the skin or mucous membrane warmer by several degrees, but imparts a sensation of cold, since it affects the psychrophoric dendrites most. Aconite is distinctly analgesic. Volatile oils (cloves) relieve the pain of an aching tooth by paralyzing the exposed nerve-ends after preliminary irritation (Cushny). Guaiacol is a powerful analgesic and antipyretic. A fine spray of any volatile substance (ether, ethyl chloride) produces cold by rapid evaporation, and so benumbs the skin. Except nitrous oxide, all anesthetics belong to the alcohols or simple or haloid ethers. When a subject has acquired a tolerance for alcohol, he requires a larger quantity of hypnotics or anesthetics. Ether and chloroform are absorbed and excreted almost wholly by the lungs, according to the ordinary physic laws of absorption of gases by fluids (Cushny). The greater the concentration of vapor in the lungs, the more is absorbed into the blood, and overconcentration at any time, rather than the total amount inhaled, may give rise to dangerous symptoms. Chloroform enters into a loose combination with the lecithin of the red cells and the brain, causing slight coagulation of the protoplasm of the ganglion cells; Pohl has found much more chloroform in the brain than the liver. Nitrous oxide, when inhaled, behaves as a molecular depressant (like chloroform or ether) to the central nervous system. In relation to the blood it behaves as an indifferent gas (like H or N), causing asphyxia, since it is not a supporter of combustion at body temperature.

SOME RECENT DEVELOPMENTS IN CLINICAL PATHOLOGY.[1]

BY FREDERIC E. SONDERN, M.D.,
OF NEW YORK.

THE chemical and microscopical examinations made as an aid in diagnosis and prognosis are matters which have been receiving a large share of attention during the last few years, as shown by the many recent publications on the subject. The *refinements* of this work require a rather expert knowledge of chemistry and of chemical laboratory technic, somewhat beyond that usually acquired in the medical school even at present, and a more elaborate working outfit than the clinician has been in the habit of maintaining. An added difficulty is the amount of time required by this work, and interruptions are likely to jeopardize the accuracy and consequently the utility of the investigation. As a result of this, much of the work has been done by beginning practitioners often insufficiently equipped with knowledge and apparatus, and by chemists without clinical knowledge and consequently not able to appreciate the direction in which to pursue an investigation, a direction apparent to the clinician by developments early in the examination. Publications on the subject are oftentimes faulty from the physician's point of view; either the technic has not been described with sufficient minuteness to tempt the practitioner to make the investigations, or the article has been burdened with graphic formulæ and technical description without a clear statement as to the absolute clinical value of the procedure.

Most men appreciate that clinical pathology is a factor of more or less value as the case may be, in diagnosis and prognosis, but as in all other questions there are extremists. It is reasonable to claim that the practitioner who makes every diagnosis in the laboratory is as short-sighted and liable to grave error as the man who ignores microscope and test tube. The laboratory finding should be considered one of the supports in diagnosis and only in exceptional instances the diagnosis itself.

[1] Read at the Annual Meeting of the New York County Medical Society, Oct. 24, 1904.

While it is impossible to review in the few minutes at my disposal all the advances made since the subject has had more careful attention, I hope you will allow me to allude briefly to a number of points which are, or promise to be, of undoubted clinical merit.

The aids given by careful blood examination in the differential diagnosis of chlorosis, secondary anemia and pernicious anemia are well understood, generally appreciated and need no further comment. The present methods of determining the amount of coloring matter in blood are crude and need replacement by more scientific determinations of the actual amounts of hemoglobin and iron. Detailed examination of leucocytes and the differential count of the same in cases of acute and chronic leucemia lead to general dissatisfaction with the present clinical classification, which is as much in need of revision as was that of Bright's disease twenty years ago. Since blood examinations have become a routine matter, the details of many cases of acute lymphatic leucemia have been published; cases where death would probably have been ascribed to other diseases had the examinations not been made. In recent literature one also finds careful records which would seem to indicate an acute myeloid leucemia, a hitherto undescribed disease.

Concerning the Widal clump reaction in typhoid, prolonged use demonstrates that positive reactions are rare before the fifth day in bed. This makes the test of less diagnostic value early in the disease than we had hoped at first.

A method for the use of sterile suspensions of typhoid bacilli instead of fresh live cultures has been revived. Widal reactions in non-typhoid cases are often due to inaccurate rather than to deliberately insufficient dilutions, and to the use of improper cultures. On a recent visit to some military and civil hospitals in Japan, I was pleased to find the dilutions made in accurate blood pipettes with carefully prepared bouillon cultures, and not as one sometimes observes at home, with dried drops of blood of unknown size, an old agar typhoid culture and water, the dilution judged by the color of the resulting mixture. It is not my object to condemn the use of dried blood for the Widal test, but if it is used, my experience teaches that a bouillon culture and a careful attempt at volumetric dilution are far better than a mechanical mixture of bacilli and a colorimetric dilution. The administration or urotropin has been known to give a Widal reaction in the usual dilutions.

In suspected malaria it is well to remember when searching for *Plasmodia*, that the characteristic evidences of a decided secondary anemia and an increase in the relative percentage of large lymphocytes, are corroborative factors.

Blood changes as an indication of inflammatory lesions have recently been the subject of much discussion and promise a valuable aid in diagnosis. The presence and degree of leucocytosis is the feature on which most conclusions are based, and present day literature is still largely occupied with this problem. Many monographs have appeared in which the authors attempt to fix the degree of leucocytosis at which an inflammatory lesion without exudate may be suspected and that at which a suspicion of the presence of a purulent exudate is justified. Leucocytosis is, however, largely dependent on body resistance toward infection; thus good resistance will occasion pronounced leucocytosis in slight infections, and poor resistance little or no leucocytosis in grave infections. As there is no method of determining this body resistance with sufficient accuracy, the inference drawn from a leucocytosis of given degree must remain questionable except perhaps in unusually excessive counts.

For the past few years I have been impressed by the fact that the differential count of leucocytes offers a far better guide as to the status of the inflammatory process, one which is not influenced to a perceptible degree by body resistance, and furthermore, that the leucocytosis with a given differential count may be an indicator of this body resistance. I cannot here enter into the details of this subject, but I hope to lay the matter before you with the necessary clinical and laboratory data at an early date.

Cytodiagnosis in cerebrospinal, pleuritic and peritoneal transudates and exudates has been the subject of extended research, and some advances of practical value have been made. In the differential diagnosis of exudate and transudate, the older chemical methods are still very much in use.

Careful urine analysis and attention to the evidences of faulty metabolism are important in the differential diagnosis of nephritic eclampsia and that due to puerperal toxemia, and of neurosis and definite gastro-intestinal lesions, and present distinct therapeutic indications in the diseases classed under the headings of rheumatism and gout.

In the different varieties of nephritis the urine offers much information of clinical value in addition to albumin and casts. While extensive records tempt me to resent Cabot's statement in a former lecture at the New York Academy of Medicine, that the knowledge of the daily excretion of urea is useless, still it is time that the quotations of " grains per ounce " disappeared from our hospital charts.

In diabetes the urine also presents facts which give a much better insight to the patient's actual condition than the mere knowledge of the percentage of sugar.

Examination of specimens of urine obtained by ureter-catheter, cryoscopy of blood and urine, and the phloridzin, methylene blue and indigocarmine methods of estimating renal functional ability are of much value to the surgeon, give clearer indications and contra-indications in contemplated renal surgery and have thus contributed to improved statistics.

MEDICAL PROGRESS.

SURGERY.

Congenital Absence of the Tibia.—This subject is interesting principally from the standpoint of its etiology, which may be considered as still unsettled. The condition is viewed from a new point of view by J. K. YOUNG (*Univ. Penn. Med. Bull.*, November, 1904), who reports four cases which have been under his observation, making a total of 51 thus far known. The theories as to the cause for the deformity may be summarized as follows: Heredity, prenatal disease, or musculonervous theory; arrest of development, or osseous theory; mechanical pressure, or intra-uterine pressure theory; and amniotic adhesion theory. The author is inclined to the latter theory and believes that the amniotitis, which is the cause of the amniotic adhesions, is a traumatism occurring in the early months of fetal life. Five cases are known in which the effect of injury upon the loss of parts could be traced. The fact that the tibia suffers more frequently than other parts is due to two factors—first, the position of the fetus is such that the pressure upon the abdomen would force the lower extremities against the sacrum and produce an injury to the amnion directly overlying the tibia, and second, the centers of ossification of the tibia are deposited very early,—during the seventh week, which accounts for the loss of the shaft of the lower extremity. After the attachment of the part to the amnion, the inflammation present produces an acute polyhydramnios which, making traction upon the attached portion of the amnion, pulls the skin and the underlying structures from their places, separating them from their vascular and nervous connections, or by the formation of amniotic bands, cutting them off entirely and producing their absorption. The author's cases lead him to think that a sudden and violent pressure upon the uterus which would be sufficient to cause inflammation of the soft parts, but not of sufficient force to injure or fracture the bones, would lead to an amniotitis, followed by a hydramnios which would produce the exact conditions which are found in these deformities. The traumatism probably occurs about the third month of fetal life.

A Case of Thymus Death from Local Anesthesia.—This took place in a woman, aged thirty-one years, who presented a goiter of moderate size, the removal of which was undertaken by the aid of Schleich's method of infiltration anesthesia. H. NETTEL (*Archiv f. klin. Chir.*, Vol. 73, No. 3) who reports the case, states that the patient suddenly lost consciousness, went into rapid collapse and died apparently with paralysis of pulse and respiration. The autopsy showed the presence of the status lymphaticus with enormous hyperplasia of the entire lymphatic apparatus, especially the lymph follicles in the tongue, spleen and intestines. The author thinks that the immediate cause of death was the operative procedure combined with the mental excitement of the patient. This is similar to the sudden death which individuals afflicted in this manner often meet by being subjected to comparatively trivial irritants, such as taking a bath. Nettel thinks that the best method of anesthesia in these cases is by means of ether given in the smallest possible amount and for the briefest possible period.

Sarcoma and Carcinoma in the Same Individual.—An instance of this kind is described by H. HABERER (*Archiv f. klin. Chir.*, Vol. 73, No. 3), in a man, fifty-four years of age, who presented a rounded growth on the border of the epiglottis. It was shaped like a mushroom and was readily removed by the cautery loop. Microscopical examination showed the tumor to be a spindle-celled sarcoma. A year and a half later the patient presented himself with an infiltrating, indurated tumor at the base of the tongue. Total extirpation of the tongue was performed, together with excision of the epiglottis and the hyoid bone. Two days after the operation he died from pneumonia. The tumor was found to be a carcinoma. The author considers the case as one where two independent malignant growths presented themselves, each arising from separate organ and tissues, a number of similar cases being known.

Contribution to the Technic of Nerve Suture.— A method for bringing about union between the ends of divided nerves is suggested by C. FORAMITTI (*Deut. med. Woch.*, Vol. 73, No. 3), who proposes to insert these ends into sections of fresh or hardened arteries. The tubes may be prepared from the fresh arteries of animals, or sections of the latter may be drawn over glass rods the exact size of the caliber of the vessel, and then hardened in formalin, washed with water, boiled, and then preserved in alcohol. The extremity of the divided nerve is caught with a thread of catgut which is passed through the lumen of the tube. The latter may then be shoved over the end of the nerve. The same catgut thread may be then attached to the other end of the nerve and this likewise drawn into the lumen of the tube. Both ends are then held in place by this foreign body. The experiments have been successfully conducted in dogs without producing any reaction, and the author suggests that the method be given a trial in the human subject.

Diagnostic Value of Blood Examination in Surgery.—TUFFIER is reported in the (*Gazz. deg. Osped.*, November 29, 1904, as follows: Cryoscopy of the blood is now a method of value in the diagnosis of renal disease. Whenever the increase of molecular concentration of the blood shows a persistent insufficiency of the kidneys, nephrectomy ought not to be performed. Unfortunately this method does not give constant results in renal disease; the increase of molecular concentration does not always indicate a bilateral lesion, and even in insufficiency or uremia, the point of molecular concentration may be normal or sub-normal. The hemoglobin index is valuable. Mikulicz does not operate if it is below 38 per cent, except by means of local anesthesia. Bloodgood and Cabot do not believe in general anesthesia if the hemoglobin is below 40 per cent. The study of the red corpuscles is of less importance to surgery. The iodophil reaction of the leucocytes in suppuration is interesting. Locke in 800 cases claimed great value to the test in demonstrating the existence of a focus of suppuration. It has been obtained however in gonorrheal rheumatism.

The presence of leucocytosis is valuable in pointing to hidden purulent inflammation, especially in appendicitis, and a disproportion between the temperature and the leucocytosis is even more important. In rupture of one of the viscera following a contusion of the abdomen, Cazin has demonstrated a rapid increase of leucocytes. In intestinal perforation in typhoid fever, the hypoleucocytosis suddenly changes to hyperleucocytosis. In carcinoma, a gradual diminution of the red corpuscles, an equal decrease of hemoglobin and a polynuclear leucocytosis is suggestive of malignancy. In gynecology may or may not assist in diagnosis.

Treatment of Cancer.—It is not at all certain that Koch's laws will be valid for the forms of parasites

other than bacteria, which are gradually being shown to take a prominent place in the infections of the human body. MAYO-ROBSON (*Lancet*, December 3, 1904) states that we know nothing at present conclusively as to the etiology of cancer. Councilman has shown that vaccine bodies form one phase of the life history of the protozoan said to cause smallpox, and Roswell Park regards the cell inclusions in cancer as being of the same nature. At the Royal Institute, a microscope was exhibited, which showed objects distinctly under a magnifying power of 10,000 diameters. In order to understand what this means, a nouse-fly under this magnification would appear 24 feet long by 13 feet broad. This instrument will undoubtedly bring to light many hitherto absolutely unknown and unthought of conditions. As to the infectivity of cancer, the author states that it is both contagious and innoculable. So positively is this now known that all dressings from cancer patients should be burnt and that common use of beds and utensils should not occur. Preventive operations should be practised on precancerous conditions. Most of these are found in the skin, occuring as warts, eczematous patches, sebaceous tumors, ulcers, scars, etc. When these occupy such a position that they are liable to irritation, they should be excised, and under any conditions, the mere enlargement, without any other significant signs of malignancy, should constitute sufficient grounds for their immediate excision. The precancerous conditions in the mammary glands, such as eczema of the nipple, chronic inflammatory enlargements, cysts, and induration from traumatism. In the presence of these lesions, delay is inadmissible. Precancerous conditions of the stomach are considered under the one general heading of ulceration, the conclusion being that ulcers should be removed. The precancerous conditions of the pelvic organs of women, particularly those who have had lacerated cervices, old ulcers, leucorrhea and other forms of endometritis are discussed. Conditions which are termed precancerous in the intestines, are considered by the author and he urges the use of the electric sigmoidoscope as the only means of determining papillomatous conditions which may reasonably be looked upon as precursors of malignant change. As to the radical treatment of cancer, he quotes Halsted's ultimate results in 161 cases. Of these $42^8/_{10}$ per cent were positively cured, $51^9/_{10}$ per cent survived the three years' limit. Cancer of the stomach, according to the statistics of Kocher, is by no means hopeless. He has performed 97 resections of the stomach. Of these 52 cases or $65^4/_{10}$ per cent. recovered; $34^6/_{10}$ per cent. died. From 1898 to August, 1904, 45 cases have been operated on with $82^2/_{10}$ per cent. recoveries. As to definite results, 51 of the whole series died later, living up to six years. The average being $18^7/_{10}$ months. Twenty cases are still living, the oldest one of the series having been operated upon 16 $^1/_4$ years ago. Nineteen are in good health. Of Mayo's 43 operations, several are well more than two years after the operation. The statistics are given of the results of radical operation for malignant disease of the tongue, the larynx, the intestine, the rectum, the gall-bladder and liver, the lip, the penis, and the uterus. Some crusade, the author urges, should be taken against the neglect of the well-known early symptoms of early form of cancer, but of uterine malignant growth in particular.

Modern Bullet Wounds.—The Russian-Japanese war will undoubtedly cause a revision of the entire subject of bullet wounds. The old-fashioned lead bullet has been displaced by the small caliber nickel-jacketed missile, driven by smokeless powder. The Japanese bullet is smaller, has greater penetration, flatter trajectory and greater range. FRANK W. FOXWORTHY (*Annals of Surgery*, December 4, 1904) believes that the difference between these and the Russian wounds will be very little, as all high-velocity bullets give practically the same wounds. The increased velocity has no bearing on wounds in the soft tissues, its most obvious ill effects being found on the nervous system. The one exception to this rule is in the case of brain wounds. Heads struck by modern bullets frequently have a small wound at entrance, while the entire opposite side of the skull is blown off together with more than half the cranial contents. The track of a normally flying bullet through the body is straight, no structure in the body being dense enough to interfere with its direction. It bites out pieces of nerves and blood vessels, comminutes dense bone and perforates cancellous bone. English and American surgeons place abdominal wounds in the following fatality order: (1) Spleen wounds, most fatal of all; (2) perforating wounds of the small intestine and mesentery; (3) wounds of the stomach; (4) wounds of the large intestine; (5) wounds of bladder; (6) wounds of liver; (7) wounds of kidney; (8) non-perforating wounds of the intestine; the least fatal of all. Treves has formulated the following rules; In penetrating abdominal bullet wounds, he advises operation if (1) patient is seen before seven hours have elapsed; (2) patient has had an empty stomach when wounded; (3) patient has had a short and easy transport. He advises non-interference if (1) patient not seen until seven hours have elapsed; (2) there has been a long and tedious transport; (3) patient has been wounded soon after a meal; (4) the liver, spleen, or kidney be wounded; (5) it be a transverse or oblique wound above the umbilicus; (6) the bullet is retained; (7) the wound be below umbilicus, as in this locality the patients generally get along all right. (8) the colon alone be implicated (except the transverse).

Closing Wounds of Larger Arteries.—No one can operate many times without inadvertently wounding an important artery. GEORGE EMERSON BREWER (*Annals of Surgery*, December, 1904) recites the history of a case in which he, while doing an ordinary Bassini operation, he cut the femoral artery with a Hagedorn needle, and after ineffectual attempts at suturing, was obliged to tie the artery. This experience forcibly presented to him the desirability of perfecting some technic of closing such wounds. At the Surgical Laboratory of Columbia University he carried on a series of experiments on large dogs, during which he evolved the technic which is singularly successful and practical. The technic depends upon the employment of an elastic arterial plaster, which is wound around the artery, extending well above and below the wound. Such material must be thin, elastic and capable of maintaining its elasticity for several days after being imbedded. No suture will hold in a sclerosed or calcified wall, but such a preparation should work equally well irrespective of the condition of the artery. The vessel to be experimented upon is brought to the surface of the wound and compression is then made approximally and distally. The part is then thoroughly cleaned with sponges saturated with ether. A strip of the plaster is then passed beneath the vessel and the two corners are held by artery clamps. The elastic is then gently stretched and the lower

extremity placed in contact with the vessel, while the upper is drawn upward. This causes the vessel to rotate so that the surface of the plaster come in contact. A rotary motion of the thumb and forefinger completes the technic. The most important point in the successful application of this method lies in the employment of exceedingly thin and adhesive plaster, and second, in the obtaining of perfect asepsis.

The Present Status of Prostatic Surgery.—This department of surgery has made tremendous strides in the last decade. Ten years ago J. WILLIAM WHITE (*Annals of Surgery*, December, 1904) reviewed the conditions of prostatic surgery up to that date and again to-day he dwells upon the same topic. It is well known that a decade ago he regarded castration as curative of prostatic hypertrophy for the reason that he believed it to be the result of a persistance of the testicles after the need for these organs had disappeared. The theory seemed logical, but has unfortunately not been supported clinically. In his present article, however, White states that Robsing has recently reported five cases of double castration. In three of these, there was no history of previous gonorrhea, and the results were extremely favorable. The two remaining cases showed no improvement, but it is interesting to note that both were gonorrheal. Referring to palliative treatment, the author states that it still consists, as it did ten years ago, either in the use of steel sounds or in the employment of the catheter. He considers that the attitude of the professional should be rather toward early operation than toward palliation. He concludes that the objections to habitual catheterism are: (1) the risk of vesicle infection; (2) the production of vesicle atomy. He considers that the section of the neck of the bladder by Bottini's method and its modifications should in fairness be regarded as still on trial. It may be that surgeons are correct in dismissing castration and vasectomy from consideration. Neither of these methods have been given suitable trial by the profession. Since Robsing in 1902 reported 40 cases of vasectomy, of which 27 were cured, 9 relieved and 4 unimproved, there have been no notable papers on the subject. In the last ten years, White has found but 15 cases in which he considered castration justifiable and 37 in which he has performed vasectomy. The results were gratifying. The extraordinary results of total extirpation by improved technic have cast into unreserved shadow more conservative methods which still deserve recognition.

PHYSIOLOGY.

Ethyl Alcohol Considered as a Food.—There is probably no question before physiologists and practising physicians which has remained longer in an unsettled condition than this one. W. H. GODDARD (*Lancet*, October 22, 1904) gives a history of a large number of experiments on dogs from the study of which he reaches a number of interesting conclusions. The animals weighed each about ten kilograms and they were thoroughly purged and subsequently starved for twenty-four hours. Sixteen grams of alcohol was then given, after which the animal was placed in a respiration chamber and the expired air as well as the urine passed during the time collected. The animal was then killed and the body examined for all the carbon compounds, with the exception of the carbonates previously enumerated as derived from alcohol. Another dog of similar weight was then used, the amount of alcohol being doubled. The examination of this animal was made identical with that of the first. Lastly, double the quantity of alcohol to that in the last instance was given and the same methods pursued. The author concludes from his experiments that when alcohol to the amount of $1/100$ part of the body-weight was administered a little more than five per cent. of bad alcohol was excreted, and since no aldehyde or other alcoholic derivatives were found in any part of the body or in the excreta of the animal after death, one may conclude that 95 per cent. is used as a food. When double the quantity of alcohol is given a little more than 65 per cent. is excluded and here, for the first time, acetic aldehyde makes its appearance in the expired air. This may perhaps justly be interpreted as an indication of a failure on the part of the animal system to deal with so large a quantity of alcohol, and more especially so since at the same time there is no aldehyde in the urine or elsewhere in the body. When as in the last set of experiments, very large doses are given, nearly 50 per cent. of alcohol or its equivalent is excreted. There is thus to be noticed an absolute failure on the part of the body to utilize half of the alcohol administered. The compounds into which the alcohol has been formed are aldehyde, alkaline acetates, alkaline carbonates and probably carbon dioxide and water. Other carbon compounds excreted from the animal may exist in addition to these, but they are not distinguishable by the chemical methods employed. In small doses, therefore, alcohol is most undoubtedly a food, but inasmuch as half of it is excreted from the system when large doses are given, it cannot then be considered a food in the proper sense.

The Function of the Tonsil.—An interesting contribution to this subject is made by G. B. Wood (*Univ. Penn. Med. Bull.*, October, 1903), who has made careful histological studies and brings forward three propositions for discussion. These are (1) the older forms of leucocytes are derived by a continuous development from the younger lymphocytes. He thinks the lymphoid cell must be considered to be a young form of leucocyte capable of growing and undergoing certain morphological changes. (2) The lymphocyte is originally derived from the epithelial structures. In this connection the thymus gland plays the most important rôle. Recent research has practically established the fact that there is a direct conversion of the epithelial cells into lymphocytes in the center of the ingrowing sprout of epithelium in the thymus, before any outside structures could have influenced this metamorphosis. (3) There exists a strong histological evidence that lymphocytes are directly derived from the epithelium of the tonsillar crypts. In the development of the tonsil there is an ingrowth of epithelium into the mesodermic tissue before any lymphoid cells can be seen in this region. The first lymphocytes in the tonsil are found directly around this epithelial ingrowth and are characterized by fine anastomosing processes of protoplasm. A careful histological study has convinced Wood that the epithelium of the crypts exhibits a marked tendency toward constant growth. This is shown by the penetration of the epithelial cells into the parenchyma of the tonsil and the formation of keratoid masses in the lumen of the crypt. There also exist transitional cells by which all stages may be traced between the epithelial cell and the lymphocyte and the variation of types in the latter is most marked in the region of the cryptal epithelium. The degree of infiltration of the epithelium holds no relation to the cryptal contents. On the other hand, the ingrowing sprouts of epithelium possessing no lumen, show as much, if not more infiltration than the true crypts. The complete destruction of the cryptal epithelium is a rare occurrence, almost always a sufficient number of epithelial

cells being left to provide an intact barrier along the surface toward the cryptal lumen. The author thinks he is justified in saying that the truth of his three propositions has been established, and that an affirmative answer must be given the question, "Is the tonsil a primogenial source of leucocytosis"? If to the tonsils is accorded the function of leucocytic primogenesis, their presence in the human economy is explained. The leucocytes are intimately connected with various tissue changes, and the tonsils are the largest and most fully developed at the time of life when tissue changes are most active,—in childhood. The tonsils take up the function of the thymus gland after this atrophies earlier in life. Furthermore the author thinks that the adenoid tissue in the adult may be carrying on the same work which was accorded the tonsils in childhood.

Venous Valves in Relation to Varicose Veins.— That the venous valves play a less important rôle in the mechanism of the circulation than is usually taught, is the opinion of LEDERHOSE (*Deut. med. Wochenschr.*, Oct. 20, 1904). He does not believe that the valves support the column of blood in the veins of the lower limbs, or that these are a feature in accelerating the blood stream or prevent regurgitation in sudden changes of position in the limbs. It is also known that the number of veins decreases with increasing years. The author's theory is, that in most cases the valves play no part in adjusting the circulation, but that this is effected by retrograde stasis and variations in speed. The writer applies this theory to the cure of varicose veins by the Trendelenburg method of ligating the saphenous vein. The aspirating effect of the movements of the large joints on the vessels causes blood from the femoral vein to be drained out more rapidly in the act of walking, and if the saphenous vein has been ligated, the varicosities can more easily discharge their contents into the deeper vessels without receiving any additions from the long column of blood in the saphenous vein.

Action of Ammonia Compounds of Some Metals. —J. BOCK (*Arch. f. exp. Path. u. Pharmak.*, Vol. 52, Nos. 1 and 2) has carefully studied the action of certain ammonia compounds of metals on animals with the following results: In frogs the hexamin cobaltic salts behave as strong poisons, giving rise first to a paralysis of the peripheral motor nerves, later to clonic muscular switchings and convulsions owing to irritation of the medulla spinalis. In guinea-pigs, tetanic convulsions are very typical. The aqua-pentamin compounds (one ammonia group replaced by water) possesses much less toxicity, but gives rise to the same train of symptoms. With still more water in the molecule, the poisonous qualities are gradually lost. The chloropentamin compounds show, in addition, a decidedly narcotic action upon the brain and the same diminution of toxicity is observed if radicals of water are introduced. The carbonatotetramin compounds are almost innocuous. Though metallic cobalt, and its simpler inorganic compounds, possess distinct toxic properties for cold and warm-blooded animals, nothing of this is observed in the more complex ammonia salts. The cation alone seems to be active, in proportion to the amount of ammonia it contains. This observation is also borne out by the fact that the corresponding salts of other metals, such as rhodium and chromium, have the identical action, though the metals themselves and their simpler salts behave differently.

Action of Hexamin Cobalt on Motor Nerves.— The action of hexamin cobalt (a base consisting of one atom of cobalt combined with six molecules of the radical ammonium) is peculiar since no other known substance behaves similarly. J. BOCK (*Arch. f. exp. Path. u. Pharmak.*, Vol. 52, Nos. 1 and 2) finds that if injected into frogs in small, non-fatal doses, general, fascicular, clonic, muscular twitchings will appear, owing to irritation of the motor nerve-trunks. Similar compounds of rhodium and chromium show the same symptoms, hence the specific action resides within the cation (the six molecules of ammonium).

PATHOLOGY AND BACTERIOLOGY.

Experimental Streptococcus Arthritis.—It has been found by R. I. COLE (*Jour. of Infect. Dis.*, November 5, 1904) that arthritis and endocarditis may be produced by the intravenous inoculation of rabbits with steptococci from various sources, and the results obtained are quite similar to those described as resulting from the so-called *Micrococcus* or *Diplococcus rheumaticus*. Therefore, the description of a distinct variety or species of streptococci based on this property of causing endocarditis and arthritis is unwarranted. Whether the evidence is sufficient that acute rheumatic fever is simply a form of streptococcus septicemia is not discussed by the author.

The Dangers of the Microscope in the Early Diagnosis of Pulmonary Tuberculosis.—H. C. CLAPP (*Am. Med.*, December 10, 1904) calls attention to the fact that even now many physicians, no matter what their theoretic belief, practically often act on the supposition that absence of tubercle bacilli in the sputum on two or three examinations means absence of tuberculosis. This comforting assurance from their trusted medical advisers often induces patients to neglect proper treatment until the stage of incurability is reached. Cases are quoted from his records in the Massachusetts State Sanatarium, at Rutland, showing that when tubercle bacilli have been found in the sputum of patients, they are not by any means uniformly present at each examination, but often fail to appear for long periods, or are irregularly present. So that microscopical examinations, which happen to be made only at such times, would be very misleading in diagnosis. Cases are quoted, undoubtedly tuberculous, in which the microscope failed to disclose tubercle bacilli. If the physician should wait until the microscopical evidence was conclusive, the patient might sometimes lose the golden opportunity for recovery. Not always, but often the skilled diagnostician ought to be able to recognize the disease before enough ulceration and cavitation (surely not the very earliest stage) have occurred to allow the escape of the bacilli from the lung substance into the sputum.

Piroplasma Hominis and Certain Degenerative Changes in the Erythrocytes.—CHARLES F. CRAIG (*Am. Med.*, December 10, 1904) publishes the results of his investigations concerning *Piroplasma hominis*, claimed by some investigators to be the cause of "spotted" or "tick" fever, and concludes that no such organism can be demonstrated in the blood of patients suffering from this disease. Dr. Craig is convinced that the phenomena observed in the red blood cell were not due to a parasite but to certain changes, especially in the hemoglobin of the red cell, produced by disease. He believes that future research will prove that peculiar areas occurring within the red blood cell, chiefly those devoid of hemoglobin and occurring in human diseases, have been mistaken for a protozoan parasite by the investigators who have demonstrated *Piroplasma hominis*. The author refers to the report of Stiles, who was also unable to demonstrate the parasite after a thorough investigation of ten cases.

PRESCRIPTION HINTS.

Treatment of Dysmenorrhea.—Every practitioner knows how painful and troublesome dysmenorrhea is, and the following counsel given by M. Dalché on the affection may be useful. The first thing to be done is to discover the cause of the malady. Constipation should be avoided as well as intellectual and physical fatigue. To ease the pain, simple means may be at first enjoined—rest, warm applications, belladonna suppositories. An enema may be given in the morning with:

R Antipyrin ....15 grs.
Laudanum ....20 drops.

Or the following ointment:

R Extract of hyoscyamus................½ dr.
Extract of belladonna................½ dr.
Vaselin ....1 oz.

As to applications of ice, recommended by some, they are dangerous, for if they ease the pain they may arrest the flow of blood. A German author, Fliess, having found that there existed regions of the mucous membrane of the nasal fossæ constituted of erectile tissue, remarked that when the ovary became turgescent the mucous membrane of the nose was similarly affected. Hence he wanted to endeavor to calm the pain of dysmenorrhea by touching the nasal cartilage with a solution of cocaine and with some success.

M. Dalché tried the method of Fliess with satisfactory results in some cases. When the blood is normal in quantity at each period, antipyrin should be prescribed in 15 gr. doses, associated with 10 grs. of bicarbonate of soda, or 6 grs. of pyramidon. Dr. Huchard recommends:

R Tincture of piscidia erythrina.........10 grs.
Tincture of viburnum prunifolium....10 grs.

Twenty drops four or five times daily.

For lumbar neuralgia, ichthyol externally is very efficient.

R Ichthyol ....2 dr.
Chloroform ....3 dr.
Camphorated spirits....................2 oz.

Between the periods cannabis indica should be prescribed.

If the flow was excessive (menorrhagia), the fluid extract of hydrastis canadensis is indicated (20 drops three times a day). If, on the contrary, the flow is insufficient or slow to appear, general tonic treatment should be ordered with ovarian opotherapy. Where the menses are entirely irregular, cold bathing, corporal exercise, gymnastics, and ovarian opotherapy will render good service. Marriage might also be recommended.

Neuralgia.—For anemic and debilitated cases the following is worthy of a trial:

R Ferri reducti..................gr. c   (6.00)
Acidi arsenosi................gr. iv   (.26)
Phosphori ....gr. i   (.065)
Extracti nucis vomicæ........gr. xxv   (1.60)

Misce. Fiant pilulæ No. c.
Sig. One pill after each meal.

Chilblains.—Used when red and inflamed, but skin remaining unbroken:

R Ichthyoli ....f℥ ii (8.00)
Unguenti potassii iodidi......... ℥ iv (16.00)
Olei terebinthinæ................f℥ i (4.00)
Adipis lanæ hydrosi.....q. s. ad ℥ ii (64.00)

Misce.
Sig. Spread upon new unbleached muslin and apply.

THE MEDICAL NEWS.

A WEEKLY JOURNAL
OF MEDICAL SCIENCE.

COMMUNICATIONS in the form of Scientific Articles, Clinical Memoranda, Correspondence or News Items of interest to the profession are invited from all parts of the world. Reprints to the number of 250 of original articles contributed exclusively to the MEDICAL NEWS will be furnished without charge if the request therefor accompanies the manuscript. When necessary to elucidate the text, illustrations will be engraved from drawings or photographs furnished by the author. Manuscript should be typewritten.

SMITH ELY JELLIFFE, A.M., M.D., Ph.D., Editor,
No. 111 FIFTH AVENUE, NEW YORK.

Subscription Price, Including postage in U. S. and Canada.

PER ANNUM IN ADVANCE $4.00
SINGLE COPIES 10
WITH THE AMERICAN JOURNAL OF THE
MEDICAL SCIENCES, PER ANNUM . . 8.00

Subscriptions may begin at any date. The safest mode of remittance is by bank check or postal money order, drawn to the order of the undersigned. When neither is accessible, remittances may be made at the risk of the publishers, by forwarding in *registered* letters.

LEA BROTHERS & CO.,
No. 111 FIFTH AVENUE (corner of 18th St.), NEW YORK.

SATURDAY, JANUARY 7, 1905.

SHOULD OUR PRIVATE HOSPITAL SYSTEM BE CHANGED?

THE "Hospital Trusts" of New York are warmly attacked by an anonymous "M.D." in a recent issue of the New York *Sun*. In the opinion of this redoubtable champion of equal rights, it is a debatable question whether the management of large private hospitals in New York is "along lines which are productive of the best results." The *Sun's* correspondent thinks that the much-advertised annual deficits (which, by the way, since the hospitals are not actually in debt and do not get into debt, are really only arbitrary expressions of the amount of work that hospital managers would like to do) would speedily disappear if the hospitals were made a free field for the entire medical profession of the metropolis.

It is no doubt true that empty wards could be filled by opening wide the doors of hospitals to the general profession; but it is by no means certain that such a course would result in increasing the relative incomes of the institutions practising it. Elsewhere, in his argument, the *Sun's* correspondent points out that the great private hospitals often refuse admission to needy patients because the care of such patients would add to their deficits.

The deficit, however, real or imaginary, is not the subject which chiefly interests us here. We are particularly concerned with the proposal that hospitals be made free to all practitioners, first on the theory of equal rights, and second in order that patients entering hospitals may be enabled freely to choose their physicians. Is this proposal a practical one, worthy of the serious consideration of hospital managers, or is it an unwarranted and mistaken application of a mere social theory?

Outside of New York there are many hospitals, both municipal and private, in which "every physician in good standing is accorded the privilege of attending his own patients in both wards and private rooms." We cannot agree with the writer in the *Sun*, however, when he states that such hospitals are to be found "in many of the large cities of this country." In large cities the typical hospital is a large hospital, and large hospitals cannot be managed in the same manner as institutions of less size. In the smaller towns a large proportion of hospital patients pay for their support as hospital inmates, and hospital managers therefore find it profitable to keep their beds full. If in order to do this it becomes necessary to open the doors of the hospital to the general profession, this is done; and since the total number of physicians in the locality is small, no disorder follows. But can any one who knows intimately the work of a large metropolitan hospital seriously maintain that this method can be applied in an institution of the latter class with similar results? Imagine the nurses and house officers of St. Luke's, with its two hundred or more beds, maintaining professional relations with and receiving orders from one hundred or one hundred and fifty non-resident physicians of unknown antecedents, irresponsible to the trustees of the hospital, free to order and to use in their discretion expensive medical and surgical supplies, enjoying the right to transfer or discharge patients at will, permitted to operate with or without suitable previous experience, and owning no credentials but a license to practise medicine in the State of New York! Imagine two hundred and fifty physicians rioting uncontrolled in the wards of Mount Sinai Hospital; or six hundred clamoring for the use of the operating rooms at Bellevue! Are such conditions thinkable? Would such a system justify itself in a city like New York?

It is truly a pity that in Manhattan and the Bronx scarcely one physician in ten enjoys the privilege of an up-to-date hospital. It is indeed an arduous task for the remainder to achieve professional or scientific eminence; hence we are prepared to welcome and approve any associative or philanthropic measure which promises relief to the excluded majority. But such relief never can be obtained by the means proposed in the *Sun*, and it is idle to waste effort in agitating the impossible.

If the middle and lower classes in New York ever choose to organize benevolent or cooperative societies which shall establish small hospitals in which members may be treated by their family physicians without restriction; or if groups of physicians in the various city localities find it worth while to band themselves together in associations for the purpose of equipping and operating small clinics, a change in the distribution of professional opportunities will result. Thus far neither the laity or the profession in Manhattan have found it worth while to take such steps; and until they do, the majority of our physicians will have to be content to be received in New York's hospitals as guests.

IN A YELLOW LIGHT.

FAMILIARITY breeds not only contempt but tolerance as well, and deplorable conditions constantly before our eyes are far too apt to be taken as a matter of course. Under such circumstances we should be grateful for anything that may serve as stimulus to a fresh point of view and show us the familiar evils in all their essential menace. Such a service has been rendered, albeit with a light and entertaining touch, by the chapter on "The American Doctor," in "As a Chinaman Saw Us," reprinted in this week's issue of the MEDICAL NEWS.

The Chinaman "saw" nothing new, nothing that we do not see ourselves, but he saw it as one sees new phenomena, undulled by use, and enables his American readers to share, temporarily at least, his point of view. It is not necessary to accept all his conclusions as to the comparative superiority of his own country, nor even to believe the anecdotes of individual gullibility on the part of American patients and blundering on the part of American surgeons, many of which tales bear the hall-mark of the Yankee joke-smith. The actual facts, as we know them, supply quite sufficient food for reflection, and the records of the daily " Saunterer About Town " furnish incidents that are more

startling than any the Chinaman reports, if not quite so artistic in finish.

It is, as has been said, in the presentation of a fresh point of view that the value of his service lies. We have all seen the advertisements of the patent medicine man monopolizing acres of hoardings in town and country, and, in the aggregate, acres also in the newspapers. We know in a general way that these nostrums are worthless and worse than worthless, and that such enterprises are not only supported but enriched at the expense of the people in general. Once in a while, stimulated by the dramatic discovery of fatal effects in some given case, a brief crusade is directed against such evils, but it invariably dies out, as a result of the apathy of the public. The same thing is true of the various " fake " cures and cults of a pseudomedical nature. Those who are involved in them naturally shut their eyes to criticism, and those who see their absurdity content themselves with seeing that and ignore their dangers. We have accepted as regular concomitants of American life Blank's Universal Panacea, Prof. Gullem, Hypnotist and Oriental Magnetic Healer, and all the innumerable multitude of that ilk. Secure in the carelessness of the American public they reap their harvest merrily and only occasionally come to grief at the hands of the Board of Pharmacy, or some similar organization.

It is axiomatic that in this country the only effective, if somewhat slow weapon is the " campaign of education." The impossibility of enforcing laws which are not actively supported by public opinion has been repeatedly demonstrated, and this fact makes more threateningly significant the appalling proportion of persons in the toils of the spoiler and the indifference of those who are not his victims.

The physicians of the country can do little, unsupported by the people at large, and their efforts must therefore be directed to awakening and securing this support. To further this object, the Chinaman's chapter alluded to might well serve as a tract. Anybody could tell funnier or more extravagant stories of the vagaries of Christian Science and " Kickapoo Liniment," but he has given us a positively startling impression of the mass effect of all these empty pretenses upon an unprejudiced observer. The bulk of this incubus in American life is what strikes the Chinaman and the Chinaman's reader. With a sort of refined selfishness we are apt to tolerate an evil which owes its existence to an ignorance or prejudice to which we feel ourselves superior. *We* know better than to take irresponsible patent medicines, *we* know better than to try to cure pneumonia by " absent treatment " or musical tones. Why then trouble ourselves about those who do? But when we read the Chinaman's summing up we cannot but recognize the gravity of the situation. " It is not overstating facts when I say that three-fifths of the people buy some of these patent nostrums which the real medical men denounce, showing that the masses of the people are densely ignorant, the victim of any fakir who can shout his wares loud enough. In China such a thing would be impossible ; the block would stop the practice."

There seems to be no reason to doubt his statement of the proportion of victims, and how shall we combat his conclusion that " the masses of the people are densely ignorant? " It is almost enough to make us long for the Chinese method of settling the question, but in default of the block we can only have recourse to the " campaign of education." Obviously, the " three-fifths " cannot be expected to assist, except as each one cries up his own favorite delusion by crying down the others, and it therefore devolves upon the sane remnant to hold up the hands of the physicians who are striving to combat this evil.

Whether the prognosis is hopeful or not it might be hard to say, but let us choose the part of the optimist, and believe that common sense will eventually triumph and make it possible for even a Chinaman to find our people enlightened and civilized.

A CONTRIBUTION TO CANCER ETIOLOGY.

AFTER many years of almost persuasion on the part of pathologists that malignant disease of all kinds was due to a parasite, there has come the inevitable reaction, and now the trend of thought is back toward the original opinion that it is a tissue fault.

Recent investigations have pointed particularly to two conditions in tissues which seem to indicate the basis of malignant degeneration. One is a reversion apparently to the reproductive type of cell, so that multiplication and a certain independence of generation become the most characteristic feature of cell life. The other partook more of the reversion to the embryonal type of which so much was to be heard twenty years ago. It seems as though some irritant of very powerful character is required to send cells back

to these reversionary types, and it may possibly be that this irritation is supplied by a parasite.

There are, however, a number of indications in recent literature that would seem to emphasize the fact that a merely mechanical irritation frequently repeated and sufficiently prolonged may under favorable circumstances, prove quite sufficient to account for the origin of cancer.

At the last meeting of the New York State Medical Association, New York County Branch, held November 21, 1904 (see Society Proceedings, MEDICAL NEWS, page 40), during the discussion of the dangers of the X-rays, attention was particularly called to the fact that in a considerable number of reported cases, cancer had developed in the midst of a scar due to a deep burn by the X-rays. In some of these cases, the burn has been not on the patient but on the physician. In one case the most notable feature of the affection was that the malignant neoplasm was multiple. Amputation was required first of one hand and then of the other, and subsequent amputations in the arm had to be performed and the end of the case remains to be seen. This is a most interesting feature of X-ray work, since the very agent which it had been hoped would lessen the mortality from cancer, has added to the incidence as well as the fatality of this dread affection.

It has been a constant search for many years to find some agent that would produce cancer. Now it has been found masquerading under the guise of what was hoped would be, and has actually proven to be, in certain cases, a most efficient remedy for the disease. It is not easy to conclude as to the significance of these facts. One thing, however, seems to be very clear, that the persistent irritation of scar tissue constantly contracting, as is so typically the case in the healed deep burns, produced by the X-rays, forms the most suitable condition for the development of malignant disease. Of course, this has been known before. It is at the pylorus, in the stomach and at the flexures in the intestines, that is, just at those parts of the gastro-intestinal tracts which are most liable to injury and most likely to be the location of persistently contractile scars that cancer develops. With the X-rays, however, these effects have been produced experimentally under conditions, all of which were perfectly open to observation.

It is easy to say that the scar tissue, owing to its lowered resistive vitality, may well have presented a favorable nidus for the growth of a cancer parasite. The mechanically irritant effects of contracting connective tissue upon tissues of higher orders have ever been considered to have a prominent place in the etiology of the disease. Pigmentary irritation as by moles, or the frequently repeated irritation to which warts are subjected, furnish further confirmatory examples of this fact. It would seem that parenchymatous tissues, especially of the epithelial variety, when subjected to constant irritation for prolonged periods, revert to that embryonic activity, and reproductiveness, which constitute the very essence of cancer. Unfortunately, it appears probable that there will be further opportunities for the study of such conditions as productive of cancer in the very near future. Let us hope that the chances thus afforded for actual observation will not be lost.

The cost of the precious lesson that physical energies, whose scope and limitations are not well determined, cannot be employed with impunity in medicine, falls on physician as well as patient in this case. Its warnings and its teachings must not be neglected.

ECHOES AND NEWS.

NEW YORK.

Appointment at Bellevue Hospital.—Dr. Edwin Sternberger has been appointed assistant visiting physician to the Fourth Medical Division of Bellevue Hospital.

Quacks and Newspapers.—On January 23, 1905, before the Medical Society of the County of New York, at its regular meeting in the Academy of Medicine, Mr. Champe S. Andrews, counsel for the Society, will deliver an illustrated lecture entitled "A Century's Criminal Alliance Between Quacks and Newspapers." It will be an exposure of the methods used by the so-called "Specialists in Diseases of Men Only," and their corrupt relations with some of New York's newspapers.

Spitting in the Subway.—The conspicuously dirty condition of the roadbed of broken stone, in front of the station platforms, already indicates the justice of the Health Board's criticism. The more dangerous, although less obvious, defilement of this germ trap by spitting and by secretions from the nose and lungs, which cleaners ostentatiously disinfect on some of the station platforms and stairways, is constantly occurring with no apparent attempt to prevent it. There are no signs prohibiting either smoking or spitting in the stations. Nine men out of ten will expectorate on the roadbed rather than the platform, and feel that they are showing special breeding and thoughtfulness by doing so. As a matter of fact, they are depositing the material in a more dangerous place, as the platform is occasionally cleaned.

Death-Rate Higher.—November deaths for the fifteen years preceding 1903 in this State averaged 280 a day. November, 1904, had an average of 339. This increase is in excess of the birth rate, the death rate being 16.0 against 15.2 for the last five years. Acute

respiratory diseases, 72 per cent. of which were from pneumonia, caused 250 more deaths than the average of the month; diseases of the circulatory system 200 more; those of the urinary system are 15 per cent. above the average, 8.0 per cent. of the deaths of the month have been from Bright's disease. There is also a large increase this month in the cancer mortality. The chief cause of increase in the mortality of the month is pneumonia, which caused 1,220 deaths, against 800 in October; 12.0 per cent. of the total mortality was from this cause, against 9.4 per cent. last November, and 8.0 per cent. in October of this year.

Beth Israel Hospital's New Property.—At the annual meeting of the Beth Israel Hospital Association, held last week, the report of the board of directors was read by President Joseph H. Cohen. During the current year the six-story building on Jefferson Street, adjoining the present hospital building, has been purchased for the sum of $71,000, so that the Association now owns the entire block between Jefferson and Cherry streets. The number of free patients during the year was 1,435; the number of pay patients was 194. The number of applicants approved, but who were refused admission for want of room, amounted to 902. The average length of stay for each patient was 23¹/₆ days, and the death-rate was about 10 per cent. In the dispensary 40,022 patients were treated. The total receipts were $95,742, and the expenditures $62,781.54. The present membership is 3,112, an increase during the year of 1,208.

School War on Disease.—The proposition to teach public school children about consumption, how it is spread, and how to avoid catching it, which, it is said, Governor Higgins strongly favors, is a step in the right direction, but only a step. There is no reason why the teaching should be limited to tuberculosis. The other infectious diseases, diphtheria, pneumonia, typhoid fever, etc., questions of eating, of clothing, and of ventilation, are of first importance in determining the health and comfort of the individual. There is no practical instruction whatever at present given in the schools regarding the majority of these subjects, and even the modicum of physiology provided is a perfunctory and almost useless study. Every child ought to be taught enough to enable him to avoid the most obvious dangers, and to keep him out of the hands of the great army of quacks, which exists and flourishes only through the ignorance of the people regarding the elementary laws of health.

Lecture of Dr. Flexner.—Professor Simon Flexner, of the Rockefeller Institute, on December 21, delivered a lecture previously announced in these columns, "On the Action of Snake Venom." Dr. Herter introduced the speaker in a few well-chosen words, the audience applauding for fully five minutes after Dr. Flexner arose. The most important work on snake venom was done in this country by Weir Mitchell to be followed later by that of Reichert. This work was basic, it has been added to but has never been controverted in its details. Some snake-bites are very poisonous which seems to depend upon the different kinds of venom, these differences are more pronounced the larger the quantity introduced. The cobra and the vipers may be taken as types, some of the poisons are intermediate in character between the cobra and rattlesnake venoms, the character of the local lesion in poisoning by the rattlesnake is the hemorrhage developed there. The symptoms of cobra poisoning are an anxious expression, interference with respiration, and death. It kills chiefly by the action of the poison on the respiratory center in the medulla, no clot formation takes place. The symptoms caused by rattlesnake bite are almost *nil*, since death is instantaneous. On post mortem the heart is still pulsating, the right heart being occupied by solid red clots,—the poison has little effect on the respiratory center. In experimental work rapid injection gave almost instantaneous coagulation, while slow injection showed absence of coagulation. All venoms can destroy animal cells but the cells destroyed are by no means always the same. The cobra poison acts chiefly on the blood cells and those of the central nervous system and contains an energetic hemolysin for red blood cells with a neurotoxin for nerve cells; both cause solution indirectly. The hemolysin attaches itself to cells through the amboceptor and the venom is inactive in 'absence of a complementary substance, which may be single or multiple. Lecithin is the most stable complementary substance. Injection of venom into the peritoneal cavity causes thrombosis of vessels, and also a neuro-intoxication which was proven experimentally on the rabbit, the venom attacks the endothelial lining of blood vessels and gives extravasation of blood into the cavities. Animals poisoned by venom quickly putrefy because of destruction of normal bactericidal powers of blood. Snake venom produces antibodies and therefore an animal can become tolerant of it. Antivenine against vipers cannot be prepared because immunization cannot be effected on account of local effects and destruction of tissue by bacterial invasion and death of animal from secondary causes. Venom is modified by heating or by treating with hydrochloric acid, but by so doing its combining power is somewhat destroyed and good results are difficult to obtain.

PHILADELPHIA.

Inquests During 1904.—According to the statement issued by the Philadelphia Coroner, 3,467 autopsies were made during the year just ended. The 'number of deaths due to alcohol was but one-half as great as during 1903; there were 43 murders which is 15 less than during the preceding year; the number of deaths due to tetanus was also less. Deaths as a result of heart disease and suicide were increased.

A New Hospital.—The United States Steel Corporation has decided to erect a hospital at Donora for the care of the injured mill workers. It will be maintained merely for emergency work. So soon as the patients are able they will be removed to their homes or to some hospital in Pittsburg. All modern appliances will be provided. The hospital will have a trained nurse, and a physician and a surgeon will be within easy reach.

To the Tropics.—Dr. McFarland, Professor of Pathology and Bacteriology at the Medico-Chirurgical College, Philadelphia, has left for Panama to attend the fourth meeting of the Pan-American Medical Congress. After the meeting he will go to Havana as a member of the American Public Health Congress, from which place he will visit Santiago to investigate the recently reported outbreak of yellow fever at that place. Neither Dr. McFarland nor Dr. Coplin, of the Jefferson Medical College, give credence to Dr. Nelson's view that the yellow fever germ lives or may live in the subsoil.

Cold Street Cars.—The Rapid Transit Company, of Philadelphia, is being taken to task with reference to this matter not only by the physicians but also the business men of the city. The Downtown Business Men's Association decided to send committees to all downtown organizations, secular, charitable and social, to ask them for their support in the health campaign. The physicians are calling the company's attention to the dangers to which the public is exposed by riding in their overcrowded, cold and dirty cars. A Harrisburg

physician intimates that the officials of the Philadelphia Rapid Transit Company could learn much by studying the conditions of the street cars of Harrisburg.

Philadelphia County Medical Society.—At the last meeting W. W. Smithers, attorney, read a paper entitled, "Defects in Pennsylvania Food Legislation." During the course of which, he said, the pure food act of 1895 is a clear violation of the Constitution of 1874. Some of the definitions under the act of 1895 seem to aim at protection to health and others to prevent fraud from being practised upon purchasers, but every one of them can be used successfully not only to interfere with lawful commerce, but to subject citizens to punishment for acts which in no sense should be deemed crimes or even open to criticism. While the statute may be valid and even just as to some cases, in many it invades and impairs individual property rights, prevents the use of many desirable food preparations and needlessly interferes with trade. But the incongruities, imperfections and absurdities of the language of the law pale before the system for its enforcement. In concluding, Mr. Smithers advocated a new pure food law which would simply provide that every article sold should be guaranteed to be what is called for. Dr. H. W. Wiley, chief of the Bureau of the United States Department of Agriculture, read a paper upon "Food Preservatives and Food Adulteration." Dr. Thomas L. Coley read one upon "The Evaluation of Evidence as to the Pharmacological Action of Food Preservatives."

The Meeting of the American Association for the Advancement of Science.—Monday evening the American Physiological Society gave a smoker at the University Club. The American Society of Naturalist and Affiliated Societies gave one on Tuesday evening at the same place. The annual dinner of the American Society of Naturalists was held at Hotel Walton, Wednesday evening, on which occasion the President delivered his address. The retiring president of the American Association for the Advancement of Science, Hon. Carroll D. Wright, gave his address in the University Gymnasium at eight o'clock the same evening. Dr. Chapman entertained the American Physiological Society at luncheon on Wednesday, in his home, No. 2047 Walnut Street. A reception was given to the members of the American Association of Scientific Societies in the Free Museum of Science and Art on Wednesday evening. The smoker of the Psychological and Philosophical Association was given at the Colonnade Thursday evening. The Lady Members of the Committee on Reception and Entertainment gave a reception to the American Association and Scientific Societies, at the Acorn Club, Friday evening.

Cerebral Morphology.—Dr. E. A. Spitzka, of New York, in discussing brains, said that persons possessing great intellectual capacity and excelling in creative arts and in science are apt to have heavier brains than ordinary individuals. Criminals should have correspondingly light brains, but this is not always the case. The study of criminals by anthropological methods does not necessarily tend to establish a criminal type, nor does it tend to describe crime as equivalent to infantilism, epilepsy, atavism or anything else as maintained by the Lombroso school. Many criminals do not show a single anomaly in their physical or mental make-up, while many persons with marked evidences of morphological aberrations have never shown criminal tendencies. Dr. R. B. Bean, of Johns Hopkins University, spoke of the negro's brain. His remarks were based principally upon the studies of 100 negro brains. He found that the anterior portion of the brain, the seat of will power, of esthetic and ethical feeling, of the negro much inferior to a corresponding portion of a white man's brain, therefore, he said, the negro by his physical conformation is prevented from being as strong of will and is less fine in his perception of right and wrong. The posterior portion of the brain, which is the seat of artistic sense and emotion, he found as well developed in the negro as in the white man.

Diet.—Before the section on Chemistry Dr. Wiley, of Washington, D. C., read two papers, one on "Diet in Tuberculosis" and the other on "Proper Diet for the Tropics." In the course of the first paper, he said, in many maladies whisky and brandy have apparently been used to great advantage and doubtless such is the case in tuberculosis. He further stated that alcohol, like a true oil, is readily and quickly absorbed and before it becomes oxidized into water and carbon dioxide produces gentle stimulation which seems to favor the general metabolic process. He inclines to give the patient what he likes to eat if the food stuff called for be nutritious, and does not deem it essential to force the patient to take what is positively distasteful to him. Dr. Wiley recommends fruit as the best food in the tropics.

Radium.—In a paper entitled "Future Development of Physical Chemistry," Dr. Wilder D. Bancroft said of radium that many people thought radium was to be the catalytic agent which would change all elements, but the recent work of Rutherford seems to have put an end to that idea.

The Ability of Bacteria to Ferment Sugars.—In his paper A. I. Rogers, Department of Agriculture, says the best test for this is accomplished by filling the cavity of a hanging drop slide with a sugar-free litmus bouillon to which a small amount of sugar is added. A cover glass is sealed over the solution. Fermentation is indicated by reddening of the litmus and the appearence of gas bubbles.

Germ-Proof Filter.—F. P. Gorham, of Brown University, calls attention to a filter which consists of a porcelain tube encased by a layer of aluminum hydroxide which is bound together by mineral wool. The effluent, he says, is of excellent quality chemically, is free from odor and is germ free after running continuously for one year. The flow is seven times as rapid as an uncoated filter at the start and twice as rapid after running continuously for fourteen days.

Bacteria Encountered in Suppurations.—D. H. Bergey, of University of Pennsylvania, notes that in pus bacteria are found which are not to be classed as the ordinary pyogenic organisms. In order to verify his opinion he examined the pus of 30 surgical cases and found, aside from the ordinary pyogenic organism, such as the *Bacillus pyocyaneus, Bacillus coli communis,* the streptococcus and the staphyloccocus, an organism belonging to the group of pseudodiphtheria bacillus and another belonging to the proteus group. These bacteria do not appear to him as being accidental contamination, but he is not yet able to state the extent to which they are capable of producing suppuration, as his work has not been completed.

Gelatin as a Substitute for Proteid in the Food.—Murlin found by experiment that when an amount of gelatin equivalent to one-quarter or one-half of the nitrogen necessary to maintain the nitrogenous equilibrium was given to an animal the percentage

of sparing nitrogen was the same as when all meat was fed to the animal; if, however, two-thirds of the amount of nitrogen necessary was substitued by gelatin the percentage of sparing nitrogen was reduced. After the second period of fasting when one-half of the nitrogen necessary was substituted by gelatin the sparing nitrogen was 85 per cent., while, if two-thirds of the amount was substitued by gelatin, the sparing nitrogen was 100 per cent. or perfect equilibrium. Murlin obtained almost identical result when after fasting he substitued a certain amount of gelatin for an equal amount of proteid.

The Pharmacology of Ethyl Salicylate.—Dr. E. M. Houghton, of Detroit, says it is an irritant to the mucous membrane and is a substance very similar to the methyl compound. The minimum fatal dose of ethyl salicylate is .0014 gm., while the methyl compound is just one-half or .0007 gm. When administered to an animal emesis soon occurs, due to the irritating action of the substance upon the mucous membrane of the stomach. It is eliminated by the kidneys in from five to ten minutes after intravenous injection; when taken by mouth it appears in the urine in from fifteen to forty-five minutes after administration and is completely eliminated in eighteen hours. The respirations in the first hour after administration are slowed, but later become increased; the pulse is increased and the temperature is at first raised but afterward falls. When ethyl salicylate is given to animals for some time continuously, they waste and finally die. Death is due to paralysis of the respiratory center.

Psychic Secretion.—W. Koch being deeply impressed with the work of Paltauf carried out a series of experiments in the same line. He succeeded in producing secretion in the stomach of dogs by showing food to them and this could be produced at irregular intervals. He also succeeded in producing gastric secretions when the dog's eyes were bandaged and the animal was allowed to smell the food only. Koch also found that those foods that were not palatable failed to produce the secretion either by smell or by sight. He closes his paper by stating that an animal must possess some acute power of perception in order to produce the secretions through psychic influences.

Tumor of the Fourth Ventricle with Cerebellar Symptoms.—Dr. F. P. Knowlton, of Syracuse, N. Y., presented the report of this condition observed in a cat. He called attention to the peculiar attitude of the animal; she seemed to dread to be lifted, although the dread could not have been due to pain, for she seemed to be totally void of such phenomena. The cutaneous sensibility for touch and pain were normal and hearing appeared to be unimpaired. There was present a tremor and nystagmus. The hind legs were widely separated; the occiput was drawn to the right and the body bent toward the left. At the autopsy he found the left half of the cerebellum depressed, the convolutions obliterated to a certain extent, the restiform bodies were bulging, and a tumor occupied the floor of the fourth ventricle. Upon microscopical examination it was discovered that the restiform bodies and a part of the cochlear nucleus were destroyed. The degenerations were due to pressure of the glioma.

The Presence of Soaps in the Organism.—Dr. O. Klotz, of Montreal, Canada, calls attention to the fact that if in such a disease as arteriosclerosis sections of the vessel are stained with sudan III many granules take the stain with a moderate degree of intensity but if silver nitrate be applied before the sudan III the granules assume a black tinge and there is evidence of the pink hue of the sudan III. In calcified fibromyomata of the uterus the central zone is composed of calcareous substances while in the intermediate zone are many granules which assume the yellowish-pink due when sudan III is applied. In these areas he says there is fatty substance and calcium or soaps, which can be demonstrated in all areas of calcareous infiltration. To verify these observations he injected bichloride of mercury into a kidney in which cloudy swelling and later fatty changes occurred, so that when sudan III was applied to sections granules were found which had stained reddish-brown, and if silver nitrate was applied they were stained black. He succeeded in extracting soap from the tissue showing such changes. These soaps, he says, attract the calcium salts from the blood. In a mixture of albumin, potassium salts and carbonates he found granules which stained with sudan III like those already mentioned.

CHICAGO.

Officers of the Chicago Medical Examiners' Association.—At a meeting held December 19, the following officers were elected: President, Dr. Walter A. Jaquith; Vice-President, Dr. Liston H. Montgomery; Secretary, Dr. Morton Snow; Treasurer, Dr. U. J. Grim. Councilor of the Chicago Medical Society, Dr. Walter A. Jaquith.

State of Chicago's Health.—After three weeks of unusually low December mortality, the seasonal increase has set in sharply. The 548 deaths from all causes reported during the week represented a 7.6 per cent. increase over the previous week and nearly 4 per cent. more than the corresponding first winter week of 1903. In themselves none of the important causes of death shows any increase sufficient to create alarm; consumption only six more, cancer seven more, diphtheria three more, pneumonia nine more, smallpox four more, and whooping-cough three more than the previous week. But the revelations of the laboratory indicate a serious increase of atmospheric impurity, only temporarily checked by the snowfall. The germs of all the air-borne diseases are rife and the influenza bacillus or "grip" germ is endemically prevalent in many sections of the city. The department renews its warning against all unnecessary exposure to those suffering from any of the contagious and infectious diseases, and especially to pneumonia and influenza.

Dr. Wood Sentenced to Imprisonment.—Dr. N. News Wood, President of the Christian Hospital, and the medical institution itself were recently held in contempt of court for the violation of an injunction restraining them from using the name of Dr. John B. Murphy in connection with the hospital. The decision of the court, after the two days' hearing, was brief and very scathing. Judge Holdom, among other things, said that "judging from the record in this case, Dr. Wood is a dangerous man in the community. I am not free from the suspicion, and it is a grave one, that the manner in which Dr. Murphy's name appears upon these documents, being written there, is a forgery and a criminal offense. This must weigh in my decision and I shall fine the Christian Hospital $250, and fine Dr. Wood $100, and order him to the County Jail for ten days as punishment." Dr. Murphy's name appeared in the advertising of the hospital as a member of its staff, as previously stated in the columns of THE MEDICAL NEWS. His name was said to have been used in selling "certificates of membership" to medical students and young physicians throughout the country.

Memorial of the Iroquois Fire.—Chicago sat in sackcloth and ashes on the last day of the old year, the anniversary of its most fearful tragedy, and paid honor to the hundreds that perished one year before in the Iroquois Theater fire. Though time had assuaged the violence of grief, the memory of a common sorrow enshrouded the city, and the general heartache found expression in a memorial service at Willard Hall, where bereaved and survivors gathered to mourn the victims "lest we forget." At the cemeteries friends and relatives visited the graves of the 575 victims and strewed the tombs with wreaths and flowers. In some extremely pathetic cases one survivor placed the offering on a long row of graves containing all the other members of a family circle. As a prelude to the services, the Iroquois Memorial Association held a business meeting at which President J. J. Reynolds submitted a report on the progress of the emergency hospital plan. Within sixty days it is expected that $50,000 will be raised as a nucleus for a building fund, which will be placed in the hands of fifteen trustees. Officers for the ensuing year were elected as follows: Honorary President, R. T. Crane, Jr.; President, D. R. Martin; First Vice-President, C. M. Bickford; Second Vice-President, J. P. Hoyland; Treasurer, Phelps B. Hoyt.

Physicians Responsible for Victims of Morphine Habit.—Superintendent Sloane of the Bridewell says that prisoners unanimously claim that they fall into the morphine and other habits after being excessively doped by physicians. After hearing confessions from 970 "dope fiends," the Superintendent says in his annual report that the alarming increase of slaves to drugs among the prisoners of that institution this year is due to a careless and too liberal use of the deadly stuff by physicians. Leading medical men of this city were not a little indignant when the contents of the report and the prisoners' alleged confessions were read to them. Several physicians were interviewed regarding the subject, and among them Dr. G. Frank Lydston, who said that he failed to understand how the Superintendent of a prison, a man who is supposed to have some insight into human nature, can swallow the silly excuses of the unfortunates in his care. No drug fiend is a criterion on any important matter. Increase in the number of victims should not be laid at the door of the medical profession, says Dr. Lydston. The report of Superintendent Sloane further states: "The many cocaine, morphine, opium, paregoric, codeine, phenacetin and other victims thronged the cells everywhere. Many were women, and they almost unanimously blamed their physicians for getting them into the habit. They fell through despondency and bad associations."

GENERAL.

Cossacks Surround Plague District.—The plague district in the Ural region has been cordoned by cossacks and the disease has been localized. The mortality has slightly decreased.

Gift to Syracuse Hospital.—The Syracuse Hospital of the Good Shepherd is the recipient of a New Year's gift of $50,000, the donor being William B. Cogswell, general manager of the Solvay Process Company of that city.

Big Donation to King's Hospital Fund.—Baron Mountstephen, president of the St. Paul and Manitoba Railway, has donated £200,000 in Argentine bonds, producing £11,000 yearly, to the King's Hospital fund.

Sanatorium Afire.—The New England Sanatorium, formerly the Langwood Hotel, situated on the shore of Spot Pond, two miles from the village of Stoneham, Mass., was burning at an early hour Christmas day, and it was feared would be a total loss. So far as known no lives were lost, but there was a panic among the patients.

Pan-American Medical Congress Opens.—The Pan-American Medical Congress opened its session at the theater in the City of Panama last Tuesday. Sanitary Officer Gorgas and Chief Engineer Wallace delivered addresses. President Amador received the delegates this afternoon.

Massage As An Employment for the Blind.—In Japan the blind have a practical monopoly over massage. There massage is cheap and within the means of all classes. The blind, protected by the government, are self-supporting, and contented with their lot. This condition has existed for centuries. In four countries—Russia, Belgium, England, and Germany—there have been well-organized and successful attempts to teach selected blind people massage. Here in America the only definite series of attempt in this direction were made by Mr. Allen.

Medical Society of the Missouri Valley.—In response to a cordial invitation from the Jackson County Medical Society, the semi-annual meeting of this association will be held in Kansa City, Thursday, March 23, 1905. Those desirous of presenting papers should send their titles to the secretary not later than the first of February. Papers will appear upon the programme in the order in which they are received. An invitation has been extended to the presidents of the State associations within the territory embraced by the Missouri Valley and to the profession in general, and an interesting and profitable meeting is expected.

The National Association for the Study and Prevention of Tuberculosis.—The first annual meeting of The National Association will be held in Washington, D. C., at the New Willard Hotel, on Thursday and Friday, May 18 and 19, 1905. There will be general sessions, and division of the work into the following three sections: 1. *Sociological,* of which Mr. Homer Folks is the chairman, and the secretary Miss Lilian Brandt, United Charities Building, 105 East Twenty-second Street, New York. 2. *Pathological and Bacteriological,* of which Dr. Mazyck P. Ravenel is chairman. The secretary is Dr. D. J. McCarthy, Phipps Institute, Philadelphia, Pa. 3. *Clinical and Climatological,* of which Dr. Norman Bridge is chairman and Dr. S. G. Bonney is secretary, Stedman Building, Denver, Colo.

Institute for the Study of Blood Infection.—Before the meeting of the American Association for the Advancement of Science, held last week in Philadelphia, Dr. P. A. Maigneu, of that city, said: "From a careful study I have become convinced that it is of paramount importance to the public health that an institute be founded in this country for the special study of blood poison, particularly as regards the first step of infection. A sterilizing agent should be discovered which would be applicable in every case, and the dressing of wounds should be thoroughly gone into. We know practically nothing of the immediate phenomena which appear at the beginning of the disease. There are eighteen known ways of infection, which constitute a very large programme for study."

Brains Bequeath to Science.—Brain anatomists throughout the United States have begun a movement which they hope will bring about a condition of affairs more favorable to the study of that most wonderful organ of the human body. It is for the formation of a society, modeled on the plan of the Mutual Autopsy Society of Paris, the members of which after their death contribute their brains and other

organs to science. A committee, consisting of Dr. Alexander Hrdlicka, Dr. E. A. Spitzka and Professor B. G. Wilder, three of the best known brain experts and anatomists in this country, has been appointed for the purpose of preparing a general form of brain bequest, which will hold in law and not to be rendered null by any action that may be taken by relatives of the person making the bequest.

Rabies on the Increase.—Rabies has been more prevalent in New York during the past year than ever before, according to the State Department of Agriculture. The annual report says: "Action has been taken promptly upon notice or information reaching this office that the disease existed. Notices have been issued in each geographical district where the disease existed, as required by statute, and such surveillance has been given as could be with the men and means at command. It is believed that the disease in these localities has been practically suppressed. This belief is based upon the fact that there has been no manifestation of the disease since enforcement of the quarantine, except in one instance in the town of Halfmoon; in this case the dog was immediately killed. Rabies has been found in the following counties: Sullivan, Ulster, Saratoga, Broome, Tioga, Tompkins, and Chautauqua.

Health in the Navy.—The annual report of the surgeon general of the navy for 1903 contains some interesting statistical material. The average strength of the active list was 37,248. There were 28,569 admissions to the sick list; that is, of every 1,000 men 782 were at some time during the year incapacitated by disease or injury. The admissions for injuries, 4,024, were less, and those for disease greater than during 1902. The total number of sick days, 470,496, was equivalent to 12.88 days for every man in the navy and marine corps. The deaths during the year numbered 224, 164 of which were from disease. Of the total number of sick days 114,571 were caused by venereal disease, which shows a marked increase over 1902. One of the recommendations made by the surgeon-general is that a corps of skilled dentists be added to the medical service. This has recently been done in the British army, where "military" dentists are now stationed at the largest barracks.

Yellow Fever.—During the past week there has been an unconfirmed report that six cases of yellow fever have been found in the canal zone at Panama. The news has caused some surprise but no alarm, because it had been expected that there would be a recrudescence of the disease there until the sanitary measures which are being adopted by the commission, under the supervision of Dr. Gorgas, can be carried out. In the Public Health Report, issued by Surgeon-General Walter Wyman, on December 30, 1904, is a report of the yellow fever situation at Guayaquil, Ecuador, which discloses two deaths from the scourge. The steamship Limari, bound from Panama to Valparaiso, stopped at Guayaquil with a case of yellow fever on board. The patient had been in Colon before boarding the ship. There has been constant communication between Panama and Guayaquil, at which place yellow fever always exists, but in the present instance the fever went from the isthmus to Ecuador, instead of the reverse. At Santiago de Cuba one undoubted case and one suspicious case occurred during the latter part of last October. Neither patient succumbed and no evidence that infection is lurking in this ancient stronghold of yellow fever could be detected by Dr. Nelson, whom the New York *Herald* commissioned to report on Cuban sanitation.

The Sale of Poison.—The *Globe* recently printed n interesting editorial under the above caption vhich is given below without comment: "Recently he Illinois Board of Pharmacy sent out 139 prescriptions to Chicago druggists to be filled. Analysis howed that twenty-three of the bottles contained no race of the drug called for, sixty-six were 80 per ent. impure, ten were 20 per cent. impure, and only hirty-one were pure. The revelations in the New York bogus pill case, not to speak of the slaughter n one part of the city by wood alcohol whiskey, show that Chicago has no monpoly of the adulterators and poisoners. There are bogus drugs in our prescriptions, aniline dyes in our jellies, sulphuric acid in our wines, sulphate of lead in our mustard, copperas in our olives and canned vegetables, and oxide of iron in our chocolate. Yet it seems probable that the coin-clutchers who thus play havoc with health will succeed in preventing the enactment of the protective legislation that the researches of Dr. Wiley of the National Bureau of Chemistry have shown to be necessary. It is a remarkable commentary on the boasted intelligence of the American people that they permit themselves not only to be defrauded but in many cases to be poisoned. It can no longer be said that there has not been sufficient exposure, or that it is impossible to provide a remedy.

The Hook-Worm in Porto Rico.—Mayor L. L. Seaman, M.D., who has recently visited the island in the interest of the New York *Herald*, reports a most serious state of health among the inhabitants the true nature of which has only lately been understood. He says, "the dreadfully anemic condition of the rural population of the island, embracing as it does nine-tenths of its inhabitants, has long been a matter of common knowledge. It has been accepted as a necessary evil, being attributed to poverty and poor food, and no special measures were taken for its prevention and cure until it forced itself upon the attention of medical men after the hurricane in August, 1899. Then an unusually large number of people came under medical and surgical treatment, and the astounding fact revealed itself that no less than eighty per cent. of the white victims suffered from this illness, thought to be pernicious anemia. The great prevalence of the disease excited much discussion among the attending physicians, for, they argued, if anemia is the consequence of insufficient food practically all Porto Rico must be on the verge of starvation, which, as a matter of fact, they knew was not the case. Hence they concluded that the disease was not anemia from deficient nourishment, and this conclusion has now been verified and the real exciting cause has been discovered. Captain Bailey K. Ashford, who was in charge of the field hospital established after the hurricane for the relief of the suffering poor, learned through biological and microscopical examinations that practically all sufferers from "anemia" were infested with a parasite, a so-called hookworm or nematode, which is known to the scientific world as *Anchylostoma duodenale*. On the authority of Dr. C. W. Stiles, zoologist of the Public Health and Marine Hospital Service there is a slight difference between the Porto Rican variety and the above species known in the Old World and which has been christened "*Uncinaria Americana.*" But the parasite is a bloodsucker all the same—that is, if the majority of the authorities on the subject can be believed. On February 16, 1904, the bill providing for the appointment of a commission "for the study and cure of the disease known as 'tropical anemia' in Porto Rico" was approved. Even then it was supposed that the anemic conditions confronting the commission constituted the disease instead of being the result of a totally different trouble, the nefarious effects of that silent but terribly efficacious bloodsucker, *Uncinaria Americana.*

The obstinate official adhesion to the theory of malnutrition, coupled with the unquestionable poverty of the Porto Rican land toiler, gave rise to that story of starvation which recently made the rounds of the American press. As a matter of fact, there is no starvation in Porto Rico.

The report is headed "Uncinaria in Porto Rico—Report of Commission on Anemia," and gives expression to the following: "About ninety per cent. of the rural population in all parts of the island are infected. If remedies are not taken the disease will continue to reduce the white and mixed inhabitants forming a country class in the island to a lower and lower grade, mentally, morally and physically, until the very existence of the class will be threatened. The inhabitants of Porto Rico belong to the poorer classes and seventy-five per cent. are agriculturists. Unicinariasis is a disease of the poor; the poorer the man the more exposed is he to infection. Here, again, poverty alone is a considerable cause of 'anemia,' whereas it is really a predisposing element. This is the reason why, when a gibaro (countryman) comes to a town where infection is not possible, or at least rare, he often gradually gets better of his 'anemia,' his multiple reinfections cease and the parasites he brings with him die as they reach the limit of their natural existence. Persons treated in Utuardo (excluding our special case), not more than three hundred of whom were ever rationed even for a short time by the commission, living in their homes as they had always lived, extremely poor and generally with an illy balanced, often an insufficient, dietary, were radically cured, expelling their uncinaria and leaving the clinic with normal blood tested by instruments. It is the imperative duty of the insular government to take hold of this work with decision and energy. The government should cooperate with the municipalities to fight the disease."

The therapeutic measures which experience has indicated are summarized by Dr. Seaman. The drugs first recommended were male fern and thymol, with a distinct preference of the latter. More recently beta-naphthol has been administered, which the former advocates of thymol state is not only more efficacious, but less irritating and less expensive. The statistics do not give a clear picture of the efficacy of the treatment, inasmuch as in the grand total of 5,490 treated cases, 1,029, or eighteen per cent. are included which did not return and the results of which were not recorded. As it is, however, eighty per cent. have been cured or improved, and if it is assumed that the majority of the eighteen per cent. above mentioned did not return on account of their improved condition the percentage of successes would come very near the hundred mark. As a matter of fact, in less than three per cent. of the total number of cases no improvement occurred or death supervened. But effective treatment of the infected alone will not save the situation. It is the preventive measures to which we have to look for an eradication of the disease. Of course, it is patent even to the layman that if arrangements could be made for preventing the infection of the soil, and practically enforced, the disease would be completely stamped out in a short time. and the bugbear of Porto Rican economist, "anemia," would soon be relegated to the annals of history. as uncinariasis is pre-eminently a filth disease and the general use of latrines would lead to its complete eradication.

SPECIAL ARTICLE.

BYWAYS OF MEDICAL LITERATURE.—XXIII.

THE AMERICAN DOCTOR—AS A CHINAMAN SAW HIM.[1]

"At a dinner in Manchester in the summer I had as my *vis-à-vis* a delightful young American, who, among other things, said to me: 'It is astonishing to me that so many of your people live long, considering the ignorance of your doctors. I assured her that this was merely her point of view, and that we were well satisfied with our doctors or physicians. I wished to retaliate by telling my fair companion a story I had heard the day previous. An American physician operated on a man and removed what he called a 'cyst,' which he displayed with some pride to a doctor of another school. 'Why, man,' said the latter, 'that isn't a cyst; it's the man's kidney!'

"The Americans have made rapid advances in medicine and surgery and they have some extraordinary physicians. From two to four years of study completes the education of some of the doctors, and hundreds are turned out every year. Some are of the old and regular school of medicine, but others are called homeopathic, which means that they give small doses of the more powerful medicines. Then there are those who practice in both schools. Indeed, in no other field does ignorance, superstition, credulity and lack of real education display itself as among the American doctors and healers. I believe I could fill a volume by a mere enumeration of the diabolical and absurd nostrums offered by knaves to heal men who profess to hold in ridicule the Chinese doctors. I mention but a few, and when I tell you, as a truth beyond cavil, that the most extraordinary of these healers, the most impossible, have the largest following, you can see what I mean by the credulity of the people as a whole. Christian Science doctors have a following of tens of thousands. They combine so-called science with religion; leave their God to cure them at long or short range, through the medium of so-called agents. The head of this faction is an ignorant but clever woman, who has turned the heads of perhaps thirty-three and a third per cent. of the American women whom she has come in contact with.

"Then come the faith curists, who rely upon faith alone. You simply are to *think* you will get well. Of course, many die from neglect. As an illustration of the credulity of the average American, a Christian Science healer was once treating a sick woman from a distant town, and finally the patient died. When the bill was presented the husband said, 'You have charged for treatment two weeks after my wife died.' It was a fact that the healer had been treating the woman after she was buried, the husband having failed to give notice of the death. One would have expected the 'healer' to be thrown into confusion, but far from it; she merely replied, 'I thought I noticed a vacancy.'

"Next come the musical curists who listen to thrills of sound, a big organ being the doctor. Then there is the psychometric doctor who cures by spirits. The spirit doctor cures in the same way. The palmist professes to point out how to avoid the ills of life. Magnetic healers have hundreds of victims in every city. The advertisements in the journals of all sorts are of countless kinds. Some cure at short hand, some miles distant from the patient. They are equaled in number by the hypnotists or hypnotic doctors, who profess to

throw their patients into a trance and cure them by suggestion. I heard of one cure in which the guileless American is made to lie in an open grave; this is called the 'return to nature.' Again, patients are cured by being buried in hot mud or hot sand. I have seen a salt-water cure where patients were made to remain in the ocean ten hours a day. The plain water cure has thousands of followers with hospitals and infirmaries, where the patient is bathed, soaked, filled, washed and plunged in water and charged a high amount.

"Then there is the vegetarian cure, no meat being eaten; and there are the meat eaters who use no vegetables. There are over fifty thousand *masseurs* and osteopaths in the country, who cure by baths and rubbing. You may have a bath of milk, water, electricity or alcohol, or a bath of any description under the sun, which is guaranteed to cure any and all ailments. Perhaps the most extraordinary curists are the color doctors. They have rooms filled with blue and other colors, in whose rays the patient victim, or the victim patient sits, 'like Patience on a monument.' I could not begin to give you an enumeration of the various kinds of electric cures; they are legion. But the most amazing class comprised the patent medicine men, who are usually not doctors at all, but buy from someone a 'cure' and then advertise it, spending in one instance which I investigated one million dollars a year. Every advantageous wall, stone or cliff in America will be posted. You see the name at every turn, and the gullible Americans bite, chew and swallow.

"It is not overstating facts when I say that three-fifths of the people buy some of these patent nostrums, which the real, medical men denounce, showing that the masses of the people are densely ignorant, the victim of any faker who can shout his wares loud enough. In China such a thing would be impossible; the block would stop the practice; but my dear ——, the Americans assure me that China is a thousand years behind the times, for which let us be devoutly thankful.

"I have not enumerated a tenth of the kinds of doctors who prey upon these unfortunate people. There are companies of them who guarantee to cure anything, and skilfully mulct the sick of their last penny. There are retreats for the unfortunate, farms for deserted infants, and homes for unfortunate women carried on by villains of both sexes. There are traveling doctors who go from town to town, who cure 'while you wait,' and give a circus while talking and selling their cures; and in nine cases out of ten the nostrum is an alcoholic drink disguised.

"In no land under the sun are there so many ignorant, blatant fakers preying on the people, and in no land do you find so credulous a throng as in America, yet claiming to represent the cream of the intelligence of the world; they are so easily led that the most impossible person, if he be a good talker, can go abroad and by the use of money and audacity secure a following to drink his salt water, paying a dollar a bottle for it and singing his praises. Such a doctor can secure the names and pictures of judges, governors and States, senators, congressmen, prominent men and women, officers of the volunteer army, artists, actors, singers,— in fact prominent people of all kinds will provide their pictures and give testimonials which are blazonly published. These same people go to a Chinese drug shop and laugh at the 'heathen' drugs, and wonder why the Chinaman is alive. America has a body of physicians and surgeons who are a credit to the world, modest, conscientious, and with a high sense of honor, but they are as a dragon's tooth in a multitude to the so-called 'quacks' who take the money of the masses and prey

---

[1] By the courtesy of D. Appleton & Co., N. Y., publishers of "As a Chinaman Saw Us." This is a reproduction of one of the chapters.

upon them, protected in many cases by law. No one profession demonstrates the abject credulity of the great mass of Americans as that of medicine.

"One other incident may further illustrate the jokes which these so-called doctors play upon the common people. In a country town was a 'quack' doctor who professed to be a 'head examiner,' giving people charts according to their 'bumps,' a fad which has many followers. 'This, ladies and gentlemen,' said the lecturer, holding out a small skull, 'is the skull of Alexander the Great at the age of six. Note the prominent brow. This (holding up a larger skull) is the same at the age of ten. This (holding up another) at the age of twenty-one; (then stepping to the front of the stage) this is the *complete* skull of Alexander at the time of his death.' All of which appeared to be accepted in good faith.

"Of the best physicians in America one cannot say enough in praise. I was most impressed with their high sense of honor. They have an agreement which they call their 'ethics' by which they will not advertise or call attention to their learning. Consequently the lower and ignorant classes are caught by the blatant chaff of the patent-medicine venders and the 'quack' doctors. What the word 'quack' means in this sense I do not quite know; literally it means the cry of a goose. The 'regular doctor' will not take advantage of any medicine he may discover or any instrument; all belongs to humanity, and one doctor becomes famous over another by his success in keeping people from dying. The grateful patient saved tells his friends, and so the doctor becomes known. In all America I never heard of a doctor that acted on the principle which holds among our doctors, that the best way to cure is to watch the patient and keep him well, or prevent him from being taken sick. The Americans in their conceit, consider Chinese doctors ignorant fakers; yet, so far as I could learn the death rate among the Chinese, city for city, country for country, is less than among Americans. The Chinese women are longer lived and less subject to disease. In what is known as New England, the oldest well-populated section of the country, people would die out were it not for the constant accession of immigrants. On the other hand, the Chinese constantly increase, despite a policy of non-intercourse with foreigners. The Americans have, in a civilization dating back to 1492, already begun to show signs of decadence, and are only saved by constant immigration. China has a civilization of thousands of years, and is increasing in population every day, yet her doctors and their methods are ridiculed by the Americans. The people have many sayings here, one of which is, 'The proof of the pudding lies in the eating.' It seems applicable to this case."

MODERN SPIRITUALISM AS IT IS.

Spiritualistic séances have so often been enlivened by skeptics who seized "materialized" visitors claiming to be from another world, that accounts as to just what world it was to which the visitors turned out to belong, long ago lost even the value of confirmatory evidence, and it has been known for years that anybody who wanted the excitement of catching a flesh-and-blood spook could not possibly go wrong in selecting his hunting ground, no matter where he went among the places devoted to the materializing industry. New interest has been added to this old sport, however, by a variant of it just developed in Brooklyn, writes the *Times*. There, it seems, the business of "raising" Indian chiefs and big and little maidens of assorted kinds has been so vigorously followed, that bitter jealousies

have grown up among the "mediums," and they are engaged in the work, admirable in some ways, but a bit treacherous in others, of proving each other to be humbugs. The first reported effort in this novel campaign was a complete success. The three " investigators " posed convincingly as—well, as believers, and to them trustingly appeared as fine a specimen of the Indian ghost as any reasonable collector could demand. The three seized "Fallen Water," and immediately several other things and persons fell in a general scrimmage the very reverse of spiritual. Suits for assault and battery have now been instituted, and the situation is most promising of joy. Exactly what there is in it for people themselves in the ghost trade is not easily seen. Such internal warfare threatens the very existence of their industry, for even to Brooklyn's credulity there are limitations, and "exposures" planned and carried through by "mediums" will be sure to have a deplorably retroactive effect. What these enterprising folks should do is to combine, to form a trust. Then only will they be able to charge monopoly prices for ghosts while paying competitive prices to their workmen. Involved in this amusing episode, however, is one very serious feature. In the house where "Fallen Water" did his turn the so-called spirit of a little child often floated airily out of the cabinet. Now, can anybody conceive of more harmful surroundings for a child than these or use of a child more deeply reprehensible? Speaking on this general topic of Spiritualism, Dr. I. K. Funk, of New York, has some interesting experiences. He writes (*Literary Digest*, October 8, 1904) that the subject is one that belongs to the "sphere of influence" of the clergy, and he urges upon ministers the duty of fitting themselves to take the leadership in this new series of investigations. With a view to clearing the ground for intelligent research, Dr. Funk has himself made extensive inquiries into the nature of spiritualistic phenomena, the results of which he has embodied in book-form. In *The Homiletic Review* (October) he recounts a "unique experience" of his brother, Mr. B. F. Funk, in contact with the seamy side of Spiritualism. It seems that a business card bearing the words "Radium, Medium's Paraphernalia," and advertising "crowns, belts, hands, heads, veils and full-size figures illuminated with the new radium light" which would "appear, gradually float about room and disappear," recently came into Dr. Funk's possession. The card carried a Chicago address, and it was handed by him to Mr. B. F. Funk with the request that he investigate and report the facts of the case. This report is now incorporated in Dr. Funk's article, and opens as follows:

"On my first call I was informed that in order to see this radium expert it would be necessary for me to make an appointment. The appointment being duly made and kept, I found the proprietor to be a youngish, gentlemanly sort of fellow, apparently refined and educated. The card served as an open sesame, somewhat stiff, gaining for me the desired interview. In reply to my question whether he sold outfits for mediums, he said, eyeing me closely: 'I sometimes sell things that are of interest to mediums and—to other people.' After a moment's silence he continued: 'What do you wish? What are you *after?*'

"Then followed much verbal fencing, when he finally said: 'I always insist, as a mark of good faith, that at the outset an order be given with payment for an outfit.' This outfit, he told me, varies in price from $50 to $1,000."

Mr. Funk went on to say that a lady friend in an Eastern city wished to equip herself as a Spiritualistic medium. "I do not wish her to do wrong," he concluded. To this the young man replied:

"'Certainly not, certainly not; I understand. I have many such among my clientele. It is my business to help mediums make a good show. They do not do wrong; on the contrary, they are doing a great deal of good in getting people to believe that their friends who have died are really alive. I have seen mothers made happy at the sight of their dead children, husbands at the sight of their departed wives. It has often brought tears to my eyes to see the simple faith of these people. If a man is a philanthropist who can multiply blades of grass, surely I or a medium should be entitled to praise if we cause rejoicing where there are tears. Why, my dear fellow, Spiritualists are the happiest people in the world. Why undeceive them? They are in heaven. It does them no hurt, but much good to believe these things. My business is to put clever people in the way of making the world happier.' The man grew quite eloquent in dilating on his philanthropic calling."

The report of the conversation continues: "He finally asked: 'What kind of phenomena would you prefer that your friend should produce?'

"I replied: 'I wish her to give physical manifestations, such as materialization of hands, of the entire human form, spirit voices, illuminated stars, sparks, rays of light, floating balls of fire, floating musical instruments, trumpet talks, slate-writing, mind-reading, etc. Are these things within the scope of your art?'

"He smiled at the modesty of my wish, then said: 'All this is merest child's play, provided your lady friend is apt, quick-witted, and has nerve. I am furnishing help after this sort to the mediums of Chicago—they all come to me; I know them all.'

"'Do good, genuine mediums use this kind of help?'

"'All mediums are *good* mediums and genuine mediums. I don't know any other kind.'

"'Is there no difficulty in manipulating this machinery or paraphernalia?'

"'It is so simple you will wonder why it is that people do not at once detect it. When you understand it, and understand the *modus operandi* of handling it, you will be much amused.'

"'How about slate-writing?'

"'Perfectly simple.'

"'With the tied slates, glued and sealed?'

"'Yes, oh yes. I have laughed until my sides ached after a séance at the remembrance of how easily and completely the d. e.'s ('dead easies') were fooled. To see a doting father take the materialized form of his dead child on his knee and pet it and kiss it, and then hear the little one say, "Now, papa, I must go; I feel I am getting weak," and then see the child slip from his lap and disappear, to the infinite surprise of all the faithful—it is more laughable than an Artemus Ward "wax-figger show."'

"'But is there no danger of getting caught?'

"'No, there are two hundred mediums in Chicago. How seldom you hear of an exposure.'

"'But I have been where I was permitted to touch the hand of a form. It seemed warm, as if flesh and blood.'

"This seemed to amuse him greatly. Finally he said: 'Yes *it does feel precisely like flesh.* But this is another phase of the business. It is all explained when the outfit is sent.' . . . . .

"After some more interchange of this kind of talk

I said: 'Speaking seriously, do you mean to tell me that no mediums possess occult or abnormal powers; that it is all humbuggery and trickery?'

"After a few moments' thought, his face growing serious, he said: 'There *is* something mysterious, something that puzzles me at times about some mediums. I have seen phenomena that I cannot explain. At times an outside influence seems to come over the medium, taking possession of her. What it is I don't know. Possibly telepathy will explain it, possibly spirits.'"

In his comment on this report, Dr. Funk admits "the abundance and the disgusting nature of the frauds which attend many spiritualistic séances," as well as the dangers that attend this line of investigation. He adds: "I have seen psychic cobwebs—if cobwebs they be—tangle the feet of even intellectual giants; and the shrewdest experts—to change the simile—need to sail these mystic seas with sharp eyes and level heads, for these seas are almost wholly uncharted, and in sailing over them, at times, the ship's compasses exhibit inexplicable variations. Yet these investigations must be made and these seas must be sailed and charted." The criminologists, be it interpolated, have been charting these seas for decades, but the clergy rarely ever meet the true criminal, and more rarely understand how much akin he is to the rest of mankind.

SOCIETY PROCEEDINGS.

NEW YORK STATE MEDICAL ASSOCIATION, NEW YORK COUNTY BRANCH.

Regular Monthly Meeting, held November 21, 1904.

The President, Francis T. Quinlan, M.D., in the Chair.

Dangers of the X-Ray.—The first part of the scientific business of the evening consisted of a paper by Dr. Milton Franklin on the dangers commonly met with in the employment of the X-rays for diagnostic and especially for therapeutic purposes. Dr. Franklin said that while the most important and serious danger is that of localized burns, there is a certain amount of risk of producing general depression with even a tendency to cachexia when patients are exposed frequently and for prolonged periods to the influence of the X-rays. This is only what might be expected considering the influence that such radiations have upon living tissues. It emphasizes for care in the use of the X-rays and for experience in the operator, so that such unfortunate sequelæ may not result.

Protectors.—Dr. Franklin suggested that parts which are unaffected should not be subjected to the influence of the X-rays. Consequently the need of having metallic protectors usually made of sheets of lead, so that only such parts as are desired may be submitted to the influence of the X-rays. When the seance is at all prolonged, slight movement of the patient is likely to cause the rays to act upon portions sometimes at quite a distance from the lesion to be treated. Sheets of lead may be arranged, however, in such a way that only the lesion itself will be exposed. The neglect of this precaution has probably done more to bring the X-rays into disrepute than almost any other feature of their employment. Dr. Franklin considers that one of the most crying needs at the present time is for a radiometer, that is an instrument that will measure the radiation strength of the rays. Tubes are sure to differ, not nly among themselves, but also from time to time nd it is important for the operator to know exactly /hat radiation strength he is employing. Dr. Frank- n has made use of the principles employed in the iscovery of radium to construct a radiometer which ells exactly the strength of the X-rays employed at ny given moment. Repeated trials have shown him that this instrument, which is construtced on the principle of ionizing effects of the X-ray, can be absolutely depended on. It is sufficiently simple to be employed by any one at all familiar with electrical measurements, and does not itself vary from day to day.

Forms of Danger.—Dr. William B. Coley, in opening the discussion, said that in the use of the X-rays there is danger first to the patient, next to the operator and then, finally, to the public mind. With regard to the patient, the most serious danger is that oi burns. With experience the risk of this decreases, but never entirely. On the other hand, the inexpert frequently meet with this complication. The use of too strong radiations may produce a breaking down of cancer tissue with rapid dissemination of the material and generalized malignant disease. At first this was mere theory. Now it is certain and is attested by the experience of many. Dr. Coley has seen a lymphosarcoma, which usually does not give generalization, breaks down under the effect of the X-rays and disappears to a great extent, but shortly afterward tumors appear in the mesentery and elsewhere throughout the body. Mammary carcinoma may be made in this way to spread to the spinal cord, to the pleura or to other inaccessible portions of the body, with a rapidly fatal result. Dermatitis frequently occurs in those who use the X-rays much and is rather expected. Not infrequently, however, ulcers are seen and these are of a very intractible type. The most curious feature about them is that they seem to have a special tendency to malignant degeneration. There has been much seeking after an agent that would produce cancer. The X-rays were looked upon as likely to cure malignant disease. In a certain number of reported cases, however, they have actually produced cancer. Dr. Coley himself has seen four cases. A very interesting feature of most of these cases is that there is a multiplicity of the malignant lesions. In one case, after the amputation of a hand, the other hand had to be amputated and then the arm on the opposite side and then eight further operations, though the end is not yet and the fatal issue is looked for. Too much stress cannot be laid on these unfortunate results, for the profession is evidently dealing with an agent whose power is very little known and witn regard to which it is extremely difficult to take proper precaution.

Danger to the Public Mind.—This consists mainly of the danger that because of the flattering reports only too often published, patients insist on being treated with the X-rays when the knife is the only proper treatment. Small nodules of carcinoma may be treated by the X-rays and apparently be cured, while lymphatic involvement is gradually producing other foci of the disease that may prove to be incurable. The X-rays therefore should only be employed in cases that are inoperable by the knife or after operation to prevent recurrence, or for the treatment of recurrent nodules. In this latter regard the X-rays are especially valuable.

No Protector.—Dr. Carl Beck said that whenever there is a question of malignant disease, the X-rays should be employed without any protection for the surrounding tissues. The old idea used to be that cancer was limited and that consequently only the nodule itself needed to be excised. Under such conditions of surgical procedure, recurrences were almost inevitable. It is important that the surrounding tissues, which are always infiltrated with cancer cells, should be subjected to the influence of the curative agent quite as well as the tumor itself. If the X-rays are employed for cosmetic purposes, for the removal of hair or some cutaneous blemish, then a protector is advisable, but never in cancer cases.

Deep Burn, Relief of Deep Carcinoma.—Dr. C. W. Allen presented a case that had been sent to him to be treated by the X-rays with the diagnosis "liver carcinoma." Because of that diagnosis, a number of treatments were given, until unfortunately a deep burn was produced. This was several years ago and before the proper limitation of the effects of the X-rays were so well known. Owing to the cachexia of the carcinomatous condition, the woman was in very poor health and it looked as though a fatal issue was not far off. The burn proved extremely difficult to heal. At the end of two years the patient returned ever so much better. Now it would seem as though her hepatic cancer had been delayed in its progress so materially that she may look forward to even years of reasonably comfortable life. Almost any one would be satisfied to stand a burning that has been experienced in this case with its subsequent discomfort for the sake of the improvement against all expectation which has resulted.

Experience with X-rays.—Dr. Morton said that any agent may become dangerous if inexpertly employed. He does not consider that the electroscope would prove of great service in the measurement of radiation. Hence, the necessity for experience rather than mechanical aid as a guide as to the way the X-rays should be employed. Dr. Morton considers that as the X-rays are useful after operation, so they should also be employed before operation. In this way the cancer will be better limited and certainly if at any time there is to be delay in the use of the knife, then it would be almost criminal to neglect the use of the X-ray.

Dr. Franklin, in closing the discussion, said that there is an idiosyncrasy to the X-rays, but this is no more important than the idiosyncrasy for other remedial measures. Special directions are not given for the employment of drugs so as to avoid the inconvenience that always results from the presence of an idiosyncrasy because it is impossible to anticipate these. The same thing must hold good with regard to the X-rays. Rules must be made without reference to such idiosyncrasy. With regard to the use of metallic masks and screens, Dr. Franklin wishes to emphasize the fact that he suggests the covering only of the area that is not to be treated. This does not mean that only the microscopical lesion is to be the subject of treatment, but also as much of an area around it as may be deemed advisable by the operator. All skin outside of this area, however, should be protected.

The Russo-Japanese War.—Dr. L. L. Seaman read a report of his personal observations on the medical and surgical treatment of the Russo-Japanese war. In the very hospitals that he visited, he realized that the Japanese had secured fresh air and sunshine to a greater degree for their hospitals than had ever been accomplished before. The toilet arrangements, owing to the fact that earth closets are employed, might be the subject of criticism, but the exquisite cleanliness of the people themselves more than made up for any drawbacks in this matter. After the cleanliness, the order that reigned was the most noteworthy feature. The mechanical precision of hospital reception of large numbers of patients was a never-ending source of wonder. Within an hour or two after the reception of hundreds of patients, the routine of the hospital was proceeding as if there had been no such call upon its resources.

No Surgery at Front.—The rule among the Japanese has been that no surgery of any importance is done at the front. In cases of serious hemorrhage, it is of course checked by whatever surgical needs are necessary. Anything else that is necessary to save life is also done by the field surgeon. As a rule, however, first aid bandages are applied and then the wounded are sent back to Japan. On their reception at the hospitals, there is as a rule very little to do. The mortality on the way is not large. Most of the patients' wounds have healed by first intention before their arrival and the only thing necessary is to make their convalescence as rapid and complete as possible, for they are all anxious to get back to the front. In the cases seen of soldiers who had shared in the attack on Port Arthur, the explosive effects of bullets of high velocity received at close quarters, was very evident.

Aneurisms.—A very interesting phase of the surgical work was the presence of many aneurisms, even in his short stay Dr. Seaman saw nearly thirty of these. Often the external wound healed by first intention, and it was only after several weeks that the development of a pulsating swelling revealed the injury to the artery. This was of course due to a true aneurismal dilatation. These lesions were treated by cutting down upon the artery, tying it at both ends near the swelling and then excising the dilated portion. A certain number of traumatic aneurisms, due to the direct wounding of an artery, were also observed. In these cases the pressure of the clot made the tissues in the neighborhood friable and lowered their resistive vitality so as to make their treatment by surgical measures rather difficult. In a certain number of cases, the wounds had produced arteriovenous aneurisms. At times the bullet seems to have passed between the vein and the artery, pushing the vessels aside but injuring their coats so that later a communication took place within them. In the case of the radial artery and in the vein, the removal of portions of both the vessels brought about a cure of the condition.

Medical Aspects of the War.—Of all the cases Dr. Seaman was surprised to find no hernia, nor were there any cases of appendicitis. Besides this, so far, there has been no record of the necessity for operations upon the biliary tract. Considering the large number of men who are under arms, Dr. Seaman considers this very striking. This freedom from medical diseases and especially from affections of the digestive tract, is a tribute to the plain digestible diet which the Japanese soldier uses. In the American experience with war, these affections were so common as to make the medical history of the war much more important than the surgical. The morale of the patients in the hospitals is excellent. No complaints were heard at all. Besides this, however, there was an air of discipline about the hospital that was most encouraging. and it was evidently maintained with very little difficulty. The Russian wounded and prisoners in the hospitals seemed to be very well satisfied. They were well entertained. Most of them were peasants from the center of Russia and they were much better off than they had been at home. There were no signs of any special effort to detain them as prisoners. Many Russians hoped to stay.

Special Medical Features.—Beriberi or kakke, which used to be a scourge in the navies of the East, was wiped out of the Japanese Navy by proper regulation of the rations served to the marines. So far, it has not made its appearance in this war, though it is possible that the Japanese may have to add lentils or pea sausage, such as the Germans use, or some other form of nitrogenous food material in order to prevent it. It is now well understood that the disease is due to the starvation of the nerves and especially to the lack of nitrogenous material for their proper nutrition. All of the Japanese sailors receive three ounces of saki, a mild spirit, every day. In cases where extra work and long hours of watching are demanded of them, this amount is doubled. Of course the well-known abstemiousness in the Japanese prevents abuse in this matter. In all his experience in Japan Dr. Seaman never saw a drunken individual either in or out of the service. The Japanese army believes in the maintenance of a canteen for its soldiers as do indeed all the governments of the world now, except the American and the Chinese.

Rank of Medical Officers.—The surgeon-general of the Japanese army has the rank of Major-General. The head of the navy has the rank equivalent to that of Lieutenant-General. There are at least half a dozen of the high medical officers of the army who have a higher rank than it is possible for medical officers in America to attain, even if they should get to the highest possible place for them. Another feature of the Japanese army medical service with regard to which comparison with America is apt to make the American feel ashamed, is the number of individuals in the hospital corps of the two armies. To a division of the Japanese army consisting of about 20,000 men, 1,200 beds are allowed. Over 600 persons are considered to be necessary for the hospital service. In the United States the number of beds is much less than this and the corresponding branch of the hospital corps consists of less than 100 men. Japan was the first nation to recognize the value of the army medical corps as a life-saving institution.

Prevention of Disease.—One of the officers in charge of the Medical Department of the Japanese army remarked to Dr. Seaman that Japan realized perfectly her inferiority to Russia in the point of numbers. Japan can put half a million soldiers in the field while Russia can put two millions. So far, in war, however, it has been the custom to consider that only one man will be killed out of the four who died during the war. Japan resolved to counteract her inferiority to Russia by saving all the men that would ordinarily be lost by disease. This, so far, has been accomplished almost to a man. The advance guard is always accompanied by medical experts who examine the water, test the food and even investigate the condition of the houses in the villages in which soldiers are likely to be quartered. Wherever there has been contagious disease within short time before the oncoming of the troops, no billet is allowed to be given for houses. The Japanese soldiers have the inherent instinct of obedience to command, and as a consequence, there are no violations of orders. In camp between marches, instructions are given by the medical staff as to how the men shall conduct themselves in order to be free from disease during the variations of the weather and the varieties of food.

Contrast with America.—The contrast with America in many points is extremely interesting. Evidently in this country pensions are preferred to prevention disease, while in Japan, sanitation and hygiene are considered important parts of the instruction of officers

These subjects are not taught at West Point at all. Though 80 per cent. of the losses in war are usually due to disease, it is only the killing part of the service that receives due recognition. In this country fanatic women deprive army officers of the power to regulate soldiers' habits, to some extent at least, by depriving them of the canteen. It is to America that Japan owes many lessons. From Japan, however, at the present time much could be learned.

American Needs.—Major John L. Phillips, United States Army, said that there is no doubt that a valuable lesson can be learned from the present conduct of medical affairs in war by the Japs. As a result of Dr. Seaman's calling attention to the matter, medical officers from the United States Army have now been detailed to make observations in the East. One of these goes to the Russian and the other to the Japanese army. It is not an easy matter, in the United States, however, for the army in case of war to secure good sanitariums, since the medical schools of the country furnish only a limited amount of instruction in hygiene, something less than fifty hours being the rule for the annual course in this subject.

Major Jarvis said that the Japanese have been preparing for ten years for this war with Russia. Comparison therefore of conditions with those which obtained in our recent war are entirely unfair.

Capt. A. E. Piorkowski of the Imperial German Army said that the Franco-Prussian war was the first one in history in which the proportion of men who died from disease was less than the number killed. It must not be forgotten that that war was not so short as it seemed, since troops had to continue in France for a considerable period after the actual cessation of hostilities. Von Moltke's plan of keeping the corps of the army separate and drawing them together whenever battle was expected did much to make sanitation easier than it would otherwise have been. It must not be forgotten that besides the preparation which the Japs had had for this war, they are members of a great military empire and are natural born soldiers.

Colonel Church, United States Army, said that one advantage the Japanese had in the present struggle has been the absence of any sentiment with regard to the disposal of dead bodies. With us there is apt to be insistence on the burying process. This is often so incomplete that portions of the dead are left exposed to become the prey of bird and beast and to form a nidus for infectious material that may be carried away by air or water. In Japan, however, there is no prejudice with regard to the cremation of dead bodies and consequently after a battle the bodies are simply gathered together and burned. This is a complete destruction of dangerous material and is eminently sanitary. Certainly this must be considered in the great battles of the future as one method of doing away with dangerous material that is eminently suited to this stage of our civilization.

HARVARD MEDICAL SOCIETY OF NEW YORK CITY.

Regular Monthly Meeting, held Saturday, October 22, 1904.

The President, Augustus M. Knight, M.D., in the Chair.

Seminal Vesiculotomy.—Dr. E. Fuller said that not a few patients, who suffer from the results of chronic gonorrhea, after having been submitted to all forms of treatment of the urethra, find that there is no relief afforded and after a time also find that their sexual capacity is becoming impaired. In a certain number of these cases, impotence asserts it-

self and the most careful examination of the seminal fluid fails to show the presence of spermatozoa. In this class of cases an examination of the seminal vesicles not infrequently reveals the fact that they are either thickened or surrounded by inflammatory products and that they are therefore evidently incapable of performing their function. For these patients, Dr. Fuller has devised the operation of vesiculotomy. Dr. Fuller said that the stripping of the seminal vesicle and massage through the rectum is often effective in mild cases of disease of the seminal vesicles. In severe cases, however, it takes too long to do good and patients become impatient, besides, for patients at a distance, it is extremely inconvenient to come as frequently as is required to the surgeon's office. Consequently the necessity for some radical procedure to which patients will be ready to submit if it promises to relieve their symptoms. The operation of seminal vesiculotomy he has now done in 33 cases without a death and as the after results have been very satisfactory, this new operation would seem to deserve a place in regular surgical procedure. With the first patients he was perfectly frank in telling them that the operation was as yet untried, but that it was not dangerous and that there was no reason why it should not be successful in affording them relief. After all the thorough opening of the seminal vesicles with drainage is only a following out of the surgical principle that has been applied to so many other cavities of the body when they have become infected.

Results of Operation.—It has sometimes been considered that operations upon the seminal vesicles might afford relief from pain and from certain of the dangers of carrying an infected area in the body, but that they could scarcely do more than this. In fact, there used to be an objection that operations upon them rendered the patient sterile and were somewhat akin to castration. One German authority, indeed, spoke of the operation as high castration. This is, however, entirely a mistaken notion. While too much was not expected or promised from early operation, the results obtained have been most satisfactory. Perhaps the most satisfying feature of the cases has been the return of sexual potency in cases where it has been absent for some time. The function of the seminal vesicle which has been lost is not infrequently regained. This is after all only what might be expected from the improvement of the local condition which takes place as a consequence of the evacuation and drainage. Dr. Fuller himself has not had a death in thirty-two cases. There seems no reason to think that in the hands of any careful surgeon thoroughly familiar with the anatomy of these parts, there should be a death. The mortality that would come would be from interference with neighboring organs, especially the rectum, the bladder, and, in certain cases, the ureter or the peritoneal cavity. Incomplete postoperative drainage might give rise to a septic condition that would easily prove serious. While the operation has its dangers, these are due to complications and are not necessarily attached to the operative procedure itself.

Contra-Indications.—In Dr. Fuller's opinion, there is just one contra-indication to the operation and that is the existence of tuberculosis of the seminal vesicles. In these cases, the sinuses do not heal well and the patients are usually in poor condition for operation and the result as regards the recovery of function is not likely to be satisfactory. Where tuberculous processes exist in connection with seminal vesiculitis, that is, in neighboring genital organs, all methods of palliative treatment should be tried and surgery avoided. It is sometimes said that such an operation will need to be done only very rarely. In recent years, however, there has come the realization that secondary infections in gonorrhea involving the seminal vesicles not infrequently, are quite common. Patients suffering from conditions of the seminal vesicles requiring operation are seen much more frequently than would otherwise be imagined. After all it is not surprising that this should be the case, since the liability of the gonococcus to wander through all parts of the male genital system is now well understood.

Differential Diagnosis.—It is interesting to note how many different affections seminal vesiculitis is taken for by those who are not familiar with its ordinary diagnostic signs. In a recent case where, as a consequence of the presence of pus in the urine, with some tendency to irritation, the affection was thought to be of the bladder, all sorts of irrigation of that viscus had been carried out by various surgeons for several years. All the known urinary antiseptics that may be employed through the mouth had been prescribed in abundance and besides the various antiseptics for irrigation had been employed. All, of course, to no avail. After a time, because of the difficulty of urination, a rather characteristic difficulty at the beginning, with inability to empty the bladder completely without special effort, the affection had been taken for enlargement of the prostate. As this could not be felt, it was thought to be an enlargement of the middle lobe. It is not hard to understand how the chronic inflammatory condition around the seminal vesicle at the base of the bladder prevents its contraction to some extent, and gives rise to such a confusion. In this case all sorts of suggestions were made to the patient. One surgeon wished to perform castration, another suggested Bottini's operation, that of burning a tunnel through the supposed enlarged prostate. Still a third surgeon suggested prostatectomy.

Real Condition.—At operation, both the seminal vesicles were found suffering from a chronic inflammatory process and filled with granulation tissue. They were slit and this was scraped out with a curette. There did not seem to be much hope that the seminal vesicles would resume their functions. They have done so, however, and the patient is well satisfied with the result. As a consequence of the removal of the inflammatory products that were hampering the action of the bladder, all the urinary symptoms have now disappeared.

Lengthy Convalescence.—In cases that have suffered from the affection of the seminal vesicles for many years, it is not surprising that convalescence may require a considerable period. As Dr. Fuller has gained more and more experience in the operation, however, and has consequently been enabled to do less and less damage to tissues in the course of the operation, the period of convalescence has grown shorter. In some of these cases, the seminal vesicle is found so filled up with physiological and pathological products as to be ballooned almost to the size of an egg. In such cases, of course, it is easier to find the offending organ, but in many patients, the seminal vesicles are enlarged little beyond their normal size and consequently care and experience is needed not to injure surrounding tissues, all of them of the greatest importance and associated with hollow viscera containing infectious material of great virulence.

Dr. Frederick Curtis, in discussing Dr. Fuller's paper, said that it is good surgical logic to open up cavities containing pus, no matter where they may be. As far as this is concerned, Dr. Fuller's new operations are an exemplification of a very old surgical principle. It seems not unlikely that these operations have been done before when considered necessary and that there is not the novelty that might be expected. Certainly before any operation should be done, the stripping of the seminal vesicles should be carefully tried. This constitutes an added means of treatment for chronic cases that resist massage and other remedial measures.

Valuable Addition to Surgery.—Dr. Follen Cabot said that Dr. Fuller's operation, of which he has had the opportunity to see several examples, is undoubtedly an important measure for the relief of conditions that have been considered intractable before. Any one who has a large experience in male venereal cases knows how many of these sufferers from chronic blenorrhagic conditions receive no relief and go discouraged from one surgeon to another. After a time they fail to have any hope and make most discouraging patients. This operation gives relief in these cases and restoring sexual power that has been lost for some time, brings with it a great measure of consolation to the sufferer.

Questions of Technic.—Dr. Fuller, in closing the question, answered some questions with regard to technic. In the older methods of performing operation upon the seminal vesicles, the patient was placed upon his back, and it was practically impossible to properly reach these organs. Extirpation might be accomplished, but relief could scarcely be afforded by any less serious operation. In the knee-chest position, the rectum can be dissected up and put out of the way by means of a wide incision that is an extension of the Zuckerkandl. Notwithstanding the fear that there might be infection preventing union in parts so liable to infection, good union is the rule. After the seminal vesicles have been incised, the interior is packed with gauze, which is pulled out on the fifth day. As the parts are very vascular, union proceeds rapidly and infective material is disposed of by the excellent vitality of the parts.

Acute Cases.—In some of these infections of the seminal vesicles an intensely acute condition develops with a formation of pus all around these organs. By means of this incision, such a collection can be thoroughly opened up and though for a time the parts may present a ghastly appearance, the result is excellent beyond all expectations. In one case the patient who developed an abscess deep in the perineal region, had a temperature of 105° F. and fatal septicemic infection was feared. Immediately after the evacuation of the pus the temperature came down and the large cavity healed completely under strapping and stitching.

Chronic Cases with Pus Formation.—In a certain number of cases there seems to be a collection of pus around the seminal vesicles, producing a condition of chronic invalidism, the pus finding an exit every now and then through the prostatic sinus. In these cases there is apt to be deep indefinite pain in the prostatic region and at times the burrowing of the pus may produce a sinus of communication between the bladder and rectum that accounts for the appearance of urine occasionally in the rectum. In these cases, thorough operation is the only sure means of giving these patients relief, and, as a rule, the seminal vesicles will have to be laid open in order to secure thorough removement of infective materials.

Functional Results.—The results obtained are especially good as regards the sexual functions after operation. There does not seem to be a common duct of the seminal vesicles and the vasa differentia. The vas deferens on each side empty directly into the seminal vesicle and the vale in the ampulla of Henle prevents all regurgitation. This has been demonstrated by careful dissections. As a result of this, if the function of the seminal vesicle is restored, the ejaculatory element of the sexual function is also restored. This is the experience with patients who usually have the function restored which they had considered lost for good.

SOUTHERN SURGICAL AND GYNECOLOGICAL ASSOCIATION.

Seventeenth Annual Meeting, held at Birmingham, Ala., December 13, 14 and 15, 1904.

(Continued from Page 1277.)

Review of the Treatment Immediately Before and After Abdominal Section.—Dr. L. S. McMurtry, of Louisville, stated that the directness and simplicity of surgical methods were proportionate to the accuracy of pathological knowledge. The marked changes which had characterized the evolution of the modern aseptic surgical technic illustrated the truth of this observation. Present methods were wonderfully simplified in comparison with those of the early antiseptic era when chemical germicides played a conspicuous rôle in every phase of the scheme of operation. The general indications for preparatory treatment in cases of abdominal section were to cleanse the alimentary canal thoroughly without violent disturbance or exhaustion; to put all the eliminative functions in the best possible condition, and to favor in every way a tranquil state of mind and body. More than a year ago he became satisfied that to put the patient to bed for three days, or even longer, as was practised by many, was not the best course of preparatory treatment. There was a positive advantage in having the bowels cleaned out in a relatively short time, as the patient was not relaxed by purgation and was less prone to suffer from toxic changes. Prolonged and irritating catharsis increased the nausea and vomiting of ether and chloroform anesthesia. A prolonged period of preparatory treatment impaired the patient's strength and depressed the nervous system. There were exceptional cases, of course, such as associated functional and organic disease of other organs than that for which the operation was proposed. If these disturbances were the result of the disease for which the operation was to be done, no good could come of delay; but when such associated conditions were distinct from the disease for which the operation was contemplated, and which might be improved by treatment, a judicious course of preparatory treatment should be observed. The same rule should be applied to cases of anemia, and in cases of acute diffuse infection which might become circumscribed, preparatory treatment might be utilized with advantage. In the cleansing and disinfection of the skin, it is an established fact that sterilization of the skin from a bacteriological standard was impossible; yet mechanical cleansing would for all practical purposes free the skin of all active germ action and provide for immediate primary union of wounds. In the effort to accomplish this, the important fact had

been overlooked that the unbroken skin was endowed with a power of resistance to the activity of its own and other germs; and when the epidermis was cracked, denuded and broken by irritating germicides, and scrubbing with hard brushes, this natural resistance was impaired, and infection occurred. Mechanical cleansing would remove germs readily from smooth and unbroken cutaneous surfaces. For these reasons the brush and chemical germicides should be discarded, and only soap and water and alcohol should be used, applying these with gauze instead of the brush. In the after-treatment only the most simple course was necessary in average cases. The routine use of purgatives here, as in the preparatory treatment, was to be avoided. The patient should be allowed to move about in bed freely, and should be given water as soon after operation as it could be retained.

Employment of Celluloid Plates for Covering Openings in the Skull in Operations for Epilepsy, Brain Tumor, Etc.—Dr. William P. Nicolson, of Atlanta, Ga., read a paper with this title. He said that celluloid was a material which remained indefinitely in the tissues without irritation or disturbance, and the physical character of it was such that it could be easily shaped with scissors to the required size and shape for adjustment to the opening to be covered. Its harmlessness in the tissues was demonstrated to him many years ago by the absence of any irritation from a celluloid testicle introduced by him into a patient's scrotum. Given such a material, one was enabled to enlarge the opening in the skull to whatever size he might desire, knowing that he could cover the opening and protect the brain from subsequent injury or from undue protrusion from want of support. In operations for epilepsy it not only protected the brain from subsequent pressure, but left an increased space, which was measured by the thickness of the individual's skull. After describing the technic of inserting the celluloid, the author reported a case of cyst of the brain which produced epilepsy. He also reported two cases of Jacksonian epilepsy, and one of exploratory operation on the brain. Although the duration of the cases reported did not give a long observation of results, the author felt safe in making the following claims for the routine application of this principle to all operations, where the surgeon was compelled to make openings of any size in the skull: (*a*) It was safe, and did not add any extra risk to the operation. (*b*) It not only removed the pressure and irritation, which the surgeon was endeavoring to combat, but by its resistance prevented a recurrence from the subsequent consolidation of the coverings in a false position due to atmospheric pressure. (*c*) It protected the patient from external influences, and not only made him feel safer, but he was actually safer. (*d*) It enabled surgeons to be much more untrammeled in the amount of bone that they could remove. (*e*) It prevented deformity, which especially, when beyond the hair line, was necessarily great in large bone removals.

Traumatic Synovitis of the Knee Joint.—Dr. Edward A. Balloch, of Washington, D. C., made a plea for earlier operative intervention in cases of traumatic synovitis, the author's contention being that so-called conservative measures should not be tried too long. The reluctance of surgeons to open the joint was ascribed in part to a fear of sepsis and in part to a lack of a precise knowledge as to the normal structure of the joint. Illustrative cases were cited showing the advantages of early operative intervention. The following conclusions were reached: (1) In most, if not all, cases of traumatic arthritis of the knee, there was an injury to some of the structures of the joint. (2) Conservative measures should not be persisted in too long. Three weeks was proposed as a fair length of time for a trial of these measures. If no improvement was manifest at the end of that time, the propriety of operative intervention should be considered. (3) Arthrotomy, properly performed, was not an essentially dangerous procedure, and might do great good. (4) Early operative intervention would give a greater proportion of useful joints in a shorter space of time than any other method.

Cases in Which Early Diagnosis of Cancer of the Body of the Uterus was Made.—Dr. Rufus B. Hall, of Cincinnati, O., read this paper. To show that an early diagnosis of primary cancer of the body of the uterus was possible, or that a diagnosis could be made while the disease was yet very limited in extent, the author reported two cases. Of the many cases of cancer of the body of the uterus coming under his observation only these two were seen early enough to make a diagnosis while the disease was limited to a very small area. Adenocarcinoma was found to be the variety of the disease in each case. It was this form of the disease that most frequently attacked the body of the uterus, and if recognized early it promised great immunity from recurrence. The disease could be diagnosed in its incipiency if surgeons systematically curretted every suspicious case and made repeated microscopic examinations of the scrapings removed from the uterus until they confirmed or disproved the presence of malignant disease.

Contribution to the Origin of Adenomyoma of the Uterus.—Dr. J. Whitridge Williams, of Baltimore, Md., after calling attention to the anatomical appearance of adenomyomata of the uterus, and the various theories which had been advanced according to the origin of the epithelial structures contained in them, described a uterus removed at autopsy from a woman who died just after delivery as the result of hemorrhage from placenta previa. At the time of its removal the uterus apparently presented the characteristic appearance of the organ immediately following delivery, except that the area of placental attachment covered two-thirds of its interior, instead of being more circumscribed and limited to the anterior or posterior wall, thus indicating in all probability that interference with its blood supply had led to a much more extensive implantation of the placenta than usual. On making a sagittal section through the uterus after hardening, numerous irregularly shaped, more or less oval areas, of a dull white appearance, and varying from a millimeter in diameter to structures five by ten mm. in their various dimensions, could be seen throughout the entire thickness of the uterine walls, which measured three cm. in their thickest parts. These areas were most abundant immediately beneath the endometrium, but could be traced outward through the entire thickness of the uterine wall to its peritoneal covering. Upon microscopic examination they were found to consist of typical decidual tissue, which was made up of the characteristic decidual cells and glandular spaces lined by cuboidal epithelium. The speaker stated that so far as he could ascertain this was the first case in which such a distribution of decidual tissue had been observed, and then proceeded to discuss the importance of such an observation in contributing toward determining the derivation of the epithelial structures contained in adenomyomata. In his specimen there could be no doubt as to the origin of the decidual areas, and everyone must agree that they were derived from the uterine mucosa. Their wide distribution throughout the uterine muscle precluded the possibility of their having resulted postpartum, and indicated most conclusively that they must have existed prior to the onset of pregnancy. Such being the case, the specimen afforded a most beautiful example of the presence of tissue derived from the endometrium being scatterd throughout the myometrium of an adult woman, and should myomata happen to develop in their vicinity, a most satisfactory basis for the development of an adenomyoma would be offered. Dr. Williams then mentioned the fact that in not a few cases the glandular elements in typical adenomyomata showed changes identical with those occurring in the menstruating endometrium, and held that the development of the decidual tissue in his case seemed to make it probable that where portions of Müllerian tissue were scattered through the myometrium, they might undergo the same changes as the normal endometrium, namely, menstruation and decidual formation. The speaker then referred briefly to the literature upon the histogenesis of adenomyomata, and pointed out that von Recklinghausen's contention that they were of Wolffian body origin, which at first had been received with great enthusiasm, had gradually lost ground, so that the vast majority of recent writers hold that such structures are developed more frequently from Müllerian than from Wolffian body elements, some even going so far as to state that only the former mode of origin was possible. The speaker, however, made it clear that he did not wish to be understood as taking so extreme a ground, but felt that while the vast majority of such growths were clearly derived from Müllerian tissue, conclusive evidence against the Wolffian body origin of certain cases had not yet been and probably never could be adduced.

Development of Fibroids of the Uterus After Ablation of the Appendages.—Dr. J. Wesley Bovée, of Washington, D. C., stated that the large number of published cases of fibroid tumors that had undergone malignant degeneration, or that had broken down, became infected or underwent other changes in structure detrimental to the lives of their unfortunate possessors had swept away the old ideas as to their benignancy. Pathologists were now searching for a distinct borderline between benign and malignant soft uterine myomata. Recurrent myomata, while not so positively dangerous as cancer, must be considered malignant. Between these and sarcomata there was not always a distinct difference. Five cases were cited. Of these, two were operated upon for non-infectious disease, two were victims of infection, and in one the condition requiring removal of the appendages was not known. Did the sudden change in the pelvic circulation incident to the ligation of the utero-ovarian blood vessels in double salpingo-oophorectomy act as a cause of the subsequent fibroid degeneration of the uterus? This question might be reasonably answered negatively, else such degeneration might logically be seen commonly instead of rarely. Yet it might be possible that hemorrhagic infarcts in the uterus might occasionally in that manner be formed that would result in hyperplasia of connective tissue and be the origin of fibromata. In considering the changes in the uterus after ablation of the appendages in the lower animals, the author quoted the experimental work of Hunter Robb and others, and stated that from these experiments and investigations, one could find but one theory upon which to base a cause for the development of fibroids after double alpingo-oophorectomy. This was the endarteritis obliterans, noted by Benckeiser. The speaker wished the relation was clearer and more cases could be cited in substantiation. In all the cases of development of fibroids of the uterus after removal of the appendages cited in the paper, the tumors were multiple, showing the existence of a number of foci, and pathologists had been interested in endarteritis obliterans in the uterus as the origin of fibroid tumors. The cases of such development of fibroids after castration were probably rare, and their existence must be due to some rare cause, such as was this form of endarteritis. In the absence of a better explanation, he was disposed to accept this one.

The Effect of Suspensio-Uteri on Pregnancy and Labor.—Dr. Joseph Taber Johnson, of Washington, D. C., in a paper with this title, contended that very few if any such injurious effects need be feared as had been frequently charged against the operation of suspensio-uteri. That it sometimes failed to cure was true, but that was not the charge. By ventrosuspension he did not mean ventrofixation. He was free to admit that the uterus should not be securely fixed into the abdominal wound or to the abdominal wall in women likely to become pregnant. It was quite certain that some of the pains of pregnancy and difficulties of labor which had been charged against suspension were really the result of fixation. In over one hundred suspensions done by himself he only knew of two pregnancies. These were both normal. In one case the labor was so rapid that the child was born before the doctor's arrival, and he knew from recent·examinations that there had been no return of the retroversion. The other case he delivered in November last after a five-hour normal labor, without chloroform or forceps. The author mentioned the number of suspension operations performed by other operators, and concluded by saying that when the retrodisplaced or prolapsed uterus was suspended, not fixed, according to the technic of the author of the operation, it appeared to him to be the best operation yet devised for the great majority of women suffering with this displacement irrespective of the fact that they might become pregnant subsequently.

Typhoid Fever and Appendicitis.—Dr. John C. Oliver, of Cincinnati, Ohio, called attention to the possibility of these diseases being so irregular in their manifestations as to be mistaken the one for the other. He cited illustrative cases in which these mistakes had been made. A case was also reported in which an attack of appendicitis was followed within a month by an attack of typhoid fever. The possibility of mistaking the perforation of a typhoid ulcer for an acute attack of appendicitis was exemplified by the report of a case of walking typhoid in which perforation of the ileum occurred. The author's conclusions were: (1) That typhoid ulcers may appear in the glandular structures of the appendix and give rise to a typhoid appendicitis. (2) That the infiltration of the ileum and cecum in typhoid fever may be so great as to give rise to a distinct tumor mass in the right iliac fossa. (3) That the Widal test is of but little, if any, value in the early diagnosis of the disease present. (4) That the leucocyte count proved in his series of cases to be of value in distinguishing between the two diseases. (5) That an exploratory laparotomy in typhoid fever is not devoid of danger. (6) That abdominal incision is imperative when it becomes necessary to establish the differential diagnosis between a typhoid perforation and fulminant appendicitis. (7) That in the absence of

perforation, cases of typhoid appendicitis should not be operated upon.

Problems Presented to the Gynecologist Twenty-Five Years Ago and To-day.—Dr. P. F. Chambers, of New York City, read a paper with this title, in which he said that the problems presented to the gynecologist of that date were entirely different from those of to-day, and as different, he had no doubt, as would be those of twenty-five years hence. To illustrate the class of diseases that patients had twenty-five years ago and were admitted to hospitals and the methods of treating them in vogue then, he gave the diagnosis of all the patients who were admitted to the Woman's Hospital of New York at that time, and the operations which were there performed for the relief of these conditions. The peritoneum was the surgeon's *bête noir*. Abdominal surgery, then in its infancy, constituted but a little part of the work of the gynecologist. This was before the days of asepsis. Antiseptic surgery was then in vogue; consequently the mortality of all abdominal work was still so great the abdomen was never opened except in desperate cases, such as for the removal of ovarian cysts, or the ovaries in cases of intensely severe dysmenorrhea, or very large fibroids as then advocated by Battery, Tait or Hegar. For other causes, for which now the abdomen was readily opened, it was then a sealed book. Except where retroversion of the uterus was due simply to an elongation of the ligaments, and when the uterus was small, was easily replaced, and the force from above was slight, the author preferred the ventrosuspension operation in all cases. Then he would perform the operation for shortening of the round ligaments either by exsecting a portion of the ligament and bringing the ends together, or by looping the tube upon itself. He never did a ventrofixation. An example of conservative surgery upon the uterus was given in the case of fibroids. The Trendelenburg posture had had more to do with the solving of gynecological intraabdominal problems than any other aid in the technic of the operating room.

(To be Continued.)

MANHATTAN DERMATOLOGICAL SOCIETY.

Regular Monthly Meeting, held November 4, 1904.

The President, I. P. Oberndorfer, M.D., in the Chair.

Bromoderma.—Dr. B. F. Ochs presented a case of this affection with large papulo-pustules, nodules and excoriations; best seen on the buttocks, lower limbs, face, scalp, and some papules on lower eyelids; the lesions followed the administration of two-grain doses of natr. brom., given to a baby, three months old, for an acute attack of bronchitis. Dr. Bowman commented upon the extreme degree of inflammatory irritation and believed this to be due to treatment. Dr. Weiss said the eruption resembled that following iodine; he likewise commented upon the grave inflammatory lesions following such small doses of bromides. Dr. Gottheil saw three other cases, and from the character of the eruption alone would make the diagnosis without the history; severe eruption will often follow the use of small doses of bromides. Dr. C. W. Allen agreed in the diagnosis made; the condition is often rebellious to treatment, but will get well; the general features of such eruptions were alike and typical; he saw bromine eruption in adult epileptics, taking the drug. Dr. Pisko also noted severe lesions after small doses of bromides; the physician usually sees the cases after the parents maltreat the child at home; hence the unusual type of inflammatory irritation as seen in this case. Dr. Blei-

man called attention to the susceptibility of young infants to certain drugs, especially quinine and belladonna.

Herpetic Chancre.—Dr. Ochs presented a young
man having a lesion on penis; when first observed the
lesion was of a herpetic character; at present a granulating slightly indurated ulcer is seen; slight inguinal
adenitis and a mild secondary (?) eruption was observed by Dr. Ochs up to two days ago; presented as
herpetic chancre. A second smaller lesion is also observed close by. Dr. Gottheil, who also observed the
case, stated that varied and indifferent treatment for the
past five weeks did not change the herpetic character
of the lesion; the presence of parchment induration, local
adenitis and mild roseola favored diagnosis of hard
chancre. Drs. Bowman, Pisko and Oberndorfer regard
them as multiple chancroids; the induration present is
that of inflammation and not the characteristic hardness
of a true chancre; besides the existence of a roseola
is in doubt.

Guttate Psoriasis.—Dr. Ochs then showed a case
of marked seborrhea involving hairy parts of face, including eyebrows and eyelashes; case under observation
over one year; recently his lower limbs presented distinct lesions of guttate psoriasis, a condition never observed before. Dr. Ochs asked if there was any connection between the two present lesions. Drs. Weiss and
Pisko recognize two distinct lesions; the members concurred in this opinion.

Urticaria Pigmentosa.—Dr. W. S. Gottheil presented
two cases. *Case I.*—Male infant, ten months old; during the past summer the body and especially the buttocks were covered with small inflammatory papules;
these disappearing leave a corresponding area of light
pigmented skin; new lesions now on chest look like
urticaria papules; the mother states at no time was there
itching. (?) Dr. Gottheil presents the case as one of
urticaria pigmentosa. Drs. Sobel, Bleimau and Pisko
agree in the diagnosis of urticaria pigmentosa. Dr.
Weiss said the lesions resembled urticaria; the skin
showed dermographia; these and other angioneurotic
conditions, such as acute outbreaks and the pigmentation
following seem to bear out the correctness of the diagnosis made; a condition closely allied was erythema
papulosum, but pigmentation following was rare. Dr.
Allen accepts the diagnosis of urticaria pigmentosa.

Dermatitis Herpetiformis.—*Case II.*—A young girl,
aged fourteen years, with grouped vesicular and bullous inflammatory lesions on the face, surrounded by
healthy skin; three years ago patient had a similar outbreak, but on the body, the character of the lesions always being the same; at present, the face, arms and
legs show these vesicular lesions; recurrent attacks
date back ten years; presented as a case of dermatitis
herpetiformis. Diagnosis concurred in.

Epidermolysis Bullosa Hereditaria.—Dr. E. L.
Cocks presented this interesting case. The patient, a
boy of nine years, has been under observation for the
past twenty months and was well up to two years ago.
There is no history of bullous eruptions in parents or
other members of the family; the eruption at present is
confined to limited parts of the face, ears and upper
and lower limbs (scattered patches); innumerable
milia are seen on face and neck; trauma to the epidermis
is followed by development of bullæ; photographs taken
recently and presented show such formations on palms,
lower arms and lower legs; serosanguinolent lesions
were observed on tongue and roof of mouth, some time
ago. Dr. Allen stated the absence of definite lesions
in the parents robs the case of one of its characteristics;
the present lesions and other traumatic bullæ undoubtedly favored diagnosis of epidermolysis bullosa.

Drs. Weiss and Gottheil stated that the history was
negative; the traumatic lesions were typical; they
concurred in the diagnosis made.

Pityriasis Rubra.—Dr. E. L. Cocks showed a man
whose entire skin was thickened and covered with slight
desquamation; four weeks ago the process began on the
back as two large erythematous patches, these extending, involving the entire interment; skin now pale and
dry and under local treatment is getting better; patient
gives history of excessive and profuse sweating upon
little exertion. Presented with tentative diagnosis of
pityriasis rubra. Dr. Bleimau said the marked induration of the skin spoke for a lesion of more than four
weeks' duration. Pityriasis rubra was characterized by
hyperemia of the skin and was progressive; he could
not agree with Dr. Cocks, but classes it as a chronic
dermatitis. Dr. L. Weiss stated the primary lesion was
obscure; the marked thickening and paleness of skin
did not favor diagnosis of pityriasis rubra; the patient's
skin was characterized by a marked keratosis, and
lichenization; for want of a better term he designates
the condition as lichen keratosis. Dr. E. Pisko quotes
Crocker on Sweat Eczema; he thought this resembled
the condition as described. Dr. Gottheil called it
chronic universal eczema; the hands show fissures and
marked lichenization. Dr. Allen was also impressed
with the marked degree of lichenization; he would not
call it pityriasis rubra and preferred to leave diagnosis
open until case could be again observed. Dr. Cocks
stated various diagnoses were made by as many derma-
tologists—chronic eczema, chronic psoriasis, pityriasis
rubra and dermatitis exfoliativa.

Favus of the Scalp.—Dr. C. A. Kinch presented
three cases of this disease: *Case I,* showing result
of treatment; a few red spots were still visible and the
growth of hair is returning. *Case II,* a more pronounced case: typical yellow favus cups still visible
and old healed lesions shows scarring. *Case III,* under
observation two years and now almost cured. The
treatment in general consisted of epilation and local
application of ointments of iodine, 10 per cent. in goose
grease or binoxide of mercury. 1 to 2 grams in 30
grams sulphur ointment; also bichloride washes of
$^1/_{1000}$ to $^1/_{200}$ strengths. Case II was conceded to be
favus, but in Cases I and III some doubts was entertained; epilation and local antiparasitic remedies were
advocated; Dr. Allen, in addition, saw good results
follow use of X-ray. Dr. L. Weiss agitated the position
taken by local health boards in excluding contagious
scalp diseases from attending public schools. Dr. Gottheil stated that a movement recently to procure suitable
isolation quarters and instruction for such cases was
not seriously considered by the present health authorities.

Simultaneous Chancres of Lips.—Dr. I. P. Oberndorfer presented a young man with lesions on upper and
lower lips, of four weeks' duration; sub- and post-
maxillary glands enlarged; the body shows a roseola; a
beginning pharyngitis and sore throat is likewise observed; presented as simultaneous chancres of upper
and lower lips.

BOOKS RECEIVED.

Vital Statistics. Department of Health, City of
Chicago. 8vo, 122 pages. Chicago.

A Text-Book of Histology. By Dr. F. R. Bailey.
8vo, 482 pages. Illustrated. Wm. Wood & Co., New
York.

The Doctor's Red Lamp. The Doctor's Recreation
Series. Volume II. 8vo, 340 pages. Illustrated. The
Saalfield Publishing Co., Akron, Chicago and New York.

THE MEDICAL NEWS.

A WEEKLY JOURNAL OF MEDICAL SCIENCE.

VOL. 86. NEW YORK, SATURDAY, JANUARY 14, 1905. NO. 2.

ORIGINAL ARTICLES.

CARE OF PUERPERAE.

BY JAMES D. VOORHEES, M.D.

OF NEW YORK.

THE discussion of the above subject will be very informal and incomplete. To insure a normal convalescence after childbirth is indeed a matter of great importance, not only from the patient's standpoint, but also on the part of the physician, for the physician cannot be too careful as to details, nor too conservative in his management of puerperal women. I make this statement at the outset simply because if any complication develops, no matter how insignificant, the patient is very prone to attribute it to some omission in the treatment and so blame the doctor. It is much better, therefore, for him to lay down the necessary rules, because in this way if his instructions are not carried out his responsibility will cease.

Everyone will grant that a properly managed labor is absolutely essential to a smooth convalescense, unless Dame Fortune smiles favorably on the accoucher when mistakes have been made. By this I mean that the case is more apt to be a normal one when the asepsis and antisepsis have been perfect, when the labor has not been allowed to drag out too long, where little damage has resulted from the birth, where injuries, if any, have been carefully repaired, where the uterus has been properly massaged with little hemorrhage, and finally when the physician has completed the delivery, positive that nothing has been left behind in the uterus.

Assuming, therefore, that our prophylaxis has been carried out according to rule and to the best of our ability, what should we do for the care and comfort of the patient during the puerperium? Certainly every physician has his own ideas which appeal to him as certain. I am only going to take up certain parts of the subject such as in my experience seem to need discussion.

In the first place and of greatest importance is a continued asepsis after delivery. This falls to the lot of the nurse. When one is selected, we must be just as sure of her asepsis as of our own. She should always regard the vulva and also the nipples in the light of clean laparotomy wounds, for then we know that all precautions will be taken against infection at these points. Her hands must be sterilized before doing the dressings, or she should wear sterile rubber gloves. The bed linen should always be clean, the douche pan scalded, and in doing the dressings the vulva should be washed by irrigation from above downward, the parts cleansed from within outward and the anus swabbed last. For the first two or three days I advocate a piece of gauze, wet with a 1-10,000 bichloride solution, placed over the vulva beneath the sterile vulva pad, which is kept tight in place by a T-bandage. These dressings should be changed and the parts cleansed with every movement of the bowels and with each urination, at any rate regularly every four hours for the first two or three days. Early vaginal examination and douching are to be condemned. These procedures should only be practised at an urgent indication. Nature is very reliable and undoubtedly more harm is often done by meddlesome douching than when we leave things alone. Later in the puerperium, after ten to twelve days, hot douches undoubtedly help the involution of the uterus.

Directly after delivery the patient demands a refreshing sleep, and all relatives and friends should be excluded. If sleep does not come on naturally, chloral by rectum seems to act most effectively. If the after-pains are severe and interfere with her rest, codeine is generally necessary. But after-pains can usually be limited by a proper massage of the uterus, by expression of clots by the physician before he departs after labor, and the administration of ergot directly after the expression of the placenta. In some cases where the uterus continues to relax immediately after delivery, I often give an intra-uterine douche of acetic acid with good results. This is justifiable for those patients who suffer almost as much or even more from after-pains than from the pains of labor.

I often doubt the efficacy of the abdominal binder. For the first two or three days it does keep down the gas and supports the abdominal walls. In short-waisted women who have carried the child high and well out in front, it certainly does prevent an anterior relaxation of the abdominal walls. But for women who carry the child low and well backward, they are more or less unnecessary. Consequently if such cases are bothered by the binder after the third to fifth day, I allow it to be discarded. Many women, however, are so anxious about their figures that they much prefer to be bound up and uncomfortable if by any chance the binder will preserve their graceful curves.

I believe that a fluid diet should be given for forty-eight hours after labor or until the bowels move. Then a soft diet is allowed for a day or so longer, for the digestion is always below par. A cathartic should always be given on the morning of the third day, followed by an enema, if necessary. The bowels should move daily by injections, if small doses of cascara at night are not effectual. I cannot agree with those obstetricians who allow their patients to sit on the commode within the first few days after labor, if there is difficulty in urination or defecation. I know of patients who have fainted in the act and others who have pleaded with the nurse not to carry out the doctor's orders on account of their weakness. Besides, there is always the risk of a cerebral embolus. One case of this complication from the procedure in 100,000 cases would be enough to contra-indicate it altogether. Catheterization, of course, is often harmful but carried out when necessary under strict antiseptic precautions ought not to result in a cystitis. A great deal of trouble could be avoided by training the woman to use the bed-pan during pregnancy.

One of the greatest sources of discomfort to the puerperal woman is in nursing. This is very annoying, not only to the patient but also to the doctor. It is difficult enough nowadays to persuade women to nurse. They are unwilling to be tied down and cannot give up the many engagements which come to a city woman. There are enough patients who naturally cannot nurse either from insufficient or poor milk, from some taint, and from inverted nipples, but to have to give it up on account of sensitive and cracked nipples seems almost to be the last excuse. How can this be avoided? During pregnancy the nipples should be cleaned and softened by cocoa butter or albolene. If the nipple is small, it should be massaged. The hardening treatment I am not altogether in favor of, because I think it makes the nipple more easily injured during nursing. Then after delivery until the milk comes in I would put the child to the breast three times the first day and five times the second day, allowing it to nurse only a few minutes. The child can be readily fed and in this way the injuries avoided which are caused by vigorous sucking. If the nipples are sensitive, I would at once use a shield before any abrasions result. The general management of the nipple should be as follows: Cleansing before and after nursing with boric acid solution and then anointed with albolene. Of course the infant's mouth should also be cleansed with a boric acid solution before and after nursing. Then, most important of all, the nipples should be covered by sterile lint dressings, which are kept in place by the breast binder. In this way and also by cautioning the woman against touching the nipples, germs can be excluded and the greatest predisposing cause to mastitis avoided

Associated with painful nipples is the distention of the breasts. Fortunately this lasts only for a few days. At the onset relief can be obtained by a strong nursing baby and by massage. At the same time it is well to put the patient on a dry diet, only allowing enough fluids to quench the thirst. In order to carry off the fluids by other channels saline cathartics are invaluable. When massage is ineffectual, breast pumps can be used, but both these manipulations are often more painful than the distention. They should be used, however, if there is caking. Locally, I think, an ice bag gives more relief than hot com-

presses. Occasionally a sedative such as codeine is necessary to produce sleep and allay the nervousness caused by the distention.

Our principal duty to the puerperal woman is to insure as complete an involution as possible. With this ultimate object in view we must commence early to accomplish it. On the second day the patient should be turned first on one side and then on the other; on the fifth day she should commence to lie on her abdomen for shorter or longer periods and be encouraged to sleep in this position if possible. This change in posture favors the escape of the lochia and allows the uterine ligaments to contract, so favoring the normal anteflexion. One of the greatest difficulties is to keep the patient in bed long enough. One should insist on at least two weeks and longer if any signs of subinvolution persist. Then she should begin to sit up, being lifted to a chair, gradually increasing the length of the period, but she should not walk till the beginning of the third week. Even at this time she should spend most of the day in the recumbent position. If there is any rebellion on the part of the patient, generally all you have to do is to tell her that her future health depends on a slow convalescence and she will willingly carry out your directions. If involution is delayed, hot vaginal douches, boroglyceride tampons, ergot, quinine and strychnine are of great service.

Finally a routine vaginal examination should be made before any case is discharged. For at this time slight erosions and inflammations of the cervix, displacements of the uterus, involvement of the adnexa, and relaxations of the pelvic floor can more easily be corrected. Failure to advise the patient or family of any abnormal condition will often bring upon the physician irrevocable censure.

150 West Fifty-ninth Street.

TRAUMA AND CHRONIC COMPRESSION OF THE EPIGASTRIUM AS ETIOLOGICAL FACTORS OF GASTRIC ULCERS.[1]

BY WILLIAM ACKERMANN, M.D.,
OF MILWAUKEE, WIS.

A GREAT deal has been written regarding the etiology of gastric ulcers, but relatively little has been said regarding the mechanical element which figures in its causation. Even at this date the opinions of various authorities as to the influence of this factor are somewhat at variance.

I therefore feel justified in bringing forward this subject. Having, through the courtesy of Dr. Paul Cohnheim, the material of his polyclinic placed at my disposal, I have collected all cases of gastric ulcers treated in the clinic for the past five years and endeavored to ascertain what influence traumatism and epigastric compression—particularly long-continued compression—exerts in the causation of this disease.

Judging from the mode of origin of decubital ulcers at the heels, nates or any other part of the

1 From the Polyclinic of Dr. Paul Cohnheim, Berlin.

body subjected to long-continued pressure, it is but reasonable to presume that gastric ulcers of like nature may be caused by chronic compression of any portion of the gastric walls. This presumption coincides with the fact that the prevailing opinion of to-day is that most gastric ulcers result from a local circulatory disturbance.

Owing to the frequency of chlorosis in the earlier years of life, females, up to the age of thirty are more often subjected to gastric ulcers, but after the thirtieth year, males are more prone to this disease. Taking into consideration the fact that men, owing to their occupation, are more liable to epigastric compression than those of the opposite sex, it is plain why ulcers occur more frequently in men than in women during the latter years of life.

The fact that the pyloric ulcers of males frequently lead to cicatricial stenosis with a subsequent gastrectasia, while the chlorotic ulcers rarely run such an unfavorable course, shows that the latter have a greater tendency to heal without subsequent complications. In all probability many cases of gastric dilatation thought to be due to perigastritis really owe their existence to cicatrices following traumatic ulcers.

Our clinical experience of gastric ulcers caused by trauma or by long-continued pressure of the gastric region without injury to the external abdominal walls is still very limited.

Many cases of complete ruptures of the gastric walls causing death in from one hour to several days have been reported, also cases in which the life of the patient was saved by immediate operation. But, excluding these cases of complete ruptures, there are a large number of traumatic incomplete ruptures, the exact location and extent of which can only be presumed by the clinician from the symptoms presented. These injuries, unless severe, have a tendency to heal, thereby excluding the verification of diagnosis by the surgeon or pathologist. This is the reason why so little is known regarding the local condition existing in ulcer produced by trauma or, in fact, caused by any other etiological factor.

Clinically, we know that constitutional diseases play a prominent etiological rôle and every physician is aware of the close relationship existing between chlorosis and gastric ulcer, but why the chlorotic subjects should be so predisposed has never been satisfactorily explained. According to Virchow's hypothesis these ulcers are caused by an interference of circulation due to thrombosis and a subsequent autodigestion. Even at the present time this view is generally accepted.

In their experiments on animals, Quincke and Dättwyler[1] found that artificially produced ulcers were much slower to heal in animals previously rendered anemic than in healthy ones. They concluded that in the presence of anemia, slight injuries of the gastric mucosa may develop into ulcers, and ulcers already existing require a longer period of time to heal.

[1] See bibliography on page 56.

Hyperacidity usually being present with ulcers, many authors attributed the ulcers to the excessive amount of hydrochloric acid while others were inclined to believe—especially in the presence of chlorosis—that the decreased alkalinity of the anemic blood was responsible. But deductions from a long series of experiments on animals, as well as clinical observation, confirm the fact that either one of these factors alone cannot be held responsible and that some concomitant anomaly must be present to favor the formation of an ulcer. There must be present some predisposing condition leading to an impairment of the vitality of the cellular structures.

That hyperacidity is not a necessary accompaniment of ulcer is proven by the fact that ulcers are sometimes associated with subacidity. Ewald, for instance, found hyperacidity present in about 34 per cent. normal, in 57 per cent. subnormal acidity in nine per cent. of all ulcer cases. Einhorn mentions two cases of ulcer with achylia gastrica. Probably this condition would be found more frequently were it not for the contraindication of the stomach-tube in any case where the existence of a fresh ulcer is anticipated.

Thermal causes, such as indigestion of hot food or drinks were at one time supposed to be quite a factor and held to be responsible for the frequency of ulcers in cooks, but there is no satisfactory statistical evidence that ulcers are more frequent in cooks than in persons following any other vocation. In fact, injuries to the mucous membrane by direct mechanical, chemical or thermal causes are of frequent occurrence but under normal circumstances heal very rapidly.

After these few remarks, we come to the subject under consideration, namely:

Trauma and Chronic Compression of the Epigastrium as Etiological Factors of Gastric Ulcers.
—Cases of traumatic ulcers following contusions of the abdomen have been reported by Leube, Wagner, Limont and Page, Duplay and a number of other authors, showing that they are not of infrequent occurrence.

After the clinical demonstration of traumatic ulcers by various authors, Ritter and Vanni investigated the existence of same experimentally on animals. For this purpose Ritter used dogs and found that severe blows in the region of the stomach often caused the formation of a submucous hematoma which later was dissolved by the gastric juice, leaving in its place an open ulcer. These results were substantiated by Vanni, who experimented on rabbits. Later Gross conducted a series of experiments, the results of which were similar to those of the above-named authors. He arrived at the conclusion that in an otherwise normal stomach, injuries to the mucosa, unless severe, would not lead to the formation of ulcers.

Traumatic injuries of the stomach, such as violent blows, may cause either a complete or an incomplete rupture of the gastric walls. Owing to the better protected position of the stomach, cases of complete rupture of this organ are not as numerous as those of the intestines, but a curious fact in this connection is that the region of the stomach usually ruptured—the lesser curvature—is the part mostly protected. Complete ruptures are usually caused by an overdistention of the gastric walls by fluids or gases at the time of injury, thereby causing the part offering least resistance to give way (rupture by contrecoup).

Injuries causing incomplete ruptures with subsequent formation of ulcers can be divided into two classes. Firstly, injuries causing an extensive lesion limited to the mucous membrane; secondly, those injuries causing an extravasation of blood or a hematoma between the mucosa and muscularis, the pressure of which, together with the injuries to the vessels, cause a necrosis of the surrounding tissues.

Clayton reports a case of a boy who, two hours after being caught between the buffers of two railway trucks, was taken with severe pains, vomiting of blood and distention of the abdomen. Death ensued within twenty hours. Post-mortem examination showed no evidence of injury to the gastric serosa. On opening the stomach it was found to be ruptured in two places, midway between the cardia and pylorus, the injuries being limited to the mucosa which was stripped off from the underlying coat. The abdominal distention was caused by a hemorrhage from the lacerated spleen.

It is but natural that the gastric juice should act detrimentally upon injured surfaces, as in the case just quoted. It certainly is remarkable, especially when the pathological changes are taken into consideration, that injuries calling forth the most alarming symptoms, such as extreme collapse, intense localized pain, and vomiting or hematemesis, should be entirely healed in from two to three weeks. Yet many cases are reported in which all these symptoms were present, lending a most serious aspect to the case and, after two or three weeks' treatment, the patients were free from all pain, dismissed as cured and in all probability never heard of again. Naturally it would be of interest to know whether or not symptoms of ulcer developed in later years.

The following case of ulcus carcinomatosum is of special interest, as the first symptoms of the ulcer appeared one and a half years after the injury:

Case I.—R., coachman, aged forty-six years; six years ago, while currying a horse, was kicked in the epigastrium. Except for slight pains in the epigastric region, which lasted only a few days, patient suffered no inconvenience. Four years later, horse fell heavily on patient's abdomen, giving rise to slight epigastric pain. After several days' duration, pain disappeared entirely, appetite was good and he continued his work without any inconvenience until six months ago. At that time he first noticed pressure in the epigastrium after eating. This pressure later developed into severe lancinating pains, especially

after partaking of course food; soups and liquids causing no disturbance. Frequently these paroxysms of pain were relieved by vomiting. Several weeks later vomiting also occurred during the night, or early in the morning before breakfast, and then vomitus contained particles of food taken the day before. Patient lost about forty pounds in weight during the last three months. No hematemesis but melena occurred twice two months ago.

Status Præsens.—Cachexia with great emaciation. Heart normal. Fine crepitant râles in apices of lungs. Abdomen sunken and palpation reveals a slightly movable tumor, about the size of a walnut, in the epigastrium. Considerable quantity of dark chocolate-colored fluid was withdrawn from stomach in fasting condition. Examination of fluid revealed large amount of food remnants, yeast cells and sarcine; free HCl + T.A = 78; blood-test negative. Patient passed about 500 c.c. urine daily, containing trace of albumin. Bile-stained sarcine, many fat crystals and encysted amebæ were found in feces.

Case being diagnosed as gastric dilatation due to ulcus carcinomatosum of pylorus, operation was advised. Three weeks later patient was operated, but death ensued within six days after operation and diagnosis was verified by autopsy.

This evidently was an ulcer due to traumata, the first symptoms of which appeared eighteen months after the last injury, the transformation of the simple ulcer into a carcinomatous one arising as a later complication.

Two somewhat similar cases of gastrectasis were reported by Krönlein. These were due to benign pyloric stenosis following traumata, one case being operated five months and the second eight months after the injury. Both patients complained of symptoms pathognomonic of gastric ulcer immediately after accident.

Ebstein mentions two cases of ulcer caused by the lifting of heavy weights. The overexertion probably caused a rupture of a gastric vessel leading to hemorrhagic infiltration of the mucosa and subsequent formation of ulcer.

Pauly reports a case of ulcer in a man who, to prevent a fall, threw his body violently backward. Slight gastric disturbance appeared immediately after accident, and six weeks later perforation of the newly formed ulcer occurred.

In an article on gastrectasia following traumata, Cohnheim cited seventy-four cases, six of which presented typical symptoms of ulcer soon after the injury, which finally led to pyloric stenosis.

From the foregoing we see that as long as the stomach is normally nourished and a sufficient quantity of blood circulates through its entire walls, the vital resisting power of the tissues prohibits autodigestion. But just as soon as there i an interruption of the circulation in any circum scribed area, gastromalacia is apt to follow. It i a well-known fact that normally, gastric juice wil not destroy the delicate layers of epithelium dur ing life, but if, at the time of death, a considerable quantity of secretion is present it will destroy the walls of the stomach. The large number of cases of incomplete ruptures of the gastric walls, which in from two to three weeks are entirely healed, demonstrate the fact that unless the mucosa is extensively damaged the disease need not necessarily take on a progressive nature, but if a considerable area of mucosa is denuded from the submucosa, or its circulation cut off by the presence of a large blood-extravasation, autodigestion will take place and, as a result, a traumatic ulcer is formed.

In the polyclinic of Dr. P. Cohnheim, from which the following cases, as well as the case first cited, are taken, a great number of gastric ulcers are treated annually. A surprisingly large number of these patients give a clear history of chronic epigastric compression, and it is subsequently found that the cause of the ulcer can be traced directly to the patient's occupation.

The frequency in which these cases came under our observation, justly led to the belief that long-continued epigastric compression is to be looked upon as one of the most important etiological factors.

Owing to the importance of this subject, I will take the liberty of reporting the following cases which I am led to regard as instances of gastric ulcers due to this cause.

Before presenting the cases, however, I wish to state how, in this clinic, the diagnosis of ulcer is made long before the appearance of hematemesis or melena.

The paroxysm of localized pain appearing some time (from one-half to three hours) after meals. the intensity of which depends entirely upon the quality of food ingested, is considered the most prominent symptom of ulcer. Liquids or soups cause little or no distress, while solid foods bring on the most excruciating pains, often lasting until the patient vomits or takes either warm drinks or sodium bicarb.

These pains invariably begin in the epigastrium, are of a crampy, burning or lancinating character and have a tendency to radiate toward one or both sides into the back or upward toward the sternum. Of the remaining symptoms hematemesis. melena, hyperchlorhydria and the epigastric and dorsal painful pressure-points are of importance. The epigastric pressure-point is usually situated in the median line or a little to the left of it, immediately below the ensiform process, while the dorsal, as a rule, can be found to the left of the vertebral column, between the tenth and twelfth thoracic vertebræ. When present with other symptoms, hematemesis is of particular diagnostic value but, according to Hemmeter, occurring in only about one half of the cases, its absence is of no significance. Ehrlich lays special stress upon the so-called "painful emptyness" of stomach (Boas' schmerzhafte Magenleere) which usually disappears after ingestion of foods, especially liquids, and he believes it to be one of the important symptoms.

According to Cohnheim's teaching, the severe cramp-like pains occurring regularly from one-half to three hours after meals, especially after ingestion of solid foods, is the most characteristic symptom of any lesion in the region of the pylorus—whether it be ulcer, fissure or erosion. The pain is due to the passage of the chyme over the eroded pyloric surface, causing a mechanical as well as chemical irritation, thus producing severe spasmodic contractions of the circular muscles of the pyloric end of the stomach. In the following cases this is the symptom most frequently found.

Case II.—J. L., female, forty years of age, seamstress. Patient was obliged to sew heavy garments, the work causing her to assume a stooped position most of the time, thereby producing constant pressure of the epigastrium.

After undergoing treatment for ulcer four years ago, patient was in good health until several weeks ago. She now complains of anorexia and nausea. Liquid foods give rise to a burning sensation in the stomach. One or two hours after ingestion of solid foods, she is attacked with severe crampy pains which begin in the epigastric region and then radiate toward the right side into the back. Appetite impaired. No hematemesis or vomiting.

Status Præsens.—Patient pale, anemic and emaciated. Has lost 30 pounds in the past few months. Abdomen sunken and abdominal walls relaxed. Heart and lungs normal. Epigastric and dorsal pain-points present. Examination of stomach contents one hour after the Ewald-Boas test breakfast shows contents well chymified, free HCl +, T.A. = 54. Aloin test negative.

Case III.—P. S., male, twenty-seven years of age, stonemason. Ulcer was produced in this case by continual pressure in the epigastric region caused by the position assumed while working.

When stomach is empty patient complains of burning pains in epigastric region which are immediately relieved by warm drinks. From one-half to one hour after meals, especially after solid foods, he has severe lancinating pains which begin in the pyloric region and radiate into the back. . Hematemesis and melena present. Appetite good and bowels regular.

Status Præsens.—Patient well-nourished, heart and lungs normal. Epigastric pain-point present. Test breakfast well chymified, free HCl +, T.A. = 68.

Case IV.—H. S., male, thirty-five years of age, driller. Patient was obliged to press his abdomen against drilling machine causing a constant pressure to epigastrium.

From one to two hours after ingestion of solid foods, such as meat, cabbage, etc., patient is attacked with severe crampy pains. Soft foods or liquids cause no inconvenience whatsoever. Appetite good but afraid to eat on account of subsequent pain. No hematemesis; no vomiting; bowels regular.

Status Præsens.—Patient well-nourished.

Heart and lungs normal. Epigastric pain-point present. Was given test breakfast but on account of pharyngitis stomach-tube could not be passed.

Case V.—E. M., twenty-nine years of age, printer. This patient while at his work feeding press had constant pressure of the epigastrium from the " feed board."

Ten months ago patient was unable to work for eight weeks, having at that time crampy epigastric pains after meals. During this time hematemesis and melena occurred. At present he complains of mild attacks of pain after soups or liquids, but solid foods cause severe lancinating pains which occur from one to two hours after meals. Appetite good, but patient is afraid to eat.

Status Præsens.—Patient fairly well-nourished. Heart and lungs normal. Epigastric and dorsal pain-points present. Test breakfast not given.

Case VI.—A. G., male, thirty-seven years of age, bookkeeper. Patient while writing sat in a stooped position causing constant compression of the epigastric region. Has suffered for the past two years with gastric pains when stomach was empty. Relief was obtained by taking warm drinks. During past two months patient has severe crampy pains occurring from one to two hours after meals, especially after solid foods. These pains begin in epigastrium, then radiate toward both sides into the back. No vomiting but regurgitation of bitter tasting fluids. Slight melena four days ago. Appetite good and bowels are regular.

Status Præsens.—Patient somewhat emaciated. Heart and lungs normal. Abdominal walls relaxed and gastric region very sensitive to pressure. Epigastric and dorsal pain-points present. Test breakfast not given.

Case VII.—L. W., male, thirty-six years of age, laborer. Patient for the last eleven years has carried heavy weights, pressing same against his epigastrium. He complains of severe cramplike pains occurring regularly from one to two hours after eating solid foods. These pains begin in epigastrium and radiate toward the back. At times patient has slight pains between meals which are relieved by eating light foods. Appetite good, bowels regular. Four years ago patient had same symptoms of several weeks' duration.

Status Præsens.—Well-nourished patient, but anemic. Heart and lungs normal. Normal habits. Epigastric pain-point present. Patient refused to take test breakfast.

Case VIII.—A. Z., male, fifty-eight years of age, shoemaker. In this case the continual pressure of the shoemaker's "last" against epigastrium caused chronic compression of same. Patient gives history of previous attacks typical of gastric ulcer. For the past three months patient complained of severe lancinating pains occurring regularly one-half hour after heavy meals. These pains usually started in epigastric region and

radiated toward both sides into the back. No appetite; bowels are regular.

Status Præsens.—Patient pale and emaciated. Heart and lungs normal. Entire epigastric region sensitive to pressure. From fasting stomach 20 c.c. of bile-stained secretion was obtained containing large amount of shrunken leucocytes and pavement epithelial cells, few starch granules, no sarcine, free HCl +, T.A. = 56. Test breakfast well chymified, free HCl +, T.A. = 84.

Case IX.—R. S., male, fifty-two years of age, shoemaker. Cause was constant pressure from 'last." Since one year patient has had severe lancinating pains in the epigastric region occurring regularly three hours after heavy meals. At times he suffered slight plains when stomach was empty, which were relieved by warm drinks. During a previous attack several years ago, patient had an attack of hematemesis.

Status Præsens.—Great emaciation. Heart normal. Râles heard over apex of right lung. Normal habitus; abdominal walls rigid; no pain-points present. Owing to old pharyngeal cicatrices, it was impossible to pass stomach-tube.

Case X.—M. N., female, thirty-six years of age; acrobat. For many years while performing patient was obliged to have heavy weights press against epigastrium.

Patient complains of severe cramp-like pains occurring regularly one-half hour after meals, especially after ingestion of solid foods. Occasionally vomiting occurs at height of paroxysm of pain. Pyrosis appears after each meal. Appetite fair, bowels sluggish.

Status Præsens.—Patient fairly well-nourished. Heart and lungs normal. Abdomen slightly distended and tender to pressure. Epigastric pain-point present. Test breakfast not given.

Case XI.—P. B., female, thirty years of age, seamstress. Patient was obliged to work in a stooped position continually, causing her to have constant compression of epigastric region. She was in good health until eight weeks ago. Since then she is attacked with paroxysms of severe lancinating pains occurring about an hour after partaking of solid foods. These pains began in the epigastric region and radiated toward the left side under the border of the ribs. One year ago patient had a similar attack associated with hematemesis.

Status Præsens.—Patient is pale and emaciated. Heart and lungs normal. Abdominal walls relaxed; greater curvature of stomach extends to umbilicus. No pain-points present. Test breakfast not given.

Case XII.—A. H., male, thirty years of age, teamster. Patient's occupation required the carrying of heavy barrels, which he supported by the aid of his epigastrium. He was in good health until two years ago. At this time he complained of epigastric pains when stomach was empty, but was immediately relieved by ingestion of fluids or soft foods. Two hours after eating solid foods he was attacked with severe lancinat-.

ing pains which began in the epigastrium and radiated toward the back. Patient vomited twice when pains were at their height. Appetite good; bowels regular. Two years ago patient had a similar attack associated with hematemesis.

Status Præsens. — Well-nourished patient. Heart and lungs normal. Epigastric pain-point present. From fasting stomach 35 c.c. of bile-stained fluid was withdrawn. Examination of same showed HCl +, T.A. = 32. Test breakfast well chymified, free HCl +, T.A. = 48.

Case XIII.—M. S., male, thirty years of age, policeman. Patient for many years wore a tight belt, the pressure of which caused him great discomfort in the epigastric region. For about one year he has suffered with severe cramp-like pains in the gastric region. These pains occurred regularly one-half hour to one hour after eating, especially after ingestion of solid foods. Vomiting occurred occasionally during the height of paroxysm of pain. Appetite variable. Bowels irregular with alternating diarrhea and constipation.

Status Præsens.—Heart and lungs normal. Normal habitus. Epigastric pain-point present. From fasting stomach very little fluid was obtained, which was slightly acid and contained only a few leucocytes. Test breakfast well chymified, free HCl +, T.A. = 40.

Case XIV.—O. S.. male, thirty-two years of age, teamster. Patient was obliged to lift heavy weights and at times he rested same on his epigastrium. Some three months ago, while lifting a heavy log, patient felt a sudden pain in the gastric region. Since this incident he has had paroxysms of severe crampy pains in the epigastric region, which occurred about half hour after meals. These pains lasted from one to two hours. One month ago he vomited about one liter of dark blood and at this time had several tarry stools. Appetite good, bowels regular.

Status Præsens.—Patient anemic. Chest organs intact. Epigastric pain-point present. Test breakfast not given.

Case XV.—B. H., male. thirty-one years of age, bookkeeper. For a number of years. while writing; patient sat in a cramped position and was conscious of a pressure in the gastric region. Since three months, he has had severe cramp-like pains occurring about one hour after meals. These pains began in the epigastrium and radiated toward both sides into the back. Appetite variable, bowels quite regular.

Status Præsens. — Patient well-nourished. Heart and lungs normal. Epigastric pain-point present. Test breakfast well chymified, HCl, T.A. = 78.

Case XVI.—A. K., male, fifty-two years of age, basketmaker. Patient for many years was obliged to work in a stooped position and most of the time pressed willows against his epigastrium. For about one year he has suffered from digestive troubles. Two or three hours after meals he was

attacked with severe crampy pains beginning in epigastrium and radiating toward the back. Pains usually ceased after taking warm drinks or sodium bicarb. Appetite good, bowels sluggish. Two years ago patient had a similar attack associated with melena.

Status Præsens.—Patient fairly well-nourished. Heart and lungs normal. Greater curvature of stomach extends slightly below umbilicus. Nothing obtained from fasting stomach. Test breakfast well chymified, HCl +, T.A. = 90. Patient's father, who was employed at same kind of work, complained of symptoms similar to these.

The paroxysms of localized epigastric pain coming on regularly (one-half to three hours) after meals, and the intensity of which as a rule depended upon the quality of food taken, occur in no disease excepting that of gastric ulcer. As further evidences of ulcer in each of the above mentioned cases we either had the presence of hematemesis, melena, vomiting or hyperchlorhydria together with the characteristic findings elicited by the physical examination.

All the cases cited had constant pressure of the epigastrium due to the nature of their occupation.

I could cite a large number of other cases in substance identical with the foregoing, but I believe those briefly sketched will serve my present purpose, viz., to maintain the importance of epigastric compression in gastric ulcers.

That I am not alone in my deductions requires but a perusal of the literature of Rasmussen, Ritter, Petry and many other writers on this subject, who have in the course of their publications arrived at the same conclusions.

In the latest editions of Boas, Ewald, Rosenheim and Hemmeter, this subject is mentioned only in the merest cursory manner. Riegel, however, devotes more space to it.

In 125 consecutive cases of ulcer treated in the polyclinic, 28 occurred in males and 97 in females, the majority of the latter occurring between the ages of twenty and thirty-five years.

The greater number of these females were employed as seamstresses. Their occupation caused them to lead an indoor life, predisposing them to chlorosis or anemia, and this combined with the pressure of corsets in bending over their work, can be pointed out as being the cause of their disease.

The frequency of ulcers in the male in the later years of life can be attributed to the compression of the epigastrium caused by their occupation. As seen in the above cases, we have several kinds of "occupation compression." Firstly, the continual pressure, such as exists in shoemakers, basketmakers, etc., caused by the "last" and "willows" respectively. Secondly. the temporary pressure caused by heavy weights resting on the epigastrium, such as teamsters are exposed to, and lastly, the epigastric compression of tailors, bookkeepers, etc., who are obliged to work in a stooped position.

Knowing that a large percentage of persons following such occupations are afflicted with this disease, epigastric compression deserves more than a passing notice, and we must regard it as one of the most important etiological factors.

The situation of the ulcers in these cases also seems to substantiate this view, the ulcers usually being found near the pylorus, this part of the stomach being more exposed to pressure.

Not only is long-continued compression of the epigastric region of interest from an etiological standpoint, but of value in the prophylaxis and treatment of this disease.

If this paper serves the purpose of directing general attention to this etiological factor of gastric ulcer, thereby aiding in its prophylaxis, then my object will be achieved.

I desire to express my thanks to Dr. P. Cohnheim for the use of his clinical material, as well as for his valuable assistance.

BIBLIOGRAPHY.

Clayton, Brit. Med. Journal, 1894, No. 1, p. 634.
Cohnheim. Archiv f. Verdauungskrankh., 1899, Bd. 5, 405.
Duplay. Cit. Virchow-Hirsch, 1881, Bd. 2, p. 178.
Ebstein. Deutsches Archiv f. klin. Med., 1895, Bd. 54, p. 442.
Ehrlich. Münchener med. Wochenschrift, 1904, No. 20.
Ewald. XX. Congress f. innere Med., 1902, Wiesbaden.
Gross. Mitteilg. a. d. Grenzgeb., 1902, Bd. 10, p. 713
Krönlein. Mitteilg. a. d. Grenzgeb., 1899, Bd. 4, p. 493.
Leube. Centralbl. f. klin. Med., 1886, No. 5.
Limpnt and Page. Lancet, 1892, No. 2, p. 84.
Pauly. Aerztl. Sachverst. Ztg., 1898, No. 2, p. 25.
Petry. Beiträge z. klin. Chirurgie, 1896, Bd. 16, p. 545.
Quincke and Dattwyler. Deutsche med. Wochenschr., 1882, No. 6, p. 80.
Rasmussen. Centralbl. f. med. Wissenschaft, 1887, p. 162.
Ritter. Zeitschr. f. klin. Med., Bd. 12, p. 593.
Vanni. Lo Sperimentale, 1889, T. 64, p. 113.
Wagner. Centralbl. f. d. Grenzgeb., 1899, p. 507.

THE NERVOUS SYMPTOMS ACCOMPANYING PERNICIOUS ANEMIA.[1]

BY ROY M. VAN WART, B.A., M.D., C.M. (MCGILL),

OF NEW ORLEANS, LA.;

CLINICAL ASSISTANT IN NERVOUS DISEASES, NEW ORLEANS POLYCLINIC; VISITING PHYSICIAN TO CHARITY HOSPITAL; NEUROLOGIST TO TOURO INFIRMARY, NEW ORLEANS, LA.

THE first description of pernicious anemia and its recognition as a distinct disease we owe to Addison. His description mentions nervous symptoms which at the present time would be called neurasthenia. No mention, however, is made of organic changes until 1887, when Lichtheim published two cases, with autopsy. Other cases were published by his pupil, Minnich, in 1889, who showed that other toxic conditions would show the same anatomical lesions. Other cases of spinal cord lesions accompanying pernicious anemia were published in rapid succession. The same lesion was shown to accompany tuberculosis, carcinoma, leucemia, dementia paralytica, pellagra, septicemia, ulcerative endocarditis and Addison's disease. Still later, in pernicious anemia, degenerative changes were noted in the brain.

The symptom-complex presented by the degenerations in the spinal cord in all these cases, has been described as a separate disease under the name combined sclerosis. The cases present a certain similarity in the fact that degenerations

[1] Read before the Orleans Parish Medical Society, New Orleans, La., September 10, 1904.

are found in the columns of Goll and Burdach, in the direct cerebellar and crossed pyramidal tracts. Occasionally Gowers' tract and the anterior pyramidal tract are involved.

The symptoms presented are easily understood when we consider those relative to isolated disease of the posterior tracts and isolated disease of the lateral tracts and combine them. This does not include the not infrequent cases of tabes which in the later stages show evidence of pigmented tract degeneration.

In cases complicating pernicious anemia the posterior tracts are involved earliest and the disease may not extend beyond this. In other cases, however, the crossed pyramidal tracts may be involved simultaneously or later. These cases have been studied by Dana and Putnam in this country, and Russell, Batten and Collier in England. They developed in a few months and terminated fatally in from one to two and a half years. These authors divided this disease into three stages. The first stage showed paresthesiæ with slight spastic weakness and slight ataxia. The second stage showed anesthesia of the leg and trunk, with a spastic paralysis of the lower extremities. In the third stage the spastic paralysis gave place to a flaccid one, with loss of reflexes, anesthesia, loss of control of the sphincters and, in extreme cases, muscular atrophy. Herpes, girdle pain and irregular temperature were noticed. Paralysis of the ocular muscles occurred, but never rigidity of the pupil.

Oppenheim divides the cases into two classes: (1) Those in which the symptom-complex of spastic spinal paralysis is combined with ataxia, bladder atony, lightning pains or other symptoms of tabes; (2) those in which the symptom-complex of tabes is from the beginning combined with motor weakness.

The following case shows the difficulty of clinically classifying the forms met with:

Case.—The patient, a white male, forty-seven years of age, complained of "weakness" and inability to control the lower limbs. His family history was good. His father died at forty-seven years of some liver trouble. The mother died when sixty-seven years of pneumonia. He had two brothers, one died in infancy, the other is living and well. One of four sisters died at fifty-seven years of 'cancer of the stomach;" the others are living and well. There was no history of any nervous trouble, paralysis, epilepsy, insanity, tuberculosis or rheumatism in the collateral branches of the family. The patient was born in the Western States and had lived in Louisiana the greater part of his life. He had never been strong, and any extra work exhausted him. He had had the ordinary diseases of childhood. He had had malaria several times, as well as scarlet fever. He had never had typhoid fever, dysentery or diphtheria. He had had rheumatism when a child and for a few years slight "rheumatic" pains in his legs. They never were severe enough to cause him to leave work or to consult a physician. He had never, that he was aware of, been exposed to any metallic poison, lead, arsenic, zinc, etc. He had gonorrhea twenty years ago. He denied having had syphilis or its symptoms. He occasionally used alcohol, but not to excess. He never used tobacco. He used coffee freely, but no tea.

His illness commenced in June, 1902. While on his vacation he went horseback riding, the first time in many years, and slipped in dismounting. The horse moved, and in the fall the index finger of his left hand was hyperextended. There was pain and soreness, which disappeared in a few days and was forgotten.

In September of the same year, after a period of heavy work, he had a peculiar numb sensation in the tip of the finger of the left hand he had injured in the previous June. He paid no attention to this at first, as he was feeling in excellent health. This gradually spread until the whole finger had the same curious sensation. The four fingers of the same hand were next involved, and it soon extended to the whole hand. Soon after there appeared a sensation of pins and needles in the same region. He kept at work, but there was no improvement. Early in November, 1902, he had a sensation as if the blood left his hands with a rush, leaving them icy cold. During the attack his ability to write was impaired. The hands looked as if they were soaked in water. He consulted a physician and returned to work. He had a second attack, lasting half an hour, the same afternoon. A few days later he had a sensation as if an iron band were fastened around his waist. There was at the same time a feeling of oppression in the throat and abdomen. His appetite was good. He had no trouble with his bowels or bladder.

He remained in this condition until May of the following year, having occasional attacks similar to those above described.

He noticed, however, a gradually increasing weakness in his legs, disappearing when he walked. Shortly after he went to the mountains for a time. Here he noticed his ability to walk gradually diminishing. The numbness increased and now involved both hands and arms as high as the elbow. On returning, two months later, he was able to walk only a few blocks, and in a few weeks was confined to his house. In January of the present year he was able to get about on crutches. In April he was only able to walk from his bed to a couch with his crutches, assisted by two members of his family. He spent most of his time on the couch. Previous to this he noticed difficulty in picking up objects. There had been since the first of the year a gradually increasing stiffness in the legs. He had had no ptosis and no diplopia. His eyesight, he thought, had failed. He had had no muscular twitchings and no convulsions. He had had for many months cramps in the muscles of his legs. He had not lost in weight. He has had constipation for some months. For three weeks previous to the writer's

observation he had had some difficulty in emptying his bladder.

The patient was first seen by the writer early in May. He was sitting in a chair propped up by pillows, with his legs elevated. He was well nourished, in striking contrast with his great weakness. The skin was of a curious lemon-yellow tint. The tongue was thickly coated. The slightest movement called forth an effort out of all proportion to that usually necessary. He was unable to stand or walk without assistance. The right leg was occasionally involuntarily drawn up. His appetite was poor. Pulse, 89; respiration, 24; temperature, 98.4° F.

The examination of the lymphatics was negative. The thorax was somewhat barrel-shaped. The lungs showed nothing beyond a slightly prolonged expiration. The heart showed no visible or palpable apex beat. The dulness was within the normal limits. On auscultation a faint blowing systolic murmur was heard at the apex, loudest over the second left costal cartilage. The pulse (84) was regular, of fair volume and rather low tension. The artery wall was just palpable. The urine was of a deep amber color, acid in reaction, with a specific gravity of of 1.022. There was a trace of albumin, but no sugar; microscopically there were a few hyaline casts and much debris. The blood was thin, watery and light in color. The hemoglobin was 55 per cent. (Gowers). The red blood corpuscles 1,900,000 and leucocytes 8,000. There was slight poikilocytosis and many megalocytes. Twenty-three megaloblasts were counted in counting four hundred leucocytes. The presence of megaloblasts was constant from this time until death.

The Nervous System.—There was no disturbance of the sense of smell. The patient complained of some disturbance of vision. An ophthalmoscopical examination revealed the presence of several small recent retinal hemorrhages. The pupils reacted to light both directly and concentrically. The accommodation reflex was active. There was no ptosis, diplopia or nystagmus. There was slight tremor of the tongue. The examination of the other cranial nerves revealed nothing. The motor power was much diminished, but equally so on the two sides, and was in striking contrast to the appearance of the muscles, which presented no sign of atrophy. There was some spasticity in the lower limbs, most marked on the right side. There were, at irregular intervals, painful contractions of the calf and thigh muscles of the right leg. These were accompanied by pain and, when at all frequent, were followed by great exhaustion. The handwriting showed no affection beyond that due to the ataxia in the arms. Speech was slow; the words were spoken with much difficulty and only after considerable effort. There was no aphasia. The reflexes of the upper extremities were all very active (scapular, supinator-biceps and triceps). The knee-jerks were greatly exaggerated. There was a well-marked patellar clonus on the right side. Babinski's sign was present on both sides. There was no jaw clonus. The supra-orbital reflex and the reflex produced by tapping the facial nerve were active. The cremasteric and abdominal reflexes were active. There was a complaint of numbness in both hands and feet. Examination revealed diminished sensation in both legs below the knee and in both arms below the elbow. To pain, touch and temperature. There was no astereognosis. The deep sensations were not tested. Ataxia was marked in both upper and lower extremities.

The patient for two months past had had diffi-culty in urination, manifested chiefly in starting the flow. The bowels had been constipated, re-quiring the daily use of laxatives The course was progressively downward. The difficulty in taking food increased, owing to the condition of the mouth and the nausea induced. He occasionally had sensations suggestive of girdle pains, a feeling of an iron band encircling the abdomen. The cramps in the right leg increased in severity, and were now evident in the left leg. Several days later the patient had an epileptiform attack. The movements in his legs for several hours preced-ing the attack became more and more violent. The onset was marked by a feeling of an iron band encircling the abdomen. This was rapidly followed by slow, violent contractions in the muscles of the legs, trunk and arm. The con-traction would commence suddenly, slowly pro-gress to a maximum, and remain for five seconds, then suddenly relax. These attacks continued for half an hour, unless moderated by treatment, and gradually ceased, leaving the patient wet with perspiration and completely exhausted. The pain accompanying them was excru-ciating. There was no loss of conscious-ness. The patient had ten attacks in all. They were only controlled by morphine. He became slowly weaker and unable to move volun-tarily. The reflexes now slowly disappeared and the paralysis became a flaccid one. The disap-pearance was gradual, first the ankle clonus, then the knee-jerks, then those of the upper extremity. Babinski's sign was present until the end. The difficulty in urination increased to complete re-tention. The patient died probably from some terminal infection, as his temperature slowly rose during the last forty-eight hours to 110° F. No autopsy could be obtained.

This case corresponds in its main features to the cases of Dana, Putnam and others described in outline above, and corresponds to the type us-ually seen with pernicious anemia. It illustrates the necessity for prolonged observation in order correctly to classify them. Cases of spinal cord lesions accompanying pernicious anemia may or may not present symptoms. Nonne found that while 10 out of 17 cases showed lesions post-mortem, only two showed symptoms during life. The lesions in the cases showing no symptoms may be as marked as those presenting symptoms as severe as in the case reported.

Bastianelli has noted that the spinal cord symptoms may antedate the presence of anemia. In this case the numbness was the first symptom noticed, but there is no record of the blood con-dition, so it is not possible to say which was the primary symptom. Lapinski has shown that loss of blood without toxic changes will produce dis-appearance of the Nissl bodies in the cortical cells, of the cells of Purkinje and those in the anterior horn of the spinal cord. The symptoms produced are sensory changes and increase in the reflexes.

This may serve to explain those not infequent cases with symptoms and no post-mortem lesions. Changes in the peripheral nerves are not at all or only rarely observed.

As arsenic is constantly used in the treatment of pernicious anemia, the occurrence of sensory disturbances may in some cases be due to a peri-pheral neuritis and not to lesions in the spinal cord. As far as the writer is aware, no observa-tions have been made in this direction.

The etiology of these lesions, as well as the etiology of pernicious anemia, still remains in doubt. The generally accepted view is that ex-pressed by Bödeker and Juliusberger, that both the anemia and the nervous system lesions are due to the same cause, whatever that may be.

Charlton produced similar lesions in the cord by repeated injections of colon bacilli. Von Vofs failed to produce lesions by the injection of poisons, (pyrodin).

The method of production of the lesions and their position seems to depend on the circulatory distribution. The patches of degeneration result either from a fibrosis of the capillary wall or a true endarteritis. Lenoble considers that there is a primary thrombosis due to the altered blood condition, with stasis and rupture of the already weakened vessel wall. Hemorrhages are well-known to occur in the retina and were present in this case.

In this connection it is interesting to note that hemolysins have been demonstrated to occur in-termittently in the urine in pernicious anemia by Morris.

The condition of the mouth and gastro-intes-tinal tract suggest that the view of Hunter that oral sepsis is the etiologic factor, is supported by this case. These symptoms were, however, of comparatively late development.

Other symptoms, as optic atrophy, pupillary phenomena, convulsions and hemiplegia, have been noticed. Ziehen calls attention to the neur-asthenic symptoms which occur in this disease.

The mental symptoms seemed to have received little special attention. Nearly all writers have noted the apathy and indolence in these patient and their increasing inability to accomplish an mental work. Addison, in his description of thi disease, states that " the mind occasionally wan ders." Ziehen speaks of the occurrences of stu porous conditions and sometimes of hallucinatory excited states. Grantly, in speaking of these says that they are usually transitory and end in bodily improvement. Other writers speak of loss of memory and delirium.

Marcus has recently described a case lasting six months, in which the psychosis took a form resembling dementia paralytica, with delusions of grandeur. This lasted six months and ended in recovery.

Pickett, after describing the mental condition in five cases, concludes as follows: " A composite picture of the mental disturbance in those cases presents a shallow confusion, with impairment of ideas in time and place (disorientation) more marked on waking from sleep. Illusions particularly of identity are common. Hallucinations appear at times, pertaining to any of the special senses. Based upon these illusions and hallucinations, persecutory delusions arise. These are usually transient, but may persist for considerable periods.

The case reported showed occasionally some irritability, but apart from the apathy there was no more marked mental disturbance until a few hours before death. The disturbance at that time, owing to the high temperature, could not be called a pernicious anemia psychosis. Another case, complicated, however, by an organic brain lesion, observed by the writer, and to be described elsewhere, committed suicide by cutting his throat and throwing himself from a window.

Those interested in this subject are referred to *Des scléroses combinées de la moëlle* by Crouzon, Paris, 1904, where a number of cases are reported, and references to literature will be found.

PROSTATECTOMY IN EMERGENCY CASES.[1]

BY JOHN F. ERDMANN, M.D.,

OF NEW YORK;

CLINICAL PROFESSOR OF SURGERY IN THE UNIVERSITY AND BELLEVUE HOSPITAL MEDICAL COLLEGE.

IT is not the intention of this article to enter into the historical aspect of so thoroughly discussed a subject as the surgical procedures advocated in prostatectomy, but merely to call attention to the advantages of doing a prostatectomy in every instance possible when the prostate is in part the cause of obstruction in cases coming under the head of emergency drainage of the bladder. I cite records of eight cases in this paper that belong distinctly to this class in which relatively six different emergency indications are dealt with. They are as follows:

1. Impassable urethra due to stricture with rupture and gangrene of the entire scrotum and perineum.

2. Retrograde hemorrhage, bladder being full of clots and bloody urine, with malignancy of the prostate.

3. False passage; retrograde hemorrhage; suprapubic aspiration with infiltration of the abdominal wall extending to the thorax and to the gluteal regions.

1 Read before the New York State Medical Association, October, 1904, and The Medical Association of Northern Berkshire, December, 1904.

4. Acute obstruction due to exposure to cold and wet, inability to catheterize; trauma of the urethra.

5. Trauma of the urethra; catheterization for several days, retrograde hemorrhage, etc.

6. Deep stricture of the urethra; obstruction; catheterization cystitis with absorption.

In each case cited above drainage alone by perineal or suprapubic section would have been the operative procedure in former years and in the hands of the ultra conservative I am quite satisfied is still advised. I am of the opinion that drainage by prostatectomy in these cases is the only method of procedure and have come to the conclusion that the perineal route is the one to be selected in practically every instance. Urethral section, *i.e.*, internal urethrotomy with a Bottini operation is impracticable in all of these cases.

Suprapubic section can be considered only in those cases in which the prostate is not removable as a result of extensive malignancy. Personally I would limit the selection of the suprapubic route to cases of inoperable malignancy of this gland when obstruction to the urine outflow is complete or when the condition of urinary decomposition, etc., are such as to demand operative relief. The type of perineal operation performed by me in each of these cases and in all ordinary or elective prostatectomies is that after the method of the late Dr. Bryson and performed and advocated by Dr. Goodfellow, of San Francisco, *i.e.*, a perpendicular incision in the raphe and in the deep urethra upon a guide, when possible, then enucleating the gland by attacking it from the prostatic urethra. I never have seen the profound sepsis or symptoms of toxemia when the perineal type of operation was done that we see in suprapubic cases.

The patient is not compelled to assume the prone or almost prone position, but is ordered to sit up in bed as early as the second day, proper precautions being taken to prevent pinching or kinking of the tube, and is in the upright posture or out of bed, provided that the bladder conditions permit the removal of the tube, on the third or fifth day. There is no question but that this posture and method of treatment is advantageous, providing not only for proper drainage but also preventing hypostasis, a condition often seen in the feeble and aged when occupying the recumbent posture. As a secondary matter the patient is not lying constantly in wet dressings risking early decubitus, etc. A much earlier flow of urine by the anterior urethra is insured by this posture as a constant state of apposition of the buttocks is produced while the patient is sitting, thereby insuring a more rapid adhesion of the surfaces of the wound and repair of the incised floor of the urethra.

Of the eight cases reported in this paper, six have made recoveries. The two deaths should have no bearing for argument from a statistical standpoint upon the justifiability of the emergency operations as can be seen by reading the histories, but they are included in this paper to show the type of cases one has occasionally to contend with.

Case I. Impassable Urethra Due to Stricture with Rupture of the Urethra, Gangrene of the Entire Scrotum and Portion of the Perineum, etc.—Unfortunately an overzealous house surgeon assumed responsibility in this case for two days before reporting the patient, although daily visits were made by myself to the wards. David G. sixty-two years of age, admitted September 3, with a history of having had difficulty in voiding his urine for eight days previous to admission noticed considerable difficulty in passing his urine, then that the scrotum and tissues roundabout began to swell and continued doing so until the day of his admission. On this day it was observed that the scrotum and perineum were in a foul and gangrenous condition. The house surgeon made numerous free incisions inserting gauze drain. The cause not having been understood by him no attempt was made to give free exit to the urine. When seen by me on September 5, owing to the complete destruction of a portion of the bulbous and deep urethra no instruments could be passed. A filiform was finally made to pass into the bladder and a perineal operation was then done upon this as a guide. The prostate was found enormously enlarged and was readily removed, tube inserted, bladder irrigated. The patient, in addition to having the gangrenous condition mentioned, was also suffering from a delirium which we were led to believe was due to alcohol, as some of his friends stated that he had been rather a hard drinker. The condition of delirium deepened, the patient dying on September 9, four days after the operation. The sloughing area did not extend after the operation.

It will readily be understood that in this case, although from a statistical standpoint it must be included in the mortality rate of prostatectomies, the conditions were such that death would have followed without question had a simple perineal section been done as the prostatectomy did not take more than six minutes and the hemorrhage was not of any extent whatever.

Case II. Retrograde Hemorrhage, Filling the Bladder with Clot and Bloody Urine.—Patient, seventy-one years of age, in a miserable physical condition, seen by me on September 16. Had been a sufferer from frequent urination for ten years, arising at night two or three times and voiding quite frequently during the day. For several weeks before he had had a diarrhea, which was finally controlled by quinine, he having given a distinct malarial history. Ten days before being seen by me he had a slight hemorrhage from the urethra. This latter portion of his history was obtained three weeks after the operation. The day before being seen by me he had a complete obstruction for which he was readily catheterized by his physician. Again, on the fol-

lowing morning, it was necessary to catheterize him. As a result of these two catheterizations, a very large amount of bloody urine was passed and accompanied by straining and expelling of clots and blood by the urethra. When seen by the family physician on the 16th, ordinary catheters could not be introduced. When seen by me, prostatic catheters passed without any difficulty but no urinary outflow followed. The bladder was found to extend fully five inches above the pubis, rather firm and painful to sense of touch. A diagnosis of a retrograde hemorrhage with, in all probability, clot filling the bladder was made. Irrigations were made, washing away blood clot and some bloody urine. Operation was advised and was done at eight o'clock that evening.

At the time I opened the bladder, no difficulty was met with in introducing an instrument. Perineal section was done with practically no hemorrhage. A large quantity of clot was extruded; a dull uterine curette was then used to evacuate a still greater quantity of clot. The bladder was irrigated and the prostate removed. Upon examination at the patient's house, the prostate was found to be as large as an orange, hard, stony in character, with evidence of invasion of the sides of the pelvis. A tentative diagnosis of malignancy was made at that time.

At the time of the operation it was found that the prostate, although the tissues were pretty thoroughly invaded, could be removed; feeling that the patient's condition demanded free outflow of urine, we decided upon its removal.

Upon opening the capsule of the prostate a very vigorous hemorrhage took place; in fact, so profound that for a time it was felt that no further interference should be made. By packing for two or three minutes, however, and continuing the enucleation from above and then removing the packing, the hemorrhage was found to be controlled; in fact, after the first three minutes there was no further hemorrhage worthy of mention. The prostate by microscopical examination was proven to be carcinomatous. The tube in this case was removed upon the fourth day, the patient sitting up each day following through a period of one-half to two hours, October 19. This patient still has complete atony of the bladder, having 12 ounces residual urine on October 18, and a very foul bladder, said to be due to sloughing carcinomatous tissue.

Case III. False Passage, Retrograde Hemorrhage, Suprapubic Aspiration with Extravasation of Urine into the Space of Retzius, also in the Abdominal Wall up to the Costal Arch, upon the Back down to the Gluteal Region. Complicated by Delirium Tremens.—Patient, sixty-five years of age, hard drinker, occupation, outside man, suffering from delirium tremens. Was seen by the family physician two days before calling me, at which time he was unable to catheterize the patient, so aspirated him with a trocar and canula, entering about five inches above the symphysis. When I saw the patient his condition was one demanding an immediate drainage of the bladder. Owing to the suprapubic extravasation, I deemed it advisable to recommend free incisions of the abdominal wall, also of the dorsum and gluteal regions to open the space of Retzius and to drain the bladder by means of the perineum. This latter step seemed advisable owing to the conditions of delirium from which the patient was suffering. This was done three hours later; the prostate, readily palpable, was removed within six minutes; five large incisions were made upon the abdominal wall, the median one entering the space of Retzius, the others simply going down to the aponeurosis of the external oblique, while posterially several incisions were made through the cellular tissues. The hemorrhage was slight from these wounds while the elimination of urine was considerable. A tube was introduced into the bladder and gauze packed in the abdominal and dorsal incisions. The condition of delirium, which was exceptionally great before the operation, was progressive afterward, the patient dying within two days.

This was the second case of death and also from a statistical standpoint increased the mortality rate, but, from the moribund condition of the patient previous to the operation, should not be included under the head of death due to prostatectomy.

Case IV. Acute Obstruction Due to Exposure to Cold and Wet, Inability to Catheterize, Trauma to the Urethra.—Patient, sixty-seven years of age, laborer by occupation, constantly exposed to the changes of the weather, became wet and chilled and could not void his urine as a result, this being the first manifestation of any bladder trouble whatever. When seen by his family physician and another in consultation both found it absolutely impossible to catheterize; as a result of the efforts trauma was induced and bloody urine overflow followed. On examination the prostate was found somewhat enlarged, chiefly involving the left lobe, bladder extending within two inches of the umbilicus. The patient was prepared for operation by the family physician. When under the anesthetic an instrument passed into the bladder without difficulty. Some bloody urine withdrawn, perineal section made, prostate removed, tube introduced, bladder irrigated, tube removed on the second day, patient made a recovery.

Case V. Trauma by Catheter. Catheterization for Three Days. Large Prostatic Obstruction, Retrograde Hemorrhage.—Patient, seventy-four years of age. History of relatively little or no bladder trouble. Sudden onset; first attempt at catheterization readily accomplished by the family physician but followed by some blood; second attempt at catheterization obstructed evidently by spasms of the urethra, passing some amount of urine, patient suffering now from overflow. When called to see him found to have an overflow of bloody urine. Catheterization readily accomplished. Suggested opera-

tion; interference refused. Catheterization continued by the family physician for three days, obstruction at the end of the third day was well marked with inability to catheterize. Operation accepted.

Patient large, well-preserved person for his age. Prostate size of an egg, perineal section made, prostate removed within a few minutes, fair amount of hemorrhage, tube introduced, bladder irrigated, tube removed on the fourth day and patient sitting up. Discharged from the hospital on the tenth day. Perfect recovery recorded later.

It was observed while doing the prostatectomy that a false passage had been made between the rectum and the neck of the bladder of an extent sufficient to introduce a large English walnut. This in all probability accounted to a degree for the moderate amount of hemorrhage at the time of the removal of the gland.

Case VI. Deep Stricture of Urethra, Obstruction, Catheterization, Cystitis with Pronounced Absorption.—This case demanded drainage and washing due to infection. Patient's age 68 years, admitted on March 4, history of having been catheterized, etc. For two days before admission he could not urinate, was catheterized by his family physician. For thirty-six hours previous to his admission to the hospital no urine was removed or passed. Bladder was aspirated suprapubically on date of admission. On March 6, the patient presented symptoms of absorption. Rectal examination showed that the patient had quite a large prostate. Suggestions were made to him that it would be to his interest to have his prostate removed at the same time that his bladder was drained. This was accepted. A filiform guide was passed into the bladder, perineal section done through which the prostate was removed. Patient sitting up in bed the third day, although his tube owing to the condition of the bladder was retained until a week later. He was finally discharged from the hospital cured within about eight weeks.

Cases VII and VIII were obstructions with slight trauma to the urethra in which it was advisable to operate for reasons both of trauma and for drainage.

Case VII was a patient sixty-five years of age; admitted August 18. Conditions were such that a perineal drainage was demanded. Prostate found enlarged and removal advised at the same sitting; accepted. Patient made a recovery.

Case VIII was a patient sixty-eight years of age with obstruction, cystitis, impassable urethra, perineal section done without guide. Prostate removed at same sitting, patient recovered.

This emergency operative procedure is recommended because: (*a*) Only a few minutes more are required to remove the gland, the hemorrhage as a rule is not excessive, and the operative procedure itself does not increase the shock to any degree. (b) The removal of the prostate gives proper exit to the urinary outflow and admits of easy drainage. (c) Washing the bladder is much facilitated.

The perineal route is recommended in emergency operations because: (a) The opening is practically at the lowest point of the bladder and complicated devices for drainage such as are necessary in suprapubic sections are not required; (b) The old, being irritable and feeble and requiring to be moved frequently, the drainage in the suprapubic method is constantly interfered with, while in the perineal method it is readily controlled. (c) The after soiling, when the tube is removed, is slight and easily controlled in the perineal method as compared with the suprapubic. (d) Bladder irrigations are more readily done with less soiling to the bed, etc., by this method.

OBSERVATIONS ON THE BLOOD PRESSURE IN DISEASE.[1]

BY ROGER S. MORRIS, A.B., M.D.,

OF ANN ARBOR, MICH.;
INSTRUCTOR IN MEDICINE,
AND

CHARLES W. EDMUNDS, A.B., M.D.,

OF ANN ARBOR, MICH.;
INSTRUCTOR IN PHARMACOLOGY IN THE UNIVERSITY OF MICHIGAN.

THE present tendency in medicine is to substitute methods of precision for methods of approximation, using the terms in a relative sense. The greater the accuracy attained in studying the various phenomena of the human organism, the better will be our insight into not only physiological but pathological manifestations. Among the most recent of the unexplored fields to be examined is that of the blood pressure. It was as late as 1887 that what might be termed the first practical sphygmomanometer was introduced by von Basch. Other workers since then have described modifications of the von Basch idea or have themselves constructed new instruments, but it is only within the past six or eight years that the subject of blood-pressure determination has awakened general interest. Although the various pieces of apparatus made for this purpose should not supplant digital estimation of the arterial tension, they should be used for purposes of greater accuracy and control. The problems which present themselves for solution in the field of arterial pressure are many and offer abundant opportunity for investigation. The next few years will in all probability yield apparatus of greater utility than we now possess, but at present not the least vexing of the questions one is called upon to decide is the choice of a sphygmomanometer.

Instruments of various forms have been devised but it seems unnecessary to enter into a detailed description of them. It may be said, however, that in general those now most in use may be divided into two groups. One is, per-

1 From the Clinic of Internal Medicine, of Dr. Dock.

haps, best represented by the Gärtner tonometer, in the application of which a finger is rendered anemic and the artery supplying it occluded by pressure which is slowly lessened until the first flush is seen under the nail. The pressure is then read on the manometer. This gives the systolic arterial pressure. This instrument, while it possesses several advantages, such as ease of application, has also some disadvantages, among which may be mentioned the difficulty of seeing the flush in cases of marked anemia and in negroes. In cases of either very low or very high tension the instrument is not satisfactory, according to Cook and Briggs.[1] The fact that only one band or ring for compressing the finger is supplied with each instrument is also a drawback, for the diameter of the ring cannot be altered and there are cases in which it can be applied to none of the fingers. This objection could, of course, be overcome by ordering rings of different diameters. The rubber of which the rings are made is also peculiarly lacking in durability, in this climate at least. There are many observers, nevertheless, who prefer this form of instrument, for such reasons as ease of application and the avoidance of any considerable amount of soft tissue overlying the artery, to the Riva Rocci sphygmomanometer which may be taken as an example of the second class. With this instrument the brachial artery is compressed by the pressure of a rubber band or cuff around the upper arm, the cuff being hollow and connected by tubes to a mercury manometer; the pressure inside the tubes is raised by means of a hand bulb. When the pressure inside the cuff is great enough to occlude the artery, the radial pulse disappears and by gradually lowering the pressure, the pulse reappears, the point between these two being taken as the maximum or systolic pressure.

The important question with any of these instruments pertains to their accuracy, and upon this point much work has been carried out. The first factor which one might think of is the influence of the tissues overlying the artery. This is of especial importance in connection with the Riva Rocci apparatus. What effect, then, has the size of the arm upon the pressure in the manometer? Hensen[2] considered that it had none if we take the precaution of having the arm muscles relaxed. Gumprecht,[3] on the other hand, believes that the pressure exerted on the brachial artery may be 30 to 50 mm. lower than that in the cuff, basing his opinion upon experiments carried out upon the cadaver; the error, as a rule, increases, the higher the reading. H. von Recklinghausen[4] believes the amount of soft parts of the upper arm to be a negligible factor, if we modify the apparatus slightly, as will be pointed out shortly. Cook and Briggs,[1] who have done considerable clinical work with the Riva Rocci, say that they regard the size of the arm as of little importance unless in cases of extreme cachexia, when the absence of the cushion of tissue may give a reading which is too high. On the other hand, excessive muscular development or an excessive amount of subcutaneous tissue may give a high reading, as was indicated by the Research Committee for the Division of Surgery, Harvard Medical School.[5] This observation was confirmed in a striking case of our own. We tried to take the blood pressure of a woman whose arm measured 37.5 cm. in circumference. We raised the pressure until the mercury had reached the top of the glass tube (graduated to 350 mm.) and almost filled the small funnel-shaped enlargement on the top of the tube, but could get no obliteration of the radial pulse. With the Gärtner instrument we found a pressure of 135 mm. Aside from these extremes, however, it would seem that the amount of soft parts of the arm may not be as great a factor as would appear at first sight.

So closely connected with the size of the arm that a discussion of one is almost impossible without a consideration of the other is the effect of the different widths of the cuffs used to compress the artery. There is no more unanimity on this point and there can be no doubt that the narrower bands (4.5 cm.) give higher readings than the broader ones. To von Recklinghausen[4] belongs the credit, we believe, of first drawing attention to this subject. He found that a cuff 10 cm. broad sufficed for the average arm (24 cm. in circumference), while a cuff 15 cm. wide answered for practically all cases, though the most accurate results were obtained from a band covering the entire upper arm; such a band as the latter, however, would be cumbersome and inconvenient for clinical purposes. Erlanger,[6] in some work upon dogs, found that with a narrow cuff (3.5 cm.) an error of 50 mm. mercury might be made by the resistance offered by the tissues, while with a 9 cm. cuff he thinks the error would never be greater than 10 mm. Hg. Groedel and Kisch,[7] investigating the same subject on an arm measuring 30 cm. in circumference found that the Riva Rocci instrument with a 4.5 cm. band showed a pressure of 168 mm. Hg.; with a 12 cm. band 128 mm.; with one 15 cm. wide 118 mm. Hg. Stanton[8] contrasted the pressures given by 5 cm. and 10 cm. bands on a series of five cases in which the arms measured from 19 to 23 cm. in circumference and found in two cases a difference in the readings of 20 mm.; the smallest error in the five cases was 8 mm., the average being 15 mm. As a comparison he also made observations with the two bands on thighs measuring from 29 cm. to 35.5 cm. and found in some of these cases differences as high as 120 mm.; the smallest difference in this instance was 45 mm. It seems to us, however, that his work would bear out what we have said above, viz., that while the size of the arm is undoubtedly a factor to be reckoned with, it may not be of great importance in the majority of cases. How wide the cuff should be remains

a question. The Harvard Research Committee, referred to above, report that they found that the 10 cm. band gave practically the same readings as wider ones. In two of Stanton's cases the 10 cm. band gave the same readings, whether taken from the arm or the thigh, while in the other three cases the differences ranged from 10 to 25 mm. Erlanger has adopted a cuff 12 cm. wide. Although we have only recently begun to inquire into this phase of the subject, we are convinced that von Recklinghausen's recommendation has thus far received too little heed, and that a wide cuff will in the future give the most satisfactory results. In every case in which we have made determinations with both narrow and broad cuffs, the former has given the higher reading. We believe, therefore, in view of the experience of others, as well as from our own limited experiments, that a band 12 cm. wide or, preferably, one measuring 15 cm., should be used in connection with the Riva Rocci apparatus, and that such a cuff would give fairly accurate results.

It must be acknowledged, however, that thus far we have no absolute proof that any of these instruments are correct. True, many of them have been tested upon animals or fresh cadavers, but none have been controlled by actual experiments on human beings. As a matter of fact, there are very few cases in medical literature in which human blood pressure has been taken directly. In 1857 Faivre found, acording to Hensen,[2] in an amputation case, a pressure of 120 mm. Hg. in the femoral artery of a man aged thirty. In a man of sixty the pressure in the brachial artery registered the same. In another case (man aged twenty-three) a pressure of 110 mm. Hg. was found in the brachial artery. Albert[9] in 1882 found a pressure registering from 100 to 160 in the anterior tibial artery; the pressure varied 10 to 20 mm. when the body was changed from the horizontal to the vertical position. As the results of these experiments agree fairly well with those given by the various sphygmomanometers, it would appear that we are justified in believing that the instruments now in use give approximately correct readings.

Besides the size of the arm and the width of the cuff used there are other factors that must be taken into consideration in estimating the blood pressure. First, the condition of the blood vessels is of some importance, but this can be discussed to better advantage under the various diseases modifying the pressure. The posture of the patient must be considered as of some importance, as a difference of 10 to 15 mm. is found between the recumbent and the upright position, so that in making estimations a rule should be followed always to have the patient in the same position. Most of our readings with the Riva Rocci apparatus have been taken with the arm relaxed and the patient in the recumbent position. This avoids not only the effect of gravity but, as pointed out by Goldwater[10] the arterial system is subject to reflex variations which will alter the arterial tension, but, as he also points out, by following a routine method in our estimations we may overlook these changes caused by different postures.

There is some evidence to show that the pressure as given by the various instruments is higher on the right side if the person is right-handed, while if he is left-handed the pressure is higher on the left. Jellinek[11] examined 532 healthy soldiers in this respect and found such a condition present in many cases. Hecht and Langstein[12] in 63 cases found that in right-handed persons the tension was 5 to 20 mm. higher than on the opposite side, or if left-handed, it was higher on that side. Contrary to these results are those of Goldwater[10] who could find no rule of difference between the two sides. Our results, though few in number, agree with his; while in some cases we found slight differences, yet we could not see that there was any definite rule in the matter. From theoretical reasoning such a condition should not exist, as it is well known that the pressure in all the large arteries is practically the same when the influence of gravity is excluded. The subject is of practical interest as well as theoretical, because differences between the two sides may, if found, be of some aid in the diagnosis of an aortic aneurism or mediastinal tumor. Other factors which must be considered but which require no lengthy discussion are exertion and psychical influences. It is recognized by all that exercise causes some change in the blood pressure. The influence of the mind, such as mental effort or excitement, is known to raise the pressure, showing that observations should be made with as little disturbance to the patient, physical or mental, as possible.

What, then, may be considered a normal blood pressure in an individual? The answers to this question are many, making the literature of blood pressure very confusing, especially on first glance. Further study of the subject, however, seems to show that there is not as much diversity about the normal as at first appears and we might add that the small differences we do find between the machines appear to lose some of their importance when we consider the number of factors that enter into our estimations to change them. Considering then, first, Gärtner's tonometer we find the standard for the normal adult, as given by Gärtner himself, to range from 100 to 130 mm. Hg. Grebner[13] gives 110 to 130 mm. as a standard, while Weiss,[14] with the same instrument considers 90 to 130 mm. as normal for men and 80 to 100 for women. For this apparatus, then, we may take the figures of Gärtner as being approximately normal.

With the Riva Rocci sphygmomanometer Gumprecht,[3] using the narrow cuff (4 cm.) gives the normal for children as 90 to 110 mm. Hg.; for adult men 140 mm.; for women 120 mm.; and

for old and hard working men he considers readings of 160 to 200 to be within the normal. Hensen[2] gives a rather wide range to the normal limits for adults under 30, i.e., 100 to 160 mm. Hg. In our work we have adopted Gumprecht's standard, realizing at the same time that the narrow band used (4.5 cm.*) gives readings that are a little too high. Referring to the high pressures found in old and hard-working men, Gumprecht[3] says that among these laborers he has found them to be common and that if these men are confined to bed in a hospital for a time, the pressure rapidly falls. Cook and Briggs[1] say that with increasing age there is a rise in blood pressure which runs parallel with, if it does not depend upon, changes in the vessels.

A question might arise with the Riva Rocci type of instrument whether the finger is delicate enough to register the earliest return of the pulse, or whether some form of apparatus could not be devised which might give more accurate results. Grödel and Kisch[7] investigated this subject and on comparative readings they obtained closer results with the finger than with Gärtner's pulskontroller, Oehmke's turgoskop, or Jaquet's sphygmograph, so they concluded that the finger is more accurate than any of these instruments.

In the observations we have made upon patients in the wards of the University Hospital, almost all of our readings, as above stated, were made with the patients in the recumbent position, and with as little disturbance to the patient as possible. The arm was bared and we took a number of readings to avoid errors, whether caused by physical or mental effort. All of our readings were made in the morning when, as has been shown by several observers, the pressure is lowest, there being a rise of 10 or 15 mm. during the afternoon. We have in very many patients made daily readings over considerable lengths of time and in some instances have been able to follow the changes in condition by variations in the arterial tension. In studying the cases in this way we have become very much impressed by the fact that arterial tension in both health and disease is a fairly constant quantity, for we were able many times to get readings on successive days that would vary only a few mm. On the other hand, as has been pointed out by Gumprecht,[3] after we have obtained these uniform readings for a time, we may suddenly find a variation of 20-30 mm. Hg. and may not be able to account for it in any way. These variations are usually greater the higher the pressure.

The pathological condition which seems perhaps more than any other to affect arterial tension is a diseased condition of the kidneys. Very few cases of acute nephritis are reported in the literature. Weiss[14] says that in recent nephritides of short duration he found normal or sub-

*In our work we have used Cook's modification of the Riva Rocci sphygmomanometer.

normal pressures. He cites a case of acute hemorrhagic nephritis with no accentuation of the aortic second sound in which pressures of 90 and 60 mm. were recorded with the Gärtner tonometer. Carter,[15] using the Hill-Barnard apparatus found in his cases that those which showed no complication other than a mild degree of sclerosis gave an average increase of tension of 7 to 10 mm. Hg.; with an increase in the amount of albumin he observed an increase in pressure. Orr,[16] of Montreal, reported seven cases of acute nephritis, three showing high pressures. He used the Gärtner apparatus. We were able to make observations upon two interesting cases of acute parenchymatous nephritis. The first patient was a boy, aged fifteen years who, while performing the duties of orderly in the hospital, was being treated for a fibroma of the nasopharynx. He was suddenly attacked with almost complete anuria and a typical case of acute nephritis followed. The urine at all times contained a large amount of albumin, which early in the disease formed a solid coagulum on heating in a test tube. The sediment showed very large numbers of all kinds of casts. At this time his arterial tension registered 177 mm. with no accentuation of the aortic second sound and the heart apex in the normal position. Under treatment it decreased so that for a period of two weeks it varied between 168 and 170 mm. During this time the second aortic became accentuated, the apex remaining in the normal position. At the end of this time symptoms of uremia appeared and the · sphygmomanometer showed a pressure of 187. On the day following this reading the patient felt better and examination showed a pressure of 170, but for the next week it varied between 175 and 177. At this time symptoms of uremia again appeared and after three convulsions the pressure was 192. For the next two days the patient was very weak and exhausted and had a pressure of only 155 mm. Hg. During the next week the readings varied from 166 to 176 at the end of which time exitus occurred very unexpectedly from uremic convulsions. Our second case was one of acute parenchymatous nephritis occurring during the course of a very severe attack of typhoid fever. No increase in pulse tension took place; on the contrary, there was a steady decrease following the course of the fever, the pressure becoming subnormal toward the end. Four days before death a reading of 58 mm. Hg. was obtained. The clinical diagnosis in this case was confirmed by autopsy.

In chronic interstitial nephritis the universal clinical observations have been confirmed by the sphygmomanometer. All workers on the subject report finding in this disease high pressures. Weiss[14] considers high pressure the rule in chronic parenchymatous, as well as interstitial, nephritis, in cases where there is hypertrophy of the left ventricle with accentuation of the second aortic sound. Hensen[2] reports marked and fairly constant elevation of pressure in fifteen cases, all being above 175 mm. Hg. with one exception (145 mm.), and in ten cases readings of 200 and over were recorded. Gumprecht[3] gives pressure of 260 and 270 mm. Hg. in contracted kidney. Both Hensen and Gumprecht used the Riva Rocci apparatus. Czyhlarz,[17] though preceded by the writers quoted above, claimed the distinction of being the first to report high pressures in chronic nephritis. Using the Gärtner apparatus, he gives his results in 12 cases, the readings being high (210 to 225 mm. Hg.) on admission to the hospital but falling gradually under rest in bed and a strict milk diet. In 19 cases reported by Orr[16] the average pressure was 208.5 mm. Hg., the highest reading being 260. Jackson[18] made observations upon cases in which decapsulation of the kidneys was performed. In five of six cases he found a rise in blood pressure even with marked improvement. In one case the pressure was 125 mm. (Gärtner) at operation. At the end of two weeks it had risen to 210 mm. Hg. Digitalis was now administered because of failing pulse and the pressure took a most unexpected fall to 130 mm. As the condition of the patient improved, the arterial pressure again rose and was 190 mm. three months after the operation. In a patient examined by us, etherization had lighted up a chronic process in the kidneys. The patient, a woman just past the climacteric, had been given nitroglycerine every four hours for a day previous to entering the clinic, at which time (10:30 A.M.) her blood pressure was 158 mm. In the afternoon (3 P.M.) after a hot air bath, during which the patient perspired freely, her pressure fell to 150 but at 6:45 P.M. it had gone up to 178 mm. During the following days the patient improved, her pressure decreased to 150 and she was finally discharged. In the parenchymatous form of chronic nephritis Hensen[2] examined eight cases and reported the following pressures: 135, 160, 130 to 155, 130, 142, 120, 115, 155. We had a case of this kind in which the pressure varied from 166 to 182 mm. The diagnosis was, however, based purely on clinical manifestations, together with the typical findings in the urine. Hypertrophy of the heart was not present. An interesting observation made by Vickery[19] on two adolescents with constant albuminuria, but without any casts, showed that both had a low tension as opposed to the hypertension of nephritis. In cyclic albuminuria Erlanger and Hooker[20] have shown that an increase in pulse pressure is accompanied by an increase in amount of urine but with a diminution in the amount of albumin.

To summarize the effect of renal disease on pulse tension, it may be said that an acute inflammation or degeneration may or may not raise the pressure, but that a chronic interstitial nephritis practically without exception causes an increase, which, if it terminates in uremia, may give still higher readings. As the uremic symptoms disappear, the pressure becomes lower, as shown in the cases of Gross[22] and in our own cases. Chronic parenchymatous nephritis probably does not cause elevation of pressure as a rule.

In chronic valvular disease of the heart, results, which in the present state of our knowledge appear anomalous, have been obtained. Whereas in chronic interstitial nephritis, as we have just shown, one may expect to find high pressures, there is a striking lack of uniformity in chronic endocarditis, as Weiss[14] pointed out. Goldwater[19] remarks, " Frequent and forcible cardiac contraction is recognized as one of the chief elements in the production of a high-tension pulse; and hence it is very easy to say that in valvular disease tension is high in proportion to the degree of compensatory hypertrophy and that in uncompensated cases pressure is low. But there has been no satisfactory experimental demonstration of such a rule." Our own cases offer strong clinical evidence against this supposition, as we shall presently show. In ten cases of mitral regurgitation the same author found pressures below the normal, ranging from 80 to 106, exclusive of one case which had a pressure of 128 and another, mitral in-

ively. We obtained, as did Hensen, the lowest pressure, 133 mm. Hg., in a recent case in which compensation was good and hypertrophy had not taken place. The highest pressures were recorded in a case with incompensation in which the readings varied from 186 to 222. Moderate sclerosis existed. Incompensation also was present in the case in which the average pressure was 151, while in the remaining case the pressure of 164 mm. existed with fair compensation. In two cases of combined mitral and aortic insufficiency the pressure averaged 138 and 170, incompensation being present in each instance. In the latter a pressure of 182 on admission fell to 120 under the influence of rest in bed and liquid diet. The high pressures obtained in some cases of incompensation bear directly upon the statement of Goldwater, quoted here. It should be added that the arteries, with the exception just noted, were palpably thickened in none of these cases. In mitral insufficiency we are unable to agree with the findings of some observers. In one case, that of an athlete intending to enter the Navy, who was examined by one of us, characteristic signs of mitral regurgitation were found. The patient had never complained of cardiac symptoms and, in fact, sup-

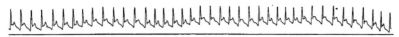

Dicrotic pulse; systolic pressure [Riva Rocci-Cook] 194 mm. Hg. in a case of mitral insufficiency with good compensation.

sufficiency and aortic insufficiency and stenosis, in which the pressure varied between 138 and 148. Hensen[2] had fifteen cases of mitral insufficiency with practically normal pressures. He obtained the same results in mitral stenosis. Orr[16] reports eight cases of mitral stenosis, six being normal; fourteen of mitral stenosis and regurgitation, eleven being normal. Carter[15] reports low (diastolic) pressures in aortic regurgitation. Norris[21] found normal pressures in mitral insufficiency to be the rule, with an occasional subnormal pressure and more rarely one above normal. In stenosis of the mitral orifice he obtained somewhat higher values than for insufficiency. In aortic regurgitation he stated that the systolic pressure is high when compensation is good. Hensen[2] says that high pressure is the rule in this lesion (15 cases), though sudden variations are both greater and more frequent than in health. According to Vickery[10] all varieties of valvular lesions may show high pressures, but the majority of those with very high tension were cases in which compensation was broken. Our results have been comparable in a way to those of the last named author. In four cases of aortic insufficiency the pressure averaged 198, 151, 133 and 164 respect-

posed his heart to be normal. His pressure, with full compensation and moderate hypertrophy, was 195 mm. Hg. This seemed incredible, for previous to the pressure determination we had noted dicrotism of the pulse, which was proven to be present by sphygmographic tracing. In another case of mitral insufficiency with broken compensation—marked dyspnea and cyanosis, with edema of the extremities—the pressure varied from 120 to 127. In a third case to which we may call attention, readings of 125 to 159 were obtained, the average being 141. The case was complicated with pulmonary tuberculosis and two points of interest may be brought out in connection with it; first, a fall in pressure from 141 to 129 following hemoptysis in which about five ounces of blood were lost; two days later the tension had reached 159; second, palpable dicrotism was determined with a pressure of 145 mm. In our remaining case, that of a boy aged four years, with compensation the pressure averaged 116. In one case of combined stenosis and insufficiency of the mitral valve, the pressure averaged 121. In a case of pure mitral stenosis a pressure of 137 mm. was found, compensation being good.

We offer no explanation at present for the

findings which we have obtained in these cardiac cases. It should be remembered, however, that our observations record simply the maximum or systolic pressure. It is particularly important not to lose sight of this fact in connection with the cases of aortic insufficiency. It seems highly probable to us that considerable advance may be made in the study of this particular group of cases, not to mention others, by determinations of diastolic as well as systolic pressures, a point upon which we are at present engaged.

Next to nephritis, there is probably no disease which excites greater interest in connection with observation of arterial tension than exophthalmic goitre. In seven cases examined by Gross[22] with the apparatus of Riva Rocci an increase of arterial pressure was found almost without exception. At times he was able to show that an increase in pressure was synchronous with increased frequency of the pulse. Orr[18] obtained normal pressures in two cases. Jackson[18] recorded pressures of 120 to 160 mm. Hg. All of his patients were females. He followed the cases for two years and no diminution in pressure accompanied improvement in the condition of the patients; in fact, in those without symptoms he found the pressure increased. In the main our results are similar to those of Gross and Jackson. Our series consists of eight cases, two males and six females. In the males the pressures averaged 164 mm. and 153 mm. Hg. respectively. In the female patients pressures were on the whole somewhat lower, half of them being normal. With two exceptions all of our patients had well developed cases with the appearance of the secondary manifestations. Of the two, one has had the disease for about two years, and the pressure at the end of a year of teaching was 161 mm. Hg. Her symptoms were mild. The second case first developed symptoms of Basedow's disease about six years ago, though at present, after a recent pregnancy which went to full term, she shows little evidence of the disease; the pressure was 133. In three of the remaining four cases the pressures averaged 179, 135 and 132 (the last with an arm band 15 cm. wide) respectively, the eighth case showing variations from 112 on admission, when the symptoms were most severe, to 138. This patient gained rapidly in weight and there was marked improvement in all symptoms. About five weeks after admission the pressure rose to its maximum, 138, a week later it was 119, at the end of seven weeks 131, and when the patient was discharged nine weeks after entering the clinic, her pressure registered 116 mm. Hg. The cause of the usual high pressure is not evident. None of the patients showed sclerosis of the arteries, except one of the men (pressure 164) in whom a slight thickening of the radial existed. In the two cases in which the highest pressures were obtained, the evidences of cardiac hypertrophy were most plain. It cannot

be stated, however, whether the hypertrophy is the cause of the high pressure or whether the converse is true. The latter seems the more likely. Again it might be supposed that the elevation in tension is in some way related to hypersecretion of the thyroid; this view appears to be untenable, for Vamossy and Vas[28] and Roos[24] found no rise in blood pressure after administration of iodothyrin. Among our cases is one of myxedema bearing upon this point. This patient's pressure, previous to the administration of thyroid extract was 166 mm. Hg. Since beginning the treatment, the patient has received 1,095 grains of thyroid extract in seven weeks and yet the pressure at the end of that time registered 150 mm. Hg. That vasomotor action may explain the alterations in tension seen in exophthalmic goiter, at least in part, seems not improbable.

In anemia, whether primary or secondary, the earlier work has shown that the pressure is lowered. The work of Orr is an exception as he reports on six cases, all with normal readings. In our series of eleven cases of pernicious anemia we had only three which showed a normal tension; all of the rest being subnormal, one very markedly so, having a pressure of only 87 with a mild sclerosis of the arteries. Another case with very marked sclerosis showed a pressure of 98. The highest reading we obtained in this class of cases was 152, the patient having very marked thickening of the arterial walls. The average tension of the whole series of cases was 120.

One of the most important fields for blood pressure estimations is without doubt in typhoid fever. Carter, Orr, Norris, Crile and Gumprecht all report that in this disease there is a tendency toward a lowered pressure. Vickery, however, cites the case of a woman in whose urine no casts were found, but who had a pressure of 152. He also mentions three other cases, one having chronic nephritis, all with a pressure of over 160. Our cases, five in number, with only one exception showed a lowered pulse tension. The readings from day to day were fairly uniform in most cases but some rather large variations, even as high as 20 mm. Hg. were found. In general, it may be said, the readings averaged lower as the disease progressed. In one very severe case (mentioned above), which later terminated fatally, the patient suffering a relapse, with intestinal hemorrhages, nephritis, a dilated heart and pneumonia as complications, we obtained during the latter days of his life the lowest readings we have found in any case, a pressure of 58 mm. being found at one time, four days before exitus. In perforation and in the stage of peritoneal irritation Crile[25] and Briggs[26] have reported a sudden rise in arterial tension. If further work confirms their observations, the changes of blood pressure will be a very great aid in making a diagnosis of this complication and it seems to offer one of the most important and promising fields for blood pressure work. As will be gathered from the statement in regard to Vickery's cases, we cannot count on a subnormal pressure in typhoid and it is necessary to make repeated observations upon each case during the course of the disease to ascertain the average height

The rôle which arteriosclerosis plays in the production of high arterial tension has probably been much exaggerated. Von Basch[27] showed, in some experimental work performed on fresh cadavers, that it required about 1 to 3 mm. Hg. to bring about collapse of the wall in medium-sized normal arteries, while in those which pre-

Disease.	Sclerosis.	Av. Pressure in mm. Hg.	Remarks.
Proctitis	none	126	
Senility (age eighty-four years)....	slight	184	Slight gastric symptoms.
Cyst of broad ligament	none	135	Before tapping.
Acute artic. rheumatism	none	111	Three weeks later, 158; heart negative.
Acute artic. rheumatism	none	133	Aortic diastolic murmur.
Gonorrheal arthritis	none	112	
Arthritis and mitral insufficiency (age four years)	none	116	Heart lesion chronic; compensated.
Arthritis deformans	moderate	162	
Tuberculosis, lungs	none	131	No fever, early stage.
Tuberculosis, lungs	slight	108	Hectic; cavity.
Tuberculosis, peritoneum	moderate	150	Before withdrawing fluid.
Tuberculosis, pleurisy	none	114	Temperature irreg.
Tuberculosis, pleurisy	none	107	Hectic.
Tuberculosis, lungs	none	124	Early stage.
Adhesive pleurisy	none	132	Irreg. low fever.
Neurasthenia	rather marked	147	
Neurasthenia	none	213	Enormous panniculus on arms.
Hysteria, enteroptosis	none	123	
Cardiac arrhythmia (neurotic)	none	134	
Locomotor ataxia	moderate	112	During gastric crisis, 118 and 110.
Cerebellar tumor	slight	134	Slow growing tumor.
Syphilis of brain	moderate	155	Hemiplegia.
Angioneurotic edema	none	133	
Hypochondriasis, chr. gastritis	?	112	
Ulcer of stomach	none	167	
Ulcer of stomach	moderate	163	
Dilatation of stomach	none	88	Benign.
Dilatation of stomach	none	130	Benign.
Chronic gastritis, (morphinism)....	slight	128	
Cancer of esophagus	none	134	
Amoebic dysentery	none	152	
Amoebic dysentery	none	113	Also anchylostomiasis.
Perivesical abscess	none	128	Fever.
Chr. jaundice	slight	167	Cause not clear.
Chr. jaundice	rather marked	163	Malignant.
Diabetes, mellitus	slight	198	Large arm.
Diabetes, insipidus	moderate	113	Syphilis.
Aneurism, thoracic	moderate	r. arm 140 l. arm 138	Never a marked difference on the two sides.
Aneurism, thoracic	moderate	r. arm 175 l. arm 204	Confined to bed.
Bradycardia	very marked	172	Pulse 18 to the minute.
Erysipelas	none	117	Fever.
Influenza	none	138	Mild attack.
Influenza	none	134	Mild attack.
Influenza	none	122	Mild attack.
Secondary anemia	marked	120	
Lymphosarcoma	none	l. arm 140 r. arm 126	Dulness under upper end of sternum.

for that individual. As some one has pointed out, the important point is not the height of the curve from the base line but the change in direction of the curve. As no case of perforation occurred in our small series, we are unable to give any additional data upon this question.

sented the most marked sclerosis, 5 mm. Hg. sufficed to produce the same result. Weiss[14] looks upon arteriosclerosis as a cause of high arterial tension, but considers the heart as the chief factor in bringing this about. He reports cases of marked sclerosis with hypertrophy of the left ventricle in which, the heart being competent, high pressures are obtained, whereas in cases with the same apparent degree of sclerotic change in the arteries, but with weak heart action he finds low (subnormal) pressures. Hensen,[2] in his investigations, found high pressure to be the rule. In nineteen cases of sclerosis of the arteries of moderate degree he found the pressures, with one exception, to be above 155, while with marked grades of sclerosis the blood pressure was 172 or more in all but one of eight cases. Orr[16] examined twenty-seven cases, the highest pressure being 210 mm. Hg.; in sixteen cases the pressure registered 150 mm. or over; in four cases from 130 to 145; in three cases from 110 to 135; in four the pressure was subnormal. Carter[15] says that slight and moderate degrees of arteriosclerosis cause very little departure from the normal pressure and that it is only with marked sclerosis that we obtain any considerable increase of tension. Norris[21] does not consider sclerosis of the arteries a very important factor in influencing the blood pressure, for he found normal pressure in some cases with marked thickening. Goldwater's[10] results show wide variations in the different cases. One case of marked sclerosis is reported with a pressure of 80 to 82 mm.; another, in which renal disease coexisted, had a pressure of 160 to 174, though it is impossible in this case, it would seem, to ascribe the high tension solely to the condition of the arteries. This author agrees with Weiss in looking upon the heart as the most important factor in determining the height of arterial tension. Jackson[18] says, "We know . . . that in arteriosclerosis the blood pressure is high," but that this statement needs qualifying is shown by the work of Weiss, Orr, Norris and Goldwater, as well as by our own. One of our most marked cases of sclerosis occurred in the patient with pernicious anemia, referred to above, in whom a pressure of 98 mm. Hg. was found. From our rather small number of cases, we believe that the pressures found in arteriosclerosis are influenced little by the condition of the arterial wall, but rather are dependent upon not only the heart but also accompanying conditions, possibly the result of disturbances of metabolism, which are as yet little understood.

In a subject which is in its infancy, as is the case in the determination of blood pressure, it is important to obtain numerous estimations in various diseased conditions. Although our remaining cases are not sufficient in number to warrant their separate consideration, we feel that they may ultimately be of some value, when taken in conjunction with the results of others. Therefore, the foregoing table of blood pressure in miscellaneous diseases is given.

Testing the effect of certain drugs upon the arterial tension is another important field for the use of the sphygmomanometer. Some work has been done along this line, as with digitalis for example. We have not thus far attempted

to study this subject, but consider a few observations which we have made upon the effect of amyl nitrite of sufficient interest to make a brief report justifiable, especially in view of the findings of Weiss.[14] This author reports an increase in arterial tension of 10 to 20 mm. Hg. after inhalations of amyl nitrite, and cites the following cases: (1) Dr. Robert R. Pressure (Gärtner) 140 mm. Inhalation of two drops of amyl nitrite; two minutes later, pressure registered 150 mm.; three minutes later, 140 mm. (2) Johann K. Pressure 140 mm. Hg. Inhalation of two drops of amyl nitrite; one minute later, 160 mm.; after five minutes, 140 mm. In our observations upon the effect of this drug on arterial pressure we have repeatedly and without exception found a very prompt, though

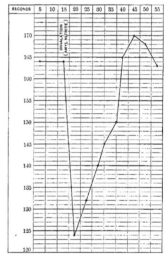

Showing effect of amyl nitrite upon blood pressure.

extremely transient, decrease in the systolic pressure amounting to as much as 43 mm. Hg. in the most pronounced cases. The accompanying chart will serve to illustrate this fact. It will be noted that within a minute a sudden fall in arterial tension occurs, with a return to the former level. We explain the results obtained by Weiss by a failure to take the pressure immediately after the inhalations. With the Gärtner tonometer it is manifestly impossible to take consecutive readings upon the same patient as rapidly as with the Riva Rocci sphygmomanometer and even with the latter the rapidity required to register the extremely sudden variations in pressure produced by amyl nitrite gives rise to certain inaccuracies, which, however, amount to no more than a few millimeters mercury, in all probability. Simultaneously with the fall in pressure, flushing of the patient's skin occurred.

In conclusion, we can only urge the necessity for a more widespread use of the sphygmomanometer, with the publication of results. The instruments are too little employed by those in active practice, not to mention hospital workers, and the results obtained from them too frequently underestimated. It would be folly to say that every case, to be successfully treated, should have blood pressure determinations made, but that there are *some* cases—and their number will doubtless increase—in which the treatment can be *most successfully* carried out when we know accurately the height of the arterial tension, is a statement which needs no amplification. We cannot refrain from emphasizing the necessity upon those who use the Riva Rocci type of apparatus for obtaining a broad cuff, one 15 cm. wide.

To Dr. Dock we wish to express our thanks for many valuable suggestions and for his lively interest in the work.

REFERENCES.

1. Cook and Briggs. Johns Hopkins Hosp. Reports, Vol. 11, p. 451, 1903.
2. Hensen. Deutsches Archiv f. klin. Med., Bd. 67, p. 436, 1900.
3. Gumprecht. Zeitschr. f. klin. Med., Bd. 39, p. 377, 1900.
4. H. von Recklinghausen. Archiv f. exp. Path. u. Pharm., Bd. 46, p. 78, 1901.
5. Research Com., Harv. Med. School, Bost. Med. and Surg. Jour., Vol. 150, p. 255, 1904.
6. Erlanger. Amer. Jour. of Physiol., Vol. X, p. 15, 1904.
7. Grödel H. and Kisch, Jr. Münch. med. Woch., Bd. 51, p. 698, 1904.
8. Stanton. Univ. of Penn. Med. Bull., Vol. XV, p. 466, 1903.
9. Albert. Wien. med. Jahrbücher, 1883 (quoted by Hensen).
10. Goldwater. MEDICAL NEWS, Vol. 82, p. 926, 1903.
11. Jellinek. Zeitschr. f. klin. Med., Bd. 39, p. 447, 1900.
12. Hecht and Langstein. Deut. med. Woch., Bd. 26, p. 513, 1900.
13. Grebner. Wiener med. Blätter, Bd. 22, p. 878, 1899.
14. Weiss. Münich. med. Woch., Bd., 47, p. 69, 1900.
15. Carter. Amer. Jour. of the Med. Sci., Vol. 122, p. 854, 1901.
16. Orr. Jour. of Am. Med. Ass'n, Vol. 39, p. 789, 1902 (Reported in abstract).
17. Czyhlarz. Wiener klin. Rundschau, Bd. 16, p. 299, 1902.
18. Jackson. Bost. Med. and Surg. Jour., Vol. 148, p. 223, 1903.
19. Vickery. Ibid., Vol. 150, p. 480, 1904.
20. Erlanger and Hooker. Amer. Jour. of Physiol., Vol. X. Proc. of Am. Phys. Soc., p. 16, 1904.
21. Norris. Amer. Jour. of the Med. Sci., Vol. 125, p. 888, 1903.
22. Gross. Deutsches Archiv f. klin. Med., Bd. 74, p. 297, 1900.
23. Vamossy and Vas. Münch. med. Woch., Bd. 44, p. 667, 1897.
24. Roos. Ibid., Bd. 49, p. 1607, 1902.
25. Crile. Jour. of Am. Med. Assoc., Vol. 40, p. 1202, 1903.
26. Briggs. Bost. Med. and Surg. Jour., Vol. 149, p. 343, 1903.
27. von Basch. Zeitschr. f. klin. Med., Bd. 2, p. 79, 1881.
Note. Janeway's valuable book on Blood Pressure appeared too late to be of service in the preparation of this article.

MEDICAL PROGRESS.

PEDIATRICS.

The Physiology of Nursing.—In the case of an ideal breast, during the first few minutes of a meal, every suck is followed by an act of swallowing, according to J. Süsswein (*Arch. f. Kinderheilk.*, Vol. 40, Nos. 1 and 2). The greater half of the meal is finished in the first five minutes. If the child drinks with many interruptions and if the act of swallowing occurs but seldom, then the breast is unsuitable or insufficient for the child. In judging of the suffi-

ciency of the breast, weighing the child is a still better help than the above observations.

The Value of the Finding of Diphtheria Bacilli i Nurslings.—A thought frequently arises in the min of the practitioner that perhaps, after all, a cas from which a culture has been taken with a positiv finding, is not one of diphtheria. L. SCHAPS (*Arc f. Kinderheilk.*, Vol. 40, Nos. 1 and 2) agrees wit Ballin that the finding of the bacillus alone give no assurance that diphtheria is present, that rathe the greater emphasis should be placed on the clini cal impression. Bacteriology can furnish an aid t the latter. In supporting his contention the autho reports his interesting experience in the Infant Hospital of Dresden. Nine cases of rhinitis simul taneously presented themselves among his charge and owing to certain repairs that were going on i the hospital, it was impossible to isolate them. Ther was a serosanguinolent secretion from the nostril and excoriations of the upper lip. There was n temperature, but all the cultures gave a positive re port. From 21 other and normal cases in the hos pital cultures were taken, and some of these als revealed the presence of diphtheria bacilli, althoug there were absolutely no clinical symptoms of diph theria. None of the patients at any time had feve in spite of the positive finding, in one of which th bacilli proved to be virulent on inoculation int animals. No membrane was discovered either i the nose or elsewhere. There were no pharynge or laryngal symptoms, no nephritis, or nervous man ifestations. All the cases received antitoxin, but i had no effect upon the rhinitis. The conclusion i that no diphtheria was present. The diphtheri bacilli in the above cases played simply the rôle o relatively harmless saprophytes, which, howeve may at times give rise to a genuine diphtheria.

Spontaneous Rupture of the Heart in Infants.— William Harvey was the first to observe a case o rupture of the heart, and at no time has a case bee seen in a child less than one year old until recentl when a case came under the observation of 1 SCHAPS (*Arch. f. Kinderheilk.*, Vol. 40, Nos. 1 an 2). The most prominent cause of cardiac ruptur is arteriosclerosis, but in this case it was a septi embolus that lodged in the heart muscle. This cas is of considerable interest, as it furnishes a ne cause to that long list of causes of sudden death i infants. The case of four months was brought to th hospital, badly nourished and presenting small, di crete, subcutaneous abscesses in the back, head, an extremities; there was a maculopapular exanthen the bridge of the nose was depressed, the child ha snuffles and excoriations about the nose. The splee and liver were enlarged and there were small papul about the arms. A swelling of the lower end of th left forearm proved on radioscopy to be a swellin of the epiphysis of the radius. The case was clear one of congenital syphilis and was given inunctior of one-half gram of ung. cin. pro die, and wa nourished by means of expressed woman's mil Four days later there occurred a sudden rise of ten perature, the next day a few fine râles were hear over the pericardium and in the afternoon, one-ha hour after feeding, the child died suddenly. At a topsy the pericardium was found filled with th blood and dark necrotic fragments. There was fibrinous exudate over the pericardium. In the mi dle of the left ventricle there was a perforation 3 mi in diameter, in the neighborhood of which the hea muscle was soft and friable. Here was an absces ½ cm. long in the wall of the left ventricle, sharp circumscribed, dark red in the periphery and yellow in the center. There was also a small abscess near the apex of the heart. Microscopical examination showed that the muscle in the neighborhood of the rent was quite necrotic and the nuclei did not take up the stain. Staphylococci were found. The case was one of staphylococcus sepsis (independent of lues), originating in the subcutaneous abscesses. The frequent occurrence of septic processes in infants originating like the above must be borne in mind.

The Passage of Bromide into Woman's Milk.— If bromide be given to the mother in customary doses it passes into the milk, but only in traces, according to H. ROSENHAUPT (*Arch. f. Kinder-heilk.*, Vol. 40, Nos. 1 and 2). It can thus have no therapeutic value if administered by this route. Yet the possibility that pathological processes in infants may come from the administration of bromide to the mother, is suggested by the case of acne in an infant immediately disappearing upon the mother ceasing to take bromide.

Phosphorus in the Milk.— Only an increased casein-content, according to A. SCHLOSSMANN (*Arch. f. Kinderheilk.*, Vol. 40, Nos. 1 and 2), has the effect of increasing the amount of phosphorus in the milk. The prolongation of lactation, menstruation or fever has no effect on the amount of phosphorus. A part of this is held in organic union in the milk, particularly in casein; the content in other nucleones and in lecithin has not ben thoroughly worked out.

Intestinal Tuberculosis in Children.— A type of tuberculosis occurring among the children of coal miners in Germany is described by R. RICHTER (*Berl. klin. Woch.*, November 7, 1904). It affects principally the intestinal lymph glands, and though rarely fatal, may constitute a grave illness. The children become emaciated, pale, suffer from abdominal pain and tenderness around the umbilicus, headache, insomnia and slight rise of temperature in the evening. The cervical and submaxillary glands are frequently swollen. The disease may progress very rapidly for a time and then take on a chronic type, which is more apt to be prolonged in the older children. After the subjective symptoms disappear, anemia. and general weakness persist for a considerable period. The author describes the disease to the fact that the local milk supply is of very poor quality and the hygienic conditions are also bad. In view of the fact that Behring states that tuberculous infection in childhood protects against reinfection later in life. it is interesting to note that tuberculosis is very rare among the adult inhabitants of the district.

History of Pediatrics.— This subject, together with its relation to other sciences, was ably presented at the recent Congress in St. Louis by A. JACOBI (*Am. Med.*, November 5, 1904), and the conclusions at the end of the address are well worthy of note. He states that "pedology is the science of the young. The young are the future makers and owners of the world. Their physical, intellectual and moral condition will decide whether the globe will be more Cossack or Republican, more criminal or more righteous. For their education and training and capabilities, the physician, mainly the pediatrist, as the representative of medical science and art, should become responsible. Medicine is concerned with the new individual before he is born, while he is being born and after. Heredity and the health of the pregnant mother are the physician's concern. The regulation of labor laws, factory legislation, and the prohibition of marriages of epileptics, syphilitics and criminals, are some of his preventive measures to secure a promising progeny. To him belongs the watchful care of the production and distribution of foods. He has to guard the school period from sanitary and educational points of view, for heart and muscle and brain are of equal value. . . . And in the near future the pediatrist is to set in and control school boards, the health departments and the legislature."

The Lymphoid Affections of the Upper Air Tract of Children.— W. F. CHAPPELL (*Med. Record*, Nov. 12, 1904) describes the anatomy, functions and diseases of the pharyngeal and faucial tonsils. Adenoids may be hard or soft, and often decrease in size between two examinations, owing to change in the patient's systemic condition. The relative degree of development or dimensions of the nasopharynx is an important factor in determining the danger line of the pharyngeal tonsil, as is also the temperament of the child. An acute pharyngeal tonsillitis of a catarrhal nature is quite common in small children, without any other part of the lymphoid ring being affected. It is usually the result of a cold, and attacks the vertical clefts of the gland. The chief symptoms are high fever, the temperature rising to 105° F., extreme prostration, and some enlargement and tenderness of the posterior cervical glands. He believes that an affection of the pharyngeal tonsil causes more systemic disturbance than similar affections of any other lymphoid tissue. Conditions requiring differential diagnosis from adenoids are (1) Lymphatism, (2) syphilitic and gonorrheal rhinitis, (3) congenital occlusion of the nares, (4) digestive disturbances, (5) congenitally high-arched palate, (6) small or occluded nostril, (7) unusually small postnasal space, (8) anterior projection of the bodies of the cervical vertebræ, (9) some malformations of the soft palate, and (10) hypertrophy of the tongue. In deciding whether the faucial tonsils are sufficiently enlarged to require removal, care is needed not to overlook so-called buried tonsils which lie hidden between the lateral pharyngeal wall behind and the opercular fold in front, and extend high up into the lateral pharyngeal vault. This is sometimes a more dangerous condition than the marked hypertrophy of the gland which occupies a large part of the pharyngeal space. If small, adenoids and tonsils not causing symptoms may be treated by non-operative means; but large tonsils and large lymphoid masses in the nasopharynx should be removed, even if they do not produce symptoms. The author prefers to operate at an early hour of the morning, and usually under general anesthesia. Gas and ether is the anesthetic of choice for children over three years old; for younger patients, chloroform may be used to start with, followed by ether. Chloroform alone is considered very unsafe.

OBSTETRICS AND GYNECOLOGY.

The Hematom Mole.— Hematom moles have been considered exceedingly rare, a fact probably dependent upon careless observation or insufficient description. F. J. TAUSSIG (*Am. Jour. Obstet.*, October, 1904) says that they are found most frequently in young women who have born several children. Often there is a tendency to miscarriage. Endometritis is probably a precursor to their formation. Patients usually have a history of "missed abortion." After several months of apparently normal pregnancy the abdomen ceases to enlarge, there may be a slight bloody discharge accompanied by bearing-down pains, but nothing is expelled and the symptoms subside. Later the irregular bleeding continues, becoming more persistent from the sixth to twelfth month. There is rarely any offensive odor to the discharge. On examination the uterus will usually be found enlarged, not tender and somewhat harder than a pregnant uterus of the third month. A delayed abortion may be differentiated by the presence of fever and an odorous discharge. Hydatid moles may be recognized by the more rapid increase in the size of the uterus, the profuse bleeding and the finding of hydatid formations in the discharge. The irregular shape and the history of menorrhagia will help differentiate a myomatous uterus from a hematom mole. The prognosis is favorable. The treatment consists in evacuation of the uterus, which can usually be accomplished by cervical and vaginal tamponade. Pathologically the main characteristic feature consists in the presence of amniotic cavity greatly out of proportion to the embryo and encrouched upon by numerous subchorionic hematomata. Two classes may be distinguished: In one the hematomata are found scattered about the entire surface of the ovum and are polypoid. In the second class the hematomata are limited to the placental site and have broad bases. Examination of the fetuses in these cases has thus far revealed no reason for their premature death. The formation of the mole is explained by an increase in the fetal membranes and amniotic fluid after the death of the fetus in the first or second month. The fluid is subsequently absorbed, the ovum shrinks and by the negative pressure thus produced folds of the membranes arise which became filled with blood from the intervillous spaces. The continued absorption of the fluid together with a stretching of the membranes by the blood clots eventually forms the hematomata. In this process the insertions of the villous stems act as fixed points, the formation of a broad-based or polypoid hematoma depends upon the proximity of the stems to one another.

The Act of Labor Observed on the Isolated Uterus.—Very interesting physiological and pharmacological experiments on the contractions of the uterus are reported by E. M. KURDINOWSKY (*Archiv f. Gyn.*, Vol. 73, No. 2). He removed the uterus of rabbits under ether narcosis, after injecting it from the aorta with Locke's fluid and thus removing all the blood. The uterus, together with the adnexa, was then placed in a special chamber and kept moist with Locke's fluid. It was found that the isolated organ responded to stimuli for two or three days and from these contractions a curve could be constructed. In two cases the author was able to watch the act of labor in a pregnant rabbit uterus from beginning to end. The contractile wave began at the cornua and extended toward the body of the uterus. The result is the gradual separation between the uterine wall and the embryo. After the separation is complete, the embryo is slowly pushed through the horn into the corpus. The same takes place in the other horn and the two fetuses meet in the general cavity. The body of the uterus is then subjected to ring-like contractions which gradually press its contents into the vagina. The broad ligament take an important part in this act and so soon the embryo is in the vagina its action ceases until the second is ready to be expelled. From this it seems quite certain that the uterus can fulfil this expulsive function without the intervention of any stimuli from the central nervous system. Thermic and chemical stimuli strengthen the contraction, but often make them tetanic in character while electric stimuli have apparently little effect. An interesting feature is the part which the broad ligaments take in the process. Ergot was found to affect the uterus in a peripheral manner, and produce contractions independent of any contractions of the vessels. Narcotic poisons, such as chloral and alcohol, have little effect. Adrenalin in dilute solution (up to 1:20,000,-000) increases the contractions more than the so-called specifics and demands further investigation.

Nephritis in Pregnancy.—Pregnancy occurring in a subject with chronic interstitial nephritis must always be considered a serious complication. These cases rarely terminate in eclampsia but the renal lesions may become so aggravated as to cause uremic poisoning. The most common result of nephritis is seen in the so-called placental red infarcts. G. N. DOBBIN (*Maryl. Med. Jour.*, December, 1904) is of the opinion that these infarcts, through interference with fetal nutrition, are the cause of the high fetal mortality in nephritis, second only to that caused by syphilis. Many theories have been advanced as to the essential nature of the poison giving rise to the toxemia peculiar to pregnancy. The source has been attributed to products of fetal metabolism; inadequacy of the maternal thyroid system; the presence of an organic acid, readily changeable into various compounds which attack the epithelium of the parenchymatous organs. Whatever the cause, it is indicated by urinary changes that can always be recognized. The presence of albumin in the urine and diminished urea excretions, while of prognostic value, should be considered only as adjuncts to the clinical manifestations. The eliminative functions of pregnant patients in whom renal complications are suspected, should be closely observed. Fetal death in cases of interstitial nephritis is common at about the seventh month, hence from the fifth month maternal elimination should be carefully observed and appropriately treated by saline infusion, diuretics, sweats, cathartics and diet, as may be indicated. Cases are on record in which nitrogenous elimination was markedly increased by the use of thyroid extract.

Operative Intervention in Cancers of the Cervix Uteri.—Thus far all bacteriological and pathological researches pertaining to the etiology of cancer have been absolutely negative. Clinically the outlook is less discouraging. In considering operative measures in cancer of the cervix uteri the most encouraging reports come from Germany. The tendency of American opinion is that cancer of the cervix usually comes to the notice of the surgeon when operation is useless. E. A. BALLOCK (*Am. Jour. Obstet.*, December, 1904) explains the difference in results reported here and abroad by the fact that German operators do not draw any sharp distinction between cancer of the cervix and cancer of the body of the uterus, the latter being far less malignant. German surgeons also consider that two years' freedom from recurrence usually means a permanent cure. American surgeons are convinced that any such two- or three-year limit is not justified by after-histories of these cases. English operators, a fair proportion of French and German surgeons and a few Americans favor vaginal hysterectomy. This is the easiest and quickest operation for the disease but the remote results are far from satisfactory. The radical abdominal operation with wide removal of the parametrium and glands together with the upper part of the vagina is by all means the best procedure. Vaginal hysterectomy is of value only as a palliative measure. Starvation of the disease by cutting off its blood supply is a palliative measure worthy of trial and a valuable addition to the radical abdominal operation. In inoperable cases the judicious use of the actual cautery, zinc chloride, calcium carbide and other caustics may afford marked relief. Early diagnosis is of great importance. Any irregular hemorrhage, at or after the menopause, or any persistent ulceration about the cervix should raise the suspicion of cancer. Any unusual friability or vascularity of the tissue should be regarded with suspicion. In some cases an acrid watery or brownish discharge occurs as a prehemorrhagic symptom. The value of a microscopical tissue examination depends upon the competency of the pathologist. The fact that there will in all probability be recurrences at the site of operation or elsewhere in spite of the utmost care in dissection, tempts the consoling thought that a general disease must have antedated the appearance of the local lesions.

The Effects of Castration on the Phophorus Content of the Female Organism.—It has been proved that osteomalacia is accompanied by a lack of phosphates in the bones and the observation has also been made that castration has resulted in a cure and the administration of phosphorus is followed by favorable effects in this disease. This has prompted numerous investigations of metabolism, which have also included the changes brought about by castration. The final results have varied greatly. Investigators who have experimented with healthy animals (dogs) have sometimes observed an increase, sometimes a decrease and occasionally no change at all, while those who made their observations in women, the subject of osteomalacia, usually found a diminution in the amount of phosphorus excreted. Their results, however, are not beyond the sphere of doubt. F. HEYMANN (*Archiv f. Gyn.*, Vol. 73, No. 2) now presents the results of his researches made for the purpose of deciding whether any differences existed betwen healthy individuals, subjected to castration and those which had not been thus treated, with reference to the chemical constitution of their organs. Both classes were selected with regard to equality of race and size, and kept under the same conditions as regards their life and nourishment. The animals employed were rats, as being most suitable on account of their size and ease of procurement. His results are as follows: He is certain that the castration of healthy mammals is not attended by any permanent retention of phosphorus. On the contrary there is apparently a diminution in the phosphorus content of the organism, which decrease seems to involve the soft parts as well as the skeleton. The lecithin is apparently not affected. Heymann accounts for the favorable effects which follow castration in osteomalacia by assuming that in this disease the ovaries are primarily diseased and that the softening of the bones which subsequently occurs, is a secondary trophoneurosis.

Pyemia Treated by the Production of Artificial Suppuration.—Fochier proposed some time ago a plan for the production of local suppuration in cases of general pyemia, for he had observed that in severe cases the general condition improved if local suppuration occurred either as a pelvic abscess, subcutaneous phlegmon, etc. For this purpose he injected turpentine subcutaneously and reported favorable results in six cases. Other observers have tried the method with equal success, others have found it ineffective. BROSE (*Deut. med. Woch.*, October 27, 1903, reports a case of puerperal septicemia of four weeks' duration, with septic temperature, a pulse of 140 and great prostration. He injected 5 c.c. of rectified turpentine into the calf of the leg and the temperature began to fall. She kept on improving and on the tenth day there was no longer

any fever and the general condition was better. On the fifth day after the injection, the leg was incised and a quantity of pus evacuated. The suppuration continued, however, and a second incision was found necessary. The wound took a long time to heal and the author is of the opinion that the dose of turpentine injected was larger than really necessary and produced too great a local reaction. The author believes that the good result in this case was due to the method employed.

Benign Character of Chorio-epithelioma.—Although at first regarded as a universally malignant class of neoplasms, it has been found that many cases recover without recurrences after operation. The distinction between the two groups has never been fully determined, however, and an attempt to differentiate them on a histological basis has now been made by D. V. VELITS (*Zeitschr. f. Geb. u. Gyn.*, Vol. 52, No. 2). He reports an advanced case in which a complete cure resulted after total extirpation, and compares his microscopical findings with those cases where after incomplete operation, curettement, or the appearance of vaginal metastases, the patients nevertheless recovered. The author considers these cases as relatively benign. Clinical experience teaches that a chorio-epithelioma together with its metastatic deposits may heal spontaneously. The latter process depends on a necrobiosis, which can be perceived by the naked eye alone in advanced cases. The microscopical picture shows the following :—diminished vitality of the Langhans cells, manifested in the partial or complete absence of mitosis, and the appearance of migrating cells, which are indicative of the dissolution of the syncytium and are the degeneration products of the disintegrating chorio-epithelium as well as of the cystic mole.

Treatment of Complete Rupture of the Uterus.—That the question of the proper treatment of this condition is still open to discussion, is the opinion of R. KÜSTNER (*Deut. med. Woch.*, September 22, 1904). The former idea that laparotomy or vaginal hysterectomy was necessary has been succeeded to some extent by the notion that more conservative measures were indicated. Caution is necessary in drawing conclusions from statistics, for this accident, more than any other must be judged by the merits of each particular case. The writer reports seven cases treated by laparotomy and although only two of his patients recovered, he still expresses himself as in favor of this plan. He advises free incision whether the laparotomy is demanded for the mere checking hemorrhage or not. A careful search for all pools of blood, meconium and liquor amnii in the peritoneal cavity is necessary, especially in the upper parts. The abdominal cavity should not be flushed by any solution. Bleeding points should be controlled by ligature and the rent in the uterine wall sutured. The bladder, if torn, may also be repaired. Hysterectomy can only be done in exceptional cases, as the patients are not in fit condition for this procedure. In some posterior ruptures, it may be better to drain vaginally, instead of suturing the uterus and a large Mikulicz tampon should in all cases lead from the uterine tear out through the abdominal incision.

Spinal Anesthesia in Obstetrics.—Good results have been obtained by A. MARTIN (*Münch. med. Woch.*, October 11, 1904) from the injection of cocaine, preceded by adrenalin, into the subarachnoid space in women about to give birth. The anesthesia frequently lasted up to three hours and not rarely extended as far as the clavicles. After-effects with the exception of vomiting, were not noticed. Hypodermic injections of caffeine have recently been recommended to prevent vomiting, but in the author's hands, they were without effect. It seems that patients weak and advanced in years, possess a special tolerance for cocaine, so that this may often be substituted to advantage for chloroform. Application of forceps, version and perineal suture can be done without inducing pain but it is undeniable that the contraction of the womb and of the abdominal muscles is somewhat retarded. Involution of the uterus and the formation of milk are not interfered with.

A Case of Quadruplets.—It is rare for the human female to give birth to four children at once. Fothergill gives the ratio as one in 387,000. ANNIE C. GOWDEY (*Lancet,* October, 1904) reports the case of a woman, aged thirty-six years, who, while lifting a heavy weight felt something " snap " inside her. Typical labor pains developed within a few hours. On admission to the St. Pancras Infirmary, she gave the following history: She was pregnant 5½ months and had noticed that she was unusually large; otherwise, she had had no discomfort whatsoever. The physical signs were: The abdomen was greatly distended, the uterus reaching to within three fingerbreadths of the ensiform. The fetal parts were not satisfactorily palpable. The os was dilated and the cord prolapsed. The pains subsided and the next day a hand prolapsed and could not be returned. The child was delivered by the forceps. It weighed one pound, four ounces and survived thirteen hours. Within the next twenty minutes, three other children were expelled. These were all stillborn. The placentæ are described as follows: Two were quite separate, the remaining two had coalescing margins with separate chorions to each. There was no post-partem hemorrhage, the recovery of the patient being without incident. Two of the presentations were transverse, one was vertex and the other breech. The presence of the separate chorions indicating the uniovular development of each child is interesting inasmuch as it is the most common mode of development in twin pregnancies but most unusual in multiple pregnancies.

Treatment of Tumors During Pregnancy.—That vaginal removal of tumors may be done as readily during pregnancy as at other times, is the opinion of DUHRSSEN (*Deut. med. Woch.,* October 20, 1904), who describes a number of such cases. He considers that the attempt to replace incarcerated ovarian or parovarian cysts during pregnancy, is unsafe with any method of forcible manipulation, with or without anesthesia, and it should never be resorted to on account of the danger of injury to the pedicle with consequent internal hemorrhage. In such cases the proper treatment is vaginal ovariotomy, supplemented if necessary by laparotomy, which if the proper preparations have been made, does not increase the dangers to the patient. During labor, abdominal removal of the tumor is to be preferred only if the genital tract or the contents of the tumor have become infected. During pregnancy, tumors which can be pressed down to the anterior or posterior vaginal vault, should be approached by this means. Those which cannot be reached in this way should be left untouched during pregnancy, provided that they do not increase in size and that the general condition remains good. After the uterus has involuted, vaginal extirpation may also be done. Myomata which block the parturient canal and are not drawn up by the uterine contractions may be excised either by anterior or posterior colpotomy, combined with Cæsarean section.

Serum Treatment of Puerperal Fever.—The failure of antiseptic methods in labor cases to be followed by as good results as in other operations, is due, according to E. BUMM (*Berl. klin. Woch.,* October 31, 1904), to the difficulty of carrying out the various details, especially in private practice, rather than to any increase in operative procedures, etc. Surgical operations last a short time as compared with labor cases, and are carried out in suitable quarters as a rule and with skilled assistants while a woman may be in labor for days and subjected to numerous or indiscriminate examinations. The genital region, moreover, is very hard to disinfect properly and germs also find a ready soil in the parturient canal especially after labor. The ideal solution of the problem would be to provide a sufficient number of obstetrical hospitals in which all could be accommodated whose home surroundings militate against surgical cleanliness. Bumm thinks that the general treatment employed in cases of puerperal infection is insufficient and efforts should be made to further develop an antistreptococcus serum. In spite of all its shortcomings he has adhered to this method for ten years with extremely favorable results. He has used various sera, beginning with Marmorek's from the Pasteur Institute, then Merck's, Tavel's, Menzer's, and finally Aronson's. Septic puerperal infection may be divided into the following clinical pictures: (1) The localized streptococcus endometritis, due to infection of puerperal wounds of the vagina and perineum; (2) the extension of the infection along the mucous membrane into the tubes, leading to a septic salpingo-oöphoritis and pelvic peritonitis; (3) the extension of the germs into the broad ligament, septic parametritis; (4) extension of the infection over the entire peritoneum, septic puerperal peritonitis; (5) the extension of the infection from the placental site through the venous channels, leading to phlegmasia, pyemia, endocarditis, or septicemia. Fifty-three cases divided among these anatomical and clinical groups were treated with serum injections, with a mortality of 11 per cent. The latter figure, however, is not conclusive, as about 80 per cent. of women who present a streptoccocus endometritis, eventually recover. The value of the serum lies in the fact that a more serious class of cases have recovered than would otherwise have been the case. Bumm admits that at present there is no serum which exerts any effect on tissues which have been infected by an invasion of streptococci beyond the original point of entrance. Where there is developed a general peritonitis, parametritis, pyemia, endocarditis, etc., the injection of the serum is ineffectual and useless. On the other hand there is no doubt that where the infection remains localized in the endometrium, or where the streptococci are circulating in the blood in moderate numbers without having produced any lesions in other organs, the administration of the serum will serve to overcome the infection and its use is to be recommended. The comparative harmlessness of the subcutaneous injection prompts him to give the serum whenever the labor has been severe, the placenta adherent, so that it required removal, the liquor amnii decomposed, and fever present during labor,—as a prophylactic measure and he firmly believes that in this way many an infection may be avoided, or if not, at least made much less virulent. He considers Aronson's sera the strongest and best.

Intrapelvic Hematomata.—Subperitoneal hematomata, in which the collection of blood lies beneath the peritoneum, but above the pelvic floor are usually due to incomplete rupture of the uterus or deep cervical tears. In a small number of cases the hemorrhage results from the rupture of vessels within the broad ligament in the neighborhood of the supra-vaginal portion of the cervix or about the base of the bladder. A similar condition may follow rupture of a pregnant tube between the folds of the broad ligament. In non-pregnant women sub-peritoneal hematomata may follow injuries to blood vessels in curetting the uterus or removing tumors. In considering intra-pelvic hematomata following labor, J. N. WILLIAMS (*Am. Jour. Obstet.*, October, 1904) thinks the concensus of opinion to be that such an accident does not result from injury of the large vessels, but is due to the tearing through of smaller ones as a result of the tissues of the birth canal being dragged from their attachments by the friction caused by the oncoming presenting part. The symptoms of such an accident are severe pains about the rectum, the absence of any visible lesion, shock, and the high position of the fundus. In most cases the treatment should be expectant, employing a saline infusion if indicated. If the tumor rapidly increases in size and collapse becomes pronounced, laparotomy should be resorted to, and appropriate means adopted for checking the flow of blood.

Papillary Tumors of the Ovaries.—The histological structure of cysts and papillary tumors of the ovary is the same. The presence or absence of a limiting cavity is a temporary and accessory morphological difference. There are two important features which belong to these tumors: ascites and disseminated growths over parietal and visceral peritoneum while the omentum may or may not be infiltrated. T. POZZI · (*Am. Jour. Obstet.*, October, 1904) says that the prognosis in connection with these tumors is often too severe, they are not always malignant and can often be completely removed, even an incomplete operation may be followed by improvement, if not permanent recovery. It is important to make a careful destinction between carcinomatous generalization and simple grafts which result from contact or plain growth upon the peritoneum of detached papillary vegetations of the ovary. This latter process is benign. In the absence of positive symptoms of· malignancy (cancerous cachexia or visceral metastasis), the tumors should be treated as benign. The frequency of successive invasion of both ovaries by papillary tumors constitutes indication for removal of the adnexa of both sides, even if the one side appears healthy. In young women only should a conservative operation be performed.

The Electric Treatment of Uterine Myomata.—In spite of the shortcomings of this method, it has been further studied by E. WITTE (*Deut. med. Woch.*, November 3, 1904), who has perfected a method which apparently gives satisfactory results. His plan is to produce firm uterine contractions by strong faradization, with the idea of causing the blood vessels to contract, and thus to check hemorrhage, while at the same time the nutrition of the tumor is interfered with, and it diminishes in size by a process of absorption. He passes one electrode through the cervix into the uterus, while the other is applied to the abdomen. If possible the treatment is continued daily for from twenty to thirty minutes, and the current is used as strong as the patient can stand it. Both the strength of current and the frequency of application must be carefully regulated at the beginning of treatment in order not to overtax the patient. The author has never observed any bad effects from the treatment, and has found that the metrorrhagia is entirely controlled and the tumors are greatly reduced in size.

Rubber Gloves in Manual Extraction of the Placenta.—The comparative results obtained in a series of cases of retention of the placenta treated in the Woman's Hosiptal at Basel, with or without rubber gloves, are published by WORMSER (*Deut. med. Woch.*, November 3, 1904). The conditions of delivery were practically the same, but in the service of one of the attending obstetricians the gloves were worn and in the service of the other they were omitted. Forty cases were done without gloves, thirty with, and the mortality was nothing. The patients treated with the gloved hands showed less febrile reaction, however, during the puerperium than the others, and the author warmly recommends the gloves for this reason. This is still more advisable in private practice, where there is more chance for infection, and where haste may be necessary on account of the hemorrhage.

Inversion of the Uterus.—The treatment in cases accompanied by necrosis of the inverted part, together with the report of such a case, is discussed by B. M. ANSPACH (*Am. Med.*, November 26, 1904). The patient in question had two labors in which the placenta was delivered with difficulty. Three months after her confinement, a slight irregular hemorrhage from the vagina was noticed, which continued for over six months, after which there was a free flow of blood every ten days. One of these hemorrhages was quite severe, with backache and bearing-down pain, and followed by a very offensive discharge. On examination a spherical mass was made out which filled the vagina, semifluctuating and gangrenous. Under ether the diagnosis was made of complete inversion of the uterus. Removal was indicated, but vaginal hysterectomy was rejected on account of the danger of infection, and the plan of amputating the necrotic mass was adopted. The pedicle of the mass was caught with a large hysterectomy forceps, the tumor being first incised in the middle line in order to avoid a mistake in diagnosis or a knuckle of small intestine which might have been caught in the funnel of the inversion. The necrotic mass was cut away beneath the forceps, which were left in place and then pushed back somewhat and the region packed with gauze. Forceps seemed safer than sutures on account of the danger of infecting the peritoneum. There was left the lower third of the endometrial cavity and' the ovaries. The forceps sloughed off on the fifth day and convalescence was uneventful. The inversion probably began during the puerperium and continued· until three months later it gave rise to symptoms.

Thrombosis and Embolism in the Puerperium.— This subject has been studied from the material of Leopold's clinic, including 16,000 maternity cases, by A. RICHTER (*Archiv f. Gyn.*, Vol. 74, No. 1). He found 20 instances of embolism. 78 of thrombosis and 18 of puerperal pulmonary affections. Sixty per cent. of the cases of emboli ended fatally with the first attack, in a few instances a milder attack preceded the fatal one. As careful prophylaxis may avoid embolism, it is important to be acquainted with an early symptom which may direct the attention to the existence of a thrombosis. The rise in the maternal pulse, first described by Mahler, was demonstrated by Richter without any doubts, in 63 per cent. of his cases, with some doubts, on account of the presence of fever, in 34 per cent. In the cases of pulmonary embolism it was plainly evident in 42 per cent., but doubtful in 52 per cent. Richter thinks that this rise in pulse rate is more important than other .symptoms of hidden thromboses, which are accepted as characteristic. *e.g.,.* rise of temperature, variable hyperemia in the affected thigh and the skin of the abdomen, pain in the hip and side. The increased pulse rate is due to the fact that the necessity for the production of new collateral channels around the obstructed vein brings about increased cardiac resistance and the heart of a pregnant woman, being more or less subject to degeneration, can only accomplish the additional task by an increased number of contractions. Richter thinks that thrombosis in the pelvic veins is less dangerous than that of the lower extremities, because in the latter, larger fatal thrombi may be freed, while in the pelvic veins much smaller thrombi are formed which are caught in the capillaries and collaterals. When these smaller emboli reach the lungs they give rise to sharp pains in the side, which may be followed by pleurisy, pneumonia, bronchitis, or infarct. The prophylaxis when a suspension exists of the presence of a thrombosis, consists of absolute rest and careful nursing, together with bandaging of the varicose extremities.

NEUROLOGY AND PSYCHIATRY.

Intermittent Lameness and Other Symptoms of Peripheral Arterial Disease—These conditions, which were formerly ascribed to lesions of the peripheral nerves or the spinal cord, are now acknowledged in many instances to be due primarily to disease of the arteries of the extremities, and that nervous lesions, when present, are secondary. The best known effect of peripheral obliterating endarteritis is intermittent lameness, described by Erb as dysbasia angiosclerotica, and more common than ordinarily supposed. C. W. BURR (*Am. Med.*, September 17, 1904) reports a fatal case in which gangrene developed but not all cases are as severe as this. The typical case may be described as follows: The patient, while walking, is seized with a pain or numbness, localized or diffuse, in one or both legs, and at the same time there is a feeling of stiffness or even distinct cramp in the calves or thighs. If the patient sits down, relief comes quickly, but very soon after beginning to walk the symptoms return, and soon he is unable to walk at all, on account of the pain and muscular debility. Examination at this time shows that the arteries of the feet, and even the femoral, may be pulseless, their walls are distinctly thickened, and the feet may be warm or cold, cyanosed or normal in color. The attack may vary from several minutes to hours and come on almost always during muscular exertion. The legs are more frequently affected than the arms, and rarely the arm and leg may be seized in a manner resembling transitory cerebral hemiplegia. Glycosuria is a frequent complication, but the one constant symptom in intermittent lameness is chronic arteritis.

The Classification of Hydrocephalus.—Various conditions have been described by different authors as examples of this disease, without, however, bearing any definite relation to one another. There follows consequently confusion as to the different forms and a misconception of the true relationship existing between them. W. C. KRAUSS (*Medicine*, October, 1904) has attempted a classification based on the pathological standpoint in such a manner as to meet all the different views taken on this subject. Hydrocephalus may be either acute or chronic. The acute or inflammatory form may be either external, due to an inflammation of the meninges, or internal, due to an inflammation of the ependyma. The chronic forms may be either congenital (developmental) or acquired (obstructive). Each of these is described. Cases of alcoholic pseudotabes are not so rare among women as to call for reports of cases except where unusual sequelæ are present. The case reported by the author terminated in death through an intercurrent serous meningitis or

acute internal hydrocephalus. The patient was a pronounced alcoholic and suddenly developed ataxic symptoms which grew gradually worse until she finally presented the type of paraplegia characteristic of alcoholic neuritis or false tabes. The mental symptoms were well marked, but there were no disturbances of the vesical or rectal reflexes until a few days before death, which occurred practically without symptoms or external evidences of dissolution.

The Paradoxical Flexor Reflex; its Diagnostic Value.—A. GORDON (*Am. Med.*, December 3, 1904) describes a reflex which, in his opinion, by its novelty and diagnostic value in organic diseases of the nervous system ranks alongside of exaggerated knee-jerks or the phenomenon of extension of the toes. He claims that it is of great value, particularly in those obscure cases, in which other symptoms are vaguely manifested, also in those in which the diagnosis between organic and functional disease is doubtful. He says that in the latter case especially this new reflex renders great service and consequently may give an entirely different orientation in regard to the prognosis and treatment. Gordon cites one case among many others, in which the foregoing is well illustrated. He examined 30 cases of various organic diseases and for the purpose of control he examined several hundred normal individuals and about 50 cases of various nervous diseases in which the new reflex could not be expected. The reflex is elicited by pressing upon the flexors of the legs in a certain manner which must be followed strictly and for which the reader is referred to the original article. Gordon calls it paradoxical, as excitation of the flexors gives extension instead of flexion. The article also gives Gordon's view concerning the relationship of his reflex to other reflexes, particularly those which are manifestations of involvement of the motor tract.

Tachycardia and Injuries.—U. F. MARTIN (*Med. Rec.*, December 3, 1904) terminates an extended exposition of the literature of tachycardia by the report of a case of his own. The patient was caught by his coat in a rapidly revolving wheel and whirled about till the throwing out of a cog stopped the machinery. He was deeply asphyxiated when cut down, though he had not lost consciousness, both feet were crushed, and several ribs were fractured. Amputation of both legs was necessary, and during the operation the pulse varied from 144 to 175. He was delirious for over a week, during which his pulse remained at 150. In the course of the next four weeks it gradually dropped to 112-120, but rose again to 150 after a secondary operation on the flaps, and was still 112 on discharge over seven weeks after the injury. During his stay in the hospital no murmurs or abnormal signs other than the rapidity and a slightly accentuated second sound could be detected about the heart. The author places the case under the head of pure cardiac neuroses following injury to the neck and chest.

Cerebellar Localization.—PAGANO (*Rivista di Patologia Nervosa*, Vol. IX, 1904), published a study of cerebellar localization. The cerebellum is not functionally a homogeneous organ, but depends for its activity on definite and distinct parts. It should be possible to develop a true and definite localization. Pagano has been able to define the location of certain centers, even motor centers. These motor centers are not situated on the surface of the organ but within quite different cerebral cortical centers. Luciani says it is not possible to exclude from the cerebellum participation with psychical centers. An original theory (Luciani) considered that force emanated from the cerebellum. The theory of Flourens and Ferrier considered chiefly the method of its distribution. Pagano combined the two and held that some impulses, capable of causing a muscular contraction arose from some parts of the cerebrum but are rarely derived from the cerebellum where ultimate nervous ganglia exist. The cerebellum exerts a tonic, static, and sthenic function, and acts as a regulator between motor impulses. Clinical observations cannot exclude the psychical activity of the cerebellum. An important part of the work of the cerebellum is its influence on the reflexes. It is certain that lesion of the cerebellum increases the activity of the knee-jerk and diminishes certain reflexes.

Hysterical Pseudotetany.—The great simulator, hysteria, may even closely mimic that peculiar clinical entity, tetany, according to H. CURSHMANN (*Deut. Zeitsch. f. Nervenheilk.*, November 9, 1904). This simulation is so well marked that well-known students of tetany in France, have fought the conception of tetany as a disease *sui generis*, and have classed it with the diatheses of contracture. Hysterical pseudotetany is a disease corresponding to the polymorphic and genuine disease. It has manifold varieties and yet it is a distinct clinical entity. It is not merely an imitation of the grosser convulsive manifestations of tetany, but closely apes nearly all the objective and subjective aspects of this disease. It displays the same pathognomonic phenomena as tetany. Trousseau's sign, which is partly sporadic and quickly disappears after the attack; also the facial phenomenon and the mechanical irritability of the motor nerves are present. One sign, however, is absent, namely, the rise in electrical excitability of the motor nerves. This is the cardinal symptom in the differential diagnosis between the two diseases.

Polyneuritis.—DeRENZI says (*Gazz. degli osped.*, September 25, 1904) mixed types are most common; pure motor cases are occasionally met with, with inappreciable sensory changes. The upper extremities are more commonly affected than the lower, especially in cases of lead poisoning. In studying the motor paralysis note that while normal subjects lying on their back hold their feet at right angles to the leg, the cases of neuritis hold the feet at an obtuse angle. In polyneuritis the muscles are usually attacked. Notice the gait of the patient, and how closely it simulates that of the cerebellar ataxia, the titubating, drunken or zigzag gait, with a tendency to fall to one side. Recall the gait of a tabetic, which presents the so-called "stamping" phenomena. The gait is quite different from that of cerebral hemiplegia. In multiple neuritis the patient cannot lift the foot, and consequently must make a movement of flexion of the thighs, like horses made to trot in sand, or the so-called "high school gait." Of the question of localizing the paralysis three types are distinguished: Antibrachial type, Aran-Duchenne, and brachial type. In the first, the radial nerve is chiefly affected, which ennervates the triceps, forearm, muscles and extensors; this is seen in lead poisoning. The second type, less common, affects muscles ennervated by the median nerve, affecting the pronator muscles of the thenar eminence, adductors of the thumb, and some of the short flexors. It causes the so-called monkey's hand. The third type, still rarer, affects the deltoid biceps, brachialis anticus and long supinators. The supra and infra spinatus muscles are sometimes affected and also a portion of the pectoralis major. The reflexes may be normal or lost. Usually there is considerable muscular atrophy. Fibrillary twitching of the affected muscles may be present. Both faradic and galvanic excitability may fail, or faradic fail and the galvanic be increased to the point of reaction of degen-

eration. Test the excitability of both nerve and muscle. Glossy skin is a common trophic disturbance. Gluber's symptom is an indolent swelling of the back of the hand, sometimes reddened of variable extent. The complication of polyneuritis and psychical symptoms has been studied under the name of Korsakoff's disease. The chief etiological factor is some form of intoxication, infection or diathesis.

Tremors as Physiological Phenomena.—BLOCH and BUSQUET (*Presse Med.*, No. 11), offer a study of physiological tremors, as measured by accurate apparatus in normal and diseased subjects. The different portions of the human body present tremors varying in rhythm and extent. Pressure of strain applied to any part experimentally produced an increase in the intensity of the oscillation, but did not influence the frequency of the movement. Cold water varies these tremors. The different types of tremor—occurring in paralysis, Basedow's disease, alcoholism, lead poisoning, mercurial poisoning, each have their own characteristics. The camera can be used in distinguishing these types. Nearly all these tremors are symptomatic rather than pathological entities.

A Case of Multiple Sclerosis Following Whooping-Cough.—GUSTAVO MINCIOTTI (*Gazz. degli osped.*, October 2, 1904) contributes to the study of multiple sclerosis a rare case of the disease in a child. The etiology is an infectious disease, pertussis. In some published cases the interval between the pertussis and the attack of multiple sclerosis was too long to make the connection sure. In the author's case the interval was very brief, and the symptoms of multiple sclerosis appeared before those of the whooping-cough were entirely finished. The clinical history showed change in the speech of the scanning monotonous type, intention tremor, nystagmus, exaggerated reflexes and other symptoms. The diagnosis of neoplasm of the brain was regarded as impossible from the absence of pain, vomiting and other pathognomonic symptoms. Friedreich's disease does not develop earlier than ten years, the nystagmus is inconstant, the reflexes should be lost instead of increased, and the speech changes of Friedreich's disease do not resemble those of multiple sclerosis. The course of multiple sclerosis may be remittent or intermittent, the symptoms may improve or disappear. The tremor varies at different times and in different cases. The gait is distinctly cerebellar, paretic, spastic, the speech disturbance is subject to great variation.

EYE, EAR, NOSE AND THROAT.

Esophagismus.—HUCHARD (*Gazz. degli Osped.*, September 27, 1904) discusses the two great causes of esophageal dysphagia: (1) Parietal lesion, carcinoma, scars from caustic agent, syphilis; (2) Functional disturbance characterized by a spasm of the walls of the esophagus (esophagismus). The same result is produced by both these causes, the calibre of the esophagus is altered. The spasmodic conditions are similar to the urethral. Except that functional activity of the esophagus is more apt to cause the spasm than passing a sound or other foreign body, which is rather the reverse of the usual action of the urethra, where urine will freely pass but a sound be resisted. The diagnosis of esophagismus is often difficult; it may depend on some slight lesion. Pain may be present in some portion of the esophagus. Sounding is often dangerous. The use of X-ray is of most valuable assistance. If the sound is arrested one day and not another a spasmodic condition is probable. If X-rays are used, the patient should be made to swallow a capsule of bismuth, to locate the stricture; or the bismuth may be used in suspension in water. Esophagismus is due to hysteria or other nervous causes, and to arteriosclerosis. To treat the stricture, electrical methods may be used, applied locally by a sound.

Exophthalmos in the Newly Born.—Ordinary variations in the infant's head, which result from the pressure incident to birth afford little more than transient interest. When, however, exudations are of such nature as to produce exophthalmos or some such serious lesion, they certainly merit the closest attention. HUGH H. BORLAND (*Lancet*, November 12, 1904) recites the history of a case in which the vault of the cranium showed evidence of protracted pressure; presenting a squashed appearance, the frontal and parietal bones being practically at right angles. The labor had not been instrumental. The child's face was pallid and both eyes were so markedly exophthalmic that the organs protruded like goggles. This was so marked that the sclerotic coat was seen above and below the cornea and the eyelids were unable to meet. There was no ptosis. The pupils were equal and fully dilated. A few hours after birth, an effusion of blood under the conjunctiva of the right eye was noticed. Paralysis of the recti followed but this was confined to the right eye in which the hemorrhage had been seen. On the third day an ecchymotic patch was observed on the external surface of the right upper lid. On the fifth day the paralysis of the superior rectus became less marked. On the seventh the effusion under the conjunctiva had diminished and did not encroach beyond the upper margin of the cornea. On the ninth day when the child raised the eyeball, one-third of the cornea was above the level of the inner canthus. On the tenth day the exophthalmus was no longer evident. On the nineteenth day a clot of coagulated blood came down the nostril. Three weeks after birth there was still soon a slight degree of paralysis in the superior rectus. Three years later the child was normal in every respect. The question arises whether the pressure causing this lesion was intra-uterine or not. There was no history of hemophilia. There was absolutely no caput succedaneum although the labor was moderately long. The mother's pelvis was normal. No instruments, it must be remembered, had been used, and it is difficult to understand how sufficient pressure could have arisen either from the head impinging upon the promontory of the sacrum or upon the pelvic floor. Whatever its origin, the bulk of the pressure had fallen on the right side of the cranium, there being little or no hemorrhage in the left conjunctiva. The discharge of the clot from the right nostril is perhaps to be accounted for by the fact that in children there is almost always a communication between the nasal vein and the superior longitudinal sinus in the antrum. Altogether the case was a difficult one to explain. It might arise from extreme hyperemia behind the eyeballs, or possibly to the fact that the child, on being delivered, fell to the floor, the small friable bones of the face having possibly been broken. Damage to the cavernous sinus might possibly be the cause of the trouble, but whether this was due to pressure or to inherent frailty of the blood vessels or to the condition of the blood is indeterminable. The fetal blood in that of the newly born differs in quantity and quality from that of the adult, the young infant having less blood in proportion to the entire body-weight. The author's experiments go to show that infantile blood has a higher specific gravity and higher hemoglobin percentage than the maternal blood. That the coagulation power of infants' blood is, first, very much below that of an adult's blood, and second, that this degree of coagulability is very variable.

PRESCRIPTION HINTS.

Dysmenorrhea.—The following has been found efficient in relieving spasmodic dysmenorrhea:

℞ Ext. hyoscyami fluidi	.f℥ ii	(8.00)
Ext. cannabis indicæ fluidi	.. ...f℥ i	(4.00)
Ext. cimicifugæ fluidi	.........f℥ iv	(15.00)
Spiritus camphoræ	.............f℥ i	(4.00)
Spiritus ætheris comp...q.s.ad f℥ iii		(90.00)

Misce.
Sig. Teaspoonful in water three times a day several days prior to and during menstrual epoch.

Synovitis.—Used in acute conditions. This solution may be employed hot, and joint surrounded with hot water bags; or, if more agreeable to patient, may be employed ice cold, and joint surrounded with ice-bags. The rubber bandage firmly applied frequently relieves pain and swelling.

℞ Liquoris plumbi subacetatis..f℥ ii		(60.00)
Tincturæ opii	...............f℥ ii	(60.00)
Aquæ bullientis......q. s. ad f℥ xxxii		(960.00)

Misce.
Sig. Apply upon soft cloths saturated with solution, and place joint at rest.

Epistaxis.—The following has been found efficacious in this affection:

℞ Adrenalini chloridi	...........gr. ½	(0.03)
Acidi borici	..................gr. xlv	(3.00)
Aquæ cinnamomi	.............f℥ x	(40.00)
Aquæ camphoræ	.............f℥ x	(40.00)
Aquæ destillatæ	.........q. s. f℥ iii	(90.00)

Misce.
Sig. Warm gently and instil with a dropper.

Fissure of Anus.—As a laxative the following has been found to have merit:

℞ Sulphuris loti	....................℥ vi	(24.00)
Potassii bitartratis	...............℥ ii	(8.00)
Pulveris sennæ	...................℥ i	(4.00)

Misce. Pone in cachetas No. xii.
Sig. One each night at bedtime.
To relieve pain and promote healing:

℞ Iodiformi	.....................℥ i	(4.00)
Acidi carbolici	....gr. xx	(1.30)
Petrolati spissi	................℥ i	(32.00)

Misce.
Sig. Apply once daily with hard rubber pilepipe after evacuating bowel with enema.

Prostatitis.—In acute conditions of this affection with vesical irritation and tenesmus, or with slight prostatic hemorrhage, the following is useful:

℞ Tincturæ veratri viridis.....♏ xxiv		(1.60)
Morphinæ acetatis	...........gr. iii	(.20)
Syrupi acidi citrici	..........f℥ iv	(15.00)
Liq. potassii citratis..q. s. ad f℥ vi		(180.00)

Misce.
Sig. Two teaspoonfuls in water every two hours.

Prurigo.—In anemia and debility use the following:

℞ Olei amygdalæ amaræ	.........♏ iii	(.20)
Olei morrhuæ	................f℥ vi	(180.00)
Acaciæ	......................℥ i	(32.00)
Extracti pancreati	............℥ ii	(8.00)
Liquoris calcis	........q. s. ad f℥ xvi	(480.00)

Misce. Fiat emulsum.
Sig. One to two teaspoonfuls two hours after meals.

Blepharitis Marginalis.—For eczematous forms:

℞ Hydrargyri oxidi flavi	.........gr. i	(.065)
Olei amygdalæ expressi } aa ♏ x		(.60)
Aquæ destillatæ }		
Lanolini	......................℥ ii	(8.00)

Sig. Apply to margin of lids night and morning.

THE MEDICAL NEWS.

A WEEKLY JOURNAL
OF MEDICAL SCIENCE.

COMMUNICATIONS in the form of Scientific Articles, Clinical Memoranda, Correspondence or News Items of interest to the profession are invited from all parts of the world. Reprints to the number of 250 of original articles contributed exclusively to the MEDICAL NEWS will be furnished without charge if the request therefor accompanies the manuscript. When necessary to elucidate the text, illustrations will be engraved from drawings or photographs furnished by the author. Manuscript should be typewritten.

SMITH ELY JELLIFFE, A.M., M.D., Ph.D., Editor,
No. 111 FIFTH AVENUE, NEW YORK.

Subscription Price, Including postage in U. S. and Canada.

PER ANNUM IN ADVANCE	$4.00
SINGLE COPIES	.10
WITH THE AMERICAN JOURNAL OF THE MEDICAL SCIENCES, PER ANNUM . .	8.00

Subscriptions may begin at any date. The safest mode of remittance is by bank check or postal money order, drawn to the order of the undersigned. When neither is accessible, remittances may be made at the risk of the publishers, by forwarding in *registered* letters.

LEA BROTHERS & CO.,
No. 111 FIFTH AVENUE (corner of 18th St.), NEW YORK.

SATURDAY, JANUARY 14, 1905.

PERIPHERAL NERVE REPAIR AND THE NEURON THEORY.

THE recent appearance of a work (Ballance & Stewart) the chief inspiration of which was a desire for a correct understanding from the surgical standpoint, of the process of repair in the peripheral nerves, has emphasized the importance of this subject; while the more recent revival of surgical work along this line has made this interest acute.

From the time of Ranvier, whose positive ideas regarding the mode of regeneration in the peripheral segment of a divided nerve deviated radically from that of some of his contemporaries, opinion and demonstrated fact have diverted first to one side and then to the other of a warm controversy, with able advocates for each new theory and each modification of the old.

We seem now in a better position to answer the various questions incident to the controversy than ever before, and, as usual, we find some elements of truth clinging to each of the various theories of the past. Whether the nerve heals by a growth of the axis cylinder from the central stump into the distal segment, which latter in turn remains passive during the repair process (Schiff, Ranvier, Stroebe) or whether the peripheral segment takes an active part in the process of healing through

the peculiar activity of the neurilemma cells belonging to it (Bowlby, Ziegler, Weir Mitchell, Howell and Huber, Bethe), have been the main questions. As corollaries to these questions, discussions regarding the behavior of the axis cylinder in repair, the origin of the myelin, its function and time of appearance, comparison of the first signs of repair in the proximal and distal segments, the peculiar features of repair following compression, and other similar discussions have appeared from time to time. Now that we are in a position to settle more or less definitely the two chief questions, a review of the evolution of our present knowledge is of considerable interest and reflects in no small degree the advance of neurological knowledge incident to the last decade.

Shortly after the publication of the neuron theory, there appeared as more or less corroborative of it the work of Stroebe (1893) who, since he described in extensive detail the growth distalward of the axis cylinder from the central stump of a divided or compressed nerve, was supposed to have placed an important stone in the foundation supporting Prof. Waldeyer's theory. The publication of the author's stain for the axis cylinder gave it added weight and since the work seemed to emphasize the primacy of the neuron body and the essential unity of all its elements, it fitted admirably into the trend of thought of the period and was quickly accepted and found its way into many text books. The views of Phillipeaux and Vulpian, as well as those of Hjelt, and Tent of an earlier period, who maintained opinions opposed to Stroebe's, were supposed to have been effectually and finally answered in the body of his thesis, while the meager facts supporting the neuron theory at that time gave his contention further support. But the reign of undissenting peace was short lived. There was already appearing in Hungary, a quarter where it attracted little attention, a publication destined to be followed by others from a versatile and persistent investigator which struck at one of the essential elements of the neuron theory, the independent unity of the neuron. Apàthy's subsequent writings, appearing in the Italian and German languages, attracted more attention. By means of his staining method, he was able to demonstrate in clear and sharp contrast the neurofibril, or primitive fibril conceived of years before by Schaefer. He not only proved the fibrillary structure of the axis cylinder process and the fibrillary arrangement existing in the body of the neuron, but he also called attention to the fibrillary communication between different neurons (a fact undemonstrated up to that time) and in some of the lower forms of animal life an actual communication between the dendrites and collateral branches of the neuron itself. He regarded the neurofibril as the conducting element of the neuron, a point, however, which he failed to prove.

Apàthy's first work remained unnoticed. His subsequent work was received with more or less indifference until the recognition of Held and Bethe and Nissl on the continent of Europe, and of Barker in our own country, accorded him a place among the best workers of the period. And now both his work and the conclusions that he drew from it are quite generally accepted. It seems we may accept the neuron theory as a fact with this as its corollary;—that actual continuity between neurons does exist and is maintained by means of the primitive neurofibril. This is accepted unreservedly by Nissl (1904) who has lately published several communications regarding the fibrillary structure of the intercellular substance of the cerebral cortex. But the most important and most conclusive thesis comes from the work and able pen of Bethe (1903). One of the most important portions of the work of this author is that bearing upon the repair of the divided nerve after section and the behavior of the peripheral segment during the process. He not only shows the importance of the peripheral segment during the repair process, but the prime importance of the reestablishment of the fibrillary structure of the axis cylinder before the nerve can conduct cerebral impulses. This forms a distinct addition to our knowledge and forges the last link in the chain of evidence in favor of Apàthy's original contention that the neurofibril is in fact the conducting element of the neuron, a contention which he failed to substantiate, as noted above.

Bethe furthermore demonstrates the great importance during the repair process of the cells of the neurilemma belonging to the peripheral segment. In very young animals he succeeded in bringing about an almost complete repair without allowing the peripheral and central stumps to unite. This "autogenetic" power of the peripheral segment of a divided nerve to regenerate diminishes, however, with age; moreover, regeneration up to the point of the formation of fibrils in the axis cylinder does not take place independent of the central segment. The power of the axis cylinder to grow peripheralward (recognized by Bethe) exhausts itself after a growth in length amounting to about two centimeters. Thus we find in this work of Bethe's the principles by which we may justify and harmonize the divergent views of other investigators of an earlier period.

BIOLOGICAL INHERITANCE.

"Natural Selection" and "the survival of the fittest," familiar terms, which the genius of Charles Darwin has long since made almost household words, are receiving blow after blow in recent years from the accumulative effects of which they can scarcely recover. Soon these notions, too, in their original forms, will probably be relegated to the numerous company of the departed—in Bacon's phrase, outgrown "idols of the theater." It is not so much that the principle of teleology, which so long has appealed to man's ethical nature, is losing support and being cast aside in this age of religious iconoclasm, as that newer facts and truer theories are threshing over the foundation-hypotheses of biological evolution as set forth by Darwin and by Lamarck, and not urgently casting out the chaff. Teleology, far from being discredited, is only set further back into the basal philosophy of life and given its truer place in the principles rather than in the details of the natural order.

The latest substantial contribution to the destructive criticism of natural selection as Darwin defined it ("the preservation of favorable individual differences and variations and the destruction of those that are injurious"), is to be found in Morgan's essay "Evolution and Adaptation," a book as simple as it is argumentatively convincing. It serves especially to set forth even for the busy physician the becoming mutation theory of inheritance as opposed to the doctrine of selection, so many years the generally accepted theory of at least the amateur biologist.

It is to Gregory Mendel's work in 1865 that we owe the facts underlying the mutation theory, although the importance of it only the last few years have recognized. This work was discussed in the Congress of Arts and Science at St. Louis and said to be "one of the most prominent papers ever published in biology," as is undoubtedly the fact, for it seems to be the basis of a theory of heredity much more substantial and scientific than any other which now is current. Its recall to life is due to the similar discoveries of de Vries. The general principle involved in Mendel's law of mutation may be best stated by a theoretical case: "If *A* represent a variety having a certain character, and *B* another variety in which the same character is different, let us say in color, and if these two individuals, one of each kind, are crossed, the hybrid may be represented by *H*. If a number of these hybrids are bred together, their descendants will be of three kinds; some will be like the grand parent *A* in regard to the special character that we are following, some will be like the other grandparent, *B*, and others will be like the hybrid parent *H*. Moreover, there will be twice as many with the character *H*, as with *A*, or with *B*. If now we proceed to let these *A's* breed together, it will be found that their descendants are all *A*, forever. If the *B's* are bred together they produce only *B's*. But when the *H's* are bred together they give rise to *H's*, *A's*, and *B's*. * * * In each generation the *A's* will also breed true, the *B's* true, but the *H's* will give rise to the three kinds again, and always in the same proportion." It is the exact numerical relation between the different varieties which here constitutes the striking fact, for heredity thus becomes an exact relation based on the calculus of probability for any series.

The explanation of this exact relation appears to be in short that every hybrid, in practice then every animal and plant, produces in its reproductive cells both male and female germs, each of which is the bearer of only one of the alternative characters, dominant or recessive as the case may be. Such being the case and it being true that on the average there are the same number of female and of male germs in a given generation, each having one or the other of these kinds of characters, then on a random-assortment meeting of these female cells and of male cells, the results of Mendel's law would follow. For 25 per cent. of dominant germs would meet with 25 per cent. of dominant germs; 25 per cent. of recessive germs would meet with 25 per cent. of recessive germs; while the remaining 50 per cent. of each kind would meet with each other, and form hybrid mutations.

So far as variation is concerned then, change, evolution, takes place by steps each at once produced *de novo*, and not by gradual and continuous variations as Darwin's theory of natural

and sexual selection implies. Inheritance is by mutation based on the chance meeting of different mixed inherited germs. Such is the evidence of most of recent researches on heredity, such, for example, as that of Castle with guinea pigs.

The bearing of these mutations according to the doctrine of probability on the theory of biological evolution is obvious. It may explain the essential problem of that theory, namely the origin of the experienced variations and the causes of the changes from generation to generation. This really important question the Darwinians appear to have neglected for the very different problem as to the causes of the survival of a changed species after it has been produced. The mutation theory, unlike that of selection, accounts for the origin of useless or even harmful variations, and many instances of these are, of course, to be found in the brutes, while one in man, the vermiform appendix, will readily occur to nearly everyone these days. On the other hand, demonstration that adaptations occur merely because of their usefulness is not complete. Teleological natural selection not only presumes and asks rather too much *a priori*, but the underlying principles bid fair to be more or less disturbed by the numerous and very various actual researches recently completed and now going on. It is only the normal condition of progress—a rich but too inclusive hypothesis giving way to the more exact facts of a somewhat later period, controlled by the theory they supplant.

QUACKERY AND ITS DEFEAT.

DOCTOR A. T. SCHOFIELD of London recently published in the *British Medical Journal* a brief article, embodying a suggestion very significant to all who wonder at the prevalence of quasi-medical humbugs or worse,—and who forsooth does not! This suggestion is in direct line with one of the strong medical tendencies of the times, namely, the more adequate recognition of the mental aspect of the individual. It recommends, in fine, that our future physicians be instructed systematically in the power of mental influence over the minds and bodies of all sorts of people, for it is by practically this means that the charlatan gains his livelihood.

The quack is nearly always a clever fellow with insight far-reaching into the common human nature. Fond of money and that which it will buy, yet afraid of the vigorous labor by which alone scientific medical knowledge can be acquired, he looks within his own self as type of other selves to see how the game may best be played. He finds there a weakness of judgment based on lack of knowledge which, not unnaturally, he accords to the great multitude of his brothers and especially to his sisters and his cousins, and his aunts,—and these he can reckon not by " dozens " but by millions all over the world. A weak judgment (in other words a relative lack of commonsense), whether or not based on ignorance, is the natural prey of suggestion from a mind allowed to come in contact with it. This contact is brought about, as we all too well know, by wide and omnipresent, persistent advertising, and usually, through this agency, as the mere repeated categorical statement that maladies, even the most incurable, have been and may be cured, and will be cured therefore in the reader's particular case. Aware that the art of medicine is not as yet, alas! certain master over all the multifold adverse conditions of human health and life, even the somewhat intelligent man or woman listens to these claims (which he cannot but " hear " if he uses eyes at all) and patronizes the quack who makes them. Either the latter uses modified scientific medical methods and manages to confer real benefit on a real disease but at a large price and under unpleasant conditions; or he works upon the subconscious mind of his victim, and cures an hysterical or imagined disease, claiming it organic, or, more commonly than either, he does neither of these,—but collects unfailingly large and unearned fees, perhaps month after month, just the same, reluctantly leaving the patient only when the latter begins to realize that he is buying experience at much more than the current rate. In what proportion of cases the quack benefits " organic " disease by mental influence which the physician or surgeon would have treated more radically, it is difficult to say, but there are certainly signs of a growing belief among many excellent scientists that, be it mistaken diagnosis or be it something harder to explain in physiological terms, the mind can dictate more to the body than the more materialistic of our profession can be made to believe.

In all of these cases, except the out-and-out robbery of collecting fees where no fee is even remotely due, there are conditions which the average quack seems to appreciate better than the average physician,—and this need not, as it

should not, be. It is the privilege of the medical profession to minister to the whole and not to a part only of his fellows, for to him belongs by education the best of human knowledge concerning life and the conditions of its maintenance. All that the professional man demands in opposing the ever growing horde of quacks of every sort is *knowledge* based on real and truly Christian science, dug out of nature by centuries of toil, thought out of normal and vigorous minds, collected, compared and systematized into the science and art all men recognize as Medicine.

The part of Medicine so understood, which is today the most neglected of all the many branches, is the science of the mental aspect of the individual. Indeed, in speaking of it as a branch we belittle it unduly for in a sense, like physiology, it underlies many other branches, is one of two or three foundations of the whole. If nothing else, quackery shows us that what the medical student needs most as addition to his curriculum, is a wide and detailed *knowledge of the individual* as an unit at once mind and matter, " fire and clay." We hear much of this of late, but not yet enough so that more than two or three of our best medical schools out of the hundreds in the land include it in their subjects of instruction. The charlatan has little else than this knowledge of humanity oftentimes and he uses it, often wrongfully to be sure, but in a way none the less to show to the physician what benefit to humanity might accrue did the medical schools generally recognize its force. They, too, should learn that oftentimes ideas and emotions and beliefs and many abnormal conditions similar to these in substance have more influence over the man and woman than some of the agents which pathology describes. On the other hand, therapeutically, these factors of the psychophysical organism may be used sometimes as instruments more fitting and more adequate than medicine or even occasionally than surgical procedure. These means the physician could apply better than the quack, for the former has the ability to truly diagnose where the latter can usually only guess. Did the medical practitioner inspire invariably the confidence which the quack by mere force of suggestion often compels, how much greater still were his success! But too often he thinks of his patients as little more than organic machines best controlled by means which never range outside of narrow mechanical effects. Even the average quack knows better, and thrives largely on this

.ntuition. The whole fact is, the human individual is a far more complicated being than the
average physician is apt to realize, however familiar he may be with the bodily nature of men
and women. Every patient is like the circle's
circumference,—convexity is inseparable from
concavity, yet some of us see him only in his outer
aspect, ignoring that the circle is the part within.

ECHOES AND NEWS.

NEW YORK.

The Society of Medical Jurisprudence.—The 186th
Regular Meeting was held on Monday evening, January 9, 1905. The following addresses of the evening
were read: "The Society of Medical Jurisprudence,
ts progress, prospects and importance," by the re-
iring President, Theodore Sutro, Esq. "The Importance of Medical Jurisprudence for the Phy-
ician," by the President-Elect, Carl Beck, M.D.

City Hospital, New York.—At the annual meeting
of the Medical Board of the City Hospital, Black-
wells Island, Dr. Edward S. Peck resigned the posi-
ion of Visiting Ophthalmologist, held by him for
over twenty-five years. With one exception this is
the longest service rendered by any Visiting Surgeon
o the City Hospital. Dr. Peck has been appointed
Consulting Surgeon to the Eye Division of the
Hospital.

New York Neurological Society.—The following
officers were elected for 1905: President, Dr. Joseph
Fraenkel; First Vice-President, Dr. J. Arthur Booth;
Second Vice-President, Dr. Smith Ely Jelliffe; Re-
cording Secretary, Dr. J. Ramsey Hunt; Treasurer,
Dr. G. M. Hammond; Corresponding Secretary,
Dr. F. K. Hallock; Councillors, Dr. B. Sachs, Dr.
Adolph Meyer, Dr. Joseph Collins, Dr. Pearce
Bailey, Dr. E. D. Fisher.

New York Hospital.—Several additional physicians
are needed in the Class of Genito-urinary Diseases
n the Male, which meets every Tuesday and Friday
night at 8 o'clock. The number of patients averages
over 75 each night, and constitutes a very instructive
clinic for the study of this specialty. Physicians
who are interested in Venereal Diseases, and who are
willing to attend faithfully, will receive regular, but
unofficial appointment upon application to Victor C.
Pedersen, M.D., 16 West Sixty-first Sreet.

Pneumonia's Grip on City Tightens.—New York
City is threatened with an epidemic of pneumonia.
At Bellevue Hospital it was said last week that the
week ending with Saturday night was almost a record
week for pneumonia cases. The record from January 1
showed that fifty-nine persons had been taken to the
hospital up to Saturday night, while during the day
before many other cases which the doctors said might
prove to be pneumonia were registered for observa-
ion. Bellevue is provided with six medical wards of
wenty beds each, where pneumonia patients together
with others may be treated. There is usually enough
sickness among the poorer classes in the city to
keep these wards pretty well filled, but with the
extra number of pneumonia patients received during
the last week every one of the medical wards is
now overcrowded, and many of the patients have
.een transferred to the surgical wards, where they
are occupying cots which at any time may be needed
or patients requiring surgical treatment.

The Governor's Message.—The recent message of
Governor Higgins contains a number of sound
statements bearing on medical topics. It gives us
pleasure to call attention to some in this place.
Speaking on the subject of *Public Health*, he says:
The best methods of preventive medicine and public
hygiene should be adopted by the State and the
civil divisions thereof. Germ diseases may be
classed as preventable diseases, particularly those
that are caused by the contamination of the water
supply. All sources of public water supply should
be examined and analyzed by the State commissioner
of health as rapidly as possible and at frequent
intervals. The private water supply of public resorts
should also be subjected to State analysis and the
results should be made public. I recommend that
the Legislature devise a system of State inspection
of domestic water supplies, to be maintained at the
cost of the municipalities, corporations, and private
owners affected thereby.

The growing demands for additional water supplies in the greater cities and for adequate supplies
of pure and wholesome water for domestic purposes
in other municipalities indicate that in the not
distant future the problem of water supply for municipalities will be a most serious one. It seems
doubtful whether all the centers of population can continue indefinitely to rely upon a natural supply of
pure and wholesome water without recourse to artificial methods of purification. The question presents
itself whether it is not feasible to develop some
plan whereby the municipalities may be insured a
water supply at a minimum cost under State supervision through State conservation of the waters of
the Adirondacks and other sources. The Legislature of 1904 enacted a law creating a water storage
commission which has for its object practically the
conservation of water for power purposes. A State
commission, having also for its object the supply
of water to the cities, might be of great service.

Study of Pneumonia.—The pneumonia commission
of the Board of Health, authorized recently by the
Board of Estimate to expend $10,000 to secure spe-
cific knowledge concerning pneumonia, and to ascertain what measures can be taken to decrease the
rapidly growing percentage of deaths by that disease, has mapped out its work in a way that
by the middle of next summer a comprehensive report will be turned in. While the greater part of
the work is to be done in this city, bacteriologists
and pathologists are working along parallel lines
in Boston, Philadelphia, and in Dr. Trudeau's sanitarium at Saranac Lake. In this city data are being secured at the Board of Health laboratory at
the foot of East Sixteenth Street; at Bellevue, Mount
Sinai and the Babies' hospitals, and in Dr. Prudden's
laboratory. Twenty men in all are engaged, eight
of whom are in the Board of Health laboratory.
The commission expects to learn why the death rate
from pneumonia has increased from 7 per cent.
twenty years ago to 17 per cent. at the present time,
although there has been an actual decrease in fatalities from all other diseases. It hopes to propose
measures for the prevention of the disease which
will enable the Board of Health to treat pneumonia
as scientifically as tuberculosis is now treated.
Probably the most important part of the work is to
be done at Bellevue Hospital, where a new pathological laboratory has been fitted up at considerable
expense. Dr. Charles Norris, for many years assistant to Dr. Prudden, pathologist at the College of

Physicians and Surgeons, was recently appointed pathologist at Bellevue at a salary of $5,000 a year. Bellevue's contribution to the work of the commission will be to determine, after death, the distribution of pneumonia germs in the upper part of the nose and head, as well as in the bronchial tubes and lungs and the deeper cavities. Autopsies will be made in every case of death from pneumonia where permission can be secured, and a complete stenographic report of each autopsy will be made. The history of each case will be complete, in order that some idea of the effect of social conditions upon pneumonia can be secured. Aside from the aid to be given to the pneumonia commission, the new Bellevue pathological laboratory is expected to make valuable contributions to medical knowledge in other fields. In the past, when the cause of death has not been clear, and the course of a disease unusual, the pathological examinations have been made in various medical colleges, and by the members of the Bellevue surgical staff. For this reason the reports have not been as complete as they will be when the examinations are made under the supervision of one pathologist. While the reports at Bellevue will be mainly for the aid of the hospital staff, they will be published by the board of trustees annually. "The great amount of material available for pathological and bacteriological research at Bellevue has been wasted for many years," said Dr. John W. Brannan, President of the Board of Trustees. "In securing the appointment of an able pathologist we can now save this to science, and Bellevue can take the part it should have taken long ago in adding to the world's medical knowledge. We will now secure a complete history of every interesting or unusual case where we can get permission for an autopsy." The Bellevue laboratory occupies two rooms in the old boiler house, and is fitted up with complete bacteriological and pathological apparatus. Besides a stenographer, Dr. Norris will shortly have two assistant pathologists.

Insane and Charities.—On this vexed question made obnoxious by the late Governor Odell, some hope may be seen in Governor Higgins' message. He says: "The management of the State hospitals for the insane, fourteen in number, with a total number of patients on October 1, 1904, of 25,019, was completely centralized by legislation in 1902, abolishing the boards of managers of the various hospitals and leaving with the Commission in Lunacy complete jurisdiction, both as to financial control and internal administration. The advantages of centralized control of the financial operations of the hospitals are evident. It is of the utmost importance, however, that this great system of hospitals, involving the expenditure of so large a sum of money annually and the care of so many thousands of peculiarly unfortunate and defenceless persons, should rest upon a broad basis of public interest and public confidence, and should retain the cooperation of philanthropic citizens throughout the State. In my opinion this can best be secured by leaving the control of all financial matters, as at present, in the hands of the commission, and by providing for each hospital a board of managers, in general charge, through the superintendent, of the internal affairs of the hospital.

" The present overcrowding of the State hospitals, the large increase in the number of the insane each year, and the expiration—next September—of the lease of the buildings now occupied by 1,200 patients at the Long Island State Hospital at Flatbush, makes it imperative to take action during the coming session for a material enlargement of State hospital accommodations.

This can probably best be met, in part, by additional accommodations in existing hospitals, and in part by the establishment of a new State hospital. In increasing the accommodations in existing institutions the importance of providing for each State hospital a building especially adapted to the treatment of acute insanity should always be borne in mind.

"It is not the duty of the State to maintain in the State hospitals for the insane at the expense of the State, any insane person who has property or who has relatives legally chargeable with his support who are able, in whole or in part, to pay therefor. While the attorneys for the various State hospitals have in many cases been able to collect the charges for support of inmates from the persons and property liable therefor, no effective check is placed upon the commitment as dependent insane of those who are not properly State charges. The rapid growth in the population of the insane hospitals since the adoption of the State Care act is not entirely due to the increase in insanity in the State, but may to some extent be attributed to the practice of commitment of senile or feeble-minded relatives to the State institutions at the instance of those who are properly chargeable with their support. I recommend that before any insane person is permanently received as a State charge, the question be judicially investigated and determined whether such person is a pauper without relatives chargeable with his support and able to contribute thereto. The crowded condition of the State hospitals would, in my judgment, be relieved if they were maintained strictly as institutions for the pauper or dependent insane. Mild cases of insanity in a purely technical sense, due to old age or other cause, where there is no more need for State treatment than in other cases of illness, should so far as possible be excluded from the State hospitals and the patients cared for in the home or elsewhere as persons afflicted with other diseases are cared for.

" The most urgent need in connection with the State charitable institutions appears to be that of additional accommodations for the feeble-minded at the institutions at Newark and Rome. A substantial increase in the capacity of these institutions would make possible a transfer of many adult inmates from the School for Feeble-Minded Children, at Syracuse, and the reception there of many feeble-minded children who cannot now be accepted. The additional accommodations at Newark and Rome should be sufficient to provide also for the admission of many feeble-minded adults now in county poorhouses.

"Great progress has been made during the past few years in improving the reformatory system of the State, and in providing proper buildings and equipment for the best reformatory work. With this end in view, the commitment of girls to the House of Refuge on Randall's Island and the State Industrial School, at Rochester, has been discontinued, and the former House of Refuge for Women, at Hudson, has been converted into a State Training School for Girls. The State Industrial School, at Rochester, is being transferred to a country site, and a commission has been appointed to select a new site for the boys' department of the House of Refuge on Randall's Island.

"It would seem that some additional safeguards should be provided looking toward more public competitive bidding in the purchases made by the hospitals and State charitable and reformatory institutions, either by amendment of the law or by some set of rules and regulations to be adopted pursuant to statutory authority granted therefor. Purchases wherever possible should be made in bulk and in large quantities and from the lowest satisfactory bidder, after public advertisement for bids. I recommend that all appropriations to enlarge or improve the State charitable and reformatory institutions be included in one bill with such provisions as will in every instance insure the most careful and economical expenditure of the moneys appropriated.

"I also recommend that suitable legislation be enacted to enable the State Board of Charities to transfer in proper cases inmates from one charitable or reformatory institution to another, where it appears that such persons more properly belong in an institution of the State other than the one to which they were originally committed. Different classes of defectives should not be allowed to remain in the same institution if by proper system of transfers they can be so distributed as to receive the best and most scientific care."

PHILADELPHIA.

State Board Examination.—Of the 126 candidates who came up for the examination 39 failed to obtain the average grade required to pass. Of these three failed to complete the examination. The students present were graduates from colleges of this country, Germany, France, Italy, Spain, Russia and Japan.

Oncologic Hospital Opened.—This event was marked by the presence of such members of the Board of trustees, as George H. Stuart, Jr., President; William H. Scott, Vice-President; C. Wilson Roberts, Secretary; Richard T. Cadbury, Treasurer; also The Rev. Dr. Perry S. Allen. There were many surgeons and physicians present, among them, Dr. G. Betton Massey, Dr. Addinell Hewson and Dr. Howard Swayne who are the Attending Surgeons and Dr. Boardman Reed, Attending Physician; Dr. William S. Newcomet, his Assistant, and Dr. J. Solis Cohen, Consulting Laryngologist.

Elections.—At the annual meeting of the Board of Trustees of the Samaritan Hospital the following officers were elected: President, The Rev. Russel H. Conwell; Vice-President, Cyrus S. Detre; Treasurer, John Little; Secretary, William B. Craig. Fifteen members of the Board were elected; Charles A. Gill was appointed, as Superintendent of the hospital and Miss Margaret J. Maloney as Chief Nurse. Alfred Moore, of the Board of City Trust, was elected a member of the Board of Trustees of the Jefferson Medical College and Hospital, to fill the vacancy caused by the death of Judge Arnold. The following officers have been elected at the meeting of the College of Physicians: President, Dr. Arthur V. Meigs; Vice-President, Dr. James Tyson; Censors, Dr. Richard A. Cleemann, Dr. S. Weir Mitchell, Dr. Horace Y. Evans and Dr. Louis Starr; Secretary, Dr. Thomas Neilson; Treasurer, Richard H. Harte.

Academy of Surgery.—This meeting, on January 2, was the occasion of their annual address, which was given by Dr. J. Chalmers DaCosta upon "The Surgeon." In opening the address he reminded the society that this was the 25th annual address of the Academy and that the first one was given by the late Samuel D. Gross and the second by Dr. Agnew. He first dealt with the question "Why does a man become a surgeon?" Many men have the desire from early youth, and he gave instances of several great men whose surgical aspirations date back to an early period in life. Then, he said, family influence determines it in many instances and he noted that Abernethy wanted to become a lawyer, but through the influence of his father he turned his attention to surgery. Others, he said, were induced to take up the profession after having seen an operation, or having visited a hospital or from seeing an ambulance. Few great men become surgeons, as men with

broad, philosophic minds, incline to research work and confine themselves to laboratory work. Because medicine is not an exact science, he said, quackery is stimulated. He then compared the profession with the trade; the latter is merely working to obtain the almighty dollar, while the profession has greater consideration for the good that it does than for the financial recompensations derived from his work, and the surgeon who does not entertain those views is not doing his duty to his profession, and the surgeon who does not do his duty is mixing profession with trade. The commission-paying surgeon DaCosta places in a low social order. He said, surgeons are divided into two groups, the conservative and the radical. The first, he said, looks upon new things unfavorably, follows customs blindly and progresses in a circle. The conservative is rarely brilliant and dashing. The radical surgeon is an original thinker, has broad ideas, he may jump at conclusion and often falls short of his mark. He has a contempt for authority and is constantly discovering new things. A good surgeon must first be a good physician. He then discussed the relationship between the specialist and the surgeon. The surgeon must not take the findings of one specialist to come to a diagnosis. He must take the chain of findings and compare them with the clinical deductions and then make his diagnosis.

Meeting of the Philadelphia Medical Examiners.—This was held Tuesday, January 3, and the first paper was read by Dr. Wilmer Krusen, upon "Gynecological Diseases in Relation to Life Insurance." He called the attention of the Society to the fact that of those examined the blanks of but two companies referred to the examination of the pelvic organs. The bimanual examination is required to determine disease of these organs. He informed the society that renal disease is frequent in primipara above 35 years, therefore it is probably better to wait until after the first labor before insuring them. Since about 95 per cent. of cancer of the genital tract occurs at the cervix, he is inclined to believe that the injuries incident to labor in some way predispose to the production of this disease. The triad of symptoms of cancer are pain, bleeding and offensive discharge, two of which may be absent. Post menopause bleeding must be looked upon as with some suspicion of the presence of cancer. To diagnose cancer physical examination is necessary. Dr. Krusen does not believe the displacement of the uterus increases the risk, but he does believe that applicants with tumors of the breast should not be insured. He maintains that a patient in good health after an abdominal operation can be insured with safety, provided there is no evidence of hernia two or three years after the operation. He is of the opinion that applicants who refuse a pelvic examination should not be insured. In opening the discussion, Dr. Bradford said he was at loss to know why the companies neglect to put a space for examination of the pelvic organs on their blanks. Dr. Wolf asserted that a medical examiner should prognosticate the liability to disease and the outcome of the disease with which he predicts the applicant is likely to be afflicted. He inclines to the belief that it would be better for the company not to print a blank with a specified set of questions, but hold the examiner responsible for a thorough examination of the applicant's condition. Dr. Hammond states that a woman over fifty is a better risk than a man. Dr. Barnes called the attention of the society to the difference between the relation of the physician to the patient and the relation of the physician as examiner to the applicant. Dr. H. M. Christian then read a paper upon "The Macroscopic Appearance of the Urine in Relation to Venereal Diseases." In speaking of syphilis, he stated that if a patient admitted having the disease he should not be rejected at once but should be questioned closely as to whether he has been under treatment; if the applicant has been under treatment for two or three years, he believes the risk is a perfectly good one. He then spoke of the shreds in the urine, and said they are not as significant as is generally held. If the urine contains shreds about ⅛ inch long which sink to the bottom of the vessel quickly the presence of a stricture should be suspected. If the shreds float they are due to some catarrhal condition of the urethra and are of no importance. When the stricture is above 20 caliber the risk is good, but when it is 18 or 16 then it is liable to produce surgical conditions in the kidneys. In speaking of hypertrophy of the prostate gland, Dr. Loux calls attention to the fact that often an applicant is insured in whom there was present, at the time of the examination, a tuberculous focus in the epididymis which may travel along the vas deferens to the seminal vesicles, then to the prostate and so involve the bladder and then kidneys. The mortality of hypertrophy of the prostate is not great if the case was properly treated. Infection of the bladder is nearly always due to the use of the catheter. Malignant disease of the prostate is often overlooked by Medical Examiners, also gonorrheal infection of the seminal vesicles. In such a condition intervals occur when the urethra is free from infection, then there is a discharge from these organs which infect the urethra anew. If the applicant should present himself during the interval when the urethra is free from the infection he would be insured while there is present a disease which vitiates the risk. Dr. Brick, in speaking of conditions of the rectum in relation to life insurance, said that carcinoma and fistula in ano are the two which attract attention. Many fistulæ are tuberculous.

Perforation in Typhoid Fever.—This paper was read by Dr. J. Allison Scott, at the meeting of the Section of Medicine at the College of Physicians, January 9. His article is based upon the 50 perforations that occurred at the Pennsylvania Hospital during the last four years. He said the greater number of cases occurred under the age of 30. Twenty-seven of the cases were severe, accompanied by delirium, chills and hemorrhage. In 86 per cent. of the cases the perforation was in the ileum; in the third foot of this part of the intestine there were no perforations, but in the fourth there was one. In four cases the appendix alone perforated and in one case the same ulcer was perforated at two points. Pain, tenderness and rigidity are the three cardinal symptoms. The pain is sudden, sharp and severe; in some of the cases there was no pain and in 21 cases it was on the right side; in one it was over the bladder and in one it began in the testicles and extended over the abdomen; in few it was generalized. Distention, he says, is a late symptom. In one-half of the cases there were no record of the leucocyte count; in 10 there was a rise and in three a fall in the number of leucocytes. He regards the leucocyte count as of very little aid in the diagnosis and says the obliteration of liver dulness is an unreliable sign. The diagnosis of perforation was made in 37 cases of the series. Thirty-nine of the cases were subjected to operation, of which 12 recovered, 11 were not operated upon, all of which died. He notes that one out of every third death from typhoid fever is due to perforation and that recovery after operation occurs in one of every four cases operated. Perforation during typhoid fever is less frequent on the continent of Europe than in the countries of English speaking people. In opening the discussion on this paper, Dr. William Osler says that of the 1,500 cases of enteric fever at the Johns Hopkins Hospital 39 perforations

had occurred, 20 of which were operated upon and 7 recovered. In one other case the death occurred about seven days after the operation but was due to toxemia. In 7 of the 39 perforations hemorrhage was present. In three other patients hemorrhage took place some time before the perforation. Dr. J. C. Wilson maintained that the slightest suspicion of perforation should induce the surgeon to operate and he believes hemorrhage will engage the attention of the surgeon more in the future than it has in the past. Dr. Le Conte, during the discussion, said he could account for the absence of pain in some of the instances by the dulness of the sensibilities of the patient; he also believes the involvement of the parietal peritoneum gives rise to more intense pain than when the visceral peritoneum alone is involved.

Pneumonia in Philadelphia.—Pneumonia now heads the list of fatal maladies in this city, with consumption in one form or another a close second, according to the official report of the deaths in 1904, issued to-day by the Bureau of Health. The total number of deaths from pneumonia during the past year aggregated the alarming total of 3,360, as against 3,107 deaths from consumption, which, owing to its high death rate, is known to the medical profession as "the great white plague." Exposure to the cold, such as riding long distances in cold, damp trolley cars, where the atmosphere is vitiated by a lack of fresh air which is excluded in view of the absence of heat, is held by physicians, to be in the main responsible for the fatal prevalence of pneumonia. Contributing causes, colds contracted in places which are not sufficiently heated, the victim being unable to recuperate quickly, relapses follow, which usually result fatally. From now until the last of March these diseases are expected to increase. Notwithstanding death has been busy with pneumonia and consumption, the health of the city as a whole, is regarded by the authorities as being good. The total number of deaths during 1904 reached 25,972, which is only twenty-five more than the figures for 1903. These figures are viewed in a favorable light by the officials, who say that with the usual growth in population, an increase in the number of deaths is looked upon as a matter of course. The statistician of the Bureau of Health figures it out that the death rate per 1,000, last year, was 18.44, as compared with 18.82 per cent. in 1903. The official report giving the number of deaths from principal causes during 1904, compared with the record for 1903, is as follows:

Diseases.	1903.	1904.
Pneumonia	3,180	3,360
Consumption	3,053	3,107
Typhoid Fever	957	744
Small-pox	278	229
Diphtheria	521	458
Scarlet Fever	189	201
Membranous Croup	84	84
Sunstroke	23	6
Malarial Fever	3	11
Heart Disease	2,008	2,289
Apoplexy	965	937

The report of contagious diseases in 1904 compared with that of 1903 follows:

Diseases.	1903.	1904.
Small-pox	1,637	821
Diphtheria	3,043	3,456
Typhoid Fever	8,650	6,613
Scarlet Fever	3,200	3,659
Totals	16,530	14,549

The decrease in contagious diseases is attributed to the system of medical inspection introduced by the appointment of fifty physicians during the year, whose heroic measures under the direction of Director Martin have in many instances kept contagion from spreading.

CHICAGO.

New Superintendent of Chicago Baptist Hospital. —Joseph Purvis, for several years Chief Clerk and Assistant to the Warden at Cook County Hospital, has been appointed Superintendent of the Chicago Baptist Hospital, and will enter upon his duties shortly.

Report of Visiting Nurses' Association.—Nine hundred patients have been cared for, and 4,228 visits were made by this Association in December, according to the report of the Superintendent, made at the meeting of the Board of Directors, held January 4. It was added that financial limitations compel the refusal of calls daily.

Improvement in City's Health.—Mayor Harrison, in his annual report, states that the health department of Chicago has made a record for highest degree of healthfulness and lowest *per capita* expenditure for health purposes among all the cities of the world having populations of more than 300,000 each. Thanks to the intercepting sewer system, the water from all tunnels has been found, by rigid tests, to be as good as the samples taken twelve miles from shore, which is the department standard of purity or safety. The result is seen in the lowest typhoid fever death rate in the history of Chicago. To the improved quality of the milk supply, caused by the work of the department, aided by various volunteer agencies, is largely due the reduction of mortality among children of the milk-feeding period. The city is to be congratulated on the present condition of the public health and the promise of its further improvement. A gold medal has been awarded to the department by the Louisiana Purchase Exposition.

New Educational Methods.—Superintendent Cooley, of the Chicago public schools, put the present educational problem in a nutshell in his address before the Illinois State Teachers' Association, held at Springfield. He said that the mind must be trained through the hand; the playground is as important as the schoolroom; school athletics must be freed absolutely from all taint of professionalism. The child cannot be rightly educated without play. The playground, to use his words, "is and always has been one of the important moral as well as physical agencies of the schools." On the playground the boy sees real life. Its standards are most likely to be the standards of honor and morality, that he will take with him into actual life when school days are over. There seems to be a tendency on the part of the high schools to imitate the athletic vices of the colleges and universities. This Mr. Cooley calls the dangerous side of the reaction in favor of sports and games. When this is done, athletics, instead of being a vital factor in the training of hand, head and heart, become a demoralizing influence, not only to those taking part in the games, but to the entire school. In the training of the whole boy and the whole girl, in improving and developing the mind through the hand, the moral standards of the playground and the gymnasium must be kept as high as those of the schoolroom. Supt. Cooley has clearly outlined the new educational methods. He has the support of the most influential educators of the country. The course he defines is certain to govern eventually, and it will be in every way distinctly advantageous to our future citizenship.

Cook County Coroner's Report.—In the annual report of Coroner John E. Traeger, it is stated that "The State maintains at enormous cost penal correctional institutions for men and boys who have committed crime, but permits them to buy, unrestrained, the means of committing it. When the State strikes at the root of the crime instead of devoting all its attention to punishing offenders, it will greatly reduce the cost of maintaining its penal institutions and prevent hundreds of murders and shooting affrays." Suicides by carbolic acid have decreased from 63 in the first half of the year to 43 in the last half, as a result of the ordinance regulating the sale of the poison, passed by the City Council last March, the Coroner says. Of the 3,821 inquests held during the year, 575 cases were due to the Iroquois fire, 426 were suicides, 382 due to railroad accidents, 208 to alcoholism, 140 to street car accidents, 228 to falls. Accidental drowning caused 83 deaths within the county, undetermined drowning 86 deaths, and burns 86 deaths. Of the 382 railroad fatalities, 141 occurred at crossings, and 144 of the number killed were railroad employes. Forty deaths occurred from tetanus, 17 of the cases being due to stepping upon a rusty nail or wire splinter. Suicides were greatest in July and August, there being 42 in each of these months. Suicides by poisoning numbered 146, and 97 of these were from carbolic acid. On the charge of murder, 96 persons were held to the grand jury. The total number of cases investigated in the year was 5,960.

Increase in Capacity of Cook County Hospital and Dunning Institutions.—Mr. Henry G. Foreman, retiring President of the County Board of Commissioners, says, in his report, that Cook County has completed nearly all the new buildings authorized by the bond issue of $500,000 in the year just closed. These buildings increase the capacity at the Cook County Hospital more than one-third, and at the Dunning Institutions more than one-quarter. To state the results of this work in brief form he presented the following table:

Estimated capacity.	Buildings.	Cost per capita.
220	Cottages for Consumptives,	$182.18
160	Contagious diseases hospital,	722.25
120	Children's Hospital,	634.35
164	Three cottages for insane,	440.45
55	Farm ward for insane.	423.80
160	Pavilion (3 cottages) for insane.	331.86
879	Total and average,	$432.80

SUMMARY.

599	Dunning, new buildings,	$315.06
280	County hospital, new buildings,	684.70

Of these new buildings the only ones not completed at the beginning of 1905 are the pavilion for the insane at Dunning and the children's building at the Cook County Hospital. But the others are well advanced and soon will be in service. The old hospital for consumptives at Dunning has been remodeled into a splendid hospital for the physically sick insane. In addition, the county erected at Dunning, at a cost of more than $16,000, a morgue and pathological building, so that the bodies of the claimed dead may be kept decently until moved, and so that the study of perplexing diseases may be carried on for the benefit of humanity at large. Taking up the charity work, the Cook County Hospital treated during the year more than 22,000 patients, and the county agent gave relief to 7,650 families.

GENERAL.

Sanitation in Cuba.—The first act of the House on the resumption of the session of the Congress, January 9, in Havana, was the passage of the appropriation for the immediate sanitation of Cuban cities, the amount of which was raised by the Senate to $326,000. The vote on the passage of the bill was 23 to 15.

Tuberculosis in Vermont.—The new state tuberculosis commission will hold meetings in the principal towns in every county at which special information for the benefit of physicians will be given and addresses explaining methods of preventing the disease made to the public. The commission also will employ speakers to attend the meetings held throughout the State by the state board of agriculture.

Fifty Years a Subscriber.—Dr. Joseph W. Edwards, of Mendota, Ill., writes: " I am compelled now to discontinue my subscription to the *Americal Journal of the Medical Sciences* and the MEDICAL NEWS. You will see I have been a subscriber for fifty years. I have discontinued active practice of my profession—a country practitioner. I am indeed sorry to discontinue their weekly and monthly visits after so many years. However the time has come." Dr. Edwards graduated at the Rush Medical College a half century ago and since that date has stood for the most worthy traditions of medicine in his State. To expressions of our regret at the loss of so esteemed and loyal a patron we wish to add congratulations upon the accomplishment of a long and honorable career and wish Dr. Edwards many years of happy life in which to enjoy the well-earned rest from his professional labors.

To Improve Medical Corps.—President Roosevelt sent to the Senate last Monday a message urging the passage of two bills providing for the reorganization of the medical and ordnance corps of the army. " I am satisfied," said the President, " the medical corps is much too small for the needs of the present army, and therefore very much too small for its successful expansion in time of war to meet the needs of an enlarged army, and, in addition, to furnish the Volunteer service a certain number of officers trained in medical administration. If the medical department is left as it is no amount of wisdom or efficiency in its administration would prevent a complete breakdown in the event of a serious war. " It is reported to me that the ordnance corps is in a position of disadvantage ; that its personnel is inadequate to the performance of its duties with which it is charged, and that, under existing conditions, it is unable to recruit its numbers with officers of the class necessary for the conduct of its very technical work." Both bills referred to by Mr. Roosevelt have passed the Senate and are now in the House.

Public Health Association.—More than a hundred professors, physicians, sanitary officers and experts, the large majority of them from the United States, have arrived in Havana to attend the annual meeting of the American Public Health Association. Owing to the cool wave which prevails at the present time the Northern visitors are not finding their winter clothing uncomfortable. The sessions of the main association began Tuesday last.

The first meeting of the Laboratory Section opened last Monday with fifty members, presided over by the chairman, Dr. V. A. Moore, of Cornell University. The session was devoted to " Water and Sewage." Mr. G. W. Fuller, of New York, Chairman of the Committee on Standard Methods of Water Analysis, submitted an elaborate report on the changes and improvements in the methods being used in bacteriological tests of water. The report was ordered to be distributed to bacteriologists in Europe and America. In the afternoon the Laboratory Section discussed the Water Analysis Committee's recommendations, listened to an address by the chairman, Dr. V. A. Moore; heard reports of committees on the variety of technical subjects and several bacteriological papers, witnessed some demonstrations and inspected the work of the General Wood Laboratory, in which the sections were held. The election of the laboratory section resulted as follows : Chairman, Dr. W. H. Park, New York; Vice-Chairman, H. W. Clark, Boston, and Recorder, Dr. H. D. Pease, Albany.

Cancer Research Reports.—We learn from the daily press that a further report of the Harvard Commission has been issued in which the opinion is expressed that cancer is not hereditary and that it can be best cured by the knife. The research has been made with a fund of $100,000 left by Mrs. Caroline Brewer Croft to Harvard, for this specific purpose. A member of her family died of cancer and this caused her to leave money, hoping to benefit mankind by having a corps of experts thoroughly investigate the subject. Those who form the commission are Dr. E. H. Nichols, Dr. F. B. Mallory, Dr. Edwin A. Locke, Dr. Charles J. White, Dr. W. H. Robey, Jr., Roxbury; Dr. Tyzzer and Dr. Weis, now of New Orleans. Dr. Nichols, who has charge of the laboratory work, which was done at Harvard Medical College and Massachusetts General Hospital, said : " Our work thus far has been to find the cause or origin of cancer, and we have been unable to do so, although we have exploded popular theories. When we know what life is I think we will then know what cancer is. No more is known about its origin now than at the beginning of the Christian era. It is a supreme mystery. On present lines of investigation the cause of true cancer will never be learned. Our only hope is in some new method. No discovery has been made which offers any hope of cure of cancer which begins to compare with the surgeon's knife."

Tuberculosis in Boston.—In a long and convincing letter to the Boston *Herald* of January 9, Dr. W. T. Councilman spoke on the tuberculosis problem in Boston. He said that during the past year more than 1,227 deaths had occurred from this disease, and that 2,100 cases had been reported to the board of health. He then discussed, in a manner to be clearly understood by every one, the cause of tuberculosis, the pathology of the disease, its insidious character and its dangers even while there may be no symptoms. The disease has existed so long that it has come to be looked on as a necessary evil and as a part of the general scheme of nature. He dwelt on the three factors to be employed in fighting it, fresh air, sunlight and food. He said that although Boston had an excellent hospital, though small, for treating the tuberculous, at present one had to be either a pauper or a criminal to be admitted. He went over in detail the present state of things at Long Island Almshouse and Hospital, and spoke of the crying need of a large plant where the sick and respectable poor, who could pay a part at least of their expenses, could be sent and treated. Long Island, in his opinion, was an ideal place for a large hospital. By removing the paupers at present in the almshouse to the almshouse in Charlestown, which could easily be arranged, two buildings now used as dormitories would be left empty

hich could easily be altered into hospital wards. The
ict that this island is only one-half hours' boat
ide from Boston, that it is large, and completely
iolated made it a splendid locality for the carrying out
f some such scheme as he proposed. At present the
'ards are overcrowded and a separation of acute from
hronic lung cases was impossible.

Tuberculosis in Maryland.—A state association for
ie prevention and relief of tuberculosis in Maryland
'as organized December 13, at the close of a mass
ieeting held in McCoy Hall, Johns Hopkins Univer-
ity. This association may be accounted one of the
ingible accomplishments of the state commission, which
as been working for almost three years to cultivate
popular interest and sense of responsibility in regard
) the subject of tuberculosis. By its bills before the
egislature, by its admirable report on the prevalence
nd economic aspects of tuberculosis in Maryland, and
erhaps most of all by the tuberculosis exhibit which
'as held last winter in Baltimore and has since
een copied on a smaller scale in other places, the
ommission prepared the way for a cordial response
o the invitation it sent out for the meeting this month.
)r. William Osler, the recently appointed Regius Pro-
essor of Medicine in Oxford University, presided at the
ieeting. The principal addresses of the evening were
y Dr. Edward O. Otis, of Boston, who described the
iethods of the Boston association; Dr. W. S. Mayer
nd Dr. William H. Welch, both of Baltimore, who
poke of the need for organized private effort in Mary-
and, the results to be accomplished and the way to ac-
omplish them; and Dr. Henry Barton Jacobs, Secretary
if the National Association for the Study and Preven-
ion of Tuberculosis, who gave an account of the origin
nd hopes of that body. The audience was a represen-
ative one, composed of physicians, social workers, and
nany men and women with a less professional interest
n the subject discussed. Before the meeting, member-
hip cards were distributed; many of these were re-
urned signed at the close of the evening. A constitu-
ion was adopted and the following officers elected:
'resident, Dr. Henry Barton Jacobs; Secretary. Dr.
'oseph S. Ames; Treasurer, David Hutzler; Vice-Presi-
lents, Governor Edward Warfield, Mayor E. Clay
limanus, Cardinal Gibbons, Lloyd Lowndes, of Cumber-
and; John Walter Smith, Snow Hill; Dr. D. C. Gil-
nan, Michael Jenkins and Eugene Levering.

Boston Medical Library.—The last meeting of the
3oston Medical Library in conjunction with the Suffolk
)istrict Branch of the Massachusetts Medical Society,
vas held last Wednesday at the Library. Dr. F. B.
Harrington was in the chair; the subject for discussion
vas "The Treatment of Appendicitis." Dr. Harrington
poke on the "Choice of an Incision." By means of
harts and diagrams he illustrated all the well known
nethods of precedure, dwelling briefly on the advantages
)f each. In his own practice he always tries to have the
lrainage canal outside the coats of intestines so that
)ne wall at least is made up by the parietal peritoneum;
ilso he never cross-cuts a muscle or a fascia if possible
o do otherwise; his favorite incision for anything but
he so-called interval operation was the modified Mc-
3urney or extended McBurney incision. The dangers
)f hernia from the cut in the median line were dwelt
)n. In cases of doubtful diagnosis he advised going
hrough the right rectus muscle. Dr. Fred. Murphy
lescribed some experiments he had done on cats with
'egard to peritoneal drainage. Under full anesthesia,
in incision was made low down in the abdomen and
lrains of various kinds inserted in the different cases—
jauze, cigarette, rubber and glass tubes, etc. A variable

time after this a higher opening was made and a solution of carmine-colored melted gelatin poured into the
abdominal cavity; at autopsy some time later it was
then ascertained how far the drain previously inserted
had been walled off and how far it acted as a drain of
the entire peritoneal cavity. His results led him to believe that only for a short time were the drains of any
value as regards general peritoneal drainage.

Dr. Brewster spoke on the subject of "Immediate
Operations vs. Delay." He was strongly of the opinion
that in all cases save in strictly "internal operations"
immediate operation was indicated in almost every instance; the mortality of mild acute cases was very low,
while no one could tell what would happen in case of
a delayed operation; the more cases he saw, the less
was he willing to wait. Tables made from 1,000 cases
of Ochsner and his own cases, show low mortality
figures.

Dr. C. A. Porter said that he thought the tendency
to delay was rather on the increase with a consequent
danger of misapplication of the Ochsner treatment.

Dr. M. H. Richardson spoke in favor of immediate
operation and cited personal cases and statistics.

Dr. R. H. Fitz spoke on the general subject of appendicitis; in the early days of this disease he mentioned Dr. Honans, of Boston, and Dr. Cutter, of Waltham, as men who were pioneers in the operative treatment and to whom too little credit was given. He
thought the term "immediate operation" a misleading
one; he, while favoring operative measures thought
there were cases in which a few hours careful observation in the hands of a good man was wiser than operating at the earliest possible moment.

Alcohol and Tuberculosis.—In an urgent letter to
the *New York Times,* Dr. S. A. Knopf writes: "Alcohol for Tuberculosis. 'Whisky, Beer, and Wine Useful for Consumptives, says Dr. Wiley.' Under this
heading, in your esteemed issue of yesterday, I read a
report of the meeting of the Americal Association for
the Advancement of Science. In this report it is alleged that Dr. W. H. Wiley, the distinguished Chief
Chemist of the Department of Agriculture, had said
that 'among the food material which had justly attained a high place as nutriment for persons troubled
with tuberculosis was alcohol.' That 'alcohol was most
commonly used in the forms of beer, wine, whisky, and
brandy,' and that 'in many maladies whisky and brandy
had apparently been used to great advantage, and doubtless such was the case in tuberculosis.'

"Whether the distinguished scientist has been reported
correctly or incorrectly, the harm that is done by such
announcements in the public press seems to me incalculable. As one interested in the solution of the tuberculosis problem, I feel it my duty to protest and, if
possible, correct an erroneous impression before it takes
a stronger foothold in the minds of the people.

"Extensive experience in the treatment of tuberculosis
has convinced me that alcohol can never be considered
a food for the consumptive. There is so little food
value in alcohol, and it is so easy to overstep the amount
that can be assimilated by the system, in which case
the deleterious effects far exceed the benefit derived,
that it is not safe to recommend it as a food at all. It
may be possible to apparently arrest the disease in a
consumptive by making a drunkard of him, but this will
not be lasting; on the contrary, the disease will soon
break out again, and the general system (liver, kidney,
heart, etc.), will have suffered by the secondary effects
of the excess of alcohol to such an extent that all the
natural resisting power to the new invasion of the
tubercle bacilli will have been destroyed.

"To preach to the masses that alcohol is a food in tuberculosis is to my mind an error so grave, so fearfully dangerous, that I repeat that I cannot let it pass without the strongest possible protest. The average person will say that if good whisky will cure consumption, it will certainly also prevent it. Alcoholism, with its fearful consequences, will be on the increase. A statement praising alcohol as a food in tuberculosis, if really made by that distinguished Government official, will be used as a means to advertise all brands of strongly alcoholic beverages as 'sure cure for consumption.'

"We are only just beginning in our anti-tuberculosis campaign to educate the people to the fact that alcohol never was a food for consumptives, never cured and never will cure tuberculosis. We are cautioning all our consumptive poor against the use of alcohol, and urging them to spend their money for milk, eggs, and meat instead. Not only will the poor consumptive himself derive no benefit from taking alcohol as food, but often the children must suffer for it. It has happened again and again that because some one had said that alcohol was good for consumption, wife or children were in want of food because the consumptive husband and father needed so much money for 'the sure whisky cure.'

"No unbiased physician will deny that in a few isolated cases a judiciously prescribed dose of alcohol may do good to combat certain symptoms in consumption.

"Large doses, often repeated, are absolutely harmful in tuberculosis, and I venture to say, in all other diseases as well. In my private and hospital work alcohol is prescribed for consumptives with the same care and prudence as if we were dealing with poisonous substances, and I know that the colleagues known to me, who are engaged in this kind of work, follow the same rule. Alcohol does not cure tuberculosis! Used in excess and injudiciously administered, it surely retards recovery. Alcohol used in excess predisposes to consumption! Statistics in hospitals for tuberculosis and scrofulous children show that the majority of them had parents addicted to the excessive use of alcohol."

OBITUARY.

Dr. CHURCHILL CARMALT died last Sunday afternoon at his home No. 130 East Thirty-sixth Street, of acute pneumonia following the grip after an illness of three days. Dr. Carmalt was born in Susquehanna County, Pennsylvania, and was educated at Harvard University, from which he was graduated fourth in his class in 1887. He received his medical education at the College of Physicians and Surgeons, from which he was graduated in 1891. In his practice Dr. Carmalt was associated with the late Dr. T. Gaillard Thomas. Dr. Carmalt was but 39 years of age and was one of the most promising of the younger surgeons of New York City.

Dr. GEORGE V. CONVERY, for many years a sanitary inspector for the Brooklyn Health Department, died last week at his home, No. 47 Fourth Avenue, in that borough. His duty was to inspect the vessels on Brooklyn's long water front.

EDWARD H. WEIL, who has been a member of the Board of Trustees of the Jefferson Medical College and Hospital, died at his home, 1720 Pine Street, Philadelphia, January 3, of carcinoma of the liver.

Yellow Fever from Panama.—There arrived in New York harbor this week a patient with yellow fever from the Canal Zone. He had contracted the disease from his wife, who died from the malady.

CORRESPONDENCE.

OUR LONDON LETTER.
(From Our Special Correspondent.)

LONDON, December 23, 1904.

THE MEDICAL SERVICE OF THE ARMY—MEDICAL OFFICERS AND THE MILITARY CLUBS—THE STUDY OF TROPICAL DISEASES—THE STERILIZATION OF THE UNFIT.

THIS day the appointment is announced of Surgeon General Alfred Henry Keogh, Commander of the Bath, as Director General of the Medical Services of the British Army. This appointment means that the party of progress in the councils of the Army has triumphed over the "old gang," as Randolph Churchill would have called them, who have been striving to keep the medical service under the military jackboot. For weeks past there have been alarms and excursions on the stage of officialdom. The Secretary of State for War has been harrassed on both sides; military officers of the highest position have threatened to resign and influential ladies have put forth their powers of fascination in favor of undoubted seniority but less indubitable merits. The King was known to be on the side of progress, but the military people felt that the matter was one of life or death to them and stuck to their guns with a courage worthy of a better cause. The tangle seemed hopeless when the Prime Minister intervened and told the Secretary of State for War that if he could not manage to unravel the knot, the Cabinet would have to do it for him. So in defiance of tradition and wirepulling and the feminine influence which was all powerful with Lord Roberts, a comparatively junior man has been placed at the head of the medical service of the British army. Keogh is only forty-eight years of age but he has had an exceptionally wide range of experience. His work in the South African War was so conspicuously good that it won for him not merely commendation but promotion, rapid almost, if not quite beyond precedent. He was made Deputy Director-General with the official rank of Surgeon General while still only a Lieutenant-Colonel. Naturally in a body like the Royal Army Medical Corps, which is still largely composed of men who entered the Army under the old order of things, when an officer had only to keep in good odor with his military superiors to be carried automatically to the highest posts, the advancement so far out of his turn of a brilliant young man, was viewed with dislike and jealousy. Keogh's administrative ability and strength of character tempered by tact have to a large extent silenced the grumblers. He may be trusted to work well and loyally with the Advisory Board whose Chairman he is ex officio. This in itself will make for progress and efficiency, for under the present system a Director-General, who is wedded to militarism in the medical administration of the Army can, if he be so disposed, practically burke the recommendations of the Advisory Board.

In my last letter it was stated that in a recent election at the Junior United Service Club a number of medical officers had been blackballed by a small clique. A special meeting of the members was held on December 11 at which some two hundred were present. The wholesale blackballing of classes of officers was unanimously condemned in words of no uncertain sound, and a full and graceful apology was tendered to the Royal Army Medical Corps and to the profession to which its officers belong. The act was all the more gratifying because it was entirely spontaneous, the doctors not having moved at all in the matter. The incident may therefore be looked upon as closed in an entirely satisfactory manner.

The establishment of chairs of protozoology and helminthology in the London School of Tropical Medicine which has just been announced marks an important step forward in the study of tropical pathology in this country. The new departure is largely due to the action of Mr. Lyttleton, the Secretary of State for the Colonies, who has inherited the enlightened sympathy shown by Mr. Chamberlain in the development of tropical medicine. The funds have, owing to his influence, been provided by subsidies from Colonial Governments. I understand that a still more important step is in contemplation. Mr. Lyttleton hopes to induce the home government to found and endow a chair of protozoology in the University of London. At present British workers have to look for the most part to Germany and France for guidance in that province of research. The new chairs may be taken as an indication that a sense of the importance of the subject has at length been awakened in those who have the destinies of our colonies in their hands. The salaries offered—$1,250, rising by annual increments rapidly to $2,500—compare favorably with those paid to teachers of purely scientific subjects in most of the medical schools of London, and should attract competent men to devote themselves to original work in a field of research which there has hitherto been little inducement to cultivate. The London School of Tropical Medicine which was called into being by the Seaman's Hospital Society on the inspiration of Mr. Chamberlain some five years ago is now a thriving institution. About forty students pass through its courses every session. Each session lasts two months and there are three in the year. The annual output of men and women specially trained for medical practice and research in the tropics is therefore considerable.

Some time ago mention was made of a suggestion put forward in a pamphlet by Dr. R. R. Rentoul, of Liverpool, that the true means of preventing degeneracy, physical and mental, was to be found in surgical sterilization of the unfit. The proposal was received with indifference by the public and the profession and with ridicule by the medical press. Dr. Rentoul, who is one of our medical "cranks," has the dull pertinacity of a man to whom the saving sense of humor has been denied. He brought his proposal forward again the other evening before the Medicolegal Society. It met with little favor. The opinion was pretty generally expressed that before anything could be done some agreement must be arrived at as to the cases in which the remedy should be applied. The remedy itself was considered neither efficacious nor practicable. Mr. G. Bernard Shaw, the dramatist and social reformer, with whom I do not often agree, seemed to me the one to go to the heart of the matter. He held that the difficulty they were in was that they did not know what a degenerate was. It was nonsense to include in the table which Dr. Rentoul had prepared epileptics and backward children, who sometimes turned out very well. One gentleman had said that soon there would be one lunatic to each sane person. There would be no difficulty then, for in time there would be nine lunatics to one sane person, and then, of course,

the nine persons would proceed to shut up the one sane person as a lunatic. Insanity was an extremely relative term. The medical profession did not know yet what heredity was. There was no question which was so important as population, but what they had to do with was the quality of the population. If they thought they could settle this population question by going, as it were, into a flower garden and snipping off all unlikely-looking buds, they were greatly mistaken. Lord Russell said he feared that a good case had been spoiled by overstatement. Sir William Collins, who is a physician as well as one of the leading spirits of the London County Council, said, the ethical aspects of the proposed treatment had not been dealt with by Dr. Rentoul. What he asked would be the conditions in society with sterilized criminal lunatics hovering about at large. The methods proposed might be criticized from the surgical point of view. Sir William Collins concluded by saying he would lift up his hand against compulsory mutilation.

SPECIAL ARTICLE.

AN ANTI-CARCINOMA SERUM.

By Harvey R. Gaylord, M.D., G. H. A. Clowes, Ph.D. and F. W. Baeslack, B.A.,

OF BUFFALO, N. Y.

PRELIMINARY REPORT ON THE PRESENCE OF AN IMMUNE BODY IN THE BLOOD OF MICE SPONTANEOUSLY RECOVERED FROM CANCER (ADENO-CARCINOMA, JENSEN) AND THE EFFECT OF THIS IMMUNE SERUM UPON GROWING TUMORS IN MICE INFECTED WITH THE SAME MATERIAL.

In the latter part of February one of us (Gaylord) visited Copenhagen and received through the courtesy of C. O. Jensen, Professor in the Veterinarian and Agricultural High School in Copenhagen, two white mice with actively growing tumors, inoculated from a strain of mice infected with adenocarcinoma, described by Jensen in the *Centralblatt für Bacteriologie*, Erste Abt., Vol. XXXIV. These mice were brought successfully as far as New York, but between New York and Buffalo both died. One of them was used on the day following death for the inoculation of twelve mice. The second mouse was placed on ice and on the third day following death the tumor was used to inoculate twenty-five white mice obtained from a source outside of Buffalo. All of the inoculations from the first mouse were unsuccessful. From the second mouse 60 per cent. of the inoculations were successful, thus giving us the material for further inoculation. From that time to the present we have succeeded in having constantly on hand a number of infected mice in various stages of the disease. Our transplantations were uniformly successful, the percentage of "takes" varying from 20 to 70 per cent.

In September and October we noted, for the first time in a number of mice that the tumors which had grown to a demonstrable size, ceased growing and underwent a form of spontaneous retrogression which terminated in the disappearance of the tumor without recurrence. Shortly after the observation of these facts a combination of circumstances resulted in our having, for a period of time, but a few available tumor mice. For this reason certain experiments in immunity which had been previously commenced were suspended. In the latter part of November the supply of mice was sufficient to resume the immunity experiments. In the meantime we had succeeded in getting a large number of mice in which the transplanted tumor grew with unusual rapidity and great virulence, showing no tendency to retrogression. For the purpose of determining whether the blood of the mice that had recovered spontaneously possessed any immunizing qualities, a series of experiments was carried out with the following results:

The blood-serum of mice which had recovered spontaneously from tumors possessed a power, when injected into mice infected with growing tumors of inhibiting the growth of large tumors and causing the retrogression of smaller tumors, leaving the animal possessed of an immunity which prevents recurrence of the growth. The degree of immunity in the mice thus far tested varies within considerable limits, the most marked illustration of its activity being found in one mouse whose blood-serum injected in a single dose of .2 c.c. caused the rapid retrogression and entire disappearance of two tumors in one animal and one in another, all of which were as large as peas, in the space of three days. The same serum injected into a mouse with a tumor the size of a small cherry (about two grams), caused a noticeable reduction in size of the tumor, which remained stationary for ten days, when an operation for the removal of a portion of it resulted in a return of activity to the growth. The latter part of this experiment will be dealt with in our final publication.

All of these experiments were controlled with mice inoculated at the same time, the tumors of which were smaller than those of the mice treated with the immune serum. These control mice received doses or normal mouse serum equal in volume to the doses of immune serum referred to above. In every case the tumors in the control mice developed rapidly and led in the course of three or four weeks to the death of the animal. In spite of the fact that the control tumors were invariably smaller than those used for the immune serum at the commencement of each experiment, in the course of a week or ten days the control tumors were found to be larger, and up to the date of making this announcement, while several control mice have died of their tumors, not a single mouse treated with immune serum has so far succumbed. In those cases in which the tumor was too large or the immune serum too weak to effect a cure, the marked retardation in the development of the tumor was always associated with a diminution in the cachectic symptoms invariably exhibited by the tumor mice in the last stages.

The second stage of our work has shown that the mice cured by injection with the immune serum referred to above, possess in like manner active immune qualities in their serum, which thus far have proved capable of causing the disappearance of small tumors and the inhibition of larger ones.

The test tube experiments carried out to determine the nature of this serum, and such information as we have been able to obtain as to the mechanism of its activity from sections of tumors inhibited and cured, lead us to the conclusion that in all probability we are not dealing with a cytolytic serum. We wish, however, to reserve our opinion until we have accumulated more data. Sections of tumors which have undergone partial spontaneous retrogression show that the changes in the epithelium are closely allied to simple atrophy. The connective tissue stroma of the tumor increases greatly in amount and in the last stages nothing is found but a connective tissue nodule with occasional pseudogiant cells produced by coalescence of the remaining rests of epithelium, similar to those described by Becker and Petersen as an evidence of spontaneous healing at the margin of cancer in human individuals. The changes in the tumors inhibited in growths show about the periphery a marked increase in the connective tissue stroma with extensive round-celled infiltration, characteristics which are not found in the growing tumors. At the margin of these tumors one finds an actual disintegration of cancer nests, atrophy of the epithelium, giant-cell formation and final disintegration. The remains of the small tumors, which have disappeared under the influence of the immune serum, consist of minute masses of connective tissue which in the later stages present the characteristics of ordinary organizing connective tissue. A tumor which received but one injection of immune serum from a mouse cured of a small tumor by the activity of serum from a spontaneously cured mouse and which decreased from the size of a small pea to that of a grain of rice within thirty-six hours, and which remained stationary for ten days, was found on examination to consist of a mass of newly-formed connective tissue surrounding the remnants of atrophied and disintegrating epithelium. In this case the evidence of disintegration of the epithelium was greater than that found in the tumors spontaneously recovered. A description of the histological characteristics will show that the changes in the epithelium are similar in principle, differing only in the rapidity of the process. The changes found in the spontaneously cured tumors and in those inhibited or cured with the immune serum, correspond to the changes already described by several authors as an attempt at spontaneous cure in human cancers.

A review of the literature shows that authentic cases of spontaneous cure of cancer in human beings are not unknown and the correlation of our histological findings with those already noted in man lead us to the conclusion that a similar immunity undoubtedly exists against human cancer. Although our work thus far has shown us that great difficulties will undoubtedly be encountered, it is perhaps not too much to hope that a careful analysis of the facts obtained in our experimentation on mice may ultimately lead to a practical application of these facts with a solution of the question of the curability of cancer in human beings.

SOCIETY PROCEEDINGS.

SOUTHERN SURGICAL AND GYNECOLOGICAL ASSOCIATION.

(Continued from Page 47.)

UNVEILING EXERCISES.

The monument erected by the Association to its founder, the late Dr. W. E. B. Davis, was unveiled in Capitol Park, with fitting ceremonies, Wednesday, December 14, at 11 o'clock. About five thousand people attended these exercises, including the members of the Association. After an invocation by Rev. Dr. L. S. Handley, Dr. Chas. M. Rosser, of Dallas, Texas, was introduced, and delivered the address of presentation. The statue was unveiled by Elizabeth and Margaret Davis, the little daughters of the beloved physician. Dr. R. M. Cunningham, Acting Governor of the State of Alabama, accepted the statue in behalf of the State in an eloquent address. The statue, in behalf of the city, was accepted by Hon. John C. Forney, the representative of Mayor Drennan, who was unavoidably absent.

The Management of Acute General Peritonitis.—Dr. J. Garland Sherrill, of Louisville, Ky., considered two forms of infection: (1) Acute septic peritonitis, in which the poison was so intense that the patient died from a profound toxemia before the local changes had progressed to the point of pus formation. (2) This type was general suppurative peritonitis, in which pus was found free in the peritoneal cavity without any localization of the process. The two forms resulted from infection following perforations of the alimentary canal, rupture of the urinary or gall-bladder, ileus, abdominal operations, puerperal infection, and disease of the ovaries and tubes. Many cases, especially of the septic type, resulted fatally regardless of the time they were seen or the treatment employed, while some responded to medical and more to promptly applied surgical measures. The various methods of medical treatment were considered, and the position taken that these cases were surgical, except where operation was refused and the patient's condition would not permit surgical interference. Under such circumstances the medical treatment should be planned with reference to the causative condition, if this could be determined, and a distinction should be made between perforations of the stomach and those of the intestine, and also those cases in which there was reason to believe the intestinal wall was intact. In the first, emphasis was laid upon absolute rest of the stomach to limit leakage; rectal lavage and nutrient enemata were advised. In the second class (intestinal perforations) gastric lavage, small rectal enemata to unload the lower bowel could be employed, and opium used freely while the patient was nourished per rectum. In the third class with an intact intestine, lavage, gastric and rectal purgation and nutrient enemata were recommended. Heat and cold were considered the best topical applications, and the patient's position should be suited to the location of the causative lesion. In considering the surgical treatment of this disease, much stress was placed upon early operation as a measure for the prevention of general peritonitis, while the process was yet localized. The outcome of a given case would depend upon the following factors: (1) The virulence of the infection; (2) the quantity of the infecting medium; (3) the resistance of the patient; (4) the activity of the organs of elimination; (5) the time at which the patient came to operation; (6) the rapidity and thoroughness of the surgical procedure. It seemed to the writer that the special technic of the operation was of less importance than the dexterity of the surgeon and the care with which he did his work. The author found that by flushing he could best free the peritoneum of infectious material, and usually drained. The patient should have the usual treatment given all abdominal cases.

Some Further Advances in Renal Surgery.—Dr. John B. Murphy, of Chicago, made a forcible plea for more conservative surgical work on the kidney and ureters in the future, saying that surgeons must consider the importance of preservation of any portion of a kidney that was still in a condition to functionate, on account of the enormous mortality associated with the removal of this organ. The mortality in the past following the removal of a kidney that was secreting practically the normal amount of urine varied from 29 to 35 per cent. He reported six cases of conservative operations on the kidney. In all of them the enlargement of the pelvis of the kidney was almost equivalent to, and in many instances larger than, the kidney itself. In cases of great dilatation of the pelvis of the kidney, formerly it was his custom to remove the kidney until he realized that it was practically a normally secreting

organ, and that the dilatation of the pelvis was due to ureteral obstruction, and that there was no good reason for taking out the kidney when the sac was removed, regardless of the position of attachment of the ureter to the sac, as this varied in every case. He believed in connection with surgery of the kidney, that surgeons were coming to a time when they would examine the kidney carefully, cautiously, and then decide, as in certain lesions of the stomach, that this or that portion shall be removed and the remaining portion husbanded.

Four Cases of Vesical Diverticula Requiring Operation.—Dr. Hugh H. Young, of Baltimore, Md., read a paper on this subject. He said that a patient died after obscure bladder symptoms, and autopsy showed seven diverticula, the largest about five inches in diameter, communicating with the bladder by small orifices. Both urethers were compressed by the diverticulum, and hydro-ureter and hydropelvis had resulted. The patient died of uremia. Since then the operator has had four cases of vesical diverticula where operation was advisable, and was performed with success in each case. In two cases the diverticula were larger than an orange, in the others smaller. In one case the ureter was compressed by the diverticulum and intermittent attacks of renal colic resulted. In one case the diverticulum lay in the urachus and became constricted at its orifice several times a week, producing severe tenesmus in the region of the umbilicus. In three of the cases the disease developed early in life, and in only one was an enlarged prostate the cause of the diverticulum. Careful study of the literature showed that only three cases had been operated radically, namely, one by Czerny—excision by transverse abdominal incision, transplantation of the ureter, development of pyonephrosis, nephrectomy, and final cure. One by Riedel, suprapubic incision, death from collapse. One by Pagenstecher, parasacral extirpation, resection of ureter, kidney involvement, result improvement, with fistula. The writer's four cases were all living and in good condition. In three cases the diverticula were completely excised, but ureteral transplantation was avoided by a plastic method. Renal infection was avoided, and no fistulæ resulted. Study of autopsy specimens showed that diverticula might be congenital or acquired, the latter due to obstruction, stricture or enlarged prostate. They developed most commonly near the ureteral orifices, and by pressure caused dilatation of the ureters and kidneys, and death followed from uremia. In many cases removal of an enlarged prostate or stricture was all that was necessary, but if the diverticula were large or pressed upon the ureters, or were congenital, and independent of obstruction, excision should be performed; suprapubic extraperitoneal, extravesical enucleation of the saccule, with suture of the bladder at the site of the diverticular orifice being the best method.

Ultimate Results Obtained by Conservative Perineal Prostatectomy in Seventy-five Cases.—Dr. Young also read a paper with this title. In this series there were 5 cases over eighty years, one eighty-seven years of age, with one death five weeks after the operation in a man aged eighty-four years. Two other deaths, neither attributable to the operation, occurred, each in the third week, one in a patient walking about and ready to go home, from pulmonary thrombosis, and the other in a man, seventy-seven years of age, who had been uremic for several weeks, and autopsy showed double pyohydronephrosis. The innocuousness of the operation was thus shown. The use of the author's double-bladed metal tractor was of great help in steadying the prostate for the incisions, drawing it down for a complete enucleation, enabling the operator to deliver and remove even large middle lobes without tearing away the mucous membrane of the bladder or urethra, or the ejaculatory ducts. The advisability of preserving the floor of the urethra, the vera montanum, and the ejaculatory ducts in men whose sexual powers were well preserved (and these represented over 50 per cent. of the cases), was shown by the impotence which followed in nearly all cases those operations like Albarran's and Murphy's, in which the floor of the urethra and duct were deliberately destroyed, and the results obtained in these seventy-five cases in which in a large proportion of them the sexual power and ejaculation were preserved, and even spermatozoa present in the semen afterward. The preservation of the prostatic urethra intact did away with the necessity of postoperative passage of sounds, greatly hastened the closure of the perineourinary fistula (all urine passing through the penis after the sixth or eighth day in many cases), and was possibly responible for the absence of incontinence, and the early establishment of normal urination. The frequent presence of epididymitis in Albarran's cases led to the routine ligation of the vasa deferentia in the groins after he had finished perineal prostatectomy by his method. The great rarity of testicle infection after the author's technic showed the advisability of not tearing away the terminal valvelike portions of the ejaculatory duct. The absence of mortality from the operation showed that the advantage gained by a nice exposure of the prostate by blunt dissection, through an inverted V cutaneous incision, and proper traction of the prostate by an intraurethral tractor with the consequent ability to enucleate the lobes without morcellement, and spare useful and non-obstructive structures—prostatic urethra, and ejaculatory duct—was well worth the slight addition to the length of the operation as performed by a blind, tear-out-what-will-come-out technic.

When Shall We Resect in Tuberculous Disease of Joints?—Dr. C. H. Caldwell, of Cincinnati, Ohio, read a paper on this subject. His judgment as to the advisability of resort to resection in a given case of tuberculous joint disease would be influenced by many considerations, and among them the following: (1) The joint itself, its anatomy and general characteristics. (2) The part it bore as a weight-bearer. (3) The degree of disability incurred by its involvement. (4) The relation of the joint to surrounding soft parts (its accessibility, and the readiness with which it admitted of grainage. (5) The degree of severity and progress of the disease as influenced by the function of the joint. (6) The results to be expected from conversative treatment. (7) The results to be expected from excision. (8) General considerations. As to the joint under consideration, somewhat would depend on whether it was a single large isolated joint, such as the knee for instance, or whether it be a smaller joint, such as the carpal or tarsal, in immediate continuity with other joints. A single tuberculous focus in the epiphysis of a long bone which was susceptible of complete immobilization stood a much better chance to undergo reparative change than would such a focus in the spongy bones of the wrist in the close proximity of synovial and ligamentous structures which favored dissemination and persistence of the disease. To this close approximation of the surfaces primarily affected in these joints, he was inclined to attribute the frequent resistance of disease in the elbow joint even when completely immobilized, and in the hip, where traction was not carried to the point of distraction of the diseased surfaces. Only when direct traction in the latter instance was supplemented by lateral traction was it at all likely that distraction of these surfaces occurred. In the

case of the elbow, he knew of no method by which distraction of the surfaces of the sigmoid cavity of the ulna and the inner condyle of the humerus could be effected. Taking it for granted that the vast majority of cases of joint tuberculosis had primary epiphyseal bone lesions, there was but little doubt that could we but see these cases before the stage of fibrillation of cartilage, a condition which preceded erosion for some time, conservative treatment might be sufficient to effect a cure. The part which a joint played as a weight-bearer, or the degree of pressure to which it might be subjected in manual occupations undoubtedly influenced greatly the development of the disease. The absence of both factors, weight-bearing and pressure, accounted for the comparative immunity of the shoulder-joint. In disease of joints at the upper extremity, immobility and protection might be effected with but little difficulty, and the disability was such only as was incurred by the disease of the limb. The result to be expected from conservative treatment might be divided into three classes—ideal, satisfactory, and unsatisfactory. An ideal result was where after a reasonably long period of treatment a cure was obtained with no limitation or but slight limitation of movement, and no deformity. Under satisfactory results might be classed those which after a reasonable period of treatment were cured with a stiff joint, or one in which a slight range of motion was possible, without shortening or malposition, and in which if there had been abscess or sinus formation, the sinuses had healed. Under satisfactory results might be classed those which after a reasonable period of treatment either showed no tendency to get well, or might be said to have recovered with sinuses still weeping, with a tendency to fatigue on exertion, with more than an average amount of shortening, and with deformity to a greater or less degree. The absence of any active symptoms of disease, pain, increased temperature or muscular rigidity, placed these in the category of cured cases, but cured with unsatisfactory results. The results from the resection of the hip were of necessity unsatisfactory when complete, as with ablation of the head and neck of the femur, one left no point d'appui for the femur, and there must be a greater or less amount of give to it under the weight of the body. It was questionable whether resection of the hip should be undertaken except in cases of rapidly destructive epiphysitis of the femur, with possible or present involvement of the acetabulum; cases of abscess of an acute and painful nature associated with high temperature; and cases of chronic abscess which failed to get well after repeated aseptically conducted aspirations when there were obstacles to the proper drainage of the joint, such as acetabular complications, the presence of a detached head, or gelatinous tuberculous débris. The great objection to the operation in any case was the difficulty of removing all affected structures, and the unsatisfactory prosthetic results. In tuberculosis of the knee one was confronted with an entirely different problem. There was but little use of wasting time with a knee-joint in which marked osseous changes were already present, and which in spite of conservative treatment over a period of six months had shown no improvement. Resection of the knee in cases which had passed the period of adolescence had much to recommend it and but little could be said against it. In those cases too prolonged delay often meant amputation. As to resection in elbow cases, one was again confronted by the fact that results were at the best far from what one might desire. In the smaller joints, such as the wrist and carpal joints, excision must depend on individual judgment. Ankle joint and tarsal excisions were, s a rule, very unsatisfactory. The deficiency in weight-earing capacity rendered the results far more gratify-ig, and amputation was, as far as his observations rent, too frequent a sequel to these operations. Several kiagrams were exhibited, illustrating the tuberculous joints, and the results of resections.

Obliteration of the Stomach by Caustic.—Dr. Samuel J. Mixter, of Boston, stated that doubtless other urgeons had seen cases of constriction of the esophagus fter the ingestion of acid or strong alkalies, and also jome cases of constriction of the pylorus from the same aause. It was very rare, however, to find practically ne whole stomach destroyed, and this was the reason or putting the cases he had seen on record. He reorted three cases in which the stomach was almost enrely obliterated by caustics.

Vaginal Cæsarean Section.—Dr. C. Jeff Miller, of lew Orleans, read a paper on this subject, in which he eported a case and summed up the advantages of the nethod as follows: (1) In severe eclampsia, when the roman is unconscious between the convulsions, the cerix rigid and elongated, and delivery imperative, it i always preferable to abdominal section, and, under roper surroundings, may be preferable to metal dilators r manual dilatation. (2) In severe cases of accidental emorrhage, when the cervix is closed, it is safer than ne other method of accouchement forcé, owing to the apidity with which the uterus can be emptied, and nould be given preference over abdominal hysterectomy, *hich is generally advised. (3) It may be considered n other conditions where Cæsarean section is indicated, xcept in contracted pelvis or dystocia, arising from naternal or fetal disproportion. It has not the disadantages of an abdominal operation; the peritoneum eed not be opened unless hysterectomy is to be preerred for malignancy, and there is less shock than jllows abdominal operations. (4) It is not more danerous than attempting to deliver either by version, or orceps, when the os is not fully dilated, if done under trict aseptic precautions.

Dermoid Cysts and Fistulæ of the Sacrococcygeal tegion.—Dr. Lewis C. Bosher, of Richmond, Va., uring the past few years had had occasion to operate n seven cases of dermoid cysts or fistulæ of the sacrooccygeal region. The patients sought relief either on ccouut of the presence of annoying exudation or after jome traumatism had given rise to the formation of bscess, with the usual train of inflammatory symptoms. he cases operated on by the writer were all in male dults. After referring to the diagnosis and prognosis, ne author said that the usual methods resorted to for reating inflammatory fistulous tracts would seldom esult in permanent cure. Complete extirpation of the stula and sac must be performed to prevent a recurence. It was to be noted that this was not always possble, as in a case reported by Wette, where complete xtirpation would have involved opening the spinal anal, with serious injury to the nerves.

Hematoma of the Ovary.—Dr. Magnus A. Tate, f Cincinnati, Ohio, in a paper on this subject presented study of the cases which he had collected from the terature. These cases showed that three periods of fe markedly predominate as a predisposing factor in ne causation of hematoma of the ovary: (1) Before r during birth; (2) At or near the first menstrual flow; 3) Early adults or child-bearing period. In studying nis variety of cases collected, he presented a few facts f importance. Klob had stated that in frequency the ollicular variety was by far the commoner. Scott, in perating for ovarian disease, stated that hematomas rere frequently found. In this the author concurred

and did not believe that hematomas were so rare as the paucity of case reports in literature would lead one to believe. Hemorrhage might collect in small dark patches or he so diffuse as to destroy the parenchyma or even the ovary itself. In size, hematomas varied from that of a hazelnut to a good-sized orange. In no case reported was a diagnosis positively made before section, except the one reported by Edebohls, and this diagnosis was questioned by everyone who took part in the discussion. The cases uncomplicated were free from fever, but pain was almost a constant symptom. Vaginal examination disclosed almost constant tenderness. Sometimes the ovary was fixed, and the pain frequently severe. Schultze and Riedel reported hematomas in newborn infants. Winckel saw the follicular variety of hematoma following petroleum burns, phosphorus poisoning, typhoid fever, cerebral hemorrhage. tuberculosis and heart failure. Edgar reported a case where the hematoma ruptured and caused a pelvic hematocele; and Boldt a case where the hematoma ruptured and peritonitis resulted. Two cases of hematoma were reported in which the hematomas became cystic and had twisted pedicles. Garrigues gave the history of a case associated with vicarious menstruation; Janvrin, a case of dysmenorrhea where on section there was salpingitis of both tubes, abscess of right, hematoma of left ovary; and Murray, a case of abscess of left ovary and hematoma of right. Kramer reported a case associated with purpura and epilepsy; and Edehohls, one where hysteroepilepsy complicated. Wylie had a case where electricity was the probable cause. Tate, a case following a long, tedious labor; Reamy, one where one ovary was removed and a portion of the other, and subsequently the patient had two children. Ricketts reported one associated with a large ovarian tumor, one with a dermoid, one with a suppurating appendix, one where the left hematoma was removed, the right being normal, and in one year later the right ovary had to be removed for a hematoma. Wenning operated upon a case of double hematoma, the patient suffering from excruciating pain when an examination was made. The age of child-bearing women who were afflicted with hematoma of the ovaries varied from fifteen to forty years, and the left ovary seemed more affected.

Pathogenesis and Surgical Treatment of Tuberculous Peritonitis.—Dr. William E. Stokes, of Salisbury, N. C., after dwelling on the pathogenesis, divided tuberculous peritonitis into four forms—the adhesive, suppurative, tympanitic and ascitic. He quoted extensively from the literature of the subject, referred to the modes of infection, gave synopses of cases, histological examinations, and reported six cases. After describing the surgical technic, he said that operation was contraindicated in cases of tuberculous peritonitis, whenever there was an advanced tuberculosis of the liver, lung, kidney, intestines, glands, or when the exudate within the peritoneal cavity was solid. What the actual changes in this infection of the peritoneum were, or what reaction was brought about in the local lesions and the peritoneum itself by the mere abdominal incision, remained problematical. Was it the mechanical action brought about by the air and sunlight; the increase of the peritoneal resistance, or whether after the operation a local reaction in the periphery of the tuberculous nodes took place, or an increased phagocytosis brought about absorption of the tuberculous product, with the formation of new connective tissue, as had been shown in experiments on animals, still remained unsettled. However, through this process, it was claimed that a local reaction was thereby induced, and the absorptive power of the peritoneum increased.

Treatment of Uterine Bleeding.—Dr. H. J. Boldt, of New York, read a paper with this title, in which he supplemented his former report on the use of stypticin, the name applied by its introducer, Dr. Martin Freund, to cotarnine hydrochlorate, in various cases of uterine hemorrhage, his opinion of the therapeutic value of this agent being based on seven years' experience with it. He first briefly described stypticin, which was a base obtained from narcotin by oxidation. It occurred as a micro-crystalline yellow powder, was soluble in water, and had an intensely bitter taste. A resumé of its physiological action followed. The author then cited a number of cases in which he used stypticin with marked effect, and gave also those in which it was ineffective. In 35 cases of fibromyomata, 11 were more or less benefited, while 24 were not. In one case of excessive menstruation due to an interstitial fibroid, the relief was very marked. In nine cases where hemorrhage was due to cancer of the uterus, the result was negative. Complete cure· followed in from two to six days in five cases of postpuerperal bleeding after removal of retained placenta particles. In conjunction with curetting stypticin was found effective in hyperplastic endometritis, but in the glandular form results were negative. In one case out of five of retroversioflexiouterus with endometritis, the menorrhagia was relieved without resort to surgical intervention. In chronic retro-endometritis, five of nine cases were more or less benefited. In various forms of noh-suppurative pelvic inflammation, only three out of 23 patients were not relieved by stypticin. In irregular bleeding during pregnancy stypticin had been found very beneficial, and no unfavorable symptoms had been noted. In profuse menstruation in virgins, without changes being found in pelvic organs, only five of seventeen patients were not benefited. In atypical bleeding during the climacteric period, if no pathological cause was found, stypticin usually gave a satisfactory result. The author remarked that while stypticin was not a panacea for all cases of uterine bleeding, he had found it better than any other remedy. In some instances it had practically served as a specific. If no effect at all was produced after three large doses had been given (from 2½ to 5 grains), it was useless to continue the drug. Likewise, in fibroid, it was not recommended to continue its use if two hypodermic injections of five grains each at intervals of four to twelve hours did not cause a diminution of the hemorrhage. An important fact was that the author had never noted any harmful results from stypticin, even when administered in such large doses as five grains every three hours. In some instances it also relieved the patients of pain associated with the profuse bleeding. In instances of too profuse menstruation, the author found the best plan was to begin with one grain doses, three times daily, about one week before the expected flow, and as soon as the flow began to let the patient take 2½ grains every three hours, to be continued during the entire period. In instances of metrorrhagia, from 2½ to five grains might be given at intervals of from two to three hours until the bleeding was lessened; then the dose might be decreased to from one to 2½ grains, at intervals of three to four hours. If a quick result was important, it was best to give three to five grains in a ten per cent. solution subcutaneously into the buttocks, using the customary antiseptic precautions. Because of the disagreeable taste of stypticin, it was best administered in the form of capsules, the pharmacist being ordered to put the powder dry into the capsule. It might, however, also be given in tablet form.

Some Points in the Technic of Aseptic Operating. —Dr. Henry T. Byford, of Chicago, in this paper said

he did not offer any new methods, but emphasized t necessity of more thoroughness in those already use The method he employed consisted in (1) twenty mi utes' scrubbing with green soap and water; (2) thr minutes' in dilute acetic or citric or oxalic acid; (five minutes in strong alcohol; (4) five minutes in ¹/₂₀₀₀ solution of mercuric chloride in water. T author considered the use of rubber gloves open to t objection of macerating the cuticle with danger of th· being punctured and allowing septic sweat to escaj He deprecated the mixing up of the steps of the prepai tion by using a combination of green soap and alcoh or by dissolving the mercuric chloride in alcohol, sin aqueous solutions were more efficient than alcohol He advised disinfection of the hands one or more tim during the course of long operations. Attention w called to the necessity of unusual care in the preparati of the field of operation in operations about the put and vulva. He recommended absorbent rather th occlusive dressings in the dressing of the wounds aft the operation.

Suprapubic Prostatectomy.—Dr. W. H. Dough· Jr., of Augusta, Ga., reported a case of suprapul prostatectomy, and described an improved method after-treatment. He also narrated an unusual case intraperitoneal hydatids.

Tracheotomy for Gunshot Wounds of the Trach· —Dr. J. McFadden Gaston, of Atlanta, Ga., discuss the subject of gunshot wounds of the trachea, and t complications that were likely to occur from septic inf· tion or laryngeal stenosis. He reported a case of gu shot wound of the trachea in a female child, eight yea of age. The position of the incision in the trachea w lateral rather than on the anterior surface of the win pipe. The patient made an excellent recovery.

Rupture of the Diaphragm.—Dr. Geo. S. Brow of Birmingham, Ala., contributed a paper on this su ject, in which he reported an interesting and instru tive case in a fireman, twenty-seven years of age, ; feet tall, and weighing 190 pounds. The patient h hurt or strained his side slightly about two years hefc the rupture occurred. Although an operation was p formed, the case terminated fatally.

Encephalomeningocele.—Dr. W. D. Haggard, Nashville, Tenn., reported an unique case of encepha meningocele, in a male child, four months of a Operation was performed July 16, 1902. The ch weighed six pounds. The tumor weighed five poun and measured 23 inches in diameter one way, and inches another. Dr. Haggard also described an e method of instituting peritoneal gauze drainage throu the cul-de-sac.

Dr. J. B. Murfree, of Murfreesboro, Tenn., read paper on Strangulated Hernia, and Dr. E. Dene Martin, of New Orleans, reported two cases of can of the appendix.

BOOKS RECEIVED.

Blood Pressure. By Dr. L. F. Bishop. 12mo, pages. E. B. Treat & Co., New York.

The Art of Cross-Examination. By Dr. F. L. W man. 8vo, 404 pages. The Macmillan Co., New Y·

Practical Physiological Chemistry. By Drs. J. Milroy and T. H. Milroy. 8vo, 201 pages. Illustra Longmans, Green & Co., New York.

A Manual of Experimental Physiology. By W. S. Hall. 8vo, 245 pages. Illustrated. Lea Brotl & Company, Philadelphia and New York.

A Treatise on Bright's Disease and Diabetes. Dr. Jas. Tyson. Second edition. 8vo, 381 pages. lustrated. P. Blakiston's Son & Co., Philadelphia.

THE MEDICAL NEWS.

A WEEKLY JOURNAL OF MEDICAL SCIENCE.

VOL. 86.   NEW YORK, SATURDAY, JANUARY 21, 1905.   NO. 3.

ORIGINAL ARTICLES.

PRECAUTIONS USED BY THE NEW YORK CITY DEPARTMENT OF HEALTH TO PREVENT THE SPREAD OF CONTAGIOUS DISEASE IN THE SCHOOLS OF THE CITY.

BY THOMAS DARLINGTON, M.D.,

COMMISSIONER OF HEALTH OF NEW YORK CITY.

THE medical supervision of the schools of the City of New York was adopted by, and has been under the control of, the Department of Health since March, 1897. The condition which led to the adoption of the medical inspection of schools was the frequent epidemics of measles, scarlet fever, and diphtheria among school children, sometimes of so great a degree as to necessitate the closing of an entire school.

During the month of October, 1896, an Inspector of the Department was assigned to investigate the part that the aggregation of children in the schools of the city played in the spread of contagious disease. The plan of the work was as follows: Those schools were visited from which cases of contagious disease had been reported to the Department; the classes where the sick children had been accustomed to attend were examined, and an examination made of all the children present. All children who were absent from this class, or even absentees from other classes of the school, were visited at their homes to ascertain the reason of their absence. The result of this investigation showed that a great number of these absent children were sick with contagious disease, and were directly infected in the school rooms, where conditions were favorable to infection, viz: heat, stuffiness, overcrowding, and the presence of contagion. Children continued to attend school while some member of the family was at home sick with contagious disease.

In cases of diphtheria, the child attending school might have been a little sick but not sufficiently ill to cause prostration; after a day or two at home it would return to school with slight sore throat, and when it was examined at the school and a culture taken from the throat, the bacteriological examination would show the presence of Klebs-Löffler bacilli. So also in cases of scarlet fever; cases would return to school desquamating after an absence of one or two weeks; it is related that one child amused himself and schoolmates by peeling the skin off his hands and passing it about the classroom for inspection. In such cases and in children's homes, numbers of cases of the disease were found to have developed directly traceable to schools.

The investigation of measles cases was conducted in a similar way,—that is, the homes of children sick with measles were visited, if other children of the family were attending school; the class which the patient attended was visited, all absentees from such classes were visited, and a high percentage of children sick with measles was found.

These facts were embodied in a special report and forwarded to the Board of Estimate and Apportionment by the Board of Health who at once appropriated a sufficient sum to appoint one hundred and fifty sanitary inspectors at the rate of $30 per month, assigned to the daily inspection of schools.

In March, 1897, these inspectors were instructed in their duties and to each inspector was assigned one or two schools. The duty of the inspectors was to report to the schools to which he had been assigned about 9:30 A.M. each school day, and examine all children whom the teacher had sent to his office in the school suspected of having any contagious disease. Any case of measles or scarlet fever was telephoned at once to the Central Office of the Department of Health, which case was visited at once by a diagnostician of the Department; further disposition of the case was according to the diagnosis of the diagnostician; if the diagnosis was confirmed, instructions were given at the home of the child to insure the proper isolation of the child during its illness; a postal was sent to the principal of the school which the child attended informing him of the presence of contagious disease in the family of the children, with instructions that all children of that family must be excluded from school attendance until the termination of the case, and that these children must not be readmitted to class attendance until the child could show a properly signed certificate that the premises had been properly fumigated, and, in the opinion of the officers of the Department of Health, were now free from contagion. If the children attend different schools, a postal card is sent out by the inspector to the principal of each school and course of procedure is the same as above described. If the diagnosis is not corroborated, the school inspector is notified, and the child ordered back to school. During the course of the disease, a district inspector has charge of the case. He will visit the case at its home at least once a week, and oftener, if for any reason he may believe that proper isolation of the case is not observed. On his first visit, the district inspector instructs the family in the method of proper isolation of the case and pastes a placard on the door of the apartment, warning all the occupants of the house or apartment of the nature of contagious disease in the family. He then visits every apartment in the building and informs the other tenants, verbally or by special card, of the presence of contagious disease in such a family on such a floor.

If the child is ill with contagion in the rear of a store or other place of business, either the store must be closed and no business transacted, or the child may be removed to the hospital, the premises fumigated, business resumed, and the other children of the family given proper certificates to return to school.

If, due to some perversity on the part of the people in evading the requirements of the Sanitary Law, the proper isolation of the case is not observed, as, for instance, the child is not kept in its own room, and is allowed to run out on the street or into public halls, or the store is opened for the transaction of business, or the placard is removed from the door of the apartment, a police officer of the Health Squad is assigned to the case. The officer puts up another placard and warns the people that a repetition of the offense will necessitate a removal of the case to the hospital. Forcible removal of a case is rather an infrequent occurrence.

If a child suspected of having diphtheria is seen at the school, the inspector in charge of the school is required to take a culture from the throat or nose and forward the same at once with special blank on which the following data is written:
1. The number of the culture—Whether the first, second or third. 2. The school number. 3. Date on which culture was taken. 4. Name of the child. 5. Address of the child. 6. Whether exudate is present in the throat. 7. How long sick. 8. Address, name, and telephone number of the school inspector. The child is excluded at once from school attendance until a report is received from the Bacteriological Division. These cultures are left at a culture station before 2 P.M. of the day on which they have been taken. The culture slips are made out in duplicate and both slips wound and fastened about their respective tubes. These cultures are later in the day collected by members of the Department assigned to that work and placed in the incubator over night. The next morning these cultures are examined and the slips reporting the cases are marked " L present," or " No L," or " Doubtful, another culture required." If the Klebs-Löffler bacillus is present, or the case is doubtful, the school inspector is notified, and the case is looked after by the district inspector. If the bacteriological report is negative, the school inspector is notified and it is the duty of the school inspector to visit the home of this child and order him back to school, provided, of course, nothing new has developed in the case.

Although this method of school inspection was superficial, depending for its efficacy upon the acuity of a school teacher for the detection of disease, nevertheless, a great deal of good was accomplished.

The presence of a medical inspector in the schools each day was a source of great reliance to the principals and teachers; whereas, before the advent of the medical inspector, a number of cases of doubtful nature would be allowed to continue in the class; these cases were now sent for diagnosis to the medical inspector, who always gave the school the benefit of doubt by excluding any case suspected of having any contagious disease.

To assist the principals in keeping record of all cases of contagious diseases existing in the families of the children attending the school, and reported to the Department of Health from all sources, a daily list of all contagious diseases is sent each day to each school in the city. This list is now arranged in districts so that the principal can see at a glance the residences and names of all cases reported to the Department, and from her knowledge of these children and their addresses she can at once send home from school any child from a family where contagion is reported. This is a most potent factor in keeping down the number of cases of measles, diphtheria and scarlet fever found in the public schools.

The method adopted by the principals is as follows: During general assembly of all classes, which is the first exercise in the public schools each morning, she reads off the names of all children reported ill with contagious disease who she thinks may attend her schools and inquires if any other members of the family are in school. Thus the first work of the principals and teachers is to exclude any possible carrier of contagion. Then the report of cases to the principal by the district inspectors' postal card insures other principals against the possibility of allowing a member of a family from a distant district to attend school and become a source of contagion.

The following table shows the results obtained by this system of school inspection in the Borough of Manhattan for the school year, September, 1897, to June, 1898, and school year September, 1901, to June, 1902:

	1897-1898	1901-1902
No. of school days.........	196	194
No. of schools visited......	294	266
No. of visits to schools....	45,754	47,679
Average attendance........	236,677	260,182
No. of children examined..	118,811	87,730
No. of children excluded...	7,086	9,703

Table showing diseases for which children were excluded:

	1897-1898	1901-1902
Measles	107	85
Diphtheria	138	94
Scarlet fever	28	34
Whooping cough	135	174
Miscellaneous	456	526
Contagious eye diseases......		3,470
Pediculosis of head and body..	4,163	4,125
Chicken pox	302	354
Skin diseases	483	841
(Miscellaneous includes croup, tonsillitis, mumps.)		

The work, however, was entirely unsatisfactory and it became necessary to devise some method of school inspection in which the physician had entire charge of the work and was held directly responsible for the condition of his schools.

Such a system was adopted and put in operation in September, 1902, and consisted in the regular morning and routine. inspection of the schools.

The schools of the city which were not numbered were given arbitrary numbers, and the site of each school was placed upon a map of the Borough of Manhattan. This scheme facilitated matters in assigning groups of schools to the inspectors.

The schools were so grouped that each inspector had under his charge about 5,000 children, whom he was required to inspect once a week. If the distance between his schools was considerable, the number of the children assigned to the inspector was less.

The following is a resumé of the rules governing the inspection of schools: Inspectors must visit all public schools assigned to them before 10 A.M. each school day. The first visit is called the morning inspection and consists in calling at the schools to inspect (1) all children isolated by the principal as possibly sick with some contagious disease; (2) all children who have been absent from school for a few days; (3) all children excluded from school attendance.

After the morning inspections have been finished the inspector returns to some one of his schools to make routine inspection. The routine inspection consists of a class to class examination of each child present. The inspector enters a class and stands with his back to a window and has the children pass before him. Under no circumstances is an inspector allowed to touch a child in a classroom. The children march by the inspector, pull down their own eyelids, and open their mouths wide. As the children pass, the inspector examines the eye, throat, hair and hands of each child. If a child is suspected of having any trouble which is not quite evident, the inspector orders the child to his office in the school for a more thorough examination. Children showing signs of measles, scarlet fever, diphtheria, smallpox, varicella, rötheln, whooping cough, mumps, acute catarrhal affections of eyes, nose and throat, are excluded forthwith.

Each child excluded from school is given a properly filled without exclusion card giving the name, age, residence of child, the number and location of the school. This exclusion card is given to the principal, who gives it to the child in a sealed envelope furnished by the Department of Health.

It may not be clear why the Department requires all exclusion cards to be put in sealed envelopes, but the following experience shows the wisdom of the procedure. Before this means was adopted, it was not uncommon to learn that a little " tot " excluded from school for pediculosis would run along the streets exultantly showing this card to all her friends thinking it a good ticket from school. Imagine the chagrin of the

parents when they read this card excluding their child from school for pediculosis capitis.

In cases of pediculosis, contagious eye diseases and skin diseases, the child is allowed to return to class and is excluded at the next occurring recess. The date on which they should return to school is marked on the back of the exclusion card.

Cases of measles and scarlet fever are telephoned by the school inspector to Central Office of the Department of Health and each case is visited by a special diagnostician of the Department for the purpose of verifying the diagnosis. If the case is considered a true case it is looked after by the district inspector. If false,—it is so reported to the school inspector, who visits the child at its residence and orders it back to school.

Daily reports are to be made out in duplicate. These reports state the school number, location of school, the number of children examined, the number excluded, and the time at which the inspector arrived at the school. One report is forwarded to the Central Office of the Department of Health for each school. At the Department of Health office the information on the report is transcribed to the card corresponding to each school in the borough. This card gives the number examined and excluded and the reason for exclusion of each child. The name and address of each child and reason for its exclusion is put on file card and filed away in chronological order behind the weekly history card for each school.

The inspector must ascertain from the principal the names and addresses of all children absent from school for a few days for no known reason. These addresses must be visited each day by the inspector to ascertain the cause of absence. There has been found by this means a great number of contagious diseases unreported to the Department of Health.

Table showing the number of contagious diseases found unreported, by visiting absentees, from November 2, 1903, to May 12, 1904:

Measles	561
German measles	107
Scarlet fever	70
Chicken pox	81
Diphtheria	19
Whooping cough	25
Mumps	24
Pneumonia	2
Typhoid fever	3

I believe that this rigid investigation of all cases of absence from school, and the discovery of unreported cases of contagious diseases thereby, together with the fact that this administration is very exacting in forcing observation of the Sanitary Code requirements from physicians in regard to reporting contagious disease, is the chief reason why there are on record so many more cases of measles, diphtheria, scarlet fever, etc., than ever before in the history of the Department of Health. I do not for an instant believe that the ratio of measles, scarlet fever and diphtheria, to the population, is any greater than it has been in other epidemics, but a more willing disposition on the part of physicians in general to report all their cases of contagious disease and the discovery of cases unattended by physicians at their residences by school inspectors, and the fear of discovery of cases if not reported by the physicians in charge, gives stimulus to physicians who otherwise might be negligent in reporting cases, and gives us at the present time the approximately true number of cases of contagious disease that have occurred in the Borough of Manhattan from January 1, 1904, to date. Tenement house inspectors find many cases of disease which they report to our Department for investigation.

I have here a table showing the results of this later method of school inspection for the year 1902 and 1903:

Daily attendance of schools...........	287,592
No. of school days....................	188
No. of schools........................	263
No. of visits to school...............	62,298
No. examined..........................	6,236,336
No. excluded..........................	41,826

Janitors and their families are not allowed to occupy apartments in school buildings.

Table showing the diseases for which children were excluded:

		True Cases
Diphtheria	510	416
Scarlet fever	45	22
Measles	168	94
Varicella	673	528
Pertussis	201	
Miscellaneous	4,728	
Pediculosis	8,676	
Contagious eye diseases......	25,264	
Contagious skin diseases.....	1,561	

On the first day of school there were turned out of schools some 1,886 children for pediculosis. The indignation was twofold: 1. Those whose children were excluded. 2. Those whose children were not excluded and who were indignant that such conditions were allowed to exist in the public schools where their children attended.

After a short time an investigation was required to ascertain what facilities existed in the schools for the care of children's outer garments. The facilities were not the best and recommendations were offered that each child would have a separate locker for its clothing or each child take care of its own clothing in his or her own desk. There has been some improvement in this regard but not enough.

Later investigations were made as to the means adopted by the school principals and teachers in caring for the writing and drawing utensils of the children. A number of cases of trachoma have been known to be contracted by putting pencils in the eyes.

The following form of blank, which was to be filled out and returned to the Central Office, was given to each inspector for each public school under his care:

School number.
No. of classes in school.
No. of classes using envelopes.
No. of classes using antiseptic pencil holder.
No. of classes using individual boxes or bags.
No. of classes in which each pupil has his or her own pencil; no collection or distribution at all.
No. of classes in which pencils are marked for identification but collected in a common box.
No. of classes in which pencils are collected and distributed indiscriminately each day.

The result of the investigation was astounding. Not 50 per cent. of the principals and teachers took the slightest interest or concern about the matter of sanitary precautions in caring for these utensils. Some of the teachers used in their own classes some up-to-date means of keeping each child's writing utensils separate. The cheapest and best means, and the method later endorsed by the Department of Health, was a large manila envelope, the face of which was marked with the child's name. The envelope was given out at the beginning of class, and the pencils, etc., of the child were handled only by the child itself, who removed the contents and replaced the same and clasped the envelope. These envelopes were then collected at the end of the class. It would be better to allow each child to place its own envelope in his or her desk and thus avoid any possible contact.

These envelopes were later furnished by the Board of Education to all schools, and all teachers were required to keep themselves supplied with them.

The old custom of sending a child to the home of an absentee to learn the cause of such absence was ordered discontinued.

School books at the homes of children who have been ill with contagious disease are always destroyed by fire.

Public library books, when at the homes of children sick with contagion, are disinfected before they are returned to the library. A daily list of all contagious diseases reported at the office of the Department is sent to each public library, whose authorities require from clerks an observance of these residences before books are allowed to be loaned out.

This list is also sent to Sunday schools throughout the city. The practical utility of this procedure, however, is very doubtful when you consider that these children congregate for only one hour once a week.

It is a fact worthy of mention that in those schools where the principals are alive to the up-to-date sanitary and hygienic precautions, the greatest welcome was extended to the medical inspection, and there also the medical inspector received the most interested cooperation.

It is evident from the tables here given that

this wholesale exclusion of children was not just right. The office of the department was besieged with mothers and children berating inspectors, and some funny stories are related of the experiences of inspectors with parents. A parent came one day to the office of the Department and said she thought the Department had gone crazy. Her child was excluded for "pediculus cap." The poor woman said she hunted in about six drug stores and they never heard of such a cap. Another one, an irate mother who thought she was imposed upon because she was a widow met the male inspector at the school and berated him very strenuously. Finally, as a culmination of her indignation she said, "Ye spalpeen, may you live to see your own children fatherless."

However, as much as the Board of Health bemoaned the fact that schools are depopulated, they still maintained it was their strict duty to exclude from school attendance any child found in a communicable condition and thus protect from contagion children who were clean.

In regard to acute eye diseases and pediculosis, it was decided that as long as the children could show signs that they were under treatment they might be allowed to attend class. Children with live pediculi were sent out at once. Cases of nits, for practical purposes, were considered non-contagious, while in the embryonic stage, and allowed to attend class as long as they shampooed the hair with kerosene and olive oil, followed by thorough washing and drying of the hair, and later, the application of hot vinegar to the hair to dissolve nit shells and then have the hair brushed with a stiff brush. A pamphlet with these instructions was given each child found with pediculosis and placed in the envelope.

The number that had to be excluded, however, was so great that they could not be attended by dispensaries and in private, and they could not get schools until under treatment. To overcome this condition, a nurse was loaned to the Department of Health by the Nurses Settlement to work in the school to see what might be accomplished. After a six weeks' trial it was decided that a system of school nursing could be advantageously established and would accomplish what was so desirable: the regular care of all cases of communicable condition, as pediculosis, conjunctivitis and skin diseases, while they attended school.

The nursing system was established in 1902. In the Borough of Manhattan eight persons were appointed for this work, who were under the immediate control of a supervising nurse.

The supervising nurses arranged the schools in groups and assigned the nurse to these schools. The supervising nurse was held responsible for the efficiency of the work performed and was required to visit each of her nurses at school at least once a week. Each nurse was responsible to the supervising nurse for the condition of her schools. She was required to keep a record of all cases treated by her at her schools; she was to visit at their homes all children excluded from

school when they did not return to school for reinspection on the day appointed by the school inspector; also to instruct parents in the proper way of caring for children's heads at home and thus clear up the sources of contagion.

The following cases are the ones that are attended by the school nurse: Pediculosis, conjunctivitis, ringworm, favus, molluscum contagiosum and scabies.

Definite rules are given to the school nurse as to how to treat these cases sent to her for treatment. The diagnosis is sent to the nurse by the school inspector and she treats the case as directed. Under no circumstances will a nurse treat a case of trachoma.

The supplies required for such treatment are furnished by the Department of Health on requisition to the principal of the school.

Table showing work performed by nurses in the Borough of Manhattan for the year 1903:

No. of treatments for pediculosis......	156,886
"　　"　　"　　" contagious eye diseases	106,257
No. of treatments for eczema.........	3,379
"　　"　　"　　" ringworm	8,498
"　　"　　"　　" scabies	335
"　　"　　"　　" miscellaneous (including favus, impetigo, molluscum contagiosum)	10,438
Total number of treatments...........	285,793
Visits to tenement houses.............	12,891
Visits to schools......................	11,098
Miscellaneous visits	293
Total visits	24,282

From January 1, 1903, to February 8, 1903, there were eight nurses, and one supervising nurse. From this latter date there were sixteen school nurses and one supervising nurse for the Borough of Manhattan. At the present time, there are nineteen school nurses in the Borough of Manhattan.

It was now evident with the nurses in the schools that the following ends could be attained: (1) A great reduction in the number of children excluded; (2) the obviation of any serious interference with the opportunity for the education of the children; (3) the eradication, if possible, of the source of infection of these school children by a visit to their homes and a demonstration of the means necessary to keep the family free from these conditions; (4) strict observation of all children excluded by the medical inspectors to see that they get and keep under treatment, and that they return to school and not become truants.

Now that the number of exclusions was reduced by the method described above, it was necessary to adopt some system of record by which all children who were found in the classes of the schools with some communicable condition could be followed and watched closely to see that the instructions given to them by the medical inspectors were observed. Such a system was adopted March 23, 1904, and known as the "card index system."

This system provides a card for each class in each school. It is identified by the school number, class number and room number. The name of each child found in a class room with any communicable condition is entered on the class card and the code number of the disease is called out to the teacher, who, seated at her desk, writes the child's name and code number of the disease on the class card. If there is a nurse assigned to the school, all cases, with the exception of trachoma, measles, etc., are sent to the nurse for treatment. Either from the class card or from a special piece of paper, the nurse learns the diagnosis of the physician and treats it according to the rules adopted by the Department of Health. All cases are treated and advised individually as it has been found that directions given to large numbers of children at a time, do not accomplish so well the desired end.

On the class card is put the date on which the child was ordered under treatment; on a subsequent visit to the class, the inspector calls out the names of all children ordered under treatment on a previous visit. Under the heading "Under Treatment," is put the date on which the inspector found the child under treatment. If the children can show no evidence of having had treatment it is excluded forthwith and is not allowed to return to school until readmitted by the school inspector, who requires some evidence that bona fide treatment has been established. When the child is admitted to school, the date of this event is put on the class card. Under the heading of "Remarks," is put the date of termination of the case and in cases of trachoma, whether an operation has been performed or not.

The code number of diseases is as follows:

1. Diphtheria.	12. Varicella.
2. Pediculosis.	13. Pertussis.
3. Tonsillitis.	14. Mumps.
4. Pediculosis.	15. Zero.
5. Ac. Conjunctivitis.	16. Scabies.
6. Pediculosis.	17. Ringworm.
7. Trachoma.	18. Impetigo.
8. Pediculosis.	19. Favus.
9. Zero.	20. Molluscum contagiosum.
10. Scarlet fever.	
11. Measles.	21. Ac. Coryza.

The reason for having more than one number for pediculosis and zero numbers is this: When the system was first adopted, No. 6 meant pediculosis. It was only one week after it had started when every child in the schools knew No. 6 meant pediculosis. Now each child as it passes by the physician in the classroom, is given a number. The teacher knows that "9" and "15" means "no disease." It was hoped by this means to confuse the children, but I believe the system should have been changed each week to fool the young American in public schools of the city.

Under this nursing and card system the number of excludable diseases is seven, viz: Diphtheria, scarlet fever, measles, varicella, pertussis, mumps and acute coryza.

For the quarter ending December 3, 1903, we have the following table of exclusions:

Measles	18
Diphtheria	140
Scarlet fever	13
Pertussis	61
Mumps	9
Trachoma	12,647
Pediculosis	8,994
Chickenpox	172
Contagious skin diseases	661
Miscellaneous	1,823
Total	24,538

Under the new system the cases that would absolutely be excluded are:

Diphtheria	140
Scarlet fever	61
Measles	18
Mumps	9
Chickenpox	172
Total	400

Therefore, the number of children allowed to continue attendance at school as long as they were recorded as under treatment each week, would be 21,138. Therefore, this system nullifies the charge that the medical inspection of schools causes truancy and illiteracy.

Each week, as far as possible, the classes are reinspected to see that treatments have been persisted in by the old cases, and to find any new cases. Under this system it is possible to find out, within 24 hours, just how many cases are under treatment in all schools, and the disease the case is treated for, and thus we can ascertain how much good is being done by this systematic care of children.

The following table shows the number of cases recorded on the school index card for the school year 1902 to 1903 and 1903 to 1904:

Census taken.	May 31, '03	Sept. 25, '03	Dec. 19, '03	April 23, '04
Diphtheria	42	2	0	24
Measles	37	3	2	33
Scarlet fever	4	3	1	2
Pertussis	38	4	9	5
Varicella	138	4	19	11
Mumps	426	3	27	7
Pediculosis	52,571	20,888	25,256	25,288
Trachoma	17,710	9,605	8,709	7,818
Acute conjunctivitis	3,066	2,364	2,642	2,074
Acute coryza	1	6	0	2
Scabies	82	56	53	51
Ringworm	602	181	353	542
Impetigo	238	180	403	227
Favus	39	14	51	51
Molluscum contagiosum.	21	14	20	57
Tonsillitis	457	39	31	21

After the first few months a condition arose which could not be anticipated. A number

parents were pleased that their children were excluded from school inasmuch as they could use them at home and they would neglect getting children under treatment that they might not be returned to school. This condition was ably met by the City Superintendent of Schools and District Superintendents of Schools, in conjunction with the District Attorney's office. An extract was made which is as follows: "Any parent who refuses to put its child under proper medical treatment that it may return to school is violating the compulsory educational law and is guilty of a misdemeanor punishable by a fine." A test case was tried and the parent of a child fined $10.

In the spring of 1902, some five oculists were appointed for the purpose of determining the prevalence of trachoma among school children. The report of these gentlemen showed that about 17 per cent. of the school children examined were afflicted with trachoma to some degree.

The regular inspectors were required to take special instruction in the New York Eye and Ear Dispensary for the purpose of becoming better qualified in the diagnosis of this special disease. Each inspector was required to spend two hours one day a week for two weeks. If it was found that the inspector made very many errors of diagnosis he was given another assignment at the Eye Dispensary.

The number of trachoma cases was so great and surveillance of these cases so rigid, that the children were excluded and not allowed to return to school until they could show evidence, either objective or by a card that they were under treatment. The result was that all the dispensaries and hospitals were so congested with trachoma cases that almost no other class of cases could be attended to. The authorities of the dispensaries and hospitals would not treat these cases. If they did treat them, the surgeons in charge would not take the trouble to stamp the cards showing that the children were under treatment and exclusion of the children would be continued by the inspector. This abominable state of affairs continued until the facts were brought before the Commissioners of Bellevue Hospital and Allied Hospitals. After some discussion it was decided to fit up the old portion of the Gouverneur Hospital as an Eye Hospital and Dispensary of the Department of Health. The following table shows the results of the work performed at the Trachoma Hospital for 1903:

No. of cases treated by operation..... 4,337
No. of cases treated without operation. 11,599
Total number of children treated...... 15,936
No. of visits made for subsequent treatment 129,830
Total number of treatments............ 145,766
No. of children examined not having trachoma 3,121

During the school months there were four operators and four clinicians, also two anesthetists. During the vacation months, the staff was reduced one-half.

The nurses were furnished to this hospital from the training school at Blackwell's Island.

When it is considered that these 4,337 operations have been performed under ether anesthesia, the fact that not one death or one serious accident occurred is a source of great gratification to the officers of the Department of Health.

Trial Cultures.—On January 10, 1903, the school inspectors were required to take cultures from the throats of all children showing the slightest redness and an hypertrophied condition of the tonsils. The following results were obtained:

No. of cultures taken.......... 11,451
No. showing Klebs-Löffler bacilli...................... 757
No. showing no Klebs-Löffler bacilli 10,376
No. showing doubtful bacilli.... 318

Total 11,451

Two inspectors are assigned to the work of vaccinating school children. The work is so arranged that each public school is revisited for the purpose of offering vaccination once in four years. Any child who has not been successfully vaccinated within these five years must be vaccinated. Physicians' certificates are accepted when they state definitely that the vaccination was successfully performed by the giver of the certificate on a certain date.

During the year 1904 there were performed:

BY MEDICAL INSPECTORS.
No. of visits to tenement houses..... 22,952
No. of visits to schools............. 55,293
No. of visits miscellaneous.......... 3,690

Total 81,935
No. of vaccinations performed, primary 16,952
No. of vaccinations performed, revaccinations 183,271

Total 200,223
No. of school children examined...... 8,261,733
No. of school children excluded....... 12,289

BY NURSES.
No. of visits to tenement houses..... 19,524
No. of visits to schools 16,155
No. of visits miscellaneous.......... 607

Total 36,286
No. of children treated.............. 515,505

There were 53 inspectors and 20 nurses.

Only very occasionally is a primary vaccination performed at the school. When it does happen it signifies that the vaccination performed so as to admit the child to school was not a "take."

No child will be accepted in the public schools of this City of New York unless it can show either a white certificate stating the date on which vaccination was performed or a yellow certificate to successful vaccination. This certificate is good for five years.

While the Department does not directly compel a child to be vaccinated, it does enforce the law that if the inspector in charge of the school deems vaccination necessary, the child must be vaccinated, or it will not be allowed to attend school.

All children vaccinated at school, of which about 90 per cent. are "takes," are furnished with a certificate of successful vaccination if reinspection of the arms shows the vaccination a "take." The efficacy and potency of this work, is at once manifest when it can be truthfully stated that not one case of smallpox occurred in a public school child during the severe epidemic of 1901 and 1902, in the Borough of Manhattan, although about 10 per cent. of these cases of smallpox were in children of school age, six to sixteen years.

I believe that as far as the medical inspection of schools, *per se,* can accomplish good results, the work, as conducted by the Department of Health of New York City, is obtaining its end, but there are so many considerations over which our Department has no control, as for instance: (1) The proper care of the children's outer garments at schools; (2) the proper aeration of the classrooms; (3) the proper lighting of the classrooms; (4) ample accommodation for each school child; (5) sufficient playground facilities; (6) establishment of baths in the public schools; (7) Examination and compulsory care of the children's teeth and oral cavities. Examination and correction of error of refraction. About 30 per cent. of 981 children examined showed refractive error in one or both eyes. (8) Correction of deformity of locomotive apparatus. (9) Exclusion of all nervous diseases from class attendance. (10) The segregation of children with inferior mentality.

I certainly do feel hopeful, however, that while all the good that we would wish for may not be realized in the present generation of school children for the reason that they, too, are powerless to change their environment, the labor bestowed upon them now will so dissatisfy them with their present condition and surroundings that they will demand and they must have, for no power can gainsay public indignation and dissatisfaction, better homes for the bringing up of their children and the latent pride that is in their breasts will become active and exhibit itself in the better hygienic care of their children.

Then, as far as bodily cleanliness and disease are concerned, there will be no lower classes. Education will have made us all equal and the purpose of medical inspection of schools established by the Department of Health in the City of New York will have been realized.

Western Hospital, Montreal.—The Board of Governors of the Western Hospital, Montreal, has decided to erect a three-story addition to that institution, for the accommodation of 36 extra patients. During the month of November, 1904, there were 44 patients in this hospital and there were 543 consultations in the outdor departments.

THE CYSTOSCOPE AS AN AID IN GENITO-URINARY SURGERY.

BY FOLLEN CABOT, M.D.,

OF NEW YORK;

VISITING GENITO-URINARY SURGEON TO THE NEW YORK CITY HOSPITAL; INSTRUCTOR IN ENDOSCOPY AND CYSTOSCOPY, NEW YORK POST-GRADUATE MEDICAL SCHOOL AND HOSPITAL.

IN this paper I do not intend to make an exhaustive study of the cystoscope and its various uses, but to touch upon different conditions in genito-urinary surgery when I have found it of value and also to refer to other instances where the contrary has been the case.

However enthusiastic we may be in regard to the cystoscope we must always remember that it is but one means of aiding us in this special branch of surgery. The various other methods should be used with as much care and thought as before. Consideration of the patient's past and present history, with study of the urine, microscopically, chemically and bacteriologically, may be of more aid than the use of the cystoscope alone. The condition of the urethra and bladder should be carefully considered before we attempt an examination of this kind. My rule is to prepare the patient for the cystoscope by preliminary treatment. By this I mean the use of sounds, washing out of the bladder, etc., before the examination. This preliminary treatment should be given at least a week before the cystoscope is to be used, and in many cases even earlier. It will accustom the patient to instrumentation and allow us to judge how he will react to it. In elderly people and in those who are highly nervous, rest in bed during this preliminary treatment is desirable. In chronic cystitis, thorough washing of the bladder is essential to a good cystoscopic view. Otherwise thick tenacious mucus will obscure the view of the bladder walls and ureteral openings.

Cystoscopy will never become an easily accomplished method of examination. Large experience, great patience and plenty of time are among the primary needs. Another question to be considered is the operator's eyesight. It must be excellent and in addition, to be unusually skilful with this instrument, he must have a perfect perception of color. The lack of this latter quality, I have become convinced in teaching others, is the frequent cause of failure to accomplish much with the cystoscope. A steady hand and freedom from all sudden moves while the instrument is in the bladder is of importance. I have frequently seen the object of the examination entirely defeated by the operator making useless movements in looking for the ureteral opening. Each motion should be prompted by reason and the fewer we have to make the better for all interests. In many patients cocaine is the source of much comfort and in a one per cent. solution I have never seen any serious harm follow its use. I usually introduce a soft rubber catheter, drawn off the urine from the bladder and then with a small syringe introduce about one-half ounce of a one per cent. solution into the bladder.

A little is placed in the deep urethra as we with-draw the catheter. Three to six minutes is allowed before the introduction of the cystoscope.

I do not intend to describe in this paper any particular variety of cystoscope. I have found the direct view instrument the easiest to handle and to teach to students. I believe though that the other type, the indirect view or angular instrument, should be understood by all of us who do much work of this kind. I have been using the Bierhoff instrument in my service at the City Hospital, and believe I shall find it an excellent instrument. In examining the prostatic region the angular and retrograde telescopes are necessary. For ureter catheterization I prefer the straight view telescope.

A word more before describing the various surgical conditons which to my mind call for a cystoscopic examination. I believe that we should try to fill the bladder with about the same amount of fluid each time. In other words, it should be carefully measured. My reason for this statement are, first, that the bladder varies in color and general appearance under varying amounts of fluid, and second, we can judge better of the amount of pressure necessary to fill the bladder. I try to place in the bladder about six to eight ounces. This amount cannot always be introduced, but we should at least measure the amount. I am convinced that a piston syringe is the best method of measuring the fluid. This matter is of still more importance when the patient is under a general anesthetic. Here it is quite possible to rupture a bladder by overdistention. Such cases have been reported. I have in mind one of my own cases where the bladder was adherent to neighboring organs and also contracted. By great care I avoided this complication but the bladder could very easily have been ruptured from too much pressure. The position of a patient during a cystoscopic examination is of importance. A table devised by Dr. Tilden Brown is an excellent one. The patient should be made as comfortable as possible while at the same time the ureteral openings and other parts of the bladder must be brought into view.

No exact rules can be laid down for the position of the ureteral openings. They vary very much in normal individuals. The amount of distention of the bladder also influences their relative position a great deal. We should always first study the mucous lining of the bladder and the ureteral openings. We can often gain much information by this careful inspection.

Let us now consider conditions in genito-urinary surgery where the use of the cystoscope is usually of advantage. 1. Calculus. If present in the bladder we generally find it without ·the aid of the cystoscope. However, in cases of encysted stone of the bladder, of stone in diverticula or sacculations and in other instances where litholapaxy has been performed, the cystoscope will sometimes be of service in detecting such stones or particles of stone.

If present in the ureter, they can frequently be detected by the aid of the catheter dipped in wax, after the method of Kelly. I have been experimenting for the past year with metallic sounds and catheters, and with these I believe I shall be able to detect calculi in the ureter and renal pelvis.

If the stone is in the renal pelvis we can often detect its presence by aid of the wax tipped catheter. The advantages of the metallic catheters I have just spoken of are, first, they can be boiled, and, second, since they are made of metal a stone can be more readily detected.

The X-ray will also have to be used in many of these cases and will often help in clearing up obscure points in the diagnosis.

Case I.—Man, aged thirty-seven years, complained of pain in region of neck of bladder, some frequency in urination. One month ago had attack of what was diagnosed as renal colic, right side. Five years ago a similar attack. Case referred to me by Dr. Schram. Rectal and urethral examination negative. Region of right kidney sensitive to pressure. I cystoscoped the man and passed a catheter into right renal pelvis; no obstruction. The urine drawn from this side was examined by Dr. H. T. Brooks, who reported as follows:

"I find no evidence of renal (parenchymatous) lesion aside from the hyaline and granular casts which, in my opinion, indicate rather an irritative state. The presence of large numbers of red cells (isolated) and much urates would, it seems to me, point to mechanical irritation (provided the hemorrhage was not caused by catheterization), and suggest a calculus."

I suggested that an X-ray picture be taken, but I have not yet heard of the result. In this case I took three separate specimens from this right kidney covering a period of one hour. I believe from my experience that the catheter should be left in place much longer where possible, say as long as six hours in some cases, the instrument being removed and the patient put to bed. In this way we avoid mistaking blood produced by the instrumentation for a pathological condition. The patients I cystoscope are given urotropin in full doses and occasionally sandalwood oil.

New Growths. Bladder.—The cystoscope is frequently of aid in detecting new growths in this organ. We must be extremely careful, however, in using this method of examination. Some large growths, of villous type, bleed freely and the bladder is often intolerant to instrumentation. I have in mind one case I saw in the City Hospital a year ago, where I was unable to inject into the bladder (even with the patient under a general anesthetic) more ·than two to three drams of boric acid solution. I tried adrenalin $1/_{5000}$ to control the hemorrhage, which was profuse, but with no effect. He refused operation. We must also bear in mind the danger of infection in these patients and be usually ready to operate immediate after an examination of this kind. In another case of villous growth of bladder, which occurred in a man, aged twenty-four years, and was referred to me by Dr. Buchler for diagnosis, I found a growth the size of a small peach atached by a single pedicle three-quarters of an inch long to the anterior wall of the bladder slightly to right of median line, an unusual position. Dr. Eliot removed it at the Presbyterian Hospital by suprapubic cystotomy. The examination caused no bleeding, as the instrument did not touch the growth. The view was so clear that even the contraction of the vessels could be distinguished. This man had been bleeding for two years and had received much treatment, but of course it did no permanent good. He was very anemic, had lost much weight, and was gradually getting worse.

New growths of the ureter I have not seen. But I have seen three or four cases of narrowing of the canal. In one case in which I was at first unable to introduce a ureteral catheter the patient had symptoms of hydronephrosis. These symptoms disappeared gradually as I dilated the ureteral stricture. This was performed once a week for six to eight times.

New growths of the kidney are not rare. I have seen several. In one, a man of sixty, the disease apparently was the result of a severe injury several years before the patient came under my observation. When I first saw him he had a tumor which half filled the right belly. In order to test the condition of the other kidney and determine the origin of the blood in the urine I catheterized both ureters. I found the left kidney healthy. The patient was operated on and the tumor was found to be adherent on all sides. It was removed but the patient died in a few hours from shock and loss of blood. Diagnosis sarcoma. The ureter was unobstructed. In the cystoscopic examination constant irrigation was necessary to keep the field clear. Adrenalin would of course have been useless as all the blood came from the kidneys.

In some instances we find pus in the urine and the three glass test shows that the trouble is not urethral. We have perhaps a cystitis chronic in character. The question arises, Is the pus entirely from the bladder or is it partly or wholly of renal origin? The microscope will help and will often clear up the diagnosis, but not always. I have had a young man, twenty-four years old, under my care; symptoms of vesical calculus at fourteen; operation suprapubic cystotomy two years ago, a large stone removed. Relief from all symptoms. Urine remained cloudy. Bladder washed out for several months three times a week for cystitis. No relief. Cystoscopic examination showed a practically healthy bladder but jets of pus coming from right ureter. No tubercle bacilli found in urine and he never had gonorrhea. Lavage of the kidney and pelvis has been considered but as the patient is improving on cod-liver oil, urotropin, etc., it has not yet been resorted to. The ureter is free, but no

X-ray picture has been taken of the kidney for possible stone. The *prostate* in connection with the cystoscope has received much attention. It has not helped me much in determining the size of the prostate or the presence of a so-called third lobe. In some cases I have been unable to use the instrument at all and in others I have thought it better not to. In a few cases of prostate hypertrophy it has been of service. In a man of fifty-four years, left kidney removed eight years ago; I did a perineal prostatectomy two months ago, after determining condition of the left ureter. I found it and put a catheter into it for nine inches. I did this because some of the patient's pain had been directed to region of old nephrectomy. The kidney when removed eight years ago by Dr. Lange was the size of a child's head. Apparently hydronephrotic. I found this left ureter stump healthy, so I removed a large prostate and the patient got absolute freedom from his old pain and urinary urgency.

In another case in which I did a suprapubic prostatectomy the cystoscope enabled me to diagnose a diverticulum which held eight ounces and had been caused by years of straining. The ureteral openings in the case were large enough to admit my thumb and directly back of the left one I found the opening to the diverticulum, which was about the size of a quarter. The whole bladder was tremendously hypertrophied and distended; capacity 32 ounces.

Foreign Bodies in Bladder.—The cystoscope is frequently of assistance in locating foreign bodies, particularly in the female. I have devised a forceps to be used in grasping a foreign body and removing it. In this connection I will refer to a curette I have devised for removing a piece of a new growth in the bladder and then with the forceps removing it for microscopical examination. In all kinds of surgery it is desirable to know the condition of the kidneys, but in operations on one or the other, the importance of determining the presence and condition of a second kidney is of great moment. I have not done enough lavage of the renal pelvis to be able to state definitely my views on the subject, so I shall say little about it. I believe, however, that it has a place and one of much importance. The kind of cases in which it will be of value is the point to determine.

In tuberculosis of the urinary organs the cystoscope is frequently of use, particularly in involvement of one kidney or the other. In some cases tuberculosis of the bladder may be determined in this way. I am inclined to believe, however, that in many tuberculous conditions, particularly of the lower genito-urinary tract, instrumentation tends to aggravate the condition and we should therefore use the cystoscope as little as possible.

In a considerable experience with cystoscopy and ureteral catheterization I have seen no severe symptoms follow its use. I think its dangers have been much magnified. I do, however, believe that it should be used in selected cases and with careful technic.

THE RELATION OF CHOLIN TO EPILEPSY.[1]

BY DR. JULIUS DONATH,

OF BUDAPEST, HUNGARY;
DOCENT AT THE UNIVERSITY OF BUDAPEST; CHIEF OF THE DIVISION OF NERVOUS DISEASES AT THE ST. STEPHEN HOSPITAL, BUDAPEST.

I.

IT has already been pointed out in a previous article,[2] that whatever the real cause of the epileptic attack may be, a mechanical factor can always be discovered. This may be a trauma affecting the skull, or a tumor of the brain which increases the intracranial pressure by its growth and thus irritates the cortex. The irritation may also be reflex in nature and act upon the periphery; to this class belong painful scars, neuralgias, errors of refraction, insufficiency of the internal muscles of the eye, iridocyclitis, affections of the nose, intestinal disturbances, worms, etc. In all these conditions, an increased irritability of the cortical substance and, consequently, of the psycho-motor area, is present. The same holds true for epilepsy of chemical origin whether of infectious (encephalitic processes, syphilis) or purely toxic nature (alcoholism, saturnism, uremia, eclampsia of pregnancy and probably also the eclampsia of children). It will be shown later that chemical irritation also plays an important rôle in the epileptiform attacks of paralytics and probably also in senile epilepsy. Despite its psychogenous origin, an increased irritability of the cortex is probably also present in the hystero-epileptic attack, especially when we consider that rigidity of the pupils and every symptom of genuine epilepsy may be present in transitional forms of this disease during the height of the attack, so that a differentiation is hardly possible.

In contrast with these forms of epilepsy, of known etiology, we have the large class of genuine or idiopathic epilepsy. In some these infectious or toxic influences are inherited, in others, hypoplastic or encephalitic processes are acquired during intra-uterine or early extra-uterine life. Up to the present, however, a constant and definite anatomical lesion has not been discovered. L. W. Weber[3] states in his recent important article, based upon 35 autopsies on epileptics, that the various lesions found by him (proliferation of glia tissue, fibrous thickening of the vessels, gradual disappearance of the nerve-elements, atrophy and sclerosis of the cornua Ammonis, in six cases; subependymal hemorrhages throughout the entire extent of the gray lining of the ventricle, in eight cases, etc.) must not be looked upon as the anatomical cause of epilepsy, but merely as lesions which predispose the tissues for the real epileptic changes. These latter are still unknown to us. He does not believe that the anatomical diagnosis "epilepsy" can be made at present, since the findings, particularly those of the cortex, are not sufficiently characteristic. to permit us to conclude that epilepsy has existed.

That very strong irritation alone, without increased irritability of the cortex, is quite sufficient to induce an epileptic attack, follows from the curability of traumatic epilepsy, if the cause is removed and from the fact that typical convulsions are seen if the animal brain is irritated experimentally by electrical, mechanical or chemical means. In genuine epilepsy, however, increased irritability of the brain is always present, but in addition to this, we must assume a second factor, which, though not necessarily active at all times, must certainly be present in severe and frequently repeated attacks. A healthy individual will experience no ill effects from a full meal or the ingestion of a moderate amount of alcohol, whereas the epileptic will react with an attack of convulsions since mechanical or chemical factors of slight intensity (normal toxic products liberated by the metabolic activity of the organism) have proven themselves quite sufficient to irritate the hyper-sensitive cortex. If on the other hand, the frequency of the attacks increases when irritation of any kind is carefully avoided, and in addition, the sensitiveness of the cortex is diminished by means of therapeutic measures, it is likely that some definite chemical substance plays an active part. Cabitto[1] discovered that the perspiration of epileptics is poisonous and Krainsky[2] proved the same thing for the blood. The latter author removed some blood before and during a status epilepticus, by means of wet cupping, defibrinated it and injected one to three cubic centimeters subcutaneously into rabbits. Periodical convulsions followed with paralysis of the hind limbs and death within four to eight days.

Roncoroni[3] found that the urine of the post-epileptic or intermediary stage was generally no more poisonous than the urine of normal individuals if injected subcutaneously or intraperitoneally into animals. The toxicicity was increased only in a few cases particularly in one epileptic where the intraperitoneal injection killed three animals and rendered a fourth one very ill. Convulsions, however, were never seen. Bratz[4] comes to the same conclusions. He extirpated the gyrus conciatus in a dog, in order to set up a scar in the brain and thus bring about an epileptic pre-disposition. Injections of urine or blood of epileptics obtained during the attack were never followed by convulsions or epilepsy but only by general symptoms of intoxication.

The cerebrospinal fluid protects the central nervous system against concussion, but probably also facilitates the removal of excretory products. Hence the chances of detecting a toxic substance here should be very favorable, provided one comes into play during an attack. Dide and Laquepe[5] injected the cerebrospinal fluid of epi-

1 Craig Colony Prize Essay.
2 B. Donath. Bestrebungen und Fortschritte in der Behandlung der Epilepsie, Halle a. S., 1900; also Psychiatrische Wochenschrift, 1900, Nos. 8 to 10.
3 L. W. Weber. Beiträge z. Pathogenese u. pathologische Anatomie der Epilepsie. Jena, 1901.

1 G. Cabitto. Riv. speriment. di freniatr., xxiii.
2 N. Krainsky. Allg. Zeitsch. f. Psychiatrie, 1897, X. p. 612. 1901.
3 Roncoroni. Archivo di Psychiatria. Ref. Neurol. Centralbl., 1901.
4 Bratz. Die Rolle der Autointoxication in der Epilepsie. Ref. Neurolog. Centralbl., 1901, No. 10.
5 M. Dide et E. Laquepeé. Notes preliminaires sur la toxicité du liquide cerebro-rachidien dans l'epilepsie. (Société de neurologie de Paris. Seance du 18 Avril, 1901).

leptics into the brains of guinea-pigs in amounts of 0.3-0.5 cubic centimeter; the fluid did not contain any particular cellular elements and was free from bacteria.

The fluid obtained during the intermediary period was not toxic, but if withdrawn after a number of attacks one-fourth cubic centimeter generally set up intense general convulsions, while half a centimeter killed the animal in a few hours, sometimes even in a few minutes. If the fluid was injected after a single epileptic attack, less severe symptoms were observed, such as lassitude, numbness, occasionally a few general twitchings. The cerebrospinal fluid of epileptics was also found highly toxic by Pellegrini,[1] especially if it was withdrawn directly after an attack. If injected into guinea-pigs, convulsions were observed by this author.

Stimulated by these observations a thorough chemical and microscopical examination of cerebrospinal fluid obtained by means of Quincke's lumbar puncture was made and it was generally found to contain cholin in epilepsy. Animal experiments have then convinced me that this cholin is chiefly responsible for the convulsions.

Mott and Halliburton[2] have discovered this alkaloid in the blood and cerebrospinal fluid in diseases of the nervous system which are accompanied by breaking-down of nervous tissue, particularly in general paresis and tabes, combined sclerosis, disseminated sclerosis, alcoholic polyneuritis, beriberi and after the experimental division of both sciatic nerves in cats. They believe that the cholin results from the decomposition of lecithin, which is set free as the medullary sheath disintegrates. It was identified chemically by extracting the blood[3] with alcohol and then converting it into its double salt with platinum, which crystallizes in the form of octahedra from a saturated solution in 15 per cent. ethylalcohol.

The physiological test was also resorted to for verification: the residue of the alcoholic bloodextract dissolved in physiological salt solution and injected into the external jugular vein of cats, dogs and rabbits, diminished the bloodpressure chiefly by dilating the visceral vessels.

Mott and Halliburton also found that the cerebrospinal fluid of paralytics contained three times the normal amount of albumin and some nucleo-albumin, which does not occur in health. The latter is supposed to come from the broken-down Nissl bodies.

I shall now give an account of my own investigations of the cerebrospinal fluid, chiefly of epileptics and of the animal experiments which I made with cholin.

II.—EXAMINATION OF THE CEREBROSPINAL FLUID FOR CHOLIN IN EPILEPSY AND SOME OTHER DISEASES.

After many preliminary experiments, the following method was adopted: The cerebrospinal fluid is carefully collected in sterilized test tubes. The slightly alkaline fluid is rendered weakly acid with dilute hydrochloric acid and then evaporated to dryness on the water-bath. Owing to the precipitation of albumin, the fluid will froth and become slightly turbid. The residue is always dark (orange-yellow up to dark-brown) even though the fluid was usually clear as crystal and did not contain any blood. In the presence of the latter, the residue will be black. This change in color probably depends upon the presence of an easily oxidizable substance which has not yet ben definitely isolated. The residue is now extracted with alcohol which must be absolutely free from water if the experiment is to succeed. The absolute alcohol does not dissolve the chlorides of sodium, potassium and ammonium which are always present, but only the hydrochlorate of cholin. If platinum chloride, also dissolved in absolute alcohol is now added to this alchoholic extract, the chloroplatinate of cholin will precipitate out. This can be identified by two important properties: (1) Its easy solubility in cold water as contrasted with the very slight solubility of potassium and ammonium platinochloride and (2) its very characteristic form of crystallization. The crystals are usually serrated and lanceolate or leaf, wreath or rosette-shaped, the latter with three or four leaves. Occasionally one meets with radiate needles or needles arranged in sheaves (obliquely cut prisms) or hexagonal or rhombic plates. They are generally tinged yellow, but if very thin (particularly the needles), appear colorless. The crystals are best obtained, by allowing a few drops of the aqueous solution to evaporate on a slide. The alkaline platinochlorides can be easily detected by the presence of octohedra or tetrahedra, which may have blunt angles. With the above method not even traces are seen. Absolute alcohol will thus completely separate cholin from the alkalies[1] while 99 per cent. alcohol will not suffice.

The above reactions are more practical than those mentioned by Mott and Halliburton. If the chloroplatinate of cholin is crystallized from 15 per cent. alcohol, the serrated leaf or rosette-shaped crystals mentioned above, will always be found together with the incomplete octahedra. If the precipitate of chloroplatinate be dissolved in hot 15 per cent. alcohol, further reactions for octohedra can be made.

1 R. Pellegrini. La tossicita del liquido cerebrospinale negli epilettici. Riforma medica, 1901, No. 55.
2 Mott and Halliburton. The chemistry of nerve degeneration. The Lancet, April, 1901.
3 They generally isolated the cholin from blood obtained by venesection; less often they employed cerebrospinal fluid from the cadaver and only rarely fluid obtained by lumbar puncture from the living.

1 I have convinced myself by two experiments, that by means of alcohol dehydrated by anhydrous copper sulphate and kept over this substance, one can completely separate cholin chloride from potassium and ammonium chloride. (a) 0.1675 cholin chloride, together with some potassium, ammonium and sodium chloride were dissolved in 50 c.c. of water. The alcoholic extract precipitated with platinic chloride 0.3355 gm. cholin platinochloride corresponding to 0.1521 cholin chloride. On microscopical examination, no octohedra, but only forms characteristic "for cholin" were found. (b) In another experiment 0.0707 cholin chloride, gave 0.1534 cholin platinochloride, corresponding to 0.6955 cholin chloride.

Another delicate reagent for cholin in aqueous solution is phosphowolframic acid. In dilute solutions, a white precipitate will form which appears under the microscope as small hexagonal plates or rhomboids. Chloride of potassium and ammonium will also give precipitates with phosphowolframic acid, hence the extract in absolute alcohol should be filtered, the alcohol evaporated and the residue dissolved in water. Less delicate reagents are potassiomercuric iodide (sulphur-colored or greenish-yellow precipitate) iodopotassic iodide (dark-red, flocculent precipitate). Both precipitates are easily soluble in an excess of either reagent. The delicate physiological test—fall of blood-pressure after intravenous injection—is usually not necessary.

All attempts to discover some characteristic color-reaction for cholin such as are found for the vegetable alkaloids, have failed. This is not surprising in view of the fact that this body belongs to the fatty compounds with low percentage of carbon.

Owing to the fact that the alcohol employed during the first experiments was not absolutely free from water, some chloride of potassium and ammonium was also taken out, and formed compounds with platinum chloride whic! d, however, be detected by the presence of ' ·dra.[1]

Since the platinochloride of cho... is entirely insoluble in absolute alcohol, a quantitative test is possible. Mott and Halliburton[2] claim to have detected cholin in about 20 c.c. of blood obtained by venesection from a case of beriberi, by treating the blood with alcohol, drying the filtrate at 40° C., dissolving the residue in physiological salt solution and then observing a fall of blood-pressure on injecting the solution into the external jugular vein of cats. According to my own observations, there can hardly be any doubt that the alcoholic extract of the blood contained some potassium and possibly also some ammonium salts besides the cholin. We know that potassium salts when injected into the circulation behave like cholin in that they first raise the blood-pressure, and then lower it, while ammonium salts raise the blood-pressure. The presence of these salts is therefore apt to interfere with the accurate determination of pressure.[3]

1 Before the separation by means of absolute alcohol was used, experiments were made with gold chloride instead of the platinum salt. It is well known that the double salts of gold with potassium and ammonium are readily soluble and thus do not contaminate the precipitate. On the other hand, the cholin-gold chloride is readily reduced and is not insoluble in alcohol, so that a complete separation is impossible and traces escape detection. Phosphowolframic acid is excellent for qualitative but not for quantitative work, owing to the complicated process necessary to isolate cholin from its combination.
2 Mott and Halliburton. Notes on the blood of a case of beriberi. Brit. Med Jour., July 29, 1899.
3 In an article received after this paper was finished, Mott (A discussion on the pathology of nerve-degeneration, Seventieth Meeting of the British Medical Association, Manchester, 1902) avoids this error by separating cholin from the alkalies of the blood according to the following method: The blood is treated with six to eight times its volume of absolute alcohol, filtered and dried at 40° C. What remains is extracted three times with absolute alcohol, filtered and evaporated. The alcoholic solution of the residue is precipitated with 10 per cent. alcoholic platinum chloride and the precipitate decanted from absolute alcohol. The precipitate is finally dissolved in 15 per cent alcohol, filtered and evaporated in a watch-glass at 40° C. with low magnifying power, the octohedral crystals of platinochloride of cholin may be seen. Five c.c. of normal human blood only rarely give rise to such crystals so that the result is practically negative.

In the following, I shall give an account of my examinations on cerebrospinal fluid. The lumbar puncture was done for diagnostic or therapeutic purposes. In the former case, the collected fluid was centrifuged and then examined for cellular elements and bacteria. Cultures were also made and one of my pupils will shortly report on this work. The therapeutic indication consisted in diminishing the increased intracranial pressure or in removing the toxic excretory products during repeated epileptic attacks or to supply drainage for the infected liquor in acute infectious forms of meningitis or encephalitis. In epilepsy, the fluid was withdrawn soon after the convulsions. Lumbar puncture was thus performed altogether in 80 cases under strictly aseptic precautions and no accidents were observed. Rise of temperature never followed, but headache, lasting several hours up to two days, was regularly complained of, especially if the fluid was permitted to flow out rapidly or in larger quantities. This headache is, however, easily treated by several doses or morphine (up to one centigram) or dionin (up to two centigrams).

The cerebrospinal fluid was generally absolutely clear and only rarely slightly discolored by blood. Slightly turbid fluid was obtained in cases of meningitis basilaris tuberculosa, meningo-encephalitis gummosa and abscessus cerebri; very turbid fluid in one case of meningitis after purulent otitis.

The quantities obtained usually varied between 12 and 85 c.c. In one case only 5 to 6 c.c. of a bloody fluid could be withdrawn. Rarely even repeated punctures at different levels of the lumbar vertebral column, were unsuccessful even though the needle reached the subarachnoidal space. Possibly the cauda equina is in the way, in these cases.

For the qualitative test for cholin, 10 to 20 c.c. were employed; for quantitative estimation, at least 30 c.c.

From Table I it follows that in 18 cases of genuine epilepsy, cholin was found 15 times;[1] in three cases of Jacksonian epilepsy, three times;[2] in one case of syphilitic epilepsy, once; in three cases of dementia paralytica, twice; in two cases of tabo-paralysis, once; in 15 cases of tabes dorsalis, 10 times; in three cases of lues cerebralis, three times; in two cases of tumor cerebri, twice; in two cases of abscessus cerebri, twice; in one case of encephalomalacia, once; in one case of hydrocephalus chronic, once; in one case of sclerosis cerebrospinalis multiplex, none; in one case of spina bifida, once; in one case of compression myelitis, once; in one case of polyneuritis alcoholica, once; in one case of coccygodynia, none; in three cases of neurasthenia, once; in two cases of hysteria, none; in three cases of hystero-epilepsy, once.

It is a significant fact that in genuine, syphilitic and Jacksonian epilepsy cholin was found as frequently (in 19 out of 22 cases), as in organic

1 Five patients were punctured two or three times, making a total of 11, with 9 positive results.
2 Among these, lecithin was found once.

TABLE I.—CEREBROSPINAL FLUID.

No.	Name.	Diagnosis.	Amount of Cerebrospinal Fluid withdrawn in c.c.[1]	Microscopical Examination		Cholin ($C_5H_{15}NO_2$) Percentage[2]	Remarks.
				of Platinumsalt.	of Precipitate with Phosphowolframic Acid		
1.	N. N.	Hydrocephalus chronicus		Needle and rhombic prisms.			
2.	Rosa V.	Epilepsia genuina...	57	Serrated crystals.			
3.	"	" ...	32	Serrated, simple, 3 and 4-leaved crystals and hexagonal crystals.			
4.	Joseph K.	Tabes dorsalis (Crises gastriques)	54	No cholin found.			
5.	Stefan N.	Epilepsia genuina...	23	Serrated and 3-leaved crystals.			
6.	Alexander H.	Epilepsia Jacksonia..	36	Serrated crystals (fig. 2)			
7.	"	" ..	60	Lecithin platinum chloride-round, concentrically layered bodies[4] like starch grain.			
8.	Joseph N.	Epilepsia genuina...	52	Serrated, 3-leaved and hexagonal crystals.			
9.	"	" ...	33	Serrated, simple and 3-leaved structures and hexagonal crystals.			
10.	Irma R.	"	60	Serrated crystals.			
11.	George N.	Tabes dorsalis (Crises gastriques)........		No cholin.			
12.	Aranka K.	Tabes dorsalis......	85	Lecithin platinum chloride.			With gold chloride flocculent yellow precipitate.
13.	"	"	37				
14.	Ludwig N.	Epilepsia syphilitica.	46	Serrated, lanceolate structures and leaf-shaped forms as well as four-leaved and hexagonal crystals.			
15.	Karl M.	Dementia paralytica..	33	Four-leaved and amorphous forms; hexagonal crystals.			
16.	Johann G.	Epilepsia genuina ...	26	Serrated, lanceolate and 3 and 4-leaved forms; hexagonal crystals.			
17.	Regine D.	" ...	35	Serrated, lanceolate crystals and leaf-shaped forms, four-leaved rhombic and hexagonal crystals.			
18.	Johanna F.	Hystero-epilepsia ...	74	Serrated, rhombic and hexagonal crystals.			
19.	Mrs. Sch.	Tabes dorsalis	19				With potassio mercuri iodide gives a slight yellowish turbidity which dissolves on warming and reappear on cooling; and with phosphowolframic acid a slight flocculent turbidity.
20.	Eva P.	Epilepsia genuina...	43				With iodopotassic iodide potassiomercuric iodide phosphomolybdic and phosphorwolframic acid and gold chloride no precipitate.
21.	"	" ...	36	Serrated, lanceolate and four-leaved forms, rosettes with needle.			
22.	"	" ...	24	Radiating crystals or sheaves and tufts. Also four-leaved forms.			
23.	N. N.	Spinabifida	10	Serrated, lanceolate and 3-leaved forms.			Behavior toward reagent like No. 20.
24.	Karl Sz.	Tabes dorsalis	28				" "
25.	Stefan N.	Hysternepilepsia	38				No precipitate with iod potass, iodide, potassi mercuric iodide or gol chloride.
26.	Irma D.	"	12				
27.	Mrs. Alex. Sz.	Hysteria	22				Slight turbidity with phosphowolframic acid
28.	Julius B.	Sclerosis cerebrospinalis multiplex.....	32				Behavior toward reagent like No. 26. No precipitate with potassio-mercuric iodide phosphomolybdic acid phosphowolframic acid and gold chloride

TABLE I.—(Continued).

No.	Name	Diagnosis	No.	Crystal structure	Plates	Value	Remarks
29.	Joseph N.	Tabes dorsalis.......	41				Yellow crystalline precipitate with gold chloride.
30.	Joseph T.	Epilepsia genuina...	32				Potassio mercuric iodide and gold chloride give no precipitate, phosphowolframic acid a yellowish-white precipitate.
31. 32.	Rudolf S.	" Myelitis e compressione	60		Hexagonal plates.		Yellow flocculent precipitate with gold chloride.
33.	Zolten J.	Tabes dorsalis.......	10 / 23				"
34.	Adolf K.	Gummi cerebri......			Hexagonal plates.		Cerebrospinal fluid turbid, contains fibrinous coagula but no bacteria.
35.	Stephen H.	Epilepsia genuina...			Square and hexagonal plates.		
36. 37. 38.	" Joseph H. Katherina S.	" Encephalo-malacia .. Tumor cerebri......	38		Hexagonal plates. Hexagonal and rhombic plates.	0.036	
39.	Joseph K.	Polyneuritis alcoholica			Hexagonal plates.		
40. 41.	Eugen H. Michael K.	Neurasthenia .... Lues cerebralis	24	Indented lanceolate and vineleaf-shaped structures, hexagonal and rhombic plates.			No cholin.
42.	Samuel G.	Lues cerebrospinalis hereditaria	56	Hexagonal and rhombic plates and vine-leaf-shaped structures.			
43.	Susanna C.	Tabes dorsalis	30	Irregularly indented and branched structures.			
44.	Mrs. Andress B.	"	20	Hexagonal and one and four-leaved forms.			
45.	Mrs. Alexander P.	"	31	Rhombic and hexagonal plate, needles.			
46. 47.	Joseph N. Anton B.	" ...,.... Dementia paralytica..	22 / 75	Vineleaf-shaped forms. Vineleaf-shaped forms, needles arranged in sheaves and clusters.			
48.	Adolf G.	Tabes dorsalis	17				Slight yellow turbidity with platinum chloride (probably owing to the small amount of fluid).
49. 50.	Elizabeth H. Bertha W.	Epilepsia Jacksonia.. Hysteria	11			0.039	No precipitate with platinic chloride.
51.	Ladislaus Cz.	Tumor cerebri?.....		Dentated lanceolate crystals and 3 and 4-leaved forms.			Slight precipitate with platinic chloride.
52.	Julius Gy.	Epilepsia genuina....	23				Slight slimy precipitate with platinic chloride.
53.	Martin K.	Tabes dorsalis......	42				Slight slimy precipitate with platinic chloride.
54.	Karl R.	Taboparalysis	50				
55. 56. 57.	Franz Sch. Friedrich L.	Epilepsia genuina... Abscessus cerebri.... "	60 / 27 / 28	Serrated crystals. Chiefly needles. Serrated, lanceolate forms, leaf-shaped structures, needles and chiefly hexagonal plates.		0.021 / 0.046	Fluid somewhat turbid.
58.	Mrs. Johann B.	Tabes dorsalis.......	25	Vineleaf and four-leaved forms, needles, single and in sheaves.		0.037	
59.	Maria M.	Epilepsia genuina...	29	Serrated, lanceolate structures, wreath-shaped and branched crystals.		0.028	
60. 61.	Leopold R. Stefan P.	Coccygodynia ...... Taboparalysis	18 / 28	Vineleaf forms, four-leaved, fibrous and dentated structures.		0.028	Slight yellowish turbidity with platinic chloride.
62.	Johann G.	Dementia paralytica.	29	Irregularly branched, indented forms.		0.042	
63.	Michael M.	Neurasthenia	23	Traces of needles arranged in sheaves.		0.025	
64.	Israel H.	"	60	Indented, lanceolate and leaf-shaped forms.		0.025	

1 Only a portion of the cerebrospinal fluid obtained was employed unless the amount was small or a quantitative estimation was made.

2 Determined from the amount of cholin platinochloride $(C_5H_{14}NOCl)_2PtCl_4$ obtained.

3 I am indebted to my friend, Prof. Johann v. Brókay for this fluid. It came from a boy, two years old, on whom 15 lumbar punctures had been made in two years; in all 660 c.c. of cerebrospinal fluid had been removed.

4 For comparison, pure lecithin was prepared from the yolk of eggs, dissolved in alcohol and precipitated with platinum chloride. The precipitate was insoluble in water, alcohol or ether and gave the same microscopical appearance as above.

5 The positive reaction with the latter reagent is not conclusive for cholin since absolute alcohol was not used in this experiment and the presence of potassium and ammonium chloride could not be excluded.

diseases of the central nervous system, where we must assume a breaking-down of nervous tissue and a splitting-off of cholin from the increased amount of lecithin set free. The amount of cholin present in the cerebrospinal fluid is probably proportional to the degree of nerve disintegration. This fact may not be evident from the ten quantitative estimations given above, but this probably depends upon the small amounts with which I had to deal (8 to 15 milligrams of cholin). For this reason, the cholin could not be identified by means of platinum and the behavior toward reagents mentioned above and the microscopical appearance was resorted to instead.

The case of encephalomalacia deserves special mention. The patient exhibited a severe status epilepticus of Jacksonian type owing to an acute, destructive process in the central and Broca's convolutions. The status epilepticus lasted for days and the cerebrospinal fluid which was withdrawn for therapeutical purposes during this period, showed well-marked cholin crystal with phosphowolframic acid.[1]

On the other hand, no cholin was found in two cases of simple hysteria and only once in three cases of hystero-epilepsy and neurasthenia.[2] In coccygodynia and multiple sclerosis, negative results were also obtained.

These observations correspond with the fact that anatomical changes cannot be detected in hysteria. Even the most severe hystero-epileptic (more properly termed convulsive) attacks are not accompanied by complete loss of consciousness, since the patients can still be influenced by suggestion and since, when placed in the hypnotic trance, the patients will recall what has happened during the attack, even though they may not be aware of it when awake. Directly after the hysterical attack, the patients feel fresh and wideawake and not a trace can be found of the stupor and somnolency and the markedly altered psychical state which characterizes the true epileptics, so that it is hardly proper to assume an auto-intoxication. There are, however, exceptional cases of hystero-epilepsy, which form the connecting link between both diseases and which can hardly be distinguished from idiopathic epilepsy.

The reason why I consider cholin responsible for the convulsions, will be evident from the animal experiments. It will also follow from these that chemically pure cholin is by far more poisonous than generally stated in the text-books. Indeed, no experiments have been hitherto made to show that it is particularly irritating to the cerebral cortex.

III.—OTHER CONSTITUENTS OF THE CEREBRO-SPINAL FLUID.

In connection with my investigation of the cerebrospinal fluid, a few qualitative tests for other ingredients were made.

By far the most abundant solid ingredient is invariably chloride of sodium. Potassium (intense flame reaction) and ammonium are also present and phosphoric acid may be detected by means of the nitric acid salt of ammonium molybdate (it is probably a decomposition product of lecithin). Though ammonia is a fairly constant ingredient, it cannot be looked upon as a decomposition product of cholin. The tests for potassium, ammonium and phosphoric acid were always positive, except in two cases (Nos. 7 and 8) where ammonia could not be detected by means of Nessler's reagent. Strangely, both of these cases where epileptics, hence it is hardly probable that ammonia induces the attack. It is also unlikely that the ammonia is derived from the decomposition of cholin since dilute solution of this substance, when boiled alone or with potash lye or barium hydrate do not evolve ammonia or trimethylamine.[1]

In two cases (tabes dorsalis and Jacksonian epilepsy), lecithin was found. This substance has not been found hitherto and is probably pathological, indicating a rapid breaking-down of nerve-tissue.

Marked reduction was obtained on boiling cerebrospinal fluid with alkaline copper solution, ammoniacal silver nitrate and alkaline bismuth subnitrate. On the other hand, ferricyanide of potassium plus ferric chloride does not yield Prussian blue.

Halliburton believes this reducing substance is pyrocatechin, Nawratzki[2] thinks it is glucose. The latter author found 0.0461 per cent. glucose in the normal fluid of the calf, which is somewhat less than the amount in animal blood (0.1-0.2 per cent). The occurrence of glucose does not, however, seem to be constant. Quincke[3] found it regularly with cerebral tumors, Lenhartz,[4] on the other hand, could never detect it. With inflammatory processes, Quincke's examinations were also negative. Covazzini[5] reports positive findings in hydrocephalic fluid, while others were less successful.

Without discriminating between the different forms of dementia, Schäfer[6] obtained a positive Nylander's reaction in all cases where he examined the fluid. Zdarek[7] as well as Panzer[8] found one per cent. dextrorotatory sugar.

The albumin test with acetic acid and ferrocyanide of potash was always positive.

There was no occasion to test the cerebrospinal fluid for neurin, a substance which is closely allied to cholin in chemical and toxicological properties (see later). Cholin (trimethyloxethyl ammonium oxyhydrate, $CH_2(OH)CH_2 N (CH_3)$

---

[1] This case is also remarkable in that trepanation over the central convolutions, incision of the dura and removal of the trephined portion of the skull (about the size of the palm) caused disappearance of the Jacksonian epilepsy and the hemiplegia for quite a while and also brought about a remarkable improvement in speech and psychical condition. The correctness of the localization was verified later at autopsy.

[2] In this respect the observation of F. Z. Bosc (Du degré et des caractères de la toxicité urinaire dans l'hystério-épilepsie. Compt rend de la soc, de biolog, Séance du 30 Janvier, 1897) is very interesting. This author occasionally found the urine in hystero-epilepsy hypertoxic before the attacks. When injected into the veins of rabbits and dogs, respiration was slowed, the heart-action increased, the temperature reduced and the pupils contracted. An abundant discharge of urine and severe convulsions were also noticed.

[1] The ash of cerebrospinal fluid has recently been analyzed by E. Zdarek (Ein Beitrag zur Kenntniss der Cerebrospinal-flüssigkeit. Hoppe-Seyler's Zeitsch. f. physiol. Chemie, Vol. 35, No. 3). The water-soluble portion consisted of carbonic acid, chlorine, small amounts of sulphuric acid, traces of phosphoric acid; potassium and sodium. The insoluble portion was made up of carbonic acid and calcium, with traces of magnesium, phosphoric acid and iron. The ammonia contained in the original fluid seems to have escaped detection. It may also be mentioned here that Neuthner did not notice any decomposition on boiling a 1.4 per cent solution of cholin. Nothnagel made the same observation with a 4 per cent. solution. Hoppe-Seyler's Zeitsch. f. physiol. Chemie, 1897, Vol. 23, page 532.
[3] Quincke. Berl. klin. Woch., 1895, No. 41.
[4] Lenhartz. Müuch. med. Woch., 1896, p. 89.
[5] Covazzini. Centralbl. f. Physiolog., 1896, Vol. 10, No. 6.
[6] Schäfer. Ueber das Verhalten der Cerebrospinalflüssigkeit bei Dementia paralytica und einigen anderen Formen des Schwachsinns. Allg. Zeitsch. f. Psychiatrie. Vol. 59. No. 1, pp. 96 and 97.
[7] Zdarek, loc. cit.
[8] Panzer. Zur Kenntniss der Cerebrospinalflüssigkeit. Wien. klin. Woch., 1899, No. 31.

$_3OH=C_5H_{15}NO_2$) merely differ from neurin, (trimethyl ammonium oxyhydrate $CH.CH_2$ N $(CH_3)_3$ $OH=C_6H_{13}NO$) in containing in addition the elements which make up one molecule of water.

Both bases were formerly considered identical and were frequently mistaken for each other. Bayer and Brieger, however, pointed out the difference between the two. According to the exact investigations of Gulewitsch,[1] the fresh brain of the ox does not contains any neurin, but its aqueous extract as well as the alcoholic extract, treated with sodium alcoholate, will yield cholin exclusively. This author also pointed out, that the protagon discovered by Liebreich will not yield neurin, but cholin, when boiled with baryta. He also proved that neurin-platinum-chloride, when recrystallized from hot water will remain unchanged and will not take up one molecule of water and change into cholin, as Liebreich has stated. It is also possible to evaporate solutions of cholin chloride, acidified with hydrochloric acid or to boil dilute solutions of cholin with barium hydrate or treat them with sodium alcoholate, without the formation of neurin. According to Brieger, neurin appears rather late during the process of putrefaction by the splitting off of one molecule of water from cholin, which is already present at the very beginning, but this process cannot be regarded as analogous to what goes on in the cerebrospinal fluid. It is a fact that Halliburton could not detect neurin in the latter and Sowton and Waller[2] came to the same conclusion from the physiological experiment. Neurin removes the electro-motor conductivity of nerves, while cholin does not, and the cerebrospinal fluid behaves like cholin and not like neurin in this respect, hence does not contain any neurin. If really present, neurin could be easily detected in the precipitate thrown down by platinum chloride. After dissolving the chloroplatinate of cholin in a small amount of water, the platinochloride of neurin would remain behind, together with the corresponding potassium and ammonium salts. If these salts are dissolved in hot water, decomposed with sulphureted hydrogen, filtered, evaporated and rendered alkaline, the neurin will readily pass over into chloroform.

IV.—PRESENCE OF CHOLIN IN URINE AND BLOOD.

Experiments were made, to detect the presence of cholin in the urine after intracerebral or intravenous administration. Platinic chloride is not suitable on account of the large amount necessary to bring about precipitation. Even if the urine is treated with absolute alcohol, the extract will require a large amount since it contains many substances in solution which are precipitated by platinic chloride. A more suitable reagent is phosphowolframic acid.

The urine is acidulated with hydrochloric acid and evaporated to dryness, the residue extracted with absolute alcohol, filtered, again evaporated, taken up with water and finally completely precipitated with hydrochloric acid and 10 per cent. aqueous solution of phosphowolframic acid. As a rule, a greenish-violet discoloration will appear. The precipitate is now washed on a filter with water acidulated with hydrochloric acid, then washed into a high breaker and treated with finely powdered barium hydrate. After a short time, the mixture is filtered and the filtrate saturated with carbonic acid. After again filtering, the liquid is evaporated to dryness, taken up with absolute alcohol and finally precipitated with alcoholic platinum chloride.

Cholin could be detected microscopically by means of this process, after two milligrams of the hydrochlorate had been added to 100 c.c. normal urine. When as much as 3 to 7 centigrams of hydrochlorate of cholin were injected into the brain or the veins of four dogs, no cholin appeared in the urine.

It seems, therefore, that cholin is completely burnt up in the system. Mott and Halliburton have had a similar experience, and could not detect cholin in the urine.

Similarly, cholin could not be found in 45 c.c. of normal urine. The pressure of cholin in so small an amount or even in less serum, must therefore be looked upon as pathological. In progressive paralysis, Halliburton frequently found large amounts of cholin by chemical means in 10 c.c. of blood obtained by venesection. With the general distribution of lecithin, the mother-substance of cholin, in the body (not only in the brain and nerves, but also in blood, spermatic fluid, etc.) it need not surprise that cholin may be obtained from large amounts of ox blood. Marino-Zucco and F. Martini[1] have succeeded in this, for it follows from their account that the platinum salt of the isolated substance was easily soluble in water and hence was identical with cholin and not with neurin, as they stated.

V.—THE CONVULSIVE ACTION OF CHOLIN AND NEURIN.

Since cholin could never be detected in the urine after it had been given to animals, it is safe to assume that this substance is rapidly burnt up in the blood.

In order to study the immediate action of cholin and neurin upon the central nervous system, both substances were injected directly into the cortex or under the dura.[2] The results indeed surprising for the most severe tonic and clonic convulsions, often leading to paresis, made their appearance. The convulsions usually occurred over the entire body but occasionally predominated on one side. Thus in some instances, the extensors were chiefly affected in the con-

1 Gulewitsch. Ueber Neurin u. einige Verbindungen. Zeitsch. f. physiol, Chemie, Vol. 26; also, Ueber Leucomatine des Ochsenhirns, ibid., Vol. 27.
2 Sowton and Waller. Jour. of Physiol., Supplement.

1 Atti. d. R. Acc. de Sincci. I Sem. 396 to 399. Ref. Bericht der deutsch. chem. Gesellsch., 1894. Referate, p. 240.
2 Occasionally the deeper injections reached the medullary substance, leading to slight separation of the fibers. The symptoms were, however, the same. Where a hemorrhage took place into the lateral ventricle, the symptoms were very severe and fatal.

tralateral extremities, while on the same side, the motions were those of running or else (in guinea-pigs), a rotation in the same direction around the long axis. Sometimes a jar would start these rotating movements again, after the limb had already come to rest. After the convulsions, the paresis also appeared first on the contralateral extremities probably on account of the more intense irritation and more rapid exhaustion of the corresponding motor center. This is soon followed by paresis of all extremities but occasionally a general paresis is seen at once after severe muscular convulsions. From time to time the tonic or clonic spasms may be repeated in the paretic extremities. Trismus and spasm of the muscles of the back of the neck are pronounced.

General tremor is very marked directly after the injection and between the convulsions. It is rather odd that during the entire duration of the tremor, even guinea-pigs and dogs do not utter a sound.

The injections were never made into the motor center, but the frontal or occipital lobe was usually selected. In most cases, the same amount of physiological salt solution (0.7 per cent.) was injected so as to make sure that the symptoms were not referable to the pressure of the fluid introduced. At most a tonic spasm of the muscles of the neck was observed here, the head of the animal being drawn to the opposite; sometimes, however, to the same side. Sometimes a slight paresis of the contralateral extremities was seen, but all these symptoms were transient. Occasionally the intracortical injection of salt solution was not followed by any symptoms whatsoever. Cholin and neurin frequently render respiration difficult, sometimes with spasm of the respiratory muscles. In one dog, respiration ceased altogether after five c.c. of a 10 per cent. solution of cholin were injected into the crural vein, but reappeared with artificial respiration. The heart action could not be recorded during this experiment on account of the constant convulsions and tremor. Usually, however, the heart is stimulated at first, later depressed. Other constant symptoms are marked salivation, leading to frothing of the mouth, lacrimation, increased intestinal secretion and peristalsis (gurgling of the intestines) and frequent discharge of urine and stool. The urine passed during the attack was found free from albumin. Vomiting was noticed in a few instances. The palpebral fissure and the pupils are dilated, but sometimes miosis is observed. With dogs, a reaction to light could always be obtained, but with guinea-pigs accurate observation is rendered difficult on account of the dark iris. The background of the eye was rendered decidedly anemic by both cholin and neurin. After the spasmodic dilatation of the palpebral fissure has abated, a continuous blinking observed. Consciousness was perfectly retained during the convulsions in dogs for these animals readily reacted when called, by turning their head, or wagging their tail, no matter how severe the attack.

Though chemically pure cholin and neurin were used,[1] very little quantitative or qualitative difference in action were observed after intracerebral or intravenous application. Both are strongly toxic toward the nervous system, but this action is much less intense after intravenous than intracerebral injection.

(To be Continued.)

SOME OCULAR REFLEXES—(PSYCHOSES).[2]

BY S. W. S. TOMS, M.D.,

OF NYACK-ON-HUDSON, N. Y.;

LATE INSTRUCTOR IN OPHTHALMOLOGY, N. Y. MEDICAL SCHOOL AND HOSPITAL; MEMBER OF VISITING STAFF, NYACK HOSPITAL.

IN preparing this paper I have concluded to submit some observations made in the course of a busy general practice: the cause of many symptoms from which nervous patients frequently suffer—the importance of these symptoms correctly interpreted, and the indications for treatment.

I wish to state at the outset that I do not approach the subject from the standpoint of the specialist, and that I disclaim any extremist's or prejudiced views on the subject. I have tried to study my cases most thoroughly, and in doing so have examined all other organs as carefully as I have the eyes—in fact, in many of them, their eyes were the last thought of, after other therapeutic measures had been tried in vain.

It is a fact that every general practitioner is called upon to treat more derangements than diseases; the ' Neurotics " are a very considerable portion of his clientele. Do we regard this class of cases " as sufficiently interesting " to claim our best thought and care? I fear they are often " treated on general principles," because our text-book authorities have not yet given us *all* the etiological factors for *hysterical* and *neurotic* states; and in consequence there is a resort to hap-hazzard therapeutics instead of selective measures. I believe I have found through a systematic examination by exclusion, indications that lead to the employment of rational measures in a pretty large percentage of these cases. These patients do suffer without doubt. They go from one physician to another and often we are glad to get rid of them—they vainly seek relief until eventually loose faith in regular medicine and turn to quackery in one form or another. My plea is that we take hold of these cases and study them as we would those entering a hospital to report their history for the visiting staff's inspection. A *thorough* examination is usually very fruitful and always " interesting." My last series of one thousand

[1] Both substances were obtained from the chemical factory of E. Merck, Darmstadt. The cholin had been prepared synthetically, according to Wurtz, by the interaction of ethylenchlorbydrin and trimethylamin. The following test gave evidence of its purity: 0.278 gm. of the hydrochlorate were dissolved in 50 c.c. of water, acidified with hydrochloric acid and evaporated to dryness. The residue was then dissolved in absolute alcohol and precipitated with alcoholic platinum chloride. Dried at 100° F. the precipitate of platinochloride of cholin weighed 0.6105 gm. on incinerating 0.1910 gm. = 31.29 per cent. platinum were obtained (theoretically = 31.63 per cent).
[2] Read by invitation at Twenty-first Annual Meeting of New York State Medical Association, New York, October 17 to 19, 1904.

eye examinations—most of which were made as part of routine work—convince me that many patients who complain of symptoms, other than those directly referable to their eyes, would have gone unrelieved had I not made eye examinations.

· There are no text-book types of this class of sufferers—and it must be understood that I am not referring to, or including those patients with organic disease whose eye conditions are only part of their systematic malady. The reflexes from which these cases suffer, and their symptoms, are often very anomalous and curious.

The conditions found on examination may be equally so; as we rarely detect relationship between the amount or kind of eye defects and the disturbances produced; in fact, it is often in inverse ratio—a slight visual defect may create serious and profound nerve-racking disturbances of one kind or another, depending not upon the kind of defect, but on the peculiarity of the individual idiosyncrasy; for instance, a slight astigmatism or hyperopia may cause, (as recently witnessed by me in a young woman,) uncontrollable hysterical emotions which develop shortly after removing the patient's glasses. Another condition: that of puzzling muscular anomalies as an exophoria in distance with an esophoria in accommodation—or conversely. Careful studies of duction of all the muscles, rotations in all directions, and the study of the principal meridians in relation to the horopter are absolutely necessary in attempts to solve these apparently contradictory conditions. The ocular defects mostly productive of nervous disturbances are astigmatism in oblique or unsymmetrical axes (and usually the hyperopic types), anisometropia or unequal refraction of the two eyes, astigmatism against the rule and mixed astigmatism. Muscular imbalances are quite as potent in their influence as those of ocular defects and often exist independently of the latter. The symptoms complained of are frequently legion, and a catalogue of them would carry me far beyond the time-limit of this paper. The more frequent and common symptoms are the different types of headache, vertigo, nausea, vomiting attacks, "bilious spells," nervous dyspepsia (so-called), symptomatic migraine, cardiac neuroses, "nervous spells," clonic muscular twitchings symptomatic of chorea and epilepsy, insomnia, neurasthenia, lassitude, sea- and car-sickness, night terrors in children, and others which simulate organic nervous diseases.

Frequently a lowered state of the system from disease, overwork or worry, will rupture a compensated eye defect, and eyestrain will follow with its train of nervous phenomena. Pregnancy or miscarriage, I have observed to be conditions that unmask eye defects. Occasionally the eyes themselves suffer from peripheral irritation, producing styes, blepharitis, meibomian cysts, watering and suffusion, pains in eyes, etc. Certain anomalies of the ocular muscles induce malposi-

tions of the head, as wry-neck with compensatory scoliosis from hyperphoria (where one eye is in a higher plane than its fellow). Both eyes being too high causes a "ducking" of the chin against the chest; but where they are too low the opposite condition may result. Esophoria causes an *intense* expression, with wrinkled forehead and "crowfeet" at the outer canthi. Exophoria often produces a "blank" expression.

"Whether physiologic of pathologic, the eye is necessarily actively functional during every instant of the waking hours. It is bound up with every emotion and guides every concept; our thinking is by photographic images, even the letters of the alphabet are conventional pictures. When vision is morbid, there is therefore no limit to the kind and extent of the resultant harm to the organism and to the life."[1] I have not neglected general hygiene and occasionally the temporary employment of drugs in the treatments of my cases—as a crutch would be used to assist in regaining strength and function for a disabled limb. The nervous system is often depleted of its reserve, and requires every means of assistance together with the removal of the cause of depletion, in our efforts to assist recuperation. Right here I want to put myself on record with the statement that no absolute refraction of the eyes can be accurately determined under presbyopic age, without the employment of a mydriatic. Ciliary spasm often precludes a correct retinoscopic test and a minus glass occasionally will be preferred instead of a plus glass; but where the pupils are paralyzed the true condition is revealed.

Case I. Nervous Prostration.—F. L. W., female, aged twenty-six years, school teacher, single, father living, strong and vigorous (mentally and physically) mother neurotic, has been a martyr to headaches, bilious attacks, insomnia and dyspepsia all her life. (Has had to wear glasses for some years). Two brothers have visual and muscular defects. Patient came to me June, 1900, after suffering some weeks from a nervous breakdown which compelled her to give up her school. At first she noticed that she became very tired and exhausted early in the afternoons, with restless nights, and was unrefreshed in the mornings. Severe occipital headaches ensued and a tender spine developed. A trembling sensation in the epigastrim, indigestion, uncontrollable hysteria and depression followed so that she had to stop work and go to bed. This was her condition when she came to me. I carefully examined her, finding her physical condition good, and apparently nothing existed to account for her symptoms. Her visual tests were negative. She would not accept any lenses whatever —her vision being $20/20$ for distance, and she read No. 1 Jager at 8 to 20 inches without effort. The muscular anomalies were $9°$ of exophoria in distance, with abduction of $15°$. She had diplo-

[1] Preface to first series of Biologic Clinics.—Gould.

pia at six inches and both eyes deviated outward under the exclusion test. After she had worn 2° prisms bases in, for two weeks, with much relief, I did a partial tenotomy on the left externus, which reduced the exophoria to 2°. On the fourth day I operated on the other eye, slightly overcorrecting. Two weeks after she had 2° of esophoria, with abduction of 5°, adduction 34°, without diplopia in convergence. On the completion of the second operation she remarked that she felt as if the "World had been lifted off her shoulders." Her insomnia, nervous and dyspeptic symptoms were magically relieved and she left for home within a month, free from all her symptoms except some nervous dread if she exerted herself. I examined her two years later when she stated she had not had any return of trouble and her eye tests showed perfect balance—adduction 30°, abduction 7°, sursumduction 2°. (I have operated on her brother for exophoria within a few months and another brother is using prisms for muscular asthenopia.)

Case II. Cardiac Neurosis.—B. F. G., aged thirty-four years, married; clergyman. I have known patient for fifteen years. I have seen him faint and carried out of his church. He has been treated for heart disease by several physicians. He never had complained of eye symptoms or headaches, but some blurring after prolonged use of the eyes, frequent bilious attacks (monthly), pain in stomach and indigestion. Has been of a nervous disposition and has fainting attacks when overworked, nervously excited or in a close room. These attacks are accompanied by cold extremities, feeble pulse, vasomotor paresis, unconsciousness and slight clonic convulsions. Physical examination is negative excepting for an indistinct aortic first sound. Pulse normal and of good tension. Vision $^{20}/_{20}$—accepts+75 axis 90°=$^{20}/_{15}$; this he has been wearing for years. Muscular tests show homonomous diplopia with red glass with an excessive convergence esophoria of 10° in distance, and 24° in accommodation—adduction 40°, abduction 0°. A 2° prism over each eye (bases out) relieved him of much nervous tension. These were increased gradually to 4° over each eye. He has worn these for over a year and reported only a week ago that he had not had any return of his trouble, had gained 10 pounds and has felt perfectly well, but cannot go without his glasses. He was so well pleased that he brought a friend 150 miles to me, hoping I might find ocular defects as the cause of some similar nervous trouble.

Case III. Spasmodic Type.—W. A. J., aged twenty-seven years, married. Freight conductor. Father alive and well. Mother alive, has eye defects and belongs to a pronounced neurotic family. Patient came to me September, 1903, with a spasmodic tic, affecting the facial and cervical muscles of the left side, mostly. His present attack has lasted three months. He had been treated for chorea with arsenic until his eye-

lids were edematous and conjunctivæ suffused. He had his first attack two years before and subsequently slight recurrences at different times. There was no rheumatic, syphilitic or alcoholic personal history. He had a maternal uncle die of epilepsy and a maternal aunt of some nervous disease. The patient is a strong healthy looking and well-developed man, his manner not indicating a nervous temperament. I at once tested his eyes, finding a compound far-sighted astigmatism—against the rule, with 9° of esophoria; adduction excessive and abduction deficient. I deemed it necessary to employ acyclopegic which revealed a deficiency in vision of $^{20}/_{200}$ but with + 2.75 D.^{s} + .75 cy axis 180° = $^{20}/_{15}$. One-half of the hyperopic correction was prescribed with full astigmatic lenses for constant wear. Two hours after the atropine had been instilled into his eyes these spasmodic twitchings were much lessened and he slept during the night without an hypnotic, a thing he had not done before for weeks. I was enabled on the second day to complete the examination without difficulty, whereas the first attempt was unsatisfactory and tedious. His glasses gave him immediate relief and after two weeks he attempted to go without them. A recurrence followed, and as he had to lose sleep with night runs, I found it necessary to administer bromide for a week to assist the work of the glasses. I would have used the mydriatic again instead of bromides, had it been possible for him to stop work. He has had no recurrences since. None of the textbooks on nervous disease that I have consulted have given eyestrain as an etiological factor in producing facial tic or any other spasmodic affections simulating chorea.

Case IV. Nervous Insomnia.—On September 12, I was called to see a colored woman suffering from an uncompleted abortion in the fourth month. I found she was excessively nervous and sedatives and hypnotics failed to relieve her. After she had been affected this way for several days and nights, she told me my medicines were ' no good,' I asked her what made her nervous since her suffering had terminated. She could give me no information in her reply. I noticed she had put on her spectacles and that her head was tied up. These observations gave me a clue. I looked at the lenses, finding one of a different refraction from the other. I noticed also that she received the light from the windows directly into her eyes and at night a lamp burned on the mantle in front of her. When the hypersensitive retinæ are irritated by rays of light imperfectly focused, the brain often is affected through the optic nerves and headaches result. I had her bed turned around so that she faced the wall, the shutters closed and the lamp removed, *with the result that she fell asleep within an hour and no more medication was required.* Next morning at ten o'clock I found her asleep, and she told me she dad had a full night's restful sleep, which she had not had for some time.

REPORT OF A CASE OF POSTDIPHTHERITIC PARALYSIS.[1]

BY WILLIAM J. BUTLER, M.D.,

OF CHICAGO.

THE various changes observed during the course of acute infections and subsequent thereto, the comparative frequency with which they occur, and the peculiar predilection exhibited by some acute infections for certain organs and tissues, have always formed an interesting study for the clinician and pathologist. The earlier authors seemed scarcely clear as to these conditions and their explanation. Among the older writers some attributed all cases of sudden death in diphtheria to extension of the membrane into the larynx, maintaining this in the face of tracheotomy. Trousseau suggested that some cases of sudden death in diphtheria were due to disturbance of heart function, the result of changes in that organ. The earliest recorded pathological observations were made by Louis, Gunsburg, Wunderlich, Androl and Stokes. They commented on the appearance and consistency of the heart. Gunsburg, in describing the heart of typhoid fever, said it is easy to recognize, having an almost pathognomonic appearance. Stokes emphasized that the changes in typhoid heart were less frequent and less marked than in the acute exanthema and diphtheria.

Virchow, in addition to the macroscopic changes, mentioned a parenchymatous inflammation in which there was a fatty and granular degeneration of the muscle fibers. Following this came the works of Bottcher, Stein, Waldeyer and Hoffman, who struggled over the origin and significance of certain fusiform cells found in interstitial tissue of the heart.

Whereas these earlier observations concerned the cardiac changes in various infectious diseases, especially typhoid, those of diphtheria now occupied chief attention. Among the notable investigators in this direction was Birch-Hirschfeld, who described a high grade of interstitial inflammation. Hayem found parenchymatous and interstitial inflammation and endarteritis of small arteries of heart, with resulting thrombosis and cicatrization. Martin and Barrie confirmed Hayem's findings.

Landouzy and Siredey reported practically the same changes. Romberg, after an exhaustive study of the pathology of hearts in fatal cases of acute infections, stated that parenchymatous and interstitial inflammation is never absent in diphtheria, seldom in scarlet fever, and in little less than half the cases of typhoid. He expressed the opinion, which is not at all improbable, that the sclerosis of the coronary arteries is not the only cause of chronic myocarditis. A second cause might be found in an earlier acute interstitial myocarditis. This might also explain cases of idiopathic hypertrophy of the heart in children.

Although much had been done up to this time in the pathology of the subject, apparently little

1 Read before the Chicago Medical Society, October 26, 1904.

advance had been made clinically, as indicated by Leyden, in 1880, who wrote that the symptoms and course in the heart changes in diphtheria were not yet clearly defined, nor widely known. Richardson's description of cardiac weakness during the height of an attack of diphtheria is as follows: A peculiar dyspnea and restlessness, a pale face, and a small pulse, point toward heart weakness and asphyxia. Such cases are not seldom fatal.

Oertel stated that in stormy septic diphtheria the face is puffy, pale and waxy. Pulse small, irregular and very slow. Temperature slight or subnormal. Marked exhaustion present. Mentally clear up to death from heart paralysis or pulmonary edema. If process is slow, you get a gradual exhaustion, anorexia, vomiting of nourishment taken, skin cold and clammy. Pulse 40 to 50; irregular and intermittent. Sudden death in such cases may follow quick movement, or the patient may be seized with vomiting and syncope and die in attack.

Mosler stated that such cases of fatal syncope could occur in advanced convalescence, especially when pulse remained slow, small and irregular.

In contrast to slow pulse, mentioned by Oertel, Lubadie and Largrave described the pulse as small and frequent.

Leyden, in 1880, made an effort to harmonize the clinical signs and symptoms with the pathological findings. He regarded vomiting as an important symptom, and considered it the result of reflex action from the diseased heart along the vagus. Indeed, he thought vomiting an ominous symptom, which should cause fear of heart paralysis. From the pathological study of his cases he concluded that there was an acute myocarditis and fatty degeneration of muscle fibers. He reasoned that such changes exerted marked influence on the function and tone of heart muscle, that on account of diminished tone dilatation occurred, and galop rhythm resulted. Disturbed function was expressed in the small frequent pulse.

In the same year Leyden, by a close study and analysis of the symptoms and electrical reactions of the paralyzed muscles, with tendency toward early regeneration and recovery, concluded that in the majority of cases of postdiphtheritic paralysis a trophic disease of the motor system existed, which attacked nerve and muscle in varying extent, probably occasionally extending to the motor area of the cord. A year later Paul Meyer found extensive parenchymatous changes in peripheral nerves of postdiphtheritic cases. Similar results were later described by Eichhorst and Preisz, who also described changes in the pneumogastric.

Bikeles and Koliski noted degeneration in posterior columns and nerve roots, to which they attributed the ataxia sometimes seen following diphtheria.

Not a few of the more recent investigators along this line, including Veronese, Klimoff and Thomas, believed that changes in the nerves of the heart, analogous to those of the peripheral nerves, were the cause of heart paralysis.

Returning to the clinical features, Hibbard analyzed 21 cases of heart paralysis in diphtheria, and found that the first symptoms pointing to the heart occurred in the vast majority of cases in the first and second weeks, and that the greatest number of them died in the second and third weeks, and seldom in the first week, seeming to indicate that while we speak of sudden death in diphtheria, it is invariably preceded by symptoms extending over a period of one to several days, pointing to cardiac changes; as was long ago pointed out by Leyden and others. And some of these cases live on for several weeks. Among the symptoms noted by Hibbard as pointing toward cardiac paralysis was rapid, feeble, intermittent, irregular pulse, or a slow pulse. Vomiting was frequently present. Occasionally abdominal pain. Sometimes systolic murmur at apex. He noted galop rhythm in six cases, five of whom died. Collapse occurred eight times and death followed within two days in every case. Thomas made a pathological study of these cases and reported degenerative and interstitial changes of more or less severity in the pneumogastric nerve in every case. His work, however, did not include the myocardium. Cardiac thrombosis was noted in four of Hibbard's cases.

Eppinger, of Gratz, in 1903, wrote that since the introduction of antitoxin, interest in the diphtheritic process has subsided, and still there occur consequences that have not yet been definitely explained, especially that which concerns sudden death. From 1882 to 1901 he had in his wards 380 deaths from diphtheria, distributed as follows: 186 from pneumonia, 87 from asphyxia, 43 from sepsis, 24 from pure diphtheria, 22 from tuberculosis, and 18 from postdiphtheritic paralysis of the heart. All these 18 cases had occurred since introduction of antitoxin in 1895, and only one was uninjected with serum. Prior to serum therapy, it was a rare occurrence. This would seem true from the fact that Leyden's work was based on three cases only, and Romberg's investigation in 1882 covered nine cases.

Eppinger, in his clinical analysis of the 18 cases, which he states varied very little, found that from the first to tenth days after patient had entered the stage of convalescence there occurred suddenly, probably after apathy, restlessness and abnormalities of the heart, the most threatening heart symptoms, which with vomiting and collapse lead to unexpected death.

Pathologically, Eppinger found a disintegration of the muscle fibers and termed the process myolisis cardis toxica in diphtheria.

White and Smith's clinical study of the heart complications in diphtheria included 24 fatal cases. They found galop rhythm in all these cases. Late vomiting (with relation to beginning of illness); epigastric pain, and tenderness. In their 36 cases of serious heart complications, with 24 deaths, only one recovered that presented the above symptom and signs. In but two of these

fatal cases from heart paralysis bradycardia was observed. The majority of their cases developed in the second and third weeks.

In regard to the later frequency of postdiphtheritic paralysis, Meyer, in his statistics, taken from Park Hospital, London, for 1899, reports in 1,316 cases, 275, or 20 per cent., of postdiphtheritic paralysis. Of these, 80 died; 64 from cardiac paralysis, and 11 from paralysis of the diaphragm, usually associated with other paralysis. In referring to the symptoms and signs of cardiac paralysis, he states that the appearance of a galop rhythm indicates that the patient is near the end.

Possibly it might be well at this time to introduce the generally accepted explanation for increased frequency of postdiphtheritic paralysis, since the introduction of antitoxin. This is practically that many of those severe cases that formerly died early from asphyxia, rapid sepsis, etc., now live to show the various subsequent complications of heart and peripheral nerves.

The following case seemed of interest, because it presented what would appear to be a typical clinical picture of cardiac paralysis:

Case.—Dora W., aged twelve years; second youngest of five children, all living and well. Was never sick, with the exception of an attack of gastros-enteritis at two years. She had eczema capitis from second week of life to end of first year. Weighed 91 pounds before taken ill, about June 15, when she complained of sore throat, headache, chills and fever; also vomited. Submaxillary swellings appeared on both sides. The mother considered it mumps and treated patient with linseed poultices and a gargle, consisting of potash and borax. About ten days after onset another member of the household complained of sore throat, when a doctor was called in, and pronounced the disease diphtheria. By this time liquids had started to return through nose of first patient on effort at swallowing them. He gave her 2,000 units of antitoxin at once, after which she seemed better for a couple of days and sat up in bed. While in this position she was taken with severe epigastric pain and vomiting. Complained of dizziness, and seemed very short of breath. Face grew pale, and lips blue, and she lost consciousness. This lasted several minutes, and on arousing she again complained of abdominal pain, vomited, and fainted. On recovering from this she had a similar third attack. Thereafter she complained of pain in chest, and was very restless. Her breathing was labored and rapid, and she had to be elevated during the night to breathe. During the same night she had two or three attacks of great pain, vomiting and syncope, cyanosis and coldness of extremities. She now began to cough and expectorated a bloody, frothy sputum. The spells of syncope recurred from few to several times in twenty-four hours, frequently preceded by pain or vomiting, or both. At other times she vomited or complained of severe epigastric pain only.

In the course of four or five days the pain localized itself over precordial area and lower part of sternum. Syncope now became less frequent, but severe attacks of angina, with great difficulty in breathing, occurred several times every twenty-four hours. Frequent cough and bloody expectoration continued. About July 3 it was noticed she not only had difficulty in swallowing liquids, but could not swallow solids.

I first saw patient about July 1, and found the following: Patient was apathetic; coughed frequently and hard, expectorating a bloody sputum. She complained of pain over lower part of sternum and precordia. Face pale, with cyanosis of lips. Eyes negative. Tongue moist, slightly coated. Soft palate immovable. Complete aphonia. Neck: No swelling of glands noticeable at present. Marked venous pulse extending into lobe of ear; carotids not palpable. Chest: Breathing labored and rapid, 40 per minute; at times of Cheyne-Stokes type. Respiratory movements entirely thoracic and confined to upper part of chest. Excursion equal on both sides. Percussion gave hyperresonant sound anteriorly on both sides, lower border on right side terminating on sixth rib, and immovable on inspiration. On left side it extended to third rib. Auscultation gave vesicular breathing, accompanied with dry râles over both lungs, but almost inaudible in lower and lateral parts of chest.

Examination of lungs posteriorly gave resonance above, but dulness on right side from midscapular region down, and on left side from angle of scapula to lower border. Auscultation gave vesicular sounds above with dry râles, disappearing over dull area. No visible apex beat or impulse of chest wall. Heart: Dulness above commenced in second interspace, becoming absolute on third rib. Toward right, absolute dulness extended two fingers' breadth to right of right sternal border. To left, dulness commenced just inside anterior axillary line. Auscultation gave feeble heart tones, with galop rhythm over entire heart. No murmurs. Pulse was 120 per minute, irregular in quality, intermittent, very feeble, and small. Abdomen: Retraction of epigastrium on inspiration. Liver extends three fingers' breadth below rib arch in mamillary line, and is painful to pressure. Lower border palpable.* Spleen not palpable. No ascites or edema of extremities. Patellar reflexes absent. Gave strychnine, gr. 1/60; codeine, gr. 1/8.

After a few days slight improvement was noted. The pulse was a little less irregular and intermittent, and of slightly improved tension. Had had only one spell of syncope and attacks of angina were less frequent. Cough did not seem so troublesome, and expectoration was diminished. Heart tones were a little louder, but galop rhythm continued. July 16 she had two attacks of syncope, preceded by severe precordial pain. July 17' Dr. Stein examined larynx, and found paralysis of the tensors. Swallowing of solids still difficult. On morning of July 19, found cough much increased, copious expectoration of red-colored sputum. Respirations 40 and la-

bored. Conditions of swallowing and speaking unchanged. Numerous dry and subcrepitant râles heard over lateral surfaces of chest. Galop rhythm marked. Sounds feeble. Pulse 130; of lower tension, and smaller volume than on previous day.

On inquiry, found patient had not received any medication for sixteen hours. This suggested the possibility that her previous improvement might have been influenced to some extent by therapy, and therefore ordered the strychnine and codeine given every three hours during that day.

Saw patient same evening and found cough less frequent. Respirations 32 per minute. Auscultation of lungs unchanged. Heart area unchangd, except dulness to right of sternum was less intense. Heart tones stronger, and galop rhythm hardly distinguishable, although it was observed the next day.

From this on, improvement was maintained, and on July 27 found the following:

Face pale; mucosa cyanosed; voice sounds moderately loud; soft palate moves slightly; swallows solids, but with difficulty; venous pulse noticeable only in lower part of neck. Carotids palpable. Respiration still thoracic. Lower lung borders the same, with slight clearing on inspiration. Respiratory sounds more distinct in lower and lateral surfaces of chest. Posteriorly, the dulness below angle of scapula previously noted faded into a dull tympanitic resonance on right side, and at lower level on left side. Respiratory murmur more distinct and accompanied by occasional râles. Heart area the same, with dulness less distinct to right of sternum. Heart tones moderately loud, with galop rhythm heard chiefly over apex and base. Epigastric retraction on inspiration. Liver dulness about two fingers' breadth below costal arch. On August 8: Diminished heart area, and louder second pulmonic than aortic tone. Galop rhythm still continues. Strabismus is present. there being paralysis of both external recti.

Saw patient about September 10, now out of bed. Physical signs about same as at previous examination. She walks with an ataxic, paretic gait. Patellar reflexes still absent. Pulse 104; fair tension, and not intermittent, but accelerated on slight exertion, with complaint of palpitation.

The diagnosis in the above case seemed clear, namely, a postdinhtheritic paralysis of unusual extent. involving the external recti of the eyes, the soft palate, the pharynx, the abductors of the larynx. the diaphragm, and peripheral nerves. Acute cardiac dilatation, with pulmonary hypostasis, and edema; also liver stasis.

It will be noted that among the 270 cases of postdiphtheritic paralysis reported by Meyers, in only one was the larynx involved.

The conditions which specially interested me in this case concerned the heart and diaphragm. In the fatal cases of cardiac complication during or following diphtheria, various writers on the subject lay special stress on the galop rhythm, vomiting at height of attack of diphtheria, or in convalescence; the pallor of face, cyanosed lips, the rapid, feeble, irregular and intermittent pulse; the syncope; more recently the much emphasized epigastric pain—all of which were present.

The point that particularly interested me was to attempt to decide clinically how much the pneumogastric nerve, and how much the myocardium were pathologicaly involved in the change. The size of the heart, which, according to the percussion findings, was increased on both sides; the feebleness of the heart tones; the presence of a galop rhythm; the rapid, feeble, irregular and intermittent pulse; the marked dyspnea; the pulmonary hypostasis, and edema; the enlarged and painful liver; and the frequent attacks of angina and syncope permitted the diagnosis of acute dilatation of the heart of a high grade.

During the subsequent course it will be observed that after withdrawal of the codeine and strychnine for sixteen or eighteen hours, a previous improvement in heart status was now replaced by a condition approaching its earlier stages, and that there was a prompt improvement on resumption of medication. It would, therefore, appear as though the therapy had had some influence on the cardiac condition in this case. We could hardly attribute to codeine such effects. If either had any bearing, I would consider strychnine as the probable cause. This would imply intact vasomotor and vagus centers, and likewise, at least in great part, intact vagus. It is, therefore, probable in this case that the dilatation was due to a change in the myocardium, that is, an acute myocarditis, concurring in Romberg's statement that all cases of diphtheritic heart paralysis presented changes of acute myocarditis.

At the same time, this case would seem to fulfil the early theory of Leyden, namely, that the changes in the hearts, even in his cases, that died from cardiac paralysis, were not so extensive that they might not have healed, for if the inflammatory process subsided, the heart would tend to return to a normal state, and the small contracting foci resulting from the myocarditis would not exert any material influence on its functions. However, this process is not capable of being checked, and when once established, proceeds to an independent course. Is it beyond the range of speculation that the inflammatory process was arrested by the use of antitoxin in this case, and thus we had a material demonstration of Leyden's opinion. This would seem more in sympathy with our conception of the merits of antitoxin, than to accept the inference conveyed by Eppinger, that heart paralysis is more frequent since the employment of antitoxin. However, it is not improbable that the latter is true, as von Leyden's study involved only three cases, and Romberg eight cases, while Meyer's statistics for the year 1899, in London Park Hospital alone, cover 64 cases, or 4.7 per cent. of the entire number of cases of diphtheria handled. Hibbard and Thomas' work, in 1898, embodied 21 cases. More recently White and Smith reported 24 fatal cases of heart paralysis in diphtheria.

Reverting to the case in point, it would appear that on account of the changes in vagus branches to the palate, the pharynx, and the cricothyroid muscle (which latter is supplied by external branch of superior laryngeal, and which in turn sends a branch to the cardiac ganglion), one might naturally expect the same in the cardiac branches, sent direct from the vagus or its branches, or in the vagus itself. Indeed, this seems more than probable; at the same time, if it occurred, we had no evidence that it exerted any material influence on the heart; that is to say, we did not have a bradycardia, nor did we have an excessive tachycardia following a previous bradycardia, signs which, in this condition, are referred to vagus changes. On the other hand, an acute myocarditis would explain all the physical signs and clinical symptoms. It would account for the feeble, irregular, intermittent and rapid pulse, the dilatation, the galop rhythm, the resulting stasis, the syncope, the angina, etc. There can, however, be no doubt that a small percentage of the fatal cases, where a marked bradycardia is observed, or excessive tachycardia following a bradycardia appears, die as a result of vagus paralysis. However, it is more than likely that the vast majority of these fatal cases result from an acute myocarditis; that their clinical features as pointed out by Eppinger, are very similar, namely, small, rapid, irregular, intermittent, feeble pulse; vomiting, often epigastric pain, more or less cardiac dilatation, galop rhythm, and facial pallor and puffiness. It is very probable that there are usually changes in both myocardium and vagus, and that according as one or other predominates, the clinical picture will vary.

The future prognosis in such cases that result in recovery, or even in those that have had only moderate heart complications, is well illustrated in a case reported by von Jaksch, in 1880. A woman, twenty years old, had sore throat four months before admission to the hospital with typhoid fever. Temperature at the time was high; pulse rapid. After one week in the hospital increase in size of the heart was noted. Pulse small, and 132 per minute. Following day she had a chill, vomited, and complained of abdominal pain. Pulse arrhythmic, small and frequent, and 80 per minute. Heart enlarged. Thereafter, subnormal temperature, cyanosis, great dyspnea, liver stasis, and some edema. Pulse was less frequent, 120 per minute. About a week after the onset of the symptoms the patient sat up, and shortly thereafter died in collapse.

Post-mortem:—Intestinal findings of typhoid; acute myocarditis. As regards the reported case, it is likely that any severe acute infection might result disastrously, should it occur in the next several months in this case. Again, sudden strain might precipitate another attack of acute dilatation.

The treatment employed in this case consisted of codeine to allay restlessness and cough, and strychnine, which latter seemed to exert a favorable influence on the heart tone from the beginning of its use.

MEDICAL PROGRESS.

MEDICINE.

Observations on Coal Gas Poisoning.—The question as to whether death in any given case is due to the inhalation of gas or whether the individual was already dead when placed in this atmosphere, has been made the subject of a series of practical experiments by F. STRASSMANN and A. SCHULTZ (*Berl. klin. Woch.*, November 28, 1903), for the purpose of determining the degree of absorption of the gas which can take place after death. It has always been believed that the presence of carbonic oxide gas in the blood was evidence of the fact that the latter had entered the circulatory system through the lungs during life. But at the present day this view is no longer tenable and it has been shown that gases may penetrate the tissue of the dead body, as well as other poisons. Gas in the pure state, and also when mixed with air or smoke, can penetrate into the interior of a dead body through the skin. The experiments here detailed were made on seven dead bodies which were exposed to illuminating gas in a closed box for varying lengths of time. The findings substantiated the claims of other observers and it was proved that the gas could penetrate all the parts if the exposure were long enough. Dilution with air did not interfere with the absorption, nor did it make any difference whether the gas was quiet or in motion. The authors state that a useful diagnostic sign is the marked difference in color between the outer and inner layers of the superficial muscles, such as those of the chest, when the gas is absorbed from without, the hemoglobin of the outer layer being more saturated, in proportion to the amount of gas taken up, than the inner layers. The palladium test was found more satisfactory than the spectroscope.

Blood-Pressure in Arteriosclerosis.—The result of over a thousand estimations of blood-pressure with Gärtner's tonometer, are embodied in an article by T. DUNIN (*Zeitsch. f. klin. Med.,* Vol. 54, Nos. 5 and 6). The general impression is that arteriosclerosis is always accompanied by increased vascular tension, but this is by no means the case. Among 420 patients (not including any cases with loss of compensation on part of the heart), 120 gave evidence of normal or diminished pressure. Some of these patients were not aware of their vascular lesion and complained of only few symptoms referable to it, but in the great majority angina pectoris, arrhythmia of the pulse, dyspnea and swelling of the feet were present. Cases with increased tension may be divided into several groups: (*a*) those without subjective symptoms, constituting about 30 per cent. The usual complaint was here referable to nervousness, obesity or renal or biliary calculi. Some of the severest cases (240 to 290 mm. pressure) belong to this category and the absence of symptoms can only be explained by a healthy conditon of the heart, which was able to overcome the increased resistance in the capillaries. Accentuation of the second aortic sound and a systolic aortic murmur were common. (*b*) In this group the subjective symptoms were slight or very marked, but the kidneys were usually affected. (*c*) Here angina pectoris was very common. Angina is much more common with low pressure but no difference between the two forms concerning general course or prognosis could be detected. The lowest figures obtained (65 mm.) were in cases of angina, and during the attack, the pressure often fell 30 mm. Improvement may be accompanied by either increase or decrease in pressure. The last group (*d*) includes five cases of intermittent claudication. It seems that obesity is very common with arteriosclerosis and that reduction of obesity also lowers the pressure. The second aortic tone is of no value in determining the pressure, since it may often be accentuated with subnormal tension. The physiological law, that the frequency of the pulse is less, the higher the pressure, does not apply to pathology.

Alcohol in the Tropics.—CHAS. E. WOODRUFF, *Med. Rec.,* December 17, 1904) earnestly urges a reconsideration by the profession of the long-established dictum that total abstinence is an essential to the preservation of health in the tropics. This is a conclusion without logical foundation, and the statistics of our army in the Philippines show that in that climate the moderate drinker is better off than the total abstainer. The enervating effect of tropical climates requires the stimulus of a certain amount of alcohol to counteract it, and it is a serious error to denounce its use in moderation by those compelled to live in such latitudes. Total abstinence among the people of the country at large is the ideal condition, and everything should be done to encourage it, but with the army in the Philippines alcohol is a necessity. The W. C. T. U. has played into the hands of the liquor dealers in causing the canteen to be abolished, and in the horrible dives which have sprung up about all the barracks drunkenness flourishes to a degree far in excess of what was formerly the case. The author's object is to induce recognition of the fact that a moderate amount of alcohol is essential to health in the tropics, and that the abolition of the army canteen is fostering alcoholism among the soldiers.

Estimation of Diastolic Blood-Pressure.—Since the usual blood-pressure instruments only register the systolic pressure of the blood-column, J. STRASBURGER (*Zeitsch f. klin. Med.,* Vol. 54, Nos. 5 and 6) gives the following simple method for determining the diastolic pressure. The modified Riva-Rocci apparatus is applied to the arm the usual way. As the arm is compressed by the cuff, the radial pulse can be felt to retain its original height for a time, then a marked decrease will follow, after which it will disappear completely. The height of the manometer during the first decrease, perceptible to the palpating finger, denotes the pressure in the vessels during the diastole. Normally, the difference between systolic and diastolic pressure corresponds to about 30 mm. of mercury. By dividing the systolic pressure into the difference between the systolic and diastolic pressure, the "blood-pressure quotient" is obtained. This figure will give a good idea of the work done by the heart and its relation to the resistance in the arterial system. If of medium height, heart action and resistance are about normal, if above normal, the resistance is low, if below normal, high. In order to determine the actual work of the heart, the absolute height of the pressure and the frequency of the pulse must alsobe taken into account. If all the factors are normal, we may safely say that heart action and adaptation of the vessels are also normal and that sufficient blood flows through the vessels. In healthy individuals, the quotient is usually 0.25. In aortic regurgitation, the average value of the quotient was 0.40; in mitral or muscular disease of the heart, however, it was generally below normal. It may be stated that fall of systolic pressure with stationary quotient means less work on part of the heart and stationary systolic pressure with fall of quotient, also diminished cardiac activity, accompanied, however, by contraction of the smaller arteries, so that less blood flows to the periphery. Despite the proportionately high pressure, the tissue will here receive less blood. With both factors below normal, the heart action is deficient. The quotient will explain a large number of cases where normal systolic pressure is accompanied by marked signs of cardiac weakness, hence the quotient is an extremely delicate test for detecting beginning decompensation. In nephritis, the systolic pressure and quotient both are generally high, showing that there is no increased resistance at the periphery but that the vessels have actually dilated. Cardiac hypertrophy in nephritis is therefore not caused by increased peripheral resistance but by irritation of the heart itself or by anomalies in the viscosity of the blood. In arteriosclerosis, on the other hand, the resistance is higher, hence the quotient is frequently of normal height. During the first stage of pneumonia, the quotient was increased, owing to vascular dilatation.

Tumor of the Hypophysis.—In an interesting case observed by A. BERGER (*Zeitsch. f. klin. Med.*, Vol. 54, Nos. 5 and 6) all the general symptoms of brain-tumor were present with anomalies of growth such as short stature, persistence of infantile habitus, increasing obesity, falling out of the hair and dryness of the skin. A diagnosis of hypophyseal tumor seemed justified since the eyes and eye-muscles were seriously affected. At autopsy, an epithelioma was discovered behind the chiasma which had compressed and flattened an otherwise normal pituitary body.

Anchylostomiasis in Europe.—Underground work seems to offer conditions particularly favorable to the contraction of this disease. THOMAS OLIVER (*Lancet*, December 10, 1904), studying the conditions in Westphalia stated that in Dr. Tenholt's company he had an opportunity of studying the conditions presented in this great center of infection and also of observing the methods in vogue of giving special training to the physicians in the mining districts. Already three hundred young men had been educated to combat anchylostomiasis. So grave had the condition become that not only the Mining Association, with 265,000 members, but the German Government as well have taken every means possible to stamp out the disease. Before any miner is allowed to work he must first pass through the hospital where his excreta are examined, after which he receives a certificate of health. The spread of the disease throughout Westphalia is attributed to the rapid opening of the mine. In one year 20,000 new miners have come from East Germany, Hungary and Italy. Hungarian miners are now never engaged. The Miners' Association has paid almost a million dollars in connection with its work on anchylostomiasis. The proportion of the cases per 10,000 miners at work infected by the disease has risen from 6.4 in 1896 to 52.9 in 1892. Tenholt depends on felix mas in large doses. In Hungary, Goldman observed that in one mine with a temperature averaging from 104° to 113° F. a very large proportion of the men are infected, the temperature seeming to favor it. A ground for tolerance, however, seems to have been established and now instead of 95 per cent., only 30 per cent. of the men are infected. The mine is so hot that the men are able to work but four hours a day and they drink on an average five liters of water acidified with one per cent. of citric acid. It has been very difficult to teach the men habits of cleanliness in the mines. In Cornwall anchylostomiasis has appeared in one mine, worms probably having been brought to it from Europe by an infected miner. The larvæ gain entrance to the alimentary canal through eating with unwashed hands but, as Looss has shown, they also enter through the skin.

SURGERY.

On the Possibility of Increasing Peritoneal Resistance to Operative Infection.—A series of experiments has been made on guinea-pigs for the purpose of determining the possibility of increasing the resistance to peritoneal infection with the colon bacillus. For this purpose, BORCHARD (*Deut. med. Woch.*, December 1, 1904) issued injections of nucleic acid, a horse-serum, and physiological salt solution. Subcutaneous injections of the two latter were sufficient to protect the animals against subsequent injections of fatal doses of the colon bacillus. The nucleic acid was not only inefficient, but gave rise to a severe local reaction. The solutions were also injected into the peritoneal cavity, and all three substances applied in this way were efficient in increasing the resistance of the subjects, so that two or three times the ordinarily fatal dose of bacteria could be survived. It was found that the highest point in the resistance occurred about forty-eight hours after the injection, which is much later than the highest leucocytosis. The protection was found to last about four days. The author believes that the possibility of infection from laparotomy may in this wise be considerably diminished.

Treatment of Duodenal Ulcer.—The subject of duodenal ulcer is beginning to receive as much attention as that of ulceration in the stomach itself. D'ARCY POWER (*Brit. Med. Jour.*, December 17, 1904), concludes that there are two classes, of which he draws the following composite pictures: The subject in the first class is usually a man in the prime of life who is suddenly seized with severe abdominal pains; within a hour he is lying on his back, afraid to move, showing all the evidences of perforation. He cannot locate his pain but complains of its being worse along the upper half and down the right side of the abdomen. The abdomen is not distended but is not entirely motionless. It is everywhere tender and tympanitic. Liver dulness may or may not be present. Such is the picture of a patient whose ulcer has perforated. That of a man who has a pronounced ulcer but who has not yet suffered perforation is more interesting because more difficult to interpret. The patient is often between fifty and sixty years. He has been a martyr to indigestion and has had atrocious pain which is relieved by vomiting. He has gone from place to place seeking a cure; he is usually constipated; has cold extremities and extreme mental depression; the abdomen is loose; the subcutaneous veins may be enlarged; the stomach is dilated. Twenty-five or thirty years ago, if the history can be obtained, he vomited considerable quantities of blood; he recovered slowly and has never been well since. This is a case of a patient who has partially recovered from the cicatrization of an old ulcer. How many have been allowed to die of such a condition in the belief that they had malignant disease of the stomach! Duodenal ulcer is usually single, small, conical in shape, situated in the first part of the duodenum near the pyloric fold. Adhesions to the parts contract, reducing the duodenum and at the same time involve the liver, the gall-bladder, the pancreas, or the great blood vessels and the portal system. The means of distinguishing between these cicatricial conditions and malignant growth have developed in recent years, the operation of gastrojejunostomy done for temporary help only, having turned out not uncommouly to give permanent relief. The author concludes: (*a*) Duodenal ulcers are not very uncommon; (*b*) so far as he has seen them, duodenal ulcers are single and more frequent in men than in women; (c) duodenal ulcers may penetrate and cause acute symptoms, or they may heal, and by cicatrization lead to symptoms of chronic duodenal obstruction; (d) the sequelæ of a healed ulcer may be so remote that the symptoms are mistaken for those due to cancer of the pylorus, and the patient is allowed to drift from bad to worse under the erroneous notion that he is bound to die. (e) there is no means of recognizing the existence of a duodenal ulcer, in a great many cases, until it perforates or until the results of its cicatrization becomes manifest.

Surgical Treatment of Chronic Indigestion.—Even to-day the treatment of the greater number of digestive derangements still remains in the hands of the physician. GILBERT BARLING (Brit. Med. Jour., December 17, 1904) states that the conditions for which surgical treatment may be required, exclusive of perforation, may be classified into the four following groups. (1) Chronic gastric ulcer, frequently relapsing despite proper dieting and rest. (2) Hemorrhage from gastric ulcer under certain conditions. (3) Mechanical obstruction to the emptying of the stomach from pyloric stenosis, hour-glass contraction, or external adhesions. (4) Ulcer or stenosis of the duodenum. The author considers Gunsberg's test the best for free hydrochloric acid. A further proof that if hydrochloric acid is present the stenosis is simple, that is cicatricial. If it be absent the obstruction is more likely to be due to malignant growth; further than this the test does not carry us. An important factor in establishing a diagnosis lies in determining whether or not there is "gastric stasis." By this is meant the presence of food remnants in the stomach after the period of digestion. Saundby, together with the author, resorted to the following method: Meat, bread and milk with a few currants and raisins are given at 8 P.M. Twelve hours later the stomach is emptied with a tube and washed out. Any food remnants indicate "gastric stasis." The addition of the currants and raisins makes the test more complete, as they are notoriously rather tough objects for the gastric juice to deal with, and they cannot easily get through a much-narrowed pylorus. If the test is not conclusive the same meal should be given and removed in nine hours. If there are particles in this, operation is indicative; if not, operation is contraindicated and the patient should be handed over to the medical division.

Duodenal Ulcer.—Since Robert F. Weir presented his paper before the American Surgical Association in 1900, in which he analyzed the cases of duodenal ulcer reported, many observers have given their attention to this important subject. WILLIAM J. MAYO (Annals of Surgery, December, 1904) states that until very recently duodenal ulcers have been regarded as secondary to gastric ulcers and that the two are usually combined in one case. This has not been borne out by the experience of himself and his brother, they having found that the gastric ulcer if present, has not been of the same grade and character as the duodenal. Within the last year the percentage of duodenal ulcerations, which have been recognized by these operators, has arisen from 12 per cent. to 27 per cent. The author believes that typical round ulcer of many years standing may exist without involvement of the outer coats, a condition which is well known to exist in the case of gastric ulceration. Most duodenal ulcers, however, are probably of a cicatricial type and are more prone to perforate than the gastric lesion. The form of perforation is usually a

chronic one, as is evidenced by great masses of adhesions. All the cases of duodenal ulcerform of adhesions. All the cases of duodenal ulcer occurred within the first 2½ inches of the bowel, well above the entrance of the common duct. The causation depends on the irritating gastric secretion and the treatment consequently is gastro-enterostomy, the food will pass out by preference through an unobstructed pylorus by muscular action, the apparent gravity advantage of a low point gastro-enterostomy being equalized by intra-abdominal tension. For this reason, when the ulcer does not cause at least partial obstruction, it may be necessary to artificially block the pyloric outlet. There are three ways of closing the pylorus. Infolding after the plan of Scott, a continuous suture turns the periphery of the intestine into the lumen. Fowler accomplishes the same result by the use of silver wire. Lastly, the blocking may be effected by section and invagination. This is the slowest but the most certain.

GENITO-URINARY AND SKIN DISEASES.

Chronic Prostatitis.—This disease may be the cause of many serious consequences, according to E. G. BALLENGER (Am. Med., November 12, 1903), such as sexual neurasthenia, sterility, impotence and reinfection, as it forms a favorable nidus for lingering gonorrhea. The symptoms, until recent years, have been placed under the headings spermatorrhea, azoospermatorrhea, prostatorrhea, etc., and were claimed to be of neurotic origin. The literature, except in the last few years, has been inadequate and misleading because the pathology was unknown. Before giving consent for a patient with an apparently cured gonorrhea to marry, the secretions of the prostate and appendages should be examined. There is no disease in which more information can be obtained from a careful examination of the prostate and its secretions. Treatment in prostatic disease should be directed to complications as well as to the establishment of proper hygiene for the patient. The prostate should be treated by massage, or by heat and cold variously applied. The brilliant results of prostatic surgery should stimulate increased interest in the rational medical treatment of chronic prostatitis.

Primary Lupus Vulgaris of the Oropharynx and Nasopharynx Treated by X-Rays.—H. S. BIRKETT (Med. Rec., December 24, 1904) describes a case of extensive primary lupus of the oropharynx successfully treated by X-rays. The patient was a boy of fifteen years, otherwise well, with a family history of tuberculosis. The diagnosis was confirmed by the histological examination of excised portions of the growths, by the identification of tubercle bacilli in sections and by inoculation of a guinea-pig, with positive results. An injection of tuberculin caused a general and a local reaction. Treatment of the condition by excision under ether, with subsequent curettage and local applications of lactic acid and the galvanocautery, were not very satisfactory. After an interval of several months the patient returned for treatment and the use of the X-ray was begun. After three months of intermittent treatment the local conditions entirely disappeared and the patient was considered cured, but six months later there was a slight recurrence in the oropharynx and a small ulcer had appeared in one nostril. These are improving under the X-ray, and the author believes that the condition will give way entirely to this method of treatment as it did on the former occasion.

Scleroderma With Atrophy of the Tongue and Ulceration.—M. ANTONY (*Gaz. Med. de Paris,* August 6, 1904) relates the case of a patient, aged forty-three years, showing scleroderma that has lasted sixteen years, following an attack of polyarticular rheumatism. Some improvement followed massage and electric baths. Atrophy and ulceration of the tongue are present.

Treatment of Catarrhal Pyelitis.—The local treatment of this condition by means of lavage of the renal pelvis is described by W. AYRES (*Am. Jour. of Urology,* October, 1904). He believes that this condition is more frequent than is generally supposed and that it is very often a cause for a prolonged discharge. He has found local treatment rational and feasible, and believes that beginning nephritis due to pyelitis, may be cured by lavage of the pelvis, and that its development may be guarded against by the same means. The straight view, Tilden Brown cystoscope is to be preferred, and the catheters must be passed slowly and gently. Silver nitrate, protargol and argyrol have always been successfully used, but the author's preference is for silver nitrate. He begins with a solution of $^1/_{10,000}$, and slowly increases its strength to $^1/_{5,000}$. After the catheters are in place and enough urine collected for observation, a small quantity of fluid is injected into the catheter and allowed to flow out again. This is repeated five or six times. He begins with half a dram at a time, and later increases this to half an ounce if the patient does not complain of pain. It is essential that a careful microscopical record be kept of the urine as a means of directing the medication.

The Use of the X-Rays in Diabetic Patients.—That this disease is no contra-indication to the employment of the rays for malignant skin disease is shown by the case reported by LEVY-DORN (*Berl. klin. Woch.,* September 19, 1904). A man, aged fifty-nine years, presented an extensive lupus patch of the buttock of over twenty years standing, which had lately grown rapidly and undergone malignant changes (epithelioma). The presence of diabetes for the past six years, with about seven per cent. of sugar in the urine, contra-indicated surgical interference and the patient was given short, mild exposure to the X-rays, with excellent results. The first applications were followed by great improvement, and then there was a stationary period, with complete healing after the treatment had been pushed to the production of a mild reaction.

Eosin Phototherapy.—A preliminary communication is published by F. J. PICK and K. ASAHI (*Berl. klin. Woch.,* September 12, 1904) concerning 22 cases of skin disease treated by sunlight after the application of eosin by the method of Tappeiner. These comprised 12 cases of lupus, 1 of tuberculosis cutis verrucosa, 5 of trichophytosis, 1 of rodent ulcer and 3 of scrofuloderma. The affected areas were daily painted with a special one per cent. solution of eosin and exposed to the sunlight. The results even in lupus, were very favorable, but complete cure cannot be spoken of. The procedure in its present form is not as yet sufficiently developed.

"Some of My Opinions."—An interesting contribution to journal literature consists of a review (by himself) of the opinions advanced at various times, by JONATHAN HUTCHINSON (*Berl. klin. Woch.,* September 12, 1904). In discussing the nature of syphilis, he adheres to his first conception, that this should rank as a specific fever, and that the primary symptoms were local, the secondary as implying blood contamination, and the tertiary as being sequelæ which resulted from toxic elements left behind by the inflammations which had occurred in the secondary period. For this reason he claims that the administration of mercury, which

must be accepted as a true antidote, should be commenced as soon as the diagnosis of the chancre becomes reasonably certain. The most convenient method of administrating mercury is in the form of a pill in frequently repeated small doses (Hydrarg. cum Gretæ, grs. 1 to 2). In order to prevent diarrhea, opium should be combined with the mercury. As regards marriage, he allows it after the expiration of two full years from the date of the chancre. He has had no cases to convince him that syphilis had been transmitted by inheritance to the third generation, and does not believe in the possibility of such transmission. The protection against second infection is not permanent and varies much in different persons.—*Molluscum contagiosum* he defines as a new structure which is evolved as a result of the implantation of a still unidentified parasitic germ and is the exact analogue of the galls found on plants.—Syphilitic teeth and interstitial keratitis may be accepted as trustworthy evidences of inherited syphilis.—Leprosy, he thinks, can nearly always be cured, if the patient be given a liberal supply of good food and made to abstain absolutely from fish. Recovery is also by the internal and external use of Chaulmoogra oil. The bacillus of leprosy and tuberculosis are differentiated forms of the same organisms, as they are similar in many features and their clinical results are closely parallel. He still thinks that the eating of badly cured or decomposing fish is the sole cause of leprosy and that it is not contagious by either touch, breath or insect bites. It may be communicated, however, by an infant taking milk from a leprous mother or by persons eating food which has been contaminated by leprous hands.—Gonorrhea in all stages is best treated by parasiticide injections and the more acute the symptoms, the more essential is the injection of the chloride of zinc solution. Gonorrheal rheumatism occurs almost solely in those who inherit gout.—Alopecia areata is usually a sequel of ringworm and is common in a ratio with the prevalence of the latter. The fungus in the different forms of *Tinea* is probably the same.—When tertiary syphilis simulates lupus, it is because the patient is tuberculous as well as syphilitic.—The various forms of malignant disease depend not upon parasitic infection but upon hereditary proclivities of tissue which are essentially the same for all and that the different forms are transmutable in inheritance. The long-continued use of arsenic, whether externally or internally, increases the tissue proclivity for all forms of new growth. Certain other mineral drugs may share with arsenic as tending to increase the liability to cancer.

The Treatment of Lupus by the General Practitioner.—The use of the X-ray or the Finsen light requires the employment of costly apparatus and special qualifications which lie without the means or abilities of the general practitioner. An efficient substitute for these methods is recommended by DREUW (*Berl. klin. Woch.,* November 21, 1904), who implies commercial hydrochloric acid to the affected surfaces with a cotton tipped tooth tick, after the area is well frozen with the ethyl chloride spray. The action seems to be accentuated if the acid is saturated with free chlorine gas. From the cases which he reports and the histological examinations made, it appears that the acid, when brought into contact with tuberculous tissue, causes a prompt emigration of white blood cells into these areas so that it is impossible to distinguish them. There is also a diapedesis around the vessels. This process does not take place in normal tissues under the same circumstances. Where the lupus involves the nose or lips, or in the presence of abscesses or fistulæ, a general anesthetic may be necessary. A gray slough forms within a few days after cauterization, and remains for several weeks. When this drops off the superficial tupus tubercles come away, and if any remain, the treatment may be reapplied once or twice at intervals of three to four weeks. In from three to six months the ulceration becomes covered with epidermis and if any isolated tubercles persist, these may be punctured with pointed capillary tubes filled with hydrochloric acid. The results obtained are claimed to be excellent, and three cases have been observed for a year without recurrence. But even if this occurs, it may readily be attacked if the patients are cautioned to present themselves every three months for examination. The method may also be combined with others, especially the Finsen light, as the tubercles are brought nearer to the surface by the cauterization process.

Dermopathy and Its Relation to General Trophic Disturbance.—RADCLIFF CROCKER (*Gazz. degli osped.*, October 4, 1904) states that physiological metabolism in its disturbances gives rise to dermatoses. Disturbances of the secretory glands, especially the thyroid gland, causes dermatoses. This is obvious in myxedema, but also demonstrable in psoriasis, pityriasis vulva, lichen and ichthyosis. Leucoderma, melanoderma, and various pigmentary lesions of Graves' disease, are also associated with the thyroid gland. The commonest skin troubles connected with the liver are universal pruritus; this and other skin lesions are due to general auto-intoxication associated with a bad liver. Xanthetasma and xanthoma are connected with glycosuria, as are furuncles and gangrene. Acne rosacea, chromidosis lupus erythematosis are usually held to be caused by autotoxemia. Brocqs in Paris, from 2,000 urinary examinations demonstrates nutritive disturbances in all kinds of skin disease.

PHYSIOLOGY.

Renal Function after Nephrectomy.—A number of experiments on the behavior of the remaining kidney after nephrectomy are recorded by T. SCHILLING (*Arch. f. exp. Path. u. Pharmak.*, Vol. 52, Nos. 1 and 2). He finds that concentrated solution of chloride of sodium, given by mouth, are excreted as rapidly as in normal animals, if the supply of water is not reduced. With less water the salt appears in the urine in less concentrated form and requires a longer time for its excretion. When compensatory hypertrophy is complete the remaining kidney can meet increased requirements, so that salt is voided like in normal animals. Large amounts of water introduced into the stomach of nephrectomized animals will dilute the urine much longer than normally. A single kidney is not able to get rid of large amounts of saline solution introduced intravenously as rapidly as two kidneys. Indigo-carmine is also voided in less concentrated condition and much less sugar is produced after injection of phlorhizin. With diabetes due to caffeine, there is no relation between polyuria and glycosuria, since the diuresis is due to direct action of the caffeine upon the renal cells, while the sugar is formed outside of the kidneys.

Action of Pituitary Extracts.—It is difficult to foresee the extent to which modern studies in the internal secretions will be of practical utility in clinical medicine. The numerous investigations on the internal secretion of the adrenal glands have been justified by the eminently practical application of the results. That the pituitary body, of peculiar interest to the morphologist on account of its embryological antecedents, has an important physiological significance in the organism,

is indicated by the recent experiments of P. T. HERRING (*Jour. of Physiol.*, November 2, 1904). Pituitary extracts have an important action on the cardio-vascular apparatus. Extracts of the infundibular portion of the pituitary body cause acceleration and augmentation of the isolated frog ventricle when perfused through it. Strong extracts, four per cent. of the dried material increase the contraction of the ventricle, doing away with the pause after diastole, and bringing about a pause at the end of systole. The heart's volume decreases as the cardiac muscle becomes more and more contracted. If perfusion of a strong extract continues for a long time the beats become irregular and weak, while the heart remains tonically contracted. Injection intravenously into a frog deprived of its central nervous system causes slowing and diminution of the heart-beat. This is abolished by atropine, and pituitary extract now brings about acceleration and augmentation. The infundibular portion of the pituitary contains some substance or substances which act on the intrinsic inhibitory nervous mechanism of the heart and also on the intrinsic accelerator mechanism, stimulating both. The action on the former is abolished by atropine. The active substance in the pituitary which brings about constriction of the peripheral arterioles acts by stimulating the vasomotor nerves, and this action is abolished by a larger dose of apocodeine.

The Physiological Action of Azoimid.—This substance, discovered fourteen years ago by Curtius, has the formula HN_3, and is the only substance giving the nitrogen anion in solution. Its sodium salt is prepared in the following manner: By the action of ammonia on metallic sodium, sodamid ($NaNH_2$) is formed, and this compound is converted into azoimid by the action of nitrous acid. Azoimid is highly explosive. According to L. SMITH and C. G. L. WOLF (*Jour. of Med. Research*, November, 1904), this substance is a protoplasmic poison resembling in its action hydrocyanic acid. Nerve and muscle are paralyzed, with a preliminary stage of increased excitability. The vapor of azoimid inhaled causes excitation of the respiratory centers with subsequent paralysis. The blood pressure is lowered. This fall is due primarily to vasomotor disturbance. The intestine and kidney take part in vasodilatation in exceptional instances only. The acid is the most powerful of the compounds containing the tri-nitrogen group. The introduction of a phenyl radical diminishes the effect of the complex. Azoimid forms a compound with methemoglobin similar to that formed by hydrocyanic acid. Neither the existence of an azoimid hemoglobin or an azoimid hematin was made out.

On the Antitryptic Action of Normal Serum.—It has been known for a number of years that blood serum prevents the action of trypsin, and it has been known for a longer time that trypsin is destroyed by contact with the tissues in vitro. E. P. CATHCART (*Jour. of Physiol.*, November 2, 1904) has discovered that the anti-action of normal serum against trypsin is found in connection with the so-called albumin fraction, *i.e.*, the fraction precipitated between half and full saturation with ammonium sulphates. Globulins do not possess antitryptic action, but are only very slowly attacked by the enzyme. This anti-action is found in all varieties of serum examined. It is effective with all varieties of proteid, whether in solid or fluid form. Absolute specificity does not exist and partial specificity is questionable. The isolated antibody—the albumin fraction—is rapidly injured by heating. Dried antibody retains its anti-ferment action very well, and dialysis, as a rule, has no apparent destructive influence.

The Oxygen Exchange of the Pancreas.—It is probable that many diseases of metabolic origin are closely bound up with aberrations of the oxidative phenomena of the tissues. The searchlight of most investigations on the origin of diabetes has been turned principally upon the pancreas. The study of the physiology of the pancreas has been richly extended within the past five years. Two recent important discoveries on the mode of secretion of the pancreatic juice are that "secretin," a substance secreted by the intestinal mucous membrane and absorbed by the blood, acts as a chemical stimulus of the pancreatic secretion, and "that there is no direct relationship between the rate of secretion of pancreatic juice and the extent of the blood supply." These two facts furnished a basis for the experiments of J. BANCROFT and E. H. STARLING (*Jour. of Physiol.*, November 2, 1904), in the oxygen exchange of the pancreas. The authors found that the pancreatic secretion is accompanied by an increased oxygen absorption from the blood by the pancreas. This is shown both by the chemical method and by the pump. This increased oxidation takes place irrespective of increased blood flow through the organ. The normal oxidation of the pancreas is much greater than that of the body generally and about the same as that of the submaxillary gland.

The Heat Contraction in Nerves.—A number of facts have been established by the researches of T. G. BRODIE and W. D. HALLIBURTON (*Jour. of Physiol.*, November 2, 1904), which indicates a biological adaptation of the tissue proteids of animals in relation to their normal temperatures, and to the rise of temperature to which they may be safely subjected. When a nerve is heated it shortens very considerably; this is especially the case with frog's nerves, and is true for the spinal cord. This shortening, as in muscle, takes place in a series of steps, and the temperatures at which these successive contractions occur coincide with the coagulation temperatures of the proteids contained in saline extracts of nervous tissues. The temperatures of the first contraction in nerves or spinal cord correspond closely with those in muscle. They further correspond with those in liver, the method being applicable to tissues like the liver, where the histological elements show no longitudinal arrangement. The death temperature of muscle is that at which the first proteid coagulates. The same is true for nervous tissues. Conduction and electrical response are abolished then.

The Effect of Poisons on Enzymes.—That the various activities of the cells of the body are largely controlled by enzymes, is one of the leading thoughts of the newer physiology. An inquiry into the manner in which enzymes are influenced by poisons, would be of undoubted importance from the standpoint of rational pharmacology. Such an investigation was pursued by G. SENTER (*Proc. Royal Soc.*, November 1, 1904). A year ago the author discovered in defibrinated blood, a new ferment which he called "hemase," which like other ferments, decomposes hydrogen peroxide but, unlike them, it does not give the guaiac reaction. Enzymes are all soluble in water, are precipitated by alcohol and are destroyed by heating to $60°$ to $70°$ F. Their activity is influenced by small traces of foreign bodies. The author conducted his investigation on hemase, using various classes of poisons. Acids have a retarding effect, while alkalis retard the action of hemase but not permanently. The effect of hemase disappears on neutralization. Alkaline salts with oxidizing properties, such as $KCl\ O_3$, have a depressing effect, which is partly dependent on the oxidation of the enzyme and partly independent of it. Reducing

agents, such as H_2S, are remarkably poisonous to the action. In this connection, as showing the analogy between enzymes and colloidal solutions of certain metal, Bredig has discovered that H_2S is poisonous to the catalysis of peroxide of hydrogen by means of colloidal platinum. Mercuric chloride, bromide and cyanide vary in this respect: while the first two are exceedingly toxic, the last has little action. Paul and Krönig have shown that the poisonous action on the bacteria diminishes from the chloride through the bromide to the cyanide, and that the electrolytic dissociation of these compounds diminishes in the same order. Carbon monoxide has no appreciable poisonous effect on hemase. It is interesting to note in this connection that CO is not poisonous to the germination of seeds, nor to bacteria, nor does it effect the fermentation of sugar by zymase. Of singular importance is the fact that aqueous solutions of iodine are only slightly poisonous to hemase, while solutions in water also containing KI (which solutions contain I in I_3 ions) are distinctly poisonous. As O_4, which is highly poisonous for the lower organisms, has a slightly poisonous effect upon enzymes. As regards the mechanism of the action of these various poisons, the author believes that hemase exists in a state of fine subdivision, but he does not believe that catalysis is due to the large amount of surface resulting from extreme subdivision, since many colloidal solutions have no catalytic effect whatever. If the enzyme is supposed to exist in a colloidal state, then the action of the poisons may be explained on any one of three hypotheses: (1) Part of the enzyme is rendered inert by forming a chemical compound with the poison. (2) Part of the surface of the particles is covered with a thin layer of the poison or its decomposition products, thus preventing further action of the enzyme. (3) The relation of the particles to the surrounding media may be altered in various ways, (change of surface tension, alteration of relative difference of potential, etc.). The second hypothesis is supported by the experience of Kastle and Löwenhart who found that the retarding action of poisons on the catalysis of H_2O_2 by metals, is due to the formation of insoluble films between the poisons and catalyzers. The author favors the first hypothesis. Some enzymes are amphoteric, which under ordinary circumstances are neutral, but in the presence of bases develop acid properties and can combine with acids to form salts.

Is Trypsin a Collection of Ferments?—The question of the unity and specific nature of trypsin was the basis of an experimental investigation by L. POLLAK (*Hofmeister's Beiträge z. chem. Physiol., etc.*, November, 1904). He found that under the influence of acids pancreatic extracts may be changed in such a manner as to lose their digestive power on serum albumin, white of egg and fibrin, and yet are able to digest gelatin. This property of trypsin is a particularly specific one, and is ascribed by the author to a specific ferment, "glutinase." It is possible to inhibit the action of the latter by means of an anti-glutinase, which is obtained by heating pancreatic infusions to over $70°$ C. This antibody is not dialyzable, it does not act like a ferment, and is not destroyed by boiling for five minutes. Its mother-substance is precipitated by ammonium sulphate and alcohol, and is present in extracts of the pancreas that contain no proteid. Its amount is variable in different extracts. It inhibits the digestion of gelatin and when present in greater concentration, it slightly inhibits the digestion of serum-albumin. It is not identical with the anti-trypsin obtained from the blood-serum. The author believes that future researches will reveal a number of ferments besides glutinase in trypsin.

THE MEDICAL NEWS.

A WEEKLY JOURNAL

OF MEDICAL SCIENCE.

COMMUNICATIONS in the form of Scientific Articles, Clinical Memoranda, Correspondence or News Items of interest to the profession are invited from all parts of the world. Reprints to the number of 250 of original articles contributed exclusively to the MEDICAL NEWS will be furnished without charge if the request therefor accompanies the manuscript. When necessary to elucidate the text, illustrations will be engraved from drawings or photographs furnished by the author. Manuscript should be typewritten.

SMITH ELY JELLIFFE, A.M., M.D., Ph.D., Editor,
No. 111 FIFTH AVENUE, NEW YORK.

Subscription Price, Including postage in U. S. and Canada.

PER ANNUM IN ADVANCE	. . . .	$4.00
SINGLE COPIES	. . . . .	.10
WITH THE AMERICAN JOURNAL OF THE MEDICAL SCIENCES, PER ANNUM	. .	8.00

Subscriptions may begin at any date. The safest mode of remittance is by bank check or postal money order, drawn to the order of the undersigned. When neither is accessible, remittances may be made at the risk of the publishers, by forwarding in *registered* letters.

LEA BROTHERS & CO.,
No. 111 FIFTH AVENUE (corner of 18th St.), NEW YORK.

SATURDAY, JANUARY 21, 1905.

TETANY.

PERHAPS in no disease is the profound effect of surgical progress more marked than upon the complex group of symptoms known as tetany. The etiology of this disease, as given in all the leading text-books, has always been too broad and inclusive to seem scientifically accurate. In other words, the widely differing conditions, which have since the days of Trousseau been chronicled as causative factors, have been so utterly different in type that it has seemed improbable that they could bring about like pathological conditions. Recent surgical findings are teaching that this supposition is true.

Take for example such widely differing etiological factors for tetany, as given by the well-known German neurologist Strümpell, in his Text-Book of Medicine,—"Catching cold deserves particular mention." "The disorder has appeared as a sequel to acute diseases." "Tetany is apt to follow the operative extirpation of goiter." "Tetany may sometimes be to a certain extent epidemic." "Endemic influences may promote its occurrence." Kassowitz attributes it to cranial tabes. Cunningham, *Annals of Surgery*, Vol. 39, page 543, recites the following etiological theories: "Kussmaul believes the

inspissation of the blood, produced by loss of fluid from the tissues of the body which results from frequent vomiting and by increased secretion of the gastric mucosa, affects the motor centers of the nervous system." Germain-See and Berlizheimer believe that the tetanic spasms are caused by reflex action produced by stimulation of the sensory nerves of the stomach. Devic considers the condition due to auto-intoxication owing to prolonged and abnormal chemical processes of digestion in certain cases of gastric retention and hypersecretion. He has isolated a substance taken from a chronically dilated stomach, which produced general convulsions when injected into animals. Mayo Robson (*Annals of Surgery*, December, 1904, page 910) is quoted as regarding auto-intoxication or gastric fermentation as a predisposing cause of tetany.

It will thus be seen that three widely differing theories as to the causation of this complex condition or group of clinical symptoms have been proposed, viz.: (1) increase of specific gravity of the blood because of diminished absorption of fluids; (2) stimulation of the sensory nerve terminations by mechanical irritation, and (3) auto-intoxication.

Largely as the clinical result of drainage operations upon the stomach, the cause and effect of which have been observed closely within the past few years, it may now be regarded as probable that the symptoms described as "tetany" have, in every case, had their primary origin in some lesion or abnormal variation of the gastric mucosa. Cases of "tetany" reported as occurring in individuals with normal stomachs have probably been erroneously so reported. In other words, surgical progress has shown that there is need of restricting the use of the vague term "tetany." In support of this may be mentioned the conclusion of James P. Warbasse (*Annals of Surgery*, December, 1904), who states that tetany in the past has been confused with epilepsy and other nervous phenomena. Is it reasonable to believe the "tetany" of pregnant and lactating women is analogous with the "tetany" described by Warbasse as occurring in a man whose stomach contained one pound of scrap iron, or that either of these conditions may even remotely be pathologically related with the "tetany" which is known to occur after total extirpation of the thyroid gland?

The time seems ripe to consider whether very widely differing pathological processes have not been erroneously grouped together simply because the clinical phenomena of the pathological lesions have borne confusing resemblance to each other.

THE HOUSE STAFF AND THE HOSPITAL DIETITIAN.

VIGOROUS young men, whose intellectual activity as well as whose firm grip on physical life have enabled them to make positions on the house staffs of our prominent municipal hospitals, are not invalids. Although the public usually believes otherwise—because of the gratuitous and merry gibes cast at these young officers by the newspapers and general public—they do accomplish an immense amount of work.

The dietetic tidal wave which is sweeping over our hospital organizations and carrying before it into deep water many old customs that were bad, as well as many positively vicious practices, cannot be expected to wash out old traditions without creating a certain moiety of disturbance. Perhaps one of the most difficult relationships to arrange in this new and very welcome dietetic departure will be that of the gentle dietitian, our modern conception of Ceres, to her relatively husky, hale and hearty brothers of the house staff.

It is interesting to picture the fair graduate of the Drexel Institute or of the Teachers' College presiding over the gastronomic functions of eighteen or twenty young gentlemen who in the past have been in the habit of depending solely upon nature's calls to regulate the quantity and quality of their foodstuff.

Now, however, by municipal command, their sugars are measured by the cube of the beet root and their fats by calorifacients. As related by a visiting surgeon who was recently belated at an Island hospital, and who elected as a consequence to dine with the staff, there is further no such thing as superfluous food in the staff kitchen. The fair graduate has estimated the number of grams which her fraternal co-workers should consume, and she allows them neither more nor less. Alas for the hapless youth who, in the possession of vigorous health and buoyant spirits, finds himself beset with the demon of hunger! Nowhere on the old Island can it now be appeased as in the good old days when a ration or two extra of ward whisky—the acknowledged unit of coinage in the Island realm—would bring forth to the hungry and weary young doctor a variety of succulent and hearty, although not weighed and calculated,

juicy, steaming viands! All this is a thing of the past!

No doubt neither the proportions of the three foodstuffs nor their quantities are as yet properly regulated for the staff. They certainly are for the patients, but what is good for the patients, wise, shy, hospital dietetic graduate, is not always to be recommended for the gentlemen who prowl the wards by day and play nefarious and energy-wrecking games by night.

A CLEARING HOUSE FOR SCIENTIFIC RESEARCH.

THE munificent endowments of Carnegie and Rockefeller for the promotion of experimental research, have, as may be seen by glancing at the vast scientific literature of to-day, already borne substantial fruit. The world has seen only a beginning in the direction of practical philanthropy, and it is comforting to reflect that at no remote time the public and private funds available for furthering scientific discovery, will be perfectly ample to repay investigators of originality and skill. Yet to one who keeps in touch with the work of that modest army, patiently toiling in the obscure recesses of the laboratories, there frequently comes the thought that in no other branch of human endeavor is there such a reckless expenditure of energy and general aimlessness as in the field of research, particularly in those sciences that are tributary to the art of medicine.

The time is ripe for the application of scientific methods to research. A great deal of this is aimless and impractical, is frequently a repetition of similar work done in the past, and often the same theme is prosecuted in two or more parts of the world. The young and inexperienced investigator depends only too frequently upon caprice and accident for the selection of his problem, without reference to its particular value from the standpoint either of what has already been accomplished or of the pressing needs of the moment. The result is that the journals are crowded with a mass of undigested and unrelated material, much of which is relegated to the limbo of the library shelves.

The criticism may be lodged against this view that no one can gauge the ultimate value of any piece of scientific work. Truth is not relative but absolute, and every fact that is recovered from darkness should be cherished without regard to its present significance or value. One may indeed cite many instances of the most unforeseen and far-reaching applications of facts which, in themselves, were dry and uninteresting.

This criticism is uncontrovertible, and yet, without disparaging the worth of any theme, no matter how impractical the latter may seem, one may ask, would it not be better that only those things should engage the attention and enlist the labors of scientific investigators, which most closely meet the requirements of the day, or which fill in some of the most prominent gaps of knowledge? In other words, a plea must be made for the more systematic and thorough tilling of the field of knowledge. The present method may be compared to that of the farmer who ploughs his acres in patches and frequently goes over the same ground twice.

How may this haphazard, hit-and-miss pursuit of truth be remedied? The mere individual guidance of the laboratory chief is not alone sufficient, for with all due deference to the comprehensive knowledge of some of the most eminent investigators, one cannot expect of them an acquaintance with all the needs of modern science and with all its enormous literature. One may then point to such monumental works, of which the *Index Medicus* is an example, and say that they supply all that can be desired. Valuable and indispensable as it must be acknowledged, the *Index Medicus* records merely by title what has been accomplished and points out neither the unexplored gaps nor the relative value of the various kinds of work. The text-books might then be appealed to, but such is the unceasing progress of the day, that the ink of these has hardly become dry before they are already behind the times. The annual and quarterly publications recording recent progress in the various sciences, testify to this deficiency of the text-books, but what is true of the latter applies with equal force to the former. .

A clearing house for scientific research should be established. Without giving the exact details for the perfection of such an institution, for time and experience alone can do this, it would not be unprofitable to suggest some of the lines along which it may be developed. This institution would demand the permanent employment of men of all but encyclopedic knowledge and specialists in their own lines,—physics chemistry, biology, physiology, pathology, etc. It would also require the services of other men. as consultants, too busy in their own separate spheres to devote all their time to the affairs of the institution. The latter would be the most eminent men of science in all parts of the world. Then there would be a large literary and clerical force to direct the enquiries and correspondence connected with the administration of this large organization.

This body would be of international scope, for it would direct all the scientific research of the world. With an immense library at its command, it would, at the height of its working capacity, represent a living, moving, and plastic index of science. An investigator, desirous of starting on some new scientific cruise, would communicate with this institution. He would then learn of some region whose exploration is urgently demanded by the present needs of science. His course would be charted out for him and he would be supplied with all the necessary data. The difficulty of his quest would be commensurate with his abilities. Various aspects of and sidelights on the same problem can thus be investigated simultaneously in different parts of the world. The journals in which the various results would be published would be designated by this central body; in this manner there would discontinue the practice, which often prevails, of publishing an important scientific paper in some out-of-the-way journal having a narrow circle of readers. A certain number of reprints of the article would revert to the clearing house, which would be an ideal repository for them to be sent at some future date for purposes of reference to other investigators, particularly if the latter reside at a locality remote from a large scientific library.

It is self-evident that the maintenance of such an institution would entail an enormous expenditure. The Carnegie Institution at Washington might find in this organization a grand extension of its sphere of usefulness. Established for the purpose of endowing scientific research, the maintenance of a bureau for the general supervision and guidance of this work, would be in line with the wise policy of its foundation.

With the establishment of the clearing house for research, the net results to scientific progress would be remarkably increased. Individual originality would not suffer, for no one who would desire to prosecute an investigation without the aid of this international bureau, could be prevented from doing so. But he who would avail himself of the collective experience and knowledge of the distinguished men connected or affiliated with this proposed institution, would receive, besides the assurance that goes with a happy start, an invaluable impetus for the accomplishment of successful work. He would feel, in a manner which no other method could make him feel, a close kinship with the scientific world;

he would become a vital part of that vast guild, working as one man for the increase of knowledge and the uplifting of humanity.

ECHOES AND NEWS.

NEW YORK.

City Hospital.—The following resolution was adopted at the last meeting of the Medical Board of the City Hospital: " That notice be sent to the members of the Medical Board calling attention to the fact that the control of the granting of vacations and sick-leaves to members of the Interne Staff is left entirely in the hands of the Committee of Inspection."

Eclectic Medical Society Election.—The New York Eclectic Medical Society reconvened January 12 and elected the following officers for the ensuing year: President, W. J. Krausi, M.D., of New York; First Vice-President, R. W. Padgham, M.D., of Geneva; Second Vice-President, F. D. Gridley, M.D., of Binghamton; Third Vice-President, M. B. Pearlstein, M.D., of Brooklyn; Treasurer, D. N. Bulson, M.D., of Rockville Centre; Recording Secretary, Earl H. King, M.D., of Saratoga Springs; Corresponding Secretary, G. W. Boskowitz, M.D., of New York. The next meeting will be held at Albany.

The Manuel Garcia Centenary Jubilee Fund.—At a meeting of the allied committees representing the Section on Laryngology of the New York Academy of Medicine, the American Laryngological, Rhinological and Otological Society and the American Laryngological Association, it was voted to appeal to laryngologists throughout the country for contributions not to exceed $5 each for the Garcia Fund. Payment should be made before February 15, to either of the following: Dr. D. Bryson Delavan, 1 East Thirty-third Street, New York; Dr. M. D. Lederman, 58 East Seventy-fifth Street, or Dr. Harmon Smith, 44 West Forty-ninth Street, New York, representing the Academy Section; Dr. R. C. Myles, 48 West Thirty-sixth Street, New York, representing the American Laryngological, Rhinological and Otological Society, or Dr. J. E. Newcomb, 118 West Sixty-ninth Street, New York, representing the American Laryngological Association.

Vereinigung Alter Deutscher Studenten in Amerika.—The last meeting (with ladies) of the " Vereinigung Alter Deutscher Studenten in Amerika " was held Wednesday, January 18, 1905, when a paper entitled "A Trip Through Manchuria " was read by Major L. L. Seaman, M.D.

PHILADELPHIA.

German Hospital.—At the annual meeting of the Board of Trustees Albert Schönhut and Otto E. Wolf were elected members to the Board of Trustees to fill the vacancies caused by the death of C. T. Wernwag and E. G. Reyenthaler. The Rev. F. Wischan, who has served on the Board for twenty-two years, was re-elected.

Polyclinic Hospital.—The treasurer's report shows that the cost to maintain that institution during the year just ended has been $71,464.17 and the receipts were $56,980.45, a deficit of $14,483.72. In the wards and in the dispensary together more than 29,000 patients have been treated and of the 20 per cent. increase 19 per cent. were treated free.

Beriberi.—The American bark Abbie Palmer arrived at the Breakwater Thursday with two well-defined cases of this disease on board. Both sailors are seriously ill but are expected to recover. The vessel came from Kaanapali, Hawaiian Islands, and was 152 days out. The crew was disembarked at Marcus Hook, where the vessel was fumigated and now will be allowed to proceed to Philadelphia with its cargo of sugar.

Purification of Water.—Dr. Mary E. Pennington claims that electricity induced into copper plates immersed in water will destroy the bacteria present. In one experiment she found that by inducing a mild current of electricity into the copper plates the number of bacteria per cubic centimeter was reduced from 42,000 in two minutes, to 2,400 in two minutes, to 900 in five and to 400 in ten minutes.

Philadelphia Bequests.—The late Henry Norris, of Philadelphia, who left an estate valued at $4,000,000, provided in his will, which has just been probated, $5,000 each for the University and Children's hospitals of Philadelphia.

Hospital in the Eastern Penitentiary.—Recently there has been completed in the prison a fully equipped hospital in which the convicts act as nurses. Six of the hospital cells are devoted to the treatment of tuberculosis. They have open fronts and have a separate yard attached where the prisoners can have out-door exercise. The tuberculous convicts have a separate dining-room and their food is prepared in the diet kitchen attached to the prison hospital. Of the 1,100 prisoners only 19 suffer with tuberculosis. In order to prevent the spread of this disease the asphalt of the exercise yard is scrubbed daily and the cells are kept perfectly clean.

Tuberculosis To Be Recorded.—The Bureau of Health sent out letters, containing proper blanks, to physicians asking them to report cases of tuberculosis occurring in their practice. This step is taken to further safeguard the public from the spread of the disease. The Bureau has no intention of placarding the houses in which tuberculosis occurs, it merely wishes to oversee the work that is being done and to extend its assistance where needed.

Portrait of Dr. Osler.—The medical graduates of the University of Pennsylvania who studied when Dr. Osler was connected with the institution have decided to present to the university a life-size portrait of their eminent friend and teacher. The painting will be done by some prominent American artist. Dr. Osler will sit for the painting prior to his departure for England.

Relationship Between the Science and Art of Pharmacy and the Science and Art of Medicine.—At a pharmaceutical meeting held at the Philadelphia College of Pharmacy, January 10, Dr. Henry Beates, Jr., President of the State Board of Medical Examiners, read a paper in which he said the pharmacist must be capable and skilful in order to perform his duties in a proper manner. To obtain these requirements a high standard of education is necessary and in order to get it there should be a cooperation of the medical and pharmaceutical colleges by establishing a rational curriculum in each. He says it is the incompetent and misrepresents only that object to a higher standard of education. Dr. Beates maintains that a pharmacist cannot serve well as a physician and a pharmacist, nor can a physician serve well as a pharmacist. Speaking upon the same topic Dr. John H. Musser, of Philadelphia, called the meeting's attention to the fact that the medical profession is making such rapid strides that the time may come when the pharmacist will no longer be necessary for very few drugs will be used as they are already being so rapidly displaced by water and fresh air. Then, too, the surgeon is relieving many conditions in which drugs were used for long periods of time. He does not consider the term " profession " applicable to medicine and pharmacy, as it permits of the encroachment of the various "pathies." He prefers to embrace them under the term "science." In order to make something of himself, of medicine or of pharmacy the individual engaged must pursue these callings as a science. It is thus, he said, that truth is elicited and character is made, for those who elicit the truth are truthful.

Evident Need of a Profession of Pharmacy.—Mr. M. I. Wilbert, Ph.M., of Philadelphia, in discussing the view, as maintained by some, that pharmacy is improperly classed as a profession, said that physicians who look upon their own calling in a true light regard pharmacy as a profession. With reference to selling of proprietary drugs he believes the pharmacist is less sinning than sinned against. He inclines to the view that higher standard of education is necessary and that the physician should not serve both as a pharmacist and as a doctor.

Meeting of the Pediatric Society.—Dr. J. P. C. Griffith reported cases and exhibited specimens of (1) Umbilical cord hernia, (2) Congenital stenosis of the bile ducts. Dr. D. L. Edsall and Dr. C. W. Miller read a paper entitled, "Dietic Use of Legume Flour, Particularly in Atrophic Infants." From the observation made they believe vegetable proteids in suitable amounts can be fed to infants. They maintain that nucleo-albumins can be supplied to the child which will aid in the development of its tissue cells without disturbing the digestion. Bean flour was used by them; it consisted of a 10 per cent. solution of very finely ground flour to which was added a diastase ferment and boiled when it became fluid. It exhibited no starch iodine reaction and was not coagulated by heat. In a series of cases in which wheat flour failed to improve the patient, they found some improvement after giving the bean flour, but they all died in time. They cited one case that had bowel derangement for two years and which had been placed upon barley and whey without improvement; after it had been fed upon the bean flour the bowel condition cleared up and the patient gained in weight and strength. From another series of observations they conclude that the amount of food value of bean flour may be substituted for an amount of milk equal in food value, and good results obtained. Digestion improves gradually while the condition of the child improves rapidly. Wheat flour, they consider, inferior to bean flour in value.

Annual Exhibition Meeting of the Pathological Society.—This was held January 11 and 12. Dr. J. McFarland, of the Medico-Chirurgical College, exhibited many microscopical sections showing how metastasis occurs in malignant tumors. Dr. M. H. Cryer, of University of Pennsylvania, exhibited many sections of the skull showing the various sinuses. Dr. W. T. Longcope and Dr. W. S. Robertson, of the Pennsylvania Hospital, showed a series of hearts and aneurisms. Dr. R. C. Rosenberger, of the Philadelphia Hospital, exhibited a series of hearts. Dr. B. M. Anspach, a series of tumors of the ovaries and uterus. Dr. Allen J. Smith, of the University of Pennsylvania, demonstrated the "Structure of the Distoma Pulmonale." Dr. J. Funke, of Jefferson Medical College, exhibited diseases of the alimentary canal. Dr. C. Y. White, of the Pepper Laboratory and Zoological Garden of Philadelphia, ex-

hibited tuberculosis of man and lower animals. Dr. C. H. Frazier, of University of Pennsylvania, showed tumors of the thyroid and salivary glands. Dr. A. F. Coca, showed peculiar bodies in the serum of artificial blisters on syphilitic eruption. Dr. D. J. McCarty, Pepper Laboratory, University of Pennsylvania, showed many specimens of cerebral arteriosclerosis. G. G. Davis, of University of Pennsylvania, showed many sections of various parts of the body. Phipps Hospital exhibited many specimens of lungs showing tuberculosis. Dr. Ludlum, of Friends' Asylum, showed neurofibrils. Dr. S. H. Gilliland, of Laboratory of State Live Stock Sanitary Board of Pennsylvania, exhibited specimens of tuberculosis and cultures of acid fast bacilli. Drs. G. E. de Schweinitz, E. A. Shumway and B. F. Bär, Jr., showed a series of sections of eyes. Episcopal Hospital exhibited a few hearts and aneurisms.

CHICAGO.

Charity Benefits By $25,000.—The executive committee in charge of the finances of the Charity Ball report that charity will benefit to the sum of $25,000. This amount will be divided pro rata among the following: Chicago Bureau of Charities, Visiting Nurses' Association, Children's Memorial Hospital, Provident Hospital and Training School, Old People's Home, Chicago Orphan Asylum, Allendale Association, Chicago Home for Convalescent Women and Children, Milk Commission of the Children's Hospital Society of Chicago, Illinois Children's Home and Aid Society, Bureau of Justice, and Home for Destitute Crippled Children.

Check to McCormick Hospital.—The proposed McCormick Memorial Hospital for contagious diseases received a setback when the Council Committee on health placed on file the amendment to the building ordinance regarding consents to be obtained for the erection of such a structure. A motion to pass the amendment was defeated by 3 to 4. The entire block bounded by Fifty-third and Fifty-fourth streets, and Calumet and South Park Avenues, has been purchased as the hospital site.

Baptist Hospital to Be Rebuilt One Wing at a Time.—Within the coming year a new wing, one-fourth the size of the present Chicago Baptist Hospital building, will be erected at a cost of $100,000, if the resolution adopted by the hospital association is acted upon. It is expected that the entire rebuilding of the hospital, which will be done one wing at a time, will cost $450,000, and will occupy many years. Seven new directors were elected, as follows: A. E. Wells, F. M. Buck, C. C. Teck, Rev. Johnstone Myers, Wm. R. Harper, John Nuveen, Geo. Burlingame. The election of officers will be held soon.

University of Chicago Crusade.—The crusade of this university for purer drinking water, which has been carried on for a year, has resulted in improved health among university students, according to Dr. Chas. P. Small, whose report for the last quarter of 1904 has just been made. Of the 3,000 students in residence at the university, there were only 355 who applied to the university physician for consultation, of which number 240 were men and 115 women. During the last quarter there has not been a single case of typhoid, and in the summer there were only three. This is the best record ever reported at the university.

Trained Service in State's Hospitals.—Miss Jane Addams and Miss Julia Lathrop presented this idea to the Chicago Woman's Club at a "civil service day meeting." They advocate educational institutions for training State Hospital employees. This may be either a feature of the civil service bill to come before the present session of the Illinois Legislature, or a development of the system when put into effect. "It has been suggested," said Miss Addams, "that a number of institutes can be founded in connection with the University of Illinois, where guards, attendants and nurses in the State institutions can receive scientific training."

High Mortality Among Cab Drivers.—The cab drivers are declared to hold the mortality record among the workers of Chicago. Seventy men out of a total average membership of the Cab and Carriage Drivers' Union are reported to have died during the last twelve months. The figures represent more than five times the normal Chicago mortality.

Staff for Cook County Hospital.—The staff of physicians for the Cook County Hospital, as recommended by an advisory committee of 25 doctors, was appointed by President Brundage, as follows: REGULAR STAFF: *Medicine.*—Drs. R. H. Babcock, W. S. Harpole, Chas. L. Mix, R. B. Preble, S. R. Slaymaker, Camillo Volini, M. L. Goodkind, J. B. Herrick, J. F. Miller, B. W. Sippy, Frederick Tice E. F. Wells. *Obstetrics.*—Drs. R. W. Holmes, Charles B. Reed, H. F. Lewis, Rachelle Yarros. *Children's and Contagious Diseases.*—Drs. W. L. Baum, I. A. Abt, E. X. Walls, E. B. Earle, F. S. Churchill, and G. H. Weaver. *Nervous and Mental Diseases.*—Drs. Sydney Kuh, Julius Grinker, L. H. Mettler, H. N. Moyer. *Surgery.*—Drs. E. Wyllys Andrews, A. I. Bouffleur, Chas. Davidson, D. N. Eisendrath, Wm. Hessert, F. A. Besley, T. A. Davis, B. B. Eads, A. E. Halstead, F. S. Hartman, C. E. Humiston, Chas. W. Heywood, O. W. MacKellar, M. L. Harris, A. P. Heineck, and W. E. Schröder. *Eye, Ear, Nose and Throat.*—Drs. Wm. E. Gamble, Frank Allport, Brown Pusey, and G. P. Marquis. *Skin and Venereal Diseases.*—Drs. L. Blake Baldwin and Wm. A. Pusey. GENERAL SCIENCE: *Pathology.*—Drs. Wm. A. Evans and E. R. Le Count. *Dentistry.*—M. J. Conley. *Pathological Chemistry.*—R. W. Webster. *Orthopedic Surgery.*—J. L. Porter. *X-ray.*—Dr. E. A. Fischkin.

Meeting of Cook County Hospital Staff.—The newly appointed staff of the Cook County Hospital met January 13, and were addressed by Mr. Brundage. In his address, Mr. Brundage made the announcement that county hospital physicians who did not visit the hospital at least three times a week, or were absent more than three successive days without an excuse of illness were to be asked by the President to resign, and their places would be filled by the Nominating Committe of 25 physicians. Greater efficiency of service is expected to result from the organization of the 78 members of the staff into one general body instead of into three separate bodies, representing the different schools of medicine. The new staff elected the following officers for the year: Chairman, Dr. W. L. Baum; Vice-Chairmen, Dr. L. Blake Baldwin, regular; Dr. H. V. Halbert, homeopath, and Dr. Hugo E. Betz, eclectic; Secretary, Dr. Chas. E. Kahlke, homeopath. New rules for the regulation of internes were drafted.

Bequests to Chicago.—The will of George E. P. Dodge, who died recently in Chicago, provides substantial bequests for a number of charitable and semi-charitable institutions. These include: Hahne-

mann Hospital, Chicago, $30,000; Central Church, Chicago, $30,000; Pacific Garden Mission, Chicago, $5,000; Selectmen, Bennington, Vt., $8,000; Beloit College, Beloit, Wis., $25,000; Chicago Commons, Chicago, $25,000; Hull House, Chicago, $15,000; American Bible Society, New York, $5,000; Gad's Hill Settlement, Chicago, $10,000. Many beneficiaries, including the kindergarten institutions, the memorial chapel at Lancaster, Mass., and the factory employees, were remembered in a private memorandum not included in the probated will.

Comparative Death Rates in Chicago and New York from Consumption and Pneumonia.—The discrepancy—so often noted in these bulletins—between the death rates of consumption and of pneumonia in New York and in Chicago is more marked in the current figures than ever. At the close of office hours in New York on January 7 there had been reported 164 deaths from consumption and 318 from pneumonia out of a total of 1,603 from all causes—proportions of 10.2 per cent. of consumption deaths and 19.8 per cent. of pneumonia deaths. In Chicago the corresponding figures are 41 from consumption and 135 from pneumonia out of a total of 542 from all causes and proportions of only 7.5 per cent. of consumption, but of 24.9 per cent. from pneumonia, or one-quarter of all deaths from this latter cause. These figures show a 36 per cent. excess of consumption proportion in New York over Chicago and a 25 per cent. excess of pneumonia proportion in Chicago over New York. Such discrepancies have never been so marked as during the present pneumonia season.

CANADA.

Ontario Medical Association.—The next annual meeting of the Ontario Medical Association will be held in Toronto, June 6 to 8, 1905. Dr. William Burt, of Paris, Ont., is the President and Dr. Charles P. Lusk, of Toronto, is the Secretary. Business and papers will be in charge of a committee for that purpose under the chairmanship of Professor Alexander Primrose, while arrangements will be in charge of another committee under the chairmanship of Professor Irving H. Cameron. Dr. Ochsner, of Chicago, will deliver an address in Surgery.

Canadian Medical Association.—The Canadian Medical Association will hold its thirty-eighth annual meeting this year in Halifax, N. S., August 22 to 25, under the Presidency of Dr. John Stewart, of that city, the General Secretary being Dr. George Elliott, Toronto. The Medical Society of Nova Scotia has decided that they will not hold their annual meeting as usual, and will act as host to the Canadian Medical Association. Mr. Francis Caird of the Royal Infirmary of Edinburgh, is coming out to deliver the address in Surgery. The address in Gynecology will be delivered by Dr. Howard Kelly of Baltimore. There will also be an address in Ophthalmology, by Dr. J. W. Stirling, of Montreal also one in Medicine and one in Pathology. The indications are that this will be a very largely attended meeting.

Trouble for Two Practitioners in British Columbia.—All has not been smooth sailing for two practitioners of British Columbia for some months past which has finally ended in the Medical Council of that Province having their names struck from the Register. In both instances the two practitioners are making an appeal to a Supreme Court judge, as the Medical Act of British Columbia provides for relief for any one who considers that he has been unjustly dealt with by the Council, may take an appeal to a Supreme Court judge, who is empowered to review the evidence upon which any such action has been taken.

Victoria Hospital, Montreal, Damaged by Fire.— At a very early hour on the morning of Saturday, January 14, fire broke out in the Royal Victoria Hospital, Montreal, which did damage to the extent of $25,000. Not a patient was hurt or even disturbed.

The Thunder Bay Medical Association.—A medical association has been organized at Port Arthur, Ontario, under the name of The Thunder Bay Medical Association. Dr. G. W. Brown, of Port Arthur, is President; Dr. W. W. Birdsall, Vice-President; Dr. H. E. Paul, Secretary, and Dr. J. M. McGrady, Treasurer.

Royal Victoria Hospital, Montreal.—The report for November of the Royal Victoria Hospital Montreal, states that the number of patients admitted during that month was 245, of whom 229 were discharged, and eleven died. In the outdoor departments there were 764 medical consultations, 407 surgical, 467 ophthalmological, 76 gynecological, 374 laryngological; total, 2,088.

Notre Dame Hospital, Montreal.—The annual meeting of Notre Dame Hospital, Montreal, was held December 14, 1904. The number of patients admitted to the institution during the last official hospital year amounted to 2,226, of whom 1,313 were men and 913 women. Of this number 1,919 were discharged cured or improved, 166 left the hospital unimproved, while 156 died in the hospital. In the outdoor services, the consultations numbered 20,458. Each patient costs this hospital $1.09 per diem. The new contagious diseases hospital in connection with this institution is well under way and will be ready for the reception of patients in April. It will have accommodation for 200 patients.

Personals.—Dr. Paul G. Woolley, late Governor's Fellow of Pathology at McGill University, Montreal, and who has been in the Government laboratory in the Philippines for the past two years, has been appointed Chief of the Serum Laboratory at Manila.

Dr. H. Wolferstan Thomas, another late Governor's Fellow in Pathology at McGill University, has been sent out by the Liverpool School of Tropical Medicine as head of an expedition to the Amazon to study yellow fever. Another McGill graduate, Dr. J. L. Todd, has been for several months in the Congo State studying sleeping sickness.

GENERAL.

Cretinism and Goiter.—Professor Grassi, of the University of Rome, lately instituted, in conjunction with Dr. Munaron, a series of researches on cretinism and goiter in the Valtellina district. According to a preliminary report of their results, the investigators have come to the conclusion that the cause of endemic goiter must be sought for in poisons derived from a specific microbe, having its habitat not at first within the body of the patient but in wet soil. They believe that those poisons gain access to the human body by the alimentary canal by means of various substances, among which drinking water may be included.

Massachusetts Medical Society.—The last meeting of the Boston Medical Library, in conjunction with the Suffolk District Branch of the Massachusetts Medical Society, was held January 11 at the library. The subject for consideration was Medical Charity. Dr. David Cheever was in the chair.

Dr. George W. Gay gave the paper of the evening. The speaker said that in spite of the fact that Boston per capita was one of the wealthiest of American cities, there was a larger number of charity patients in proportion to the population here than anywhere else. He gave the statistics of the various large hospitals and dispensaries here showing the immense amount of work done; too much, he thought, was done. The results of a canvass of the practitioners of Boston and its suburbs was given, in which questions were asked regarding the recipient's opinion about medical charity and its abuse in their own experience; the overwhelming number of replies and cases cited as regards abuse of this charity showed what the profession thought of it. He was strongly in favor of allowing the surgeon on service at a hospital to collect a moderate fee from such patients who could afford to pay, and he mentioned the leading hospitals of other cities where this is allowed, in New York, Philadelphia, Baltimore, and Montreal. In Massachusetts, outside of Boston, 35 out of 38 hospitals allow this. The real cure, he thought, lay in the increased use and the multiplication of private hospitals. In regard to the abuse of outpatient departments and dispensaries he said that in the light of his recent investigation of that department of the Massachusetts General Hospital very few patients were admitted who ought not to be; he carefully went over the system used there; the outpatient departments of the Eye and Ear Infirmary, Children's, Boston City Hospital and Boston Dispensary were still very much abused. He gave results of investigations of various patients, showing that in some of these institutions 40 to 50 per cent. could afford to pay a physician a moderate fee at least. In his opinion the system doing the best work was in use at the Rhode Island Hospital under the direction of Dr. J. M. Peters.

Dr. Hasket Derby protested against the system in use at the Massachusetts General Hospital not allowing a surgeon to collect any fee from a patient willing and able to pay. As regards the supervision of outpatients he thought it took a man of rare experience, patience and tact to successfully accomplish this.

Dr. J. W. Elliott spoke briefly on the system in use at the Massachusetts General Hospital.

Dr. Alfred Worcester, of Waltham, described conditions in London, England, compared with those here. He thought the cure lay in increasing private hospitals.

Dr. F. A. Washburn, of the Massachusetts General Hospital, strongly defended the system there used, proving by statistics and reports that the great majority of the high-priced rooms there were used by old house officers, present house officers, doctors, nurses and clergymen who were charged very little or nothing and that furthermore, of the wealthy patients sent in practically all were recommended by members of the staff who if they thus wished to sacrifice their fee, certainly should be allowed to do so.

Dr. Charles H. Cook, of Natick, and Dr. Samuel Bullard, also spoke. A committee of seven men was appointed to look further into this important matter.

Massachusetts General Hospital.—A clinical meeting of the Massachusetts General Hospital was held January 13, 1905. Dr. James Mumford presided.

Dr. John C. Warren gave a demonstration showing four patients operated on for tumors of the breast and the results.

Dr. E. G. Codman showed a case of rodent ulcer

of the nose in which he had done extensive plastic operations and secured a very satisfactory result.

Dr. Böhm read a paper on The Value of Mechanical Therapeutics describing the work being done by means of the Zander apparatus at this hospital, showing what class of cases were benefited and how they were treated.

Dr. Joel Goldthwaite spoke on sacro-iliac disease. He showed one patient whom he had treated for this condition and had obtained very great relief from pain and correction of deformity. He showed specimens demonstrating the lesions which took place and also a brace, designed by Dr. Osgood, to be used in connection with this condition.

Dr. Oscar Richardson described a case of sudden death associatel with status lymphaticus. He went over the history of this condition, the pathology and the various theories as regards its cause and origin.

Dr. Samuel J. Mixter showed a case of obliteration of the stomach and esophagus with feeding by means of a tube going directly into the duodenum. He reported three other cases and described the causes and the various operations.

Dr. H. C. Baldwin showed a remarkable case of hysterical monoplegia and aphonia of twenty years' duration with recovery. The patient was now able to speak and could walk a mile without fatigue.

Plague in Foochow.—Plague first visited Foochow in the summer of 1894, according to the British Consul for that post," states the *British Medical Journal*, " but it has reappeared annually ever since that date with greater or less severity. During the past year, however, the epidemic was the mildest in type, the most restricted in extent,' and the shortest in duration of any of its predecessors. At the beginning of July an outbreak of the disease occurred in two separate foci—in the heart of the city and in a village in Nantei, the island on which the foreign settlement is situated. It reached its height in the middle of the month, when the death-rate in the city were about 50 per day, and in Nantei about 8 By mid-August the epidemic had practically ceased, and the disease did not make its appearance at any other place in the neighborhood. In the districts lying to the south, however, between Foochow and Amoy, plague was more prevalent, and the duration of the epidemic more prolonged, but to the northward it never gained any footing. Plague has never traveled up the Min River, though cholera, which occasionally made its appearance, does so. Pagoda Anchorage, at the mouth of the river, where all the foreign shipping lies, had no cases of plague."

A City of Cretins.—According to M. Guillaume Capus, the author of a book entitled " Les Médecins et la Médecine en Asie Centrale," the population of the town of Khokand in Turkestan consists, for the most part, of sufferers from goiter and cretinism. The traveler entering the town is at once struck by the fact that nearly every person he meets is the bearer of a more or less voluminous goiter. Khokand is the only place in Turkestan in which such a state of things exists, and there appears to be nothing in the place or its surroundings to account for the prevalence of goiter and cretinism. Its sanitary condition is satisfactory. The town is situated at a height of 1,300 feet, and is abundantly supplied with water from a river which, like the others in the same region, comes from the Altai mountains. When the Russian troops occupied Khokand, in 1878, the medical officers noted that a tenth of the garrison became affected with goiter after a few months' stay. The tumors yielded to the iodine treatment; nevertheless it was decided to abandon Khokand and transfer the headquarters to Marghillan.

German Congress of Internal Medicine.—The twenty-second German Congress of Internal Medicine this year will be held at Wiesbaden, April 12 to 15, under the presidency of Professor Erb, of Heidelberg. The question proposed for discussion is heredity. Dr. H. E. Ziegler, of Jena, will present a report on the present state of the doctrine of heredity in biology; and the importance of heredity in pathology, with special reference to tuberculosis, will be dealt with by Dr. Martius, of Rostock. Among the communications promised are the following: Dr. A. Hoffman, of Breslau, The Treatment of Leucemia with X-rays; Dr. Schutz, of Wiesbaden, Researches on the Mucous Secretion of the Intestine; and Dr. M. Matthes, of Jena, Autolysis. An exhibition of instruments, apparatus, and preparations will be held in connection with the Congress. Communications relative either to the Congress or the exhibition should be addressed to the permanent secretary, Geheimrat Dr. Emil Pfeiffer, Parkstrasse 13, Wiesbaden.

The Prevention of Tuberculosis in Denmark.—"Denmark, writes the *British Medical Journal*, "has followed the lead given by Norway in attempting to deal with tuberculosis by legislation. In 1901 the law of the latter country required (1) notification of all cases of consumption of lung and larynx, and of all deaths caused by the disease; (2) that both private practitioners and public medical officers should instruct such patients as to hygienic precautions, while the authorities undertook the disinfection of dwellings and utensils. The Health Commission had the right of removing to a hospital any person whom they considered dangerous on account of infection. The law further provided against the employment of tuberculous wet nurses and children's nurses, and enjoined especial precautions as to the conditions of hotels, factories, workshops, railways, etc. Sweden introduced a less radical law, making notification of deaths by tuberculosis and disinfection compulsory.

This law came into force on January 1, 1905. Denmark has been considering a proposed new law which has in it many highly interesting points. The proposals emanate from a commission consisting of two medical men, Drs. K. Faber and C. Lorentzen, and a government official. The report of this commission deals very fully with the incidence and spread of tuberculosis in Denmark, with tuberculosis in prisons, etc., with the hygiene of tuberculosis, with the consideration of foreign legislation regarding tuberculosis, and with the means taken in other countries for the prevention of the disease. The commission puts forward two sets of proposals and the government has adopted these recommendations with but trivial changes. The first set of suggestions make notification compulsory. The cases must be notified by the practitioner in attendance on a special form. Notification of all deaths from tuberculosis is also compulsory. Disinfection is to be carried out by the public authorities if it is thought necessary. The carrying out of hygienic measures is placed into the hand of the 'Health Commission,' as is the compulsory removal of any patient into hospital. In this particular the law is limited, and only reserves the right to interfere if the circumstances appear to necessitate it. Schoolmasters are bound to notify the School Commission any case of tuberculosis among the scholars which come to their knowledge, and the commission then decides whether it is necessary to remove the patient from learning together with other children. Schoolmasters, when applying for posts, must certify that they are free from any infectious form of tuberculosis. A schoolmaster suffering from tuberculosis in an infectious form is to receive a pension of two-thirds of the salary which he is drawing at the time. The penalty for contravention of any part of the law is a fine of from 2 to 2,000 crowns, or imprisonment. The commission points out that it is highly necessary that the fight against tuberculosis should not be turned into a fight against the tuberculous. This second act of recommendations deals with the help from the State in regard to the treatment of the tuberculous. All institutes for the treatment of tuberculosis are to be under the supervision of the Minister of Justice. The minimum number of beds and the maximum daily fee charged to the patient must be stated, and are controllable. Even private sanatoriums may be brought under this part of the law. Certain classes of patients receive assistance from the State; this assitance is not to exceed half the fee charged by the institute where they are treated. This assistance is under no circumstances to be given in such a way as to pauperize the patient. The State further undertakes to assist in building new sanatoriums. The yearly amount which the State will pay for the tuberculosis movement is to be fixed, but will be revised after ten years. Such is briefly the basis on which the Danish government is prepared to deal with the problem of the consumptives, and the results of the law will be carefully watched by other countries."

Paris Academy Prizes.—The British Medical Journal states that at a sitting of the Paris Académie de Médicine, held on December 14, the names of the successful candidates for the various prizes offered for medical researches of one kind or another were announced. The Audiffred prize of £960 for the best work on tuberculosis was not awarded, but sums varying from £60 to £20 were given, by way of encouragement, to Dr. Armand Delille, of Paris, for an investigation of the part played by the poisons generated by Koch's bacillus in tuberculous meningitis and tuberculosis of the nerve centers; to Dr. Nathan-Laurier, of Paris, for a research on mammary tuberculosis; to Dr. Pautrier, of Paris, or one on atypical forms of cutaneous tuberculosis; and to Dr. Lalesque, of Arachon, for a memoir on the sea and consumptives. The Baillarger prize for £80 for researches on mental diseases was awarded to Dr. Paul Sérieux for a series of reports on the treatment of insanity and the organization of asylums. The Adrien-Buisson prize of £420 was awarded to MM. E. Leclainche, professor in the Veterinary School of Toulouse, and H. Vallée, professor in the Veterinary School of Alford, for researches on symptomatic anthrax and gangrenous septicemia. The Campbell-Dupierris prize of £92 was awarded to Dr. J. Tissot, of Paris, for an experimental investigation on the exchange of gases in the arterial blood, the ventilation of the lungs, and arterial pressure during chloroform anesthesia. The Baudet prize of £40 was awarded to Professor Monprofit, of Angers, for a memoir on tumors; to the same surgeon also fell the Huguier surgical prize of £120 for essays on the surgery of the ovaries and Fallopian tubes, and on salpingitis and ovaritis. The Theodore Herpin (de Genève) prize of £120 was awarded to Mrs. P. E. Launois and Pierre Roy, of Paris, for a biological study of giants. The Jacquemier obstetrical prize of £68 was warded to Dr. Bouchacourt, of Paris, or a series of memoirs on the applications of radiography to midwifery; while Dr. Briquet, of Nancy, gained the Tarnier prize of £120 for a work on tumors if the placenta. The Laborie surgical prize of £120 was awarded to Drs. J. Hennequin and R. Loewy, of Paris, for a monograph on the treatment of fractures of the long bones. The Louis prize of £120 was awarded to Dr. Victor Balthazar, of Paris, for a memoir on the serumtheraphy of typhoid fever, and the Saintour prize

of £172 to Drs. Fernand Bazançon and Marcel Labbé for a treatise on hematology. A considerable number of prizes of smaller value was awarded to various competitors.

OBITUARY.

Dr. HENRY MARTYN WELLS, a retired medical director in the navy, died last week in New York. He was born about sixty-nine years ago at Northampton, Mass., and was a graduate of Darthmouth College. In 1857 he entered the navy and served through the Civil War. Dr. Wells was retired in 1897, after forty years of service. He was a member of Northampton Post, G. A. R.; the Loyal Legion, and the Reform Club.

Dr. LOUIS C. D'HOMERGUE died at his home, No. 494 Vanderbilt Avenue, Brooklyn, on Thursday last, in his seventieth year. He served in the Engineer Corps of the Sixty-ninth New York Infantry during the Civil War. After the war he became a clerk in the United States Navy Department, and for a number of years had been a clerk in the Bureau of Vital Statistics of the Health Department. He was a member of the memorial and executive committee of the Grand Army of the Republic of Kings County.

Dr. THOMAS H. MANLEY, visiting surgeon of the Metropolitan and Harlem Hospitals, died January 13, at his home, No. 115 West Forty-ninth Street. He was fifty-four years old, a member of the Democratic Club, and of various medical societies.

CORRESPONDENCE.

MEDICINAL PRERARATIONS AS ALCOHOLIC BEVERAGES.

To the Editor of the MEDICAL NEWS:

SIR:—I was very much interested in the article, Quacks, Their Methods and Dangers, by Champe S. Andrews, Esq., of January 7 issue of the MEDICAL NEWS. It was particularly interesting to me because I have had an opportunity of seeing a use made of quack preparations that is not often reported. By this I mean the use of preparations containing a large percentage of alcohol, as an intoxicating beverage. This practice of the laity is especially notorious in small rural communities where there are no hotels. The physicians in these communities are frequently asked for prescriptions for whisky, the patient (would be) feigning all sorts of symptoms. Failing in securing whisky, I have known men to go to the drug store and purchase Peruna, Munyon's Paw Paw, Hostetter's Bitters, Dr. White's Bitters and many other preparations of a similar character. I have been called in to see men sick from intoxication who confessed that they got drunk on these preparations and bought them for that purpose. I know of men (temperance men?) who would be ashamed to frequent a hotel, yet they use these preparations as beverages.

I have under my care at the present time a clergyman, a man of eloquence and of the best moral character, who consumes immense quantities of Hostetter's Bitters simply for their intoxicating effects. This man claims to have a craving for alcohol, but don't dare to frequent a hotel, or trust any one to purchase whisky for him. I have seen this man so bad that it was necessary to give him a hypodermic of apomorphine and place a guard over him. Yet this man's moral character, as far as the laity is concerned, is above reproach, and he is simply regarded by them as a chronic dyspeptic. I have interviewed druggists on this question and they claim that there is absolutely no law

to stop them from selling these preparations, knowing at the same time the use to be made of them. They even claim that they have a perfect right to sell Duffy's Malt as they don't sell it as a whisky, but a tonic. It has always seemed strange to me why prominent people, senators, congressmen, actors, educators, etc., lend their aid to such a pernicious system of quackery. It also seems very unjust to men who have spent years in hard study, and thousands of dollars, in order to become members of what is justly termed the Noblest Profession (a physician), while ignorant charlatans are swarming about the country not only robbing the people, but disseminating a cowardly and hypocritical method of intoxication.   Yours truly,
                              S. CLIFFORD BOSTON, M.D.
WEST GROVE, January 10, 1905.

SOCIETY PROCEEDINGS.

NEW YORK NEUROLOGICAL SOCIETY.

Regular Meeting, held December 6, 1904.

The President, Pearce Bailey, M.D., in the Chair.

Case of Exophthalmic Goiter, Associated with Scleroderma and Alopecia Areata.—This was presented by Dr. Frederick Peterson. The patient was a single woman, twenty-five years old, a music teacher by occupation. She enjoyed excellent health until the age of twenty years, when she developed a goiter. This was the first symptom noted, and subsequently the exophthalmus and tachycardia appeared. When she first came under Dr. Peterson's observation, early in November of the present year, the proptosis was marked. The pulse ranged from 90 to 120. About eighteen months ago a patch of scleroderma developed over the right hypochondriac region: this was 6 by 12 cm. in dimensions. Soon afterward, a second patch appeared on the right breast, which now involved a considerable portion of the skin of that organ. Subsequently, a third patch appeared under the left axillary space, a fourth in the left supraclavicular region and a fifth in the left lower abdominal region. There were no sclerodermatous patches on the face or extremities. About three years ago she developed a bald spot on the top of her head, about 5 cm. in diameter. She now had three such patches of alopecia areata. There was no specific history and no hereditary taint. Möbius states that von Leube, about 1875, was the first to record his observations of scleroderma of the face and hands in a patient with Graves' disease. Von Leube, in his book on "Medical Diagnosis," New York, 1904, says that in Graves' diseases scleroma of the skin has often been observed by himself and others. Kahler, in 1888, reported a case of scleroderma with exophthalmic goiter. Jeanselme, in 1894, reported cases of scleroderma in Graves' disease. G. Singer, in 1894, stated that scleroderma frequently occurred in connection with diseases of the thyroid gland. He found that organ was usually affected in ordinary scleroderma. Beer, in 1894, reported four cases of scleroderma, in all of which there was tachycardia, and the volume of the thyroid was diminished. Ditisheim, writing on Graves' disease in 1895, said that 45 per cent. of the cases observed by him in Zurich had scleroderma in addition to Graves' disease. Grünfeld, in 1896, reports a case of Graves' disease with scleroderma. Ord and Mackenzie, writing on Graves' disease in 1897, said that the association of scleroderma and Graves' disease has been recorded by several observers. Also, that alopecia has been recorded. Osler, in 1898, reports a case of a man with Graves' disease and scleroderma. Raymond, in 1898, in a lecture on scleroderma, presented

two patients with scleroderma and Graves' disease. Dupré and Guillain, in 1900, reported the case of a man with Graves' disease, scleroderma and sclerodactylia. Kriger, in 1903, reports a case of a woman with sclerodactylia and Graves' disease. As regards the relation of alopecia areata to Graves' disease, there was not so much reference to it in literature. It was mentioned in one of the cases already cited, and Doré, in 1900, writing on cutaneous affections occurring in the course of Graves' disease, refers to the frequent loss of hair, and says: "Alopecia areata is occasionally seen; Mr. Malcolm Morris, in his book on "Diseases of the Skin," 1904, makes a casual reference to the association of Graves' disease with alopecia areata, in considering the pathology of alopecia. Luithlen, in his "Handbuch der Hautkrankheiten," 1904, refers to alopecia as an occasional complication with scleroderma. From these citations it follows that it is not infrequent to meet scleroderma in association with Graves' disease; that sometimes scleroderma is associated with alopecia and that alopecia is sometimes met with in Graves' disease. In this patient there is a combination of Graves' disease with scleroderma and also alopecia areata.

Brain-Tumor? Two Cases of Doubtful Etiology.—This was the exhibit presented by Dr. William M. Leszynsky. *Case I.*—Sarah Z. U. S., single, twenty-eight years old; a stenographer and typewritist by occupation. When she was first seen, in December, 1903, she complained that for six months previously she had suffered from frequent paroxysmal attacks of severe frontal and occipital cephalalgia, with vertigo, nausea and vomiting. The frontal headache was continuous and often prevented sleep. Her vision began to fail, especially in the right eye, and two months later that eye became blind. Soon afterward, the sight of the left eye was also lost. There was no history of injury to the head, alcoholism or syphilis. In childhood she had measles and diphtheria, and in her second year scarlet fever and right suppurative otitis. Menstruation began at the age of fifteen years, and was regular during the first year. It then appeared at irregular intervals of from four to six months, and during the past year there had been amenorrhea. There was chronic constipation. The family history was unimportant. An examination of the blood showed 70 per cent. of hemoglobin: no leucocytosis. The pupils were dilated and rigid. The motility of the eyeballs was normal. There was no perception of light. Bilateral papillitis 5 D. No retinal hemorrhages. No evidence of a kidney lesion or renal inadequacy. There was occasional right facial paresis of the lower branches of the nerve. After remaining under observation in the hospital for one week, she was discharged. Subsequently, she was trephined by Dr. Andrew McCosh at the Presbyterian Hospital. No improvement followed the operation, which failed to reveal the presence of a neoplasm. An X-ray picture of the skull was negative. There was no improvement under increasing doses of potassium iodide. The blindness persists, the disks having become atrophic.

Case II.—Male; twenty-eight years old; a native of Russia and a photographer by occupation, was admitted to the hospital in October, 1903. For several months he had suffered from frequent attacks of severe generalized headache, preceded or accompanied by vomiting. Soon afterwards he became blind, and complained of weakness and vertigo, with the sensation of falling to the right. His father died of diabetes: his mother was alive and well. During childhood the patient had suffered from measles and scarlatina. He was addicted to the excessive use of whisky, beer and wine. He admitted having had gonorrhea, but denied syphilis.

There was no history of injury to the head. An examination showed paralysis of the right external rectus. Both pupils were dilated and rigid, and there was no perception of light in either eye. Bilateral choked disk of 6 D., with numerous retinal hemorrhages. There was left hemiparesis, and occasional flexor rigidity in the left upper extremity. Pronounced astereognosis (?) (fluctuating), and slight ataxia. No disturbance of tactile, pain or temperature sensibility. Both lower extremities were extended and rigid from time to time, with spurious ankle clonus and trepidation. Left knee-jerk exaggerated; both plantar reflexes exaggerated. No Babinski. Other reflexes normal. Urine, blood and X-ray examination negative. The patient was put on increasing doses of potassium iodide, and two months later all the symptoms disappeared, but the blindness persisted. The retinal hemorrhages had become absorbed and the disks were atrophic.

Dr. Graeme M. Hammond, in the discussion, suggested that the blindness in the second case shown by Dr. Leszynsky might have been due to wood alcohol poisoning.

Dr. Leszynsky replied that in wood alcohol poisoning the condition of the eyes was one of retrobulbar neuritis, and not of choked disk, and furthermore, that the blindness, in the former class of cases, came on very rapidly.

Dr. L. Pierce Clark said he recently saw a case quite similar to those shown by Dr. Leszynsky, and in his case the patient volunteered the statement that she had been using different sorts of bleaching hair-dyes to great excess, and to these she was inclined to attribute her loss of sight. There was in this case a papillitis, followed by atrophy.

Dr. Leszynsky said that no one could make the differential diagnosis between tumor and basilar meningitis by the condition of the optic nerve or the presence of choked disk. He recently saw a case of syphilitic meningitis where the retina was filled with hemorrhages and a high degree of choked disk was present.

Tubercle of the Cerebellum.—This specimen was shown by Dr. I. Abrahamson. This case was referred to the speaker by Dr. Samuel Lloyd, in order to determine the advisibility of an operation. The patient was a male; five years old. His family history was negative. Two years ago he had whooping-cough, and about that time began to complain of pain in the head, which his father thought was due to a blow. The pain was always referred to the back of the head, and continued for about a year. Then the left side of the body suddenly became paralyzed, and this paralysis had persisted. For the past two months there had been projectile vomiting, and for the past month the child had been having three or four convulsions daily. During the convulsions, which lasted from five to fifteen minutes, the child was apparently unconscious. He cried a good deal and complained of pain, usually in the head, but also in other parts of the body when attempts were made to move him. He frequently cried out in his sleep. He had lost considerable weight, and there was a notable increase in the size of the head. Examination showed that the patient was much emaciated. The head was retracted and flexed to the left, and all attempts at movement elicited a sharp cry of pain. The eyes were turned to the left, and upward and downward movements were impossible. The left pupil was more widely dilated than the right, and there was apparently no light nor accommodation reaction. There was no pain-reaction. Attempts to look to the right were accompanied by coarse nystagmoid movements. There was marked choked disk. There was general motor weakness, and

exaggeration of the triceps, wrist and knee-jerks on the left side. Plantar reflex was not obtainable. Sensibility and special senses were intact. There was no Kernig sign. The thighs and legs were flexed; the feet extended. All attempts to straighten the legs caused pain. The vomiting from which the child had suffered seemed to bear no relation to the food taken into the stomach. It occurred at any time and without warning, and seemed to cause no special distress. When the child was admitted to the hospital he was in a semicomatose condition, which persisted up to the time of his death. He could be roused and would answer simple questions fairly intelligently. He had only one convulsion while in the hospital; this resembled a general spastic condition rather than a clonic one. The case was regarded as one of tuberculous meningitis complicating general tuberculosis, and no operation was deemed justifiable.

On opening the cranial cavity, at autopsy, the skull was found to be very thin, even for a child of six years, although the suture lines were well and firmly united. The skullcap was easily removed and the dura incised. Immediately about eight ounces of clear fluid escaped, although the brain itself had seemed to fill the entire cavity. This might possibly be explained by the collapse of the brain, showing that the fluid had occupied the ventricles and escaped through some opening. No tuberculous process was found in the meninges covering the vertex. The brain itself was removed without difficulty. On examining the basilar portion of the dura, a number of miliary tubercles were found. A gross examination of the brain showed a nodule, about one and a half inches in diameter, situated in the left cerebellar lobe; it was round and fairly regular in outline, and quite firm in texture. No incision was made either into the brain or the tumor itself, the specimen being preserved intact. No tuberculous process was found in the lepto-meninges. Examination of the other viscera showed a general miliary tuberculosis.

Acute Dementia or Mental Stupor Following Illuminating Gas Poisoning.—This case was presented by Dr. Abrahamson. The patient was a woman, fifty-five years old; a native of Russia. Her family history was negative; the patient had always enjoyed good health, and had never had any previous mental disturbance. Six weeks ago she arose to prepare breakfast for the family on the gas range. After this she returned to bed and later was found asphyxiated. There was no suspicion of attempted suicide. She was taken to the Gouverneur Hospital, where oxygen was given and phlebotomy done. She remained comatose for two entire days, when her intelligence slowly returned. There was no resulting paralysis or other symptoms, and she left the hospital in an apparently normal condition. Two weeks ago, however, her intelligence became affected. She would remain in one position for hours without a word or sign, apparently entirely oblivious to her surroundings, evincing no emotion whatsoever, and making no complaints. There were no delusions nor hallucinations. She did not resist being moved about, and did things automatically. Her facial expression was apathetic. She did not ask for food, but when it was placed before her and she was urged very strongly, she was able to feed herself. She answered one of many questions addressed to her briefly but to the point. When once outside the house, even but a few steps from the door, she lost her way. There were no lamentations, no profanity, no spells of restlessness and no excitement, no breach of ordinary decency, no undue exposure. When strongly urged, she recognized individuals, things and places.

Dr. Clark, in the discussion, said that three cases like the one shown by Dr. Abrahamson had been seen at the Vanderbilt Clinic. In one of them in which the course and the symptoms were particularly similar to the one presented, a diagnosis of paramnesia following illuminating gas poisoning was made. This patient recovered entirely in the course of three or four months. The speaker said he did not think the automatism and stupid state in the case shown were sufficient grounds upon which to base the diagnosis of acute dementia.

Dr. Harlow Brooks said that in fatal cases of illuminating gas poisoning, where the patients had survived four or five days, the autopsy occasionally revealed areas of softening in the anterior lobe of the brain, and sometimes in the striate body.

Dr. Smith Ely Jelliffe said that illuminating gas contained carbon monoxide (CO), and it was known that this substance was an active hemolytic poison; hence there might be actual agglutination of blood in the blood-vessels, and the production of functional disturbances, such as were presented in the case shown. These lesions were also allied to those spoken of by Dr. Brooks.

Dr. Charles L. Dana said that some years ago he reported a case of illuminating gas poisoning followed by what was described by him as double personality, which persisted for nearly a year. There was a form of memory disturbance, but the patient could talk intelligently, and was in no sense demented. He had forgotten almost everything concerning his previous life. He did not know his parents nor where he lived, but he was able to carry out a number of common, automatic things, and went about his ordinary duties fairly well. He was also able to take care of himself. Dr. Dana said that a number of observations had been made, particularly by French writers, showing that the poison of illuminating gas had a distinct effect on the memory and that children who were more or less constantly exposed to air contaminated by this gas were apt to have defective memories. The case shown by Dr. Abrahamson was suggestive more of memory disturbance than of true dementia.

Dr. Abrahamson, in closing, said that according to the statements made by the family, his patient had improved somewhat during the past week. Clinically, the symptoms were those of dementia rather than amnesia, as the patient had never been restless or excited, nor had she had any delusions or hallucinations.

Bilateral Cervical Sympathectomy for the Relief of Epilepsy.—Paper read by Drs. William P. Spratling and Roswell Park. The authors stated that cervical sympathectomy as a therapeutic measure for the possible relief of epilepsy had been tried in enough cases to create a fairly extensive literature on the subject. In 1902, Winter collected all cases operated on up to that date, including nine of his own, and his extensive consideration of the subject comprised 213 cases. In March of the present year, S. D. Hopkins reported five cases. According to Winter, 122 of the cases he had collected were well observed, and of these, 66 per cent. were cured; 13.9 per cent. were "preliminarily" cured; 18.9 per cent. improved; 54.9 per cent. not improved, while 5.7 per cent. died. The term "preliminarily" was probably used by Winter to include cases in which the earlier effects of the operation were favorable, but in which the cases were not kept under observation long enough to permit a positive statement of a permanent cure. As to the rationale of this therapeutic procedure, as based on anatomical and physiological facts, it might be twofold: First, by cutting off a certain amount of sensory stimulation from the viscera, i.e., preventing

these stimuli from reaching the brain; second, by influencing directly the circulation of the brain by changes in the caliber of the blood vessels through the action of the vascular nerves. The first case, reported by Dr. Spratling, was a male, twenty-four years old, a native of New York; single; a clerk by occupation. His father and mother lived to be forty-six and forty-one years old, respectively. His father had convulsions when younger, which were claimed to be uremic. The mother had frequent headaches, with "a feeling of weight in the head." A brother of eight years had chorea. Maternal grandparents died at ages forty-eight and forty-six respectively, the cause of death in both being apoplexy. The patient was the first in line of birth of six children. He was born at full term after instrumental delivery. The mother reported that he received slight cuts over the cheek bones at that time. He was breast-fed, and began teething at the ninth month. Had night terrors during childhood, and began to walk at the nineteenth month. He was subject to frequent attacks of epistaxis without apparent cause. When he was eight months old he fell from a chair, striking on his face. The first epileptic convulsion appeared when he was fifteen years old, the supposed cause being fright; a second attack occurred a week later. His aura consisted of severe headaches, and "spots before the eyes." A ball of fire, he stated, appeared between the eyes; when long lines of color were seen, and everything appeared to pass from left to right. Diplopia occurred and the seizure began. He had marked convulsive movements of the face and right arm, which had been present since the age of eight or nine years. They were choreic in form and became more pronounced previous to a seizure, and were especially marked when he became excited. He was admitted to the Craig Colony for Epileptics in June, 1903. He had one seizure in that month, one in August, two in September, and two in November. He was operated on by Dr. Roswell Park on November 16, 1903, and had a seizure the day after the operation. He had no further seizures until the following April—a period of four months—when he had two, after which they again ceased and had not recurred up to the present time, a period of seven and one-half months.

The second case was a female, twenty-two years old; no occupation; single. Both of her parents were living. Her mother was subject to headaches. Her father was a moderate drinker. One maternal aunt was insane, and one maternal grandfather rheumatic. A maternal grandmother died of tumor; grandfather of cancer, and paternal grandmother of heart disease. The patient was fourth in line of birth of five children. The birth was normal and at full term. She was said to have been a strong child. Teething commenced at the eighth month. There was no history of spasms or convulsions at that time. She commenced to walk at about the fifteenth month. Her first epileptic seizure occurred at the eighteenth month, when she had a series of them, the cause being unknown. The aura consisted of vertigo, with marked flushing of the face. She had a left hemiplegia, indistinct in character, and probably due to a cerebral hemorrhage that was caused by the first series of convulsions. She was admitted to the Craig Colony in May, 1902, and had a seizure that month; another in July and five in October. During the following year she had four attacks only. Her cervical sympathetics were resected by Dr. Park on November 16, 1903. In this case, as well as in the third one reported by Dr. Spratling, there was marked improvement following the operation. The speaker said that while the report of these three cases would not add

1uch to the casuistry of the operation in the way of ercentage, it might be of value from the fact that one f the patients presented an additional condition, a ronounced "tic" of the head and right arm, which /as radically improved by the operation. A second actor in the case was the thorough histological in-estigation of the parts of the sympathetic nerves that /ere extirpated. This was made by Dr. B. Onuf, and he changes found by him in the nerve sections re-1oved in the three cases were in essence as follows: 1) Pigmentation of a greater or lesser number of nerve ells of the cervical sympathetic ganglia in all three ases. (2) Presence in every one of the three cases f at least one nerve cell with double nucleus in some ne of the extirpated ganglia. In one of the cases about alf a dozen such cells were found. (3) Degenerative hanges in the medullated nerve fibers in the sympathetic ord and ganglia of the excised portion. (4) In one ase a focus of inflammation, *i.e.*, of perivascular round-ell infiltration.

Dr. B. Onuf, in the discussion, thought it would be vorth while to examine the excised portion of the ympathetic nerve in all cases where a sympathectomy vas done, although if any pathological changes were ound in it, it might be difficult to say whether they vere primary or secondary.

Dr. Clark said that the first case reported by Dr. ipratling had been under his care for a time. This iatient was the first in line of birth of six children: 1e was a "blue baby," the labor having been instru-nental and extremely difficult. The inflammatory :hanges found in that case might have been due to rauma, and the speaker thought there was some doubt vhether the case was really one of true epilepsy or iomething else.

Dr. Pierce Bailey thought it was rather remarkable hat so little attention had hitherto been given to the :ervical sympathetic in connection with these cases. 1ts importance was shown by the result of the patho-ogical findings of Dr. Onuf in the cases reported by)r. Spratling.

Dr. Spratling, in closing, said that while there was iome doubt in the beginning as to whether the case re-erred to by Dr. Clark was one of true epilepsy, the pa-ient subsequently developed typical *grand mal* attacks. Γhe speaker said he was still a little skeptical in regard ɔ the use of the knife in general in the treatment of :pilepsy, and he was rather doubtful whether the im-Irovement in the cases he had reported would be last-ng. He had always inclined to the view that epilepsy vas a condition usually beyond the aid of the knife, ilthough in many instances, even a simple surgical ɔperation, no matter what, seemed to prove at least :emporarily beneficial, perhaps by its effect on the gen-:ral metabolism. This, if nothing else, might render :ertain operations justifiable in some cases.

Traumatic Epilepsy in its Medicolegal Relations.— Γhis paper was read by Dr. Arthur Conklin Brush. Γhe author stated that although the clinical phenomena ɔf the epileptic condition had been recognized since /ery ancient times, yet when one comes to the con-;ideration of the medicolegal questions involved in the itudy of this subject, we again encountered the oft-'epeated difficulties in medicolegal situations, namely, 1at the nature and limitations of the condition under :onsideration were as yet unsettled questions, for it :learly appeared in evidence from the works of the :ecent writers on medicine that we were even at the 1resent time unable to give an undisputed definition of :he condition. It appeared that the weight of evidence vas in favor of considering epilepsy as an organic dis-

ease of the cerebral cortex, which weakened the inhibi-tory power of the cortical cells, and it was further al-leged that this degeneration and epileptic discharge only occurred from the presence of certain unknown toxins. If this latter theory was accepted, it would appear that injury and disease of the cortex could only produce epilepsy in persons predisposed from the presence of this toxin. This theory could not be accepted until it could be shown that this toxin really existed. Much confusion still surrounded this entire subject, and at the present time our real knowledge consisted in the fact that a certain type of convulsions could originate from a great variety of causes producing disease of the cerebral cortex. The situation was often made worse by the confusion that existed in some medical minds between true and hystero-epilepsy. Epilepsy was one of the most common diseases, occurring in one of every 500 persons, and the larger number were truly idio-pathic.

The influence of neurotic heredity was unquestioned: it was stated to be present in one-third of all the cases, and a direct inheritance in one-third of these. The effect of chronic alcoholism in the parents was also undisputed. Other predisposing causes mentioned by different writers were chronic lead poisoning, syphilis, tuberculosis, rheumatism, scrofula, rachitis, morphine, diabetes, etc. In the vast majority of cases, idiopathic epilepsy developed before the age of thirty, and in three-fourths of the cases before the age of twenty. There seemed to be no conflict of medical opinion that trauma could produce epilepsy, and according to Starr it did so in 11 per cent. of all the cases. When the evidence of the injury was so slight as not to produce a fracture of the skull, or severe cerebral contusion, or gross or-ganic brain disease, it was a matter of grave doubt whether such trivial injuries could cause epilepsy in non-predisposed persons. When epilepsy followed slight injuries, there was usually a strong neurotic here-ditary predisposition present. It appeared then that in those cases assigned to slight cerebral contusions in persons predisposed, where the symptoms were slight, and where a considerable interval of time intervened between the injury and the onset of the epilepsy, and where the two were not connected by any mental or physical symptoms, that is could not be said that the disease would not have developed without the occur-rence of the injury. In cases of more serious injury to the head, as in fracture, especially depressed, or of injury to the brain, such as laceration, meningitis or hemorrhage, the evidence of the causal relationship of the trauma to the epilepsy seems to be undisputed, and the disease to be due to an irritation of the cortex from localized thickening of the cranium, splinters of bone invading the cortex, meningeal cicatrices or localized inflammation. Traumatic epilepsy might develop at once after the receipt of an injury, or not until after a period of months or years, but the largest number of cases developed within a year.

Dr. Edward D. Fisher, in the discussion, said that Dr. Brush's large personal experience with this class of cases rendered his views on the subject of value. The speaker thought the fact was fairly well established, both by clinical observations and animal experimenta-tion, that direct injury to the brain could cause epilepsy even in the absence of any marked hereditary predis-position.

Dr. Spratling said he entirely agreed with Dr. Fisher. While the occurrence of true epilepsy as the result of a trauma, and independent of any hereditary taint or auto-intoxication was rare, such cases had come under his observation.

NEW YORK ACADEMY OF MEDICINE.

SECTION ON ORTHOPEDICS.

Stated Meeting, held Friday, November 18, 1904.

The President, Homer Gibney, M.D., in the Chair.

Congenital Torticollis.—Dr. Whitman presented a patient, a boy ten years of age, showing the secondary effects of a very severe congenital torticollis in the irregularity of the skull, the eyes, nose and mouth. The contractions had been entirely overcome by a division of the shortened tissues and by force with subsequent fixation. There was in addition a small meningocele of the neck and two supernumerary ribs. On either side one can feel resistant projections which are short ribs running outward and forward and downward, apparently to the anterior extremities of the first true ribs. The X-ray picture confirming the diagnosis had unfortunately been mislaid.

Congenital Hip Dislocation.—Dr. Whitman exhibited an X-ray illustrating one treatment that may be necessary for congenital dislocation of the hip. As we know, 50 or 60 per cent. of the cases cannot be anatomically cured by the Lorenz operation or any of its modifications. Of this 50 or 60 per cent. a large portion of the failures is due to an anterior twist of the upper extremity of the femur. In such cases the joint should be opened and if on inspection it appears that the femur is so distorted that the head cannot be placed in the acetabulum without inward rotation of the limbs, an osteotomy is indicated. The dislocation is first reduced and the limb is fixed in the necessary inward rotation for a certain number of weeks or months. When repair is complete a long drill is put through the trochanter and neck, and if desired into the acetabulum. An osteotomy is then performed at the lower third of the femur and the limb is rotated outward to the proper degree. The X-ray picture presented showed the drill in position and the point at which the bone was fractured. The limb being placed immediately in a close-fitting plaster spica bandage in which the drill is imbedded, the part is held in position until repair is complete.

Dr. Myers said that when Dr. Lorenz was here, he had just had one of those cases with very marked anterior rotation of the head, and to get it into the acetabulum, the leg had to be inverted to fully ninety degrees. Subsequently, they had performed subtrochanteric osteotomy in the upper part. In speaking to Dr. Lorenz about this, Dr. Lorenz had asked whether it was necessary at that time, as there was too much outward rotation in the socket as shown by palpation and X-ray. He said that he very infrequently performed that operation; that the neck was inclined to twist backward as time went on. Dr. Myers said he simply repeated what Dr. Lorenz had said.

Case for Diagnosis.—Dr. Myers presented a boy, sixteen years of age, who for the past two years has complained of great pain in plantar surface of both heels. Dr. Myers brought him, because there seemed to be so little cause for the pain. Taking into consideration the boy's rapid growth and increase of weight and the fact that the pain was bilateral, Dr. Myers supposed it to be weak foot of some sort, but the diagnosis was not clear. There had been no injury of the plantar fascia or tendo Achillis, no swelling of the bursæ in front or back of that tendon or the one occasionally found on

the plantar surface of the os calcis. The longit dinal arch is well preserved, also the transverse arc and there is no pronation of the feet. The boy cor plains of pain in the heel, and only in the heel. I is not able to do any work. He had worn plates a: his feet had been strapped before he came to ! Luke's, but without relief. Pain in heels only wh he walks.

Trauma Knee.—Dr. Hibbs presented a boy, t years of age, brought to the Orthopedic Dispensa: June 3, with the following history: July 17, 19 while flying a kite from the roof, he stumbled a fell one story through a skylight. Was taken at th time to a hospital where a wound in the front p: of his knee, just above the patella, was stitched and he was discharged in a few days with that e tirely cured. Afterward he had some pain and sti ness in his knee and he entered another hospi where he was treated with a plaster cast for a mon then given a brace and high shoe, which he wo for three or four days and then discontinued it. I had no other treatment, and limped around ur June 3, 1904, when he came to the Dispensary. that time there was some stiffness, distinct synovi slight atrophy of the thigh and calf; no shorteni He complained of pain and gave a history throu out of something very much like a loose cartila in the knee joint. When walking along the stre would have a sudden sharp pain, feel something s and feel relieved. An X-ray showed what was s posed to be a loose cartilage in the joint. Wl waiting for a bed in the hospital he came in c day with the knee immovably held at 90 degre Another X-ray was taken and the boy was tal into the hospital and the joint opened while at degrees. The supposed loose cartilage was loca but the boy kicked during anesthesia and it c appeared into the posterior part of the joint. T operator was unable to get it, and the wound v closed, and after a few weeks healed, and the l walked again. He was kept in the ward for t months, under observation. He occasionally cc plained of pain. A month afterward the fore body was found and removed. It was a bit of gl at the knee-joint. It had been there since July 1903, and was probably a fragment of the skyli through which the boy had fallen. It was inter ing to note that he boy could go about so well w out more serious trouble from July 17, 1903, u November 4, 1904.

Dr. A. B. Judson presented a man, twenty- years old, whose right hip seemed to be parti dislocated and reduced at will when he puts weight on the limb or, if lying down, when he pu: against something. It might be called a snapp hip as the motions are sudden and audible, rem ing one of the way some persons can snap the n joint of the thumb or other digits. The patient do this with his thumbs and with the right mit finger. Locomotion is not impaired except that says he walks carefully and the hips have the pearance of being loose-jointed. Has lately ha dull warm sensation in the hip but has had no p There are no signs of joint disease or of disloca of the femoral head from the acetabulum. same thing has developed in the left hip but in degree. This condition has caused him s anxiety since its appearance a few months ago.

For Diagnosis.—Dr. V. Gibney presented a of a woman, twenty-two years of age, for diagn Two years ago, about the eighth month of her p

ancy, she had severe pain—thought to be sciatic
nd produced by the fetus. Labor was brought on.
)id not give any relief, and lameness had been per-
istent. She appeared at the Clinic to-day and was
.ot examined, but Dr. Gibney was told that she had
.een going about in this way for a year or so. An
{-ray was produced and it looked a little like osteo-
rthritis. There are some bony growths. Dr. Gib-
.ey showed X-rays of a case of senile arthritis which
orresponds very closely with this.

Rheumatoid Arthritis and Sequelæ.—Dr. Jaeger
howed a case, a man twenty-eight years of age.
;ives a family history of rheumatism in both par-
nts. Was perfectly well until seven years old,
vhen he fell into a stream in the spring, and was
xposed to the cold air for over an hour, in his wet
lothes. The exposure was followed within a few
tours by a severe attack of articular rheumatism,
.ffecting many joints. Was very ill for three weeks;
.fter this period convalescence slowly set in and he
iad no further trouble until he was twenty years old.
ie then suffered another exposure to cold which was
ollowed by neuralgic pains in the neck. Soon a
tiffness of the neck began to set in and it has been
;rowing steadily worse. The pains continued, the
.pine gradually became rigid and bent forward. He
ias had, in the last seven or eight years, attacks of
heumatism in different joints, and now we find his
vhole spine absolutely stiff; there is a large rounded
iosterior curve, head is bent forward until chin
lmost touches sternum, the articulations of the ribs
re affected and the thorax is immovable. His
reathing is entirely abdominal. Up to two years
go, he had little, if any, treatment; then his physi-
ian tried to break up the adhesions in the neck,
nder slight anesthesia (chloroform). They went
rith a snap like the report of a pistol. The opera-
on was followed by pain and almost total disability;
week later, a plaster-of-Paris jacket with head
pring was applied. The head spring interfered with
is occupation, so he took it off about a year ago.
ince then he has been getting worse. A Taylor
pinal brace with chin cup has now been applied.
'atient also taking salicylates and iron with good
:sults. An X-ray picture giving a lateral view of
ie cervical vertebræ, is absolutely negative as no
ony changes can be noticed. This is a very inter-
;ting fact and corresponds with results obtained
y some observers in contradistinction to others who
ive reproduced radiographs of similar cases show-
g extensive bony changes.

**ESTERN SURGICAL AND GYNECOLOGICAL AS-
SOCIATION.**

*burteenth Annual Meeting, held in Milwaukee, Wis.,
December 28 and 29, 1904.*

he President, Charles H. Mayo, M.D., of Rochester,
Minn., in the Chair.

Kidney Stone.—Dr. A. L. Wright, of Carroll,
)wa, read a paper on this subject, in which he
'esented the following conclusions: (1) Kidney
one may occur at any time of life, from the earliest
ripe old age. (2) These stones are the most
equent, and give rise to the greatest amount of
ffering of any form of surgical disease of the
dney. The clinical manifestations of kidney stone
not depend upon its size. A small stone, just
rge enough to prevent its escape, and composed
oxalate of lime, will cause more suffering and

damage to the kidney parenchyma than a very much
larger deposit of softer formation, as well as completely disable the patient while the destructive
changes are taking place, although the clinical symptoms are not intensely active. (3) While generally
unilateral, stone occasionally occurs in both kidneys,
or the reflex symptoms may point most prominently
to the sound kidney, the stone being found not infrequently on the side free from pain. (4) Diagnosis
is not difficult in the typical cases, but owing to
the stone remaining quiescent in some for an indefinite period, makes recognition almost impossible.
(5) Owing to the fact that kidney stone may put on
the livery of infectious diseases, the diagnosis is
difficult, if not impossible, in those cases where
the classical symptoms are absent. (6) There are
few diseases of the kidney more certainly fatal,
when left to themselves, and more successfully
treated when encountered by proper surgical interference, arresting the destructive changes taking
place in the kidney, and restoring the viscus to its
physiological functions.

Dr. Alexander Hugh Ferguson said that this
branch of surgery was by no means complete from
an etiological and diagnostic standpoint, nor from
the viewpoint of treament. Pain was sometimes
very deceptive. It was both local and referred;
local in the region of kidney itself, and referred
to different parts of the body, chiefly along the
genito-urinary tract from the testicle, sometimes
toward the midline of the abdomen, at other times
toward the ensiform cartilage in the region of the
gall-bladder and duodenum, and not infrequently
it was referred to the back. Pain was caused in
nearly all cases at first, when there was no septic
urine, by stretching of the pelvis of the kidney
and of the kidney tissue, the calices, etc., this
stretching causing excruciating pain. A quiescent
stone did not always cause colic, although it frequently gave rise to referred pain. In the diagnosis
one should consider tumor of the kidney, recurrent
attacks of interstitial nephritis, and tuberculosis of
the kidney. The X-ray was one of the best aids
to diagnosis at our command. He called attention
to the dangers incident to the passage of such instruments as the segregator, cystoscope, etc. He
reported a case illustrating the difficulty in making
the diagnosis.

Dr. W. D. Haines, when acting as Coroner's
Physician, had made over two thousand autopsies,
and in about 50 per cent. of the cases he found
stones of various sizes in the kidney. In many of
the cases it was impossible to trace the history,
but in a number of them, in bringing out the
forensic aspect, he was able to trace the history
accurately. In those cases in which the history
could be traced, it was surprising to find how infrequently symptoms were complained of referable
to the kidney. In treating these cases surgically
one of the principal things to determine was the
presence of a kidney on the opposite side. An instructive case was cited.

Dr. Wright, in closing, maintained in regard to
the cause of pain, that it was inflammatory in
character, and not due, as claimed in textbooks
and by teachers, to stretching of the kidney tissue.
Many of these kidneys were opened, where the
clinical manifestations indicated the existence of
stone, but none was found except possibly a little
debris, possibly nothing. Furthermore, where the
deposit consisted of oxalate of lime the pain was
very excruciating. The stone was too large to en-

gage in the urether, but not large enough, however, to stretch the pelvis or parenchyma of the kidney, or to produce any stretching effect whatever, so that he believed the same would apply to the presence of stone in the kidney, as in gall-bladder work, in which pain was not due to the passage of gall-stones, but that it was of an inflammatory character, and that when such kidneys were opened and drained, and no stone or stones found, relief was prompt.

Newer Aids to Diagnosis in Diseases of the Urinary Tract.—Dr. M. L. Harris, of Chicago, in a paper with this title, arranged the newer aids to diagnosis in diseases of the urinary tract in the following order, according to their value: (1) The cystoscope; (2) urethral catheterization or segregation, with comparative analyses of the separate urines; (3) the X-ray; (4) the phlorhizin test; (5) comparative cystoscopy of the separate urines; (6) cryoscopy of the blood, with the necessary corrections made.

Dr. B. B. Davis had been using the Harris segregator a great deal in making tests as to the relative condition of the two kidneys, and asked whether the essayist had observed temporary anuria in any of the cases, enough to interfere materially with the value of the test. Dr. Davis then related a recent case in which there was temporary anuria following the use of the segregator.

Dr. Harris had observed temporary anuria, which lasted sometimes a few minutes, sometimes ten or fifteen minutes. He had noticed it in a number of instances. He had seen it last as long as thirty or forty minutes, but how long it would have lasted had the examination been continued he did not know. Temporary anuria, however, was not common. It was exceptional. He had also seen temporary anuria follow the introduction of the urethral catheter, which lasted for several hours, or until the catheter was withdrawn.

Methods of Exploring the Abdomen, and a New One.—Dr. Alexander Hugh Ferguson, of Chicago, stated that in the daily round of work the surgeon met cases requiring colpotomy, anterior or posterior, to remove myomata, or cysts, and these cases often gave a history of stomach, gall-bladder, kidney or bowel disturbances. An examination of the abdominal organs was highly satisfactory, although oftentimes one felt hardly justified in opening through the abdominal wall for that purpose. The problem was solved by passing the hand and entire forearm into the abdominal cavity through the vagina. In order to furnish enough space for this purpose, it was imperative to cut through the mucous membrane of the vagina its whole length on each side post-laterally. The mucous membrane being severed, the other structure would stretch at once. The bare arm being smeared over with sterile vaselin, glided in with ease. He had within the last three years, both in private practice and at his clinics passed his hand through the vagina to the diaphragm, and palpated all the abdominal organs. In one case, after detecting gall-stones, he cut down upon the gall-bladder and pushed it, full of biliary calculi, through a buttonhole incision in the abdominal wall. In another case a cancer of the rectum was present, and before removing it it was indicated to learn the condition of the internal organs. He passed his hand and detected cancer of the liver and gall bladder. Still a third case, a maiden lady of mature years, had a vaginal outlet so small that a digital examination could not be made without on anesthetic. He then found cancer

of the posterior lip of the cervix. Through an anterior colpotomy he passed his hand, after having slit the vagina on each side, and found the anterior surface of the stomach involved with a firm hard tumor, evidently cancerous, and the lymphathics were also extensively enlarged with the same dreadful disease.

Dr. R. C. Coffee asked under what circumstances the essayist would make such an exploration as he had described, inasmuch as the vagina could not be thoroughly sterilized, and an abdominal incision was fraught with so little danger?

Dr. A. L. Wright spoke disparagingly of this method of exploration, although he had never tried it. He questioned the possibility of being able to render the vagina aseptic. The mortality was so slight from the abdominal incision and the dangers attending it so small, that the method of Dr. Ferguson impressed him as being much more formidable and attended with much more danger than an abdominal incision.

Dr. C. O. Thienhaus called attention to the method employed by Ott, who introduces an electric light through the vagina into the abdomen, at the same time using one on his forehead, with which he can explore the abdominal cavity, and see diseases with the eye which could not possibly be diagnosed otherwise and dealt with accordingly.

Peritoneal Adhesions, their Cause and Prevention.—Dr. Arthur E. Hertzler, of Kansas City, Mo., stated that he had studied peritoneal adhesions by means of a small glass window sewed into the lateral abdominal wall of an animal. Peritoneal surfaces might agglutinate without a destruction of the endothelial layer. In true adhesions the endothelial layers were always destroyed. If the basement membrane was not destroyed, the adhesions might separate after a time. If the basement membrane was destroyed, the union was formed by a true growth of fibrous tissue, and was permanent. Ordinary adhesions were formed by fibrin formation, with a loosening of the cement substance of the basement membrane, and an interlacing of the fibers forming the basement layer. This formed in twelve to eighteen hours. The formation of peritoneal adhesions depended on the same factors as blood coagulation. The irritation of the surface destroyed the endothelium, permitting the escape of fibrinogen-forming fluid. The $CaCl_2$ is abundant below, and immediately below the endothelial cells, as may be demonstrated by silver nitrate. The escape of the leucocytes from the vessels which attended every irritative process activated the proferment, and made it active. The precipitate of fibrin thus formed was identical with that form in blood coagulation, as might be demonstrated by michrochemical tests. The identity was further demonstrated by the fact that those factors which prevented coagulation also prevented peritoneal adhesions. The methods most employed were phosphorus and peptone. The former prevented it by destroying the fibrogen, the latter by acting on an antiferment. The presence of a digestive ferment in the upper intestinal tract explains why adhesions formed less readily in spontaneous perforations in this region.

Operation for Undescended Testicle.—Dr. Emerson M. Sutton, of Peoria, Ill., reported the case of a boy, eleven years of age, a cryptorchild, who suffered from strabismus and nervousness, but otherwise was well. In making an incision in the inguinal canal the testicle was found above the internal ring free; the cord was retained by a band extending posteriorly toward the median line, and upward opposite the second lumbar vertebra. Blunt dissection was resorted to until the cord was freed and the testicle deposited easily in the bottom of the scrotum without tension. The retaining step of the operation consisted in a buttonhole incision through the bottom of the scrotal sac posterior to its middle, where the skin was less elastic, catgut stitches inserted through the edges of the skin, and albuginea or testicle, in a way which held the end of the testicle attached to the skin, necessitating healing by granulation. The convalescence was uncomplicated, and the testicle was permanently fixed in the bottom of the scrotum and was of natural size. He stated that many operations for this affection had been planned, as Kocher's circular stitch, sewing the cord in the canal without strangulating it; also Watson-Cheyne's retaining stitch through the bottom of the scrotal sac and then the testicle, tied to the under wire of a retaining frame, to be moved after three weeks, when the organ had become fixed in place by adhesions. Objections to attaching the testicle to the bottom of a movable sac were valid, since experience demonstrated the futility of such a method. The Katzenstein operation of making a flap from the inner side of the thigh was a step in the right direction. However, with the modifications employed in the author's case, considering the satisfactory results, the surgeon could fix the testicle absolutely.

Dr. Sutton also reported a case of aneurism of the superior mesenteric artery upon which he operated.

The Practical Significance of Certain Common Symptoms in the Upper Abdomen.—Dr. J. F. Percy, of Galesburg, Ill., read a paper with this title. These symptoms were pain from ulcer of the stomach and cholecystitis, with or without stones, and the action of the gastric juice on the open ulcer either in the stomach or duodenum. Another source of pain was the formation of gas from inhibited peristalsis, due to ulcer or adhesions arising from it. Vomiting was also referred to as one of the symptoms of disease in this region, but in the author's experience it was not as frequent as nausea. Two methods were referred to as an aid to the location of lesions in the upper abdomen, one being light finger percussion eliciting pain over the inflammatory focus, in patients not too obese, and the resistance of the costal cartilages on the right side in inflammatory conditions of the gall-bladder and in ulcer of the duodenum or pylorus, as recently pointed out anew by Eliot. The author laid special stress on the effects of chronic infections of the liver and pancreas from ulcer of the stomach and persistent cholecystitis, and cites cases in point. He stated that some of these cases were rarely diagnosed correctly. Biliousness and dyspepsia were the words most frequently used as descriptive of the diagnosis and upon which the treatment was based. The author stated further that a persistent infection would in an appreciable number of cases cause death regardless of the form of treatment which might be instituted, because of alteration in the functionating tissues of the liver and pancreas. Future investigation would show that the results of this infection were chemical through the intervention of bacteria at work in ulcerating areas in the stomach, duodenum or gall-bladder.

Dr. John B. Murphy congratulated the essayist on bringing out with greater force the fact that differential diagnosis between lesions of the pyloric area of the stomach, the head of the pancreas, and the gall-bladder was extremely difficult. He was pleased that the essayist brought out the periodicity of exacerbations in ulcers of the stomach. A large number of cases of ulcer of the stomach has pronounced exacerbations. They were practically well in the period between the attacks. Dr. Murphy detailed an interesting case corroborating the latter statement.

Dr. Alexander Hugh Ferguson stated that when a pain came on suddenly, which was referable to the epigastric region, although no tenderness could be elicited in that region, but could be over the gall-bladder, it tended to show that the seat of the trouble was within the gall-bladder, the stone or stones being engaged in the cystic duct. Pain occurring while the patient was in a quiescent state, or occurring after the patient went to sleep, pointed to the gall-bladder rather than to any other organ. A lancinating pain, only coming on occasionally and referable to the region of the gall-blader and ducts, pointed to carcinoma. Pain referred to the region of the ducts was more characteristic of gall-stones. In cases of stone or tumor of the kidney, as well as in tumor of the suprarenal capsule, pain was generally referred to the back. Pott's disease should not be overlooked. Pain referred to the testicle and radiating into the genito-urinary tract pointed towards the kidney as the seat of the trouble. Still, pain was referred sometimes to these regions from other conditions than stone in the kidney.

Dr. William D. Haggard said that while expertness and refinement in diagnosis were desiderata, surgeons must realize that many of the cases under discussion were not amenable to the niceties and refinement of diagnosis to which attention had been drawn. In reference to differences in pains and colics of which patients complained, he referred to the importance of a well-taken clinical history, saying that a great deal of dependence should be placed on it.

Dr. B. B. Davis had been struggling for years against the habit of making incisions without having made a careful and sufficient study of the case beforehand, but he had concluded that a man was more dangerous who did not make such incisions occasionally than the one who did make them before he had made accurate diagnoses. He related a case which he thought to be one of cholelithiasis from the symptoms and clinical history, yet much to his surprise in operating he found a large appendix, turned up underneath the gall-bladder, with dense adhesions around the cystic duct. There were no stones found in the gall-bladder; it was perfectly patulous, and after freeing the adhesions he could squeeze bile out without any thouble. He did nothing to the gall-bladder, simply removed the appendix, and thus far relief had been complete.

Splenic Anemia.—Dr. Palmer Findley, of Chicago, reported a case of splenic anemia in which he removed the spleen with good results. The patient was forty-five years old, had suffered for four years from a dragging sensation in the left side and uterine hemorrhage. Blood examination showed reds, 2,784,000 per cubic millimeter; leucocytes, 6,000, and hemoglobin, 42 per cent. Thirteen months after operation her blood showed reds, 4,600,000; leucocytes, 6,000, and hemoglobin, 78 per cent. In spite of the fact that the uterine hemorrhage continued, the patient refused curettage for its control. Dr. Findley offered a word of caution in the hasty diagnosis of splenic anemia without giving due consideration to other possible causes for splenic enlargement associated with a secondary anemia, such as malaria and syphilis, and advised splenectomy for only the rapidly progressive cases, reserving medical treatment for milder form.

High-Frequency Electricity as a Factor in the Treatment of Surgical and Gynecological Diseases.—Dr. E. M. Sala, of Rock Island, Ill., related his personal experience with the d'Arsonval high-frequency current, and reported several cases comprising a variety of affections in which the immediate results were gratifying, but what the permanent results were going to be, he could not predict. However, he was convinced that the d'Arsonval-Odin apparatus had a very promising future.

The Care of the Axilla after Excavations for Malignant or Infective Lesions.—Dr. John B. Murphy, of Chicago, discussed this subject, saying that extensive dissection of the axilla was not infrequently followed by contracting painful cicatrices, limitation of motion, edema, neuralgia, etc. These can be relieved or avoided by (a) line of skin incision; (b) immediate grafting or transplantation; (c) muscular implantation, and (d) muscular conservation.

Moorhof's Bone Plug.—Dr. James E. Moore, of Minneapolis, Minn., read a paper on this subject. The author stated that in January, 1903, von Moorhof reported a large number of successful results from the use of a new bone plug. This material consisted of sixty parts iodoform, forty parts spermaceti, and forty parts of oleum sesami. These ingredients were slowly heated to 100° C., and when allowed to cool formed a soft solid, which remained solid at the temperature of the body. For use it was heated to 50° C., being constantly stirred to keep the iodoform evenly distributed. At this temperature it could be poured into the cavity, where it immediately solidified. The material did not act as a foreign body, nor did it act as a culture medium. It possessed inhibitory and medicinal properties of iodoform without causing iodoform intoxication. His experience with this material, although limited, was sufficient to satisfy him that better results could be obtained in treating bone cavities than by any older method, and in illustration of this he reported four recent successful cases.

Dr. Arthur T. Mann stated that last winter he saw Moorhof use his bone plug. The first case in which he used it was one of tuberculosis of the tarsal bones of the foot, with a discharging sinus on the side. Moorhof made an incision across the full front of the ankle, catching up the tendons with sutures to be tied later, cut the tendons, turned the foot down, removed the astragalus, a third of the os calcis, and curetted away some tuberculous tissue, cut out the skin and tissue about the sinus, put the foot in its position, drew the sutures on the tendons, tied them, and filled the bone cavity with this bone plug. Moorhof told him that he expected the plug to fill in with bone. He also showed the speaker a series of X-ray pictures taken of a similar case a number of months ago, in which the result was eminently satisfactory. He mentioned other cases Moorhof had treated by bone plug with satisfactory results.

Dr. Moore, of Chicago, believed that cases could now be treated successfully with this bone plug in which formerly amputation was done, as, for instance, in cases of tuberculosis of the wrist and ankle joints.

Extirpation of the Gasserian Ganglion in the Treatment of Facial Neuralgia.—Dr. A. E. Halstead, of Chicago, stated that during the last decade the treatment of inveterate facial neuralgia had progressed mostly along surgical lines. The injection of osmic acid into the peripheral branches of the nerve, either directly through the overlying tissue or after exposing the nerve by incision, first proposed and practised by Neuber,

and lately revived and extolled by Murphy, had its physiological counterpart in neurotomy. Probably regeneration was somewhat longer delayed after its use than after simple section of the nerve, owing to its property of hardening nerve tissue, but in the end regeneration, with return of function, undoubtedly occurred. After speaking of the different methods and technic of extirpating the ganglion, Dr. Halstead reported seven cases, in which he had extirpated the ganglion for the relief of facial neuralgia. From the cases the author reviewed and from his own experience, it seemed possible to have a return of the pain after the removal of the ganglion. Nevertheless, he believed with Cushing that "the probability of non-recurrence bore a direct relation to the degree of entirety with which' the ganglion had been removed." In his own cases he had each ganglion subjected to a careful examination by a competent microscopist. In all of the specimen submitted ganglionic elements were found, and the gross anatomical characteristics of the organ were preserved.

Dr. John B. Murphy stated that in his 12 cases of removal of the Gasserian ganglion there were four deaths. This large percentage of deaths caused him to abandon the operation. Since his last report he had had one recurrence of neuralgia from the injection of osmic acid. In the entire number up to date, with this exception, he had not had a recurrence thus far.

(To be Continued.)

BOOK REVIEWS.

THE MEDICAL NEWS VISITING LIST, 1905. Lea Brothers & Company, Philadelphia and New York.

THE convenience of this pocket visiting list, in which a complete record of each case can be quickly and accurately made, is well evidenced by its general use among practitioners during the past nineteen years. A busy man demands, above all things, that the record of his cases shall be easily and quickly made. Otherwise they will be temporarily neglected and frequently entirely lost. This wallet-shaped book not only contains ruled blanks for recording every detail of practice, but also embodies much valuable information which is frequently demanded by a doctor at a moment's notice. Among other valuable things may be mentioned a scheme of dentition; tables of weights and measures; instructions for urine examinations; tables of eruptive fevers; directions for artificial respiration; tables of doses, incompatibles, poisons and antidotes and an alphabetical table of diseases and remedies. It is issued in four styles so that the requirements of every practitioner may be met and represents the results of a long experience in perfecting a book which embodies the best method of recording the daily work of a practitioner.

THE ACTION OF LIGHT AS A THERAPEUTIC AGENT. By LEONARD K. HIRSHBERG, M.D., Baltimore, Md. Fiske Fund Dissertation, No. 47. Snow & Farnham, Providence.

THIS is an excellent essay of about twelve thousand words on the use of radiant energy in medical practice. The history of the sporadic attempts which have been made from time to time is briefly considered and the generally accepted opinions of the different branches, at present in vogue, are stated with great clearness and conciseness. Every department of light therapy is considered.

The volume will appeal to all who are interested in phototherapy and especially to those practitioners who wish to gain a knowledge of just how the subject is regarded at the present day by the best authorities.

THE MEDICAL NEWS.
A WEEKLY JOURNAL OF MEDICAL SCIENCE.

VOL. 86.   NEW YORK, SATURDAY, JANUARY 28, 1905.   NO. 4.

ORIGINAL ARTICLES.

SOME IRREGULAR FEATURES OF LOBAR PNEUMONIA.

BY CHARLES KNAPP LAW, M.D.,

OF JERSEY CITY, N. J.;

ASSISTANT SURGEON TO ST. FRANCIS HOSPITAL.

ACUTE lobar pneumonia is one of the most common and most important of the severe acute diseases. On account of its sudden onset even to those most vigorous in health, its gravity and quick termination in death or recovery, its proneness to attack all grades of society, from the worthless alcoholic to the most useful and valuable citizen, its increasing prevalence and severity, this malady impresses the physician probably more than any other disease. When we enter the sick room and find a serious case, which examination shows to be one of pneumonia, we immediately bow with profoundest respect to a " foeman worthy of our steel."

The regular features of lobar pneumonia are so well known to every physician that in this paper I shall call your attention only to some of the irregularities of the disease which have impressed me during the past ten years.

One of the most common of these which a physician must meet is the sequel empyema. In my experience this occurs more frequently in childhood and early life, although it followed pneumonia on one occasion in a man about fifty years old at the City Hospital while I was interne at that institution. The patient generally passes the crisis as usual. The temperature may, or may not, go to normal. I have not yet, however, seen a case in which the pain and distress completely left the affected side. In from twenty-four hours to a week the temperature begins to rise and fluctuate, the pulse becomes weaker and more rapid, chills or chilly sensations occur, indicating the presence of pus. Why does this complication follow pneumonia? In all, or nearly all, cases of lung fever the inflammatory process involves more or less of the adjacent pleura. It is infrequent, however, that the germ finds its way through the pulmonary pleura, so the congestion and irritation of the membrane causing the pain in the side generally clears up with the subsidence of the pneumonic process. If, however, the resistance of the pulmonary pleura is overcome and the germs find their entrance to the pleural cavity, already congested and inflamed, they change a plastic or serofibrinous pleurisy to a purulent one, and empyema results. This accounts for the fact that in the pneumonia which precedes an empyema the patient is apt

---

1 Read before the Hudson County Medical Society, October 14, 1904.

to suffer more acutely with prolonged pain in the side; at least that has been my experience. I will cite two cases illustrating this.

J. M., aged twenty-two years; taken sick with pneumonia June 30, 1899, and passed the crisis July 16. During the whole process of the disease the pain in the affected side would not yield to counterirritations and but little to ordinary doses of codeine, at the crisis the temperature dropped to 99.5° F. in the mouth, the delirium subsided and the patient slept, but when awake still complained of pain. This continued for forty-eight hours, when the temperature again rose, dulness on percussion became flatness and the aspirator showed the presence of pus.

George O'R., aged four years, was taken with pneumonia the latter part of June, 1903. The attack subsided by lysis in about twelve days. The child began to improve and run about the house when the case was discharged. He would, however, at times put his hand to his side and complain of pain. I was called the last of July to see him again, and found the pleural cavity filled with pus. As I left for my vacation that day, I turned the case over to Dr. Hill for operation.

Other similar cases might be recounted, but time will not permit. We should then never lose sight of the fact that any case of lobar pneumonia may be followed by empyema, that it is likely to be so followed in children and young adults whenever the pleura is extensively involved and the pain unusually severe and prolonged. When the temperature does not subside in eight or ten days, or rises again after the crisis, when the dulness changes to flatness, when the bronchial breathing and subcrepitant râle subside, and vesicular breathing does not take their place at the lower portion of the lung, we should at once aspirate. It is a simple procedure, is not in the least dangerous, inflicts but little pain, and clears up all obscurity. If pus be found, no time should be lost before operating, unless the patient be very weak, when, I believe, the pus should first be drawn off with an aspirator, and shortly afterward, when the patient becomes a little stronger, the chest should be opened and thorough drainage established.

Another irregularity of lobar pneumonia, and one which is always obscure to the physician and often leads to an error of diagnosis, is the so-called central pneumonia, or pneumonia with late localization. You are called to see a patient who, perhaps, has had a slight chill. The temperature is probably quite high. He may have some gastric disturbance. He generally has a little cough and may have a slight pain in the side, or none at all. On examining the chest no abnormality whatever can be detected. This goes on for several days before any dulness, bronchial breathing or crepitant râle can be detected. There are cases on record which have passed the crisis before a slight pleuritic friction sound established conclusively the diagnosis. Yet the history of the case, the general appearances and actions of the patient, the cough and tenacious expectoration which are usually present, and the rapid respiration are at least suggestive. I well remember such a case in a child four or five years old whom I attended two years ago. All I could find wrong for the first six days was a temperature running from 105° to 106.5° F. with the symptoms which accompany any high temperature. There were absolutely no abnormal physical signs. There was not even a cough to help in making a diagnosis. On my way to see the little patient I used to spend my time studying how to avoid answering the parents' perplexing questions. At last I detected a little dulness and crepitant râles near the apex of the right lung. Although apparently so little of the lung was involved, the temperature was higher and more prolonged than that of any other case of pneumonia I have ever seen. In fact the amount of involvement of the lung in any case does not seem to influence the temperature.

I will next call your attention to what Osler calls migratory pneumonia. It begins in a certain lobe, runs its course there, during which time it extends to one or more other lobes. In such a case there may be a crisis for each lobe involved, indicated by a drop in the temperature and a somewhat improved pulse. But only after the final crisis does the temperature become normal. I will cite such a case which I attended four years ago.

Dorothy S., a girl of fourteen years, taken with pneumonia March 27, 1900. The lower lobe of the right lung was involved. It extended to the middle lobe about March 31. She had a temperature running from 103° to 105° F. April 3, or about a week after her initiatory chill, the temperature dropped to 101° F. and the pulse improved to correspond. It was the crisis for the lower lobe. Afterward the temperature again rose and I found the upper lobe involved while the bronchial breathing and subcrepitant râle completely left the lower lobe, and normal vesicular breathing took their place. She now ran a temperature of about 99° F. in the morning to 101° F. at night for about two weeks more, when the upper and middle lobes gradually cleared. All this time the apex of the lung was dull on percussion and showed bronchial or bronchovesicular respiration. I feared tuberculosis but a microscopical examination of the sputum showed no bacilli, only the pneumococcus. This case is also an example of delayed resolution,—a condition which happens quite frequently when the consolidation is at the apex. This girl made a good but slow recovery, spending the summer in the country and returning in the fall in the bloom of health.

Another feature of pneumonia to which the text-books and the profession have, in the past, given too little attention, is the complication of tympanites. This most grievous affection is pronounced by Gilman Thompson as much to be dreaded as the same condition in typhoid fever. It appears rather late in the disease and more frequently in those cases suffering with severe toxemia. It is caused by a partial paralysis of the stomach and bowel accompanied by fermentation of their contents,—a condition, I fear, often aggravated by too much opiate and a too copious diet of milk. The disorder has a twofold disastrous effect. First, mechanical. The abdominal viscera press upward against those of the throax embarrassing the unaffected portion of the lungs used in breathing and a heart already well nigh exhausted with overwork. Second, toxic. The products of malfermentation are absorbed and add to the toxemia of the disease. Unless this condition can be relieved in a reasonable length of time, I am convinced we cannot hope to save our patient. The abdomen should be examined with as much care as the chest at every visit by the physician and the first sign of tympanites properly combatted.

An irregularity of pneumonia which has attracted considerable attention in the medical profession during the past two years is the sensation of the initial pain of the involved pleura, not in the chest, but in various parts of the abdomen. This may lead the busy practitioner to the inference that he has to deal with a case of gall-stones, peritonitis or appendicitis. This phenomenon is explained by Herrick, of Chicago, by the fact that when there is irritation of the end of one branch of a nerve, pain may be referred to the end of another branch, like the well known phenomenon of hip-joint disease producing pain in the knee, or the passage of a stone through the ureter producing pain in the testicle. The lower six intercostal nerves supply the abdominal wall as well as part of the parietal and diaphragmatic pleura. So the involvement of these portions of the pleura by an adjacent pneumonia may, by irritating the supplying branches of the intercostal nerves, refer the pain to other branches or those supplying the abdominal wall, and the patient will feel severe pain in some portion of the abdomen. In these days, when abdominal pain suggests to every physician the possibility or presumption of appendicitis, we should never lose sight of a possible pneumonia. Herrick, of Chicago, and Griffith, of Philadelphia, cite instances where appendectomy was nearly decided upon in several cases of overlooked pneumonia. In one case the disease was only discovered by the routine examination of the chest before giving the anesthetic.

This reference of pain to the iliac region may occur at any time of life, but is more common in childhood. The muscles supplied by the nerves to which the pain is referred, have usually a certain amount of the rigidity which we expect in peritoneal inflammation. There may even be some bulging suggesting a tumor, which confounds the physician still more. I will cite two cases of this referred pain in pneumonia occurring in my own practice.

I attended Mrs. J. in confinement one evening about six years ago. At my post-partum call the next day I found her husband in bed with what he called a severe stomachache. He had returned from Pennsylvania that morning, having eaten heartily of lobster and other things the night before. He said he shook with the cold while passing through the mountains at which time he vomited the lobster and beer of the night before. I asked him to put his hand to the pain and he pointed to a spot about an inch above McBurney's point. There was rigidity of the right abdominal muscles and seemingly pain on pressure. Yet I managed to press deeply on his appendix when his attention was diverted. I diagnosed indigestion with a mental reservation of gall-stones or appendicitis and gave him a dose of calomel. I confess pneumonia was not thought of. The next day the pain had shifted to the region of the liver and breathing was painful. I now examined his chest and found a well-marked pneumonia of the lower lobe of the right lung. This proved a very serious case, being followed by empyema, the patient making a complete recovery in about two months.

My second case, with well-marked abdominal pains, occurred about three years ago. The patient was a girl nine years of age. I was called to her at night to give her relief from severe pain and tenderness in the left iliac region. The mother gave me the following history: The girl arose as usual in the morning and ate her breakfast. She then complained of feeling ill, and of a pain in her stomach. The mother gave her a cathartic, although this acted the pain continued to get worse, and she felt that she could not endure her condition till morning. On examination I found her temperature 104° F., pulse 115. On asking her to show me where the pain was she placed her hand on the left of the abdomen at a place corresponding to McBurney's point on the right. On examining the place I found the muscles rigid and the place seemingly very tender. I could find no tenderness over the appendix. I thought of peritonitis and those rare cases of appendicitis where the pain is on the left, without deciding just what it was. I did not think of pneumonia. Very much the same conditions continued the second day. On the third day I noticed a rapid respiration and examination of the chest revealed at once pneumonia of lower lobe of the left lung. In this instance I should certainly have advised an operation for appendicitis had the referred pain been on the right instead of the left side.

During the past year while I was on duty at St. Francis Hospital, two cases of pneumonia were sent to that institution to be operated on for appendicitis, one a man about twenty-five years

old and the other a girl four years of age. Both cases had fever, a rapid pulse and pain and tenderness in the right iliac region. In neither case, however, was there quite the rigidity of the abdominal muscles one would expect in a well-marked case of appendicitis. Examination of the young man's chest showed a pneumonia of the lower lobe of the right lung. The girl, strange to say, revealed a pneumonia of the upper lobe of the left lung. Why in this case the pain should be referred to the region of the appendix I have been unable to determine.

How are we to avoid such mistakes? No doubt there are occasions when it is impossible at the beginning of an attack in children to make a differential diagnosis. At the last meeting of the American Medical Association, McCosh advised waiting a few hours in such cases before operating for appendicitis, even though the indications point to that disease. Usually, however, a thorough examination of the chest will reveal the true state of affairs, for a central pneumonia rarely gives rise to such pain. It seems to me that only irritation of the diaphragmatic pleura could cause such pain without detection, and in a few hours such a pneumonia will be apt to manifest some physical sign. Certainly the lungs should be examined in every case of abdominal pain with fever and but few mistakes will be made.

EXCISION OF THE SUPERIOR CERVICAL GANGLION OF THE SYMPATHETIC FOR SIMPLE GLAUCOMA.[1]

BY COLMAN W. CUTLER, M.D.,
OF NEW YORK.

BEFORE excision of the superior cervical ganglion of the sympathetic can be given a definite place among other measures, likewise more or less empirical, for the relief of chronic simple glaucoma, two questions must be answered. These questions are:

1. Is the eye ever injured or the glaucoma aggravated by the operation?

2. Does sympathectomy offer a prospect of sufficiently prolonged relief to justify us in urging it in these desperate cases, either before or in place of iridectomy?

The first question should be answered only after the weighing of much clinical evidence. One of the chief claims made for sympathectomy is that even if it does no good it will do no harm. Actual risk to life may be eliminated, and the disordered sensation, paresthesia, pain in neck and face, paralysis of the trapezius and interference with phonation, may also be avoided by a skilful surgeon, and should not weigh against the operation if a favorable effect on the glaucoma is to be expected in a certain proportion of cases, or if the inevitable alternative is blindness.

The eye has not suffered, in any instance directly after sympathectomy, so far as the writer

1 Read at American Ophthalmological Society, July 14, 1904.

is aware. In two or three cases (Grünert, Bericht der Ophthal. Gesellschaft, Heidelberg, 1900, p. 18. Wilder, *Journal of the American Medical Association*, February 9, 1904) it has been suggested that intra-ocular hemorrhage following the later iridectomy or subsequent acute attacks of glaucoma might be attributed to the vasomotor changes produced by paralysis of the sympathetic. The two cases of Grünert and Wilder would be disquieting, but it is evident that the danger of hemorrhage following sympathectomy is not greater, nor can it predispose to an evil result of a later iridectomy, for in all the cases of hemorrhagic glaucoma collected by Rohmer and by Wilder, seven in number, no harm has been done, and all are reported as in some respects improved. The case of hemorrhagic glaucoma reported by Dr. Price (No. 33 in Wilder's list *loc cit.*) died of uremia nine months after the operation. His daughter states that there seemed to be no return of the glaucoma, that he used his eyes with comfort to the day of his death, and often remarked the improved condition.

The doubts as to the safety of the operation raised by De Obarrio and by Angeluocci may be dismissed. Wilder in his fifth case mentions mental confusion with mild hallucinations occurring in the first week. Bichat[1] mentions mental disorder occurring a year after the operation, and states that Brown-Séquard considered this to be a result of resection of the sympathetic.

So far as I am aware, this includes all that has been offered in opposition to the operation. The chief objection is that it is ineffectual or that its influence on the disease is too brief.

In a paper published in the *Annals of Surgery* in September, 1902, the case of A. J. Rogers was described at some length. A brief résumé of the history brought down to a recent date, will show the later progress of the case and will indicate that in probable cases the result of the operation may be sufficiently prolonged to justify its adoption.

In 1893 glaucoma began with severe pains in both eyes, impaired vision and erythropsia. For a year and a half before the patient was first seen by the writer, in 1897, there had been frequent attacks of cloudy vision with rings and more or less pain. Chromatopsia was frequent and distressing, red being the predominating color. These phenomena were lessened by myotics, and after anterior sclerotomy and iridectomy they disappeared for a time. Since sympathectomy the subjective sensations have remained absent.

The operation was performed June 10, 1901, vision at that time being O.D. $^{20}/_{100}$; T. + ½ to + 1; O.S. V. O.T. + 2. The retained vision in the right eye may be attributed to the iridectomy in that eye three years previously. After sympathectomy vision improved, and in two days it was $^{20}/_{30}$. The field was enlarged laterally, not

upward, where it still seems dangerously near the fixation point. In August, 1902, fourteen months later, it had approached still nearer, but in July, 1903, the field was larger than at any other time, and on April 26, 1904, vision was still $^{20}/_{30}$, the field larger in some directions, but upward it was narrower than the year before. Rogers reads with much ease for half an hour or more, quite small print. Vision, as I have stated, is $^{20}/_{30}$, that is, he picks out most of the letters of $^{20}/_{30}$, and at times some of $^{20}/_{20}$, but in a hesitating way, and if the light is changed he is easily disconcerted. In a brightly lighted place he is dazzled, and in the dusk he finds his way with difficulty.

These limitations are but natural when one considers the probable damage to the ganglion cells, and the partial atrophy of the nerve which is pale and excavated about 3 D.; but the fact remains that he had useful vision, had worked and enjoyed life without any symptoms of glaucoma in that eye, for more than three years. Tension in the left eye, which is blind, has been raised at times, with some dull pain and with the appearance of a symptom to which I would like to call attention. I refer to the retraction of the upper lids: Von Gräfe's sign was present in both eyes at first, but since the sympathectomy it has appeared only in the left eye, which has absolute glaucoma, and it has only been observed when the tension is raised. In the paper before mentioned I called attention to the occurrence of this symptom in certain cases of chronic glaucoma then under observation, especially to one case of unilateral glaucoma, in which the retraction of the lid was present only on the side with increased tension.

Recently a case has presented itself in which with glaucoma secondary to a dislocated lens, this sign was very noticeable. It may therefore be explained as a reflex spasm, a result of the glaucoma.

A second case which Dr. Dennett very kindly permits me to report is that of Mr. M., aged fifty-four years. Chronic irritative glaucoma of the left eye; incipient glaucoma of the right eye, May, 1902. The left eye had been failing for ten years, and iridectomy was advised tentatively; so that it might be tried on the right eye in case that developed glaucoma. The operation was performed without mishap, but vision in this eye was not improved. During the past year, in spite of the iridectomy, there has been a severe attack of acute glaucoma with iritis which produced a staphylomatous protrusion of the cicatrix of the iridectomy done with admirable technic and without complications several years ago. In the right eye there have been subtle indications of the beginnings of glaucoma for several years. Central vision has been normal, but the field has suffered, and there has been frequent chromatopsia, with pale green and lavender mottling. There is hemeralopia, and a large inconstant diffuse relative scotoma upward of variable limits. This has

1 La Sympathectomie dans le traitement du glaucome. p. 146.

made the adding of columns of figures difficult. June 16, 1902: Removal of right superior cervical ganglion by Dr. Hayward. August 23, 1904—V. O.D.$^{20}/_{20}$, very slight excavation, color of nerve rather pale. O.S. fingers counted. Nerve excavated and pale. Slight protrusion of scar above coloboma, which is of good size with free pillars.

The field of vision of the right eye taken in 1902, after sympathectomy was larger both for form and color and less variable, and the faint relative defects were less apparent than before the operation. In August, 1904, the same limits were retained. The eye has been more useful than formerly, but there is still complaint of lavender and green suffusion of the field, and of inability to see well in dim light.

In the third case of simple glaucoma the ganglion was removed by Dr. John Rogers, March, 1904. In April Dr. Alling found vision $^{20}/_{20}$ from $^{20}/_{20}$ before the operation, and the field 20° to 30° larger downward, and in October the improvement was retained. The patient is using pilocarpine from time to time. This improvement enables him to go about with much independence, and to read freely, whereas before the operation the field had been reduced to a horizontal slit up 3°, in 5°, down 10°, out 60°.

In this case the time that has elapsed since the operation is brief, but as the disease had progressed steadily, though very slowly, during a period of eighteen months' observation, it is fair to claim the cessation of progress and the slight improvement as a favorable result.

That simple glaucoma may remain nearly stationary during prolonged periods is well-known. The following case illustrates the error that might arise in claiming results for any method of treatment in this most uncertain disease:

J. F., colored, male, aged fifty-five years; May 25, 1902. V. $^{20}/_{40}$; T. at times slightly raised. Field normal except for nearly complete loss of inferior nasal quadrant, where green and red are within 5° of fixation point, blue 10° and white 15°. Nerve white, not excavated. Operation refused. No treatment. June 27, 1904, V. $^{20}/_{50}$ + ½. Nerve as before. Field: about 20° narrower than at previous examination. In inferior nasal quadrant, colors close to the point of fixation, white 5°.

In three recent cases of simple glaucoma the results of the operation have not been positive—that is, vision has not been improved, but the disease has not progressed, and the eye has not suffered. It is to be hoped that this operation will not be allowed to fall into disuse because of any fancied difficulties it presents to patient or surgeon. The risk and discomfort is trifling in skilful hands, and the danger to the eye itself is entirely negligible. Whether this can be said of iridectomy, especially in chronic, simple glaucoma, with the field near the fixation point, is open to discussion.

A later opportunity for a brief examination of Rogers was obtained on October 25. The right eye, to all appearances, was unchanged. Tension normal. Anterior chamber of normal depth. Cornea clear. Vision reduced to $^{20}/_{70}$ and somewhat eccentric. The examination of the field shows that the fixation point had been lost from above. There has been no discomfort in this eye at any time, but the field has gradually narrowed from progressive atrophy of the nerve. In the left eye, on which side there was no sympathectomy nor previous iridectomy, there is an acute iritis with much pain. Cornea hazy, anterior chamber of normal depth, pupil small and bound to lens capsule by numerous synechiæ.

The progress of atrophy in the right eye is what had been expected, and it is surprising only that useful vision had been retained so long, more than three years since sympathectomy, with the field at that time within a few degrees of the fixation point. Undoubtedly, sympathectomy delayed progress of the disease longer than did iridectomy, and improved the nutrition of the eye, since as in Dr. Dennett's case, the iritis occurred in the eye with absolute glaucoma, on the side on which sympathectomy had not been done. In Dr. Dennett's case a satisfactory iridectomy had been done.

HOMICIDE BY A BOY DURING A STATE OF SOMNAMBULISTIC AUTOMATISM.[1]

BY T. M. T. MCKENNAN, M.D.,

OF PITTSBURG, PA.;

PROFESSOR OF NERVOUS DISEASES IN THE WESTERN PENNSYLVANIA MEDICAL COLLEGE, PITTSBURG, PA.,

AND

W. K. WALKER, M.D.,

OF DIXMONT, PA.;

FIRST ASSISTANT PHYSICIAN TO THE WESTERN PENNSYLVANIA HOSPITAL FOR THE INSANE, DIXMONT, PA.

RECITATION OF THE CASE BY DR. MCKENNAN.

IN October, 1902, in a house at Homestead, Pa., a mother and four children were attacked and killed by blows of an ax. The deed was done at night and while they were asleep. One other child, a girl of eight years, in the same room, was struck by the ax, and notwithstanding a severe wound of the skull, recovered. There was no evidence that any one had entered the house from without. There were two sons in the house at the time—James, aged twenty years, and Charles, aged eighteen years. These brothers slept in a room directly opposite the one where the mother and five other children slept. The father and husband was dead.

The statement of events of that night as related by the two brothers will now be given.

Statement of James Cawley.—He was awakened in the night by heavy moanings, these evidently came from his mother's room; the moanings from the children sounded louder than the mother's. He heard something fall on the floor, a heavy body—might have been an ax. He got out of bed on the side toward the window, and saw Charles come out of his mother's room with an ax in his hands. Charles did not call to him, but as he approached the bed, exclaiming "Oh! oh! burglars! robbers!" struck the bed with the ax where he, James had been lying, struck at him the second time and hit him on the thumb; the third time James pushed a rocking chair in front of him warding off the blow and grappled with Charles. After getting the ax from him he quieted somewhat, so much so that James was able to put on his trousers, still holding Charles, however, by the wrist. During this time Charles was shaking as though from great fear, and would say once in a while "Burglars! robbers!" and at no time appeared to be in his right mind. James led him to his mother's door and saw the blood in the room, and heard the moaning, then led him down stairs. He noticed that the door to the cellar was open. (The ax was kept in the cellar.) James then took him outside and towards the lockup. All this time Charles was apparently insensible to his surroundings; now and then he would resist and attempt to throw James down. When he got him into the station-house Charles appeared in the same condition. When James returned an hour an a half later, Charles appeared to talk rationally, and wanted to know what was the matter and why he was there. Under questioning James says that for several weeks Charles appeared to be very nervous, and was unable to sit for more than a few minutes in any one place; that he was easily irritated and James noted frequently that Charles would suddenly change color, getting quite pale and then red. He said that Charles secreted his plans and drawings around the house, and that subsequent to the crime a number of these drawings were found behind a picture on the wall. After the crime he heard his sister Mamie say to one of the neighbors that she, Mamie, had said to her mother, a little while before the crime, that "Charles must be going daffy." Her mother denied this and said Charles was all right.

Statement of Charles Cawley.—Was awakened in the night by a noise as of a door being opened; punched his brother and told him that someone was in the house. He pulled on his trousers and went into the hall; he noticed his mother's door was closed, this door being directly opposite his own bedroom. He went down stairs to the kitchen. but saw nothing out of the way; he heard his little sister call and went up stairs. He noticed his mother's door was open, and that a lamp was burning in the room. *He heard no sound* but saw some blood on the wall or on the bed; he did not go into the room; he saw an ax lying in the doorway and picked it up; he then went into his own room, and called to his brother three times; his brother did not answer; he touched his brother on the thigh with the ax to awaken him; with this the brother jumped up and grappled with him and took him to the station-house.

He says he was not asleep, but perfectly awake; that he did not commit any crime; that he knew nothing of his mother and sisters being killed, until told of it the next morning at the station-house. Upon being questioned, he said that he had been working on some patents; that he had some drawings in a scratch-book and that one day about a month previous to his crime he found a number of leaves torn out of this book, and in the book a note unsigned, which read as follows: "If you attempt to find who did this, will kill yourself and family." He took the note to the Public Safety Building, in Pittsburg, and showed it to a detective; he was told by the detective that some of the boys were playing a trick upon him, whereupon he tore up the note and returned home. He said he told no one else about this note. His sister, Mamie, however, said that he told her about it, and upon her asking him why he did not go out of the house any more, he replied, "On account of that warning."

Charles did not vary from the above description in the many times that he told us the story. Note that he heard no sound and that he did not know that his mother and sisters were killed, until told the next morning.

The grand jury returned a true bill against Charles, and he was committed to jail to await a trial for murder. Upon joint application of the attorneys for the commonwealth and for the prisoner, the court appointed me to examine Charles Cawley, and upon my request, Dr. W. K. Walker was also appointed.

We interrogated the surviving members of the family and were unable to secure any information of value from any of them except James. His statement we have already given.

We found that the father had been a heavy drinker, that James the brother had been in the workhouse, and that an older sister had a marked speech defect. We found that Charles was a delicate-looking youth with a marked puerile expression of countenance.

He exhibited distinct anatomical stigmata most marked in the formation of the ears, and in the shape of the skull which was brachycephalic. His general development was fairly good. He conversed readily, but showed indifference to the serious and terrible accusation, and while denying all knowledge of the crimes, still he did not appear discontented with his incarceration in the jail.

His education was quite limited, but he showed a tendency to the reading of rather serious books and no taste for light or romantic literature. He had been the bread winner of the family, and had a decided taste, almost a genius, for machinery, and for sometime and up until four months before the commission of the crimes, was employed to run a stationary engine.

In June of 1902, or four months before the tragedy, he suddenly stopped work and announced to his mother that he was going to work upon a patent, that this patent would make them rich, and although the family were in dire need, and although his mother besought him to go to work, he continued to work upon this patent, and did actually take out a patent for a car-brake.

While in the jail he showed no interest in this patent and never asked what had become of it. The warden reported that he was a model prisoner, and that he was not irritable or morose. At our first visit his tongue showed evidence of having been bitten at a recent date. The only direct evidence of an epileptic attack occurred upon a day when his aunt was visiting him, when he suddenly fell and was unconscious for a few seconds, but there were no convulsive movements or, if so, they were not observed. The light manner in which the aunt treated this attack seemed to us to indicate the probability that she had seen him in previous attacks of a like character.

The commission of these homicidal acts was motiveless, and would indicate that the perpetrator was not of normal mind. The evidence that Charles was the perpetrator of these acts, while circumstantial, was convincing. His previous history, including the recital of events of that night as related by his brother James, and his own very imperfect and hazy and partial recollections of the events of that night, were sufficient to convince us that during that period of time he was in a condition of somnambulistic automatism. There is the further probability that the condition had an epileptic basis, though this is not essential to the above theory. If epileptic the condition represented a true psychical epileptic equivalent.

Our testimony was to this effect and our opinion was that he was irresponsible at the time of the commission of these homicidal acts. He was acquitted by the jury on the ground of insanity.

ANALYSIS OF THE CASE BY DR. WALKER.

Conduct, as representing "character," is of interest to everyone, from the moralist and sociologist down to the village gossip. However, we may philosophize concerning it; however great our interest in it as a factor influencing for good or ill either the life of the organism which manifests it or the lives of his fellowmen, the greatest interest lies in its being a revelation of the hidden and most complex inner processes of the human mind; of its sensations or impressions, images, ideas, emotions, and instincts, the association and intertwining of which condition such conduct. The behavior of these elements, as requisite preconditions to conduct distinctive of a particular organism, is further dependent upon peculiarities of inherited organization, and of education and environment; that is, of the stored-up "experiences" of the individual organism.

No judgment of conduct is complete, therefore, which does not take into consideration the various influencing and interacting factors which thus include not only previous physical and mental occurrences in the life of the individual, but the lives of his progenitors as well.

Behavior, as a manifestation of "will," may be regarded as a selection or "choice," on the part of the individual, of one course of conduct among several, in accordance with opportunities for knowledge of all that may be involved by such choice. In this sense "will" represents a summing up of all the higher faculties; of perception, presentation, comparison, and discrimination; in a word, of judgment; and presupposes the existence in the individual of clear consciousness.

Of the essential nature of consciousness we have no definite knowledge. We may briefly consider it, however, in its known relations with the higher mental life. Formerly believed that the boundaries of one marked the limits of the other, we now know that merely a portion of mental life is represented in clear consciousness. As the lower vegetative and organic functions of the human machine are carried on without it, so the instinctive and emotional phenomena—though influencing it—may arise, develop, and be manifested without representation in clear consciousness. Automatic motor phenomena, such as balancing and walking, are instances of the unconscious in the motor sphere of our organism; and among these may be included, not only the simpler special actions of writing, but also many of the habitual, though complex, motor adjustments of our professional activities.

Essential as consciousness is to the higher development that makes for human perfection; and useful, in enabling the organism to better adjust itself to the exigencies of its environment, we now know that, once established, many of the most complex brain-processes are carried on in the presence of a consciousness so greatly modified in degree as to appear absent altogether. From clearest thought down through dream-like and hazy states, to apparently dreamless or swoon-like sleep there are all gradations. Our clearest thoughts are normally accompanied by a consciousness which comprehends many of the various sensations and impressions which reach and influence us, whether coming in from our immediate environment or the residue of past experiences stored-up in the mind as images and ideas associated with emotions; these manifest themselves to us as *dispositions* or *tendencies* leading to, guiding, or restraining action. In dreaming and in other obscure mental states, impressions, sensations, images, and emotions, are less clear and we may be conscious only of vague ideas and ill-defined feelings which dispose us to action. Consciousness may exist in a still lower state, but with ideas, feelings, and impressions too faint and confused to be consciously perceived, or at all appreciated as parts of one's mental life. These latter have been designated as subconscious, or subliminal ideas; and just as the sensations and impressions stored up in memory are later recovered as *dispositions to action*, so these faint images of previous experiences enter into the sum total of factors which constitute our mental life, and persist as "*dispositions*," which, under favoring conditions, tend to final outlet in action.

All nervous function is conditioned upon sensation, and sensation is invariably transformed into movement or action of some kind. "Every current that runs into brain from skin or eyes or ears runs out again into muscles, glands, or viscera, and helps to adapt the animal to the environment from which the current came" (James). The brain is therefore an "organ for adapting movements to the impressions received from the environment," among which are included not only those immediately pouring in, but the stored-up impressions resulting from the previous experiences of the organism; and their elaboration and transformation occur in accordance with laws as fixed and definite as those governing purely physical phenomena.

That which is present in the mind at any given instant is therefore due to its past experiences; to previously experienced sensations, impressions, ideas, and emotions. These "stored-up" "sensations tend to final transformation into action"—that is, either action or restraint of action,—not only according to the laws governing all neural and mental manifestations in general, but, in particular, with the gradually acquired habit of reaction of the individual organism.

The most potent factor in determining the arrangement or association of these stored-up experiences is emotion as based upon the needs of the organism. These needs are represented in the instincts. The most important of the instincts are those connected with the preservation of the individual and the reproduction of the species. Of the emotions which determine the association of ideas having to do with self-preservation fear stands first in importance. What we call the instinct of self-preservation is in reality only one of the forms of fear. "Fear is a protective instinct. It serves its useful purpose for the organism in showing where danger lies; and in creating an aversion to that danger; and in either forcing us to flee from it or to initiate defensive actions against it." From the lowest psychic organism to the highest and most complex represented in man, the earliest *inner* excitations to action are those characteristic of the emotion of fear, which, in its normal forms,—with the concomitant involuntary physical phenomena,—closely approximates the primitive psychic movements of the lower organisms; and in its abnormal forms even more closely resembles them. Aiming either at the preservation of the individual or of the species, they are always *impulsive*. They are dependent upon the sensation of external object, which may be dangerous in itself, or merely suggestive,—by reason of its associations,—of danger; or upon the idea alone without external object. Either of these may be followed by immediate reaction in flight or in resistance without any intervention of the will; or, as we shall see, even in the absence of clear consciousness.

As normally experienced the emotion of fear is accompanied by consciousness. Whether wholly internal, or associated with its very apparent (though involuntary) external signs, we can usually explain this fear in some way and give an account of our experiences while under it. All, however, can recall fears which could not thus be explained; with tendency to suspicions, assumption of attitude of resistance, or attempt to escape, from what particular object we knew not.

Richet, in his "Psychological Study of Fear," gives the following from his own experience as an instance of the way in which fear is divorced from intelligence: "While in Baden I was in the habit of walking alone in the evening until late in the night. The security was absolute, and I knew very well that there was no danger; and as long as I was in the open field or on the road I felt nothing that resembled fear. But to go into the forest, where it was so dark that one could hardly see two steps ahead, was another thing. I entered resolutely and went in for some twenty paces; but, in spite of myself, the deeper I plunged into the darkness the more a fear gained possession of me which was quite incomprehensible. I tried in vain to overcome the unreasonable feeling, and I may have walked in this way for about a quarter of an hour. But there was nothing pleasant about the walk, and I could not help feeling relieved when I saw the light of the sky through a gap in the trees, and it required a strong effort of the will to keep from pressing toward it. My fear was wholly without cause. I knew it, and yet I felt it as strongly as if it had been rational."

This one instance can be supplemented by others from the experiences of most of us.

Even in waking life the emotion of fear is stronger than all arguments invented to overcome it; but, more than this, the intelligence (imagination) habitually elaborates any sensation experienced while in a state of fear and makes us see the thing expected. Anyone waiting in a dark place and expecting or fearing strongly a certain object will interpret any abrupt sensation to mean that object's presence. The boy playing "I spy," the criminal skulking from his pursuers, the superstitious person hurrying through the woods or past the church-yard at midnight, the man lost in the woods, all are subject to illusions of sight and sound which make their hearts beat till they are dispelled. In all these instances the particular sensations experienced have but faint relation with the emotions as regards their intensity. It is to the peculiar mental states that we must look for explanation;—to the ways in which the intelligence elaborates the sensations, whether of sight, sound, or of internal origin.

Most markedly favoring such cooperation of the higher faculties in thus elaborating sensations are those bodily conditions accompanied by a "clouding of consciousness," familiar instances of which are furnished by alcoholism—from ordinary drunkenness to delirium tremens and alcoholic insanity,—and other forms of poisoning; the deliria produced by the toxins of disease; and the narrowed, incoordinated, or disordinated consciousness of hysteria, and other psychoses, particularly epilepsy.

We do not have to resort to instances of these pathological forms, however, in order to understand its mechanism; for this condition of clouded consciousness is normally encountered in sleep; and some of the best illustrations are seen in the phenomena accompanying sleep, or rather, the outcome of its disturbances.

Most sleep is far from being perfect and it is probable that mental activity in some slight degree always persists, hence the saying, "to sleep is to dream." Our dreams, as our waking mental states, are always limited to the materials of our past experiences. They are developed under associative laws analogous to those of waking life, although differing from them in the details of their operation.

It has been observed that of all our mental powers it is fancy, or imagination that has the fullest play in sleep. "Fancy is the mind's power for putting together past acquisitons into all sorts of haphazard relations without reference to any definite plan or purpose, and this is the usual character of the product of our dreams." The shifting ideas of our dreams group themselves around whatever happens to be the dominant emotion, unhindered and unmodified by inconsistent ideas, which, in the waking state, would at once arise to quench them. "We therefore accept any incongruity as actual until we wake up and our better judgment shows us our mistake."

In dreams, as well as in states of hypnotic, or somnambulistic origin, all perceptions fit in with the phantasms of the dream or suggested idea, and all processes originated by the one active group tend to work out their logical results with a precision and certainty unknown in normal waking life.

There is no exception to the rule that all our sensations, images, and emotions tend to be translated into action. The higher intellectual activities of our clear consciousness normally tend to inhibit and control all lower emotional and instinctive impulses. Anything which interferes with the functioning of the higher faculties increases the tendency to resultant action. In dreaming, the higher activities are partially, if not altogether shut out, without a sufficient degree of consciousness remaining to allow of "choice" in the usual sense of the term. There is no conscious direction of the imagination, hence no "will."

When the dominant emotion in a dream state is such as even in waking life leads to involuntary action, we can readily understand how much greater is the tendency to eventuate in action of vivid fears which, by reason of the removal of the higher faculties through sleep or disease, are at once accepted as realities.

The few cases given below may be of service in illustrating the "mechanism," which I have attempted thus to indicate; of the way in which conduct, whether the outcome of the haphazard imagination of dreams, or of fully developed insanity, can be interpreted as the result of brain function which may be normal, perverted, or markedly abnormal in character. Depending upon certain peculiarities, or characteristic variations in this mental mechanism we find definite relations with known forms of brain disorder.

Case I.—I. N., twenty-four years old. On the night following an encounter with a copperhead snake, suddenly awakened to find himself hanging, feet foremost, from his second-story bedroom window. In a state of panic terror he climbed back into the room. Soon he became conscious of a violent pain in the leg, examination of which discovered a denuded and bleeding shin. Gradually he recalled the principal features of a terrifying dream in which he was pursued by snakes. He had no recollection of getting out of bed, or of making his way to the window. An overturned chair between these two not only explained the wounded shin but, in all probability, also the partial awakening before his act could terminate in the more serious accident which must have resulted from a fall to the ground below.

We here have an instance of somnambulism originating in a vivid emotion of fear experienced in a dream. The dream-ideas, with resulting emotion, are readily traced to their origin in the occurrences of the previous day, accompanied as they were by considerable emotional disturbance which left its impress in memory. These data of consciousness, recombined under the influence of characteristic dream-imagination, resulted in complicated automatic movements adjusted to effort at escape from the imagined source of danger.

Case II.—This case is of like mechanism, originating in the vague emotion of fear so commonly the result of being suddenly awakened from sound sleep. Mrs. W., hearing a noise in an adjoining room where two of her children were sleeping, left her bed stealthily in order that she might not needlessly awaken her husband, who was sleeping soundly. Leaving the gas burning dimly in her own room she passed into that occupied by the children. Finding everything right she proceeded to a room across the hall which was occupied by two other children, but, hearing her husband shifting and turning in bed, stopped on the way to note whether she had disturbed him. Not directly entering, but peering through the partially opened door, she was horrified to see him crouching. wild-eyed. in bed; but on the instant,—almost before she could realize what it might mean to her,—he sprang forward, throwing all his weight upon the door, which, in so forcibly closing, barely missed catching her by the neck. The door opened, and the husband at once appeared, by this time fully realizing the situation. He then explained how, awakening from sound sleep, he heard a noise in the adjoining room. His first thought was of burglars, and that instant, what, in the dim light, looked like a negro's head appeared in the doorway. That which followed was the result of an unreasoned attempt at defense, in appropriate action in the direction of attack, which, while carried out in a state of blurred consciousness, is clearly the outcome of automatic mental processes—sharply enough defined, however, to leave some trace in memory; to the extent in which this occurs are they capable of later introspective analysis and consequently of explanation.

Case III.—J. C. P., aged twenty-eight years. Was admitted to the Western Pennsylvania Hospital for the Insane, October 7, 1902. He presented a history of irregular epileptic paroxysms which commenced as " attacks of absent-mindedness: " These had extended over a period of three years, in which were exhibited many phenomena characteristic of epilepsy. That which I now describe led to his commitment as an insane patient. The father was awakened at three o'clock one morning by a noise as of some one falling down stairs. Upon investigating he saw his son running from the house to the barn. Following, but keeping out of the patient's sight, he saw him coming down from the haymow, a large carving knife in hand; from this point he ran to the cutting room and on through the stables as though in pursuit of some one, and thence to the carriage house. When overtaken the patient was found sitting in one of the carriages in a dazed and confused state. After some coaxing he was persuaded to go back to bed without further demonstration of violence. Upon arising the next morning his manner indicated no recollection of his violent behavior and, as he had previously manifested irritability upon coming out of earlier attacks, nothing was said to him concerning this one.

Questioned regarding this attack, he, sometime after admission to the hospital, told the following story: ",I remember all about it and everything that occurred while I was in it; but realizing what a fool I had made of myself I determined that if they said nothing about it, I shouldn't. Of course, I couldn't help what I did, for I didn't seem to know anything about it until I got awake and found myself seated in the carriage; then it all at once came to me. I seemed to remember that I had a dream, and the dream happened in this way: On the previous afternoon, attempting to collect a long standing bill, I had an altercation with the man who owed me. Returning home tired, worried, and out of temper, I ate but little supper and retired early for the night. Lying in bed studying over the occurrence of the afternoon I again worked myself into a temper and I recall the thought that if I'd only had a knife with me I'd have been mad enough to use it. I fell asleep and, of course, had no recollection of anything further until I found myself sitting in the carriage with father and my frightened brothers around me. Like a flash it all came to me. I recalled the details of a dream in which was continued the quarrel of the previous afternoon. My enemy was trying to get away from me; I was pursuing him. I dimly recall getting into my clothes. On my way down stairs I stumbled over a pair of shoes, falling headlong. On my feet in an instant, I went to the kitchen table; opening a drawer I took from it a carving knife. I thought my enemy had run to the barn to escape me. Following, I saw him go into the feed-room, thence to the haymow, and then back to the cutting room, through the stables to the carriage house. Pursuing him, as I thought, into the carriage, I there awoke. At first dazed and confused, I gradually came to realize the situation, and recalled all the details of the occurrence as I give them to you. It was simply a bad dream to me. I couldn't help acting it;—indeed, I didn't know I had done anything until I awoke and it was all over, when my chief feeling was of shame at having made a fool of myself."

Having for three years presented unmistakable mental and motor manifestations of epilepsy, this case is of special interest as illustrating the mental mechanism of a complicated automatic act, from images, or ideas, having their origin in actual occurrences previous to the epileptic dream. Dwelt upon before retiring, they were elaborated during a dream-state into ideas so vivid as to be at once translated into appropriate action. This occurred without clear consciousness, but his subsequent recollection of all the events of the dream would indicate the existence of a degree of consciousness at least as marked as in two previously cited cases, which were not manifestations of epilepsy, but merely vivid dream impressions. Undoubtedly, in this instance, a product of the epileptic psychosis, it presents, in common with the cases mentioned, the essential psychic features of somnambulism: namely, vivid mental images which are accepted as real; an accompanying and underlying emotional state of fear; with disturbed impaired or almost entirely abrogated consciousness, into actions logically the outcome of the uninhibited original idea or image.

I cite these three cases to illustrate the manner in which dreaming is " dovetailed in with waking." For the elucidation of the simplest phenomena incident upon normal sleep we must look to the data of waking life. We follow the same method in our study of the obscure and apparently unrelated phenomena of abnormal mental life, whether of somnambulism, deliria, or of fully developed insanity; and in all we discover relations with previous psychic occurrences which not only condition, but also elucidate mental phenomena which would otherwise be inexplicable.

In this brief study of the case of Charles Cawley we must therefore find what occurrences, if any, in his mental life, are consistent with the later development into the act with which he is charged; and if such are found, whether, in developing into action, they have conformed, in their principal features, to the laws governing such transformation of ideas into acts; and, in so far as this relation is discernable, are we justified in finding explanation of all which at first sight seems so obscure and puzzling.

As described by Doctor McKennan, we have the details of an act for which no motive can be found or, indeed, conceived; an act which all but one member of his family refuse to ascribe to the accused; and which, if performed by him, has left so few traces in memory as to suggest—to him—no connection of any active participation in the horrible affair.

What does linger in his memory, hazy and fragmentary as it is, however, corroborates the story related by the only living witness of his very significant behavior following the extreme violence at the height of the paroxysm: of his attitude of extreme fear as, with uplifted ax and exclamation of Burglars! burglars! help! help! he attempted to continue his earlier violent behavior of which the ghastly results are the only evidence: of his continued unreasoned resistance when once apprehended in his career of violence, with graduallv lessening manifestations of fear as the confused mental state faded away and merged into clearer waking consciousness.

Can we discover any connection between this final act of violence—from its earliest apparent cause in the consciously perceived and remembered sound as of entering burglars with resulting defensive attack upon them in a state of unconsciousness—and the previous psychic experiences of Charles Cawley: that is, earlier ideas, emotions, and tendencies which might furnish the materials, as it were, capable of being transformed during a dream-state into the phantasms and visions of terrifying content, and leading to a deed so foreign to his inner nature, or to any idea ever consciously entertained by him?

Among the earliest incidents of personal history significant from this view-point is that of his failure to attend school until past ten years of age. The reason given for this is that the "walk of six miles was too much for a small boy." In itself this would appear to be of slight import; but further inquiry elicits the fact that he did not seem to want to go: that he was timid and rather than associate with other children he would remain at home with his mother. Later, when regularly attending school, he seemed bright and acquired his lessons readily, but he further manifested this retiring, shrinking, and timid nature by refraining from entering into the games usual to bovs of his age.

From the details of earlier history (and these are obtained with the greatest difficulty), nothing further suggestive of marked morbidity is noted until some months prior to the commission of the deed. He, at this time, became interested in perfecting the idea of a brake for a trolley car which later he developed and had patented. Much absorbd in this he spent all his available time in study and work upon his drawings. Absorbed in his plans to the exclusion of all else he soon manifested an irritability, as of exhaustion. At times, puzzled over some matter pertaining to his plans he would ask the advice of his brother; but when this was proffered would show a decided impatience and intolerance of suggestions. In manner he was restive and unsettled; sitting a short while at work upon his plans, he would abruptly put them aside and move restlessly about the room. "Could not stick at one thing steadily." The remark by some member of his family (quoted by James Cawley) that "since Charlie has been working so hard I believe he is growing daffy"—was evidently called forth by this noticeable change in manner. It was at this time that the attacks occurred while walking along the street (noted and described by his brother James). If not attacks of petit mal (though they resemble nothing so much as these) they are still of great significance as indicating his mode of mental reaction. If merely momentary fits of abstraction they are further indicative of his peculiar habit of mind.—of its tendency to be dominated by a single idea, or bv anything associated with that idea. Always alert for impressions (from without or from within) in any way associated with his now soon to be completed invention, he is lost to all other impressions.

As a logical sequence there now enters the most significant element of emotion. Always secretive of his plans he grew more and more so as they neared completion. With the idea uppermost—indeed, always present (if not conciously at least subconsciously) that the results of his labors might be lost if in any way they became the property of another, he had the anonymous letter experience, related by Dr. McKennan; this most profoundly impressed and influenced him. Whether the incident be interpreted as the result of an earlier somnambulism (and it is altogether probable that this is its explanation) or an actual experience, it, to Charlie, was of sufficient importance to lead him to consult a detective. Advised to drop the matter it none the less left its permanent imprint in his emotional nature later evidenced in conduct,—that of staying in the house more closely than usual,—with his expressed reason for so doing that he feared some harm might come to him from the source of the threatening letter.

In all probability the outgrowth of the exaggerated attitude of secrecy (from the first inseparable from the method of work upon his invention) with fears of being robbed or cheated out of the fruits of his labors, this emotional element assumes an increasing significance,—becomes, in fact, the key to the solution of the problems presented by this case. Fear, always the parent of innumerable phantoms, gradually developing into the more clearly defined and vivid fears resulting from the threatening letter incident, is seen more and more to dominate his mental life as manifested in behavior or conduct so peculiar as to excite the already quoted inquiry of some member of his family regarding his reasons for not going out of doors. In this sequence of consistent mental traits we have data of decided "prophetic importance;" for, in keeping with all that we observe in the realm of ideas —gradually acquired, frequently dismissed, and apparently forgotten, but ever reappearing to influence us in present judgments, future plans, or hopes, or fears—we find them existing, not merely as isolated or unrelated mental facts; as entities to be called up and dismissed at will, but as mental habits or dispositions to action. With attitude and general behavior as proof of a waking reaction through paths worn by habitually experienced impressions of suspicions and fear, there occurs his vivid-dream experience. Suddenly awakened in a state of extreme fear, the sensation of sound (whether real or imagined) "touches off, as it were, a train already laid." Images and ideas which have been associated with his waking fears magnified in intensity by the terror of his clouded consciousness, are but continuations of these earlier manifested tendencies. The terrifying object seems real—indeed, is present to him "because his mind is full of the thought of it."

We have seen that even waking fear does not reason. As exhibited in this condition of clouded consciousness (whether the result of a dream or of disease), the vivid fear exists as an irresistible force resulting doubly; first in the increasing fright felt by him as a result of the original semi-waking impression; second, in a series of defensive motor phenomena. A state of subconsciousness now supervening which admits of no further introspection or memory the remaining links in the chain must further be supplied by inference.

We know that subconscious or dimly conscious reasoning is governed by the same laws as normal waking consciousness; that ideas, however originated, tend to work out their logical results in accordance with the laws governing normal mental action. We may infer, therefore, a further mechanism like this: Awakening in a state of fear he interprets the real or imagined noise in terms of threatened danger. Imagination running riot, all his images cluster about the idea of burglars or of threatened violence to himself or family. Upon this there follows the idea of defense,—resistance; his remembered statement to his brother upon attempting to awaken him proved this. With that of defense necessarily is associated the idea of weapon. With each accession of dream-ideas the state of fear gathers momentum, and

further transformation into action is continued without any intervention of clear consciousness, or rather, with consciousness so diminished that it is completely monopolized by the very intensity of the emotion. He automatically makes his way to the cellar where the ax is habitually kept; automatically returns to the place where he first located the noise (in his mother's bedroom). The state of fear having increased with movement or action; and with consciousness now so bedimmed that all objects which strike his senses are made to enter into the framework of his dream,—the figures of his mother and sisters are transformed by his vivid imagination into the expected burglars upon whom he makes attack with the result now so well known. Continuing in his blind fury he next enters his brother's room, but here he meets with opposition or resistance. The more forcible or powerful stimuli due to this resistance reach, to a certain extent, his beclouded consciousness, leaving impressions in memory which, vague and indefinite though they are, serve as connecting links with his later clear consciousness into which it gradually merges, bearing as permanent imprints of the events so recently transpired, blurred recollections of those of the beginning and of the ending of the paroxysm only.

The act of violence thus results from the transformation, in a dream or subconscious state, of the ideas, suspicions, and fears habitually dominating the waking life. The production of disorders of consciousness,—whether temporary or prolonged we know to be favored by long continued or intense concentration of the attention upon a single thing. This is true of even a healthy person. In states of lowered nerve tone, long continued or transient concentration,—or merely a single vivid impression,—may result in disordinated or disintegrated mental states. Resembling those cases developing upon a hysterical basis; or as brought about by hypnotism; they are also the products, in certain instances, of acute and chronic alcoholic poisoning. Such narrowing of the field of consciousness to a few ideas, with their concomitant emotions, whether resulting from ordinary or from pathological causes, needs, in the vulnerable individual, but slight disturbing circumstances to bring to the surface their logical manifestations in attitude, word, or deed. Depending upon the degree of vitality— that is "stability"—of the higher centers the cause may be slight or severe but, in a given case, must be regarded as adequate to its observed results. When these are such as, in themselves, bear the mark of the grossly morbid, we must seek the cause among those psychoses known to present, as characteristic features, such profound disturbances of consciousness as here observed. Pre-eminent among these stands epilepsy. Besides the unconsciousness of this attack there is additional evidence of the existence of this psychosis in the "spells" noted and described by his brother James: these closely conform, in their principal features, to attacks of petit mal. With the warden's description of the only other observed paroxysm, and the bitten tongue noted at the time of the second examination of the patient by Dr. McKennan and myself, we have sufficient grounds for regarding the complicated automatic act of killing of five people as a manifestation of epilepsy.

Showing from early life tendencies sufficiently well marked to be labeled as morbid—of timidity, shrinking, and fears, with these traits integral parts of his temperament and organization, as evidenced by their continuation into his later school life; and as even more plainly manifested under the unusual stress attendant upon close application to the work of his invention, we have continuous and consecutive phenomena indicative of his peculiar type of reaction to stimuli, both from without (physical) and from within (psychical). The vulnerability or "instability" is further traced to its origin in heredity from an alcoholic father. A like tendency to reversion to psychic movements of a primitive character is seen in at least two other members of the family; his next older brother—a convicted criminal—and a sister, who presents in marked degree a neurotic speech defect. These "brand-marks" of a degenerate organism complete the chain of clinical evidence which, from earliest manifested morbid trait to final act of violence, accord with the laws governing alike the physical and mental development with manifestations of abnormal brain-processes.

DIAGNOSIS OF DISEASES OF THE UPPER ABDOMINAL REGION. A PLEA FOR EARLIER SURGICAL INTERFERENCE.[1]

BY C. D. HILL, A.B., M.D.,

OF JERSEY CITY, N. J.;

SURGEON TO ST. FRANCIS HOSPITAL.

No ATTEMPT will be made to differentiate all the diseases referable to the upper abdominal region, but I shall confine myself to those diseases which are now classed as surgical. Even with these restrictions I can make only general statements in this plea to show the necessity of a differential diagnosis and the importance of early surgical interference.

Within the past five years, Mayo, Murphy, Moynihan, Mikulicz, Rodman, Robson, Roux, Kocher, Krönlein, and many others, by exploring this region, have not only verified many of the theories of the internists, but have worked out new problems in pathology, diagnosis, prognosis and treatment. In diagnosis they have substituted direct examination by sight and touch, for indirect inferences from uncertain symptoms. In treatment the procrastination of a conservative inactivity has given way to timely and rational surgical procedures.

These pioneers are now doing in the upper

[1] Read before Physicians' and Surgeons' Club of Jersey City, November 7, 1904.

zone of the abdomen what the gynecologists have been doing for fifteen years in the pelvic region. They are waging the same battles, gaining the same victories, overcoming the same opponents, as the abdominal surgeons have been doing for ten years in the right iliac region.

Before the surgeon invaded this region and claimed certain lesions as his own, the diagnosis of its diseases offered insurmountable difficulties to the physician. While the internist was hesitating and waiting to verify his diagnosis, the disease was advancing, or the patient had already met with some disaster.

In this region the stomach may be looked upon as the organ of most interest, because it is the one most apt to give prominent symptoms, not only when it is diseased itself, but, very frequently, when a disease arises in one of the other organs, it affects this viscus, both directly and indirectly. As in health the pyloric portion is the most important factor in the muscular function of the stomach, so in disease it is the principal part to be studied. In the majority of cases the pyloric end is the site of ulcer and cancer and their complications, and in gall-stone disease adhesions here produce their worst effects.

This group of organs includes the pylorus, gall-bladder and ducts, pancreas, and transverse colon, all of which lie below the right lobe of the liver and are situated very close anatomically to each other, or as Mayo says "the palm of a hand may cover a serious lesion of any one of these organs." When one organ in this group is diseased it causes a disturbance in function of one or more of the other organs and often changes their relative positions; therefore there is still greater confusion as to the true seat of the disease, especially, when only indirect methods of investigation are applied. In disease these organs are so closely related and so intimately associated, it is often difficult properly to refer the very valuable symptom of pain, or tenderness and resistance, or even a tumor.

It is no wonder that patients suffering from surgical lesions are treated for "indigestion," "stomach troubles," "liver troubles," biliousness," etc., and plied with a new favorite formula every time a different physician is consulted. In many of these cases if we would recognize the true value of symptoms, and endeavor to differentiate actual conditions, we should get better results. Oftentimes in these cases if we realized that an accurate diagnosis was not possible, but we were assured that there were sufficient pathological changes taking place in the patient's abdomen to justify an exploratory laparotomy, we could not only clear up the diagnosis, but we would be taking the preliminary step in relieving some mechanical condition or removing a new growth.

As an illustration of the confusion of symptoms, as well as confounding of medical minds, I will cite the following case, which also brings out another point in differential diagnosis:

Case I. Stones in Gall-Bladder; Movable Tumor; Cholecystostomy.—Mrs. J. W., thirty-five years old, the mother of five children, complained for years of various digestive disturbances, with a capricious appetite, and intermittent pain in the upper part of the abdomen. Was treated for two years for dyspepsia by various physicians, until the last attendant discovered a tumor in the right upper quadrant of the abdomen, and rightly interpreted it as an enlarged gall-bladder with stones, for which he sent her to the hospital for operation. The location, size, and mobility of the tumor caused some doubt among the physicians and surgeons, who examined the case at the hospital, as to whether the swelling was the gall-bladder, or a floating kidney (which also gives symptoms referable to the stomach). At the operation the tumor proved to be an enlarged gall-bladder, containing numerous small and seven large stones, one of these blocking the cystic duct and causing obstruction to the outflow of the secretions of the gall-bladder, and the inflow of the bile. The gall-bladder contained about three ounces of a straw colored fluid, and simulated a cyst in outward appearance. It is needless to say that the disturbances of digestion disappeared after her recovery from a cholecystostomy and drainage.

There are no adhesions in this case, and the stomach symptoms were probably reflex. Ordinarily, we would not expect it to be a difficult matter to make a diagnosis of cholelithiasis, if we bear in mind that symptoms, referable to the stomach, may be caused by disease in the bile passages, and if we make a thorough examination of the case, and get a history of cramps, coming on suddenly and disappearing suddenly, with tenderness at the Mayo-Robson point. We shall not often feel a tumor as in this case, for most of the cases are too fat for a tumor to be palpated. We need not wait for jaundice to appear, before making our diagnosis, for this only happens when there is some obstruction in the common or hepatic ducts. Often in operations for cholelithiasis we find the contiguous organs bound together by firm adhesions, and when this is the case it is well to extend the investigation further, for there may be other diseased conditions, such as an ulcer of the stomach, or a pancreatitis, or the perigastritis itself may cause trouble, as we shall see further on.

With the present perfection in the technic of the operations for pathological changes so frequent in the gall-bladder and ducts, and with such a low mortality, we think it very essential to make an early diagnosis, and treat these cases surgically. By early diagnosis and operative procedures we will relieve much present suffering and prevent many annoying complications and sequelæ. The literature of this subject is replete in almost every detail, and, judging from the number of operations performed in the past five years, it would seem as if these cases had been transferred from the internist to the surgeon.

Ulcer of the Stomach.—What will be said in regard to ulcer of the stomach will apply in the main to duodenal ulcer, for, as Osler says, in the great majority of cases they cannot be separated; and, besides, on opening the abdomen we find them often associated. By means of the surgeon's explorations it has been found that ulcer of the stomach is far more common than was formerly supposed. Different operators now estimate that ulcer exists in from $1\frac{1}{2}$ to 13 per cent. of the population, although the internists show statistics making the percentage below the lower estimate. In ulcer of the stomach we should expect to find a history of hematemesis, or bloody stools, pain after eating, and increased free hydrochloric acid. In 50 per cent. of the cases we do not get hemorrhages, while in other diseases as alcoholic gastritis and passive congestions in the portal system, the hemorrhages may be very profuse. I have had under treatment within the past fourteen months three cases of hemorrhage from these sources. Pain may vary as to time, or be entirely absent, and is frequently symptomatic of other diseases. Hyperchlorhydria is the rule, and consequently of great value in diagnosis, but there may be no increased acidity in ulcer, and besides we sometimes get an increase in cholelithiasis, and other conditions. If we get the combination of symptoms, mentioned above, in a young woman, we can make our diagnosis without an exploration, especially as we do not have to resort to surgery so often for their relief. Over 50 per cent. of these cases will heal under the proper diet, rest in bed four to six weeks, alkalies and larger doses of bismuth or some other powder to protect the ulcer. In the case of older subjects, especially if males, which give a clear history of ulcer, we shall not get such results by this treatment. It has been estimated by Rodman, Robson and Moynihan, and others, that over 25 per cent. of patients having ulcer will die from perforation, hemorrhage or anemia; over five per cent. of them will develop cancer on the site of the ulcer; many of them will contract pulmonary tuberculosis; while a great number of them will continue to be chronic sufferers from complications, such as perigastritis, obstruction of the pylorus and dilation of the stomach. We do not get any such percentage of mortality from the present operative procedures, and furthermore an untold amount of suffering is prevented or relieved. Moynihan gives a series of one hundred cases with two deaths, and over ninety per cent. of complete cures; Mayo reports 286 gastro-enterostomies with a mortality of five per cent. In view of these facts it is encumbent on us to make a diagnosis, and when necessary, apply the proper surgical procedures for its relief.

One would think that such a definite lesion as ulcer would give uniform symptoms, but here, as in many other diseases, the exceptional outnumber the typical cases. Of two ulcers exactly alike in size, situation, and duration, one will give the characteristic and pathognomonic signs; the second will lie dormant for years, or at least with no symptoms to enlighten the physician or warn the patient. Again, in the same patient, the symptoms vary at different periods. At one time ulcer causes the most distressing disturbances, such as intense pain, alarming hemorrhages, and the most pernicious anemia; at another time the disease is entirely latent, and the attendant and the patient may be soothed in the hope that it has healed. The differential diagnosis is at times unavoidable, unless we do an exploration. Surgeons of the greatest experience say it is often impossible to differentiate ulcer from cancer; and sometimes, as Sippey says, cholelithiasis may give all the symptoms of ulcer and *vice versa*.[1]

As an illustration of a case of ulcer of the stomach, with no characteristic symptoms except hyperchlorhydria; and also as an instance of latent and active periods, I will note the following:

Case II. Gastric Ulcer: Perigastritis; Periodical Attacks of Vomiting; Gastrolysis; Relief for Eight Months.—T. C., aged twenty-five years, who laid no claim to moderation in eating or drinking, has had annually since 1899, three to six attacks of vomiting which came on irrespective of previous excesses. During these attacks his stomach rejected everything, even water, which he drank in large quantities to allay his intense thirst. Never vomited blood, nor had he ever detected it in the stools, although he had been told to observe them closely. Never complained of pain during or after the attacks, but during the attacks had some soreness in the midepigastric region, and pressure here increased the nausea. After the attacks were over he quickly regained his strength and drove his coal wagon again. During these years he had been the rounds of the clinics. In July, 1903, he was advised to go to the hospital for closer observation.

On withdrawal of the stomach contents after Ewald's test breakfast, free hydrochloric acid was shown to be markedly increased, averaging over .75. By the Seidlitz powder inflation test dilation of the stomach to one-half inch below the umbilicus was noticed. A tentative diagnosis of chronic ulcer with adhesions was made, and operation advised. After much hesitation he consented to an exploration, but exacted the promise (to use his own words) "to do no cutting on the stomach." After opening the abdomen we found dense adhesions between the stomach, gall-bladder, and transverse colon. We found also an ulcer, about the size of a ten-cent piece, situated on the anterior wall of the stomach, about 1½ inches from the pylorus, and one inch from the lesser curvature. The adhesions were divided, and cargile membrane interposed between adjoining organs, which procedure, it was hoped, would at least stop the vomiting. The

patient made an uneventful recovery and seemed entirely relieved for about eight months. Then he began to suffer as before, and resumed his peregrinations for "a medicine to cure him." After taking many drugs from various sources, both high and low, he consented to have another operation done. He was sent to the hospital in June of this year, but just a few hours before the time set for performing a gastro-enterostomy he took a short circuit to his home.

Perigastritis.—The adhesions, which were so numerous and dense in this case, were the sequelæ of the ulcer. In such cases they constitute a perigastritis, and whereas a very common complication in ulcer, we may have them in cancer, in gall-stone disease, and in fact when any of this group is affected. A perigastritis really shows the efforts of nature to limit the diseased process; if an ulcer to put the stomach at rest, and to prevent perforation. But while the adhesions in the beginning are protective, they may be complications themselves, and cause symptoms by interfering with the mobility of the stomach; or they may cause an obstruction in the neighboring gut. According to their location they may cause pain in certain movements, as leaning forward, or backward, or kneeling. Robson and Moynihan report favorable results in over 100 cases, in which after opening the abdomen and dividing the adhesions, the right free border of the omentum was interposed. After opening the abdomen and separating such dense adhesions binding together the organs in this group, one is impressed with their intimate relations and interdependence, as Mayo so clearly set forth in his masterly oration at the last meeting of the American Medical Association. Furthermore we realize that only mechanical means will relieve such a condition as this. Before leaving the subject of ulcer and its complications, I will briefly narrate a case of perforation, which gave no premonitory symptoms before the unfortunate disaster occurred.

Case III. Perforation of Stomach; Old Ulcer; Peritonitis; Operation; Death.—W. F. L., bookkeeper, twenty-one years old, on November 17, 1903, was brought to the hospital with a history of having been attacked the previous night at twelve o'clock with sudden severe cramps. He had eaten a hearty meal about seven o'clock. No history of former trouble was elicited, except that about six months previously, he had had an attack of cramps which passed off in a few hours. We saw the case at 3 P.M., at which time he had an agonizing expression on his face, and complained of intense pain in the upper part of the abdomen, especially in the middle line. Near the bed was a basin containing about three pints of black sour smelling fluid mixed with blood clots, which he had just vomited. The upper zone of the abdomen was very tympanitic, with marked tenderness on the slightest pressure, and there was great resistance over the right rectus muscle. His pulse was 140, temperature 102.5° F., and

1 Journal of the American Medical Association, October 15, 1904.

withal his condition seemed desperate. We made a diagnosis of perforation of the stomach, or possibly duodenum, with peritonitis already under way, and an immediate operation was decided on, as giving him the only chance of relief. The abdomen was opened, and found filled with dirty fluid, similar to that in the basin, and containing particles of undigested food. All the signs of a general septic peritonitis appeared. A perforation was found in the anterior wall of the stomach, situated three inches from the pylorus and two inches from the lesser curvature. The opening was large enough to admit the operator's finger, with which it was plugged during the first cleaning of the peritoneal cavity. A double row of celluloid sutures were inserted, inverting the perforation. They were placed with some difficulty, as the stomach walls for an area of one inch around the opening were very friable. For the first twenty-four hours the patient's condition seemed much improved, but then he began to sink, and died forty-five hours after the operation, from a rapidly increasing peritonitis.

The statistics for the mortality in cases of this kind show that the prognosis is in inverse ratio to the period that has elapsed from the time of the perforation to the time of surgical interference; and that very few cases recover when this period has exceeded twelve hours, according to Robson and Moynihan.[1] Perforations occur more frequently when the ulcer is in the anterior wall of the stomach, as this surface is not so well protected by adhesions. When they occur in the posterior wall. or in the duodenum, as they are here generally limited by adhesions, they may run an acute. subacute. or chronic course. They may form a subphrenic abscess, or penetrate the pleural cavity and simulate empyema; or the pus may burrow down through the lesser peritoneal cavity and, appearing in the region of the appendix, simulate an appendicitis. Robson and Moynihan report 40 cases of perforations in which 18 were operated on for appendicitis.

Cancer of the Stomach.—While the internists have cleared up many of the problems in the diagnosis of this alarmingly frequent disease there are still many cases presenting an endless amount of difficulties. Many investigators now claim that it is often impossible to make a diagnosis of carcinoma of the stomach without an exploration. or at any rate in time to offer any prospect of relief. As you recall. the prominent symptoms of cancer are. pain (especially when the stomach is empty), "coffee-grounds" vomit. absence of free hydrochloric acid. cachexia. and tumor. in a patient beyond middle life. If you waited for this list of diagnostic symptoms to appear. the probabilities are that you would loose the golden opportunity of staying the progress of the disease. As referred to under ulcer. it is often impossible to distinguish the two diseases, and I doubt if in some cases the parallel columns, we so often see in text-books. would help us to solve

1 Surgical Treatment of Diseases of the Stomach, page 313.

the puzzle. While pain and hemorrhage are symptoms in both diseases, they vary very much, and may be absent in either case. While it is suggestive of cancer if you can palpate a tumor, yet you may detect a tumor in ulcer with peri-gastritis. Even after opening the abdomen and finding the tumor with enlarged glands, mistakes have been made, a gastro-enterostomy having been performed as a palliative measure, on the supposition that the mass felt was cancerous, and yet the sequel showed that the growth was not malignant. Absence of hydrochloric acid is a valuable symptom, yet if we wait for this symptom, there is little prospect of eradicating the disease, so far has it advanced. Mayo and others lay great stress on the importance of opening the abdomen in cases of suspected cancer, for only by early surgical interference could they get such results as they do. Contrast Mayo's report of 43 pylorectomies and partial gastrectomies with seven deaths, and the utter hopelessness of the cases usually coming to us seeking surgical aid. In many the disease is too extensive to be eradicated, while others are too weak to withstand any operation. Though there are many workers in the field, there is much to be desired in the early diagnosis and treatment of cancer of the stomach.

Diseases of the Pancreas.—The diagnosis of the diseases of this organ can be made only by a resort to surgery, for the pancreas lies at the very bottom of this valley of quondam speculation, guesswork and mysticism. Opie has thrown some light on the study of its diseases, and has shown that while the pancreas is not often the seat of disease, it is well to investigate, when operating in this region, especially if we find areas of fat necrosis in the omentum. Furthermore, he has shown that when there is disease in this organ it is almost always secondary to disease elsewhere, especially to cholelithiasis.

The limits of this paper will not permit me to dwell on the many acute surgical conditions arising in the upper abdominal region, which requires early diagnosis and surgical treatment. Indeed, I do not think there is such necessity for taking up your time, for I believe the majority of practitioners to-day have abandoned the "do nothing policy" of calling severe traumatisms of the abdomen, "internal injuries," and waiting for developments; and designating as "peritonitis," all acute conditions with fever, irrespective of the cause.

It is asking too much of nature to expect her in the one case to unite a rupture, caused by some explosion from without; in the other case to close a perforation due to some accident from within

If we realize that a disaster has occurred within the patient's abdomen, even if we have not arrived at an exact diagnosis. we cannot better assist nature than by exploring and making an effort to relieve. Delays of minutes and hours in the acute are worse than hesitating for days and weeks in the chronic cases.

As to the latter class of cases, of which this paper has taken a cursory survey, I trust I have not conveyed the idea that all cases showing digestive disturbances, or other symptoms referable to this region, are surgical; nor that all, nor even a large part of, the surgical cases will require exploration for the purpose, alone, of making a diagnosis. The majority of cases consulting us for symptoms referred to this region will still be non-surgical, and will be relieved by removing the cause, regulating the diet, advising rational measures of living, and prescribing the proper medicines.

In far the greater number of surgical cases, we ought to be able to make a diagnosis by thorough investigations, along the usual lines. But if we find by our diagnosis surgical measures are indicated, we should not hesitate to offer them; for many pathological conditions can be remedied that seemed utterly hopeless only a few years ago. I believe a much earlier diagnosis can be made than formerly, if we realize the necessity for it, and if we use all the means already at our command. This consists of taking thorough and systematic histories, noting all the subjective symptoms, making repeated and painstaking physical examinations, and in using the stomach tube, when practicable, and making chemical and physical examinations of the stomach contents. If, after exhausting all these methods, and weighing all the facts, we are still undecided as to our diagnosis, we are doing our patients and ourselves an injustice by persisting in this policy of waiting for more diagnostic symptoms to appear. In such cases a surgical lesion is often the basis for the morbid phenomena; a diagnosis should be made by surgical methods, and surgical relief attempted.

THE RELATION OF CHOLIN TO EPILEPSY.

BY DR. JULIUS DONATH,
OF BUDAPEST, HUNGARY;
DOCENT AT THE UNIVERSITY OF BUDAPEST; CHIEF OF THE DIVISION OF NERVOUS DISEASES AT THE ST. STEPHEN HOSPITAL, BUDAPEST.

(Continued from Page 114.)

By referring to the tables it will be seen that the neurin and cholin experiments were frequently preceded by injections of the same volume of physiological salt solution (see tables 2 and 3). In order, however, to determine the effect of the same concentration, separate experiments were made with 10 per cent. physiological salt solution (see table 4). The result was the same: at most a slight paresis of the contralateral extremities, but usually no symptoms. In one case only were pronounced symptoms noticed (table 4, experiment 2): 0.5 c.c. injected into the right parietal lobe caused slight clonic and tonic convulsions in the paralyzed limbs of the opposite side which soon. became general and persisted most intensely for two hours. The day after, recovery had set in and the paresis was no longer noticeable. When an autopsy was performed on the fourth day, a hemorrhage into the right

lateral ventricle was found to explain these unusual symptoms. It was interesting to note that recovery from a hemorrhage of this kind is possible.

In rabbits, paresis of the hind-limbs is not a characteristic symptom since it is seen frequently after most varied experiments. Evidently the center for the hind-limbs plays a very important rôle in these animals.[1]

A greater tendency to convulsion was not seen after cholin or neurin injections in dogs whose brain was injured shortly after birth. The entire physical and psychical development of these animals, however, shows no deviation from the normal. The ability of the nervous centers to regenerate or to assume vicarious function seems to be very marked in the early life of these animals.

In dogs the trephining was done under morphine.

The strongly convulsive action of cholin and neurin, is apparent from the above tables. Since it has been shown that cholin is as frequently found in the cerebrospinal fluid of epileptics as with destructive processes of the nervous system it will only seem logical to assume for this substance an important rôle in bringing about the epileptic attack, particularly since the cortex of epileptics is more readily irritated owing to hyperemic, chronic inflammatory or hypoplastic processes. Presumably the epileptiform attacks of general paresis are also induced by cholin acting upon a hyperemic cortex which responds more readily to irritation.

Halliburton states " The presence of cholin in the pathological cerebrospinal fluid and blood will not explain all the symptoms of general paralysis. For instance, it will not account for the fits just referred to." I agree with this author concerning the first part of his statement, that all the symptoms are not explained by the presence of cholin, but concerning the epileptiform attacks of general paresis, I believe that my experiments prove a direct connection.

Even though special stress has been laid upon the presence of cholin, it is not improbable that other products of metabolism such as ammonia and kreatinin also participate in bringing about the attack.

A short comparison of my animal experiments with cholin and neurin with those of other authors, may not be amiss.

As early as 1885, Brieger[2] discovered that cholin was toxic, yet many later text-books state that this base is without physiological action. Experimenting with rabbits and guinea-pigs, Brieger found that injected hypodermatically, it was necessary to employ ten to twenty times more cholin than neurin to obtain the same physiological action. Cats, however, were particularly

[1] If, however, a considerable portion of the cortex of new-born dogs and cats is destroyed, the uninjured hemisphere will also remain behind in development and moderate doses of alcohol will suffice to bring on epileptic attacks (Guisseppe D'Abundo, Volume in omaggio al Prof. Tomaselli, Ref. Neurol. Centralbl., 1902, No. 12).
[2] L. Brieger. Ueber Ptomaine. Berlin, 1885. pp. 27 to 38.

TABLE II.—ANIMAL EXPERIMENTS WITH CHOLIN.

No.	Animal used.	Time.	Method.	Amount and application of 10 per cent. hydrochlor.	Symptoms.	Autopsy.
1.	Guinea-pig. 580 gme.	June 4, 1901. 10 A.M.	The animal became asphyxiated during chloroform narcosis but could be revived with artificial respiration. 1.5 c.c. of a two per cent morphine solution were then injected subcutaneously, into the abdominal wall, after which hardly any symptoms were noticed. The skull was trephined, anterior to the occiput, 3 millimeters to the right of the median line. Moderate hemorrhage from the diploe was checked by tamponade. As control, 0.2 c.c. of a 0.7% salt solution were injected into the posterior portion of the frontal lobe, the Pravaz needle being inserted 5 millimeters below the level of the skin (3 millimeters correspond to the thickness of the skull, 2 millimeters to that of the cortex.)			
		10.15 A.M	....	0.2 c.c.	Very severe clonic convulsions, gradually abating in severity. Ten minutes later increased tonic spasms, severe trismus with dilated palpebral fissure, severe lacrimation. Pupils do not react and tendon-reflexes cannot be elicited. The animal cannot stand but remains lying on the side. Alternating tonic and clonic spasms. Urine and feces not passed, no salivation.	
2.	Guinea-pig. 575 gme.	June 6, 11.15 A.M.	Site chosen: 2 millimeters to the left of the median line as above. Injection of 0.1 c.c. physiological salt solution. Owing to tonic spasm, the animal turns the head to the injured side. Contralateral side somewhat naretic. After several minutes again normal.			
		11.33.	....	0.1 c.c.	The animal remains quiet for 10 minutes, then alternating clonic and tonic spasms begin, gradually increasing in severity. After these cease, the animal screams and tries to get away. After several minutes, clonic convulsions of the same side reappear. Also trismus and contraction of the muscles of the neck. The general convulsions are less pronounced on the contralateral side. Palpebral fissures are dilated. Marked lacrimation. 12 M. Paresis of all extremities, especially on the contralateral side. The animal maker vain attempts to get away but does not utter a sound. 12.10 P.M. Again severe clonic and tonic spasms in the extremities, especially on the same side. Discharge of feces and urine. 12.15 P.M. General clonus, equally strong on both sides. 4 P.M. The animal lies with extended extremities. The convulsions are repeated from time to time. 7 P.M. Death after continued convulsions	Cerebral vessels much injected. No disintegration of tissue upon the surface of the brain. The puncture begins 3 millimeters behind the olfactory bulb and 1 millimeter from the median line, penetrates the gray substance, and after extending one millimeter into the white substance, stops one millimeter, anterior to the lateral ventricle. The brain shows brownish discoloration in the surroundings. Coagulated blood is found along the inner border of the left hemisphere, over the corpus callosum.
3.	Guinea-pig. 670 gme.	June 7 10.55.	Injected 2.5 millimeters to the right of the median line and 3 millimeters before the superior semicircular line. The Pravaz needle is introduced 7 millimeters deep, and 0.05 c.c. physiological salt solution are injected.			
		11.05. 11.10	No symptoms.	0.05 c.c. at site mentioned.	Several discharges of stool. 11.45. No symptoms. 0.1 c.c. more of cholin injected. 11.50. Clonic convulsions. After a few minutes, the animal falls over on the right side. Paresis of all extremities. Vain attempts to get away. Clonic convulsions of all extremities, es-	The puncture ends within the cortical substance of the right occipital lobe.

TABLE II.—(*Continued*).

4.	Guinea-pig. 600 gme.	June 8.		0.4 c.c. (vena jugularis externa).	pecially of the contralateral side. Spasms of the neck muscles. Especially marked paresis of the right anterior extremity. 11.55. The animal turns around its long axis. Trismus. Dilatation of the palpebral fissure. Pupils immovable even with focal illumination. Increasing paralysis of all extremities. If the animal is turned to the right, rotation again begins. Toward evening death after continuous convulsions. Marked salivation and lacrimation. Moderate general clonic convulsions and spasmodic breathing. Paresis of all extremities. The animal screams.	The puncture ends within the cortical substance of the right frontal lobe.
		June 10.	Animal lively. 0.2 c.c. physiological salt solution into the right frontal lobe. Owing to tonic spasm, the head is turned to the operated side. When untied, showed no particular symptoms.[1]			
		June 13.	Animal lively	0.5 c.c. (vena jugularis externa).	No symptoms.	
5.	Rabbit 1850 gme.	June 13. 9.30.	0.4 c.c. physiological salt solution into the right frontal lobe. Tonic spasm of neck toward left. Paresis of left anterior extremity.			
		10.15.		0.4 c.c. at site mentioned.	Paresis of the hind-limbs. On running, these are dragged along.	
		10.30.		0.5 c.c.	Paresis also of the anterior extremities. 11. The animal appears excited, breathes rapidly, and grinds the teeth.	
		June 14.			Paralysis of the posterior and paresis of the anterior extremities, which remain until the end. Since the experiment, no discharge of urine. Death.	
		June 16.				
6.	Guinea-pig. 540 gme.	June 14. 10.05.	0.1 c.c. physiological salt solution into the left frontal lobe. The head is repeatedly rotated to the opposite side. No paretic symptoms.			
		10.30.		0.1 c.c. (at site mentioned).	Tonic and clonic spasms, increasing at once in severity. At first intermittent, later continuous. Attempt to get away. Slight paresis of the right extremities. Rotation around the long axis toward the left. Spasms less intense. Pupils dilated, do not react to light. 11.05. Death.	Heart stopped beating in diastole. The puncture in the left parietal lobe extends to the lateral ventricle. Some coagulated blood in the lateral ventricle.
7.	Guinea-pig. 520 gme.	June 15. 10.45.	0.1 c.c. physiological salt solution into the left frontal lobe. Tonic spasm of the neck toward the opposite side. No paretic symptoms.			
		11.		0.1 c.c. (at site mentioned).	Increasing tonic and clonic spasms, which are less intense on the opposite side. The animal turns around, several times on its long axis to, the right and canot stand upright. The palpebral fissures and pupils are widely dilated and the latter do not react. Trismus. The animal does not utter a sound. Toward evening, death.	The puncture ends within the cortical substance of the left frontal lobe. No blood in the ventricle.
8.	I. Dog. (4½ months old).	Nov. 10.	After trepanation, 3 c.c. of physiological salt solution injected into the left frontal lobe. The animal turns the head to the opposite side in tonic spasm. No paralysis.			
		10.05.		3 c.c. (at site of trepanation).	Tremor of entire body, marked fall of temperature. Discharges stool and frequently assumes the sitting posture. Does not eat food placed in front of it, but merely licks at it. Background of the eye somewhat more anemic than before the injection of cholin. 9.10. Marked tremor. Blinking of the eyes. Intermittent severe tonic spasm. Tremor, extending wave-like over the entire body and steadily getting more intense. Eyes constantly closed. The anterior extremities	On the left side, a 'subdural hemorrhage. The sulci of the left cerebral hemisphere are strongly injected. The brain was punctured between the anterior central and the anterior

TABLE II.—(Continued).

		9.20		3 c.c. (at site of trepanation).	are raised from time to time. The animal can hardly walk, but sits down with every attempt. At 9.20 3 more c.c. of cholin were injected, followed by a pronounced bleeding. Temporary spasms of the neck appeared and the right anterior limb is occasionally raised as if painful. The animal falls against the chair and if turned on the side, has difficulty in raising the hind limbs. 9.50. General tonic and clonic spasms, lasting 5 minutes. Palpebral fissures widely opened. Trismus, salivation. The dog recuperates considerably and begins to run about. On the following day the animal has recovered, takes food but still has salivation and howls frequently. At 9.25. 4.5 c.c. of 10% hydrochlorate of neurin are injected. No symptoms. 10.15. The same dose is repeated. Vomiting tremor. Eye kept closed. Salivation. Draws in the tail and falls. The animal is finally killed with chloroform.	end of the lateral c tral and sulcus and t puncture extended c millimeter into the g substance. A cav filled with blood, 8 m limeters long and millimeters deep, found beneath the tosylvian gyrus.
		Nov. 11. 9.25.		4.5 of 10 per cent hydrochlorate of neurin (intra-cerebrally).		
9.	II. Dog. (4½ months old).	Nov. 11. 10 A.M. 10.15.	Perforation of the left temporal bone at a callous site.	4.5 c.c., (left parietal lobe). 4.5 c.c. (at same site).	No symptoms except increased right knee-jerk. 10.15. Another dose of 4.5 c.c. of cholin. Tremor, fall of temperature, blinking of the eyes. Pupils react toward light. Background of the eyes much paler than before the injection.	On the vault of t skull, to the left of t median line, there an area in the bone c centimeter long and a centimeter broad, wh is transparent and d not contain any d loë. This area cor sponds to the gyi supraspleniialis a n centralis.
		10.40.	Perforation of right frontal bone.	4.5 c.c. (right frontal lobe).	10.40. 4.5 c.c. of cholin into the right frontal lobe. Pupils very small, react to light. No symptoms of paralysis.	The puncture is found the anterior ectosylvi gyrus. Directly und the cortex, a cavity, t size of a walnut a filled with serum, found here.
		11.	....	5 c.c. (at same site).	11. Another dose of 5 c.c. into the right frontal lobe. No special symptoms. Nov. 12. Though the animal was lively yesterday afternoon, it was found this morning lying on the left side. Tonic and clonic spasms were soon noticed, lasting several minutes. If the right extremities are brought into the fixed position, they remain almost motionless. When raised, the animal falls over on the left side. Salivation and frothing of the mouth.	
10.	III. Dog. (4½ months old).	Nov. 14.	Trepanation on the left side under morphine narcosis. Severe bleeding.			The vault of the sl shows the impress of the gyri and co sponds to their contou
		Nov. 15. 10 A.M.	....	1 c.c. (at site of trepanation).	No symptoms.	Upon the impress of the coronal gyru a site, the size shape of a bean, th is a membranous s which is adherent the brain. Some los
		10.30.	....	1 c.c. (at same site).	Another dose of 1 c.c. Tremor, cooling off of body. Pupils react to light.	substance at the onal gyrus. The changes are due to sions of an earlier riod.
		11.	....	1 c.c. (at same site).	Another dose of 1 c.c.. Symptoms as above.	Recent wound from phining over the c nal and anterior vian gyrus.
		Nov. 17.	The animal appears lively.	1 c.c. of 10% neurin hydrochlorate.	After an intracerebral injection of 1 c.c. neurin, the following symptoms are noticed. Frothing before the mouth, trismus, spasms of the neck in the form of "salaam"-like motions and accompanied by short barks. General tonic and clonic convulsions, with bilateral facial clonus, lasting till evening with apparently retained consciousness. The dog is finally killed with chloroform.	Much coagulated b under the dura. puncture is found the anterior ect vian gyrus and are it there is a he rhagic area 5 mil ters long and 2 meters broad. Acc designs of the upon the vault of skull. Over the onal gyrus, the bo membranous.
11.	IV. Dog. (4½ months old).[8]	Nov. 18. 9.45.	After perforation in the region of the anterior border of the left occipital lobe, injection of 1 c.c. physiological salt solution. The animal turns the head to the opposite side.			The perforation c sponds to the sit the left median ec vian gyrus. Vesse jected on the su of the hemisi corresponding to puncture. The pur
		10.	....	1 c.c. (at site of perforation).	After several minutes, strong salivation, trismus, facial clonus, general tonic and clonic convulsions, urination. 10.30. Consciousness retained. The animal is killed by chloroform.	

TABLE II.—(Continued).

No.	Animal	Date	Procedure	Dose	Symptoms	Findings
						is found at the juncture of the fissure supra-sylvia ant., media and the fissure ansata minor. A hemorrhagic area, the size of a lentil, is found at this place in the cortex. A loss of substance from an earlier experiment is found in the coronal and right median gyrus.
12.	Guinea-pig.	Nov. 25.		2 c.c. (external jugular vein).	The animal is weak, immobile and feels cold.	
		Nov. 26.		2 c.c. (external jugular vein).	As above.	
13.	V. Dog. 6000 gme.	Oct. 10.		5 c.c. (external jugular vein).	The animal feels cold and does not move. No other symptoms.	The injection was beneath the dura, without injury to the brain.
		Oct. 21.	Trepanation in morphine narcosis.			
		Oct. 23. 10 A.M.		5 c.c. (subdural).	After the animal had recovered from the trepanation, 5 c.c. of cholin were injected subdurally. Marked salivation, discharge of urine and feces, fall of temperature. Pupils react.	
		10.40.		2 c.c.	10.40. After 2 more c.c. are injected, intermittent convulsions lasting several minutes, appear. 10.45. The animal walks about, stumbles and falls on the left side. Consciousness retained. 12. The animal runs about and shows no special symptoms. Is killed with chloroform soon after, on account of severe convulsions.	
14.	VI. Dog. 6650 gme.	Nov. 6.		7 c.c. (external jugular vein).	Salivation, rumbling in the intestines, discharge of urine and feces. Accelerated heart action, difficult respiration. Tremor, lasting several minutes. After half an hour the animal walks about, but most of the time sits quietly, shivers and feels cool to the touch.	
		Nov. 11. 10.20.	Perforation.	3 c.c. (right frontal lobe).	10.25. Discharge of urine, salivation, tremor and fall of temperature. 10.30. Paresis of left extremities. 10.35. Tonic and clonic spasm lasting three minutes. Nov. 14. The animal has recovered but walks somewhat unsteadily. Nov. 25. In walking, the left extremities are somewhat unsteady, so that the animal slips occasionally; otherwise perfectly recovered.	
		Dec. 5.		7 c.c. (crural vein).	Immediately after the injection of 7 c.c. cholin into the crural vein, feces and urine are passed. Salivation. Several slight clonic and tonic spasms. Heart action retarded but strong. Pauses in respiration owing to spasm of the respiratory muscles. After artificial respiration for fifteen minutes, the animal recovers. It lies on the side but moves freely, feels cool and trembles.	
15.	VII. Dog. 9900 gme.	1902. Jan. 13.		6 c.c. (external jugular vein).	Several difficult respiratory movements. Marked palpitation of the heart. Salivation. No urination. The dog urinated while tied down. Tremor. The animal feels cool to the touch.	
		Feb. 22.	Perforation of the skull. 1 c.m. to the right of the median line. Injection of 3 c.c. physiological salt solution. No symptoms. Hereupon 1 c.c. of cholin was injected into the same location.	1 c.c.	Marked salivation. Discharge of urine and feces. Severe tonic and clonic convulsions lasting five minutes. Trismus. The animal is very irritable, barks and grinds the teeth. After several minutes it behaves as	Cerebral vessel strongly injected. An area of disintegrated tissue, the size of a lentil, and not extending beyond the cortex, is found in the region of the right coronal fissure. Lateral ventricles and the rest of the brain intact.

TABLE II.—(Continued).

				normal. The urine discharged during the attack is free from albumin. 12.50. Exceptionaly s e v e r e tonic and clonic spasms with trismus and frothing of the mouth. If several short pauses are not included, the attack lasted fifty-five minutes. The left extremities are extended, while the right attempt to get away. Several rotatory movements. Feb. 25. The animal is killed with chloroform.

1. This experiment was done to show that intracerebral injections of physiological salt solution per se, do not give rise to special symptoms. The animal was observed for three successive days.
2. This animal was trephined shortly after, birth, 4½ months ago, but not injured otherwise. This animal together with the

following three were used to study the influence of former injuries of the skull or brain upon the epileptic attack. In the three following animals by excision and Animal No. 13 chemically by oil of turpentine). The development with all four animals was normal.

susceptible and reacted promptly to several milligrams. He, too, noticed strong salivation, abundant nasal secretion, increased peristalsis leading to the discharge of watery stools, dyspnea and at first very frequent and strong heart action. The latter leads to cardiac weakness, manifesting itself by fall of pressure. Mott and Halliburton have used this sign for the physiological detection of cholin. The statement of these two authors, that cholin does not influence respiration, is in direct contradiction to my own observations and can only hold for small doses.

According to Brieger only fatal doses of cholin (0.5 gm. to one kilo body-weight) applied subcutaneously will lead to severe clonic convulsions in rabbits. The animals will die soon after their appearance. By means of artificial respiration, these convulsions could be suppressed in part and death thus delayed. Since, however, they reappear, Brieger argues that there must be more than simple respiratory spasm. Mention is also made of the weakness of the legs, appearing first in the hind limbs, and the general infirm condition, already pronounced before the onset of the convulsions. My own experiments show without question that the tonic and clonic convulsions after intercerebral injection are independent of respiration, since they appear at first on the opposite side. The same is true for the paresis. Both cholin and neurin therefore show a certain similarity in action to muscarin or curare. Aster and Wood[1] wrongly ascribe these convulsions to pain, though in the animal experimented upon (dog), they involved other muscles besides the respiratory muscles. They also noticed that the fall in blood-pressure was preceded by an initial rise and attributed this to a muscarin-like irritation of the ends of the vagus within the heart since this symptom was also seen after dividing the vagi. It is well known that muscarin is very closely allied to cholin chemically: it merely contains one atom more of oxygen and can be easily obtained by treating cholin with concentrated nitric acid. The anemia of the retina found in my animals is due to a contraction of the

cerebral vessels and agrees well with the dilatation of the splanchnics, detected by Mott and Halliburton with the oncometer. In rabbits, Brieger ocasionally found a remarkable contraction of the pupils; I generally noticed a dilatation.

Brieger[1] and Cervello[2] observed the same symptoms when neurin was substituted for cholin, but more intense. According to the latter author, the pupils are first dilated but will soon contract up to the complete miosis; weakness of the voluntary muscles up to complete paralysis of the extremities is another pronounced symptom. Adamkiewicz[3] states that the subcutaneous injection of 5 to 15 centigrams of neurin in man will lead to a tremor not unlike a chill. This he ascribes to direct irritation of the cortical centers of the pyramidal tracts. The muscles will react promptly when irritated directly but not when stimulated by way of the nerves or the spinal cord, even when the strongest currents are used. Halliburton also believes that neurin acts upon the nerve-endings of the voluntary muscles like curare. Cervello thinks the convulsions are due to asphyxia since they are said to occur only during the pauses in respiration, but the contralateral distribution of motor irritation and paralysis, seen in my experiments, disproves this. Cervello also think that the increased discharge of saliva, nasal mucus, bile, gastric and intestinal secretion, is due to nervous influences. He also states that the neurin leaves the system chiefly by way of the urine.

In conclusion, the carbaminic acid theory of Krainsky[4] must be referred to. In a very interesting and meritorious article, this author verified the observation of Haig[5] that the amount of uric acid always falls before the epileptic attack and rises to the same degre when this is over. Haig, however, also noticed this in attacks of migraine. This phenomenon was so constant that

---

[1] Leon Aster and Horatio C. Wood. Ueber den Einfluss des Cholins auf den Kreislauf. Zeitsch. f. Biologie, Neue Folge 19, Vol. 1890.

[1] Loc. cit.
[2] V. Cervello. Sur l'action physiologique de la neurine. Arch. italiennes de biolog., 1886.
[3] Adamkiewicz. Zittergift und Gegengift. Berl. klin. Woch., 1898. No. 40.
[4] N. Krainsky. Zur Pathologie der Epilepsie. Allg. Zeitsch. f. Psychiatrie, 1897, 4, p. 612.
[5] Alex. Haig. Further observations on the excretion of uric acid in epilepsy and the effects of diet and drugs on the fits. Brain, 1896, Spring, p. 194.

TABLE III.—ANIMAL EXPERIMENTS WITH NEURIN.

No.	Animal used.	Time.	Method.	Amount of neurin hydrochlorate and site of injection.	Symptoms.	Post-mortem.
1.	Guinea-pig.	1901. June 17. 11.05	0.1 c.c. physiological salt solution is injected into the left frontal lobe. Owing to tonic spasm, the head is repeatedly turned to the injured side. Paresis of the right extremities which disappears after five minutes. The animal attempts to get away.			The needle has penetrated the left frontal lobe for 2.5 millimeters, 2 millimeters from the median line. The ventricles are intact.
		11.15	....	0.1 c.c. 1% neurin hydrochlorate.	After the intracerebral injection of 0.1 c.c. neurin hydrochlorate, the animal lies restless and hardly breathes. (Later the respiration improves.) Palpebral fissures dilated, occasional blinking. Pupils do not react to light. Corneal reflexes present. Heart-action irregular, intermittent, 117 to the minute. Shivering, marked fall of temperature. Stares and moves the ears on hearing loud sounds. The right legs paretic, especially the anterior ones. The background of the eyes somewhat anemic if compared with an animal of the same color but the vessels of the papilla could not be determined since these are already very narrow under normal conditions. The animal sees, and looks around but does not utter a sound. 11.45. The animal crouched together trembles and shivers. When raised it screams and passes urine.	
		12 M.		0.1 c.c. as above	Heart-beat 160. The animal successfully attempts to get away. Repeated discharge of feces. The wound on the head is now sutured and on the following day recovery is complete. The retina appears darker than yesterday.	
		June 18. 10.45		0.2 c.c. 5% hydrochlorate of neurin at same site.	Immediately very intense clonic convulsions. The head is turned to the right and left. Paresis of all extremities, especially on the right side. The right anterior leg seems to be most paretic. Marked lacrimation; passage of urine. Does not utter a sound. Background of eye not changed. Marked fall of temperature. Heart-beat cannot be felt owing to constant tremor. On touching the animal or making a loud noise it attempts to get away, as a result of which the convulsions are exaggerated. Rotates around its long axis to the right. Trismus. 11.45. Convulsions and salivation persist. From time to time the animal cries out. Retina grayish-white. 12.10. Limbs paretic, particularly the opposite side. Slight clonic twitching in the legs. Motion hardly possible and when raised screams. Slight trismus. Pupils do not react. June 20. The limbs are paretic, especially on the right side, but the animal still runs about, screams and takes nourishment. June 21. Complete recovery. June 24. Is killed.	
2.	Guinea-pig. 420 gme.	June 19, 11.15	0.1 c.c. physiological salt solution, intracerebrally on left side. Symptoms as above.			The needle has penetrated the left frontal lobe for 3.5 millimeters, 2 millimeters from the median line. Ventricle intact.
		11.30	....	0.1 c.c. 5% neurin hydro. (at site mentioned).	Immediately severe clonic convulsions lasting about two minutes. The animal trembles, shivers and tries to get away. Paresis of the right	

TABLE III.—(*Continued*).

				limbs. If turned on the back, there is a tendency to fall on the right side. Restlessness. June 20. Has recovered, shows no paresis and takes food. June 22. Perfectly well. Is killed.	
3.	Rabbit. (albino, 1650 gme.)	1902. Jan. 20. 10.10.	0.4 c.c. physiological salt solution, intracerebrally on left side, 2 millimeters from the median line.		
		Jan. 21. 10.25	....	0.4 c.c. 5% neurin hydrochlorate (at site mentioned).	On running, droops toward the right. 10.35. Paresis of the right extremities (if the right anterior limb is pulled forward, the animal does not draw it back; this is less marked with the right hind limb). Salivation, marked tremor, can hardly stand or raise itself if laid on the abdomen. Marked tendency to fall to the right. Tendency to turn around in a circle; cannot turn to the left, except at rare intervals. No difficulty in motion forward. Vision good. 10.50. Gait is now normal. Jan. 22. Animal completely recovered. Is killed on the following day.	A wound is found at junction of left frontal and parietal lobes, 6 millimeters from the median line and extending 2.5 millimeters into the cortex. Ventricles intact.
4.	Dog.[2]	Sept. 19. 9.40.	After perforating the skull on the left side, 1 c.c. of physiological salt solution is injected. No symptoms.		On holding the skull up to the light, the impressions of the gyri can be seen upon the skull. The dura matter is adherent to brain and skull over the anterior and posterior ectosylvian gyrus and the left occipital lobe. The perforation took place at the left ectolateral gyrus. The right lateral ventricle gapes. A cavity is found in the left coronal gyrus 6 millimeters long and 4 millimeters broad, communicating with the left lateral ventricle.
		10.	....	1 c.c. 5% neurin hydrochlor. (at site mentioned).	Tremor, fall of temperature, salivation and lacrimation. Pupils react. 10.15. The symptoms have disappeared. 10.20. After a second dose, salivation, pronounced gurgling in the intestines, vomiting, repeated discharge of feces. Paresis of all the extremities. Remains lying on the abdomen for four hours. Finally killed with chloroform.	
		10.20.			
5.	Guinea-pig.	Sept. 24.			2 c.c. 10% neurin hydrochlor. (external jugular vein).	Fall of temperature, lassitude and inability to stand on the legs. No other symptoms.

1 Compare also the neurin experiments in table 2, No. 8 and 10.
2 See remark under table 2, footnote 2.

3 Compare above.
4 That is, three times as much salt solution as cholin solution.

the epileptic attacks could be foretold by one or two days by means of quantitative uric acid estimations unless they were very frequent or rapid in occurrence. Recently Caro[1] has verified this observation, for atypical as well as typical attacks. Krainsky ascribes the decrease of uric acid to carbonate of ammonia, an abnormal product of metabolism, which he discovered in large amounts in the blood of epileptics and in proportion to the severity of the epileptic symptoms. According to this theory, the urea is not converted into uric acid by the aid of organic acids, as in the normal individual, but takes up one molecule of water according to a well-known formula and changes into carbonate of ammonia. It is impossible, however, to attribute convulsive action to uric acid or the innocuous carbonic acid. The only substance which might induce spasms is ammonia and this possibility has already been debated above. Krainsky believes that the efficacy in epilepsy of the uric acid sol-

vent lithium carbonate is due to the fact that lithium carbonate and ammonium carbonate are formed, the latter then being excreted as such. Bromide of sodium is said to act in the same way, since it is excreted as bromide of ammonium.[1]

It is improbable, however, that ammonium carbonate plays any rôle in the pathogenesis of epilepsy, especially in such doses capable of inducing convulsions, since the epileptic poison is undoubtedly contained in the cerebrospinal fluid[2]. This can no longer be questioned since Dide and Laquepée have shown that 0.5 c.c. of the fluid, removed after a series of attacks, will kill guinea-pigs in several hours to several minutes. It has also been shown that ammonia is found constantly in cerebrospinal fluid, but was missed in two cases of genuine epilepsy.

1 Caro. Ueber die Beziehungen epileptischer Anfälle zur Harnsäureausscheidung. Deutsch. med. Woch., 1900, No. 19.

1 Large doses of lithium carbonate and bromide of potassium are said, however, to cause reappearance of the attacks. Despite the supposed formation of lithium carbonate, the author could not detect an increased total excretion of uric acid.
2 J. Gastaigne. (Société de biolog. de Paris, November 3, 1900) finds that the cerebrospinal fluid is poisonous in severe cases of nervous uremia. If injected into guinea-pigs, fatal convulsions will appear. The poison is naturally of different source and nature than in genuine epilepsy.

TABLE IV.—ANIMAL EXPERIMENTS WITH 10 PER CENT. SALT SOLUTION.

Number.	Animal used.	Time.	Amount and site of injection (10% chloride of sodium).		Symptoms.	Post-mortem.
1.	Rabbit. (2300 gme.)	May 5, 1902.	0.5 c.c. (lobus parietalis dexti).		Paresis of the contralateral extremities. No other symptoms. The following day, complete recovery.	
2.	Guinea-pig. (680 gme.)	May 5.	0.5 c.c. (lobus parietalis dexti).		Paralysis of the opposite side. After five minutes, slight tonic and clonic convulsions of the paralyzed side, which gradually become generalized. The animal screams constantly. The spasms persist and are so severe that the animal jumps up. Posture on the paralyzed side. The convulsions last two hours. May 11.—Complete recovery. The paralysis has disappeared. May 15.—No symptoms. Killed with chloroform.	Hemorrhage into the right lateral ventricle.
3.	Guinea-pig. (690 gme.)	May 13.	0.5 c.c. (right parietal lobe).		Paresis of the contralateral side. No other symptoms.	
4.	Guinea-pig. (700 gme.)	May 16. May 17.	0.5 c.c. (left parietal lobe). As above.		No symptoms. As above.	
5.	Dog. (5800 gme.)	May 16.	1 c.c. (right parietal lobe).		No symptoms.	
		May 19.	5 c.c. (left parietal lobe).		No symptoms.	

Even granted there is an abnormal decomposition of urea, it is difficult to understand why the amount of uric acid should rise after the attack to the same extent that it has fallen before it so that the total excretion of uric acid is really normal. This is very interesting phenomenon is probably merely a retention due to an aura-like vasomotor irritation, which does not permit the uric acid to pass through the kidneys. As soon as the attack is over, the vasomotor disturbance is then compensated for. This theory agrees with the observation of Krainsky that the excretion of more readily diffusible substances such as urea, the chlorides and sulphates does not stand in any relation to the attack. The marked excretion of P_2O_5 after the attacks probably indicates an increased breaking-down of the lecithin.

In conclusion, I wish to thank Prof. Arpad v. Bokay, Director of the Pharmacological Institute, through whose kindness I was enabled to work in the institute; also Dr. Hugo Lukacs, who assisted me with the animal experiments; my former assistant, Dr. Johann Firiczky and Mr. Ludwig Dupuis, who helped me in the chemical part.

New Medical Society.—The physicians of West Philadelphia have organized what is known as the West Philadelphia Medical Association. The following officers were elected: President, Dr. A. F. Targetts; Vice-president, Dr. George C. Shammo; Recording Secretary, Dr. William D. Beacon; Financial Secretary, Dr. A. P. Good; Treasurer, Dr. J. D. Brittingham; Directors, Dr. J. H. McConnell, Chairman; E. L. Graf, S. F. Gilpin, H. B. Smith, Frank Kirby, F. Mortimer Cleveland, F. R. Starkey, B. F. Wentz, A. P. Good, Charles E. Price, and J. D. Brittingham.

RUPTURED ECTOPIC PREGNANCY: WITH REFERENCE TO CASES OF THE ACUTE INTRAPERITONEAL TYPE.

BY GROESBECK WALSH, M.D.,
OF CHICAGO;
ATTENDING PHYSICIAN, ASSOCIATE STAFF, COOK COUNTY HOSPITAL, ETC.

THIS paper is written with the purpose of emphasizing a single point in the treatment of acute ruptured ectopic pregnancy, namely, the mistake *of wasting time in the attempted removal of the blood-clots.* This is a point which was constantly being brought forward by early writers some years ago when laparotomy for this condition first came into general use. The following brief quotations will make this fact apparent. Thus, from Harris before the Chicago Gynecological Section:

" I think the blood, either the clots or liquid, should not be removed from the peritoneal cavity. It is equivalent to so much transfusion and if no infection takes place the patient recovers more quickly and the blood is reutilized by the system by being left in the peritoneal cavity." Longyear's conclusions given with an analysis of seven operative cases are very much in the same vein: "Beyond what can be quickly removed about the seat of operation this exudate is best left within the abdomen. Much precious time which usually contains the valuable element of life to the patient may be lost in this manipulation . . . the douche may be used but the clots will mostly remain. In my first case I attempted to make a clean job of it by these methods, and I lost the only case of the seven operated upon," etc.

Prewitt in a series of six laparotomies for this

condition lost two under prolonged irrigation and saved four under the plan of sponging out only such blood as was readily accessible. It is unnecessary to quote his conclusions. The point at issue was also brought out with more or less emphasis by Henrotin and others.

From these quotations and a review of the literature of a decade ago, despite the advice of Pozzi quoted from Schwarz, " That we remove the whole of the blood clot, placing no reliance upon the absorptive powers of the peritoneum but rather fearing the depressing influence of the accumulated clots," it is evident that in this country at least the more experienced men not only left the blood untouched but even viewed it as an asset for the patient.

Of late years this principle of gynecology seems to have dropped out of sight or if known to have been disregarded. Many operators at the present time very evidently regard the fresh clotted blood which we find lying amongst the coiled intestines as a source of future danger to be got rid of at any cost, and the literature of recent operative procedures is plentifully sprinkled with allusions to attempts at its removal. Along this line the following quotation from Munro Kerr: " The ruptured tube was ligated and removed, as much blood-clot as possible was cleared away, the abdominal cavity was washed out with salt solution," etc., and in a second case, " All blood clot was carefully removed."

From C. E. Ruth: "Abdomen was found filled with blood, after removing the blood and washing the abdominal cavity with deci-normal salt solution, the abdomen was closed," etc.

Rushmore, in a description of four operative cases which had ruptured into the general peritoneum, details the " removal of large amounts of fresh and clotted blood," seemingly as a matter of course. The same technic is also referred to in the communications of Harold Mole, Heyer and Lea and F. F. Lawrence.

Similar items are also obtainable from J. A. Clarke in a paper on this subject. His article contains the following significant sentences: " She was then in extremis but was given the hopeless chance. I scooped out nearly a pailful of solid clots, the whole peritoneal cavity from the diaphragm down being distended with clots; unfortunately she died on the table." Sturmer's monograph also brings out a point as to the location of the clots which will be dwelt upon a little later. "A great deal of blood had run back to the sides of the abdomen and a considerable time was spent in removing this, the head of the table being raised to allow it to gravitate to the pelvis," etc. And in a second case, "A great deal of the blood had run up by the side of the spleen and liver; this was removed with sponges," etc. Probably the most outspoken opinion in regard to the removal of blood clots in this class of cases has come from Barton Cooke Hirst in his Textbook for 1903: " After rupture, the patient's only hope lies in an immediate abdominal section, evacuation of the blood clots from the abdominal

cavity and ligation of the blood-vessels, etc." And a little later on, " The blood has already been shed and is of no use to the patient. . . . The abdominal cavity should next be flushed with large quantities of sterile water. . . . I have practically given up douching the abdomen after abdominal section except in cases of extra-uterine pregnancy; there is no other means which so rapidly and so surely removes blood-clots from the abdomen; gallons are required," etc. These instances might be multiplied almost indefinitely. They may appear to be founded upon hair-lines of difference, and yet they all show a very definite purpose and intent. They bring us at once to the parting of the ways. It is so apparent to anyone who has watched its performance that this " careful removal" of scores of blood clots scattered through the abdomen is a time-consuming, shock-producing task, and the pursuit of the theory that if it is good surgery to remove some blood, then it is better surgery to remove it all, is very certain sooner or later to lead us to disaster. For the purpose of illustrating the argument I cite two cases which bring out the point very clearly. The two detailed are taken from Dr. Henrotin's records and occurred during the years of my assistantship with him. They are selected because they are typical, and the significant item of their history, common to both, a placid recovery with many undisturbed blood-clots within the abdomen, is one which could be reproduced from his records many times during the last decade. As the previous histories have little bearing on the subject, they are omitted.

Case I.—Mrs. E. P. C., aged thirty-two years; primipara; American. On the afternoon of October 13 patient was seized with a sudden violent cramping intra-abdominal pain, with great weakness. Slight show of blood from the vagina. Was seen by Dr. C. F. Ely, who diagnosed a ruptured ectopic pregnancy and referred her to Dr. Henrotin for operation. Operation at 7 P.M., at St. Joseph's Hospital. Small median incision. Abdomen was found filled with fresh and clotted blood. Extensive laceration of the right tube made out. The latter removed into the cornu of the uterus. Repair and coaptation sutures all of catgut. *Blood clots removed only in so far as they obscured the field of operation.* Abdomen closed in layers. No irrigation, no drain. Collodion seal. Convalescence absolutely uneventful.

Case II.—Mrs. C. G., aged thirty-eight years; multipara. Patient first seen by Henrotin on the night of May 15. During that evening while assisting a rheumatic husband across the floor was seized with the usual cycle of subjective symptoms accompanied by a great gush of blood from the vagina. Patient became almost exsanguinated but rallied a little before her operation early the following morning at the Policlinic. Usual median incision. Peritoneum distended with blood. Small rupture made out in the right tube one-quarter inch from the uterus; this opening in the tube was split down into the uterus and the cavity of the latter thoroughly curetted through this opening. Tube repaired with catgut. No organs were excised, the operation being purely reparative. A great deal of fresh and clotted blood could be seen reaching high up under the diaphragm. *Only such clots as obscured the field were removed.* No drain and no irrigation. Abdomen closed in layers, using the aluminum-bronze wire and double-eyed needle after the method of Harris. Silver foil dressing. Convalescence uneventful. Discharged June 11.

When we come to think it over, the principle of letting the blood clots severely alone is a very good principle. It has two noteworthy foundations of fact: (1) A clinical history of several hundred cases treated in the way with no untoward result; (2) the knowledge that we could not get rid of the blood even if we wanted to.

If we recall that the patient as a rule assumes the recumbent position shortly after the gestation sac ruptures, we see that it is inevitable that the fresh blood should seek the lowest possible level, the posterior peritoneal wall, and thence slowly work its way up under the liver, completely out of our reach. In all probability the clots which we discover by peering among the intestinal coils form but a small part of the actual products of hemorrhage. Hidden far down on the posterior abdominal wall are masses of blood which we could not possibly get rid of without killing our patient. If any one is at all sceptical as to this he should read Prewitt's paper. In regard to the proposition of "flushing the abdomen clear," the following interesting clinical experience will be of profit to us all. Many years ago when laparotomy for the relief of intra-peritoneal septic conditions first came into general use, the idea was proposed and currently believed and acted upon, that by washing the products of sepsis out of the abdomen with a stream of running water we would give the patient the best possible chance for his life. In elaboration of this idea Henrotin had special apparatus installed in his operating room at the Alexian Brothers' Hospital. Large tanks with a capacity of many gallons were fastened high up on the wall. These were filled with hot salt solution. Such cases as were considered suitable at that time were treated by free incision in the anterior abdominal wall and prolonged forcible intra-peritoneal irrigation. In order to leave no stone unturned in this matter, in several instances free incisions were also made in both flanks and the entire force of the stream turned in, so that the patient's abdomen was a spouting torrent of water. Yet it was discovered, even after the most prolonged treatment, that a sponge pushed with very little force indeed among the coils of intestines would disclose pockets of pus which the irrigation had not even disturbed. Since that time, in this immediate part of the surgical world, the plan of flushing the peritoneal cavity with the idea of removing all intra-abdominal deposits has been discarded.

A few conclusions to end with, then, brought home to us by the two cases detailed and the long list with which they are identical.

In operations for acute ruptured ectopic pregnancy every minute is of value.

Not a single one of them is to be wasted in doing the unnecessary or trying to do the impossible.

Remove the blood clots only in so far as they obscure the field of operation.

We cannot flush the abdomen clear of blood in the time at our disposal, and much of that precious time will be wasted in attempting to do so.

REFERENCES.

M. L. Harris. Trans. Chicago Gyn. Soc., September, 1896.
H. W. Longyear. Annals of Gyn. and Ped., March, 1897.
Pozzi, Med. and Surg. Gyn., P. 255.
Prewitt. Jour. Am. Med. Ass'n, January, 1897.
Henrotin. Trans. Am. Gyn. Soc., 1896.
Henrotin. American Jour. of the Medical Sciences, 1896.
J. M. Munro Kerr. Glasgow Med. Jour., November, 1903.
C. E. Ruth. Interstate Med. Jour., May, 1903.
Mary Rushmore, N. Y. Med. Jour., October 24, 1903.
J. A. Clark. Chicago Med. Recorder, March, 1904.
A. J. Sturmer. Jour. of Obst. and Gyn. of the Brit. Emp., August, 1903.
Harold Mole. Bristol Med-Chi. Jour., March, 1903.
F. F. Lawrence. Jour. of Am. Med. Ass'n, March, 1902.
Heyer and Lea. American Jour. of the Medical Sciences, February, 1904.
Hirst. Text-book of Diseases of Women, 1903.
M. L. Harris. Jour. of Am. Med. Ass'n, 1896.

MEDICAL PROGRESS.

MEDICINE.

On What Lines is the Treatment of Malignant Disease Advancing?—Malignant disease is the subject of much study at the present time and furnishes a great share of the material for scientific endeavor and research. Robert Abbe (*Med. Rec.*, December 31, 1904) considers the different methods which have been advanced for the treatment of cancer. Undoubtedly gain has been made in three notable directions, viz., (1) in the recognition of the principle that carcinoma and sarcoma are primarily of local origin; (2) in recognizing the value of extensive operation in advanced cases; (3) in establishing the value of radiotherapy. Three methods of treating cancer through systematic measures have commanded some attention and may be referred to as serum-therapy, antitoxin treatment and oophorectomy. The use of serum is at present *sub judice* and awaits the report of the French Surgical Commission. There have been enough reports to establish that a few tumors have been seen to diminish in size and disappear under bacteriotherapeutic treatment. It seems that the principle of bacteriotherapy on which the method is based presupposes an entirely unsettled problem of bacterial origin of cancer. One sees changes in the human body resulting from removal of the ovaries in cases of mammary cancer. The method devised by Beatson has been given a fair trial, enough to establish the fact mentioned, but not to place it among the list of surgical procedures for usual resort. In the consideration of radiotherapy for cancer photo-therapy may be dismissed. Lupus alone yields to the Finsen light, but the same disease subjected to radiotherapy is under prompt control without light rays. It remains to consider the Roentgen rays, the ionized rays, discharged from the iron electrodes with spark, and the rays from radium. The antibacterial action, which is at best very feeble, can play but a trifling part, and the feeble heat emitted by radium is insignificant. One must look to the rays, which are of negative electrons emitted by radium and to the Roentgen rays, as the power. The effects of the application of the three forms of radiation mentioned have been many tumors dissipated, some unaffected, occasional recurrences, and a few cures. Radium alone can be used in deep structural disease; it may be buried for hours or days according to its strength. From radium therefore we may expect the greatest future results.

Diseases of the Isthmian Canal Zone.—R. L. SUTTON (*Med. Rec.*, January 14, 1905) gives a résumé of the most prominent features of the various tropical and other diseases commonly encountered in the Canal region. The lit includes malaria, dengue, beriberi, infection with intestinal parasites of numerous species, lesions due to the bites of various insects, heat exhaustion and sunstroke, acute and chronic rheumatism, dysentery, leprosy, smallpox, and yellow fever. The latter is not epidemic at present in this region, and sporadic cases are rarely seen. Malaria is more widespread than any other affection, and the estivoautumnal form is the commonest variety. Quartan infections are not observed. Dengue is the disease which most frequently attacks the newcomer, and the local form is peculiar to the unreliability of the primary and terminal eruptions, which do not possess the diagonstic value usually accorded to them, as they are absent in the majority of cases. Blood counts show an early leucopenia with a normal differential count, which is later followed by eosinophilia after the second rise and lymphocytosis as convalescence begins. Beriberi assumes both the tropical and paraplegic forms, and especially affects the Chinese contingent, although the natives do not entirely escape. Uncinariasis is the most important and dangerous of the intestinal infections, and may cause extreme degrees of anemia with hemoglobin as low as 20 per cent. Eosinophilia is very high, seldom being below 20 per cent., and in one instance being over 65 per cent. Castor oil, followed by three 20 gr. doses of thymol, at two-hour intervals, cures most cases. Dysentery, both of the bacillary and amebic type, is much in evidence among the natives, but our troops suffer little from it, owing to the careful guarding of the water supplies. Hepatic abscess is seldom encountered.

Pneumonia in High Altitudes.—A. R. GOODMAN (*Med. Rec.*, January 14, 1905) summarizes the statistics of the morbidity and mortality from pneumonia in the American Hospital, Mexico City, from 1890 to 1904. Of 4,367 cases of disease treated during this period, 101 were pneumonia. A marked preponderance of the disease was observed in the first six months of the year, *i.e.*, before the rainy season. The average mortality was 39.8 per cent.

Intussusception of the Appendix Vermiformis.—GEORGE EMERSON BREWER (*Amer. Med.*, January 14, 1905) reports the case of a female, aged twenty-two years, who was admitted to the Roosevelt Hospital in the spring of 1904, suffering from symptoms of acute appendicitis. The abdomen was opened and a prolonged search for the appendix was made without finding any trace of the organ. Five months later the patient again presented herself, complaining of constant pain and tenderness in the right iliac fossa. The abdomen was again opened, the ileocecal region dissected free from the mass of adhesions and thoroughly inspected. No trace of an appendix could be found, but on palpating the cecum an elongated oval body could be felt within its lumen. The intestine was opened by longitudinal incision and the inverted appendix was found projecting from its attachment at the interior extremity of the cecum. The mass was removed and the wound. in the cecum and colon sutured. The patient made a satisfactory recovery and was entirely relieved of her symptoms. The pathological report showed the specimen to be an inverted appendix.

Inoculation of Horses with Syphilis.—Among animals the only evidences of syphilitic inoculation which have been demonstrated are those reported by Roux, Lassar and Neisser. Attempts have now been made to infect a horse by PIORKOWSKI (*Berl. klin. Woch.*, December 19, 1904). He injected the blood from patients who had been taking active mercurial treatment in quantities of from 5 to 10 c.c., either subcutaneously or intravenously. Altogether 80 patients were taken in various stages of the disease. Each was followed by a moderate rise of temperature, and as soon as this had subsided, the injection was repeated. Four weeks after the first inoculation a maculopapular rash appeared, which was examined by various experts and pronounced by them to be syphilitic in character, both in gross and microscopical appearances. The lymphatic glands became enlarged in the submaxillary region. Infection by contact with other horses who were in the same stable was not demonstrated. Blood serum taken from this horse and injected into various small animals was not followed by any reaction. No positive conclusions are afforded by these experiments and the author is now engaged in making controls in other horses.

Sciatic Neuritis with Paralysis following Malaria.—W. G. RUSSELL (*Med. Rec.*, January 7, 1905) describes the case of a man of thirty-eight who, after an attack of intermittent malarial fever, apparently cured by quinine and calomel, developed intense pain in the thighs and down the legs. At this time the pupillary and patellar reflexes were normal, but the pain continued with unabated severity, and after ten or twelve days both patellar reflexes disappeared, and there was loss of power of the left leg and some disability of the right one. Under massage and sanatorium treatment the condition gradually improved, so that he now, about three months after the malaria, has no pain, is able to use the right leg, and to drag or push the left one along if he is helped on either side.

Epidemic of Typhoid Fever.—J. D. BRIGGS (*Med. Rec.*, January 7, 1905) analyses in instructive fashion the circumstances attending a serious outbreak of typhoid fever in a small, isolated community in the Allegheny watershed. The water supply of the village came from two sources, one a reservoir at some distance, and the other a nearby spring. The reservoir water had a pronounced flavor and odor, due to the presence of algæ, but it was found that the clear and more agreeable spring water was the means of dissemination of the disease, owing to contamination by drainage from an imported case of typhoid. The author points out the necessity for great care in laying out sewerage systems in the neighborhood of water supplies, and directs attention to the importance of thoroughness in the disinfection of all excreta, linen, bath water, etc., from typhoid cases. Formaldehyde, bichloride and lime preparations are greatly inferior in effectiveness to carbolic acid, which should be freely used in five per cent. solution, and allowed to act for several hours.

Tuberculosis in Japan.—S. KITASATO (*Am. Med.*, January 7, 1905), after a thorough review of human and bovine tuberculosis in Japan, concludes human tuberculosis is as frequent in Japan as in the civilized countries of Europe and America. Primary intestinal tuberculosis is relatively common in adults and children, although cow's milk plays no rôle at all in the feeding of children. There are large districts in Japan where, in spite of the existence of human tuberculosis, the cattle remain absolutely free from the disease. In these regions it is not customary to consume either meat or milk from bovines. This is very important proof for the fact that under ordinary conditions human tuberculosis is not infectious for bovines, as the opportunities for infection certainly cannot be lacking. Among Japanese in general very little cow's milk is used, and especially is it employed but little in the dietary of children. Under natural conditions the native animals show but very little susceptibility for tuberculosis. If large doses of tubercle bacilli are inoculated into them, either intravenously or intraperitoneally, they become tuberculous to a certain degree; they do not seem to be at all susceptible to subcutaneous infection. The imported and mixed race animals are very susceptible to tuberculosis. Human tuberculosis is not infectious for native and mixed race animals.

Effects of Pilocarpine in Strychnine Poisoning.—A case was recently described in which hypodermic injections of pilocarpine were used and the patient recovered. S. J. MELTZER and W. SALANT (*Jour. Am. Med. Ass'n*, December 31, 1904) have submitted this claim to the test of experiments on rabbits and frogs and determined that pilocarpine hydrochlorate does not act as an antidote to strychnine, and that on the contrary; the addition of pilocarpine apparently supports the poisonous effects of strychnine, and by its aid an ineffective subminimum dose may have a toxic or even fatal effect. The authors think that the same conclusions may be applied to human beings, and that in the quoted case recovery was not dependent on the pilocarpine, and that the strychnine had merely a strongly toxic, but not a fatal effect, the dose not being mentioned. The indiscriminate use of the pilocarpine "as a last resort" is much deplored by the writers, who claim that in human beings each alkaloid should be employed only according to well established indications for its use and not according to theoretical notions. If the latter are well founded, they may be readily proved or tested on animals.

Tuberculosis of the Kidney, Ureter and Bladder.—J. M. BALDY and EDWARD A. SCHUMANN (*Am. Med.*, December 31, 1904) report the case of a girl of twenty-four years, whose present illness began in December, 1902, with marked frequency of micturition with burning pain. The urine was diminished in quantity and contained blood. She had occasional attacks of sharp pain in the right iliac fossa. Pelvic examination revealed upon the right side a somewhat tender, dense mass presenting all the features of a chronic adherent pyosalpinx. The mass extended apparently from the uterine cornua to the lateral region of the pelvis and was diagnosed as tubal in composition. The purine showed tubercle bacilli. A diagnosis of tuberculous cystitis, with probable tuberculous salpingitis, was made. Operation by Dr. Baldy revealed normal tubes and ovaries on both sides. The mass in the right was much thickened and distorted ureter running almost at right angles to its normal course and closely simulating an enlarged and adherent tube. The median incision was extended up toward the umbilicus and carried diagonally over the loin, ending immediately over the kidney. Through this incision the right kidney and ureter down to its vesical insertion were removed. The ureter was densely adherent throughout its whole course. The cystitis proved intractable, the bladder being studded with diffuse ulcers, revealed by cystoscopic examination. The pathological report shows both ureter and kidney to be tuberculous, the kidney being infiltrated by pus cavities.

Primary Sarcoma of the Stomach.—JOHN A. SIPHER (*Am. Med.*, December 31, 1904) reports three cases. The first had been of about two years' duration, beginning with sudden pain in the left inguinal region and later showing a hard nodular mass in the neighborhood of the spleen. At autopsy a tumor of the stomach was found, situated on the posterior surface toward the cardiac end. (Microscopically this was a round-celled sarcoma.) In the second case a gastroenterostomy had been performed a year and a half before death, for malignant disease of the stomach, the patient being much improved for a time after the operation. At autopsy a tumor was found causing complete stenosis of the pylorus. Apart from congestion the gastric mucosa was normal and the microscopical examination showed a sarcoma arising by the proliferation of the endothelium of the lymph vessels of the submucosa. There were no metastases. This is the second recorded case of endothelioma of the pylorus. In the third case a palpable tumor was present and the stomach analysis gave no free HCl and no lactic acid. A resection of the pylorus was made and the diagnosis of sarcoma was made at the operation, the mucosa not being involved. Microscopical examination showed a giant-celled sarcoma. The literature shows the total of 69 cases recorded.

Reflexes in the Diagnosis of Nervous Disturbances Following Trauma.—HENRY S. UPSON (*Am. Med.*, December 31, 1904) states that in differentiating the organic and functional effects of injury, and in excluding stimulation the reflexes are of the first importance. The reaction of the pupil to light, the knee-jerk, Achilles-tendon jerk, ankle-clonus, Babinski reflex, cremasteric and virile reflexes are those always to be tested. Others may assume importance in special cases. Absence of the knee-jerk, pupillary reflex, or Achilles-tendon jerk is according to Upson always indicative of organic disease. Some authorities have found the knee-jerk absent in one out of several hundred patients considered normal. In the absence of searching and continued observation there remains in these patients the possibility of a beginning tabes or unrecognized diabetes. True ankle-clonus is always pathological, spurious ankle-clonus and exaggerated knee-jerks are common in neurasthenics and hysterics, and at time of nervous excitement in normal people as well. The reflexes furnish the best available criterion of impotence so often alleged in damage suits. In the presence of the cremasteric and virile reflexes, with papillæ along the edge of the glans penis, in a patient suffering from no obvious organic brain or spinal-cord disease, impotence is functional, and will disappear with improvement in the general health. Absence of one, or especially of any two of these signs, makes an alleged impotence highly probable if not certain. The Babinski reflex is significant of disease of the motor tract, but its absence does not exclude such disease, as it is more often absent than present, even when the reflexes are exaggerated from organic causes.

Cause of Death in Operated Cases of Intestinal Perforation Occurring in Typhoid Fever.—ANDERSON (*Am. Med.*, December 31, 1904) reports his experience in 21 cases of laparotomy in perforation. In three the condition resembled perforation, as typhoid appendicitis, mesenteric gland infection, and obstruction from mass of round worms in the ileum; in which paralytic ileus occurred. In 12 cases the patients were operated upon under thirty-six hours from the onset of first symptoms with six recoveries. Three of these were the foregoing three cases. In the remaining nine cases the patients were operated upon from two to four days after perforation and all died. In nine cases there was special treatment by draining or irrigating the lumen of the bowel. Four of these patients recovered. In the others, the postoperative symptoms were less severe. Anderson believes that there is a danger of sepsis from the contents of the paralytic bowel, as well as from the peritonitis; that shock as a cause of death is usually rare during typhoid fever; that anesthesia and operations are well borne, if performed carefully; that the peritoneum acquires some immunity to infection during typhoid fever, but that paralytic ileus is readily produced in the inflamed and ulcerated intestine, and the natural protective function of the mucous membrane is destroyed and serious toxemia occurs early; that while perfecting our technic to cure the peritonitis, we must remember the contents of the paralyzed bowel may become a cause of death and must be removed.

Polyneuritis Complicating Typhoid Fever with Unusual Localizations.—GORDON (*Am. Med.*, December 31, 1904) reports a case in which the nervous phenomena pointed to a multiple neuritis, the associated unilateral facial palsy of peripheral nature making the case unusual from the standpoint of etiology, and leading Gordon to suspecting possible poliomyelitic nature. The case is that of a young man who on the fifteenth day of typhoid fever developed a right brachial monoplegia with a facial palsy on the same side. Gordon analyzes the rôle of infection and intoxication in diseases of the nervous system and concludes that the toxins of infectious diseases may affect a whole neuron (cell and its axis-cylinder) or several segments of it simultaneously.

Eyesight of Employees.—Since the very fatal collision which occurred about nine years ago, between the Elbe and the Craithie, the ophthalmologists of Great Britain have made effort to convince the Board of Trade that all employees upon whose eyesight the lives of passengers depends, should be subjected to the most rigorous ophthalmic investigation. JAMES W. BARRETT and W. F. ORR (*Lancet*, October 29, 1904) state that in Australia there has been similar agitation on the part of ophthalmologists. They have been met by the same rebuff as was experienced by the corresponding body in England, the Board of Trade in each case having affirmed very bluntly that there was no evidence to show that visual deficiency was the cause of the accident. It is quite evident that the reason for such failure of evidence was due to the fact that the gentlemen examining those who were held responsible for wrecks, made no effort to determine their visual conditions. After the wreck of the P. & O. steamer Australia; however, June 20, 1904, conditions were found by expert ophthalmological examination, which were of such startling nature that the advice of the medical fraternity in future is apt to be very closely heeded in Australia at least. In the case under consideration, the pilot boarded the Australia five miles from Queenscliffe. In entering the port, two lights must be kept in line or nearly so. The pilot stated that he was breathless from exertion of boarding but took charge and used his binoculars. The sea was not high, although it was blowing hard. Twenty-five minutes after he took charge, the steamer struck. The night was dark and it was raining. He subsequently stated that he recollected nothing after the first order to port the helm, although evidence shows that he gave orders to port on three distinct occasions. He had not been drinking and was absolutely sober. After the accident, he collapsed and was taken home and put under the care of his family physician. He was fifty-nine years of age, had a hypertrophied heart, high blood pressure and arterial sclerosis. His urine contained both albumin and glucose. He was obviously myopic and on examination was found not to have an entirely satisfactory discrimination of color. This same pilot ran the steamer Inraghiri aground on the northwest of the entrance to South Channel in the same harbor. The Court found

him guilty of careless navigation, his resignation was refused, and his certificate canceled. It is obvious that directly traceable to the ocular deficiency of the pilot rather than to his negligence.

PRESCRIPTION HINTS.

Medicinal Treatment in Measles.—Small initial dose of calomel, preceded by a glycerin suppository, are useful in the first stages of treatment. The severe vomiting is usually best controlled by cracked ice, lime water or bismuth, and the insomnia overcome by small doses of trional, 2 to 3 grs., in combination with chloral. Cough is usual and is best kept in check by sinapisms. The following prescription will prove serviceable:

R Potassii citratis....................ʒii (8.0)
Vini ipecac.....................ʒii (8.0)
Tr. opil camph.....................ʒiii (12.0)
Syrupi tolutani.....................ʒi (30.0)
Aquæ cinnamomi. ....q. s. ad ʒiii (90.0)
Misce. Sig. ʒv q. three hours.   STEVENS.

Whooping Cough.—Belladonna, quinine, antipyrin and bromide combinations still remain the standbyes in the treatment of the cough of this persistent affection. Antipyrin in combination with the bromides is one of the most serviceable remedies. It may be prescribed as follows:

R Sodii bromidi....................gr.l (3.0)
Antipyrini ....gr.xv (1.0)
Glycerini ....ʒii (8.0)
Aquæ cinnamomi.........q. s. ad ʒiii (90.0)
Misce. Sig. ʒi. q. two hours for one year old child.

Pain in Pneumonia and Pleurisy.—When the pain in these diseases is severe, the following combinations of opium are useful:

R Pulveris opii.....................gr.iv (0.25)
Hydrarg. chlor. mit.............gr.v (0.06)
Pulveris aromatici................gr.x (0.6)
Misce. Et fiat chart. No. vi. Sig. One powder every half hour until relieved. Or

R Pulveris ipecac et opii..... } ....aa ʒss. (2.0)
  Camphoræ monobromati.. }
Misce. Et fiat caps. No. x. Sig. One capsule. q. half hour until relieved.

The Treatment of Ozena.—The treatment of this very troublesome affection has given rise to many therapeutic combinations, which, being tried, were found to be more or less wanting: Camphor, iodoform, formol, thymol, menthol, etc., were recommended and are still used, but a permanent cure is difficult to obtain, many factors entering into the nature of the affection. Dr. Bobone claims to have obtained great success with the use of petroleum, which he considers in the dual point of view as a bactericide and a stimulant. The solution he uses is as follows:

R Refined petroleum...................1½ oz.
Nitrate of strychnine.............. ⅓ gr.
Oil of eucalyptus.................... 1 drop.

After antiseptic irrigation of the nasal cavities to remove all secretion, a piece of cotton wool steeped in the solution is applied by means of a stylet to all the surface of the fossæ once a day. In a short time all offensive odor disappears, and the mucous lining assumes a healthy appearance.

Another effective treatment consists in insufflation of the following powder:

R Collargol ....10 grs.
Sugar of milk........................ 3 drs.

THE MEDICAL NEWS.

A WEEKLY JOURNAL
OF MEDICAL SCIENCE.

COMMUNICATIONS in the form of Scientific Articles, Clinical Memoranda, Correspondence or News Items of interest to the profession are invited from all parts of the world. Reprints to the number of 250 of original articles contributed exclusively to the MEDICAL NEWS will be furnished without charge if the request therefor accompanies the manuscript. When necessary to elucidate the text, illustrations will be engraved from drawings or photographs furnished by the author. Manuscript should be typewritten.

SMITH ELY JELLIFFE, A.M., M.D., Ph.D., Editor,
No. 111 FIFTH AVENUE, NEW YORK.

Subscription Price, Including postage in U. S. and Canada.

PER ANNUM IN ADVANCE	$4.00
SINGLE COPIES	.10
WITH THE AMERICAN JOURNAL OF THE MEDICAL SCIENCES. PER ANNUM	8.00

Subscriptions may begin at any date. The safest mode of remittance is by bank check or postal money order, drawn to the order of the undersigned. When neither is accessible, remittances may be made at the risk of the publishers, by forwarding in *registered* letters.

LEA BROTHERS & CO.,
No. 111 FIFTH AVENUE (corner of 18th St.), NEW YORK.

SATURDAY, JANUARY 28, 1905.

THE X-RAYS AND STERILITY.

AFTER the preliminary period of extreme hopefulness concerning the beneficial therapeutic effects that might be expected from the X-rays following their original introduction, there has come such a decided reaction that we almost hesitate to credit the latest developments as to their possibilities for working insidious harm. We suggested editorially some weeks ago (see MEDICAL NEWS, January 7, 1905, page 31) in treating of the subject of the production of cancer in X-ray burns, that it must be constantly kept in mind that in this agent we have to deal with an extremely powerful physical energy, the knowledge of whose limitations is as yet only very vague and the possibilities of whose influence are quite beyond our ken. The X-rays have been a constant source of surprise, and the latest reported development is likely to add to this feeling.

At the last (January) meeting of the section on Genito-Urinary Diseases of the New York Academy of Medicine, a series of observations with regard to the sexual condition of physicians and patients who have been exposed to the X-rays was made by F. Tilden Brown, who makes the following communication to the MEDICAL NEWS:

" He had to announce that men by their mere presence in an X-ray atmosphere, incidental to radiography or the therapeutic uses of the rays, after a period of time—as yet undetermined—will be rendered sterile. In the last few days ten individuals who have devoted more or less time to the work during the past three years—none of whom have had any venereal disease or traumatism involving the genital tract—have been found to be the subjects of absolute azoospermia. None of the number are conscious, however, of any change or deterioration in regard to their potency."

This change had been brought about absolutely without any warning. There had been no sign of lack of sexual potency, or there probably would have been reports made along this line before, as it is only almost by accident that the present series of observations was begun. In one reported case a patient treated by the X-rays for pruritus ani was known to have active spermatozoa before exposure to the X-rays, but these disappeared after the treatment, and for several months no signs of spermatozoa could be found. There was, however, after some three months, a gradual return to the normal, and active spermatozoa could again be discovered.

This effect of the X-rays may seem surprising to those who are unfamiliar with some of the biological effects that have been known to occur as the result of the exposure of lower organisms of various kinds to the action of these radiations. Seeds, for instance, exposed for even a few hours to the action of the X-rays lose something of their ability to grow, and if planted alongside of control seeds which have not been exposed, the shoots to which they give rise may be readily picked out, because of the slowness with which they increase in size. On the other hand, exposure for a number of hours is likely to kill the seeds entirely. In general, the longer the exposure the more does the vitality of the seed suffer. Furthermore, a series of apparently sound observations have been made upon insects which usually undergo complete metamorphosis in their ordinary life cycle. If the larvæ of some beetles be exposed to the X-rays for a short time, they are not killed, but some curious vital change takes place in the tissues. The meal worm, for instance, will, after a certain number of days under ordinary circumstances become a beetle. After exposure to the X-rays, however, this normal metamorphosis does not take place, but the meal worm continues to live and eat and thrive without any tendency to go through the rest of its cycle of existence until death finally overtakes it. These " Methusalah " meal worms, as they have been called, will still be in the worm stage long after their brothers or sisters have passed through the beetle stage, laid eggs which in turn have become meal worms and then beetles, and so on for several generations.

With these facts in mind, it is not a matter for surprise that some serious influence should be exerted upon the reproductive tissues of human beings. It is of course extremely gratifying to learn that the change produced is probably not permanent. There must, however, be an uncomfortable feeling in those who have for a considerable period been indulging in the habit of using the X-rays freely. It seems not unlikely that carefully constructed protecting shields of metal may have to be invented and be constantly worn in order to prevent this unpleasant and undesirable consequence of a scientific application. In the meantime the observations made in New York will have to be confirmed in other parts of the country, and it may perhaps turn out that the question is not quite so serious as it seems to be at first sight. It is possible that some accidental circumstance has given rise to an unfortunate inference not quite justified by the actual circumstances in the cases, although the observations have apparently been made with great care and the report is not sensational, but, on the contrary, seems eminently conservative.

RECENT WORK IN CYSTINURIA.

SINCE Baumann and v. Udranszky first discovered the presence of putrescin and cadaverin in a cystinuric individual, the association of diaminuria with cystinuria has been repeatedly observed, and various attempts have been made to establish a casual relationship between the two conditions.

As diamins were then only known to be formed as the result of putrefactive changes the idea naturally suggested itself that the diaminuria might possibly be the expression of a specific intestinal mycosis, and that the cystinuria in turn was the outcome of an auto-intoxication referable to the intestinal infection. Against this hypothesis various objections have from time to time been raised. It was thus pointed out that putrescin and cadaverin are not always found together; that the quantity of diamins in the urine is sometimes much greater than the amount present in the feces; that one ptomain may be present in the urine, while the other is found in the stool. Cammidge and Garrod, moreover, were totally unable to isolate any diamins from bouillon cultures of micro-organisms which they had isolated from their patient's feces. Besides it has been conclusively established that diaminuria is not necessarily an accompaniment of cystinuria. Reasons enough therefore existed which could lead one to doubt the validity of Baumann's hypothesis.

A few years ago Simon pointed out another possible source of the ptomains. He indicated the close relationship which exists between arginin and putrescin, and suggested the possibility that the diamins in question might be derived from the body tissues. According to his ideas the diaminuria and cystinuria were merely correlated, and both the expression of a specific metabolic abnormality. This view was based upon the observations of Kossel and his pupils that the so-called bexon bases are essential components of the albuminous molecule and that arginin can be readily decomposed into urea and ornithin. This latter in turn could give rise to putrescin by loss of carbon dioxide. For cadaverin he similarly suggested lysin as a probable source. That putrescin and cadaverin may actually be derived from arginin and lysin respectively was then shown by Ellinger, who effected the transformation by means of putrefactive organisms. This of course furnished no proof that the same change could take place in the animal organism. It was rendered probable, however, by the observation of Emerson, who noted a fermentative splitting off of CO_2 in the case of tyrosin, during pancreatic autolysis, with the formation of oxyphenylethylamin.

But the strongest support of Simon's hypothesis has been recently furnished by Loewy and Neuberg. These observers have shown that following the ingestion of arginin and lysin by a cystinuric individual the corresponding diamins appear in the urine. The mechanism by which this transformation is effected has not as yet been worked out, but there can hardly be any doubt that ferment action is responsible for the process. Kossel has indeed shown that a ferment exists, which he terms arginase, and which is capable of effecting the cleavage of arginin into urea and ornithin.

In view of these facts the tissue origin of the urinary ptomains in cases of cystinuria can scarcely be doubted, and one of the numerous experimental problems which have suggested themselves in connection with the subject of cystinuria has thus found a satisfactory solution. Incidentally, however, additional problems have arisen, for Loewy and Neuberg have shown that the metabolic insufficiency in cystinuric individuals is not limited to the phenomena of cystinuria and diaminuria, but that it extends to still other components of the albuminous molecule. They were able to demonstrate the remarkable fact that the ingestion of some of the common mono-amido acids which result on proteolytic digestion of albumins, such as leucin, tyrosin and asparaginic acid, leads to the elimination of these bodies in the urine, while in the normal individual they are completely oxidized to carbon dioxide and ammonia; viz., urea. This seems the more remarkable, if we consider that the cystinuric patient does not eliminate such products under ordinary conditions, for barring the findings of Contí and Moreigne, which are probably referable to faulty technic, no amido acids have ever been encountered in the urine of such individuals.

Still another finding which was likewise not suspected is recorded by the same observers: Neuberg and Meyer had pointed out a little over a year ago that the cystin entering into the composition of cystin calculi is not identical with the cystin obtained on hydrolysis of albuminous material, and hence not with the cystin which is found in solution in the cystinuric urine. The products, however, are isomeric. The albuminous cystin is an α-amino-β thio propionic acid, while the calculus product is α-thio-β-amino propionic acid. This fact is in itself remarkable, if we consider that the calculus cystin is unquestionably of albuminous origin and primarily no doubt has its amino- and thio-groups in the same positions as in the albuminous product. Very curiously the cystinuric organism is capable of oxidizing this anomalous form of cystin just as well apparently as the normal individual can oxidize the albuminous product, while the latter is almost quantitatively eliminated by the cystinuric. We thus have an analogous condition to what is known to occur in diabetes, where the body is apparently quite well able to oxidize levulose, while dextrose escapes in the urine.

These various observations open up entirely new avenues of investigation into the general subject of metabolism, and lend still further interest to an already most interesting problem.

THE BECOMING NOTION OF PROTOPLASM.

WHILE various biologists are disputing more or less actively about the morphological structure of bioplasm, the physical basis of life, two sciences, physics and chemistry, not so distinct as formerly, are suggesting ideas as to its molecular composition or arrangement which, although vague as yet, have much interest. The reason for this better development of our knowledge of the ultra-visual structure over that of the formations which can be seen through the microscope lies both in the increasing facility in chemical analysis of at least the materials and the end-products of protoplasm and in the uncertainty of our present microscopical methods, which will seem very crude to the eyes of our children! Where something is vaguely seen, as in the nucleus of a nerve-cell, each man sees not what his eyes but what his brain perceives, and so each one sees more or less differently, but chemico-physically there is no seeing at all and one *guesses* at how that which he knows is present is arranged! Perhaps there is not much to choose between the products of these two methods after all. But at any rate our present topic is the probable structure of the molecule or unit-cluster of protoplasm without reference to the morphological theories. In lieu of facts a plausible and likely hypothesis often underlies not only knowledge but real scientific progress.

It is only necessary to suggest the quite unlimited latencies inherent in a human male pronucleus or even in an entire ovum to prove that protoplasm, whatever its molecular plan, is the most marvelous of substances this cooling whirl of burning matter has so far evolved. Only the biochemist endowed with an imagination really appreciates its unique complexity, and he only vaguely from recently gained knowledge as to the metabolic processes which occur within it.

The unit-cluster of protoplasm may apparently be conceived as a group composed of molecules of proteid, fat, carbohydrate, water, and salts, elsewhere called inorganic, arranged in some sort of characteristic relation to each other. Proteid molecules consist of from two or three hundred to two thousand or so atoms according to its variety, these being atoms of carbon, hydrogen, oxygen, nitrogen and sulphur, and oftentimes of phosphorus in addition. How these many hundreds of atoms are grouped is quite unknown, but loosely at all events, so that the instability of the substance is extreme, and in some way or other quite characteristic of life, for while living biogen is protoplasm surely enough, dead biogen is only lean meat, a very different substance chemically. This proteid molecule, huge and loosely built, with a host of interactions ever going on within itself, forms apparently the nucleus of the protoplasmic unit-cluster, and by far its greater mass.

The relation of the molecules of water to the proteid molecule is much in doubt, yet it constitutes an average of three-quarters of different sorts of differentiated protoplasm. Whether the aquatic groups of atoms are part and parcel of the proteid group or only in relation to it is still unknown. As for the so-called inorganic salts (a misnomer, since here they are organic in the extreme), there is still less knowledge, for we do not know even exactly what the salts are. Again, whether they are arranged as molecules or as dissociated ions is uncertain, the recent presumptions being, however, in favor of the ions. Whether these atoms are in relation with elements of the proteid and the water is another problem to be solved. Calcium, sodium, and iron seem to be always present, as well as potassium, magnesium, and chlorine, while excellent French chemists as well as work done in America go to prove that arsenic is an invariable constituent of biogen.

As for the fat and carbohydrate there is now little doubt that both are present in small amounts in every particle of (living) protoplasm, but whether in constant varieties or in variable forms, whether lecithin for example is always concerned, is again uncertain. But these in themselves are highly complex bodies, consisting of very many atoms, and their relations to the proteid ''molecule,'' to the inorganic salts, and to the water, form at present subject for much all too idle speculation.

Whatever the exact interconnections of all these in themselves highly complex groups of atoms, one fact is tolerably patent and of great importance, namely, that they all, and probably their constituents in turn, are endlessly in the most intricate of interaction, and that not only intrinsically but extrinsically, with the more or less similar groups of substances or of atoms brought to them as nutriment. This self-adjusting system of intrinsic and extrinsic interaction constitutes metabolism, destructive and constructive.

But the depths of this living matter are not yet reached! No longer can we say and try to believe that the perhaps thousands of atoms of more than a dozen sorts, which must group themselves so almost fantastically to produce a single unit-cluster of protoplasm, are spherical masses of something we call ''matter'' all of the same size but of different weights. Nor can we claim, as

most scientists would have claimed a few years ago, that all these multiform interactions are conducted on the strictest principle of the conservation of energy, once bulwark of all our reckonings. To discuss shape in relation to the ultimate unit of ''matter'' is already out of the fitness of recent things, and we must substitute for the imaginable atom something of the nature of a vortex of forces, or of a force with protean aspects to our phenomenalizing senses. And while the conservation of energy probably is valid for material reactions generally, the notion has certainly lost its former air of certainty and reliability since radio-activity upset the ancient law. It will trouble a man to say where the exception does *not* come, it will trouble the biologist especially to demonstrate that no exception to the law holds sway within his own domain in the stupendous '' continual adjustment'' we designate as life, the ceaseless interactions within and between the most intricate structures man's knowledge has so far bid him imagine.

ECHOES AND NEWS.

NEW YORK.

New York Skin and Cancer Hospital.—Dr. Bulkley's usual clinical lecture at the New York Skin and Cancer Hospital will be replaced on Wednesday, February 1, by a lecture by Dr. Boleslaw Lapowski, on the '' Treatment of Syphilis,'' and on Wednesday, February 8, by a lecture by Dr. Charles Mallory Williams on the '' Treatment of Acne.''

Medical Society of the County of New York.—At a stated meeting of this Society, held December 27, 1904, the following resolution was *unanimously* adopted: '' That in any directory or list other than a medical one, it is undesirable that any data should appear other than the name, address and telephone number, and that the use of more prominent type for one name than another, is to be severly deprecated.''

Century Mark for Wm. Wood & Co.—Few publishing houses in this country can boast a century of existence. In an interesting brochure before us, Messrs. William Wood & Company, of New York, trace the history of their establishment from 1804, when it was founded by Mr. Samuel Wood, to the present time, the firm now consisting of the founder's grandson, Mr. William H. S. Wood, and his three sons. During this period many monumental works have been published by them, notably Ziemssen's '' Cyclopedia of the Practice of Medicine,'' in twenty-two royal octavo volumes, and the '' Twentieth Century Practice of Medicine,'' in twenty volumes, edited by Dr. T. L. Stedman, completed in 1901. The little brochure is published with portraits of the founder and subsequent members of the firm, affording an interesting comparison in costume and personal appearance between 1804 and 1904.

Appointment of Dr. Farrand.—Dr. Livingston Farrand, professor of anthropology at Columbia University, has been named as head fo the National Association for the Study and Prevention of Tuberculosis. In making the announcement, *Charities* describes the appointment as signal evidence of the draft which the greater social movements of the day are making upon the largest resources of the universities. Dr. Farrand is at present an authority on the American Indian. As assistant curator of the American Museum of Natural History, New York, he was associated with Franz Boas in 1897 in organizing the famous Jesup North Pole Expedition, which made a study of the earliest peoples in Northwestern America and Eastern Asia. Prof. Farrand has been secretary of the Psychological Association since 1896, president of the American Folklore Society, recording secretary of the American Ethnological Society, and a member of the American Society of Naturalists, American Society for the Advancement of Science, the Washington Academy of Science, the American Anthropological Association, and the New York Academy of Science.

State Charities Report.—The annual report of the State Board of Charities, made public last week, contains recommendations for general legislation and for specific appropriations for the State charitable and reformatory institutions subject to the visitation and inspection of the State Board of Charities. After giving a list of the fourteen State charitable institutions which are subject to the visitation and inspection of the board, the report says: The board desires to renew the following recommendations for legislation: (1) That all the special appropriations to enlarge or improve the State institutions within the jurisdiction of the board be included in one bill, with such provisions as will insure in every instance the most careful and economical expenditure of the moneys appropriated, in exact accordance with the intentions of the legislature. (2) That the House of Refuge on Randall's Island be reorganized as a State institution with managers appointed by the governor and confirmed by the Senate. The board also recommends that the appointment of employees at this institution be made in accordance with the rules of the State Civil Service, if practicable. (3) That the State Custodial Asylum for Feeble-Minded Women at Newark and the Rome State Custodial Asylum at Rome be enlarged so as to enable them to receive all the feeble-minded and idiotic persons now retained in almshouses contrary to the provisions of the Poor law and the Penal Code, or provided for in private institutions at greatly enlarged cost to the various counties, cities, and towns of the State, and the adult feeble-minded now improperly retained at the Syracuse State Institution for Feeble-Minded Children.

Sydenham Hospital.—The newly elected Board of Directors of the Sydenham Hospital, located on East One Hundred and Sixteenth Street, has just received, for hospital purposes as, a New Year gift, from Isaac Guggenheim, the Treasurer of the American Smelting & Refining Company, $1,000. Mr. Guggenheim has also made a generous offer to further aid the hospital and its training school by giving monthly an amount of money equal to such sums as the Board of Directors succeed in raising each month, through donations or voluntary contributions. This offer holds good up to the sum of $10,-000 a year, should the directors raise a like amount. The recent benefit entertainment at the New York Theater netted the sum of $1,500 for the Sydenham Hospital. Announcement of Mr. Guggenheim's liberal offer and also the result of the theatrical benefit was made known to the Sydenham Directors at their

meeting last Monday evening. The Sydenham Hospital was started two years ago and has been very successful. At first only one building was used for its dispensary, but the work and the needs of the hospital grew so very rapidly that to-day three buildings are thoroughly equipped for this purpose. After May next, the two adjoining buildings will be added to the hospital plant in order to provide more room for nurses and private patients, and when complete the hospital will occupy five buildings, Nos. 339 to 347 East One Hundred and Sixteenth Street. The last report of the hospital shows that more than ten thousand treatments were given at the hospital dispensary during the past year, and six thousand hospital days were free in the hospital. The congested population in this part of the city has attracted the attention of Mr. Guggenheim and other members of the Board to the absolute necessity of an institution of this character in this quarter of the city, and for this reason Mr. Guggenheim's munificent gift is gratefully received by the hospital, and the directors are now hard at work attempting to raise sufficient funds to take advantage of Mr. Guggenheim's offer. William I. Spiegelberg, a son-in-law of Isaac Guggenheim, is President of the hospital. Lewis M. Bloomingdale, of 78 Fifth Avenue, is the Treasurer and Sanford Simons is Secretary. Among the Directors are Joseph P. Day, who is Vice-president; Samuel Strasbourger, Isaac Guggenheim, N. Taylor Philips and William Bretter.

Does Medical Education Deserve Recognition—In reply to this question the New York *Sun* honors itself and the profession in the following editorial comment from a recent issue:

"Medical science gave vaccination to mankind. This single discovery has caused practically to disappear from the earth one of the greatest scourges of the human race. It has saved countless millions of human beings from the sufferings of a most loathsome disease, which killed the majority of those attacked and left those who recovered from it disfigured for life.

"Within recent years, by the discovery of the source of infection in yellow fever, it has removed from the list of epidemics this dread disease, which formerly spread death and disaster in its tracks, closed our great shipping ports for months at a time, and in addition to the awful suffering and sacrifice of life caused the loss of millions of dollars to the commercial interests of the world.

"In the discovery of the germ theory of disease, if viewed only in its application to one single malady, diphtheria, formerly so destructive to children, now not only preventable, but when acquired curable practically in all cases by the simple injection under the skin of Behring's serum, medical science gave to mankind something of a value which cannot be estimated in dollars and cents. In the logical development of this theory the best minds of the profession believe that the time is not far distant when every disease will be subject to serum therapy.

"In surgery the demonstration of the aseptic and antiseptic method has done as much as vaccination in the amelioration of suffering and the prolongation of life. The operation of ovariotomy and the abdominal operations in both sexes which followed McDowell's initiative and the development of the science of gynecology due to the genius of Marion Sims have added millions of years to the sum of life and saved hundreds of thousands of human beings from untimely death.

" These are but a few examples of what medical science has done for mankind. They are the fruits of a higher and broadening education.

" Last month we expressed regret that the city of New York was not the medical center of the United States; that in spite of its vast preponderance in population and its financial standing as the first city of the Western Hemisphere it was outstripped by two or three cities of smaller size; for the reason that they, through their State or·municipal Governments, or by the aid of wealthy philanthropists, gave largely to the support of medical schools.

" At that time, writing on the practical education of graduates in medicine, we submitted a synopsis of an address by the president of the medical faculty of one of our educational institutions, the New York Polyclinic Medical School and Hospital, showing the work done by that institution for the twenty-two years of its existence, and concluding with the expressed conviction that such an institution deserved recognition by this community and perpetuation by endowment. We are glad to know that since the appearance of that article there seems to be an awakening interest in medical education in New York, and that this institution has just received substantial contributions from different sources which have enabled it almost entirely to cancel in so short a space of time a large mortgaged indebtedness.

" One of the contributors, a business man of large affairs, thoroughly acquainted with the management of the Polyclinic, referring to the president's report, said:

" ' The extraordinary record you were able on that occasion to lay before us, showing the results of the years of effort devoted by you and the medical staff so unselfishly to this noble and beneficent plan for giving the most arvanced medical and surgical teaching and clinical demonstration to physicians unable otherwise to obtain such practical instruction, together with the benefits of the very best treatment and care gratuitously given those of the sick and helpless poor, should prove beyond all question the usefulness of such a combined school and hospital and its just claims for the consideration and aid of all interested in the higher education and training of the members of the medical profession.'

" When we bear in mind what medicine has done for the world we may wonder that in the absence of individual philanthropy our State and municipal Governments have not long since discovered that medical education deserves a wider recognition."

Medical Society of the State of New York.—The Ninety-ninth Annual Meeting of this society will be held at the City Hall, in Albany, January 31, February 1, 2, 1905. After the President's Inaugural Address, and the customary reports of the several committees the following papers will be read and discussed: Dermatitis Seborrhoica and its Relation to Alopecia, and other Conditions, by L. Duncan Bulkley, of New York; To What Extent are Cycloplegics Necessary in Determining the Refraction of the Eye and in the Prescribing of Lenses, by Frank Van Fleet, of New York; Rheumatism and the Eye Muscles, by Francis Valk, of New York; Loss of Vision from Disuse of the Eye (Amblyopia ex Anopsia), by D. B. St. John Roosa, of New York; The Simulation of Appendicitis by Cholelithiasis, by George G. Lempe, of Albany; Biliary Drainage in Operations on the Gall Bladder and Biliary Ducts, by Eugene A. Smith, of Buffalo; Report of a Case of

Vasomotor Disturbance Caused by Exposure to Sunlight, by Samuel B. Ward, of Albany; Report of a Case of Angioneurotic Edema, by Clayton K. Haskell, of Bath; The Status of Suprarenal Therapy, by Samuel Floersheim, of New York; Aortitis, by Thomas E. Satterthwaite, of New York; The Antitoxin Laboratory, by Herbert D. Pease, of Albany; Recognition of Incipient Pulmonary Tuberculosis, by John H. Pryor, of Ray Brook, Essex Co.; Phosphaturia, by James Pederson, of New York; Pathology and Bacteriology of Cerebrospinal Meningitis, by W. T. Councilman, of Boston; Symptomatology and Diagnosis, by· H. L. Elsner, of Syracuse; The History of Cerebrospinal Meningitis in America, by Abraham Jacobi, of New York; The Treatment of Cerebrospinal Meningitis, by C. G. Stockton, of Buffalo; The Eye Symptoms of Cerebrospinal Meningitis, by A. E. Davis, of New York; Address, by Dr. Charles Harrington, Secretary State Board of Health of Massachusetts, of Boston, Mass; President's Address, by Hamilton D. Wey, of Elmira; The Correction of Nasal Deformities by Subcutaneous Operation, by John O. Roe, of Rochester; The Middle Turbinate in Diseases of the Accessory Sinuses, by W. J. Stucky, of Lexington, Ky.; Inferior Turbinated Bone, its Function, Diseases and Treatment, by Wendell C. Phillips, of New York; Treatment of Chronic Otitis Media, with Illustrative Cases, by W. Sohier Bryant, of New York; The Family Physician, by Robert P. Bush, of Horseheads; The Various Methods of Opening the Skull for the Removal of Tumors of the Brain, by Charles H. Frazier, of Philadelphia; Railway Spine, by Edward B. Angell, of Rochester; Report of two cases of Gastrectomy, with exhibition of patients, by Willis G. Macdonald, of Albany; The Relation of Pelvic Conditions to Nervous Disorders, by A. L. Beahan, of Canandaigua; The Non-Sequitur in Medicine, by H. A. Fairbairn, of Brooklyn; Poisoning by Potassium Bichromate, by Francis Eustace Fronczak, of Buffalo; The Etiology of Hypertrophied Prostate, by L. Bolton Bangs, New York; Some Observations on the Technic of Perineal Prostatectomy, by George R. Fowler, Brooklyn; Personal Experience in Prostatic Surgery during the Last Two Years, by Willy Meyer, New York; Suprapubic Prostatectomy, by Howard Lilienthal, New York; Prostatism, without Prostatic Enlargement, its Diagnosis and Treatment, by Charles H. Chetwood, New York; Has the Catheter a Place in the Treatment of Chronic Prostatic Hypertrophy, by Paul Thorndike, of Boston; Conservative Perineal Prostatectomy; Results of Two Years' Experience, by Hugh H. Young, of Baltimore; A Paper (title to be announced), by Francis S. Watson, of Boston; Concerning the Treatment of Infantile Marasmus, by Heinrich Stern, of New York; Researches on the Blood of Epileptics, by B. Onuf and Horace L. Grasse, of Sonyea; Three Unusual Cases of Aneurism, by W. C. Krauss, of Buffalo; A Few Thoughts Regarding Our Work, by H. A. Gates, of Delhi; A Case of, Extensive Carcinoma of Tongue and Neck, Presenting Points of Special Interest, by William Seaman Bainbridge, of New York; Prophylaxis in Pregnancy and Labor, by T. Avery Rogers, of Plattsburgh.

PHILADELPHIA.

Medical Notes and Queries.—This is the title of a new periodical to be issued ten times a year for $1.00. It is edited by Dr. Henry W. Cattell, of Philadelphia, and is to be devoted to the " practical side of medicine but from a scientific standpoint." May success crown the editor's efforts is our hearty wish.

Teachers Institute Postponed.—Owing to an epidemic of scarlet fever in the vicinity the local teacher's institute, which embraces Worcester, Perkiomen, Skippack township and Schwenksville borough, had to be postponed until next March. The outbreak occurred in the Sholl School, which has been quarantined.

To Prevent the Use of Poisonous Embalming Fluids.—District Attorney Bell and Coroner Dugan are preparing a bill to be introduced into the legislature making it illegal for undertakers to use poisonous fluids for embalming. They say such a measure would do away with the defense usually put up in murder trials where poisoning is suspected.

Charitable Bequests.—The executors of the estate of Selina Walker will distribute in accordance with the adjudication of the estate which has been made by Judge Hanna, of the Orphan's Court, the following: Jewish Foster Home and Orphan Asylum, $9,965.64; Jewish Hospital Association, $7,286.73; United Hebrew Charities, $7,286.73; and Jewis Maternity Hospital, $2,428.90.

Fear an Epidemic of Disease.—The residents of the suburbs and outlying sections of the city are circulating a petition to call the attention of the Bureau of Street Cleaning to the fact that in some of the suburbs the streets have not been cleaned since December 1, 1904, and that the garbage has been collected but twice in three months. Because of the foul odors emitted from the decaying material the residents fear the outbreak of disease.

Children's Homeopathic Hospital.—At the twenty-seventh annual meeting of this hospital corporation Alfred E. Burk was elected President, Dr. Augustus Korndörfer Vice-president, Dr. Walter Strang Secretary, and Joseph Clark, Treasurer. In order to meet the increasing demand for room, plans were formulated to build a new north wing to the hospital. Last year 22,464 patients were treated in all the departments at a total expense of $46,991.01.

Resigned.—At a meeting of the Board of Managers of the Wistar Institute the resignation of Dr. Horace Jayne was unanimously accepted. The Board of Managers were reluctant to take the step, but they agreed with Dr. Jayne that the resources of the institution were insufficient to pay his salary. Dr. Milton J. Greenman was elected to fill the position of director. The position of assistant director will be abolished, which will cut down the expenses $5,000 a year.

New Hospital Quarters.—To meet their increasing needs St. Luke's Homeopathic Hospital bought the home of Dr. John B. Mayer, at the corner of Broad and Wingohocken streets, and transformed it into a hospital. The opening was attended by many physicians, visitors and members of the Board of Trustees. In the new hospital there are eight beds in the male ward, six in the female, six in the children's, five in the male private ward and five in the female private ward. In the accident room three beds are provided.

Appropriations.—The State Board of Charities will send to the legislature its biennial report recommending $9,406,923.75 to be appropriated to State, semi-State and private institutions in Pennsylvania, for the years 1905-6. Of this amount $7,227,804.10 shall be applied for maintenance and $2,179,119.65 for buildings. The board suggest that if the State finances should not warrant the appropriations of the various amounts recommended, their reduction should be made proportionately and the State

institutions and the items of maintenance should be given preference.

Radium in the Sun.—In a paper read before the American Philosophical Society Prof. Snyder, of the Philadelphia Observatory, announces that his experiments with the spectroscope upon the sun, stars and nebula have shown that all these bodies contain radium and that the presence of this element accounts for many heretofore inexplicable phenomena of the heavens, particularly in the sun as the origin of celestial energy. He was inspired to his investigation by discovering that the spectrum lines of radium were identical with the spectrum lines of the corona of the sun and later of the stellar nebulæ.

Appointments.—William B. Hackenburg, president of the Jewish Hospital, announced the following appointments: Dr. Charles P. Noble, consulting surgeon; Dr. Lawrence F. Flick, consulting physician; Dr. William H. Randle, obstetrician; Dr. J. B. Potsdamer, pediatrist; Dr. Sidney L. Feldstein, radiologist. A number of resident physicians have been added to the staff. Dr. Francis D. Patterson has been elected surgeon to the Howard Hospital to fill the vacancy caused by the resignation of Dr. Charles H. Frazier. Mr. H. H. Meller has been elected secretary to the Medical Faculty of the University of Pennsylvania.

Medico-Chirurgical Alumni.—At the meeting of this almuni the following officers were elected: President, William L. Shindle, M.D.; Secretary, Stillwell C. Burns, M.D.; Treasurer, Emanuel S. Gans, M.D.; Executive Committee, Drs. W. E. Ashton, A. E. Blackburn, A. C. Buckley, L. N. Boston, J. A. Cramp, J. W. Croskey, M. P. Dickson, J. H. Egan, L. Webster Fox, Andrew Godfrey, C. H. Gubbins, S. L. Gans, A. W. Hammer, W. F. Hähnlen, J. A. McKenna, G. W. Pfromm, J. V. C. Roberts, H. J. Smith, J. V. Schoemaker, M. P. Warmuth, J. W. Wilkins, J. L. Widmyer.

Phipps Institute Course of Lectures.—Dr. A. P. Francine delivered an illustrated lecture on the "Care and Treatment of Consumptive Patients" to the Pittsburg Nurses' Association last week. Dr. D. J. McCarthy spoke on the subject of tuberculosis at the Deaconesses' Home, 611 Vine Street, January 23. Dr. Horace Carncross gave an illustrated lecture to the Glassblowers' Union of New Jersey, at Woodbury, January 27, and upon the following evening Dr. Ward delivered a lecture to the textile workers upon the "Prevention and Home Treatment of Tuberculosis." On the evening of February 2 Dr. D. J. McCarthy will speak upon the general subject of tuberculosis.

Tuberculosis in Pennsylvania.—The following resolutions were adopted by the Philadelphia County Medical Society at a business meeting held January 18, 1905:

WHEREAS, The State of Pennsylvania has not, up to the present time, provided adequate accommodation for the care and treatment of its tuberculous sick; and

Whereas, The plans now in projection throughout the State, even when succesfully executed, will provide for but a mere fraction of the number of those who need skilful care and medical direction, both for the saving of their lives and the protection of the community; and

Whereas, Experience has shown that by properly directed open air treatment the great majority of cases of incipient tuberculosis can be permanently cured, and that a large percentage of the daily new infections can be avoided if such patients are removed from close association with others not yet infected; be it

RESOLVED, That the Philadelphia County Medical Society does hereby petition the Legislature of the State of Pennsylvania; (1) for the appropriation of a certain sum of money, not less than $500,000 to be devoted to the establishment of camps, sanatoria, hospitals and dispensaries, for the tuberculous sick of the commonwealth of Pennsylvania; (2) for the setting aside of such portions of the State Forestry Reserve as may be recommended with a view to accommodate camps and buildings such as may be deemed necessary for the care of tuberculous patients, and for their scientific study and treatment, further, be it

Resolved, That the President of this Society be authorized and instructed to appoint a committee of three from the membership of the Society, to cooperate with similar committees that may be appointed from other societies in urging upon the legislature the need of State aid in the suppression of tuberculosis.

Single Service Paper Milk Bottle.—When informed that a paper milk bottle was placed upon the market A. H. Stewart, of the Bacteriological Department, Philadelphia Bureau of Health, obtained several bottles to determine their efficiency. The bottles are made in three sizes, quart, pint and half-pint; they are conical in shape and made of heavy spruce wood fiber of three-ply thickness. The bottom is made of heavy pasteboard and the edges are so locked that pressure upon the upper or upon the under surface merely serves to lock it more tightly in position. A downward pressure of two hundred pounds is not sufficient to collapse the bottle. The lid is made of heavy pasteboard and fits in the lumen of the bottle by a surface contact of about one-half inch, with protruding lips, to enable its ready removal. The bottles are placed in paraffin bath at 100 C. for one-half minute and then transferred to a hot chamber which removes the excess of the paraffin and facilitates penetration. The paraffin coating strengthens the bottle, prevents the imparting of the woody taste to the milk and also sterilizes it. He placed 25 c.c. of sterile water in several bottles, shook them thoroughly and then allowed them to stand for one-half hour when plates were inoculated from the water but no colonies developed. He then sent closed glass and paper bottles to several dairies in the city. When the milk was received at the laboratory the glass bottles invariable showed slight evidence of leakage while the paper bottles did not. The bacteriological examination of the sets showed that the milk in the paper bottles contained about one-fourth as many bacteria as the glass bottles. The milk was also found to remain sweet longer in the paper bottles than in the glass. The paper bottles can be made for about one cent a piece, so that after they have been used once they can be thrown away without materially adding to the cost of the milk. By so doing there is less danger of carrying disease.

CHICAGO.

Dr. Christopher Improving.—Dr. Walter S. Christopher, the eminent pediatrician, who, for several months, has been seriously ill, is reported to be improving rapidly, and hopes are entertained for his recovery.

Hospital for Oak Park.—A $100,000 hospital has been projected for Oak Park. Subscriptions will not be opened until the architects finish their plans and take bids. The incorporated hospital association has selected a six acre site.

New Medical Ward at County Hospital.—A new medical ward, with 100 beds, will soon be opened at the County Hospital as a result of the action by the public service committee. This committee concurred in the

report of the hospital committee that the old ward for contagious diseases at the County Hospital be changed to a medical ward. The contagious disease patients are now taken to the new hospital for contagious diseases. The alterations will cost about $4,000.

Exiled from Glen Ellyn.—Dr. O. E. Miller, owner and manager of Ruskin "University," and reputed proprietor and head physician of a sanitarium for the cure of inebriates and drug victims, has been ejected from the village of Glen Ellyn. He appeared before Justice J. F. Higley recently to answer charges brought against him by the village board of running an institution in violation of the village ordinance. He pleaded guilty and was fined $100, and given ten days in which to close the affairs of the "university," and leave the place.

Passavant Hospital Improvements.—To enlarge the institution, the Passavant Hospital Auxiliary Association has been incorporated, with James H. Eckels, President; Arthur L. Farwell, Treasurer; Arthur B. Wells, Secretary. The first gift to the new association is the lot and building to the west of the present hospital, which was given by O. B. Green. As soon as the building can be remodeled it will be used for hospital purposes. The new association hopes to raise $50,000 with which to build an addition to the present main building.

Hospitals in Residence Districts.—After full consideration, the City Council Health Committee has voted against recommending the ordinance permitting the construction of a free hospital in the block facing Washington Park, between Fifty-third and Fifty-fourth streets. The institution in question is designed for the treatment of contagious diseases of children. Under the ordinance now in effect the projectors of the hospital are required to secure a majority of the frontage consents, not only on the four sides of the block involved, but on the four sides of the four blocks adjacent. The ordinance upon which the health committee has just taken action proposed to amend this measure so as to require only the frontage consents representing the four sides of the block involved. The Chicago Daily Tribune remarks that "The hospital project in question is a most worthy philanthropy, deserving of hearty support. To place such an institution in a residence neighborhood, however, depriving the people living near it in large measure of their right to a voice in the matter, is contrary to public interests and to the principle of home rule in neighborhood affairs."

Illinois State Association for the Prevention of Tuberculosis.—This Association was organized permanently on the evening of January 19, marking the beginning of a new era in fighting tuberculosis. The general object of the association is to prevent the prevalence of consumption and other forms of tuberculosis in Illinois. Two specific objects are admittedly in the minds of those who are most prominently affiliated with it—to obtain from the legislature an appropriation of $250,000 with which to build a State sanitarium, and the enactment of a law compelling the registration of all tuberculosis sufferers in the State. The following officers were elected: Honorary President, the Governor of Illinois; President, Edmund J. James, President of the University of Illinois; Treasurer, James H. Eckels; Secretary, Dr. Arnold C. Klebs; Legal Adviser, Charles H. Hamill; Executive Committee, E. P. Bicknell, Dr. Wm. E. Quine, Dr. J. W. Pettit, Dr. Geo. W. Webster, and Sherman C. Kingsley; Central Committee, Dr. Wm. E. Quine, Dr. Frank Billings, Dr. N. S. Davis, Dr. E. P. Bicknell, Dr. Joseph E. Milligan, Dr. N. B. Delamater, Dr. N. H. Graves, Dr. Geo. W. Webster, Dr. W. A. Evans, and Dr. Robert Babcock. Any city or county interested in the combating of tuberculosis may be affiliated with the association upon application to the Central Council. The dues are $1 annually. The organization of the association was inspired by the Visiting Nurses' Association, under the direction of Dr. Arnold C. Klebs. A meeting of representatives of the various medical and philanthropic societies of the State was held a month ago at the Great Northern Hotel, and the committee appointed which drew up the Constitution and By-Laws accepted at the meeting of January 19.

GENERAL.

Monument to Virchow.—The city of Berlin offers three prizes for the best plans for a monument to the late Professor Virchow. It is to be placed at the intersection of Karl and Louisen streets, a square which will henceforth be known as Virchow Platz.

Yellow Fever in Panama.—Yellow fever is gaining hold in Panama in spite of hard efforts to check it. The public health report on January 21, shows seven cases in December and three new ones from January 1 to 10. One death only is reported since December 1. Havana reports three cases and two recent deaths.

American Physiological Society.—The newly elected officers of the American Physiological Society are: President, Prof. Wm. H. Howell, of Johns Hopkins University; Secretary, Prof. Lafayette B. Mendel, of Yale University; Treasurer, Prof. Walter B. Cannon, of Harvard University. Additional members of the council are Prof. R. H. Chittenden and Dr. S. J. Meltzer.

Quarterly Publication on Children.—Under the title of *Eos* a new quarterly periodical dealing with the recognition and treatment of abnormal children and adolescents is published in Vienna by A. Pichler's Wittwe und Sohn. The editors are Drs. M. Brunner and S. Krenberger, Director Mell and Director Dr. Schloss. The first number contains, among other original communications, a paper on the soul of the deaf and dumb child by Dr. Brunner, and one on the mental life of a blind person by Luigi Ansaldi.

Hare's Practice of Medicine.—Messrs. Lea Brothers & Co. announce for early publication a completely new work which will be welcomed by every practitioner, teacher and student. Hare's Practice of Medicine, a text-book of the practice of medicine for students and practitioners. As the student of to-day is the physician of the future, and as the physician must always be a student, a single volume can be conceived as answering the requirements both of a text-book and work of reference. To produce such a volume the author has brought to bear his experience of twenty years of active hospital and private practice, during which period he has been constantly engaged in teaching the subjects of clinical medicine and therapeutics. This didactic work has enabled him to understand the difficulties which confront the student and to present the principles and data with the utmost clearness. The book has purposely been given a clinical character. For this reason illustrations and plates have been introduced wherever an important point could be made more clear than by verbal description.

Methods of Antivivisectionists in London.—Mr. Edgard Speyer, the chairman of the Nervous Disease Research Fund, which carries on its work in the National Hospital for the Paralyzed and Epileptic, having been asked by the Hon. Stephen Coleridge, on behalf of the National Anti-Vivisection Society, whether his researches involve experiments on living animals, has sent the following reply: "Dear Sir,—As you

are already aware, the National Hospital is not a place licensed under the Act for experiments on living animals. I am informed, nevertheless, that your society endeavored to prevent subscriptions being sent to it on the ground that some members of the medical staff, in their private capacities, are licensed under the Act. The Nervous Disease Research Fund is an endeavor to provide funds for research into the origin and cure of those diseases. It will be conducted in the hospital under the advice of the medical staff. That being so, your past treatment of the hospital shows that it has nothing to expect from your society in the way of support. As this removes the only *locus standi* you might otherwise have to interfere, I do not think it necessary to enter further into the subject of your letter. Yours truly, Edgar Speyer. December 14, 1904."

Increase of Insanity in Connecticut.—The annual report of the superintendent of the Connecticut Hospital for the Insane shows that there were 2,259 patients in the institution for the year ending September 30, 1904. "It is unwise," says the superintendent, H. S. Noble, "to attempt longer to blind our eyes to the fact that all recent statistics bear witness to a large increase in insanity. It is a fact easily verified by a glance at the statistics of the State, that the foreign element of our commonwealth shows a much larger proportion of insanity than prevails among the native born. Although the native insane have increased, to some extent, they have not done so in any such proportion as is apparent among the foreign elements. In 1900 the foreign-born population of the State comprised 26 per cent. of the entire number. From 1898 to 1902, four years, 38 per cent. of the admissions to the hospital were of foreign birth and parentage. In other words, the 26 per cent. of foreign population furnished 38 per cent. of insane during those four years. Why the emigrant population should be especially prone to mental alienation cannot be discussed here; it may be remarked, however, that in most European countries, the former homes of our adopted citizens, the ratio of insane to the general population is higher than it is in this country."

Hongkong College of Medicine for Chinese.—We have received, writes the *British Medical Journal*, a remarkable and—from the point of view of human progress—even inspiring document in the calendar of the Hongkong College of Medicine for Chinese, in which is set forth how it was founded in 1887, largely through the efforts and enthusiasm of Sir Patrick Manson, Dr. James Cantlie (the earlier Deans of the College), the late Rev. Dr. Chalmers, and the late Dr. William Young. The College has its headquarters in the Alice Memorial Hospital, Hongkong, and the affiliated Nethersole Hospital is also open to students for purposes of clinical instruction. The Rector, who is the President of the Governing Court of the College, is Hon. Francis H. May, C.M.G., Colonial Secretary, and its present Dean, the third in the succession, is Dr. Francis W. Clark. Up to 1904, 87 students had been enrolled, of whom 28 had retired, 40 were engaged in study at various stages of the curriculum and 19 had passed all the examinations, had been certified fit to practice their profession, and were granted the title of Licentiate in Medicine and Surgery (L.M.S.H). The list of their names begins with Sun Yat Sen, Japan, and ends with Peter Quincey, Shanghai. The minimum period of study is five years, and all professional examinations are conducted by independent examiners appointed by the Senate, who, as a rule, have no other connection with the College. Candidates are required, after having passed a matriculation examination, to have attended courses of instruction in all, or almost all, the recognized subjects for the home degrees, including tropical diseases and infective fevers. During 1905 four medical scholarships are open for competition among the members of the school. It is not too much to say, on the strength of such a record alone, and assuming for the nonce the prophetic rôle, that the so-called Yellow Peril, if such there be, is growing beautifully less.

Our Immigrants not so Bad.—Dr. Allan McLaughlan, who is in the United States Public Health and Marine Hospital Service, at Washington, contributes to the January *Popular Science Monthly* a paper which cuts to the quick the fallacies of that large class who make of our foreign immigrants a scapegoat for a preponderant share of our social and political evils. From ten countries named, the percentage of illiteracy among our immigrants is but about one-third of our own general average. The native children of foreign-born parents, taking the whole foreign-born population as the basis, present but about one-eighth the percentage of illiteracy found in their parents; proving that our illiterate immigrants are quick to take advantage of the opportunity of education for their children. Indeed, the native children of foreign parentage make a better showing in this respect than the children of native white parentage; statistics of school attendance give a better record to foreign-born white children and native white children of foreign parentage than to native white children of native parentage. The charge of clannishness, and consequent lack of assimilation, of the more ignorant immigrants Dr. McLaughlan rejects, so far as it is regarded as a fault peculiar to them. "The Italian, or the Jew, or the Slav, do not shrink away from their American neighbors more than their American neighbors shrink from them." The apparent excess of criminals in our foreign-born population does not mean what it seems to mean at first sight. The vast majority of crimes among any people are committed by members of the male sex between the ages of twenty and forty-five years. Now seventy-five per cent. of our immigrants are between the ages of fifteen and forty on arrival, and the males are to the females as two and one-half to one. In view of these facts, the usual comparison with our entire population in the matter of criminality is manifestly unjust. The responsibility for the "slum," often charged to the immigrant, lies with money-grasping property-owners and incompetent civic administrations; the immigrant is its victim, not its parent. Naturalization frauds and kindred ills are simply our own sins, taking advantage of whatever promising material immigration may offer.

OBITUARY.

Dr. OTIS EUGENE HUNT, of Newtonville, Mass., died last week. He was born in Sudbury, in 1822. He was graduated at Berkshire Medical College in 1848 and continued in active practice until 1885.

Dr. CORNELIUS J. DUMOND died at his home in West Forty-second Street, New York, on January 21. He was sixty-eight years old, and had been in active practice forty-two years. He was a member of the Holland Society.

Dr. ODELIA BLINN, a pioneer among the women physicians of Chicago, died in that city January 21. She was sixty years old. Dr. Blinn was a graduate of the Women's Medical College of Philadelphia, and came to Chicago about the time of the great fire. She was the first person to advocate free public baths. Dr. Blinn was a member of the Chicago Medical Society and of the Woman's Press League, and devoted much time to Y. W. C. A. work. She gave freely to philanthropic undertakings.

Dr. LEONARD J. GORDON died at his home, 114½ Mercer Street, Jersey City, on Thursday last, from heart disease, after an illness of three months. He was born in New York on April 16, 1844. In 1860 he became a student at the New York University. When the Civil War broke out he enlisted in the Seventy-first New York Volunteers, and later volunteered in the Sixth New Jersey, of which he became Adjutant. For ten years he was engaged in business in New York, and for a time was private secretary to Daniel Drew. In 1872 he entered Bellevue Medical College, from which he was graduated three years later. Dr. Gordon practised medicine in Jersey City for two years, and was then appointed chemist of the Lorillard Tobacco Company, which position he held until the business was absorbed by the American Tobacco Company in 1894.

SOCIETY PROCEEDINGS.

WESTERN SURGICAL AND GYNECOLOGICAL ASSOCIATION.

Fourteenth Annual Meeting, held in Milwaukee, Wis., December 28 and 29, 1904.

The President, Charles H. Mayo, M.D., of Rochester, Minn., in the Chair.

(Continued from Page 144.)

Mortality, Disability and Permanency of Cure in Surgery.—This was the title of the President's Address, which was delivered by Dr. Charles H. Mayo, of Rochester, Minn. The author stated that a careful selection of cases, asepsis, and the kindness of Providence might give a low death rate which would cover much poor surgery. There was no general rule for computing surgical mortality at present, and it was best to accept the laymen's view that the operation had caused death where the patient went into the hospital alive and came out dead, regardless of the cause of death or time after operation. Failure to grasp the surgical opportunity at the proper moment was the cause of an increased mortality and disability, as well as a reduction in cures. The layman as well as the professional man understood that many diseases, such as appendicitis, ulcer of the stomach, and gall-stone disease, might each have repeated medical cures, and that in the same cases early operation was successful with a low mortality, the complications of delay causing the most trouble. During this year in St. Mary's Hospital, 516 operations for appendicitis were made, with 4 deaths. Their hospital detention was reduced an average of eleven days each, amounting to fourteen years' saving over the time which would have been required for the same work five years ago. In 205 hernias during the year this saving was from one to two weeks in each case. Among stomach operations, 108 gastroenterostomies gave 8 deaths (7.4 per cent.), most of these in late cancer, while 13 pylorectomies and partial gastrectomies gave no deaths because in an early stage. There were five deaths in 101 hysterectomies, more than one-half of these being due to an increased effort to cure cancer. Altogether, up to December 1, 1904, one thousand operations for gall-stone disease gave a mortality of five per cent. There were 673 cholecystostomies, with 2.4 per cent. mortality; 186 cholecystectomies gave a mortality of 4.3 per cent. The common duct cases, 11 per cent.; cancer, 22 per cent.; showing that one case in five had passed the safe time for operation, while early operation in 416 cases gave but two deaths. The brain was poorly constructed for repair, hence late operations gave only occasional permanent and complete cures.

The progress in the treatment of cancer was through a study of lymphatics involved in metastasis.

Surgical Diseases of the Pancreas.—Dr. D. C. Brockman, of Ottumwa, Iowa, stated that recent studies of the pancreas showed the importance of internal secretion from the islands of Langerhans; also the influence of regurgitation of bile into the pancreatic ducts, as a cause of pancreatic inflammation. Biliary disturbance was mentioned as the chief cause of pancreatic disease, and the author stated that pancreatic cysts were believed to be mostly due to this cause. He reported three instructive cases of cyst of the pancreas, and then gave an outline of inflammatory troubles, with special reference to the diagnosis and treatment of acute and chronic pancreatitis.

Cysts of the Pancreas.—Dr. D. W. Basham, of Wichita, Kan., followed with a paper on this subject. He referred briefly to the physiological anatomy of the gland, in order to elucidate the principles underlying the formation of a cyst of this organ. He recounted the symptomatology, and pointed out the difficulty attending the diagnosis. As to treatment, Gussenbauer was the first to marsupialize the sac, and since then this had been a favorite procedure with most surgeons. The only question regarding this method was whether to attach the sac to the abdomen and incise at once, or to operate à deux temps. If there was plenty of time and the cyst was not so large that a day or two might make any difference in the result, he thought it was better to operate in two stages, stitching the sac to the peritoneum and muscles, and opening two or three days later. Excision of the sac was not often practical, but might sometimes be attempted. Often such a course would expose the patient to the risk of contaminating the peritoneal cavity with pancreatic secretions. He reported the case of a tumor of the pancreas in a woman, sixty-two years of age. The tumor was removed. The patient left the hospital at the end of seven weeks, and he had not seen her since. The woman's dyspeptic manifestations were better after the operation than before, but were not entirely relieved. About the first of December, the patient began to have serious trouble with her stomach, and called a physician, who was able to outline a tumor in the region of the pylorus, which he diagnosed as cancer of the stomach.

Dr. William D. Haggard thought inflammations of the pancreas occupied the most prominent position in the future development of surgery. Disease of this organ was closely allied to surgery for lesions in the upper abdomen. When one stopped to think how our knowledge had been amplified in the last two years relative to this sequestered organ, and when one considered that many cases of so-called gastritis, intestinal obstruction, etc., were after all probably instances of pancreatitis, it made surgeons realize that the lesson had been appreciated, but we had not yet mastered the diagnosis of this as well as other lesions, but nevertheless more attention should be addressed to lesions of the pancreas than had been done in the past. He referred to the three types of infection, and called attention to the excellent work done of Opie, Robson, and others.

Dr. Brockman, in closing, expressed the opinion that pancreatic cysts were not so uncommon as had been supposed. He had had four such cases in the last twelve or fourteen years.

Excision of the Elbow-Joint for Traumatic and Arthritic Anchylosis.—Dr. B. Merrill Ricketts, of Cincinnati, Ohio, read a paper on this subject in which he drew the following conclusions: (1) Excision of the elbow-joint for anchylosis, due to any cause, at any age, is a most rational procedure. (2) If possible, it should be done before or at the time anchylosis is complete. (3) A posterior median incision is the most practical. (4) With care the operation can be done without injury to blood vessels or nerves. (5) Drainage should always be provided for. (6) The arm should be placed upon a right angle splint. (7) Results are better when only the articulating surfaces are removed. (8) If there is complete bony union of the articulating surfaces, much more bony tissue must be sacrificed, because disarticulation cannot be accomplished. (9) All soft structures cut transversely will unite, but new insertions are formed which destroy their function. (10) All attachments of tendons and muscles should be preserved. (11) All periosteum should be preserved. (12) If excision of the joint is complete, leaving only the ends of the shaft, flail joint can be prevented by approximating their ends with kangaroo tendon at the time of primary operation. (13) Wire or nail may be used, but their removal sooner or later will be imperative. (14) Flail joint rarely results from any form of excision, but is more likely to be found following excision of the entire joint. (15) If flail joint results, a mechanical device may be employed. (16) Injections of alcohol or one or more of the various astringents will increase fibrous tissue both in quantity and density.

The Operative Treatment of Fractures and Sprains.—Dr. A. E. Benjamin, of Minneapolis, Minn., stated that frequently fractures were not recognized, and that complicated joint fractures without operative treatment gave poor results. All fractures should be examined with the X-ray to diagnose positively and locate the injury. The ordinary form of treatment of even simple fractures often resulted in a deformed and crippled limb. The term ununited fracture was a myth; the condition was invariably due to some preventable cause. The habit of using the X-ray in all fractures led to more operative measures, although without its use diagnosis was frequently impossible and treatment uncertain. There was frequently as great a subcutaneous injury from a fracture as in a compound fracture, and it was just as essential that an operation should be performed in such cases, in order to prevent a lasting injury to the nerve and muscle tissue. By an operation upon these fractures drainage was established, pain and fever lessened, exostosis and the organization of the exudate was less permanent, and necessarily there followed less permanent injury to the soft structures. Many of the past inexact operative and exact methods were employed. Associated with fractures there was frequently a sprain or a tearing away of ligaments, cartilages and dislocations. The progress of a joint that had been sprained was often slow and discouraging, resulting in a weak and insecure union of ligaments. It was advisable to operate upon a number of sprains, especially where there was a great deal of exudate and pain. By the operative method drainage was established, pain relieved, and ligaments could be stitched in their natural place of habitation, the convalescent period was shortened, and a greater proportion of cures resulted.

The Surgical Consideration of Gastric Dilatation.—Dr. A. M. Pond, of Webster City, Iowa, after considering the etiology of gastric dilatation, stated that in the last three cases of gastric dilatation due to impairment of the stomach wall he had modified the standard operation. Sufficient time, however, had not elapsed to warrant a description of the operation. The last case was operated June 4. In each instance a very satisfactory result was obtained. The success of the operation depended upon two very important factors, patency of the pyloric orifice, and the ability of the gastric muscle to regain its normal tone. The author believed that gastric dilatation was usually a sequence rather than a primary cause of discomfort, and that it owed its presence to some disturbance of the elemental dynamics of digestion. It was, on close analysis, merely one of a symptom-complex of the upper abdomen, but a very valuable one, the importance of which should be included in the consideration for operative restoration.

Treatment of Acute Perforations of the Upper Abdominal Viscera.—Dr. Van Buren Knott, of Sioux City, Iowa, pointed out the importance of the early recognition of such an accident, saying that an accurate diagnosis as to which organ was involved was neither possible nor necessary at all times. The symptoms of gastric or duodenal perforation would usually be more intense than those of perforation of the gall-bladder. Previous history of the case was of importance in making a differential diagnosis. The treatment was successful in direct ratio to the promptness with which it was instituted. The resulting peritonitis was the most important result of the accident, and its treatment in the various cases was similar. He emphasized the value of posture in treatment.

Pneumatocele.—Dr. L. L. McArthur, of Chicago, reported a rare case of pneumatocele, saying that it was a gas-containing tumor of the cranium—very rare—there being but thirty-two recorded cases since 1741. It always originated in connection with either the mastoid or frontal sinuses. It was not to be confused with emphysema, which was gas in the cellular tissue. Pneumatocele was gas between the pericranium. Incident to the elevation of the periosteum were secondary bony outgrowths, giving the tumor a peculiar feel. In the preantiseptic era the simple benign pneumatocele became a dangerous affair, because of the frequent connection with mastoid sinuses, with the potential septic meningitis. Since antiseptic surgery had become well-established, all of these cases recovered.

The Value of Skiagraphy in the Treatment of Fractures.—Dr. H. A. Sifton, of Milwaukee, Wis., exhibited in connection with a paper on this subject numerous skiagraphs. He was of the opinion that, when it was possible, the Roentgen ray should be used in the treatment of every fracture. It had its deceptions, but these meant nothing to the physician who had made a study of the subject, and was familiar with the conditions under which the skiagraph was taken. Some urged its use in the obscure and complicated cases only, but the difficulty with this plan was that we could never tell whether or not a fracture was complicated until a radiograph of it was taken. It was the surgeon's duty to do his best for the patient, and to do this he should look upon every case of fracture as complicated, until it had been shown to be otherwise by a good radiograph. A good radiograph was of value for future information from a forensic standpoint, but no radiograph, in his opinion, should be admitted as evidence in any medicolegal dispute, unless both parties to the dispute knew the conditions under which the radiograph was taken.

Dr. L. L. McArthur said the X-ray was of immense importance to the surgeon from a forensic standpoint. He urged that the surgeon protect himself, whenever possible, by making an X-ray picture of a fracture after the limb had been put in the best possible position, and condition, and submitted to the patient, telling him that that was the best position that could be obtained, and asking

him if he was satisfied with it. In this way the surgeon allowed the patient to know that he had utilized every means in his power and all the instruments of precision to accomplish a good result. The surgeon should impress upon the general practitioner and the laity that it was not essential for a good functional result to have actual anatomical reposition of the fractured ends.

Dr. J. W. Andrews said, it was a revelation to him that several skiagraphs of the same case could show such a great difference. He concurred with Dr. McArthur that it was unnecessary to have absolute apposition of the fragments, yet the laity and some physicians, especially in the malpractice suits, felt that there must be absolute apposition, and that union must take place in that position; hence there was a growing tendency on the part of the laity to have fractures examined by someone with the X-ray after healing had occurred, and unless the result was a perfect one, there were threats of a malpractice suit.

Dr. C. E. Ruth said a number of malpractice suits emanated as the result of fractures, where the basis of the proceeding had been the supposed findings from skiagraphs. He would dislike very much to treat a case of fracture without having taken skiagraphs or having made fluoroscopic examinations of the limb in different positions. The surgeon should be careful not to tell any patient that he would get a perfect result.   •

Dr. A. I. Bouffleur stated that as a confirmatory measure the X-ray was of great value, but as a substitute for ordinary means, it was in his opinion not proper to place the reliance on it which he had heard at different times concerning it.

Dr. M. L. Harris said the Association should not go on record as supporting the statement that in the treatment of fractures the X-ray should be used. He did not think it was a necessary means of diagnosis. In nine cases out of ten it was not only unnecessary, but it did not furnish the surgeon with any information which could not be obtained in other ways. He admitted its value in showing something which one could not detect in any other way. He pointed out the fallacies of the X-ray. It was impossible in many instances for anyone to interpret correctly an X-ray picture. Skiagraphs should never be admitted as evidence in a medicolegal contest.

Dr. A. E. Benjamin said it was well to employ the X-ray as an additional confirmatory aid in the treatment of fractures.

The Manufacture and Use of Tin Splints.—Dr. Arthur T. Mann, of Minneapolis, Minn., made a plea for the general utility of tin splints. He pointed out the simple equipment necessary to make them; also the ease of making the splints and patterns for them. He described several tin appliances which were useful to the surgeon, and among them a device for regaining flexion and extension of the elbow joint after fractures and dislocations. He also exhibited a device for the protection of the line of sutures in operative cases of cleft palate.

Syncytioma Malignum.—Dr. H. C. Crowell, of Kansas City, Mo., reported a case of this comparatively rare disease, which was accompanied by a detailed pathological report of the specimen removed. He referred briefly to other cases which he had found in the literature.

Dr. Archibald MacLaren reported a case of what he had supposed to be a soft edematous fibroid from the history, which came on five months after delivery. Probably there was no growth present until after the birth of the child. There was no extension beyond the wall of the uterus. The fundus was diffusely infiltrated with this peculiar fungous mass. Sections of the mass were examined by a competent pathologist and a diagnosis made of syncytioma malignum. The uterus was removed above the internal os, in the belief that it was simply an edematous fibroid, and the case treated like any ordinary supravaginal amputation. The woman, at the present time, had had no return of the disease, and there was no extension apparently to the lymphatics or neighboring tissues. A year had elapsed since the operation was done.

Fractures of the Tarsal Bones.—Dr. Daniel N. Eisendrath, of Chicago, called the attention to the surgical anatomy of these bones, and the mechanism of fractures. He spoke of compression fractures; fractures of the neck of the astragalus following sudden dorsal flexion of the foot; fractures of both astragalus and calcaneus following forced supination or pronation of the foot; fractures of the astragalus which resulted from forcible action of the muscles of the calf; crushing fractures, and gunshot fractures. He discussed the symptoms and diagnosis together. In considering the treatment. he reported six interesting cases, after which he drew the following conclusions: (1) The astragalus and os calcis bear the entire weight of the body. (2) They are most frequently broken in falls from a height directly upon the feet (compression variety), or by tearing off of a portion of one of the bones either when the heel is fixed or sudden supination or pronation, or in forcible dorsal flexion of the foot. (3) Early diagnosis, on account of the danger of sepsis from secondary skin necrosis, is of great importance. (4) If there is no displacement of fragments, treat the case by cast for six weeks, with early massage. If displacement threatens necrosis of skin, convert into open fracture and remove the fragment or suture it.

Ptosis of the Abdominal and Pelvic Organs.—Dr. R. C. Coffey, of Portland, Oregon, read a paper on this subject, which was accompanied by numerous illustrations. He drew the following conclusions: (1) The peritoneum is attached firmly, not only to the diaphragm. but loosely by all its outer surface to the abdominal and pelvic walls by means of loose connective tissue which allows it to move freely, but holds it always in contact. This connective tissue is much increased around the attachment of the supports of each organ. The irritation underneath and back of the peritoneum is followed, first, by an exudate which fixes it immovably to the abdominal wall. This exudate is soon displaced by an increase of normal connective tissue sufficient to meet the demands. The peritoneum itself is but slightly elastic, its seeming elasticity being due to the elasticity of the subperitoneal connective tissue. (2) Two peritoneal surfaces brought together and held firmly in an aseptic state blend and become one membrane. If suppuration or other disturbance occurs, blending does not take place, but inflammatory adhesions are formed. The former is permanent, while the latter is transitory, and will be absorbed generally. This differentiation is all-important. (3) The uterus is suspended entirely by its peritoneum and connective tissue. (4) The so-called true ligaments are not true ligaments. but muscles, and therefore perform the same function as all other muscular fibers in the animal organism. which is intermittent contraction, but never

constant action. Their function is to sustain the normal poise or balance of the uterus during the changing position of the body. (5) Whatever may be the cause, the condition existing is a stretching of either or both the peritoneum and connective tissue. The condition may be local or general, and may involve the support of one, more than one, or all the abdominal and pelvic organs. (6) The treatment in a general way will be the shortening of the peritoneum at the points at fault by some method of plication, and blending, or by bringing the peritoneum back to its normal contact with the abdominal wall. (7) The method (he described) for suspending the liver is, Dr. Coffey believes, almost ideal theoretically, and so far in his experience clinically and experimentally, in that it shortens the normal suspensory ligament, supplements it by extending the ligament to one or both lobes by blending of peritoneum. (8) None of the operations for gastroptosis so far are theoretically or practically ideal for all cases. The hammock operation, stitching the omentum to the abdominal wall, is best suited to those cases due to adhesions holding the stomach out of place by its omentum, in which the condition accompanies operations on the lower abdomen or pelvis only. No discomfort has been observed by any of my patients. Posterior gastro-enterostomy is the best operation for those cases due to dilatation or pyloric obstruction of any kind, and is all that is necessary, as it is held by its attachment high up and well back to the transverse mesocolon.

Appendicitis, with Special Reference to this Disease in Women.—Dr. Archibald MacLaren, of St. Paul, Minn., said that in the light of recent experiences he believed the only safe advice both to the patient and the physician was that the appendix should be immediately removed in the early hours of every acute attack of appendicitis, and especially in first attacks, when the symptoms lasted six hours. On the other hand, he did not believe that every case of appendicitis should be operated upon as soon as the diagnosis was made, because the physician frequently did not see these cases until from the third to the sixth day. The favorable time had now passed, and, as Richardson had said, some of these cases were in such bad condition that the operation itself might be enough to take away the only remaining chance of recovery. He had made 422 appendectomies. In the first 241 there were 72 suppurative cases. Of these there were 42 men and 30 women, in spite of the fact that his work was largely the surgery of women. During the same time he had removed appendices showing chronic inflammatory changes 153 times in women and only 17 times in men. He did not quote these figures for the purpose of giving the impression that they fulfilled his idea of the true relationship of chronic appendicitis in the sexes. He did not believe that chronic appendicitis was as frequent in the male as in the female, but it probably was not twice as frequent in the latter sex. It was, he believed, only a curious accident that he had seen proportionately so many acute cases in men and so very few chronic cases.

Management of Hospitals in Cities of One Hundred Thousand Population or Less.—Dr. D. S. Fairchild, of Des Moines, Iowa, stated that the problems involved in the management of hospitals in the smaller cities were difficult and complicated, growing out of two important facts; first, the supposed self-interest of individual members of the medical profession, and, second, the lack of experience and knowledge on the part of boards of management. Public hospitals were generally of three kinds, as determined by the auspices under which they were organized and in part supported. (a) Hospitals under the auspices of some church; (b) hospitals under the auspices of some society, and (c) city hospitals supported by public taxation. The method of appointment of physicians to hospitals was liable to abuse only when piety or church zeal was mistaken for competency. The author discussed the management of hospitals at great length.

Arthrotomy.—Dr. E. Wyllys Andrews, of Chicago. described a new method of arthrotomy for old dislocations of the shoulder-joint, and after mentioning the steps of the procedure at considerable length, he presented the following conclusions: (1) It must be considered established that great force is never justifiable in old shoulder dislocations. (2) Few cases can be left unreduced, on account of pain and pressure symptoms on the brachial plexus. (3) Resection is satisfactory, but not ideal or wholly safe. (4) Arthrotomy by the old incisions is tedious, and never has been widely practised. (5) Arthrotomy by the author's method is simplified and made quicker and safer. It would possibly be as safe as resection, and much more ideal in results.

Curettage and Puerperal Sepsis.—Dr. C. E. Ruth. of Keokuk. Iowa, discussed the etiology of puerperal sepsis. the kinds of infection. prevention. dangers, as well as curettage, drainage, and hysterectomy in such cases.

Our Duty to the United States Army and its Medical Corps.—Dr. Donald Macrae, Jr., of Council Bluffs, Iowa, pointed out the importance of having a more efficient ,medical corps in the United States army. He made an appeal to the patriotic sense of the American surgeon in civil practice to stand by the recommendations of the Surgeon-General of the army, and otherwise to use his best endeavors to relieve a most deplorable condition in the most important branch of the service. He thought that the Surgeon-General should be elevated to lieutenant-general, and be equal in rank to the head of any other branch of the army. A medical officer should be added to the general staff. A resolution was introduced and unanimously adopted respectfully petitioning President Roosevelt to direct that the military authorities provide a field medical organization for our army at least equal in all respects to the best that exists in any army, and which will meet the approval of military sanitarians generally, to the end that the sick and wounded in future wars may receive adequate care and attention. The Secretary was instructed to forward a copy of this resolution to President Roosevelt at once.

Removal of the Covering of the Ovaries in Ovarian Dysmenorrhea.—Dr. George G. Eitel, of Minneapolis, Minn., presented a preliminary study on this subject, and described the technic of the operation he had performed in seven cases, as follows: The ovary is brought into clear view through a median abdominal incision; and one hemostatic forceps is placed at the juncture of the utero-ovarian ligament and ovary, and another on the upper border of the broad ligament close to the ovary (lateral). By means of these two forceps the ovary is held by an assistant in the proper position, while the operator makes an incision with a sharp scalpel from the utero-ovarian ligament to the lateral attachment to the broad ligament through the covering, and then carefully dissects one side, and then the other, down as far as cysts are encountered. The flaps of the covering of the ovary are now trimmed off, preferably by means of a pair of scissors. This having been done, the utero-ovarian ligament is shortened by doubling it upon itself in a similar manner as is in vogue in shortening the round ligaments, in order to hold the uterus in a normal position. There is generally some hemor-

rhage as the base of the ovary is encroached, which can easily be controlled by pressure forceps and fine ligatures.

The Diagnosis of Early Tubal Pregnancy.—Dr. William E. Ground, of Superior, Wis., after going into the, diagnosis exhaustively, and quoting from the literature, stated that during the last year he had operated upon ten cases of tubal pregnancy. He had operated upon 28 cases altogether. His deductions were based on the histories and the gross appearance of the uterus and appendages at the time of operation. He was firmly convinced that ample pathology was present to cause the arrest of the fecundated ovum in the tube. Five of his cases were in primiparae, who gave a history of painful menstruation and leucorrhea. Thirteen cases gave a history of a prolonged period of sterility; by this he meant three years or longer. The remaining 12 cases occurred in parous women, who had borne children or had been pregnant in less than three years. Many of these women gave unmistakable evidence of pre-existing pelvic disease. One primipara, had been married three years. one five, and another eleven years, before tubal conception occurred. Two cases occurred in unmarried women, one of whom had had a criminal abortion produced. Complications arose, and she was sent to Dr. Ground for abdominal section, when an unruptured tube containing a six weeks' fetus was found. Another case. a grass widow. was known to have had chronic appendicitis, was taken with sudden severe pain in the right lower abdomen, followed by considerable shock, but she soon rallied and ran a slight fever. At this juncture he saw her. Menstrual irregularities were denied. Tenderness was present rather low in the iliac fossa for appendicitis, uterus was enlarged, and a slight bloody discharge came from the vagina. There was an ill-defined tumor to the right of the uterus. The abdomen was opened and found to contain blood clots and bloody serum. The right tube was ruptured on its dorsum, at about the middle, but the fetus was still in the tube. Chronic appendicitis was also present, and the appendix removed. Two cases had small fibroids, and one had an ovarian cyst as large as an orange on the opposite side.

Officers.—The following officers were elected for the ensuing year: President, Dr. H. D. Niles, Salt Lake City, Utah; First Vice-President, Dr. E. Wyllys Andrews, Chicago; Second Vice-President, Dr. W. W. Grant, Denver; Secretary-Treasurer, Dr. B. B. Davis, Omaha, Neb.

Kansas City, Missouri, was selected as the place for the next meeting, with Dr. H. C. Crowell, as Chairman of the Committee of Arrangements.

CHICAGO MEDICAL SOCIETY.

Regular Meeting, held November 23, 1904.

The President, John B. Murphy, M.D., in the Chair.

SYMPOSIUM ON CRIMINAL ABORTION.

The Duty of the Medical Profession in Relation to Criminal Abortion.—Dr. C. S. Bacon contributed this paper. It is estimated, he said, that from six thousand to ten thousand abortions are induced in Chicago every year, a majority of which are in married women. To collect data on the subject, to call the attention of the profession to it, and to exercise an influence toward restraining the evil and checking the debauchment of the minds of the profession and the community, a committee of the Council of the Chicago Medical Society was appointed about a year ago. This committee has now arranged for a symposium as a feature in its work of education. From the medical and social sides of the problem, four reasons are given for repressing the practice of abortion. (1) It is an injury to the embryo or fetus destroyed, for the fetus is a living independent human being, and has the right to existence which belongs to all human beings, and it should be protected in this right. (2) It is an injury to the mother, for it is an unjustifiable risk to her health and her life. (3) It is an injury to the relatives of the unborn child and to the mother. (4) It is an injury to the State. According to the common law, the fetus is not considered a being until after quickening, and therefore it is not a crime to destroy it. After quickening, its destruction either by the mother or by a third party is a misdemeanor, but not a crime punishable by imprisonment. According to the Illinois statutes, which take the place of the common law, there is no distinction between an animate and an inanimate fetus, and the induction of abortion is punished by imprisonment from one to ten years. The consent of the mother does not absolve the third party who does the act. Intent is the essence of the crime, and the efficiency of the means employed is not considered. If the mother dies the act is murder. Notwithstanding the prevalence of the crime, there are practically no accusations or indictments for abortion unless the mother becomes seriously ill or dies. Even in the latter case her relatives and friends generally try to prevent any investigation in order to shield her reputation. The influence of the physician should be exerted to persuade the injured mother or her friends to act. In case of her death, it is his duty to report the case to the Coroner as he would any other case of homicide. If a case comes to trial, it is necessary that the physician know the rules of procedure of courts and the rules of evidence. In Illinois no communications to physicians are privileged. Attention is called to the great importance of a dying declaration which may become the chief factor in producing the conviction. It must be voluntary, made when the patient has given up hope of recovery, and should state that a certain individual has committed the act. In closing, the author called attention to the need of maternity asylums for the unmarried.

Decisions of Authority.—The next speaker was Rev. Peter J. O'Callaghan, of the Order of Paulists, who spoke on the moral and religious objections to inducing abortion. He said it was one of the triumphs of the ancient Church to have practically eradicated the crime of abortion, and that this Church stands to-day where she stood a thousand years ago. She declares that no man has the right to destroy by any direct act the life of an innocent human being. In the face of a sentiment which has persuaded a large section of the medical profession that direct abortion is sometimes not only justifiable, but even commendable, that Church has unflinchingly declared that the direct taking of an innocent human life is always murder, no matter what be the stage of its existence. In 1884 her authoritative teaching body was asked whether it was safe to teach in Catholic schools that the operation of craniotomy is sometimes justifiable. The answer was that it was not safe so to teach. In 1889 that same body was asked if any operation at all looking to the direct killing of the child in utero was justifiable. The question was also answered in the negative. Again it was asked if this

should be done when absolutely necessary to save the mother, and in 1895 this question was answered in the negative. Again, the formal question was asked, if, in extra-uterine conception, any operation be justifiable which meant the death of the child. This was answered in the negative. The Church, therefore, has constantly said that no one has a right on any occasion to procure directly by any act of his the death of any human being. It maintains the right of the unborn child to live just as much as the right of the mother to live. If one or the other must die, or both die, and if both die without act of ours, the responsibility is not ours. Such is the position of the Catholic Church. Although, he said, these are not dogmatic definitions of Catholic doctrine, they are the authoritative decisions of the Catholic Church on the question of abortion. The reason for the uncompromising position of the Church in this matter is clearly to be found in the decalogue, " Thou shalt not kill." The Church has always feared to make what she considers the word of God say less than it says or more than it says. The position of the Church cannot be appreciated by any who regard the Ten Commandments merely as a mosaic code of moral law, or as an embodiment of Jewish experiences in ethical culture. To the Church the Ten Commandments are a revelation of the essential and profoundly vital conditions of moral health. She regards as superficial the advantages that expediency may suggest in the breaking of the law. If the taking of human life is a crime only because men have found that society is impossible without the severest punishment of murder, then may the question be raised, How far is it necessary to respect life of the individual? If it is only expediency which sets down taking of human life as a great crime, then the shifting demands of expediency must be hearkened to. If the demands of expediency are cogent in determining the right to cut off human life in any stage of its existence, then we have not morality, but only an emotional empiricism. Whether the Kantian maxim that a moral law must be capable of universal application be a true definition of the essential quality of all moral law or not, it is certainly a good test of the morality of any principle of conduct. Principles of conduct cannot be arbitrarily confined to particular cases. If it is right to take human life to save the mother's life, it is right to take a human life to save a mother's honor. If it is right to destroy the unborn child in order to avoid the suffering that shame brings, it is right to destroy a child whose birth would mean for others the sufferings of poverty. If there is such a thing as therapeutic abortion that is commendable, Father O'Callaghan thinks that there is no such thing as a criminal abortion that is reprehensible. Legislators may determine that some conditions justify abortion, while other conditions do not, but their judgment will not control the consciences any more than their present laws inconvenience the most of those that are now guilty of what is called criminal abortion.

Criminal Abortion as it Comes Before the Coroner's Office.—Mr. John E. Träger, Coroner of Cook County, said that before his advent in the Coroner's office he had little or no opportunity to know to what extent criminal abortion was practised, especially in a large cosmopolitan city like Chicago. He found, after investigation, that many of the abortions were induced by midwives who made a specialty of it, and whose business cards announcing their vocation could be found in some of the houses of ill-fame in the city, being distributed by the landladies or inmates to the young men, or old men, for that matter, who might some time want that kind of service. In consulting the records of the office he found that there had been very few persons held to the grand jury and fewer still ever convicted of the crime of criminal abortion. This news discouraged him, and he made up his mind to devise some way to stop it. During the past four years, with the assistance of the State's attorney, four of those midwives were sent to the Joliet Penitentiary. The first year of his term he investigated 42 cases of criminal practice, the second year it fell off to 27; last year it was further reduced to 18; but this year it would reach 35, which is an increase of nearly 100 per cent. He held six midwives and one physician to the grand jury this year, and had already convicted two. In investigating the cases of abortion that came to his office, he finds that the cause for the act differs in most every case, that is, among married women; in some cases on account of poverty; in others on account of children coming too fast, and the society woman, who has not time to devote to maternal cares, and last, but not least the dwellers in modern flats. It has got so nowadays that a married couple with babies is denied admission to an apartment house or flat building, and it is his honest opinion that the attitude of the present-day landlord in refusing to rent to families with small children and allowing that impression to go out broadcast is indirectly the cause of much of the criminal practice in Chicago. He thinks the discussion as to the causes of the practice and its cure can be more safely left to physicians as they have a better opportunity of learning those things. All he could say is that he thinks it is the duty of physicians and his to try and check the practice—their's by advice to the women who come to them for assistance, and his by punishing the guilty who have violated the law.

Therapeutic and Criminal Abortion.—Dr. Charles B. Reed, in a paper on this subject, stated that in the advance of moral feeling, the opinion has developed that in certain cases where the lives of both mother and child are imperiled and one can be saved, the child should be sacrificed, since the value of the mother to the State is far greater than that of the unborn babe. Hence, where certain diseases or complications appear in or exist during the course of gestation and threaten the integrity of the case, a broad human sentiment now permits, nay even demands, the destruction of the fetus. When this situation eventuates before the viability of the child, it is recognized as a prophylactic or therapeutic abortion and becomes a justifiable measure in the presence of such conditions as hyperemesis gravidarum and eclampsia, which do not yield to treatment. In certain cases of beginning and advanced pulmonary tuberculosis, cardiac disease, insanity, severe nephritis or serious and irreducible uterine displacments with dense adhesions, the operation is justly performed. In cases of absolutely contracted pelvis, where the patient refuses Cæsarean section, abortion is sometimes desirable, although the relative dangers of the two operations do not greatly differ in skilful hands. The results of therapeutic abortion, when executed in a careful scientific way, are generally good, and the indications for its performance are found both in and out of marriage. Abortion in all its phases is necessarily more common in the married state,

and it has been said that almost half of all childbearing women have an abortion before the thirty-fifth year. It is also true that the medical man is most frequently approached by married women who desire the removal of the socially inconvenient egg. For this situation there is no excuse. When the product of conception is deliberately destroyed for social reasons only, and without physical justification, in a woman married or single, it constitutes a criminal offense before the human and moral law. It is ignorantly maintained by many that the dislodgment of the egg before quickening is in no sense reprehensible, because it is thought that the egg is not alive. This, the author says, is a distinction of degree only, and a species of special pleading, for the fertilized egg contains all the hopes and possibilities of a mature fetus, and while quickening usually occurs at the sixteenth week, the fetus is practically fully formed at an earlier period. The normal attitude of the enlightened professional man is hostile to abortion. It is well attested that nearly all of the desperate and fatal complications found in abortions occur in criminal cases. The deaths from such attempts are frequent and embrace a large range of causative conditions, among which, as the most important, he mentioned perforation, peritonitis, septicemia, pyemia, tetanus, endometritis, endosalpingitis, air embolism, abscesses, pneumothorax, thrombophlebitis, phlegmasia alba dolens, etc. Legal restrictions are relatively recent in origin, but none the less drastic. It is not the murder of a living child which constitutes the offense, but the destruction of gestation by wicked and unnatural means. The moment the womb is instinct with embryo life, gestation has begun, the crime may be committed. The liability of the mother in the eyes of the law is the same as that of the third person, and in many States is made equally culpable with the act. In Illinois the attempt is punishable by imprisonment in the penitentiary from one to ten years, and if the death of the mother results therefrom, it constitutes · murder. But the law, unsupported by popular sentiment, has proved ineffective, and in many cases no attempt is made even to secure its enforcement, and the abortionist rests in security. It devolves upon the physician to keep the light before the public mind, not only in general, but in particular instances. The artificial conditions which drive unmarried girls to abortion should be everywhere strenuously opposed.

In the development of the vast scheme of creation the author says it is not surprising that the one great dominant chord of humanity is the sexual instinct. Openly or disguised, it controls the mainspring of human endeavor. It drives some to the convent, and some to the gallows, but unceasingly it drives with relentless energy toward the preservation of the race at the expense of the individual, and the woman is the most frequent sacrifice in the maintainance of racial immortality. On her head fall legal, moral and physical penalties that should be more evenly distributed. Let the legal and moral enactments be what they will, a broad humanity demands the protection of the mother and the illegitimate unborn babe. Let maternities be established and maintained. Let homes and places of refuge for the woman awaiting confinement be founded and supported. Give charity for the unfortunate girl who, with unreasoning animalism, attempts to escape her exposure and humiliation by abortion. Teach chastity, teach restraint, but, above all, protect the devoted victim of her own strength or weakness from yielding to the eternal dominant impulse, and enable her to pass through her gestation and delivery free from the lofty scorn of an unsympathetic sisterhood.

Criminal Abortion in its Relation to Newspaper Advertising.—Dr. Rudolph W. Holmes discussed this phase of the question, and reported a medicolegal case of interest. After some years of close professional association with the pregnant, the author has become convinced that abortions among the better classes are essentially brought about by one group of causes which may be denominated social ones. He firmly believes that where one abortion occurs from the diverse pathological causes, many more are produced by the abortionist's instruments, drugs, or other measures. Education is absolutely indispensable to a proper realization of the heinousness of destroying the unborn child; the physician is the one above all others who may be the most influential in deterring women from having their desires fulfilled. Well-directed arguments concerning the dangers of having the operation done are to his mind more effective than too strong presentations of the moral aspect. So soon as the physician presents to the woman that she is doing a criminal offense, is breaking a moral law, he arouses her enmity from the suggestion implied that she is immoral or a criminal. The common law, which is founded on ancient and medieval customs, has fostered the belief that the fetus did not have life until quickening was noticed by the mother. To this day the States of Connecticut, Mississippi, Minnesota, Arkansas, and Oregon accept this obsolete interpretation of the common law in their statutes; other States and most countries by legislative action have removed such absurd qualifications as "quick with child" from their statutes defining criminal abortion. Although this really nonsensical belief that the fetus is endowed with life by the accidental circumstances of the mother feeling fetal movements has been done away with in medicine, law and theology, the laity still tenaciously adheres to the old idea with ulterior motives. The present law in Illinois as in nearly all other States making a great distinction between an abortion which does not destroy the life of the mother, and when she dies, the former is the felony of abortion, the latter is the felony of murder. Such a law is discriminative, as infanticide is murder, so should feticide be murder; the abortionist, directly, maliciously, with "malice aforethought" deliberately kills the fetus, while it is far from his intention to kill the woman. He is quite positive that the daily papers, magazines, and even some socalled religious papers are most fruitful means of disseminating the knowledge concerning the means for producing abortion, by covertly suggesting where the appliances may be obtained, the drugs bought, or even the instrumental methods which may be carried out. There is hardly one daily paper in Chicago which does not regularly print a list of advertisements of professional abortionists. The publishers and editors must be fully cognizant of the purport of the wording of these advertisements; in private these men would not stultify themselves by such declarations of ignorance, but as the veiled wording is an indispensable requisite for such public announcement, they hide behind a subterfuge. That a veiled advertisement may be brought in as evidence of the criminal intent of the abortionist has been

amply settled in Massachusetts, and would undoubtedly be accepted in the courts of other States. (See *Journal*, June 23, 1900, page 1612.) In connection with the laws prohibiting the advertisements of abortionists, Dr. Holmes briefly reviewed the laws concerning the sale of abortifacients. In conclusion, the writer stated his belief that the time has come for the Society to take an active part in aiding the prosecution of notorious abortionists. This may be accomplished in various ways: (1) By bringing moral suasion upon newspaper management, so that they will refuse all advertisements of a suggestive nature; a committee of this Society might act as an advisory board of censors. (2) By working in friendly conjunction with the State Board of Health, City Health Department, the State's Attorney's office, and with the Coroner. If work is carried on along these lines, he thinks an enormous amount of data would be collected which would be of inestimable value to the several legal bodies.

The Common and Statute Laws of Illinois.—Mr. J. M. Sheehan, attorney for the Medicolegal Committee, briefly reviewed the history of criminal abortion. According to the ancient English common law, fetal life was held to begin only at the quickening and until such time no offense could be considered committed by an operation. No offense of any kind, with the woman's consent, was recognized as punishable. If, without the mother's consent, abortion was induced, simple assault was punishable. This law remained until a short time prior to the separation of this country from the mother country. Then, certain statutory enactments were passed in England which did not become laws in this country, but which were followed in many of the States. It was made an offense, a misdemeanor merely, to commit abortion or to induce premature delivery, even though the child had not quickened. In adition, there was a provision, if the death of the mother resulted, murder was the crime committed by one who was either the principal or accessory. Coming down to Illinois, which State adopted the common law, so far as it existed up to the fourth year of James I., this condition was found until the first criminal code was enacted, that abortion was defined in a manner slightly different from the crime as it exists upon the statute books to-day. Until 1867 the crime of abortion in the State of Illinois was defined, as follows: "Whoever by means of any instrument, medicine, drug, or other means whatever, causes any woman pregnant with child to abort or miscarry, or attempts to procure or produce any abortion for *bona fide* medical or surgical purposes, shall be imprisoned in the penitentiary." This statute remained until the year 1867; that is, any abortion or miscarriage brought about, committed, abetted or advised by any person, unless it be for *bona fide* medical or surgical purposes, was punishable as a felony. In 1867 the legislature changed the statute, and enacted it as it now stands upon the statute books, and in lieu of the words for "*bona fide* medical or surgical purposes," the provision of the Illinois statute is, "Unless same were done as necessary for the preservation of the mother's life." In interpreting the words "necessary for the preservation of the mother's life," it has been held that it must be an actual physical necessity; that is, the mental depression which may come because of the unfortunate condition of the mother; the threats of suicide, the probability of insanity, the nervous condition in which the mother at that time finds herself because of her surroundings, because of brooding over her condition, are not within the medical law; they are not conditions that will justify a physician or surgeon in saying that it is necessary for the preservation of the mother's life that her child should be destroyed. The courts in interpreting these words have properly held, that it must be an actual physical condition which renders improbable the continued life of the mother unless the life of the child be destroyed. Whether practical enforcement of the law as it stands is to be brought about is dependent upon public desire, public demands. Mr. Sheehan said that the law itself is as far advanced as is the public conscience. Indeed, it is further advanced apparently than the public demand for its enforcement would require, and so if anything is to be accomplished, it is not by making appeals to the legislature for a modification of the laws at this time, nor in making appeals for a more stringent law, but public conscience should be so stimulated as to require and demand that the law as it stands to-day should be strictly enforced.

Shall Communications of Physicians be Privileged?—Dr. Harold N. Moyer discussed this question. Unquestionably, the privileged communication or medical secret has stood in the way more largely than any one factor in the prosecution of the abortionist. The common law never had but one privileged communication, and this was not the result of a statute, but simply grew up as a part of the practice of courts, namely a communication between an attorney and his client was regarded as privileged. Dr. Moyer quoted the Roman law, the French law and the New York statute in regard to privileged communications. The New York statute reads: " A person duly authorized to practise physics or surgery shall not be allowed to disclose any information which he acquired in attending a patient in a professional capacity, and which was necessary to enable him to act in that capacity." He said that this statute might put an onus on the physician. So far as the privileged communication is concerned, it does not apply to this State, and it seems that fact is not generally known to the profession. The comunication of a patient to a physician is absolutely unrestricted and open to the inquiry of the court, and this absolves a physician from all legal responsibility in case he goes into court with questions of this kind. Some years ago he urged a member of the legislature to obtain the enactment of a statute making the communications of physicians privileged ones. He regretted he made such a request, and is glad that it bore no fruit, and if to-day he heard of any attempt to have the legislature pass such a law, he would do his best not to have it passed. Such a law, he said, is not useful to the community, and it proposes an extraordinary burden on the profession in some particulars. This burden was clearly pointed out by citations from the laws of various States. Let us have no privileged communication in this State as applied to the medical profession. The courts will protect physicians. A communication made under the seal of the confessional is not a privileged communication in this State, yet he has never heard of a court in Illinois that has attempted to invade the sanctity of the clergyman's office. The courts are capable of protecting physicians against the wrongful use or abuse of

medical evidence, and the matter could be safely left to them.

Mr. Fletcher Dobyns, Assistant State's Attorney, said the State's Attorney could do nothing in prosecuting abortionists until he had complete evidence, and prosecutions failed frequently because of the fact that evidence has not been properly obtained. He referred to the manner in which evidence should be prepared in these cases. The court instructs the jury that every material allegation in the indictment must be proved beyond reasonable doubt. It must be proved that a woman was pregnant, and that an operation was performed to induce abortion. It must be proved that such an abortion was not necessary to save the life of the mother, and that she died as a result of it. It is absolutely necessary for a physician in making his examination to make it carefully and exhaustively and preserve his data, so that he can refresh his mind, and be able to take the stand and say with absolute accuracy and certainty that the woman was pregnant. This would help the State's Attorney in proving to the jury beyond a reasonable doubt that pregnancy did exist. The next point to prove to the jury is that it is not necessary to perform an abortion to save the life of the mother; and the physician must be able to take the stand to tell the conditions he found, the treatment of the patient, and give his reasons clearly to the jury to show why it was not necessary to induce an abortion to save the life of the mother. Furthermore, it is necessary to show that death resulted from the operation by which the abortion was produced.

The symposium was further discussed by Dr. M. O. Heckard, Mr. H. H. Hart, Mr. Chas Allen, Dr. Lucy Waits, and Dr. Rosalie M. Ladova.

BOOK REVIEWS.

THE MEDICAL RECORD VISITING LIST AND PHYSICIAN'S DIARY FOR 1905. William Wood & Company, New York.

THIS edition of the *Medical Record* Visiting List has been revised to increase the amount of matter calculated to be useful in emergencies, and eliminate such as might better be referred to in the physician's library. The most important change is in the list of remedies and their maximum doses in both systems of measurement. The remainder of the contents of this handy little book comprises collections of facts and data suitably arranged for quick reference. The blank pages are ruled and labeled for the physician's daily records.

PROGRESSIVE MEDICINE. Edited by Dr. H. A. HARE. Assisted by Dr. H. R. M. LANDIS. Vol. III, September, 1904. Lea Brothers & Company, Philadelphia and New York.

THE present series deals with Diseases of the Thorax and its Viscera, by Dr. William Ewart, F.R.C.P.; Dermatology and Syphilis, by Dr. William S. Gottheil; Obstetrics, by Dr. Richard C. Norris, and Diseases of the Nervous System, by Dr. William G. Spiller.

As in the past so in the present volume we have correctly and adequately reflected the chief advances that have taken place in these fields of medicine during the past year. The practitioner who reads Progressive Medicine thoroughly may feel that in practically all lines of medicine he is abreast of the real advance army of investigators.

THE MEDICAL NEWS.

A WEEKLY JOURNAL OF MEDICAL SCIENCE.

VOL. 86.　　　NEW YORK, SATURDAY, FEBRUARY 4, 1905.　　　NO. 5.

ORIGINAL ARTICLES.

PRESIDENTIAL ADDRESS.[1]

BY CHARLES L. DANA,
OF NEW YORK.

THE honor of being elected president of the New York Academy of Medicine is one which I receive with keen appreciation of the distinction that is conferred. It brings to me, however, a sense of responsibility rather than one of elation, for I know that where so much is given, much is rightly expected. I shall devote to the Academy my best energies, and if it does not continue to prosper during my régime, it will not be because I fail to serve it as loyally and as wisely as I am capable of doing.

This Academy, with its well-equipped building, its superb library and its efficient medical organization, is perhaps the greatest single achievement of the profession of this city. It not only makes the practice of our art more efficient, productive and enjoyable, but it gives a dignity and a wider esteem to our calling. The Academy has a history of over a half century linked with the most honored names and best traditions of our calling, and it has, I am glad to say, a prospering present, thanks to the works of its many devoted friends. It deserves to receive your active support, and to be the agent in fostering the enduring work of the physicians of New York and its environs.

The Academy, as the reports show, is growing in membership and in all of its active departments, its sections are well attended and splendidly active. I have no new and radical policies to present or innovations in method to suggest therefor, for they are not needed. Nevertheless, we must at times suppress the sympathetic attitude toward an institution so important as this, and critically inquire whether it is continuing to do all that can be done in the interests of promoting medicine and the public health, and if it is doing it in the very best way.

THE INCREASE OF MEDICAL SOCIETIES.

Looking at our work for the past few years from this point of view, it seems to me that we may not have fairly appreciated the tremendous changes which have taken place in the method of medical organization, and in the presentation of results of medical work. In the last twenty-five years there have been developed new methods of study and investigation, there has been an increased activity in medical organization, and a corresponding increase in the amount of medical talk, medical writings, medical journals and medical books. Thus, to refer only

[1] Delivered before the New York Academy of Medicine.

to medical organizations, twenty-five years ago there were about 20 medical societies in Manhattan and the Bronx. There are now 52 such organizations registered in the Medical Directory. Of these 26 are general, and more or less public, while 14 are devoted to the specialties, and this number will be increased to 22, if we include the sections of this Academy. More than half of these societies are small, and partly social organizations. They meet at least once a month, during eight months of the year, and this means that there are during each season about 450 medical meetings provided for the 4,000 physicians of Manhattan. This makes for the six week-days of the season an average of about two medical meetings every evening. Although the majority of these societies have a small membership, it is evident that the claims on the profession for society attendance are very considerable. Such figures, however, do not give perhaps quite the right idea of the situation. If one looks through the pages of our medical directories they will see that the great majority of the physicians of New York belong to only one society, and some, apparently, not to any at all. And there is, no doubt, a very large number of physicians who do not attempt to gain the advantages of actual contact with the members of the profession, of hearing the living voice and of scrutinizing the personality of the authors of papers, such as are furnished by our medical organizations. It would be worth while, perhaps, to call to the attention of this class the fact that a man cannot practise medicine in the best way at the present day, cannot keep in touch with the progress of affairs, when working by himself, even if he is a diligent peruser of good books and periodicals. Personal contact with his fellowmen, even casual exchanges of experience, and the stimulus which cannot fail to be received at a well-attended and well-organized medical meeting, is absolutely necessary to keep a man abreast of the times. It is not so much a duty as a necessity for a practising physician, if he wishes to continue to keep up his work, even to the level of the average current of progress, that he be in some way affiliated with a medical organization and attend its meetings.

It becomes all the more the duty of those who have something to do with the organization of medical societies to see that they make the meetings of such a character as will attract the members and make them feel that there is something to be gained in listening, and in speech, which is not found in the solitary perusal of the reports of the following week.

The problem of how to make a medical society attractive in this way, how to make it compete successfully with the medical journals, to secure in its transactions that kind of activity which cannot be put exactly into print, is the problem which has grown more serious of late years. With so many pressing duties and interesting occasions presented in a city like New York, the securing of large society meetings has become almost an art of itself, or we may say, a special kind of executive business. If securing such big audiences were one of the objects of the Academy, I would almost advise the hiring of a paid and specially skilled secretary to attend to this function, one who would see that the reader of a paper should read the right kind of a paper, and should have the right kind of men to respond to it, and have a sufficient audience, both critical and sympathetic, to justify the work expended. Only those who have had the experience know the difficulty of accomplishing all these ends.

It is, however, in my opinion, not the function of the Academy of Medicine to try and do this thing; or, at least, it should only be a secondary consideration. My hope and ambition for the academy would be rather to have it understood that its general meetings furnish a forum where those who have made some valuable observations or research, or have some special and useful experience, can present these things for record and criticism. I should like to have it a place in which a man who has accumulated some definite results of his work could come and report this, perhaps only in some brief memorandum, the details and larger substance of the paper to be published later. It should be the forum for the announcement, in brief, of discoveries made, illuminating clinical cases or pathological observations, notes on laboratory work, and on practical things of all the special branches of medicine. This should be the particular function of our general meetings; so far as it is practicable. Symposia on special topics are most useful, and are provided for by the sectional meetings, which take up nearly half of our time. It seems to me that we could add to the value of this sectional work by at times combining one or two sections and having them present some topic in common. Thus, general surgery and gynecology would be the better for occasionally working and discussing questions together, and the same, it seems, might be true of otology, rhinology and ophthalmology.

There is a certain class of medical literature which ought, as a rule, to go directly to the medical journals. I refer to the formal addresses and discourses, and the long monographic papers. I do not think it is sufficiently realized how entirely doctors have outgrown the habit of going to listen to addresses. Some of the best and most carefully prepared discourses of this class have been delivered to almost empty houses, and there is a reason for this which we cannot controvert. Addresses, to be sure, are necessary for the emphasizing of certain special occasions, and they cannot be done away with. But

then their chief value should be literary, oratorical and generally educational. It is indeed a delight and a benison to listen to an eloquent man, and I would not discourage this form of art. But I would almost advocate a law forbidding the introduction into active work of medical organizations of formal addresses or monographic papers which are to appear in print later. It is only when one has something momentous to prove, and must prove it in order to get out criticism, that such long articles are justifiable. There are few single observations or things for record that cannot be expressed in twenty minutes.

These facts are being rather quickly appreciated in our sections and our societies. A time-limit is always a part of the by-laws, but I do not find that medical men yet understand that time-limits may be reduced still further by a study and proper use of the art of language.

THE ART OF WRITING MEDICAL PAPERS.

This leads me to another observation, which I wish to emphasize, and that is, the importance of a speaker or writer taking always some pains, some special pains indeed, to present what he has to say in a lucid, well-balanced, and concise manner. I do not insist on the necessity for fine methods of expression, for elaborate English, or finished and artistic phrases, but only, that when the medical writer has a subject in hand, he feels bound to express it (with the needs of his audience in mind) in a way which avoids all that is unnecessary and brings out his point as quickly and as emphatically as possible. The paper read should often be different from the paper printed in form and length. By remembering this, it becomes possible to have a number of topics brought forward for criticism, and make the evening both enlivening and profitable.

There has been suggested of late the adoption of a " marking system " for Genius, and it is possible that we might, with advantage, suggest a marking system for medical papers, which could be consulted by the writer, and not necessarily applied by the executive officer of the organization to which he presents himself. Thus, supposing that we take the following characteristics: (1) Originality of observation, this might be given marks from 0 up to 75; (2) laboriousness of research, 0 to 25; (3) interest of the observation, from rarity, 0 to 20; (4) interest of the observation for its practical medical value, 0 to 30; (5) scholastic, bibliographic and historical value, 0 to 25; (6) literary form and lucid brevity of presentation, 0 to 25.

These headings cover the important points upon which the value of a paper would be estimated.

Applying these canons to a recent notable article in a medical weekly, I find: 1, 40; 2, 25; 4. 20. Total, 85. This, on a scale of 100, represents a very high mark and is what the paper deserved.

It is my aim, then, to show that the medical

rofession, in view of an increasing prolificness f its work, in the matter of articles written and ead, and in view of the increased number of ledical societies, and the demands put upon busy len, must take some measures for its self-pro- :ction, and these consist in abolishing some of le modes of procedure which have been utilized t the past, and have descended to us by tradi- on. Next, that the medical profession learn lat unless it wishes to be swamped by the ex- berance of its own fertility, it must learn to taster the art of presenting what is desired to :cord with accuracy, clearness and dispatch.

HE ‑PROPORTIONATE INTEREST OF MEDICINE AND ITS SPECIALTIES.

Another question, which comes with special im- ɔrtance before an organization such as this, is le proportionate attention which should be given ᵻ the departments of medicine. The New York .cademy has its general meetings and it has nine :ctions, representing nine different specialties. : will be interesting, I have thought, to find out, possible, about the proportionate interest hich medical men, in general, feel toward these ifferent branches, and I have taken three of le prominent medical weeklies here in this city ιd the *British Medical Journal*, of London, and ɔne over all the original articles published in ιem during the last year. There were about ooo original articles published in these weeklies . 1903. I have assigned these articles to the fferent general and special branches of Medi- ne and Surgery. Without claiming any great ːgree of accuracy for the results, it seems to ≀ that they show fairly well the varying de- ree of interest shown by general readers in .e different branches. Thus, out of 663 arti- es published in this city in 1903, a quarter of ιem were devoted to subjects of internal medi- ne; a little less than one-quarter to general ιrgical subjects, including orthopedic and rec- l surgery. Neurology and psychiatry come next, ith 8 per cent.; genito-urinary surgery, 6 per- ·nt.; obstetrics and gynecology, 6 per cent.; ιthology and bacteriology, 5 per cent.; physiolo- ⱱ and physiological chemistry, 3 per cent.; ryngology, 5 per cent.; ophthalmology, 5 per nt.; hygiene, climate and tropical diseases, pre- :ntive medicine, about 6 per cent.; X-ray, ra- um and light therapeutics. 6 per cent.; otology, per cent.; government, railway and insurance rvice, 1 per cent.

I wished to find out whether the relative inter- t in these different branches was the same in is country that it was in Great Britain; there- re I analyzed the 433 British articles in the me way. The results were nearly the same. ith two or three important exceptions: General rgery ranks in Great Britain considerably ɡher than internal medicine, in the proportion 100 to 80. Pathology, bacteriology and gen- al laboratory research seem to excite almost ⸍ice as much interest in Great Britain as they

do in New York, there being 10 per cent. of the articles devoted to these subjects. Physiology and physiological chemistry are also very much more in evidence in Great Britain than here, in the proportion of about 4 per cent. for us to 7 per cent with Great Britain. Naturally the sub- jects of hygiene, climate and tropical diseases also take a very much higher rank with the British. On the whole, it may be said that at least one-half of the articles which are published in our general medical journals, are devoted to subjects of general medicine and surgery. The other half is devoted to the laboratory sciences, and to the special branches of medicine in pro- portions ranging from 2 to 8 per cent. We do not need to fear, it seems to me, from these fig- ures, that general medicine and surgery are being pushed aside by the special sciences, and it would seem to me that a fair conclusion to be drawn would be that in the meetings in this Academy somewhat less than one-half the time should be devoted to special subjects, when they are such as bring them in touch with general medicine or surgery, and that perhaps more than half the time should be given to those subjects that are particularly important to those engaged in general practice or in those branches of in- ternal medicine and surgery which are really a part of it, such as pathology and bacteriology.

THE ACADEMY AND PUBLIC QUESTIONS.

The Academy has, during a large part of its history, had a great influence in matters of pub- lic health and preventive medicine. Dr. Fordyce Barker, in an address delivered on his inaugu- ration as president, declared that the New York City Board of Health was the result of the work; was, in fact, the child of this Academy. This Board has grown to be so efficient and so efful- gent a part of our municipal government, that it largely takes away from medical organizations the responsibility of watching and fostering local sanitary work. Perhaps this is why the Section on Public Health, which was once organized, and which throve for a time, has been dropped.

While I do not feel that we as a body need now to take initiative, or be known as actively work- ing for public health, and for all that belongs to State medicine, I do not think that we ought to be regarded as an advisory body of highest and last resort in matters of policy relating to all pub‑ lic medical questions not involving politics, from which latter we stand absolutely divorced.

But, in order to secure respect for our opin- ions and weight to our influence on these sub- jects, we will have to take a different course from that which is sometimes pursued by medical so- cieties. We should, for example, be unalterably opposed to the practice of adopting resolutions in a public meeting, involving questions of ex- pert knowledge, or requiring careful and exact investigation of facts, without such resolutions being submitted first to a committee of those par- ticularly expert on the matters involved.

We have no section on public health, or State medicine, or medical economics, and perhaps we do not need one; but we might well consider the wisdom of having the council empowered to appoint a permanent committee on public health and medical economics. This committee should be a large one, and contain the best experts in sanitation, chemistry, pathology and bacteriology, as well as men practically familiar with sanitary and educational administration.

This committee, reporting to the council, and then through it, or directly to the Academy, would bring conclusions that would arouse serious attention, and if endorsed by the vote of the Fellows, they would not fail, I believe, to have convincing force with the public, and perhaps even with our politicians.

The resolutions of medical organizations have heretofore been, as a rule, acts of pitifully small influence upon men of affairs, and in so far as they relate to matters of medical aggrandizement, or of the particular interests of the medical man himself, they will always be received with some austerity by the public. But on medical questions that concern the general public good, the sentiment of organized medical men ought always to carry the greatest possible weight. The voice of this Academy should represent the judgment of the best elements of the profession in a great city which itself naturally includes in large numbers the best men from the country at large.

This voice should only be heard when the occasion is fit, and then it should speak after careful deliberation and on the advice of those most wise and expert. It would then have a finality that would work to the good of the public and the dignity of the Academy. It would be no trumpet-toned resolution, but the serious conclusions of wisdom, expertness and experience.

THE SECTIONS OF THE ACADEMY.

The policy of having special sections of the Academy has been justified by the very successful work of these organizations, and by the increase in medical activity they have brought about. It has been said that the meetings of some sections have been better attended and brought out better work than those of the general Academy itself; but as long as the work is done we will not quarrel over who does it. I believe in the value of the sections, and if they become so lively in interest, and so superior in importance as to outshine the Alma Mater, so be it. The fittest must survive; but I shall try not to have the obscuration occur in my régime. It seems wise to have just as many sections as the Fellows will support without too much urging. We cannot have too many medical societies, if they are good societies, even if we have to sell this building and build a bigger, as some day we must. It is a constant tendency of medical men to get into routine, to prescribe the same old rhubarb mixture, the same calomel tablet, or the quinine and iron. A routine means early de-

generation. People of fixed habits die early, even if the habits are not very bad. It is the medical society that keeps us going ahead. Therefore, the Academy need have no hesitation in organizing for as much work as it can possibly do.

Now I have shown that after medicine and surgery, the special branches attracting most articles into medical weeklies are those of neurology and psychiatry. These branches would be of larger interest still, if to them were added what used to be called forensic medicine. There is now no such distinct science, it having been split up among psychiatrists, chemists, bacteriologists, pathologists and lawyers. That part of it which may be called "legal psychiatry" belongs appropriately with a section on psychiatry.

There has been in the last few years a tremendous impetus to the study of psychiatry. The improved organization of our State hospitals, the establishment of laboratories, the increased interest in the problems of the alienist and their better and more scientific investigation, has really given birth to a new medical science. We have in and about New York many men active and interested in this branch, and the Academy might well furnish to them an opportunity for the presentation of their work. I shall recommend the consideration of the establishment, then, of a section on psychiatry and neurology. In doing this, I hope I am not under any personal bias as to the larger exploitation of those branches in which I am supposed to be more particularly interested.

The analysis which I have made of the articles presented in medical weeklies by American and British journals, respectively, suggests that we are hardly interested enough in the problems of pathology, physiology and physiological chemistry, or the laboratory sciences, as they are sometimes called. There are probably at present no problems in medicine so intricate, so fascinating, and so fundamentally important as these. To a certain extent it may be said that purely clinical medicine is worked out. What more can be observed of the common phenomena of the every day diseases? They appear, it is true, in ever-varying phases and combinations, and each particular case of acute fever or heart, kidney and lung trouble has features of its own. We must study and hear about them again and again. But to make radical progress we must go deeper and deeper into the biology of disease. The problems of metabolism, of immunity, of toxins, bacteria, ferments, internal secretions, and the finer chemical changes are those which promise to enlighten and help us most richly in the future. Internal medicine, with the laboratory sciences as its handmaid, is rapidly regaining its former high dignity and rising to the great prominence it deserves.

The question may well arise, therefore, whether we should not furnish a forum for the laboratory sciences. The Rockefeller Institute cannot work all alone, and we should like to have it and the several State and college laboratories put themselves in touch with the working physician by presenting some of their results to us here. I shall suggest the organization of a section on the laboratory sciences, either independent or in connection with internal medicine.

I am not afraid of creating too many sections, but if it is considered unwise to expand numerically, there is the possibility of combining some of the sections already established, provided this seems entirely welcome to the members. As I look over the long programs of these sections and note their work, I confess it may be found unwise and unnecessary. But, as neurology and psychiatry consent to lie down together, why might not otology, rhinology and ophthalmology have some lines of union? It would give greater importance to the section and its officers, and would probably enlarge the point of view of all.

I present these questions with an entirely unbiased mind, and only desire that we do what will promote the effectiveness of the Academy and the harmonies of medical life and its larger work.

I must now draw my address to a close, lest I be accused of violating those canons of medical expression which I myself have just laid down. Perhaps I have already done this. There are certain conventions which we cannot at once do away with, however, and I have admitted that the addresses must occasionally be delivered in order to emphasize an opportunity or to lay down a policy.

In concluding, then, I wish to express the hope that during the coming year the Fellows will learn to feel more profoundly that the Academy is not merely a library and reading room, but is also an organization of men especially chosen to promote the science and art of medicine and public health; that these halls should be the forum for the effective exploitation of our work in curing the sick and seeking the causes of disease. And I should delight to find (for it is possible) that the records of the meetings of this Academy carried with them a history of the best achievements and most interesting activities of the profession.

Gentlemen, I have taken the honor you have given me with much genuine misgiving; for I felt that there were many who deserved it more and were better fitted for the task. But having had the laurel put upon my brow, I shall try and wear it as if it fitted some better conformation. I have the inspiration of the accomplishments of the past to help me; I am supported by an especially distinguished board of officers, who are devoted to the welfare of the Academy. I ask for your active support and confidence in order that we may work together for the continued success of this honorable organization and for the dignity and worth of the one as yet uncommercialized profession.

PARTIALLY AFEBRILE ESTIVO-AUTUMNAL MALARIAL INFECTION HAVING ITS ORIGIN IN NEW YORK CITY.

BY J. L. POMEROY, M.D.,
OF NEW YORK;
HOUSE PHYSICIAN N. Y. CITY (CHARITY) HOSPITAL.

THROUGH the courtesy of Dr. Charles E. Quimby, I am enabled to report the following case from his wards at the City Hospital. At the meeting of the Pan-American Congress in 1901, Dr. C. N. B. Camac called attention to the fact of the presence in the State of New York of this extremely grave form of malaria, and presented a series of eight cases in which he was able to find the parasite. No reliable statistics on this question could then be found, and because of the fact that the comparatively harmless tertian parasite abounds in our Northern States, and also because the term malaria is made to cover a multitude of ignorance, it becomes an important question of prophylaxis to prevent the spread of this dangerous tropical type of infection. The question of quarantine for such cases also becomes of paramount interest, for through the intervention of the mosquito this oftime fatal form of malaria may be quite widely disseminated.

The patient, B. G., aged forty-one years, single, an Irishman by birth, entered the hospital Nov. 5, 1904. He gave his address as Pearl Street, and stated that he had not been outside of the city since fifteen years ago, when he emigrated to America. Occupation longshoreman. His regular work was unloading vessels from all parts of the world. His family history is negative. His habits are good. He does not use tobacco; takes two or three whiskies a day, always in moderation. Measles and scarlet fever in childhood, otherwise negative. Denies venereal infection. Save for his present illness lasting over a period of four years, he has not been sick.

Present Illness.—During the fall of 1900 he began to suffer from chills and sweats. This attack lasted some three weeks, during which time he was bedridden and his skin became yellow. His physician told him he had malaria. Recovery was slow, and he did not regain his former strength. From time to time he would have chills followed by sweats, but as they were so irregular he did not return to his doctor. He states that he used some pills given him, taking one three times daily. Following a course of pills he would improve. For periods of several months he would feel stronger, but his loss in weight became quite apparent. Finally, three weeks ago, the chills and sweats recurred with renewed severity for the first time since June last. While they were very irregular they occurred some time during the hours of 5 A.M. to 9 P.M.

Physical Examination.—Patient was a man of large frame in whom emaciation was very apparent. His cheeks and eyeballs were sunken, the color of his skin sallow, and his general musculature flabby and wasted. He was very weak and compelled to stay in bed. The tongue was flabby, covered with yellowish fur, and the mucous membranes were very pale. Chest poorly developed, expansion poor, though equal on either side. Left infraclavicular space rather flat. Over left apex behind were a few persistent moist râles, but there were no other signs obtained. At the bases on either sides were a few sibilant râles. His abdomen was flat, muscle-wall flabby, very little subcutaneous fat present, and skin was loose and wrinkled. The liver was palpable about six centimeters below the right costal margin, edge firm and smooth. Spleen was easily palpable and was also quite hard. Examination of his heart revealed a soft-blowing systolic murmur at the apex, not transmitted to axilla, but heard over the pulmonic area. The second aortic was accentuated, the first sound was clear; there was no enlargement beyond nipple line.

Blood pressure taken on entrance with Riva-Rocci instrument (Janeway's modification) gave a reading of 130 m.m. of mercury in both arms; pulse 90, respiration 22, temperature 99.6° F. Knee-jerks were normal, muscles of calves soft and flabby.

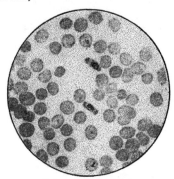

Estivo-Autumnal Malaria.

He had scarcely any appetite on entering, and suffered from a slight cough with a mucopurulent expectoration. Sputum examinations at various times were negative for tubercle bacilli. His bowels were very costive, he was extremely restless, and during the evening of his entrance he had a violent chill followed by a profuse sweat, but his temperature was normal, both before and after chill, not going above 99° F. These chills proved very irregular, appearing often without being followed by a definite sweat, and again the reverse would be the case.

Examination of his blood immediately upon entrance showed the presence of beautiful crescentic and ovoid bodies, which were always extracellular. Examinations made during the afternoon showed a preponderance of the ovoid forms. The crescentic bodies were always deeply pigmented. They seemed to be more numerous

during the forenoon. No other variety of Plasmodia was found. Slides were taken every two hours for a period of two days to determine this; Jenner's stain was used in all examinations. White blood count 7,000. The urine report showed the specific gravity to be 1.020, color amber, clear, faint traces of albumin and no sugar. Microscopical report after centrifuging revealed a few granular casts. No pus or blood cells being found.

Shortly after admission the patient was placed upon quinine sulphate in perforated capsules, grains fifteen, every four hours, and one-half ounce of Warburg's tincture, before meals, to stimulate his appetite. Saline catharsis was used to relieve his constipation and to increase elimination. After twenty hours he felt much better; his sweats became less frequent, a marked increase in strength and appetite was noticeable, and his temperature, which had previously remained normal, now ran as high as 100.2° F. In a few days more he was able to get up, and one week after the treatment was instituted he was able to be removed to his home. Examination of his blood now proved negative for malarial plasmodia.

The points of interest in this case are: (1) An estivo-autumnal infection having its origin in New York City. (2) Chills and sweats without temperature—the latter appearing only when quinine had been administered, and then not rising above 100.2° F.

SUMMER INFANT MORTALITY.[1]

BY LOUIS C. AGER, M.D.,
OF BROOKLYN, N. Y.

ALTHOUGH this paper is to deal more particularly with a study of the infant mortality of the present summer in New York City, the subject can be more intelligently treated by a brief review of past conditions, with a short report of what has been already accomplished in the way of improvement.

Although statistics are apt to be very uninteresting to all but the compiler, I will venture to present a large part of this paper in that form, —bearing in mind the adage that "while figures cannot lie, liars can figure."

In the first place we are all aware, in a general way, that the death-rate in the first years of life is much higher than in later years. Unfortunately, when we happen to give any thought to the subject, we are apt to look upon it as one of the things that cannot be helped. We give altogether too much weight to the survival-of-the-fittest idea,—considering it merely as one of the many examples of nature's superfluous fertility. This feeling is particularly common among those who come much in contact with the tenement house population of our large cities. The first thought is not, "why do so many die?" but "how do so many live?" This fatalistic mental

[1] Read before the New York State Medical Association, October 19, 1904.

attitude has undoubtedly hindered greatly the progress that we ought to expect along this line.

Taking at random the vital statistics of Brooklyn for the year ending September 30, 1903, we find that the total number of deaths was over 21,000. Of this number over one-fifth were under one year of age, and nearly one-third were under five years. Furthermore, of the 7,000 deaths in children under five years, one-fifth were caused by diarrheal diseases in children under two years, and of these about two-thirds occurred during July, August and September.

Is it not preposterous, with these figures in mind, to say that it cannot be helped? Is it not the duty of the members of the medical profession to take a more aggressive attitude on this subject and to point out to the public the economic value of sanitary and hygienic improvements in the care of our infant population? Is it not a sure proof of laziness or worse on the part of the physician who says the fault is all with the parents,—that they will not listen to advice and will not carry out instructions?

Turning to the other side of the question, What has been accomplished in the past few years in the way of improvement,—the figures for the old City of New York are presented in Table No. IV.

Considerable time might be profitably devoted to the study of these figures. They certainly present a record of improvement that any municipality might be proud of. We are all aware of the facts shown in the first column, the marked decrease in the general death-rate. But the improvement shown in columns five and seven is of even greater interest. Column five shows that while 45 per cent. of the deaths in 1881 were in children under five years of age, in 1897, only 39 per cent. were under five years. Column seven shows further that while in 1881 21 per cent. of the deaths under five years were due to diarrheal diseases, in 1897 only 15 per cent. were due to that cause. With this improvement in mind, some will doubtless wonder why I should speak so emphatically at the beginning of this paper. If New York has done so well, why make a plea for more energetic work in the future?

If, on the other hand, we put out of mind the past improvement and merely consider the facts presented in Table No. IVa, do we not see not only room for further improvement, but also good reason to expect very appreciable results from properly directed and concerted efforts? These tables show an apparent increase in diarrheal mortality since consolidation, for the reason that at that time there was a change in classification, by which more diseases are included under the term diarrheal diseases than previously.

Here we see presented statistics for the past six years, and these are not, after all, very much to be proud of. In the first place there has been no diminution in the per cent. of deaths under five years. The per cent. of deaths under five years from diarrheal diseases does indeed show a change from 27 per cent. of all deaths under five years to only 21 per cent. Unfortunately the appended figures for the summer months of 1902, 1903 and 1904 show that the summer just passed was quite the worst of the three. To present the facts in a few words the situation in Greater New York is as follows: (1) Since 1898 there has been practically no improvement in the infant mortality; (2) The deaths under five years constitute 35 per cent. of all deaths, and of these over 20 per cent. are due to diarrheal diseases. Now, there may be a wide difference of opinion among physicians as to the extent to which summer diarrheal diseases in children may be classed as preventable. The physician who still accepts " dentition " as a reasonable cause of death on a death certificate will perhaps be satisfied with things as they are. On the other hand, if we accept the logical conclusion from known facts that summer diarrheas are essentially infectious diseases, must we not go one step further and admit that they are, theoretically at least, just as much in the category of preventable diseases as typhoid, for example?

Before entering further, however, into the question of future preventability, allow me to present a few suggestions as to the cause of the very gratifying improvement in New York and Brooklyn previous to 1898, as shown in Table I, and the apparent lack of improvement since that date. The first question can be passed over very briefly. A large part of the infant mortality in the earlier days was due to easily removable causes, but those causes were outside the domain of the individual citizen, and may be summarized in general under the two heads: Lack of any adequate supervision of the milk supply, and lack of any adequate sanitary regulation in regard to tenement houses. As soon as these two matters were dealt with systematically, there resulted an exceedingly gratifying improvement in the summer infant mortality. But after a period of years the most manifest results of these things were accomplished and the infant mortality curve ceased to descend. This does not imply that the present sanitary condition is ideal, or that our milk supply is perfect, but undoubtedly the more radical changes and the more marked improvements have already been accomplished. It is probably true in some respects, in the condition of the streets, for example, that New York is much worse from a sanitary point of view than it was a year ago. Theoretically, at least, the cleanliness of the streets must have a more marked effect upon infant mortality than upon the total death-rate: first, because the streets are the children's play grounds, and second, because the children come in so much closer contact with Mother Earth than do their parents.

Investigations made in Manhattan a few years ago show that the number of bacteria in street air depends not only upon the cleanliness of the street, but also upon the height of the air above the pavement. Plates exposed on the curb developed several times as many organisms as those exposed at a height of six feet. Children on the street and in baby carriages are therefore much more likely to inhale dust-borne organisms, and their methods of play bring the organisms in the soil in direct contact with their hands, faces and mouths. The sooner the public realizes that smooth clean pavements are an actual economy

TABLE I.—Number of Deaths from Diarrheal Diseases in Children Under Five Years of Age Per 100,000 of Total Population.

Year.	Brooklyn.	Manhattan.
1881	257	297
1882	264	271
1883	214	219
1884	234	232
1885	232	205
1886	163	208
1887	180	219
1888	190	200
1889	148	200
1890	163	185
1891	179	189
1892	177	173
1893	168	164
1894	151	149
1895	159	151
1896	132	133
1897	114	118
1898	131	121

in human lives, the sooner will the infant mortality decrease.

As regards the milk supply, the improvements in the past twenty-five years are too familiar to require recapitulation here. At the present time milk of very good quality can be obtained for eight cents a quart. It does not, of course, come up to the certified milk standard, and during

TABLE II.—New Classification.

1898	224	191
1899	180	142
1900	196	160
1901	194	161

the warm weather it must be Pasteurized for infant feeding. As in the case of all other food products, the consumer who is most particular with his dealer gets the best milk, while the consumer who does not drink milk himself, and is therefore not personally interested in the milk that comes to his house, will get the milk from

TABLE III.

	Brooklyn.	Manhattan.
Population, 1902	1,166,582	1,850,093
Population under five years	28,961	46,796
Percentage under five years	2.48	2.53

the poorer dairy. The greatest value of the work of the milk commissions will be in educating the public to demand a cleaner grade of milk. In that way the improvements in production and in the rapidity of delivery suggested by the milk commissions will be introduced into all dairies.

All these things so far referred to are things

that the community has done or must do for the the individual. The future improvements must come very largely from the things that the individual can do for himself. It is at present possible in New York for parents even in very moderate circumstances to care properly and successfully for infants and children.

TABLE IV.—New York City.

Year.	Death rate.	Total deaths.	Deaths under five years.	Percentage of total under five years.	Diar. under five years.	Percentage of total deaths under five years.
1881	31.04	38,624	17,737	.45	3,710	.21
1882	29.61	37,924	17,520	.46	3,479	.19
1883	25.80	34,011	13,856	.40	2,837	.19
1884	25.82	35,034	15,272	.43	3,160	.20
1885	25.55	35,682	15,267	.42	2,892	.19
1886	25.99	37,351	16,121	.43	2,990	.18
1887	26.32	38,933	16,766	.42	3,252	.19
1888	26.39	40,175	17,356	.43	3,051	.18
1889	25.32	39,679	17,152	.43	3,135	.18
1890	24.87	40,173	16,302	.40	2,997	.18
1891	26.31	43,659	18,224	.41	3,191	.17
1892	25.95	44,329	18,684	.42	3,162	.17
1893	25.30	44,486	17,865	.40	2,898	.16
1894	22.76	41,175	17,558	.42	2,708	.15
1895	23.18	43,420	18,221	.42	2,839	.15
1896	21.84	41,622	16,807	.40	2,544	.15
1897	20.03	38,877	15,395	.39	2,296	.15

For the study of the question of ways and means for future improvements, we are fortunate in having side by side the work done and its results in the Boroughs of Brooklyn and Manhattan, and as a Brooklynite I regret to state tha

TABLE IVA.—Greater New York.

Year.	Death rate.	Total deaths.	Deaths under five years.	Percentage of total under five years.	Diar. under five years.	Percentage of total deaths under
1898	20.26	66,294	23,499	.35	6,442	.2
1899	19.47	65,343	23,801	.36	5,127	.2
1900	20.57	70,872	25,836	.36	5,747	.2
1901	20.02	70,814	24,256	.34	6,071	.2
1902	18.75	68,112	24,388	.35	5,190	.2

Deaths from Diarrheal Diseases 17 Summer Week Brooklyn and Manhattan.

1902					3,201
1903					2,735
1904					3,810

Brooklyn must be cited as an example of how n to do it.

The peculiar facts relating to infant mortali in Brooklyn were first called to my attention the spring of 1902, and my first study of t subject was published in the *Brooklyn Medic*

Journal for February, 1903. Since that time I have given considerable time to the subject and have not found occasion materially to change my views as to the probable cause of the unfortunate conditions brought to our attention every

TABLE V.—Death Rate Per 100,000 of Population, Diarrheal Diseases, All Ages, 1900.

New York County	170
Kings County	209
Queens County	216
Richmond County	228

week during the summer in the Health Department Bulletins.

Some of the statistics are presented in the tables. Table I, to which reference has already

TABLE VI.—Ages.

Under 1 month	10
1 to 2 months	15
2 to 4 months	31
4 to 6 months	61
6 to 9 months	52
9 to 12 months	42
12 to 15 months	15
15 to 18 months	13
18 to 24 months	11

been made, gives the comparative infant death rate for Brooklyn and Manhattan for the past twenty-three years. This shows that up to 1891 the difference, such as it was, was in favor of

TABLE VII.—Dwellings.

Tenements: Poor, 97; Fair, 58; Good, 45	200
Private houses	36
Institutions	14

Brooklyn. Since that time, however, with a few exceptions, the mortality in Brooklyn has been much worse than in Manhattan.

The conditions prevailing during the last three years are more clearly presented by graphic

TABLE VIII.—Analysis of Condensed Milk. Percentage by Weight.

Fat	9.6
Casein	8.5
Milk Sugar	11.5
Cane Sugar	44.0
Specific gravity	1.28

charts. In these the most noticeable fact is the difference between the first of the summer and the last. As soon as the hot weather sets in, there is a much more rapid rise in in-

TABLE IX.—Percentages—Condensed Milk Mixture and Human Milk.

Fat	.85	4.0
Casein	.75	1.5
Milk Sugar	1.02	7.0
Cane Sugar	2.87	

fant mortality than in Manhattan. After a few weeks the rate in Brooklyn comes down and meets or even crosses the Manhattan rate. This result is the product of two groups of factors,

on the one side the infants, on the other the infants' surroundings. Looked at in this way, the problem resolves itself into the question, where, among these two factors, lies the difference between Brooklyn and Manhattan?

1. Table III shows that the percentage of the population under five years of age is greater in Manhattan than in Brooklyn. The greater infant death-rate in Brooklyn is therefore not due to the presence of a larger infant population, as was at one time suggested.

2. Climatic conditions must be very nearly identical in the two boroughs, with the advantage, so far as there is any, in favor of Brooklyn's summer climate.

The logical conclusion seems to be that there must be some difference in the care that the children receive. We are all aware, I presume, of the fact that at the first blast of summer heat there is a quick harvest of those little ones that have been barely able to keep their hold on life under more favorable weather conditions. After these are gone, the death-rate settles down to its daily average among the sturdier children, who from time to time succumb to the various forms of acute hot-weather infections. There must be therefore in Brooklyn, a larger proportion of weaklings than in Manhattan. As other causes are excluded, it follows that this is due to a difference in the nutrition of Brooklyn babies,—a difference in the method of feeding and caring for them. This, at first, seems absurd, but a careful study of the statistics from the two boroughs proves this to be the case. In the report of the work of the Rockefeller Institute by Drs. Park and Holt, published in the 1903 Report of the New York Health Department and elsewhere, Tables I and II show that about one-quarter of the bottle-fed infants under observation were fed on condensed milk. In the statistics that have been collected during the past summer in connection with the milk distribution of the Brooklyn Children's Aid Society, I find that from one-half to three-quarters of the bottle-fed babies were fed on condensed milk. Two years ago, in investigating the deaths of 250 infants from diarrheal diseases in Brooklyn, I found that 60 per cent. had been fed on condensed milk, while only 27 per cent. of the fatal cases in Manhattan had been fed in that way. Drs. Park and Holt say of this subject:

" The results with condensed milk can hardly be attributed to the bacteria, inasmuch as it was almost invariably prepared with boiled water, and contained relatively a small number of micro-organisms before heating. These children were often apparently in good condition until attacked with acute disease, when they offered but little resistance, and seemed to succumb more quickly than any other class of patients. In one family three healthy infants, triplets, five months old, were taken sick on the same day with vomiting and diarrhea; one died within twenty-four hours, one within two days, and the third within a week. A bacteriological examination of the prepared milk remained in one bottle showed nothing noteworthy."

It would be a waste of time for all concerned for me to enter into a discussion of this iniquitous method of infant feeding at this time. The proper way to feed artificially an infant of normal development can be learned from any textbook. There can be no doubt that at least one-half of the infant mortality is due to the improper feeding of children that start in life with a normal stomach. A comparison of the composition of the average condensed milk mixture with that of normal human milk is found in Table IX.

This difference in infant feeding in the two boroughs is of interest, however, in another way. It indicates a fundamental error somewhere in the education of the Brooklyn mothers. How does it happen that there is this difference in two parts of the same city? There can be but one answer, The physicians must be to a very large extent responsible for it, and only to the extent that they condemn the practice can it be eradicated. It is just here that the difference between conditions in Brooklyn and Manhattan is found. There have been in Manhattan those to teach publicly and emphatically the proper methods of infant feeding, and also those to undertake the work of supplying to all willing to use it the proper food. Brooklyn, on the other hand, has not been so fortunate in her supply of medical and financial philanthropists. There has never been any free ice distribution in that borough, and there has never been any general distribution of Pasteurized or modified milk. Each summer the Children's Aid Society distributes as far as its funds will permit, modified milk to sick babies, but only on a physician's order. Moreover, a nominal charge is made for the milk unless the physician certifies that the applicant is unable to pay. Now the proper feeding of a greater or less number of infants is a very small part of the good that is accomplished by this work. The great gain is in the education of the mothers, not only the mothers of the babies fed, but also all the other mothers that see the results. The brief suggestions in regard to the general care of infants that mothers receive at the distributing stations are of the greatest value in a home of the poorer tenement class. I am firmly convinced that these facts entirely explain the difference in the infant mortality in Brooklyn and Manhattan.

The Remedy.—A realization of the cause at once suggests the remedy. We must educate the parents. Individually we can do a great deal in our contact with them. Collectively we can do even more by bringing the matter to the attention of those who are able and willing to give the financial aid required.

The details of such work are simple, and experience shows that its success is assured. It is not an expensive thing to feed properly a normal baby; expensive, that is, in money. The required expenditure is in time and brains. The cynic will say that the tenement-house mother will not give the time and cannot give the brains. The cynic, however, has no place in the practice of medicine. Dr. Kerley says, and I think that those that have had the most experience will agree with him: " Our experience with thousands of tenement mothers justifies us in reaffirming that the fault and absence of good results rest more with the doctor than with the tenement mother. When printed and written directions are used and a pamphlet of instructions given to each mother, when she learns, as she will at the first visit, that the physician is personally interested in the welfare of her baby, she will, with very few exceptions, do her best, which is usually not bad."

The experiment tried by the Brooklyn Children's Aid Society during the past summer shows little that is new. Nevertheless it may be of interest as a practical move in the right direction. There were fourteen distributing stations established in various parts of the city, each in charge of a matron. The matron, in addition to giving out the milk, was expected to visit the homes and to make whatever suggestions seemed advisable in regard to the care of the children. In addition we had a volunteer corps of physicians to visit when needed. The value of the work accomplished in this way depends very largely upon the character of the matrons, as we found by sad experience in some cases. But it is quite extraordinary how much an energetic, tactful woman can accomplish in such a position. On account of the curious working of the human mind, the mothers would pay much more attention to advice from a friendly matron than to that from a physician. The feeling is strong that the doctor is to give medicine and that his duty ends there. At the close of the season we had a few brief talks to the mothers on the home modification of milk, the babies' clothes and similar subjects. At the stations where the work of the matrons had been well done there was an intelligent interest shown in the questions asked that was very encouraging.

The financial cost of work of this kind is comparatively slight, and we have learned much from this year's experience, particularly in regard to what the matrons can do. Another year more informal talks will be given, and the mothers will be induced in various ways to attend them.

SERUM DIAGNOSIS OF TYPHOID FEVER BY MEANS OF FICKER'S TYPHUS-DIAGNOSTICUM.[1]

BY JOHANNES H. M. A. VON TILING, M.D.,

VASSAR BROTHERS' HOSPITAL, POUGHKEEPSIE, N. Y.

You all recognize the importance of the Gruber-Widal reaction for the diagnosis of typhoid fever, but at the same time you realize with how many difficulties the carrying out of the test is connected—for the general practitioner. One needs a bacteriological laboratory with

1 Read before the Semi-annual Meeting of the Dutchess County Medical Association, Poughkeepsie, October 26, 1904.

thermostat, virulent typhoid bacilli, sterile culture media, microscope, and last but not least, some practice and technical training. Therfore it is, as a rule, not possible for the practitioner to make personal use of the Gruber-Widal reaction in the way in which it has so far been customary to employ it.

Yet the aim and object of all experimenters should be to simplify all methods of investigation so that they may be made available to all practitioners; and in the Gruber-Widal agglutination test the use of Ficker's typhoid diagnosticum is certainly a great simplification.

Widal himself, as also before him Gruber and his collaborators, used to study the agglutination and immobilization of the bacilli both *with* the microscope and *without* it. Afterward it was more customary to employ the test with the microscope only; but lately several investigators, especially in Germany, have tried to simplify the method and they have again introduced the plan of carrying out the test without a microscope. Another important step forward has been the employment of bouillon culture with dead bacilli instead of living ones.

Again it was Widal who knew that the dead bacilli show the same details in agglutination as the living ones. He used for his experiments bouillon cultures in which the bacilli were killed by heat or by formalin.

During the last two years the use of bacilli which were killed by formalin or toluol, has again been repeatedly suggested. These methods, in which killed bacilli are employed, may be—just as the original Gruber-Widal reaction—carried out with or without a microscope, but the method recommended by Ficker depends only upon macroscopical observation. This Ficker's typhoid diagnosticum contains apparently ground bacilli, is absolutely sterile and looks turbid.

For the general practitioner, only this latter modification seems to be available, for, up to now, such a culture with bacilli killed by formalin one has to prepare oneself, and in the first place the practitioner is, as a rule, unable to do that; furthermore it is rather difficult to get a culture in which the bacilli are of proper virulence, in which they are not either too undergrown or too overgrown, and in which the specific gravity of the bouillon must nearly correspond to the specific gravity of the bacilli in order to keep the latter suspended.

During the last few weeks I have employed in a number of typhoid fever cases, and also as control tests in a few other cases, the method by Ficker, comparing it in each instance with the original Gruber-Widal test, and I have found the modification by Ficker to be absolutely reliable. The number of my tests is not yet very great, but since all others who have tried this test agree that the results are most satisfactory, I feel justified in recommending this modification with the typhoid diagnosticum according to Ficker.

For the diagnosis of typhoid fever in a more early stage of the disease, however, this test does not give better results than the original Gruber-Widal test.

This diagnostic fluid is manufactured and put on the market by Merck, of Darmstadt; this fact guarantees its always uniform quality. The entire apparatus needed to carry out the test is put together in a very convenient and handy way and the set can be obtained for $1.85. The test is so simple that every physician will be able to make use of the reaction without difficulty, if only he follows the description that is added to each set and also takes into consideration the modification mentioned below.

According to Ficker, to carry out the test one must obtain from one to two c.c. of blood in the regular way by means of a cupping glass, which is then to be set aside in a cool place until the serum is separated. 0.1 c.c. of this serum which must be perfectly free from red blood corpuscles, is then mixed with 0.9 c.c. of sterile physiological salt solution. This diluted serum is then mixed with the diagnostic fluid in the proportions 1:5 and 1:10 in two of the little test tubes, which therefore now contain a serum dilution of 1:50 in one glass and 1:100 in the second. Then a third glass is filled with the diagnostic fluid alone. The fluid in these three test tubes appears now about equally turbid because of the bacilli in the diagnostic fluid. The reaction is positive if after from ten to twelve hours the fluid in the first or second glass begins to get clear, for in this case the bacilli clot together and sink to the bottom. Sometimes the reaction proves positive in a shorter time, sometimes it may take twenty hours, but if no clearing of the fluid occurs within this time, the test may be taken as negative. It is hardly necessary to add that all glasses and stoppers must be thoroughly cleansed and sterilized.

This test has the great advantage of convenience, but still there is one great inconvenience connected with it for patient and physician, that of obtaining the blood by means of a cupping glass. Therefore various propositions have been made to simplify the means of getting the blood and of obtaining the serum. Among other methods it has been recommended to make a rather deep wound and to let the blood run into a test tube or to get it from a vein with a hypodermic syringe and to let it clot in the latter. However, all these modifications do not appear to me to be very ideal for the general practitioner, especially in the country, since one must, without disturbing the specimen, wait for the clotting of the blood and the separating of the serum. For this reason I have tried to make the test by catching, from a small finger wound, made by a needle prick, a few drops of blood either on a glass slide or still more conveniently on a piece of filter paper; then I have let it dry and afterward in the laboratorium dissolved it with normal salt solution in the proportion

1:10. This dilution I have mixed in the required way (1:5 and 1:10) with the diagnostic fluid, and the result was most satisfactory. Naturally the fluid, under these circumstances looks reddish, but in it the whitish flocks of agglutinated bacilli stand out very clearly, and the positive result is most easy to distinguish.

Finally I wish to say a few words about those cases in which the Gruber-Widal reaction proves negative, while all symptoms tend to the diagnosis of typhoid fever. Most of these cases probably are the so-called paratyphoid fever, caused by one of the group of paratyphoid bacilli. The serum of these patients does not agglutinate the typhoid bacilli but does agglutinate the corresponding paratyphoid bacilli. Therefore I have written to Merck & Co., and asked them to prepare in addition to the typhoid diagnosticum a paratyphoid diagnosticum from the paratyphoid bacilli, A and B, as the two types of this bacillus are called.[1] Then in those cases where the Gruber-Widal reaction proves negative, one must try to obtain a positive result with the paratyphoid fever diagnosticum.

INFLAMMATORY STRICTURE OF THE RECTUM.[2]

BY J. M. FRANKENBURGER, M.D.,

OF KANSAS CITY, MO.;

PROFESSOR OF DISEASES OF THE RECTUM, UNIVERSITY MEDICAL COLLEGE; PROCTOLOGIST TO THE ST. JOSEPH ORPHAN ASYLUM, KANSAS CITY, MO.; MEMBER AMERICAN PROCTOLOGICAL SOCIETY, ETC.

REALIZING that all that might be written about rectal stricture would require the space occupied by a goodly sized book, in this paper I will treat only of the more common varieties, and will endeavor to bring out some practical points in their management.

Under the head of " Inflammatory Stricture " must be grouped the great mass of rectal strictures, including the simple, tuberculous, dysenteric, syphilitic, etc. The exact etiology of stricture of the rectum is still an unsettled question. It is doubtful if tuberculosis and dysentery can be accepted as causes. Tuttle thinks tuberculosis quite a frequent cause, but believes it doubtful if dysentery ever is, while other authors claim dysentery as being a cause, beyond question, and doubt that tuberculosis ever is. Tuberculosis of the rectum being very rarely if ever primary, and the disinclination of tuberculous ulcers to heal explains why it so seldom occurs as an etiological factor. Allingham and Matthews both claim that fifty per cent. of all rectal strictures seen in their practice were of syphilitic origin. Other authors differ, some putting the percentage caused by syphilis higher and some lower; but this can be said in regard to the etiology—any cause that can produce a diffuse inflammation of the rectal wall must be accepted as an etiological factor, whether it be syphilitic, tuberculous, dysenteric, infectious, venereal or traumatic.

1 I have since heard that Merck & Co. have brought on the market the Paratyphoid Diagnostic Fluid.
2 Read before the Academy of Medicine, Kansas City, Mo., October 22, 1904.

This complaint is very common among the colored race. I have seen and operated upon a great many negroes in my clinic, and with few exceptions they all gave histories of syphilis, many of them having other syphilitic lesions or scars. Two-thirds of the cases occur in women. This is not hard to understand when we remember that the proximity of the female genitalia to the rectum subjects the latter to pressure from the enlarged, displaced and pregnant uterus or uterine tumors.

In studying the pathology of this disease, three places present themselves for consideration; the strictured portion itself, the portion of the bowel above, and that portion below it. The stricture appears as a bluish-white cicatrix, glistening, firm to the touch and of the consistency of a true cicatrix, with a great amount of connective tissue formation. Above the stricture the gut is dilated and the walls thinned, while it is narrowed below the stricture. Two different types of ulcer may be present. The kind present below the seat of constriction is generally of the type of the disease that produces the stricture, while above the stricture they will occur as simple infectious ulcers. Fistula is a common complication. Allingham says that fistulæ generally open below the stricture, but that is different from my observation, as in my cases the majority open above the stricture. It is generally acknowledged by all authorities that ulceration is the primary starting point of rectal stricture, independent of the original cause of the ulcers. If the ulcer is not extensive, its presence may not be noticed by the patient, and in the course of time it heals. Later there is an infiltration and deposit of plastic material in the walls of the gut, eventually to be followed by diminution in the lumen of the bowel.

The symptoms of stricture are varied, depending upon the amount of constriction present. Quite frequently it is unnoticed until obstruction to the fecal current occurs. One of the first symptoms noticed is constipation. At first this is not severe, but becomes more so from day to day; the patient is compelled to take enormous doses of cathartics to produce an evacuation, and it requires a long time, and much straining for the bowels to be evacuated. As the disease progresses constipation alternates with diarrhea, the patient sometimes spending the greater part of his time at stool. There is a constant feeling as though the bowels were never emptied, but that something is present which should be forced out. There will be a constant discharge of pus and blood. The patient's general health suffers. He loses flesh and sometimes presents an appearance of suffering from a serious systemic disease. Too much credence should not be placed upon the shape of the feces for unless the stricture is very low down in the rectum the shape of the feces may be formed by the external sphincter muscle. When the stricture is situated within four inches of the anus the diagnosis can be very easily made by the finger. Diagnosis by bougie is apt to be very unreliable as bougies may double on themselves; and if the wall of the gut is very thin it may be perforated by having the bougie trust through it. If the stricture is located too high up to be reached by the finger, the sigmoidoscope is the best instrument of precision to determine its existence. If the patient is in the proper position, a stricture located within twelve or fourteen inches of the anus can be seen and its size, etc., determined. Should the rectal walls be very much thickened, however, it may be impossible to inflate them. Should the symptoms of extreme, continuous constipation, passage of pus and blood, etc., be present, and yet the diagnosis of stricture be difficult or impossible by the hand or sigmoidoscope, an exploratory laparotomy would be justifiable.

As regards the prognosis of inflammatory stricture, it is well for the surgeon to inform his patient at the beginning that a permanent cure is impossible. By palliative treatment, operations, etc., the stricture can be kept well under control, the patient made comfortable and life prolonged indefinitely; but it is the duty of the surgeon to inform the patient that if neglected the stricture will be as fatal to life as though it were malignant. It is a favorite method with irregular practitioners to promise a patient afflicted with rectal stricture a permanent cure. After the operation the patient is delighted with his improved condition. His discharge lessens or ceases. He now has painless, normal-sized stools without straining, where before he had no evacuation without cathartics, enemas and much straining and pain. He accepts the word of the irregular that he is cured permanently, pays him his fee and gladly furnishes him with a testimonial with permission to print it if desired in the daily paper. As time rolls around, he finds his old trouble returning, and if he does not seek treatment his condition becomes worse than before the operation. He goes back to his irregular friend, and is informed that this is another condition than that for which he was operated upon. Needless to say that his fee is not returned, and his testimonial continues to be printed.

The treatment is either palliative or operative. In the palliative treatment the diet should be concentrated and nourishing. The stools should be rendered soft by laxatives. Injections of hot saline solution will help to relieve the pain and lessen the discharge. While mercury and iodides are recommended to produce absorption of the stricture, they are of very little value, as most of these cases do not come under observation until the stricture has been forming a long while and the cicatrix is too firmly organized to be absorbed.

Treatment by dilatation is probably the most popular and the one most commonly resorted to. The dilatation may be either gradual or forcible. Many cases will be benefited and relieved by gradual dilatation, and this method of treatment is more popular than the forcible dilatation, as it is done without the use of an anesthetic. When gradual dilatation is employed, no force at all should be used in introducing the bougie. One that will easily pass the stricture should first be introduced, and the size gradually increased until the size desired is reached. The patient should then be furnished with a bougie of the proper size and instructed to pass it occasionally the rest of his life. Kelsey recommends that the bougie be retained in the rectum for several hours, and if possible, all night. On the well-known surgical axiom that continued pressure produces absorption this seems to be sound advice if the continued pressure of the bougie did not produce irritation of other parts of the bowel. Should the stricture be of small caliber, and high up in the bowel, it may be impossible to introduce a bougie by ordinary methods. The proctoscope should then be inserted up to the point of stricture. Then with the aid of artificial light the opening in the stricture can be plainly seen, and the proper-sized bougie passed without danger of doing any damage to the rectal wall.

Forcible dilatation is a dangerous, unsurgical procedure, and should never be performed when it is possible to adopt any other measure. I have had no personal experience with treatment by electricity and therefore cannot tell of its efficacy. All proctologists of my acquaintance who have used it say that the results were not encouraging, and that they were compelled to adopt other methods of treatment. It would seem as though extirpation of the strictured portion of the bowel with anastamosis of the ends of the gut would be an ideal operation for this condition, but from statistics gathered of this mode of treatment, the stricture is very prone to recur at the site of the anastomosis and the condition of the patient is as bad if not worse than before the operation. This operation is mostly applicable when the stricture is in the upper part of the rectum or sigmoid flexure. The operation most generally recommended by text-books is that of proctotomy. This operation, when first introduced, was thought to be a radical cure for stricture, but like all other operations, it was found that without proper after treatment its curative properties were but temporary.

Internal proctotomy consists in making several incisions in the stricture. The incisions may be superficial or deep, as the case requires. Generally the anterior and lateral incisions are not as deep as the posterior. This operation is not as popular as it once was, as it invites sepsis, and abscesses and fistulæ are quite apt to follow as sequelæ. Matthews is a firm advocate of this operation, however, and says he has never had any unpleasant results following. I have performed it in a great many cases with satisfactory results, and yet, while I have never had any complications following afterward, I do not regard it as a good surgical procedure and am always worried about my patient for a few days after the operation, or until all danger of infection is past. In my own experience I have found external or complete proctotomy the safest, simplest and most satisfactory operation for rectal stricture. This operation consists in introducing a blunt-pointed bistoury within the anus, passing it up the rectum until well within the line of constriction, then cutting through the stricture, dividing the sphincter muscles and all intervening tissue, back to the coccyx. The incision should be made exactly in the median line, where the sphincter muscles from either side meet, for as Tuttle has pointed out, the muscular fibers here do not decussate, and by this incision very few fibers are cut. Should there be any spurting vessels they should be ligated, but this is not often necessary; irrigation with hot water, followed by firm packing, will check all oozing. The rectum should be well irrigated daily with an antiseptic solution, and dressed by laying a strip of gauze within the wound. Bougies should be passed and the incision watched carefully to see that the external portion does not heal before the internal. I have performed this operation for rectal stricture more than any other, and results have been uniformly good. I pay particular attention to the preparatory treatment of these cases, aiming to get the rectum in as near an aseptic condition as possible before operating, the operation being performed under antiseptic measures and treated antiseptically afterward. Fortunately, the great majority of rectal strictures are within three inches of the anus, hence this operation can be performed in most cases.

, Operations dealing directly with the stricture will be found inadequate and impossible in many cases, and a colostomy will have to be performed. Time is too short for me to enter into detail regarding colostomy, but the operator should use the gridiron incision and bring the gut between the oblique muscles and underneath the skin for a distance before opening upon the surface, so as to make as continent an artificial anus as possible, and if necessary a pad or truss can be worn over the bowel. Since the introduction of improved technic in the operation of colostomy, whereby the artificial anus takes on somewhat of a sphincteric action, life is made much more bearable to these patients than after the old operation where they had no control whatever over the fecal current.

Much has been left unsaid which I might say about this, to the proctologists at least, over-interesting subject, but for fear that the subject might not be as interesting to you as to myself I will close by citing three cases which have some peculiar features in connection with their trouble:

Case I.—Mr. F., aged forty years, German. Family history good; no history of syphilis. Consulted me October 2, 1902. Gave history of having had rectal trouble for sixteen years, during which time he had been operated upon four times for stricture of rectum. Examination revealed a stricture three inches up in the rectum, with a complete fistula, its internal opening being above the stricture and its external opening mid-

way between the coccyx and the anus. Patient complained of continual pain in the rectum, the pain being so severe that nothing could relieve it but morphine. Operation October 4, 1902. Anesthetic, ether. The fistula incised, the incision extending through both sphincters and the stricture. Portion of stricture removed for microscopical examination. Patient made a quick recovery from the operation, leaving the hospital in a few days. Was given a No. 12 Wales bougie to pass daily. Everything progressed favorably. ' The patient stopped the use of morphine and gained several pounds in weight. His color became much better and he resumed work at his trade. At the end of three months, the pain recurring, he was treated with the X-ray for a month, but without relief. February 26, 1903, five months after the first operation, he returned to me and said the pain was more intense than it had ever been. The fistula was found to be healed, the bowel pervious, a No. 9 Wales bougie passing without any difficulty. He demanded relief from his pain, at any cost, as life was unbearable. Operation February 27, 1903; anesthetic, ether. Did a perineal amputation of lower end of rectum, and made a left inguinal colostomy, bringing the sigmoid through a gridiron incision, running the gut between the oblique muscles and under the skin for about two inches before bringing it to the surface, so as to make the best possible anus. Patient left the hospital in a few weeks, very much improved. He was instructed to irrigate the rectum through the lower end of the sigmoid daily with a hot boracic acid solution. He discontinued the use of morphine, gained in weight and for a short time was free from pain. Six months after the operation I saw him again when he showed very plainly a malignant cachexia. He was using large doses of morphine to alleviate the pain in the rectum. The artificial anus was a decided success, he having almost perfect control over his evacuations. I did not see him again but understood that he died a short time afterward from general weakness. This case had existed for sixteen years. Tissue removed from both my operations gave negative findings as regards malignancy, yet the man undoubtedly died of carcinoma. *Query:* When did the malignancy start?

Case II.—Mrs. C., aged thirty-two years, American, family history negative, no positive history of syphilis. Stricture about two inches up the rectum; constant discharge of pus and blood. Had been operated upon by an advertiser two years previous, with guarantee of permanent cure. When informed of the nature of her trouble, she called upon the advertiser and demanded a return of the fee. He declined to return it, claiming that he had cured her of her former stricture, and that this was a new one which had developed afterward. Operation March 19, 1903. Anesthetic, ether. Internal proctotomy with forcible dilatation of stricture. Patient did not have an untoward symptom and left the hospital in a few days. Was given a No. X Wales bougie to pass. One year later she had an attack of erysipelas which lasted about three weeks, during which time she did not pass the bougie. When she recovered she found that she was unable to pass the bougie, although she had no difficulty in evacuating her bowels. One week later she called to see me, and I was only able to pass a No. 4 bougie. It was three months before I was able, by gradual dilatation, to introduce a No. 10 bougie, the same size she herself had been introducing before her illness. I cite this case merely to show how necessary it is to keep the rectum dilated by bougies. In this instance four weeks was sufficient time to allow the stricture to contract from a size large enough to pass a No. 10 bougie down to a size hardly large enough to pass a No. 4.

Case III.—Mrs. B., aged thirty years, American. Family history negative. No positive history of syphilis. Annular stricture of rectum about two inches above anus. Had been operated upon two years prior by internal proctotomy. Almost unable to have evacuation of bowels, often requiring from one-half to one hour to complete defecation, at one time fainting while at stool. Continuous discharge of pus and blood. Emaciated, weak, nervous and melancholic. Operation, April 15, 1904, anesthetic, ether. Complete proctotomy, dividing stricture and severing both sphincters. Was given a No. 10 Wales bougie to pass. Incision healed in a few weeks. Made a quick recovery and was greatly improved in mind and body. I report this case on account of the fact that never at any time since the operation has patient suffered from incontinence of the rectum although both the sphincters as well as the stricture were completely divided. Possibly the induration caused by the stricture acted as an auxiliary sphincter, and gave control of the stools.

A CASE OF SO-CALLED TRAUMATIC ASPHYXIA.

BY RANDOLPH WINSLOW, M.D.,
OF BALTIMORE, M.D.;
PROFESSOR OF SURGERY IN THE UNIVERSITY OF MARYLAND.

ON August. 10, 1904, M. C., male, aged twenty-two years, was admitted to the University Hospital and presented the following history: He is employed by a large dry goods house as conductor of an elevator and having occasion to get on top of the car to some purpose, he told an assistant to lower it, but by some mistake the elevator was raised and the man was caught between the ceiling and the top of the car. He was forcibly bent down so that he sat on his heels, while his head was forced down to the roof of the car. He was kept in this position for some moments, during which time he felt as if his head and chest would burst, and he could not breathe. He did not lose consciousness, but suffered considerable pain. The elevator was lowered, and the man was brought to the hospital. Upon admission his pulse was 120, respiration 40, and temperature normal. He was suffering much pain, and had bloody expectoration and some epistaxis. An examination of his chest revealed fracture of the fourth, fifth and sixth ribs on the left side, with some emphysematous infiltration of the subcutaneous connective tissues. There was some cough. There was no blood in the urine, nor was he unable to empty the bladder. A contusion was seen on the right ear. A lacerated wound was found around the rectum, which had evidently been made by the heel of his shoe as he was doubled up by the pressure. There was no fracture of any of the bones, except the ribs mentioned. The pupils were equal and responded to light, but unfortunately no ophthalmoscopic examination of the eyes was made. The sight and hearing were not impaired. There was an extensive extravasation of blood under each conjunctiva. The most noteworthy feature of the case, however, was a bluish discoloration of the head,

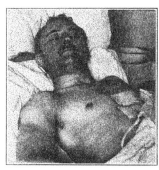

face and neck to the level of the cricoid cartilage, or the collar line. This discoloration looked as if he was cyanosed, but it stopped short at the point mentioned. It was punctiform in character, like the eruption of scarlet fever, but blue instead of red. The head and face were considerably swollen. Upon pressure the discoloration did not disappear or materially change its color. The temperature rose to 100.8° F. on the day of the injury, dropping to normal in three days, and the pulse rate rapidly diminished to 80. There is but little more to record in the after history of the case, as he was out of bed in a week and left the hospital in twelve days. The day following the injury the color of the skin was slightly pinker, and it gradually faded, but had not entirely disappeared when he was discharged. There were none of the changes seen in ordinary ecchymotic conditions, except in the bruised area mentioned, and in the conjunctiva. No special treatment was instituted except an ice-cap to the chest, and subsequently adhesive strips with enough morphine to relieve his pain.

The condition described above is one of the rare results of a forcible compression of the thorax, and has been called traumatic asphyxia by some authors. Only a few cases have been observed in the living person, though it has long been known that such discoloration was occasionally found in those who had been squeezed to death by compression of the thorax. The cause of the blue discoloration was supposed to be hemorrhage, but in a case recently reported by Beech and Cobb, of Boston, pieces of skin were subjected to microscopical examination and it was found that there was no extravasation of blood, but a dilated condition of the capillaries from overdistention. I am glad to be able to confirm this observation, as I also cut out a piece of skin from the discolored area, and requested Prof. Hirsh, of the University of Maryland, to make a careful study of its pathological histology, and I herewith append his report:

Report of skin removed from the case of Traumatic Asphyxia.—A piece of skin about one c.c. square was removed from the side of the neck and hardened in Zenker's fluid, and stained with hematoxylin and eosin, and Van Gieson's stain. Microscopically the sections show practically no alterations; the capillaries in places are more or less distended with blood, but no blood is found anywhere in the tissues outside of the blood vessels. The sections are those of normal skin.

According to Beach and Cobb, in the article quoted above from the *Annals of Surgery*, Vol. 39, page 481, April 1904, only seven cases have been studied in the living individual, two of these cases occurring in Boston and five in Germany. This case is therefore the eighth to be reported, unless others have been published since the time of the above-mentioned article.

The case herewith recorded does not present any new features, but is corroborative of the observations of other writers. The excellent photograph accompanying this paper was taken by Mr. W. B. Warthen, a student in the graduating class of the University of Maryland.

Since writing the above I understand a paper has recently appeared in the *Deutsche Zeitschrift für Chirurgie*, or some other German periodical, which I have not seen as yet, in which several cases are depicted.

MEDICAL PROGRESS.

SURGERY.

New Method of Anesthesia.—Sauerbruch has described a method suitable for operations on the thoracic cavity, in which he employs a pneumatic cabinet sufficiently large to contain the operating table, together with the surgeon and necessary assistants, while the head of the patient projects through a hole in the side of the cabinet. The air in the latter is then exhausted to the required degree and when the pleural cavity is opened, collapse of the lung is avoided. ENGELKEN (*Deut. med. Woch.* December 15, 1904) also describes a method by which it is intended to overcome the lia-

bility to pneumothorax produced under ordinary conditions. His plan reverses that of Sauerbruch and is claimed to be much simpler. The head of the patient and the anesthetizer are enclosed in a smaller cabinet in which the pressure of the atmosphere is raised above the normal. A rather complicated system of valves is required and also means for getting rid of the vapor of the anesthetic which escapes, in order that the anesthetizer may not inhale it himself. The author describes the satisfactory removal of a pulmonary tumor by the aid of this device.

Treatment of Thrombosis.—Thrombosis of the superficial veins of the lower extremity is a common and irksome complication. It is not free from danger. C. M. MOULLIN (*Brit. Med. Jour.*, December 24, 1904) states that it may be limited to one venous segment or may involve several. The usual treatment for these cases is rest in bed with the leg elevated. The author for a number of years, however, has practised the radical but eminently satisfactory method of excising the entire thrombosed portion of the vein at the very earliest possible opportunity. At first he limited this proceeding to cases in which there was merely a thrombosed loop. In one instance recently in which both internal saphenous veins were plugged right up to the opening, he cautiously explores the vein, slit it open, removed the clot and then excised the rest of the vein. A moderate degree of inflammation is prejudicial to this operation, but it is wise that, if at all acute, drainage should be free. These cases instead of lingering for a great many weeks in bed and having subsequently to wear elastic bandages, recover in ten days to two weeks.

Congenital Hypertrophic Stenosis of the Pylorus.—So much attention is being given to the pylorus at present that every reference to it should be noted. J. RUTHERFORD MORISON (*Lancet*, December 24, 1904) records the case of a male infant seven weeks old. The parents were healthy, there being no history whatsoever of syphilis. Delivery had been by forceps. The child vomited from birth. He was fed on Mellin's food. The bowels were constipated and they never acted without medicine. No treatment seemed to be of any avail. During the sixth week, the child progressively lost flesh. At the time of operation he was extremely emaciated and lethargic. The stomach was tremendously distended and every now and then could he mapped out by a peristaltic wave. No mass could be felt at the pylorus. The condition was desperate. On exposing the pylorus, it was found to appear normal on inspection, but on palpation, it felt firm and thickened. Pyloroplasty was determined upon. When the stomach was opened, it was found that the pylorus would only admit a pair of closed artery forceps with some difficulty and even they could be felt to dilate the part as they were passed through. The thickness and friability of the stomach wall rendered the operation most difficult. Two rows of sutures were used and at the end of the operation, the line of sutures looked very secure. Vomiting recommenced and the patient died thirty hours after examination. At autopsy the suture line was found secure. The pylorus was almost occluded. When the stomach was distended with water, none escaped through the pylorus. This was due to blocking by the tucked in thick pylorus ring. On the anterior wall near the pylorus, there was a small excavated ulcer one-sixteenth of an inch in diameter. Microscopical examination showed the thickening to be composed entirely of unstriated muscle, the other viscera were normal.

Removal of Large Sharp Foreign Bodies from the Upper Esophagus.—The difficulty of extracting large sharp bodies from the esophagus has long been recognized and external esophagotomy is usually the operation which is indicated for their removal. W. KRAMER (*Zentralbl. für Chir.*, December 17, 1904) states that Hacker, between 1887 and 1900 performed esophagotomy in 27 cases for the removal of foreign body. The technic of the operation is however, difficult and the results are proverbially inconstant. It follows from this that if careful extraction can be accomplished through the mouth, the results must be better than by operation, especially if this be in the hands of a not thoroughly competent surgeon. The author cites the history of two cases which showed him conclusively that the incision of the esophagus for the extraction of foreign bodies, even in apparently desperate cases may not always be necessary. The technic practised it as follows: He exposes the esophagus by the usual incision on the left side of the neck. This incision is made at least nine centimeters in length or whatever may be necessary to give the operator a full view of the esophagus. Instead of opening the organ he now practises the following manipulation: While lifting the patient's head forward and pulling the larynx up, with the left hand, he endeavored with two fingers of the right hand in the wound, to push the foreign body into a different position in the esophagus. After some effort in each case, this manipulation proved successful, and he was able to pass the usual slender esophageal forceps through the mouth, to remove the body which previously had resisted all forms of intrabuccal manipulation. He considers that inasmuch as the statistics show that of 26 cases of esophagotomy, there were 69 lethal results, any method which enables the operator to remove the body without subjecting the patient to such a very extensive risk, must be of the greatest value.

Local Analgesia.—Equal in importance with the discovery by Corning in 1885, that cocaine applied to the trunk of a sensory or mixed nerve, would abolish sensation throughout its entire (??) was the observation made by Oberst that if the circulation of the part was retarded by a ligature or by the application of cold, the action of the analgesic was maintained so long as the circulation was controlled. ARTHUR E. BARKER (*Brit. Med. Jour.*, December 24, 1904) states that although these two principles may have been realized fully, the wide application of the method has not been inaugurated for two reasons, (1) because of the fear of cocaine, and (2) because of the insufficient methods for controlling the circulation. The discovery in very recent times, however, of eucaine, which is far less dangerous than cocaine, and that of adrenalin, which fulfils Oberst's conditions without the employment of his cumbersome apparatus, has paved the way for increasing employment of local analgesia. When adrenalin and eucaine are injected, several notable effects are produced. It must not be forgotten that the anesthetic may be retained locally in the tissues for as long a time as several hours. It is, in other words, fed out into the body very slowly. This naturally is a safeguard if cocaine be used, because the organism can take care of a large quantity if supplied to it slowly enough. One of the most important questions is how best to maintain the analgesia long enough to complete an ordinary major operation. The author advises the use of the following solution:

℞ Water .... 100 c.c.
　Beta eucaine .... 2 gram
　Sodium chloride .... 8 gram
　1 per M. adrenalin, chloride solution... 10 ℳ

All this quantity can be used in an ordinary case if necessary. The author has often injected double the

amount, or six grains of eucaine. The fascial planes are convenient aids in introducing the mixture in for example the case of removal of the appendix in the stage of quiescence. The skin is easy to deal with. With the muscles, however, it is somewhat different. The author advises a long blunt hollow needle, which should be passed through the skin about two inches outside the line of incision at its lower end and to be pushed slowly between the layers of muscles. From above downward this is repeated, except that the plan of injection is deeper. In each case 10 c.c. are injected. The author presents the instruments which he has found useful in the administration of this fluid. Without the adrenalin sensation is abolished by eucaine for only about fifteen minutes. With it, however, the duration of analgesia is the same as that of the anemia, viz., fifteen minutes. Correspondingly the pain sense is lost more slowly when the adrenalin is used and it is therefore advisable to wait thirty minutes after the injection. This method has the added advantage over the older one of artificial edema, viz., that no anatomical details are masked. A cardinal point in success is to avoid dragging. This almost invariably produces pain. This is particularly true of the mesentery. If such pulling be necessary, however, or if adhesions have to be broken down, it is often convenient to give these patients a few drops of chloroform. The author closes with an enumeration of operations performed under eucaine analgesia. They number 91, 23 of them being herniæ, 8 abdominal section and 5 amputations.

New Operation for Movable Kidney.—So many methods have been employed with varying success in the effort at replacing a movable kidney that a technic which promises to give better results than those previously employed will be welcomed. ANDREW FULLERTON (*Brit. Med. Jour.*, December 24, 1904) states that by this operation the kidney is swung up in its own capsule practically in normal position. A four-inch incision is made to the vertebral side of the angle between the last rib and the rector spinæ downward and outward toward the anterior superior spine. The kidney is found and is pushed up to but not out of the wound and a small puncture is made in the capsule so that a probe or director may be insinuated and a large blister be gradually separated from the vertebral surface and outer border of the kidney. This is the portion of the organ that normally looks backward and by peeling the capsule off here, the kidney is kept as nearly as possible in its proper place. A horseshoe-shaped flap of capsule can be separated so that the base is just about the center of the horizontal axis of the kidney. The margin of the blister is now cut in a U shape, the concavity downward. To preserve the inner tilt of the upper border of the organ, the inner limb of the incision may be made a little longer than outward. The finger is now insinuated under the ligamentum arcuatum externum and the tissues on its deep surface peeled up so as to get rid of the pleura. The finger then protects the pleura and an incision is made about a third or an inch or more above the lower margin of the ligament and parallell to its fibers to the whole available distance. The last dorsal nerve should be avoided. Kocher's artery forceps are pushed through the slit and the free end of the separated capsule is drawn through, spread out and stitched down to the ligament. The wound is sutured in layers, catgut being used for the deep stitches and silkworm gut for the skin.

Ideal Method of Removing the Vermiform Appendix.—HOWARD A. KELLY (*Am. Med.*, December 31, 1904) gives interesting historic data concerning the earlier methods of removing the vermiform appendix, and describes an ideal plan which meets all the required indications and at the same time avoids the dangers often encountered. The base of the appendix is first crushed by a pair of forceps, grooved on the crushing surface and beveled above, easily managed with one hand and requiring a force of from 30 to 60 pounds in order to lock and to release them. The appendix is amputated by means of the ordinary Paquelin cautery, after which the base, held by the forceps, is cauterized and sealed by the red-hot point of the cautery, traveling slowly up and down in the groove of the crushing forceps for from forty to sixty seconds, and, on releasing the forceps, the narrow ribbon of crushed appendix is found converted into a thin translucent tissue with no lumen. The serosa is then united over this by sero-serous sutures.

MEDICINE.

The Action of the Iodides in Arteriosclerosis.—

The use of this drug in the treatment of this condition is very extensive and yet but little is known of its mode of action. MÜLLER and INADA (Deut. med. Woch., November 24, 1904) present the results of a series of observations in young men, otherwise healthy, to whom potassium iodide was administered in daily doses of from 3.4 to 0.5 gms., for periods of ten to fourteen days. It has been claimed that this drug has no vasodilating action. Examination of the blood from the experimental subjects showed that there was a marked loss of viscosity, sometimes as much as ten per cent. This apparently explains most of the therapeutic effects of the drug, as its action in increasing the fluid character of the blood, is equivalent to dilitation of the vessels, for the reason that the stream flows more rapidly. This also shows that the drug must be continued for long periods in order to produce any effects. The serum does not become fluid to the same degree as the blood en masse, and sometimes is even increased in density, so that the change appears to be governed by the behavior of the cellular elements of the blood alone.

The Rarer Forms of Rheumatism.—

Some interesting comments on this subject are made by J. SCHREIBER (Berl. klin. Woch., November 21, 1904) who believes that a sharp line must be drawn between muscular and joint rheumatism. To secure uniformity and to avoid confusion, the term muscular rheumatism ought to be dropped, and the word rheumatism applied to that inflammatory condition of the various locomotive organs and their appendages, which result from sudden changes of temperature. Persons inclined to rheumatism need not therefore fear intense, uniform cold, but rather overheating, especially that brought about by muscular exertion, followed by sudden rest and cooling. The quickest and most reliable remedy in cases of fresh or acute rheumatism, is exercise. The patient may safely indulge in all those movements which cause pain, but care should be taken to exclude joint rheumatism. Chronic rheumatism can only be cured by mechanotherapy, in which active and passive movements play an important part. Among the rarer sites for rheumatism, which are little mentioned in the literature, are the following: A rheumatic process in the periosteum of the ribs, the sternum and the long bones; rheumatism of the diaphragm, isolated rheumatism of the coccyx and the pelvic outlet; and localized rheumatism of the muscles of mastication. Instances of these are cited and good results were secured in all.

but that of the diaphragm, by forcible massage For rheumatism of the diaphragm, the faradic current gave some relief. A number of localities are mentioned which are favorite sites of the rheumatic process, mostly muscular attachments.

Occurrence of Myelocytes in Blood.—

Myelocytes are much more common in the blood of infectious cases, according to C. SCHINDLER (Zeitsch. f. klin. Med., Vol. 54, Nos. 5 and 6) than is generally believed. In pneumonia there is a moderate or marked neutrophile leucocytosis with absence of eosinophiles; after the crisis, the lymphocytes and eosinophiles are again more numerous, and a few myelocytes make their appearance. Scarlet fever is accompanied by a neutrophile leucocytosis which runs parallel with the fever-curve, but during desquamation, a second leucocytosis, affecting chiefly the mononuclear and eosinophile elements, often appears. Myelocytes may be present both during the stage of polynuclear an eosinophile leucocytosis. In cerebrospinal mening gitis and diphtheria, myelocytes were also encountered quite regularly and in the latter disease, a large number seems to signify a bad prognosis. In erysipelas the blood behaves like in pneumonia with defervescence by lysis. Myelocytes may also occur in lymphatic leucemia and in malignant tumors. There are few diseases in which the proportion of the different types of leucocytes is as characteristic as in typhoid. During the first week, the neutrophiles increase, the lymphocytes diminish and the eosinophiles disappear completely. In the stage of continuous fever, the lymphocytes gradually increase and the neutrophiles diminish and this goes on until there frequently is a crossing of the curves during convalescence. Exceptions to this rule are, however, common and there may even be a slight leucocytosis in uncomplicated cases. Myelocytes are present in all stages, independent of the number of neutrophiles. In malaria, the neutrophiles rise and fall with the temperature, but do not exceed normal figures. The lymphocytes behave in like manner while the eosinophiles are about normal during the fever and diminish rapidly in the interval. Myelocytes are rather more abundant than in other infections. The author could not detect myelocytes in the blood of patients suffering from measles, and this disease seems to be the only exception to the rule. The significance of the presence of myelocytes only the presence of a leucocytosis is very small, but if these cells persist at a time when the other white cells have become normal, they point to a functional exhaustion of the bone-marrow. This will influence the prognosis only, if the infection is still active with unabated virulence.

Sigmoiditis.—

TH. ROSENHEIM (Zeitsch. f. klin. Med., Vol. 54, Nos. 5 and 6) draws attention the frequency of benign, inflammatory processes in and about the sigmoid flexure. As separate and distinct affections these have not received the proper study and have frequently been overlooked or else wrongly diagnosed as cancer. They may be acute or chronic and productive, are frequently followed by stricture of a moderate grade, and though extremely troublesome, are generally amenable to treatment without operation. The use of the sigmoidoscope marks a very great advance in diagnosis, since a great portion the sigmoid flexure may now be inspected direct. Even exploratory laparotomy is often inferior to direct inspection, since the interior of the gut often gives more information than the exterior. It may so happen that the walls of the flexure are thickened such an extent by simple chronic inflammation, that the operator may have considerable doubt as to the true nature of the condition. The most common symptoms are pain, irregularities of defecation, and tenderness. The loop may be palpated as a thickened mass or distinct tumor. An acute sigmoiditis may be the result of simple, chronic constipation. Fever and general malaise are common here and occasionally attacks of obstruction, which yield however, to castor oil and injections. A mild general infection is probably set up from an ulceration or a diverticulum in which the feces stagnate, with secondary irritation of the peritoneum. Inspection will generally show a succulent and hyperemic mucous membrane. If the intestines are distended with air, the sigmoid will not balloon out. In the chronic cases, the patients have frequently lost so much flesh and strength, that the diagnosis of carcinoma seems probable. The mucous membranes is also very vascular here, but areas of pigmentation from former hemorrhages are very common. The stool frequently contains mucus and blood. Follicular inflammation is rare, but may also be readily diagnosed with the proctoscope. The treatment of all these conditions calls for regulation of food and stool, mild astringent irrigations and tonic drugs.

PHYSIOLOGY.

The Passage of Foodstuffs from the Stomach.— By means of the Roentgen rays, W. B. CANNON (*Am. Jour. of Physiol.*, December 1, 1904) was able to study the time it takes the various foodstuffs, mixed with bismuth subnitrate, to pass from the stomach. Fats remain long in the stomach. The discharge of fats begins slowly and continues at nearly the same rate at which the fat leaves the small intestine by absorption and by passage into the large intestine. Consequently there is never any great accumulation of fat in the small intestine. Carbohydrate foods begin to leave the stomach soon after their ingestion. They pass out rapidly, and at the end of two hours reach a maximum amount in the small intestine almost twice the maximum for proteids, and two and a half times the maximum for fats, both of which maxima are reached only at the end of four hours. The carbohydrates remain in the stomach only about half as long as proteids. These frequently do not leave the stomach at all during the first half hour. After two hours they accumulate in the small intestine to a degree only slightly greater than that reached by carbohydrates, an hour and a half earlier. Egg albumin is discharged from the stomach at about the carbohydrate speed. Doubling the amount of carbohydrate food increases the rapidity of the carbohydrate outgo from the stomach during the first two hours; whereas doubling the amount of proteid food strikingly delays the initial discharge of proteid from the stomach. The interval between feeding and the appearance of food in the large intestine is variable, but the mean for carbohydrates is about four hours, for proteids about six hours, and for fats about five hours.

The Function of the Renal Capsule.—The recent therapeutic application of decapsulation of the kidney with beneficial results in cases of colicky pains, hematuria and albuminuria, and the still more recent cures of simple Bright's disease, reported by the use of this simple surgical procedure, impart a peculiar interest to the research conducted by I. LEVIN (*Am. Jour. Physiol.*, November 1, 1904) in the rôle of the renal capsule for the function of the kidney. The fibrous coverings of the liver, spleen, pancreas and all other parenchymatous organs, when compared with that of the kidney, show the following marked difference,

namely, that while the former are very thin and rightly adherent, forming an integral part of the organ, the latter is a strong fibrous covering, easily detached from the organ. The author assumes, *à priori*, that the capsule of the kidney is functionally more important than the capsules of the other organs. By means of the oncometric method of investigation, which records the minutest changes in the size of the kidney, the author sought to discover the influence of the capsule on the kidney. He used two different agents with which to bring about a shrinkage of the kidney, adrenalin, which actively contract the blood-vessels of the kidney simultaneously with the rise of the general blood pressure, and stimulation of the vagus nerve, which causes a diminished supply of blood to the kidney through the weakening of the heart action and the consequent fall in blood pressure. Twenty-four or forty-eight hours after decapsulation of a dog's kidney, the author clasped it in the oncometer and after taking the normal tracing, either injected adrenalin or stimulated the vagus. On comparing the resulting tracing with that obtained from the non-decapsulated kidney, he finds that in the latter, immediately after the injection or stimulation, the tracing falls, then continues for some time on the same level, but always shows pulsation and returns to the old level, mostly even before the tracing of the carotid becomes normal. In the decapsulated kidney the tracing also falls immediately after the injection, then for a considerable length of time continues as a straight line, showing an absolute cessation of pulsation in the kidney, and returns to the normal much later than the carotid blood pressure. From these results the author draws the following conclusion: Any stimulus, which either by contracting the general blood pressure or weakening the action of the heart, diminishes the size of the kidney, exerts a much stronger influence on the decapsulated kidney than on the normal one, and this influence also lasts longer on the former. The capsule acts like an elastic covering. On the one hand it prevents an undue overfilling of the kidney with blood, on the other hand it does not allow the kidney to remain contracted and bloodless for a long time.

The Production of Cholin from Lecithin and Brain Tissue.—The discovery of the poisonous ptomaine in the cerebrospinal fluid in various forms of functional and organic nervous disease, has led many to attribute to cholin some causal connection with the disease. Whether this is the case or not, will be determined by investigations in the laws that underlie the production of cholin in the body. A definite contribution to this subject is made by I. H. CORIAT (*Am. Jour. Physiol.*, December 1, 1904). Cholin may be produced by the putrefaction of lecithin, and also by the putrefaction of brain-tissue. There is an enzyme present in brain-tissue capable of splitting cholin from lecithin. This enzyme acts only in neutral or slightly alkaline media, while an acid medium inhibits it. This is exactly opposite to the case with the proteolytic autolysis of brain-tissue which is favored by acid and inhibited by alkali. In the body the action of the enzyme is favored by the normal alkaline reaction of the nerve-substance and cerebrospinal fluid. The ease with which this enzyme acts is probably explained by the fact that the lecithin in the central nervous system, as in the stroma of red blood-corpuscles, is not in a chemical combination, but in an emulsiform condition and is therefore capable of mechanical solution. The enzyme can be destroyed by heating, and then, if the suspension of the brain-tissue be kept absolutely sterile, no cholin is produced; if putrefaction is allowed to supervene, cholin will be formed in a greater quantity than by autolysis alone.

As with the other enzymes, there is an inhibitory influence of reaction-products. Efforts to isolate this enzyme have so far been unsuccessful.

The Absorption and Utilization of Proteids without Digestion.—Certain writers have recently maintained that native proteids can be readily absorbed and utilized by the organism without the intervention of proteolytic enzymes, provided they are introduced in soluble form. It has, on the other hand, been recently assumed that the crystalline cleavage products of the proteids in the intestinal contents are absorbed and synthesized by the organism into the proteids peculiar to its tissues and fluids, that assimilation consists in the reconstruction of amido-acids, di-amido-acids, etc., into new molecules. A series of important experiments in this domain were performed by L. B. MENDEL and E. W. ROCKWOOD (*Am. Jour. Physiol.*, December 1, 1904), with the following results: Vegetable proteids (crystallized edestin from hemp-seed and excelsin from the Brazil-nut) slowly introduced in solution into the circulation of animals, can apparently be retained in the organism for the most part, even when the quantities introduced almost equal that of the globulins normally present in the blood. When solution of vegetable proteids are injected too rapidly or in too great concentration, toxic symptoms, including an inhibition of the cardiac and respiratory activities may be observed, especially in cats. The vegetable proteids soon disappear in considerable part when introduced into the peritoneal cavity. They do not reappear in the urine. The unaltered proteids edestin and casein are absorbed to a very small extent, if at all from portions of the living small intestine in which the ordinary digestive processes are excluded as far as possible. On the other hand, the proteoses and peptones obtained by peptic digestion of these proteids readily disappear from the intestine under the same conditions. The typical vegetable proteids show no marked difference from those of animal origin in their relation to the processes of metabolism. It is not necessary to assume that the proteids are first completely broken down by the intestinal enzyme erepsin before they are absorbed, for casein (upon which erepsin can act) may remain unabsorbed.

The Diastases and Anti-Diastases of Blood-Serum.—The manifold characteristics and adaptability of the blood are plainly indicated in the researches reported by M. ASCALI and A. BONFANTI (*Hoppe-Seyler's Zeitsch.*, October 22, 1904). The blood contains not only a diastase, as discovered by Magendie and Claude Bernard, but also several kinds of diastase, capable of converting different varieties of starch. Thus blood-serum in acting upon a suspension of only one kind of starch will not produce as much sugar as when acting upon a suspension of several different kinds of starch. The different diastases have a specific or at least a partly specific action. By means of a new method the authors have revealed a phenomenon, which by analogy with the phenomenon of selective absorption they term "selective ferment-action." After a certain quantity of blood-serum has acted upon rice-starch for twenty-four hours, and the amount of sugar produced has been measured (the further addition to the mixture of a definite amount of potato-starch will result in the formation of more sugar than if an equal amount of rice-starch had been added. It is well-known that the saccarification of starch depends upon the successive action of different ferments, dextrinase, maltase and glucase, but the researches of the authors show that these actions are still more complicated, inasmuch as there are different kinds of these corresponding to the various kinds of starch. These results correspond to those obtained with the hemolysins and precipitins. It

is, moreover, possible by means of the immunizing treat ment of rabbits with pancreatin, to produce in these animals an anti-diastase which counteracts the diastase of the pancreas. But the formation of this anti-diastase is not constant. The prolonged immunization of the animal causes the total disappearance of the anti-dias tase that has been formed. The anti-diastase unfold its activity to varying degrees with the diastases of othe animals. The authors have not been able to discove any inhibitory action upon the diastase contained in the serum of the same animal.

The Enzymes in Various Kinds of Milk.—In a series of comparative investigations on the enzymati content of different kinds of milk, A. ZAITSCHEI (*Pflüger's Archiv*, September 30, 1904) finds tha woman's, mare's, cow's, ass's, goat's and buffalo's milk contain no peptone, neither pepsin nor trypsin no glycolytic ferment, but they all contain, in thei fresh state, without exception, a diastatic enzyme.

The Effect of Surgical Operation upon the Meta bolism of Carbohydrates and upon Diabetes.—It ha been maintained by various observers that glyco suria may result from some surgical procedure. Thi conclusion has been put to a critical test by E PFLÜGER, B. SCHÖNDORFF and FR. WENZEL (*Pflüger'. Archiv*, November 4, 1904). A careful examination o the urine of 144 cases subsequent to the most divers surgical operations, was made with the following results. In spite of the employment of narcotics surgical attacks produce no glycosuria. The author's do not exclude the possibility that injuries whici cause a mechanical disturbance of the sugar cente in the medulla, give rise to sugar in the urine Narcosis, even if prolonged for 2½ hours, does no in general produce glycosuria.

THERAPEUTICS.

Antistreptococcus Serum in Puerperal Septicemi and Scarlet Fever.—The employment of antistrep tococcus serum in these conditions is endorsed by A. G. HAMILTON (*Am. Jour. Obstet.*, November 1904), who has reported a series of successful cases To obtain good results the disease must be due t the streptococcus alone or this organism must b decidedly predominant, microscopical evidence be ing solely depended upon. The serum must be ad ministered early in the onset of the disease. Th quantity given must be sufficient to produce a per ceptible change in twelve hours and be repeated a often as indications demand. For the first dos 30 c.c. should be given, repeated at twelve-hour in tervals, the dose being gradually diminished as ben efit is derived. This treatment in no way interfere with other treatment that may be demanded by pai ticular symptoms. In mixed infection the serui may be used as an adjunct to other methods, but it success is not so striking.

Roentgen Rays in the Treatment of Leucemia.- Since the publication of Senn's case, in 1903, of th effect of the Roentgen rays in the reduction of the nun ber of leucocytes in leucemic blood, the subject hi steadily increased in the amount of interest attracte GEORGE DOCK (*Am. Med.*, December 24, 1904) presen a study of the reported cases, in which the rays hav been used in leucemia. Efforts to treat leucemia wei first prompted by the results in certain tumors. Ser denied the usefulness of the rays in sarcoma and ca cinoma and thought that the action of the rays was upc certain micro-organisms which he did not doubt we concerned in the cause of leucemia. Twenty-nine cas have been studied by the author besides reports of son others which were not clearly indicated by titles. Cases of leucemia should be classified as accurately as possible according to peculiarities of blood picture and changes in the hematopoietic organs. Two cases of the acute lympthatic form died. It is said that the acute cases are not suitable for Roentgen-ray treatment, but as we have nothing better, careful treatment should be tried in all early-recognized cases. Two subacute lymphatic cases died; in one of the cases there was much improvement. Of five chronic lymphatic cases, only one has died and the others have all been greatly improved. Of twenty-one cases of mixed-cell, myelogenous, or splenomedullary cases, ten were not presented with sufficient detail to be useful. In the remaining eleven cases the leucocytes fell to normal or near it. There have been wide variations in the technic of the different operators. Some have exposed only the region over the spleen, some the epiphyseal regions of the long bones, some the shafts of the long bones and some the sternal region. The length and number of exposures have also varied widely. Exposures of from ten to twenty minutes have been the most frequent. The dosage of the ray is impossible to estimate as the language terms and even the meaning of the different operators vary, and of the many devices generally made use of none is accurate. There are differences in the results compared with length of treatment that cannot, apparently, be reconciled. Theoretically, a hard or high vacuum tube should be better in the treatment of internal organs, like spleen and bone marrow, and there is less danger of burn. In the improvement of leucemia it is necessary to consider the number as well as the kind of leucocytes. The variations of the eosinophiles, basophiles, degenerated leucocytes and nucleated red corpuscles, are not generally treated at sufficient length. The leucocytes generally decrease after the treatments; and it has been stated that the improvement continued during intervals during which the treatment had been suspended. The changes in the red blood cells do not receive as much notice as those of the leucocytes. There is generally noted a gain, and nucleated red cells have often been seen to disappear. The effect of the treatment on the diseased organs is sometimes most striking. In all chronic cases the glands diminished. The effects on the spleen were by no means uniform, and it has been shown that complete reduction of the enlarged spleen cannot always be expected. Connective tissue overgrowth may prevent the organ from resuming its normal size. Subjective symptoms were improved in most cases, and edema very often disappeared. The improvement often observed is in striking contrast to the fact that relapses and even deaths have occurred among patients apparently most improved, not only generally, but as regards the blood. Toxic symptoms have been noted in several, but toxic symptoms are so common in leucemia that it is impossible to tell how much the symptoms noted were dependent upon the Roentgen ray. The author concludes that some cases of leucemia undergo marked improvement under Roentgen-ray treatment. In no case has the treatment and observation been carried out long enough to speak of cure. It is possible that treatment in very early stages may be more effective than it has hitherto been. Roentgen-ray treatment of leucemia is dangerous on account of the usual risk of dermatitis and burns, but probably also on account of toxic processes as yet impossible to explain. No special rules can be laid down at present for treatment with Roentgen rays; great care should be taken to avoid burns; methods should be as fully described as possible in each case; the blood should be carefully examined as

fully and as frequently as possible, and if possible, urine examinations should be made, to throw additional light upon the metabolic changes.

Value of Stereoscopic Skiagraphy.—The application of the principles of stereoscopy to the art of skiagraphy was first made in this country by Elihu Thomson, and afterward abroad. MIHRAN H. KASSABIAN (*N. Y. Med. Jour. and Phila. Med. Jour.*, December 31, 1904) explains the principles and technic and presents a few improvements which he has made in the methods of practice. There is a generally mistaken idea as to the relative significance of the terms photography and skiagraphy. The photograph is made by reflected light and the skiagraph by transmitted light. A picture made with one lens seems flat as when seen with one eye, but when two pictures are taken simultaneously with lenses placed at a distance apart equal to the pupillary distance, and then viewed each with one eye, the effect will be the same as when viewing the original with two eyes. In stereoscopic skiagraphy two negatives are made of the same part. The position of the part is not changed, but the tube is moved in a line parallel with the plane of the plate, a distance equal to the average pupillary distance. The two skiagrams are afterward examined simultaneously in a special stereoscope. Usually the patient is permitted to rest on the plate, thus causing change in position of the foreign body. In the table designed by the author the tube is placed under the table and the plate upon the patient. The foreign body is carefully centered with a fluoroscope, the tube moved to one side about $1\frac{1}{4}$ inches, and the other plate exposed. The tube is then moved to the other side of the center about $1\frac{1}{4}$ inches and the other plate exposed. No two tubes have exactly the same vacuum and in any tube the vacuum changes during the exposure, so in order to have the same density in the two plates it is necessary for the operator to regulate the second exposure as his experience dictates. The development is to be carried on with care to produce equal density in the two plates. The plates may be examined in Wheatstone's reflecting stereoscope. This has the advantage that any size plates may be examined and that the negatives may be examined before any prints have been made. The right eye must view that plate which was made by the tube in the right position and the left eye that which was made in the left position. Brewster's refracting stereoscope may be used or the pictures may be reduced and examined in the ordinary method with a common stereoscope. The advantages of the stereoscopic skiagraph are that any deficiency in the one plate is easily recoverable in the other, that the anterior and posterior views are discernable. In anatomy the structure of the bones is shown. In the dry skull the grooves for the meningeal arteries are seen, the concave appearance of the processes, the frontal sinuses, etc. The exact relations in the joints, and injected soft tissues and organs are plainly shown. In surgery the advantages are numerous and new experiments are constantly being made.

Primary Lupus Vulgaris of the Oropharynx and Nasopharynx Treated by X-rays.—Primary lupus vulgaris of the pharynx and nasopharynx is sufficiently rare to warrant one's placing another such case on record, but especially when the results obtained are satisfactory and the means of treatment are new. H. S. BIRKETT (*Med. Rec.*, December 24, 1904) reports a case in a lad of fifteen years. Patient had lived an outdoor life and had always enjoyed good health. One brother and three paternal uncles had succumbed to pulmonary tuberculosis, and the patient occupied the room in which the brother had died. Two nodular growths were situated on the lateral and posterior walls of the pharynx. The nodules were the size of a mustard grain and distinct at the center but merged at the edges. The tonsils, anterior pillars and uvula were not involved. The infiltrations extended to the cushion of each Eustachian tube, involving the salpinopharyngeal folds, there being no extension into the posterior nares. Under ether the greater portion of the masses were removed. Microscopical examination showed typical tuberculous lesions. Koch's tuberculin, lactic acid, and the galvanocautery were successively tried without benefit. Roentgen-ray treatment was then commenced. The tube used was rather low and placed at ten inches from the patient. Ten minutes were given at each treatment. At the end of a week there was an inflammation of the surrounding parts and the treatment was discontinued for three weeks. Twenty-three daily exposures were then given and the cervical glands removed. The local condition in the throat had entirely disappeared and the patient was regarded as cured. At the end of three months there was a recurrence. The cartilage of the septum was alone involved and there was no involvement of the nostril on either side. The lesion was again submitted to the action of the Roentgen rays with satisfactory results. The author briefly reviews the cases that have been published.

Therapeutic Uses of the Roentgen Ray in Dermatology.—The X-ray is probably the most important therapeutic agent in the history of dermatology, and although of recent development, it has advanced with such rapidity that already sufficient material is available to justify certain definite conclusions. Louis F. Frank (*Wis. Med. Jour.*, November, 1904) gives a brief résumé of the progress made in this field of research, from the first cases reported by Schiff in 1897 to the present. Histological investigation shows that the action of the rays is to cause degeneration of the epithelium and its structure, the hair follicles, the perspiratory and sudoriferous glands, accompanied by inflammatory reaction, the extravasation of serum and leucocytes from the blood vessels. A bactericidal action of the rays is doubted by the majority of authors. Theorectically the indications for the use of the rays are in such conditions which involve the epithelial structures and clinical experience seems to bear out this theory. Epithelial new formations, benign and malignant, parasitic diseases, such as sycosis, favus, ringworm, and a third group including lupus, eczema, acne vulgaris, psoriasis, and the like, have been successfully treated. The apparent success in the eradication of epithelioma and cancerous degeneration of the skin, designated a remarkable progress in the field of surgery. Although in the majority of cases the growth will disappear without the appearance of any inflammatory reaction, a slight burn is found to hasten the process, and is generally encouraged. Although the eye cannot be protected in all cases, no deleterious effect other than a slight conjunctivitis and keratitis has been observed. It is recommended as hastening the reaction, to remove with the curette, as thoroughly as possible, all scales, crusts and broken down tissues. In the most obstinate cases of acne which have resisted all measures, a surprisingly short series of treatments will accomplish wonders. In these cases we desire to avoid a burn, and a weak soft light is to be used. Forty cases were treated. Of eczema, ten cases were treated. These were of the chronic infiltrated type seen on the palms. In none of them was the irradiation carried to the point of erythema. Experiments with cases of hypertrichosis have been unsatisfactory, and its use is discouraged. In sycosis, the results have been gratifying. The hair falls out after a few treatments and the abscesses disappear. The action

is not due to any bactericidal action but to the depilatory power of the rays. The results in lupus vulgaris and lupus erythematosus have been on the whole disappointing and the method of Finsen has given better results. The action in cases of keloids and cicatrices has been beneficial. Of cases not in the realm of dermatology, tuberculous glandular enlargement of the neck, and actinomycosis were benefited, and laryngeal tuberculosis. sarcoma of the thyroid, a large inoperable tumor, were not benefited.

PRESCRIPTION HINTS.

Treatment of Jaundice.—The radical and only satisfactory course of treatment of this condition, writes Rolleston ("Diseases of the Liver and Gall-Bladder"), is the removal or cure of the underlying condition in which jaundice is a result; for this an accurate diagnosis is essential. Syphilitic gummata pressing upon the ducts should be treated by iodide and mercury. Calculi should naturally be removed by surgical measures. In the large number of cases jaundice is due to or depends on catarrhal inflammation of the ducts. These are often benefited by copious draughts of water with Carlsbad and Vichy salts. The salicylates are also of value in the condition.

Symptomatic treatment consists in taking plenty of exercise, plenty of water, salines, particularly the phosphate or sulphate of soda, magnesium sulphate, or the natural purgative waters on an empty stomach, before breakfast. Vigorous catharsis is not advisable. A useful combination for the alleviation of the gastric irritability and to stimulate the liver parenchyma is as follows:

R Sodii bicarbonatis ....ʒi (4.0)
　Bismuthi subcarbonatis ....ʒiii (12.0)
　Bismuthi salicylatis ....ʒi (4.0)
Div. in pulv. No. xxi. One t.i.d. post. cibem.

The same prescription in combination with minute doses of calomel is efficient in the flatulency so commonly found. The following capsule may be of service in this regard as well.

R Creosoti ....♏vi
　Methyl salicylatis ....♏vi
Fiat in caps. No. vi. One morning and night.

Fresh ox bile (fel bovis) is very serviceable given in capsules, or keratin-coated pills, 5 grs. each. It makes up for the deficiency of the normal bile of the intestines.

Can Biliary Calculi be Dissolved?—Numerous drugs have been tried and recommended with a view to dissolving biliary calculi, but with little sucess. Durant's famous remedy:

R Ether ....⎫
　Ol. Terebinthinæ................⎬.....aa. ♏x.
Fiat capsulæ — q.s.

has been known to bring about some results, but the action has been one more as an antispasmodic than as a solvent. The stones have been liberated and pushed out by the peristalsis and dilatation induced. Chloroform, which enjoys some repute, acts in a similar manner. Olive oil has the best reputation. It is probably highly apocryphal that olive oil can dissolve gall-stones within the bladder, but it is conceivable that it might exert a solvent action on a calculus impacted in the actual orifice of the biliary papilla. The fatty acid and glycerin from the oil absorbed from the bowel may reach the liver and lead to an increased flow of bile in the gall-bladder. Bile acids dissolve cholesterin hence the more bile passing over a calculus, the better chance there is for it to become smaller. Olive oil i given in doses of from 6 to 8 oz. a day. Rolleston.

THE MEDICAL NEWS.

A WEEKLY JOURNAL
OF MEDICAL SCIENCE.

COMMUNICATIONS in the form of Scientific Articles, Clinical Memoranda, Correspondence or News Items of interest to the profession are invited from all parts of the world. Reprints to the number of 250 of original articles contributed exclusively to the MEDICAL NEWS will be furnished without charge if the request therefor accompanies the manuscript. When necessary to elucidate the text, illustrations will be engraved from drawings or photographs furnished by the author. Manuscript should be typewritten.

SMITH ELY JELLIFFE, A.M., M.D., Ph.D., Editor,
No. 111 FIFTH AVENUE, NEW YORK.

Subscription Price, Including postage in U. S. and Canada.

PER ANNUM IN ADVANCE $4.00
SINGLE COPIES 10
WITH THE AMERICAN JOURNAL OF THE
MEDICAL SCIENCES, PER ANNUM . . 8.00

Subscriptions may begin at any date. The safest mode of remittance is by bank check or postal money order, drawn to the order of the undersigned. When neither is accessible, remittances may be made at the risk of the publishers, by forwarding in *registered* letters.

LEA BROTHERS & CO.,
No. 111 FIFTH AVENUE (corner of 18th St.), NEW YORK.

SATURDAY, FEBRUARY 4, 1905.

ANNUAL MEETING OF THE MEDICAL SOCIETY OF THE STATE OF NEW YORK.

THE annual meeting of the Medical Society of the State of New York, which convened as usual in the last week of January, was even more largely attended than are the sessions of this always venerable organization. It is very evident that the recent unfortunate failure of union between the two representative medical bodies of this State has not lessened the interest of members of the older State organization. As to its scientific program, a glance at the report of its proceedings in this issue of the MEDICAL NEWS (see page 223) will show that this was well up to if not above the high standard set in this matter by the Society itself. The discussions were animated, the tendency to dwell on practical matters rather than theoretical considerations well marked, and the suggestive influence of the whole session as a stimulant for future clinical observation very evident.

Undoubtedly the most prominent feature of the scientific program was the symposium on "Epidemic Cerebrospinal Meningitis." Last year at this time we were here, in the East particularly (though the disease did not spare certain parts of the West), going through a rather severe epidemic of this affection. The aftermath may now be gathered with decided advantage. The cases are not so near as to be seen in exaggerated perspective and the comparison of observations and results can scarcely fail to be of service to the profession at large. We commend to the secretaries of medical organizations generally this idea of having discussions of local epidemics not only while the disease is actually in progress, when as a rule physicians are too occupied with their cases to have quite allowed their own thoughts to be clear to them, but sometime after, when knowledge gathered has simmered down into the precious residue of experience gained, which will, with all the more assurance not be lost to the physician himself or to his colleagues, if he has the opportunity for its public discussion. The other symposium on the various phases of "Prostatism and Its Treatment" was probably the fullest discussion from every point of view of this important subject that has ever been held in an American medical society apart from meetings of specialists. The interest in it serves to show how much has been accomplished mainly by American workers in a special field. There is evidence of real progress of enduring kind in a subject that seemed almost hopeless to thorough surgery only a few years ago.

The two addresses at the evening meeting of Tuesday, that of Dr. Harrington, of Boston, on the work accomplished by the laboratories of the Massachusetts State Board of Health, and that of the retiring President of the Society, Dr. Hamilton Wey, which touched a phase of a similar subject for New York, alas not in the retrospect of good work well done, but of a hopeful prospect, constituted an excellent index of the present state of medical feeling with regard to the helpfulness of the laboratory worker for public health and private practice. What Massachusetts has accomplished in a quiet unostentatious way stands as a model for every State that wants to increase the efficiency of its health department. Boston is sometimes said to be not exactly in one of our American States, but in a special state of mind. It would be eminently desirable if that state of mind could be made very generally contagious. As for New York, we sincerely hope that President Wey's suggestion that every county shall have a laboratory with an expert laboratory worker, will become an actuality within the next few years. The supply will equal the demand if a movement like this is once started, and the amount of good that may be done by keeping the general practitioner of medicine, even in distant country places, in touch with laboratory advances in clinical medicine will be almost incalculable.

Perhaps the most generally interesting feature of this meeting for the profession of New York State was the attitude assumed toward the question of reunion of the two State organizations. Before the meeting there had been rumors of a recession of the Society from its former position of willingness to encourage the union. These were dispelled by the prompt, business-like methods with which the whole subject was treated. The feelings of the profession in New York State and not individual likes or dislikes were considered and the whole matter, without a word of dissent, placed on the former plane of progress now with apparently no possible obstacle to prevent a united medical profession in New York from firmly and with a legal recognition not before possible, taking its stand for the uplifting of members and the benefit of the public health. The reception which had been arranged for Dr. Louis McMurtry, of Louisville, the President of the American Medical Association, was the best proof of the cordial feeling of the Medical Society of the State of New York toward the national body, and an index of the sincere desire once more to be in close touch with the profession of the country. This tribute was unfortunately prevented by an acute illness of Dr. McMurtry, but the feelings of cordiality inherent in the purpose were of themselves an earnest of speady and complete readjustment of all difficulties that now prevent the Empire State from taking her proper place in the medical influence she should have in this country.

THE X-RAYS AND STERILITY.—A WARNING NOTE.

In our issue of last week we discussed editorially the possible association between the Roentgen rays and sterility. These comments were based on the recent observations of Dr. F. Tilden Brown, of this city, made on a number of patients and physicians who had spent more or less time in an X-ray atmosphere. The unfortunate discovery was made that these persons were the subjects of an azoospermia without being conscious in any way of deterioration or change in their potency.

Observations of this character are of more than academic interest and would soon strike

terror into the ranks of our X-ray workers if they were found to be substantiated by further evidences of the possible havoc which this now almost universally accepted therapeutic agent could produce in the generative organs of either doctor or patient.

Albers-Schönberg, about a year ago first drew attention to the fact that in male rabbits and guinea-pigs in which the abdomen was exposed to the action of the X-ray, an azoospermia was gradually developed. Then Frieben found that this was due to the disappearance of the epithelium in the seminal tubules, which resulted in an atrophy of the testes.

Another and still more convincing series of observations is now presented in a communication by Halberstaedter (*Berliner klinische Wochenschrift*, January 16, 1905) who worked in Prof. Neisser's clinic under the latter's direction. He studied the effects of the Roentgen rays on the ovaries of rabbits and found that by exposing one side of the abdomen while the other was suitably protected, marked macroscopic and microscopic alterations took place as determined by subsequent autopsies. In order to avoid any possibility of error, the ovaries in another series of animals were first inspected by performing an exploratory laparotomy and then exposing them to the rays after the abdominal wound had healed. Any inherent difference between the two organs could thus be noted. It was proved that the marked differences between the two sides could be ascribed to nothing else than the rays. The histological change most in evidence was the complete disappearance of the Graafian follicles, in about fifteen days. Whether this loss is permanent and whether or not, regeneration can take place, has not yet been determined. It was also found that the ovaries seemed more sensitive to the effects of the rays than the outer skin of the abdomen, and when compared with control experiments in male rabbits, developed degenerative changes in shorter time and with fewer exposures.

How far these observations in animals apply to human beings cannot as yet be definitely stated, nor is it known how permanent the effects may be. Whether individual susceptibility has any influence is also unknown. Dr. Brown's observations, which are apparently the first made on the human subject, seem to be confirmed by the animal experiments of our German confrères. While further proof is still desirable, it may be just as well to take the bull by the horns and institute measures for securing efficient means of protection for both patient and physician. Well tested methods of shutting out the rays from localities where their effect is not desired are definitely known. It would seem a simple mater by the exercise of a little ingenuity to produce a suitable protectant with materials impervious to the X-rays, which we have at hand. If our fears are proved to be groundless, which now seems hardly likely, the trouble taken will not be very costly, and no restrictions will be placed on the use of what is one of the greatest of modern therapeutic and diagnostic measures.

THE " CRAW-CRAW " CRAZE.

CHICAGO, as usual, is nothing from a medical standpoint if not hustling, and now Dr. J. F. Biehan, the city bacteriologist, has climbed upon the front seat of the band wagon and is busily engaged in issuing glad sounds to the multitude at large. This is as it should be, for variety is more than the mere spice of life to a western city, and after their doleful dirge on the iniquities of bathing with the piping piccolo solo, anent the curing of inebriety by the use of glasses, already ordered, it is a comfort to hear the full orchestration of the official band merged in the soft cadences of the dreamy " Il Bacio Waltz." For Dr. Biehan gravely confirms the popular refrain that " there is no harm in kissing," at least from a sanitary standard, if only his antiseptic precautions are followed, and assures the lads and lassies that there is no need for a " body " to cry if he and she will pin their faith on a weak solution of copper sulphate or boracic acid.

The directions already published are minute and graphic in the extreme, being, it seems, furnished with a ground plan, to be supplemented by an elevation, and are as follows: " Before greeting the loved one in the hallway pause for an instant. As you gaze lovingly at her reach gracefully for your coat-tail pocket and get the vial of boracic acid. Remove the cork quickly and deftly, apply the solution to the lips with the fingers or cork; then replace the solution in the coat-tail pocket. You'll need it later. While you are thus engaged the young woman should be doing likewise. She too should carry a vial of boracic acid, or, for variety, might have one of sulphate of copper. An ornamental vial hung about the neck by a gold chain would be a pleasing novelty. When the lips of both have been

wet with the antiseptic, then kiss; kiss without fear; kiss a dozen times, for you will be safe from " craw-craw "—" craw-craw," the dread disease caused by kissing.

What this " dread " disease may be we confess we do not know. The literature on the subject seems as a thing that is yet to be, and beyond a few short notes in foreign newspapers, little has been written on the subject. According to them, however, it seems that one Dr. Dencer Whittles, who lectures on dental histology and pathology at Birmingham University, England, started the " craw-craw " panic. He declares that " the disease exists in Birmingham, having been brought from Africa, and states that ' sometimes the nematode worm is distinctly shown in the blood films.' " Now we know that the *Nematoidea* are a species of intestinal parasites, and if the indulgence in a few kisses, more or less, is to be followed in the adult by a necessity for a vermifuge, the situation has become acute and resembles that of the man who, besieged in a tree by a bear, asked his companion if he could pray? " No," he replied, " but something has got to be done."

What this " something " will be it is difficult to say, probably nothing. The kiss has existed since the days of creation and, as someone said, resembles it inasmuch as " it is made from nothing and God knows that it is good." Boys will be boys, and girls, too, will be—girls, when they are with them. As to these preliminary ablutions, these antiseptic precautions, tut, tut, youth will have its fling and its kiss too, and few, if any, with the exception perhaps of Dowie's apocryphally unkissed son, will be found ready to enroll themselves in the anointed hosts of " Dr. J. F. Biehan, bacteriologist for the city of Chicago." The American youth has never proved a laggard in love, nor a craven in war, and should he be unwilling now to run the chances taken by the classic monkey with the baboon's sister, he must indeed have been begotten of some forgotten strain derived from Joseph and the chaste Susanna.

There is, to be sure, a society of good women, located at St. Louis, the members of which wear a red button to show the world at large that they will not kiss their friends on meeting, or delay the electric cars at the street corners while they bid their fond adieux. This, however, is not a case of mixed pickles, or a scene from a problem play, but resembles rather the fight-at-Finnegan's wake, where it was simply a question of " woman to woman and man to man," and with this part of the equation we have nothing to do. Kissing proverbially goes by favor and not by legislation, and if women do not desire to kiss each other it is not only well, but it is also well enough to let alone. It was not a woman that Judas betrayed with his kiss, nor did Almansor succeed in spreading the plague in the Moorish camp with his fever-stricken lips.

There may be a worm i' the bud in the cupid's bow of fresh young lips in Chicago and St. Louis, that has not as yet reached New York or Boston, but even were this so, we do not think that our youngsters will fear to look the gift-horse fairly in the mouth. As to the older members of the community, whose clustering locks are growing gray and whose heads are bending low, they may perhaps have outgrown the halcyon days of "oats, beets, beans and barley grows," and have forgotten the delirious delights of "pillows and keys." If so, they can adopt the straight prohibition ticket of St. Louis or elect the local option (misfortunes, it would seem. never come single, even in Chicago) of the Biehan brothers. But a touch of fellow-feeling makes the whole world akin, and we doubt if one will fear to tread where his juniors have so recklessly rushed in. Should he die from the effects. then indeed has he earned the trite epitaph of the western engineer, "He did his damndest—angels can do no more."

ECHOES AND NEWS.

NEW YORK.

American Electrotherapeutic Society.—The fifteenth annual meeting of this society will be held at the New York Academy of Medicine, Nos. 17, 19 and 21 West Forty-third Street, New York, on Tuesday, Wednesday and Thursday, September 19, 20 and 21, 1905.

Medical Society of the State of New York.—The new officers of this Society are as follows: President, Dr. Joseph D. Bryant, of New York City; Vice-President, Herman R. Ainsworth, of Addison, N. Y.; Secretary, Frederic C. Curtis, of Albany, N. Y.; and Treasurer, O. D. Ball, of Albany. N. Y.

$5,000 for the Post-Graduate.—The work of the New York Post-Graduate Medical School and Hospital has been recognized by a friend of the institution, who has given it $5,000. The gift was made anonymously through a member of the corporation, and was announced by Dr. D. B. St. John Roosa.

Mount Sinai Alumni.—The eighth annual reunion and dinner of the Associated Alumni of Mount Sinai Hospital was held at the Freundschaft Society. Wednesday evening, January 25. The following officers were elected for the ensuing year: President, Dr. Fred. Mandlebaum; Vice-president. Dr. Louis Houswirth; Treasurer, Dr. Andrew Green Foord, and Secretary, Dr. Leo B. Meyer.

Work of the Hospital Book Society.—In the thirtieth annual report of the Hospital Book and News. paper Society it is shown that 6,980 books, 33,885 magazines. and 56,200 weekly and illustrated papers were distributed during the year, in addition to the 240,000 magazines and papers collected from the boxes scattered throughout the town. For the work of collection and distribution, the society asks for $500. Reading matter will be received at No. 105 East Twenty-second Street, and Mrs. J. O. Green, No. 13 Lexington Avenue, will acknowledge donations of money.

Standing Deficit of the Orthopedic Hospital Wiped Out.—That the $22,000 standing deficit of the New York Orthopedic Dispensary and Hospital had been wiped out last year, was the special announcement made at the recent annual meeting of the hospital at No. 126 East Fifty-ninth Street. The deficit was paid up, moreover, in spite of the fact that the running expenses, which amounted last year to $37,000, ran $7,000 ahead of the income. To carry on the hospital's work without debt, O. Egerton Schmidt, its president, appealed to have the endowment increased from $102,000 to $200,000. Out of the 4,017 cases treated last year, 300 were cured, 497 relieved, and 2,813 are still being treated. Only one patient was discharged as incurable. The institution founded last summer a home for convalescents at White Plains.

Bill to Restore Local Boards.—Former Charities Commissioner Homer Folks, of New York, conferred with Gov. Higgins within the last few days and showed him a brief prepared to go with the introduction of a bill into the legislature to carry out the recommendations of the Governor made in his annual message that local board of State hospitals for the insane be restored the power of management given them save as to the finances, which would continue to be supervised by the State Lunacy Commission. While the measure has not yet been put in, it is expected that it will appear in the legislature in a few days. Last week the Governor talked with President Mabon and Commissioner Daniel S. Lockwood, of the Lunacy Commission. regarding changes in the law to bring about the exercise of greater care as to commitments of persons believed to be insane.

Cornell Lectures.—The Cornell University Medical College will continue this year the courses instituted last season in lectures upon special subjects connected with general medicine and general surgery. Dr. Charles L. Gibson, Dr. Ellsworth Eliot, Jr., Dr. E. L. Keyes, Jr., will each give about six lectures on topics connected with general surgery. Drs. L. A. Conner, M. C. Schlapp, C. N. B. Camac, O. H. Schultze. will lecture on topics connected with general medicine. Dr. John McGaw Woodbury, the present Commissioner of Street Cleaning, has promised to deliver several lectures upon Municipal Sanitation. These lectures are given to the third and fourth year students. and have been found of great value in the elucidation of subjects in which the lecturer has demonstrated his proficiency. At the same time they are of value to the Faculty, who are thus able to obtain knowledge of the latest advancement made in college laboratories.

Monday Club.—At the meeting of the Monday Club, on January 30. the evening was devoted to a discussion of the tuberculosis situation. This club is composed of the paid charity workers of the city, and the problem in question is a vital one in their work. Encouraging reports were received of the seashore colony of the tuberculosis children, and also from the work of the Vanderbilt clinic in providing nursing and advice for the poor in their homes. The outdoor cure seems to be the salvation in any situation, and the nurses show infinite ingenuity in securing it for their patients. The photographs which illustrated the report showed alternately the sleeping quarters occupied by patients before being taken in charge and those devised for them since. Hammocks on the roof of a double-decker tenement are a frequent resource, and even in the deadly "Lung block" a woman had been taken from a blind cell to repose, warmly wrapped, on the fire escape.

Ophthalmic Hospital's Needs.—With the constant increase in the number of patients treated in the New York Ophthalmic Hospital, the staff has so studied the problem of making its old funds and facilities cover its new demands, that, according to the fifty-third annual report, they have decreased the cost of each house patient from $2.79 per diem ten years ago to $2.21 at present. Strict economy, moreover, in space, has enabled the increased work to be conducted in the old building at the corner of Twenty-third Street and Third Avenue, built in 1871 with the $100,000 gift of Mrs. Henry A. Keep. But the demands for special treatment of the diseases of the eye, the ear, and the throat, have at last grown so great that many applicants have to be turned away, and the patients received must be hurried out of the wards before they really ought to go, in order to make room for others. More than 15,000 patients suffering from diseases of the eye, ear, and throat, received treatment from the hospital free of charge last year. This number included natives of thirty-six countries from all over the world, the Germans and the Irish being the most numerous after the citizens of the United States. The total income for the year was $33,414.56. As the institution is not endowed, the expenses necessary to its maintenance have to be met through the efforts of interested friends through additions to the list, and through visitations by a paid solicitor.

Aural Institute's Fund.—According to the thirty-fifth annual report of the New York Ophthalmic and Aural Institute, $200,000 of the $500,000 needed for the erection of its new building at the corner of Central Park West and Sixty-fourth Street has already been raised. The change of quarters has been rendered necessary by the fact that in the thirty-five years of its existence, the Institute, in its double character of a dispensary and hospital for the treatment of diseases of the eye and ear and their accessory parts, and of a School of Ophthalmology and Otology, has completely outgrown its present quarters. The School of Ophthalmology and Otology connected with the Institute continues its important educational work in the training of specialists. It is open only to graduates of medicine, and those who take the courses are entitled to certificates of attendance, and, in case of special examinations, certificates of proficiency. The best time for the students to begin work is the first day of October. A course extending from that time to the middle of June will be sufficient for graduates of medicine to familiarize themselves with the anatomy and physiology of the visual, auditory, and olfactory organs, as well as with the symptoms and treatment of all forms of disease of the eye and ear and the parts in relation therewith, in particular the nose and the accessory cavities, also the throat and the cranial cavity, as far as they cause or complicate eye and ear disease. The course will make students proficient in physical diagnosis (ophthalmoscopy, otoscopy, laryngoscopy), the determination of acuteness of sight and hearing, the systematic examination and judicious treatment of the eye, the anomalies of retraction, accommodation, motility, as well as diagnosis and treatment of organic and functional diseases of the eye, ear, and nose, and their cranial and vascular complications, and the performance of operations. As an important accessory to its work and influence, the medical director founded an international medical journal, *The Archives of Ophthalmology and Otology*, published in English and in German. The endowment of the Institute is only $50,000, and it depends for its support largely on contributions. The total number of hospital inmates last year was 17,226, and the total number of operations 30,567. Since the institute was inaugurated thirty-five years ago, there have been treated in the hospital and dispensary 288,845 patients altogether.

PHILADELPHIA.

Ferry-House Quarantined.—Owing to the death of a colored woman upon a ferry-boat plying between Philadelphia and Camden some thirty passengers were held, because the woman's death was said to be due to smallpox.

Abortionist Convicted.—Judge von Moschzicker sentenced Mrs. Ashmead to three years' imprisonment in the Eastern Penitentiary for malpractice, but the remaining bills against her as well as those against Dr. McVicker and DeWitt Ashmead were submitted to the Judge.

Cancer Annex Opened.—The Philadelphia Home for Incurables erected a new three-story brick building expressly for incurable cases of carcinoma. The building cost $60,000; it was begun last May and finished a week ago; it has tile floors, doors without molding and accommodates twenty-five patients.

Metropolitan Surgeon Holds Clinics at the German Hospital.—Prince Skilletta, who is the guest of Dr. John B. Deaver, held clinics daily during his stay in the city. At these clinics he illustrated the "Skilletta Operation" for the cure of hernia, which was devised by his father, the famous Italian surgeon.

Lenient Standard of Drugs.—At the annual dinner of the Philadelphia Drug Exchange Prof. J. P. Remington said they would show in the new edition of the Pharmacopeia that pure chemicals and drugs were not absolutely necessary, for instance, he continued, 99 per cent. pure quinine is just as good as 100 per cent. pure, provided the one per cent. is not a non-injurious ingredient. Dr. Henry Beates, at the same dinner, denounced the "cure-alls," the Christian Scientists and also pointed out the evil wrought by handling patent medicines.

Aid for Consumptives.—A bill has been prepared by Dr. R. N. Wilson, which is to be introduced into the legislature by Senator Scott in the near future. The bill provides for an appropriation of $500,000 for the establishment of camps, hospitals and dispensaries in a section of not less than 500 acres of State Forestry Reservation in Pike County. They are to be established under a tuberculosis commission of nine and are to accommodate at least 500 patients at all times. The minimum period of treatment of each patient shall be three months.

Anchylostoma Duodenale Not a Bogy.—In his lecture before the students and members of the faculty of the Medico-Chirurgical College Dr. Rosenau, Director of the Hygenic Laboratories of the United States Public Health and Marine Hospital Service, said that while the tropical anemia due to the *Anchylostoma duodenale* is prevalent in the tropics it can be cured. He also told his audience that 90 per cent. of the Porto Rican population were infected with this disease and that 30 per cent. of them die from the anemia due to the *Anchylostoma*. Tropical malaria is the most fatal disease of the tropics, he said, and is much more difficult to cure than the ordinary quartan or tertian type of malaria.

Free Public Lectures.—The Department of Medicine of the University of Pennsylvania has announced that a series of lectures will be delivered in the new laboratories upon the subjects of hygiene and medicine. While arranged especially for instruction of the fourth year student members of the medcial profession of Philadelphia are also invited. Dr. Leonard Pearson will deliver two lectures upon the "Milk Supplies of the Cities"; one lecture will be given on February 6, the other the 13. Dr. J. F. Schamberg will speak of "Vaccination" on February 20 and on the 27 he will give a demonstration upon "The Eruptive Fevers." On March 6 and 13 Dr. Edward C. Kirk will speak upon "The Medical Relationship of Certain Dental and Oral Disorders." Dr. A. P. Francine will lecture upon the "Restriction and Prevention of Pulmonary Tuberculosis." On March 27 Dr. R. Tait McKenzie will speak upon "The Therapeutics of Exercise." Dr. Joseph Sailer will deliver the two closing lectures on April 3 and 10. He will speak on "Hydrotherapy."

Neurological Society Meeting.—This was held January 24, 1905. Dr. W. C. Pickett exhibited for Dr. L. C. Peters "A Case of Cervical Hypertrophic Pachymeningitis." Dr. Pickett informed the Society that the patient had pain in the back and shoulders which, according to the patient's story, came on seven days after the onset of peritonitis. The latter disease was probably of gonococcal origin. He also called attention to the wasting of the thenar and hyperthenar eminences, the flattening of the hands giving the "claw-hand," and the exaggeration of the knee-jerk. Dr. C. W. Burr exhibited "A Case of Epilepsy with Myoclonus." He had seen the same case in 1896 when he gathered that the patient suffered with fits at the age of sixteen months; these were minor in type. After a time the child was free from epilepsy for about twelve months, when the attacks again recurred; now the fits were more frequent and more severe. Then there was another period of latency. The child then developed twitching of the muscles of the face and shoulders, but the intellect at this time was clear. A short time ago the patient again came under his care, and when he first saw the boy he was suffering with violent choreiform movements and visual hallucinations. In the course of forty-eight hours the patient became quiet but developed major epilepsy, which was followed by muscular spasm. The myoclonus sometimes came before the epileptic attack, sometimes after it, but most frequently independent of the convulsions. Voluntary movements appear to exaggerate the myoclonus. When the patient's eyes are turned to one side nystagmus is present. The mental condition of the patient is not as bad as it was

during the first forty-eight hours in the hospital. Dr. William G. Spiller and Dr. E. U. Buckman reported "A Case of Myasthenia Gravis in which the paresis is confined to the Ocular Muscles." Dr. Spiller informed the Society that this was the first case reported in the English literature and that but three or four have been reported in the German literature. The patient first noticed in April of 1904, that things looked crooked and that he saw double, but could see all right with either eye alone. Now he finds that his eyes are not so easily opened in the morning as some time later in the day. After one eye has been used for some time the lid of the corresponding eye begins to droop, and when it reaches the pupil the other lid begins to fall. When the eyes are closed for a time the patient is again able to open them. There is no evidence of disease of the nervous system at any other point nor has the patient ever had syphilis, and antisyphilitic treatment was not followed by improvement. Dr. Joseph McCool, by invitation, reported "Four Cases of Beriberi." These cases were seen at Marcus Hook, two last summer and the other two only recently; all were from vessels that had come from the Sandwich Islands and had been on board vessel for at least 150 days. He pointed out the predisposing causes, as unhygienic surroundings, insufficiently cooked and a lack of nitrogenous foods. He noted that the disease has been attributed as being due to a specific organism. Some of the cases were of the dry and others were of the atrophic form. They all began with pains, stiffness, tingling and numbness in the ankles, feet and legs which was followed by swelling in few. There was always present dyspnea and distress in the epigastrium. Dr. T. H. Weisenberg read a paper on "The Pathology of Cerebellar Tumors." He informed the Society that the greater number of tumors of the brain in his collection were sarcoma. He noted that in some instances cerebellar tumors produce no symptoms, while in other cases there are symptoms of cerebellar tumors but no growth. He related an instance where the diagnosis of such a condition was made but operation failed to disclose the new growth and the patient left the hospital apparently cured.

Meeting of the Pathological Society.—This meeting was held on January 26, 1905. Dr. Coplin read two papers, one entitled "Some Improvements in the Petri-Dish-Plate-Gelatin Method of Mounting Gross Specimens," and the other "Celloidin Strips and Sheets for the orientation of Gross Specimens and in Such a Way as to Facilitate the Removal of Parts for Microscopical Study and Subsequent Identification of the Areas from which Such Blocks of Tissue Have been Removed." In the first paper he showed how the gelatin could be substituted by plaster-of-Paris. Dr. Loeb read a paper upon "Some Recent Contributions to the Study of the Coagulation of the Blood." He pointed out that mechanical factors are very important in aiding the coagulation of the blood. Bacteria influence the process, and this influence is especially seen in the production of thrombi. He maintains that certain bacteria are more powerful than others in inducing this change, as for instance, the *Staphylococcus pyogenes aureus* is a more powerful than others in coagulation than the *Bacillus coli communis*. Although the coagulins of the blood and the coagulins of the tissue have the same property they are not identical. He also stated that in all probability the coagulins of the blood and those of the tissues act independently upon the fibrinogen and also act upon each other. Both, he said, are derivatives of the cells. Authors who object to the latter view maintain that if such were the case, why would not fibrin formation be going on continuously, for blood cells are constantly being destroyed in the blood and then the coagulins would be present at all time. Loeb meets this objection by saying, in the first place, as these cells die they may contain very little active substances, but if they should, these substances are destroyed by antibodies, for he found agents in the serum of a dog which inhibited coagulation. Dr. H. C. Wood, Jr., read a paper on "The Clinical Means of Increasing the Coagulability of the Blood." These drugs, he said, which contract the arterioles are dangerous in concealed hemorrhages, as they may prevent the formation of thrombi. He maintained that an excess of calcium salts in the blood increases the coagulation time, and that hypodermic injection of gelatin is dangerous because this substance is so difficult to sterilize, and then, too, it may contain a tetanotoxin which is not at all destroyed by heat. When gelatin is taken by mouth and digested it does not lose its power to coagulate blood, for by artificial digestion he obtained a substance that is equally efficacious in the production of coagulation as is the gelatin itself. Dr. R. P. Reynolds read a paper on "Interstitial Fibroids as a Complication of Pregnancy." Dr. B. M. Anspach showed several specimens of fibroids which complicated pregnancy. Dr. John Funke showed a specimen of carcinoma of the gallbladder with metastasis to the liver. The gall-bladder was filled with bile sand and the common duct contained two calculi, one was located near the ampulla of Vater.

CHICAGO.

Appointment of Dr. Barker.—Dr. L. F. Barker, of the University of Chicago, has been appointed to a professorship in medicine in that institution by the Board of Trustees of Rush Medical College.

Popular Lectures for the Laity on Medical Topics. —Under the auspices of the Visiting Nurses' Association two hundred lectures on topics pertaining to medicine and sanitation will be delivered in Chicago this winter.

Warning to Hospital Staff.—President Brundage, of the County Board of Commissioners, in some prefatory remarks to the newly-appointed members of the Cook County Hospital Staff, said that they had been selected as members of the hospital staff without pull, political or otherwise. He gave them to understand that if they did not live up to the rules governing the institution, no pull of any kind would stand in the way of their resignation being asked for.

First Aid Magazine.—It is said that a 24-page magazine, under the title of *First Aid,* to be devoted to literature and science, edited by a staff of physicians and women prominent in the professional and social world, and issued monthly as the official organ of the American White Cross Aid Society, will appear early in March. Edward Howe is to be the Managing Editor. Among those who are mentioned as constituting the scientific staff are Drs. Nicholas Senn, John B. Murphy, Chas. Adams, Geo. W. Webster, Frank Billings, J. B. Herrick, John Ridlon, N. S. Davis, H. B. Favill, and Wm. E. Quine.

Invitation to Child Study Expert.—Of the multitude of college and university men who make pretensions to the title of "Physiologico-Psychological

Expert," only eight have been found in the United States who are out of jobs and competent to serve as assistants in the child study department of public schools. This fact was developed at a meeting of the school management committee, when the trustees, after reviewing the results of the canvass for candidates, that covered every large educational center in the country, finally invited Dr. Frank G. Brunner to come from Columbia University to try for the position.

Tuberculosis.—Dr. ·Arnold C. Klebs recently delivered a lecture in this course on tuberculosis, and declared that the loss in Chicago annually by consumption was enormous. He quoted experts on the extreme ravages of the disease in the United States. The total was given at 150,000 at an average age of thirty-five years. He urged his hearers not to look on the consumptive as a leper, but to remember that the victim becomes, by right living, no menace in himself, and that the distribution of germs through drying of the sputum and their propagation through lack of cleanliness and sanitation were the real dangers.

How to Live.—Dr. George F. Butler recently delivered an address on this subject under the auspices of the Chicago Medical Society, to an audience of 600 people in the Public Library Building. The address was replete with epigrammatic sentences, and may be summed up in this wise: "It has been said that it is better to be born lucky than rich, but it is in fact better to be born tough than either lucky or rich. After forty, eat less and eliminate more. Drink more pure water and keep the peristaltic wave of prosperity constantly moving down the alimentary canal. Many people suffer from too much business and not enough health. When such is the case, they had better cut out business and society for a time, and come down to mush and milk and first principles. Don't be foolish. Eat less and play more. Indulge in less fret and fume and more fruit and fun. There are people too indolent to be healthy —literally too lazy to live. Work your brains and keep in touch with people. Do something for others and forget yourselves. There is nothing so inane and detrimental to mind and health as the conversation of people on their aches and pains and troubles. The froth of whipped eggs is a tonic compared to it. All our appetites are conditional. Enjoyment depends upon the scarcity. A worker in any field, whose age is near either the shady or sunny side of fifty, should consider himself in his prime, good for another half century of temperate, judicious work. Let grandma wear bright ribbons and gaudy gowns if the colors become her, and let grandpa be as dudish as he pleases, with flashy neckties and cheerful garb. Both will be younger for it, and, besides, it is in harmony with nature. Gray hair is honorable; that which is dyed is an abomination before the Lord. Cultivate thankfulness and cheerfulness. An ounce of good cheer is worth a pound of melancholy."

CANADA.

Provincial Sanitarium for British Columbia.—Dr. Dr. C. J. Fagan, secretary of the Board of Health for British Columbia, and who is the father of the movement in that province for a provincial sanitarium, announces that the British Columbia Association for the Prevention of Tuberculosis has resolved to delay no longer, but will at once get to work and have a sanitarium ready for the occupation of patients by June 1 of the present year. Dr. Fagan will tour British Columbia in an endeavor to raise the necessary funds for the erection of the institution. In the meantime the Anti-Tuberculosis League have made overtures for renting the Royal Naval Hospital at Esquimalt, which the admiralty will shortly abandon.

Reunion of the Toronto General Hospital Surgeons.— There was held in Toronto on December 29, a reunion of the house surgeons of the Toronto General Hospital in 1892-1893. One of these, Dr. J. N. E. Brown, came all the way from Dawson, where he occupies the position of Territorial Secretary. Dr. Charles O'Reilly, the Medical Superintendent, stated that since 1876 there had been passed through the hospital 220 house surgeons, all of whom, after a period of twenty-eight years, were alive with the exception of eight. The proposal to inaugurate an Association of Ex-House Surgeons of the Toronto General Hospital met with marked favor.

Toronto General Hospital.—Mr. George Gooderham, of Toronto, after a service on the Board of Governors extending over a period of twenty years, has retired from active participation in the work of the Toronto General Hospital, and he has been succeeded by Mr. Cawthra Mulock, who a short time ago donated $100,000 to the institution. Mr. Gooderham announced that he would in the near future make a generous donation to the hospital, toward a new building. It is proposed to raise $1,000,000 by private, civic and Government subscription, and in addition to being an hospital for all classes of diseases, excepting infectious diseases, will as well provide facilities for educational purposes in connection with the Medical Faculty of Toronto University.

Results Achieved with Diphtheria Antitoxin in the Toronto Isolation Hospital.—In the January issue of the *Canadian Practitioner and Review*, Professor Shuttleworth, bacteriologist to the Toronto Board of Health, gives the results of the use of diphtheria antitoxin in the Toronto Isolation Hospital. The first experiments were made in 1894 and were continued up to the close of 1898, during which time 157 cases were treated with the diphtheria antitoxin, with a mortality of 21.6 per cent., and an average hospital term of 25.4 days for non-fatal cases. The average hospital mortality for the period was 14.3 per cent. and the term was 23.5 days. The treatment on these results not being satisfactory, it was almost abandoned in 1899, but was revived in 1900, when 62 patients were treated in the hospital, and 20 others to whom it had been given before admission. Of this series of 82 cases 20.7 per cent. were fatal. The ordinary hospital mortality for that year was 14.8 per cent. The following year there were 119 hospital and 35 outside cases, of whom 17.5 per cent. died, the annual hospital rate being 13.4 per cent. In 1902 there were only 105 antitoxin cases, most of which had been treated by their own physicians before admission. In this year the mortality was for the first time under that of the ordinary hospital rate, being 14.3 and 15.6, respectively. The total number of antitoxin cases treated since 1894 in the Toronto hospital amounted to 508, with 95 deaths, or 18.7 per cent. The average hospital mortality for the same period is 14.0.

GENERAL.

Herter Lectureship.—Dr. Hans H. Meyer, professor of pharmacology in the University of Vienna, has accepted an invitation to deliver the second course of Herter lectures at the Johns Hopkins Medical School next October.

Triumph of Jap Field Surgeons.—Statistics from the chief surgeon of Gen. Oku's army prove that the army surgeons and field hospitals have scored a triumph in surgery and medicine. There have been only forty deaths from disease in the whole army since the landing on May 6. Up to December 1 24,642 cases of disease were treated. Eighteen thousand five hundred and seventy-eight patients recovered, 5,609 were sent to Japan, 40 died, and the rest are still under treatment.

Auto Ambulances for the Army.—Plans have been prepared in the office of the surgeon-general for an automobile ambulance. If these designs can be carried out by automobile manufacturers, it seems likely that steam carriages fitted up with ambulance facilities will take the place of the present style of vehicles drawn by horses. With a view to thoroughly testing this scheme, the department has ordered Captain Clyde S. Ford, assistant surgeon, to Ormond, Fla., to hold a conference there with the automobile manufacturers. Captain Ford is charged with investigating all details of the project, and he will make a report to the Department on its feasibility. The General Staff does not favor the adoption at this time of the automobile as a means of military transportation. Major-Gen. Corbin, commanding the Philippines Division, recently recommended the purchase of an automobile for the use of military headquarters at Manila in the transportation of officers about the city and vicinity when engaged in purely military duty. The proposition was disapproved by the General Staff and the Secretary.

OBITUARY.

Assistant-Surgeon OTTO KOHLHASE died of yellow fever on the cruiser Boston at Panama. He was appointed to the navy in May, 1903, when he was made assistant surgeon. His station on the Boston was given him last November, and was the beginning of his first cruise. Prior to that time he was on the cruiser New York. Last March he was graduated from the Naval Medical School in Washington. Surgeon Kohlhase was twenty-seven years of age and married.

Dr. B. F. CORY, a veteran of the Civil War and for many years a well-known physician in southern Ohio, died at the residence of his son in Washington last week, at the age of eighty-five years. He was born in Coudersport, Pa., removed to Ohio, and in 1861 was Provost-Marshal of the Eleventh Ohio district. Resigning his office, he raised two regiments of volunteers, in one of which, a cavalry regiment, he served as captain. He served throughout the war, participating in the capture of Morgan, the Confederate cavalry leader.

The Military Secretary at Washington received a cable message from General Corbin, commanding the Philippine division, saying that Contract Surgeon JOSEPH A. O'NEILL was killed at San Francisco de Malabon, January 3, in an attack by Ladrones, and that his body will be sent to the United States on the army transport sailing from Manila on February 15. Dr. O'Neill was a resident of New York, and was appointed a contract surgeon on August 8, 1900. His entire service was in the Philippines. In the winter of 1903 he visited the United States on leave of absence, and on his return to the Philippines he was accompanied by his wife.

SOCIETY PROCEEDINGS.

MEDICAL SOCIETY OF THE STATE OF NEW YORK.

Ninety-ninth Annual Meeting held at Albany, January 31, February 1 and 2, 1905.

The President, Dr. Hamilton F. Wey, of Elmira, in the Chair.

FIRST DAY—JANUARY 31ST.

MOST of the morning session was taken up with reports of the various standing committees. Of these the following seem to be of special interest to the general medical public:

Reunion Committee Report.—Dr. Henry L. Elsner, of Syracuse, the chairman of the committee of conference for the union of the New York State Medical Society and New York State Medical Association, detailed the vicissitudes of the attempt at union and its final prevention by a legal technicality. He then read legal opinions as to the necessities for indefeasible combination of the two organizations as regards legality of meetings, special and regular, for the purpose, and made recommendations accordingly. These recommendations were unanimously adopted.

New Committee of Union.—Dr. D. B. St. John Roosa, of New York City, then proposed the names of the old committee as a new committee of conference looking to union, with power to make all arrangements, and this was unanimously adopted with applause.

Committee on Hygiene.—Dr. John L. Heffron, of Syracuse, reported the attention of the committee as having been drawn to certain subjects of public health with regard to which members of the New York State Society should keep themselves informed. The use of sulphate of copper as an antiseptic for impure water has attracted widespread interest. It would seem, if original reports with regards to it are confirmed, that its employment may serve as a protection against such dangerous water-borne contagious diseases as typhoid fever. As typhoid fever is always more of a rural than an urban disease, and as the precautions against the disease must be more individual than authoritative, the use of some such means should be in the hands of physicians in suspicious circumstances.

Food Adulteration.—Special attention was called to the fact that at the present time nearly all forms of food are packed in special packages, and that many of the forms are so prepared that there is temptation to secure their preservation by various forms of antiseptics. The United States Agricultural Department, and various special investigators, have shown that preservatives, of whose ultimate action upon the human organism little is known, are actually being used. It seems then, that for the protection of delicate individuals under their care, physicians should take special precautions and as far as possible encourage such legislative action with regard to the labeling of articles of food containing preservatives, so as to protect the public.

Wood Alcohol Dangers.—Recent events have shown that there are serious dangers to the community in the permission to make and sell wood alcohol deodorized, and under such names as may deceive the public into a failure to realize its toxicity. The occurrence of many deaths and of blindness in many cases during the past year shows how acute are the risks of negligence in this matter. The suggestion of the committee that legal regulation of the sale of such spirits be secured was adopted.

Better Situation of Medical Legislation.—The report of the committee on legislation reported a better feeling among prominent legislators of both legislative bodies, as regards the legal regulation of the practice of medicine. The committee on legislation are now consulted as to the real significance of and their position as regards contemplated medical legislation. This will make it harder to secure laws allowing the practice of medicine in parts, as is asked by the opticians or others, and will lead to the proper restriction of medical practice in all branches to the fully educated physician. The Society is to be congratulated on this improvement in the attitude of legislators, and it would seem that only a persistence of well-directed effort is needed still further to strengthen the position of the regular profession in its attempts to keep the community from being exploited by quacks and charlatans.

The Secretary, Dr. Frederic C. Curtis, of Albany, then announced the names of 115 candidates for admission as permanent members of the Society, all of whom have fulfilled the preliminary requirements including attendance at three annual meetings.

Dermatitis Seborrhoica and Baldness.—The scientific business of the session began with the reading of a paper on this subject by Dr. L. Duncan Bulkley, of New York City. He said that this disease was one of the most important the dermatologist has to treat. Statistics show that it constitutes fully 10 per cent. of all the cutaneous affections seen by the dermatologist. It follows in importance eczema, acne and syphilis in demands on his attention. It is of great importance, because it is now conceded to be at least an important contributing cause to baldness, which is growing so much more common in recent years, and the etiology and consequently successful treatment of which has been so long a mystery. The disease is undoubtedly contagious, though only mildly so. It is distinctly a barber's disease and has spread as a consequence of the universal recourse to these in later genrations. The true nature of the micro-organismal cause is not known, however. It differs from such parasitic diseases as barber's itch and favus in being due to a different form of parasite. Various cocci and bacilli have been described as specifically pathogenic, but none of these have stood the inoculation test and when in pure culture reproduced the affection.

Treatment, General and Local.—Dr. Bulkley said that the very fact that the infection is of low grade and never virulent seems to indicate that the soil in which the microbes grow is an important element in these cases. There is, however, no internal treatment that can be depended on to bring about improvement, and especially not to ward off baldness. The general health must be cared for and all digestive disturbances especially corrected, but the dependence must be on local treatment. For this the universal agreement as to a parasitic cause makes the indication for a parasiticide imperative. In Dr. Bulkley's experience resorcin and sulphur have been the best remedies. Either of them employed beyond a certain point, and especially resorcin, may give rise to a scaliness not unlike the disease itself. With care such inconvenience can be readily avoided.

Modify and Complicate Other Affections.—Dr. Bulkley said that the most important feature of dermatitis seborrhoica is its tendency to co-exist with other diseases, such as eczema and psoriasis and certain forms of syphilitic eruptions, thus complicating the problem of diagnosis and treatment. Wherever it does exist it modifies practically all other skin eruptions, and its manifestations must be carefully eliminated before the diagnosis of the case can be reached. Its frequency is not realized as a rule by the general practitioner of medicine, and this serves as an element of confusion in many skin diseases that would otherwise be easy of recognition and even of treatment.

Specific Constitutional Treatment.—Dr. Ralph A. McDonnell, of New Haven, Conn., in discussing Dr. Buckley's paper said that local treatment of the condition supposed to underly developing baldness, has been the watchword for many years, yet very little has been accomplished. The skin specialist receives a case of beginning baldness dubiously and always emphasizes the uncertainty of the prognosis. Parasiticides have not given such results as to inspire confidence. It would seem that baldness and the conditions leading up to it must be considered as of reflex nervous origin as are so many other skin affections and depending on the influence of the digestive tract. Simple acne and acne rosacea, as well as eczema and other skin conditions, are now known to depend for the most part on digestive conditions. No one thinks of treating them without proper regulation of digestion, and the same seems to be true of dermatitis seborrhoica and the other conditions preliminary to baldness.

Cycloplegics in Determining Refraction.—Dr. Frank Van Fleet, of New York City, said that the employment of substances that paralyze accommodation is much less frequent now than was the case a few years ago. Not so long since many ophthalmologists considered it almost a crime to fit glasses without the use of atropine or some similarly acting drug. Now it is never used for opthalmoscopic examinations and much of the ordinary refraction can be accomplished without it. This he considers a fortunate advance in ophthalmological practice, for their use in cases as they come was a source of certain dangers.

Seeing Not Merely Mechanical.—Dr. Van Fleet said that vision is not merely a passive quality, but requires attention. The influence of errors of vision is not limited to the eyes themselves, but invades other nervous mechanisms of the body. On the other hand, many bodily ailments are reflected in the eyes and the eye symptoms need to be treated not directly, but through the other affected organs. Hence the necessity for a physician to prescribe glasses, though it has been the custom to suggest that the fitting of glasses was more or less mechanical. Unfortunately, in many States laws have been passed sanctioning such an error, and even to some degree in New York. Further evil of this kind should not be allowed, however.

Special Cases for Cycloplegics.—Dr. W. E. Lambert, of New York City, opened the discussion by saying that in certain cases the use of cycloplegics seemed necessary. He instanced the case of convergent strabismus in children, in whom it was impossible properly to study refraction owing to the convergence without paralysis of accommodation. He, too, deprecated the evils of non-medical opticians and instanced two cases in recent practice in one of which a patient suffering from incipient cataract had been given very strong glasses, and in the other the cause for loss of acuity of vision was found not to be the presbyopia that was suspected, but a severe case of hemorrhagic neuroretinitis.

Atropine Less and Less.—Dr. Lucien Howe, of Buffalo, said that the use of atropine is becoming rarer. Personally he considers that the use of solutions of such drugs is most inexact medication. It is not known how much stays in the eye or how much is absorbed. He prefers to use these substances in disks, so as to be able to tell just the amount that may be absorbed. Complete cycloplegia, by removing the diaphragm of the camera obscura of the eye, adds some errors of its own to the problem, since the edges of any lens do not refract as well as the central portion and the rays that pass through them serve to disturb the resultant picture.

Javal's Ophthalmometer.—Dr. D. B. St. John Roosa said that the great evil among ophthalmologists in America had been the desire for overexactness of correction of the optical error. Personally he considers that the improvement of vision to useful sight without inconvenience rather than the restoration of ideal conditions of refraction is the most desirable. He has found Javal's ophthalmometer, to whose employment he was introduced by the inventor himself, a very useful instrument. After having been an advocate of the paralysis of accommodation he is now among those who, like the most distinguished European authorities, consider it rarely necessary.

Convergent Squint in Children.—Dr. Abraham Jacobi said that he considered it unfortunate that atropine should be employed in the treatment of convergent squint in young children. If time be allowed to pass, the child learns to use the originally affected muscle properly and no active treatment beyond care for the general health is needed. Haste in these cases may render permanent a condition that would otherwise be but passing. In general the forces of nature in children are much better than in adults, and due allowance should be made for this.

Rheumatism and the Eye Muscles.—Dr. Francis Valk, of New York, said that as the uric acid diathesis causes various forms of muscle trouble in the bodily muscles, so also it may be the origin of symptomatic affections of the ocular muscles. These affections are usually not of a paretic nature, that is, do not exhibit actual loss of motion in the muscles, but they do lead to symptoms of muscle weakness not unlike those seen in the so-called muscular asthenopia. The special character of these symptoms can be shown by such suitable muscle tests as those for the rotation of the eyeballs, under fusion and version. The treatment of these conditions is evidently more general than local, and it is mainly important not to think that the manifestations are local.

Cholelithiasis Simulating Appendicitis.—Dr. George G. Lempe, of Albany, described a case in which almost the classic symptoms of appendicitis seemed to be present and all the manifestations were in the right lower quadrant of the abdomen, yet on operation the appendix was found to be perfectly normal, while a search of the right upper quadrant revealed the presence of a large number of gall-stones, to account for the referred pains which had been felt in the appendical region. It seems clear that in some of these cases no differential diagnostic method yet known will enable the surgeon to decide with absolute certainty. Both conditions demand operative intervention and an exploratory laparotomy must be the deciding test.

Arteriosclerosis and the Nervous System.—Dr. B. C. Loveland, of Syracuse, suggested that some of the earliest symptoms of arteriosclerosis manifest themselves in the nervous symptoms and may thus be discovered before the occurrence of those serious conditions for which treatment is hopeless. When symptoms are found, there should be a readjustment of diet so as to keep up nutrition but throw no extra work on the organs of elimination. Too great reduction in diet is to be avoided. The habits of life must be changed, so that neither work nor recreation will be of a kind to demand stimulants. If high arterial tension is present, then the amount of water consumed must be limited. Otherwise, a good, liberal allowance of water each day should be insisted on. The iodides in some form should be given, and Dr. Loveland has found the proto-iodide of mercury in gr. $\frac{1}{6}$ to $\frac{1}{4}$ the best and least likely to cause stomach disturbance. Aconite and certain of the nitrites may be administered over months, so as to keep the arterial tension low and lessen the strain upon the heart and lungs.

Amblyopia ex Anopsia.—Dr. D. B. St. John Roosa discussed the question of the loss of vision in an eye from disuse, such as happens in cases of squint, where one eye is not equal to its fellow in visual power, the image from it is gradually so neglected that the eye loses its power of seeing. It has been said that such eye never recover their vision, and so good an authority as Dr. Priestly Smith did not hesitate to affirm that recovery of sight cannot be expected to occur in such cases. Dr. Roosa reported a case in which, though the man had lost vision in his right eye in this way and used his left eye for all seeing purposes, an accident to his left eye being followed by the loss of vision in it, he gradually regained the use of the eye, blind from early youth, from disuse. Dr. Roosa said that there were a few cases like this in the literature.

Cerebral Lack of Vision.—Dr. Van Fleet said that in these cases there seems to be a failure of the visual center for the recognition of images from the disused eye to develop. This being a basic difficulty, it is hard to get patients to exercise enough to bring about development later in life. If, as in this case, the loss of the other eye compels them to use the defective eye, the development is completed. It usually requires, as in this case, several years, but vision gradually grows better and better.

Visual Exercises.—Dr. Lucien Howe, of Buffalo, said that theory is plentiful on this subject, but the observed facts are few. Cases like Dr. Roosa's have been observed before, but only where the sight of the former seeing eye was destroyed. There seems no doubt that with enough patience and by appropriate methods the other eye may be educated. Dr. Howe uses the stereoscope for this purpose, not the ordinary instrument, but one in which the lenses are so arranged that the visual power of the seeing eye is reduced so as to adapt it to the defective visual organ. In this way an education of nerves and nerve centers may be successfully brought about.

Dr. Francis Valk said that there may be a congenital amblyopia from which any improvement seems hopeless. Other forms of amblyopia from disuse, when of high degree, are cured if vision be totally lost in the other eye.

Dr. A. E. Davis, of New York, said that amblyopia may be cured by proper exercises and then relapse from neglect. He detailed the case of a clergyman who, after operation, had taken the proper exercises and could use both eyes, yet, later, lost the power of fusion.

Biliary Drainage.—Dr. Eugene A. Smith, of Buffalo, showed by the details of some 25 cases of biliary disease, operated upon during the last two years, that drainage of the biliary region after operation always gives the most satisfactory results. Drainage is wise in at least 90 per cent. of the cases. As a matter of fact, it lessens the tendency to relapse and to the persistence of low grade symptoms that may lead to unfortunate pathological developments. Deaver insists that biliary cirrhosis is due to biliary obstruction. If this has continued for some time, drainage serves as a derivative to prevent further damage to liver tissues and enable the organ to throw off offending material. In Dr. Smith's experience cholecystectomy, though spoken of as the ideal operation, is not so good an operation in the long run as cholecystostomy. The latter can be accomplished without so much risk, the mortality being 6 per cent. for cholecystectomy and 2 per cent. for cholecystostomy. In this the gall-bladder can be stitched to the abdominal wall and drainage is easily obtained.

The symposium on cerebrospinal meningitis was opened by Prof. W. T. Councilman, of Boston, who read a paper on pathology and bacteriology of disease.

Pathology of Epidemic Meningitis.—Dr. Councilman called attention to the fact that the inflammation involves not only the serous membranes of the brain, but also the brain itself. The disease therefore deserves the name of meningo-encephalitis. The infection may take place by the blood or by extension from some other organ. The possibility of infection from the eye or from the nose has been discussed by many pathologists, though the definite mode of entering is not yet known. All of the cord and brain may be affected, but in most cases the spinal cord is more affected and in consequence the symptoms from it are more noticeable.

Cause of the Disease.—There seems to be no doubt now that the cause of the disease is the *Diplococcus intracellularis*. A corresponding affection may be caused by the pneumococcus or by the streptococcus, but these are distinct diseases and are much more fatal as a rule than epidemics or even spinal meningitis itself. The *Diplococcus intracellularis* was discovered by Weichselbaum, who found it as a quasi-inhabitant of the mucous membranes of some parts of the body. In the epidemic of the disease, studied in 1897 in Massachusetts, 31 of the 35 cases proved to have this as the causative agent when examined for this purpose. The micro-organism was found in the fluid taken from the spinal canal by means of lumbar puncture. It was found in all the acute cases. It was absent only in the chronic cases. All the patients whose symptoms had lasted less than seven days had the micro-organism in their spinal fluid. In those in whom it was not found the symptoms had been present for more than seventeen days.

Culture Peculiarities.—One reason for the absence of the diplococcus of Weichselbaum in the chronic cases is that the micro-organism has a tendency to die out quickly on any kind of culture medium, and that evidently the comparatively favorable location in the fluids of the spinal cord and the surface of the brain is not sufficiently appropriate to prolong their existence. In the laboratory it is rather difficult to grow the micro-organism successfully. It has not much effect as a rule on the ordinary laboratory animals.

Endemic and Epidemic.—The present status of the knowledge of the disease seems to show that it occurs in epidemic form at more or less regular intervals, it is more or less endemic in this country and sporadic cases are constantly occurring. The first epidemic of the disease in this country was described by Danielson and Mann, and occurred in Massachusetts during 1806. The epidemic may last a short time and yet may prove very fatal. Some of the epidemics had a fatality as high as 75 per cent. Nearly all of them have a mortality of over 50 per cent., and even sporadically the disease seems very fatal. During epidemics, however, it seems to possess a special virulence. It is probable that more frequently the disease is missed than is thought, while only rarely does it happen that some other affection is taken for it.

Comparative Fatality of Meningitis.—In all cases in which the pneumococcus and streptococcus have been found in the spinal fluid after lumbar puncture the disease has ended fatally. It is evident then that on the delicate tissues of the central nervous system these micro-organisms are more severe even than the diplococcus of cerebral spinal meningitis. It has been thought that the diplococcus may live on the nasal mucous membrane and a number of instances of its being found there have been reported. It seems very probable that there has been a mistake in this. The *Micrococcus catarrhalis* of Pfeiffer occurs very commonly in the nose and is rather easily mistaken for Weichselbaum's coccus. There are a few cases, however, in which there seems to be but little that it was present in the nasal secretion. Probably these cases will serve as the basis for the explanation of the mode of entrance of the micro-organism into the central nervous system.

Symptomatology.—Dr. H. L. Elsner, of Syracuse, said that the affection now known as epidemic cerebrospinal meningitis is nearly always present in and around Syracuse. Through the Board of Health in New York he has obtained statistics which show that cases of the disease are occurring practically always in New York City. In 1904, as a consequence of the epidemic there, 1,010 deaths from the disease were reported. This epidemic did not reach Central New York. There has been an epidemic within the last two years, and, curiously enough, though cases of the affection turn up at the hospital rather often, none were admitted to the wards during the epidemic. It is clear that the disease deserves the name of endemic more than epidemic, though there are times when it becomes epidemic.

Surroundings of Disease.—It usually occurs in the homes of the poor, but may be found under good sanitary conditions. It may exist among a large crowd of men, and yet fail to affect many of them. A typical example of this is the epidemic of the disease which occurred on board the U. S. S. Minneapolis ten years ago. One thousand four hundred and fifty men were on the vessel, which was supposed to have accommodations for only about 500. Notwithstanding this crowding, which was evidently one of the underlying reasons for the outbreak of the disease, only 23 men became infected, and of these only six died. The epidemic was not of great virulence. German observers have insisted that the epidemic meningitis is more benign than other forms of meningitis, especially those due to the pus cocci or to the pneumococcus.

Association of Nervous Affections.—Other infected diseases of the central system seem not infrequently to run their course alongside of epidemic cerebrospinal meningitis, bearing some sort of relation to it. It has been noted, for instance, that a series of cases of acute anterior poliomyelitis has occurred simultaneously with epidemic meningitis. Landry's paralysis, which is an ascending affection of the spinal cord, has also been known to occur in groups in association with epidemic meningitis. House epidemics of the disease are not infrequent, though it is usually the case to have only one patient in the household. A predisposing cause of the disease seems to be a state of mental fatigue. Occasionally the disease does not confine itself to the central nervous system, but produces metastatic lesions, especially in the joints.

Kernig's Symptom.—This is present in a great majority of the cases, probably more than four out of every five. At times, however, it is not present in typical cases, and it cannot be depended upon for absolute diagnosis. On the other hand, it is occasionally seen in patients suffering from other affections, as for example, typhoid fever, in which there is some irritation of the central nervous system. An important diagnostic help is lumbar puncture. It used to be considered that the appearance of the fluid as it issued from the spinal canal, gave important information as to the diagnosis. If fibrin and flocculi were present the disease was considered to be tuberculous. These gross morbid appearances are now known to be pathognomonic, and are not to be depended upon. The important factor for absolute diagnosis is the demonstration of the *Diplococcus intracellularis.*

Treatment of the Disease.—Dr. Charles G. Stockton, of Buffalo, said that it is a difficult matter to secure any form of treatment for a disease which is self-limited, or which has a very varying mortality in various epidemics. For preventive treatment a sanitarium is needed rather than a therapeutist. The disease undoubtely occurs as the result of crowding and filth and insanitary surroundings. Surprisingly enough, it is sometimes found under the best sanitary conditions. It would seem as though the disease acquired virulence enough in the slums to enable it to invade even the homes of those who live under better conditions. The old treatment of the disease was by means of blood-letting and mercury, with liberal doses of opium. Besides this, ice was used locally and ergot was administered internally. It is questionable whether these remedies will have to be given up, or whether any newer method proves to be more efficacious in checking the disease.

Present-Day Remedies.—Three forms of more or less novel treatment have been suggested within the last decade or so. The first of these is the hot bath suggested by Aufrecht. The second is the puncture of the spinal canal to reduce the pressure within the cord, and then also to inject various remedies that may have a local antiseptic action. The third method of treatment is by injections of bichloride of mercury beneath the skin in the neighborhood of the spine. All of these methods are supported by statistics, which seem to show their effectiveness in certain epidemics. Nearly all of them have failed to give satisfaction in the hands of others, besides those who originally introduced them.

Hot-Bath Treatment.—According to this method the patient is put into a hot bath, considerably above the normal human temperature, and this is nearly always followed by a relief of symptoms. In the original cases the baths were repeated twice daily at the request of patients. In certain number of cases the relief has been very marked. This method of treatment has been successful in many parts of the world. It produces a decided lowering of temperature and often gives the patient quiet instead of the restlessness that existed before. Whenever new symptoms develop the baths should be repeated. When this method of treatment is combined with lumbar puncture the attending physician is always impressed with the idea that he is accomplishing something for the relief of the patient. While the hot bath has been used very commonly in Europe, it has not been employed very much in this country.

Lumbar Puncture and Injection.—This method of treatment has in very recent years secured quite a number of followers. Some mild antiseptic is used as the injecting material. Lysol has been employed with good effect. According to the usual experience the patient becomes more quiet after the injection and sleep results In a certain number of cases very strong injections have been used at first by mistake, and afterward repeated deliberately because of success in the first case yet without producing a lessened mortality. In general it may be said that it is too difficult a matter as to decide as to the value of remedies because of the difference of mortality in various epidemics.

Bichloride Injections.—These are given in th muscles along the spine and are repeated daily, unti the disappearance of the fever. Sometimes only a fev injections are needed, and in most cases, according t the original report, the course of the disease is favor ably modified. As a matter of fact, however, in spit of all forms of treatment in certain epidemics the mor tality is very high.

Combination of Therapeutic Suggestions.—Dr. Stockton himself considers that the first and most important element of treatment is that the patient shall be kept in a quiet, dark room, so as to avoid all reflex excitation of the central nervous system. Hot baths should be given, and if there are symptoms of intracranial pressure, then the puncture of the cord should be undertaken with the removal of all the fluid under pressure. This should be repeated if necessary whenever the symptoms indicated. In all cases where there is fever antipyrin should be given partly with the idea of reducing the temperature, but also with the idea of making the patient less restless and therefore less capable of resisting the further invasion of the disease. Mercury should be employed freely as a laxative or for purposes of elimination. Beyond this there seems nothing except that in severe cases the injection method may be employed as a sort of forlorn hope.

Eye Symptoms of Cerebrospinal Meningitis.—Dr. A. E. Davis, of New York City, said that the eye symptoms of this disease are extremely prominent. They naturally fall into two groups, local and visual. By its local effect upon the eye, the disease may produce affections of practically every portion of the eye-ball and of the nerves. The visual symptoms are mainly due to affections of the nerve itself, but also to pressure upon centres in the brain. The eye symptoms of the disease are very various, differing in different epidemics, and including nearly every form of ocular manifestation. Nystagmus occurs quite frequently. Lagophthalmos is seen quite commonly. In this case corneal ulcers may develop as the result of the exposure of the conjunctiva, and in these cases precautions must be taken to protect the external tunics of the eye by means of vaselin and a protective bandage. All of the nerves to the eye may be affected. Ptosis, unilateral or bilateral, may occur. Optic atrophy may be seen not infrequently, but the most interesting thing about it is that in spite of a hopeless appearance of atrophy in the nerve head vision may be restored. In one case, seen by Dr. Knapp, he said to the patient, "According to all rules of ophthalmology, you should be blind." In spite of this, however, the patient had reasonably good vision in one eye. This is very surprising, as the characteristic white atrophy would seem to preclude any such favorable result. In the same case, the patient had also been deaf for some time, and yet his hearing was restored.

Eye Symptoms Suspicious.—Certain forms of eye manifestations may lead the general practitioner to suspect the presence of epidemic cerebrospinal meningitis in a given case, whenever he knows that the disease has come into epidemic form in the neighborhood. An inequality of pupils, for instance, especially if it occurs with a squint, must set the doctor on his guard. In certain epidemics some eye symptoms constantly recur. A form of conjunctivitis, not unlike that seen in pinkeye, may be the initial symptom in a whole group of cases; on the other hand, pus in the anterior chamber has been the characteristic in a group of cases seen in another epidemic. With regard to lesions of the nerve due to cerebrospinal meningitis it is wonderful how long the usual vision may seem to be retained, notwithstanding the destructive process at work in the nerve.

Brain and Meninges.—Dr. Morris Manges, of New York City, said that to remind the practitioner of how serious the condition is, Dr. Councilman's expression that it is not alone a meningitis but also an encephalitis is significant. Hence the hopelessness of any treatment of the disease in a great many cases. Any one who has seen the tenacious false membrane which occurs over the cord and brain in a number of the cases, and which develops with wonderful rapidity, will not expect to save a large proportion of his patients. Then it must not be forgotten that long after the supposed danger of the disease has passed there may be sudden death from acute dilatation of the ventricles, so-called acute hydrocephalus. This may occur as long after convalescence has been established as the sixth week. Eichhorst has reported three such cases. Lumbar puncture may be of avail in these cases if the foramen of Magendie is open; otherwise of course it would be of no avail.

Experience in Lumbar Tapping.—Dr. Manges said that any one who has used lumbar puncture in a number of cases will not want to abandon it. In some cases, because of the needed reduction of pressure there is an immediate and striking reduction of symptoms. In all cases, because of its diagnostic value, it is not a method for the specialist only but also for the general practitioner. He must acquire the technical details, and then he will not find it difficult. On the other hand, he must expect certain cases of dry tapping, that is, apparent failure of the procedure, though he can find no defect in his technic. These dry tappings are due oftenest to the fact that the thickened meninges allow themselves to be pushed before the examining needle, refusing to allow it to penetrate the subarachnoid space. In some cases the form of inflammation is such that there is no fluid to find its way out of the canal.

Tolerance of Spinal Canal for Drugs.—The experience of recent years shows how marvellously tolerant the spinal canal, formerly considered likely to be extremely sensitive, is to many forms of irritant drugs. Lysol has been employed in strength up to 10 per cent. solution without doing harm. Such drugs as guaiacol and even the milder silver salts have been employed without serious symptoms of any kind. The French have employed orthoform, and in a case treated at Bellevue argyrol was found distributed, not only over the spinal canal, but also over the cortex of the brain. These facts give promise that some new development of therapeutics may yet be possible in this direction. The use of the hot bath is easy in mild cases, but in instances of rigidity attempts to put them into a bath is to arouse a sense of pain and create a discomfort more than the bath will relieve. If this undue irritability is not present then the hot bath should always be used.

Early Differential Diagnosis.—Cerebrospinal meningitis may in its early stages simulate the coma of nephritis or that of diabetes. As a rule, in the epidemic cases of meningitis there is apt to be albumin in the urine early in the affection. This symptom taken with the comatose condition that so often develops early. may seem to indicate for sure the presence of nephritis. On the other hand, intracranial pressure may bring pressure to bear on the floor of the fourth ventricle with the consequent appearance of sugar in the urine, when, of course, the case will look like diabetic coma. Undoubtedly some of the sporadic cases of the disease masquerade under one of these two forms, and opportunities for infection and for the continuance of the disease are afforded.

Resistive Vitality in Confined Quarters.—Dr. De Lancey Rochester, of Buffalo, said that the *Diplococcus meningitidis* of Weichselbaum seems to be with us all the time. Opportunities are sometimes afforded it of securing a foothold in the human tissues beyond its existence as a saprophyte because of the lowered resistive vitality of individuals living in poor squalid confined quarters. The microorganism, having passed through a certain number of human beings, acquires intensified virulence and so there comes an epidemic of the disease that invades even the houses of the well-to-do where reasonably good sanitary conditions have prevailed. It seems clear now that like the pneumococcus the diplococcus of Weichselbaum may be present on the mucous membranes of healthy persons, until some lowering of their resistive vitality gives a favorable opportunity for the entrance of the microorganism.

Diagnosis and Treatment.—No one symptom is pathognomonic. It is the group of symptoms that points to the diagnosis. The Kernig symptom is of value, but may occur in typhoid fever or other febrile conditions producing irritation of the central nervous system. The injection of materials into the spinal cord can, in Dr. Rochester's opinion, only produce irritation but no curative effect. The warm bath with bromides in liberal doses, as well as such materials as antipyrin, has seemed to him most effi-. cient for the relief of symptoms. He feels that local treatment should be employed more and uses leeches to the base of the skull and along the spine as a routine measure.

Spread of Cerebrospinal Meningitis.—Dr. E. Libman, of New York City, said that one of the most interesting problems with regard to the disease is its mode of distribution. It has been found in the mucous membranes, but the reports in most cases are not trustworthy, since it is comparatively easy to confuse it with the *Micrococcus catarrhalis* of Pfeiffer. There is some evidence, however, that it may be on external mucous membrane before its invasion of the serous membranes of the nervous system. In one case studied at Mount Sinai Hospital in New York City the first symptom of the epidemic of cerebrospinal meningitis was an acute conjunctivitis from which the characteristic organism of Weichselbaum was obtained in pure culture. Later the same micro-organism was found in the spinal fluid. In this case the disease would seem to have spread inward along the ocular tissues to the nerve and thence to the membranes of the brain. At times it must not be forgotten that this form of micro-organism may cause joint complications and even general sepsis, and it must be looked for wherever other more usual types of pus cocci are not found.

Kernig's Symptom.—In Dr. Edward Fisher's (of New York) experience the Kernig sign is not constantly present as has been claimed. In many cases indeed there are few symptoms before the severe even comatose condition develops. Sometimes there is only a tired feeling, and after a few hours the disease in fulminant form declares itself. With regard to the nervous sequelæ of the disease the same theory holds as for the optic nerves. Curious and often almost inexplicable recoveries may take place against all expectation.

Dr. Thomson, of New York, in closing the discussion said that with regard to the eyes it is extremely important to guard patient's from the reflex irritation of light. They must be kept in a darkened room. Optic neuritis may progress to a considerable extent without reducing the visual power. As far as possible then the patients must be spared all strain of the eyes lest some latent pathological process should be thereby exaggerated.

SECOND DAY.—FEBRUARY 1ST.

The General Practitioner and the School.—Dr. Robert P. Bush, of Horseheads, gave some of the reasons why the general practitioner of medicine, in spite of the growth of specialism, must still continue to be a main feature of medical work. He gave the details of medical influence that the family physician may have not only in the home but also in the community, and especially in the school. With regard to children so much of protective medicine must affect their school life that every physician must take an interest in this. Scoliosis and various eye diseases find their beginning in the school, and only the physician can prevent them. There are many other phases of this sanitary education which must be the physician's duty. The physiology of alcohol is taught in the schools, but the physician must insist that constipation may cause as much suffering as dissipation, and that ill health may predispose to those cravings which seek satisfaction in stimulants.

Dr. Abraham Jacobi, of New York City, said that the general practitioner of medicine occupies a place in the profession that the specialist cannot fill, and the recurrent calling attention to this fact cannot fail to do good. The family physician must continue to stand between his patients and the fads of the specialists as well as the guardian of public health.

Subcutaneous Correction of Nasal Deformities.—Dr. John O. Roe, of Rochester, showed a series of photographs illustrating how much may be accomplished by careful patient operative work even in very bad cases of nasal deformity. These were usually the result of injuries, but some of them were also for syphilitic processes in which the ulcerative conditions were yet present. Notwithstanding this excellent results were obtained. Even where exostoses came as the result of chronic irritation, these were subcutaneously removed or portions of them used to fill up defects, the results of the injury. In one case, after the kick of a horse, the columna of the nose was torn from its place but was left hanging to the injured soft tissues. Instead of being replaced it was cut away. A new columna was formed by tissues taken from the upper lip. All the tissues beneath the skin were taken and by means of a buttonhole brought through to the nose. After a couple of months the mucous membrane by exposure to the air took on the character of skin and replaced the columna nasi very well.

Middle Turbinate and Accessory Sinuses.—Dr. W. J. Stucky, of Lexington, Ky., said that in recent years the significance of the middle turbinate in diseases of the nose itself and the accessory sinuses has become much clearer than heretofore. Undoubtedly affections of the middle turbinate are oftener missed than those of the lower turbinate. Much original work has been done in this line in recent years, and it is realized that the so-called grippe complications of the accessory sinuses often have their origin in some pathological condition of the middle turbinate. Dr. Stucky condemns escharotics and the galvanocautery. The scissors and snare should be used for its removal, careful asepsis being important.

Inferior Turbinate Surgery.—Dr. Wendell Phillips, of New York City, said that the inferior turbinate in pathological conditions brings about interference with respiration and drainage. It may cause infection of accessory sinuses and thus be the source of very serious conditions. As true erectile tissue it is especially subject to reflexes of various kinds, and if it becomes boggy or, in the expressive phrase, waterlogged, it is a fruitful case of hay-fever. Malformations and deformities from injury are quite common. Hence the necessity for frequent surgical intervention. Operations, however, must only be undertaken where positively indicated and when there are serious disturbances of function, never otherwise.

Technic of Operations.—Dr. Phillips said that the use of escharotics, especially of chromic acid, is no longer considered to be quite justifiable unless for small lesions. It produces serious reaction and gives rise to unfortunate sequelæ. The galvano-cautery is open to the same objection almost to a greater degree. It should practically never be used, unless in the submucous reduction of size of the turbinate by means of needles introduced beneath the skin surface before the current is turned on. Even this method is now very little employed. Electricity in the nose is now relegated to the past. The operative methods that are advisable are the wire snare for the posterior portion of the middle turbinate, while the scissors is best for the anterior and middle portions. A heavy scissors will accomplish this purpose very well.

Postoperative Technic.—Dr. Phillips said that he never plugs the nose after operation. The plug gives pain; sometimes causes sloughing; rather tends to increase the risk of infection and is unnecessary as regards the danger of hemorrhage. He uses a thin piece of absorbent cotton, which has been soaked in a 12 per cent. solution of acetotartrate of aluminum with the addition of suprarenalin if there is danger of hemorrhage. This prevents infection, and the results since its use was begun have been so favorable that Dr. Phillips would not now wish to operate and leave the open wound that some consider justifiable.

Treatment of Chronic Otitis Media.—Dr. William Sohier Bryant, of New York City, said that the cure of cases of chronic discharge from the middle ear is not impossible to cure by palliative treatment. The principal feature of this treatment must be cleanliness. All irritating materials must be carefully removed in such a way as not to leave further irritative momenta. All culture media must be removed so as to prevent the continuance of growth of infective agencies. For carious bone Dr. Bryant has found the use of 10 to 20 per cent. of nitrate of silver as the most useful remedy. It removes carious material without producing irritative reaction. Gentle and mild agents must be employed. or harm rather than good will result. Irritation may cause the discharge to become inveterate. Dr. Bryant then gave some illustrative cases showing that true chronic otitis media with discharge may be permanently cured. Patience is needed and the greatest care not to hurry the treatment, for this will surely lead to added risks and inveteracy of the condition.

Non-Syphilitic Deformities Curable.—Dr. Phillips, in discussing the papers on the throat and nose, said that he had seen the worst one of Dr. Roe's cases before operation and it seemed absolutely hopeless, yet much had been accomplished. Dr. Roe's secret is the taking of tissue from places where it is redundant and thus adding to deformity to transfer it to the tissue defects. The best results are obtained in non-syphilitic cases. With regard to the palliative treatment of middle-ear disease, Dr. Phillips is sure that in conservative, careful hands it may do good, but there is danger in allowing the discharge to continue, since the infective agents may invade other and more delicate tissues with fatal results. Life insurance companies refuse to take risks on individuals with discharging ears. and with reason. The risk of serious complications is always present.

Galvano-Cautery of the Past.—Dr. Snow, of Buffalo, said that all the cauterizing agents have no place in nasal surgery. They have done harm rather than good. There is danger, in his opinion, that Dr. Bryant's cleansing methods may in other hands than his own be a source of danger. A discharging ear needs most careful watching and radical operation whenever symptoms are threatening.

Over-Operation in Nose.—In the recent past there has been, in the opinion of Dr. Stucky, of Lexington, Ky., too much operation on the nose and there is now a fortunate swing of the pendulum the other way, though of course it may swing too far. Rhinologists reamed the nose until it was smooth as a gun barrel. Personally he believes that the septum should be always respected and that the inferior turbinate should be let alone much oftener than it is. The question is not how much may you remove, but how little can you take away and yet benefit your patient. The lower turbinate is a real bone, and if too much is removed the bothersome crusty condition develops that is a source of much inconvenience. Dr. Stucky thinks that the enlargement of the lower turbinate is often a sign of systemic disturbance and should be treated by general remedies more than local measures.

Dr. Wm. Sohier Bryant, in closing the discussion, said that the middle turbinate is oftener at fault than is thought, and he would add to Dr. Stucky's incrimination of it the fact that it is not infrequently the cause of obstinate trifacial neuralgia for which no treatment will avail except local measures for this structure.

(To be Continued.)

THE SOCIETY FOR EXPERIMENTAL BIOLOGY AND MEDICINE.

Ninth Regular Meeting, held December 21, 1904.

The President, S. J. Meltzer, M.D., in the Chair.

Members Present.—Atkinson, Auer, Burton-Opitz, Dunham, Ewing, Flexner, Gies, Herter, Jackson. Lee, Levene, Levin, Lusk, Mandel, Meltzer, Murlin, Park, Richards, Salant, Wadsworth, Wallace, Wolf.

Members Elected.—John Auer, F. G. Benedict, Ludwig Hektoen, G. G. Huber, H. S. Jennings, Jacques Loeb, Leo Loeb, A. B. MacCallum, J. H. Pratt, Torald Sollman, J. C. Torrey.

ABSTRACTS OF REPORTS OF ORIGINAL INVESTIGATIONS.[1]

Radium and Some Methods for its Therapeutic Application, with Demonstrations.—By Hugo Lieber (by invitation). He gave an account of the discovery of radium by Mme. and Prof. Curie, and demonstrated many radio-active phenomena. Special attention was drawn to recently discovered facts bearing on radium emanation. For a time it was thought that radium discharged directly, (a) The so-called "*emanations*," which had practically no penetrating power and which, like a gas, were readily carried from one point to another by an air current; and (b) the so-called "rays"—*alpha* rays of very low penetrating power. *beta* rays of considerably greater penetrating power, and *gamma* rays of enormous penetrating power. Later investigations have shown, however, that radium discharges primarily *cmanations* and *alpha rays* only. However, the emanations soon disintegrate and the disintegration products yield the beta rays and the gamma rays. Consequently, these powerful beta and gamma rays are the products of a decomposition product of radium.

[1] Proceedings reported by the Secretary, William J. Gies, Ph.D., of New York. The authors of the reports have furnished the abstracts. The Secretary has made a few abbreviations.

The proportions of the radiations given off by a certain quantity of radium and its disintegrated emanations are about 95 per cent. alpha rays and about five per cent. combined beta and gamma rays. Because of their nearly negative penetrative power, the alpha rays as well as the emanations are practically unavailable for therapeutic purposes when the radium is used in glass tubes or similar containers. Even the superficial layers of a given radium preparation are relatively impervious to both the emanations and the alpha rays proceeding from the underlying portions of the preparation. Therefore, it is essential, in order to obtain the full radio-active effects of a given quantity of radium, to have the radium in such a form (1) that the surrounding walls of the container will intercept neither the alpha rays nor the emanations, and (2) that the given quantity of radium should be spread out so thinly that, practically speaking, an upper layer does not exist.

Aschkinass, Dantzig, Caspari, Scholtz, Pfeiffer, Friedberger and others have shown that radium radiations exert very beneficial effects upon certain diseased tissues, as in sarcoma, lupus, carcinoma, etc. Marckwald states: "The radium rays have, besides a dilating effect, an elective effect upon the cells of quickly growing tissues as well as also bactericidal properties, three powers which are known to be very effective therapeutic factors." Germicidal effects of the radium rays have been shown repeatedly. Thus, Scholtz lately demonstrated that even typhoid bacilli can be destroyed with radium radiations. It is not surprising, from what was stated above regarding the low penetrative power, etc., of the emanations and the alpha rays, that disappointments have frequently resulted from the therapeutic application of radium. The author believes that in all probability many such disappointments have ensued solely because the practitioner has not had available in such cases just those radiations of radium which are required for therapeutic effects. Then, too, the radio-active powers of each radium preparation should be definitely ascertained in the first place, not taken for granted.

This opinion of past therapeutic failures led the author to conduct some experiments designed to discover a method of applying radium more advantageously. Such a method seemed to require a disposition of the radium in very thin layers, so as to yield the maximum proportions of alpha rays and emanations, and its application in a container permeable by the rays and emanations. These experiments finally led to the production of what the author terms "radium coatings."

Radium coatings are made in the following manner: Radium is dissolved in a proper solvent and into this proper solvent a proper material is dipped. This material is then withdrawn, with radium solutions adhering to it. The solvent quickly evaporates, leaving the material covered with an exceedingly thin film of radium. The kind of solvent to be used is determined by the nature of the material to be coated. Such solvents are employed as have a tendency to soften and permeate the material which is to be coated. Thus, if celluloid rods, disks, or similar instruments are to receive a radium coating in order to be used for the treatment of certain diseases, solvents such as alcohol, amylacetate, etc., may be employed. These solvents have a tendency to soften celluloid. When the solvent evaporates, the radium has been uniformly distributed over the celluloid and has also been incorporated on its surface. In order

to prevent accidental removal of the radium in such coatings, the celluloid instruments produced in this way are dipped into a proper collodion solution and are promptly removed from the same. In this process the whole radium coating is covered with a very thin film of collodion. In the course of a few days this film of collodion becomes so tough that it will strongly resist destruction even when considerable force is used, thus affording ample protection for the underlying radium. This thin film, however, permits the alpha rays as well as the emanations to penetrate freely.

In the preparation of these coatings both the radium and the collodion solutions are colored with an aniline dye. This is done to show the part that has been coated. Besides, if the radium happens to be removed by accident or otherwise, as by scraping, etc., the disappearance of the color makes such removal evident.

The great difference between radium used in containers composed of even exceedingly thin aluminum, and radium used in the form of the coatings here described, was demonstrated. Thus, in their relative influences on the electroscope it was seen that a delicate rod coated at its tip with radium bromid of 10,000 activity, and holding therefore very little radium, compared very favorably in its effects with a gram of radium bromid of 10,000 activity in a glass tube or with 10 milligrams of radium bromid of 1,000,000 activity in a very thin aluminum tube.

As is well-known, when we observe the effect of uncovered radium upon a zinc sulphide screen, such as is shown in the spinthariscope of Crookes, we see a large number of brilliant scintillations. It has been proved conclusively that these scintillations are produced solely by the concussion of the alpha rays upon the zinc sulphide. If what has just been said is correct, that is, that the alpha rays can penetrate the collodion coating of the author's celluloid rods, disks, etc., then the latter should yield evidence of these scintillations when placed upon a zinc sulphide screen. Such scintillations were abundantly demonstrated with various forms of the coatings.

As has already been stated, radium emanations will always follow the air current. Consequently, if some uncovered radium is placed in an air current, the current will carry with itself the emanations, which emanations will ionize the air and discharge the electroscope. The author demonstrated these phenomena with some strips of celluloid coated with radium and covered with collodion. The same phenomena were demonstrated with a tube which had been similarly coated with radium and collodion on the inside. When air was blown through this tube, toward the electroscope, the latter was discharged instantly.

The radium coatings make it possible to apply radium directly to practically any part of the body. The radium thus applied would be practically equivalent in radio-active effects to the same amount of uncovered radium in the same thin layer. Any instrument could be conveniently coated with radium at a proper place, by the method indicated, and the radiations could be brought into action wherever desired.

It has been stated that radium radiations destroy tubercle bacilli. Rutherford and Soddy, and others, have accordingly advised that radium emanations be blown into the lungs in phthisis. The author believes that the difficulties in the way of such a therapeutic application of radium are solved by the apparatus depicted here. It consists of a celluloid tube *A*, with a complete coat of radium on the inside, and a collodion covering on the radium coating. By means of a tightly fitting rubber stopper *B*, a small glass tube *C* is inserted, which at its end has a large perforated bulb in order to produce a uniform air current throughout all parts of the tube. This glass tube *C*, has a glass stop-cock *D*, and connected with the latter is a rubber bulb *E*. By means of another rubber stopper *F*, a glass tube *G*, with a glass stop-cock *H*, is inserted into the other end of the tube. With the loose end of the last glass tube *G*, may be connected by means of a narrow rubber tube, etc., any desirable apparatus. If we now close the two glass stop-cocks and allow them to remain tact, especially moist surfaces. If, therefore, we permit these emanations to slowly pass into or upon a diseased tissue, they will doubtless adhere to a considerable extent to the tissues treated in this way, especially if the applications are made under proper plasters, coverings, coatings, etc., to prevent the ready escape of the gaseous emanations. During their retention in this way the emanations disintegrate, as was stated above.

A very great advantage of these radium coatings is that all instruments, etc., coated by the method described, can be readily sterilized without loss of radium, for the protective coat effectually resists even continued boiling. The author demonstrated the radio-activity of a strip of celluloid which had been coated with radium and thereafter had been

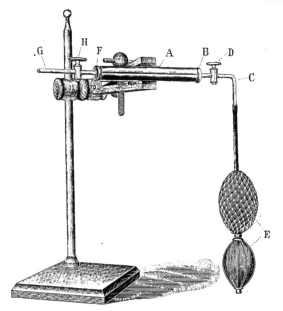

closed for several hours, a considerable quantity of emanations will collect within the glass tube. If we now blow up the rubber bulb *E*, and slowly open the exit stop-cock *H*, and then slowly open the entrance stop-cock *D*, the compressed air will enter the coated celluloid tube *A*, the emanations which have collected within the celluloid tube will follow the course of the air current, and on inhaling this air, the patient will receive the full charge of radium emanations in his lungs. A cancer of the throat or of any other part of the body may be treated by the application of a proper radium rod directly, and besides that, by blowing the emanations, if necessary, directly into the seat of a cancer through a finely-pointed hollow exit rod. It is a well-established fact that these emanations are readily deposited upon surfaces with which they come in con-

covered with collodion. The strip was then placed in water in a test tube and the contents vigorously boiled. Both the radium and the collodion solutions used for the preparation of the coatings had been colored with a soluble, blue aniline dye. That the collodion protected the radium ·in this experiment was shown by the fact that the water, after boiling, was entirely free from color. The strip also retained its original radio-activity.

The availability of the radium coatings for many kinds of biological investigation is so obvious that nothing need be said here on that point.

On Muscular Fatigue, with Demonstration of Tracings.—By Frederic S. Lee. The investigation of the subject has been continued by the employment of a method by which the isotonic curves of all the contractions of the muscle stimulated at regular intervals, are superimposed upon a recording surface. The differences which were previously pointed out in the mode of fatigue of the muscles of the frog, the turtle and a mammal, have been confirmed. Lohmann's work, in which a frog's muscle on being heated to a mammalian temperature, shows a course of fatigue similar to that of mammalian muscle, has been repeated and found in general correct. But turtle's muscle, similarly heated, continues to give its characteristic curve of fatigue.

Kaiser's method for determining the point on the isotonic curve where the contractile stress terminates, has been employed for the frog's gastrocnemius, and it has been found that as the height of the curve diminishes in the course of fatigue, the contractile stress terminates at progressively lower and lower points. The lowering of the latter does not, however, seem to keep pace with the lowering of the summit of the curve. Hence the two points seem to approach one another.

A New Form of Float for Water or Alcohol Manometers, with Demonstration.—By Haven Emerson (by invitation). The float consists of an aluminum cylinder with very thin wall, supporting a writing arm of fine aluminum wire. For manometer tubing of ⁵/₃₂ inch inside diameter, ³/₁₆ or ¼ inch aluminum tubing 2½ inches long is used. This is bored out until the walls are sufficiently light. In the upper end is forced a solid cap of aluminum with a small hole in the center into which the wire for the writing lever is driven. The lower end is plugged with cork. Both ends are painted over with hot paraffin to prevent possible leaking. For use in alcohol a somewhat longer tube is necessary. Three crossed hairs held in place across the open arm of the manometer tube by a strip of adhesive plaster keep the writing arm centered with sufficient accuracy.

The value of the float consists in its cheapness, the ease with which it can be made; its very slight inertia, and its convenience in estimating delicate changes in pressure for which a water or alcohol manometer is needed.

Gelatin as a Substitute for Proteid in the Food.—By J. R. Murlin. In a series of experiments on dogs, the nitrogen requirement of the body was determined by fasting periods. Varying amounts of gelatin containing from one-fourth to two-thirds of the required nitrogen were fed, the remainder of the nitrogen being supplied in meat proteid. The calorific requirement was estimated from Rubner's tables and was fully covered in each experiment with fats and carbohydrates. Results show an equal sparing of the body proteid with one-fourth, one-third and one-half gelatin nitrogen, the coincident sparing of fats and carbohydrates being the same. When the coincident sparing of proteid by non-nitrogenous food is increased by feeding a larger percentage of carbohydrate and less fat, two-thirds of the nitrogen requirement may be given in gelatin and perfect nitrogenous equilibrium maintained at the starvation level.

The same result was obtained on man. The bare requirement in nitrogen was obtained by analysis of the urine and feces during a fasting period of three days, and equilibrium was established at this level on a mixed diet containing two-thirds of the nitrogen requirement in meat. Then for two days the meat nitrogen was replaced by gelatin nitrogen and the potential energy supplied was increased from 40 to 48 Cal. per kg. of body weight by giving

more cane sugar, which served at the same time to make the gelatin more palatable. The nitrogen equilibrium was not disturbed during these two days nor on subsequent days when the diet was exactly the same as before the gelatin period.

The Reductions in the Body in Fever, with demonstrations.—By C. A. Herter. He called attention to the influence of temperature on the activity of reduction in the living organism as indicated by intra-vital infusion of methylene blue. Elevation of the body temperature greatly accelerates the rate of reduction in the tissues. This was demonstrated by means of an intra-vital infusion of methylene blue in a rabbit whose body temperature had been elevated to 42° C. through the external application of heat. Simultaneously with this infusion another infusion was made in a rabbit of approximately equal weight in which the temperature was maintained at about 39° C. In other respects the conditions of the infusion were as nearly alike as possible in the two animals. A definite contrast was noted at the close of the infusion between the organs of the two animals as respects their color, the normal rabbit showing more color than the one in which the temperature had been elevated. The differences in the nervous system and the muscles were particularly striking. Even during life an inspection of the muscles indicated that the reduction was carried on with greater rapidity in the heated rabbit than in the normal. Previous observations on the reducing action of the animal body under the influence of cold were referred to.

The Measurement of the Reducing Processes of Cells in Vitro, with demonstrations.—By C. A. Herter. An apparatus was demonstrated which had been devised for the purpose of measuring the reducing process of the different kinds of cells *in vitro*. Definite quantities of organ pulp were placed in specially constructed tubes and anaerobic conditions were established by the passage of nitrous oxide gas. Definite quantities of methylene blue of known strength were then added. The rate of reduction was indicated by the disappearance of the blue color owing to the reduction of the animal cells. It was shown that *in vitro* the influence of temperature is the same as that observed in the living organism. The influence of alkali in accelerating reduction was also shown. The action of salts and various poisons is at present the subject of investigation.

Some Medical Applications of the Naphthaquinone Sodium Monosulphonate Reactions, with demonstrations.—By C. A. Herter. Dr. Herter demonstrated a substance of singularly great powers of condensation with other organic substances, this condensation resulting in the formation of colored bodies. He demonstrated especially the reactions of naphthoquinone sodium monosulfonate with anilin and various amines, with nicotine, conine, piperidine, and finally with indol, skatol, and pyrrol. The reactions with indol, skatol, and pyrrol possess unusual physiological and chemical interest and will form the subjects of future publications. The reaction with pyrrol occurs in the cold and is evidenced by the deepening red which on the addition of alkali changes to purple, violet, blue, and finally reddish brown. The addition of acid to the red solution obtained without alkali is followed by the development of a green and finally a brown color. These color reactions (and particularly the one dependent on acids) occur with such rapidity if one uses concentrated heated solutions of pyrrol, that the characteristic color stages may be of extremely short duration. This reaction with pyrrol is a highly characteristic one, and should prove of service to chemists.

Among the biological and medical applications of the naphthoquinone sodium monosulfonate reactions Dr. Herter mentioned the study of various aromatic compounds in the organism, the occurrence of certain intravital syntheses, the detection in the urine of organic compounds, such as, para amido phenol, and the development of a method of staining the bile capillaries by means of intravenous infusion of the derivatives of the naphthoquinone compound. Dr. Herter also stated that these substances facilitate the study of the relation between the chemical constitution and distribution of poisons in the body.

On the Rate of Absorption from Intramuscular Tissue, with demonstrations.—By S. J. Meltzer and John Auer. In physiology no distinction is made between absorption from the subcutaneous tissue and absorption from muscles. In experimental infection and immunity, injections of virulent toxic and antitoxic material is being extensively employed, but intramuscular injection has not yet even been thought of. In therapeutics it is practised promiscuously, and for the reason, as pharmacologists and clinicians expressly state, that it gives less pain and causes less frequently the formation of small abscesses.

The authors came upon the observation that absorption from the muscles is incomparably more rapid and efficient than from the subcutaneous tissue and tested the matter with several substances. With suprarenal extract it was tested in three ways: (1) By the effect upon blood pressure. A subcutaneous dose of 0.6 c.c. or less per kilo (in rabbits) exerts no effect, and the variable effects of larger doses consist in a rise of pressure from about 10 to 20 millimeters of mercury, which sets in late and develops slowly. An intramuscular injection of 0.5 or 0.4 c.c. per kilo, or even less, invariably causes on the other hand a considerable rise of pressure, which sets in after a very short latent period and reaches its maximum in a few seconds. The curve obtained after intramuscular injection is very similar to that after an intravenous injection. The increase has been as high as 50 or 60 mm. of mercury and may go even higher. The course of the curve is frequently interrupted by "vagus-pulses." (2) The question was further tested by the effect upon the pupil on the side from which the superior cervical ganglion had been previously removed. An intramuscular dose of 0.5 or 0.4 c.c. of adrenalin per kilo caused dilatation of the pupil in less than a minute, while such a dose, given subcutaneously, rarely produced any effect. The effect of a larger dose sets in only after ten or fifteen minutes. (3) By prostration effects. A dose of 0.5 c.c. per kilo will prostrate a rabbit in a minute or two, after intramuscular injection. In cases of subcutaneous introduction, prostration does not occur until after twenty or thirty minutes, and even then is induced only by much larger doses.

Further tests were made with curare. A dose can be found which will have no apparent effect after subcutaneous injection, but which, after intramuscular introduction, will cause the paralysis of the voluntary muscles in a few minutes.

The authors have also established striking differences between the effects of the two modes of application for morphin and fluorescin.

PAN-AMERICAN MEDICAL CONGRESS.

The Fourth Meeting of this Congress was opened January 3, 1905, by President Amador, of the Republic of Panama. The formal opening, however, took place in the evening at the National Theater.

President Amador was introduced by Dr. Julio Icaza. President Amador thanked the Congress for the distinguished honor that had been conferred upon him in being selected to preside over the deliberations of the meeting, which included among its members so many illustrious colleagues. He expressed the hope that great benefit would result from the papers that were to be read. With these few remarks he declared the Fourth Pan-American Medical Congress open for scientific work.

Remarks by Mr. John F. Wallace.—The Chief Engineer of the Isthmian Canal Commission, Mr. John F. Wallace, was introduced, and, among other things, said it was unnecessary to dwell on the five hundred years since the Canal's early and original conception. It was also unnecessary to dwell upon the progress which had been made so far under the grants and franchises to attempt its construction. He called attention to the fact that the first real proposition to construct the canal emanated from America, and while the results of the French companies were failures, this work simply laid the foundation of its future construction. It would seem fair, then, that the Americans should have another trial, and it was the hope of all that it would be the last. It was a difficult matter when one passed over the line of the work to-day to realize the extent of the work done and the enormous amount of machinery purchased by the old and new French companies. It was only by a study of the situation on the Isthmus of what had been accomplished, that one could realize how much the work that had been begun before should contribute to the present success. The former operations on the canal had pointed out what to do and what not to do. The original idea of Mr. De Lesseps was a sea level canal. The reason why this project was abandoned was not one of engineering difficulty, but entirely for a different cause. His plans were changed simply because he did not have the means to put them into execution, not because he discovered anything impracticable in the undertaking from an engineering standpoint. In following in his footsteps, or, rather, in picking up the enterprise, the Americans had commenced at the opposite end of the problem, and all the plans that had been accomplished, the estimates that had been made as to time and progress, were based on the reports of the former Commission from the United States to investigate this question. In making a comparison of the Nicaragua route, with an elevation of 190 feet above the sea level, he desired to make a fair comparison with the Panama route. It was proposed to create a canal with an elevation of the same height, and it was also proposed to create an artificial lake, and create the same conditions, as nearly as possible, as existed at Nicaragua. The construction of the Panama canal was one of the problems of the new world. There was hardly any branch of the civil engineering profession that would not have to be called upon to assist in the problem. The construction of the canal might be divided into three parts: (1) The sewerage proposition, which was the excavation by ditches of the sea level portions of the canal. (2) Excavation for a short distance where the material might be excavated and wasted immediately adjacent to the canal. (3) A type of construction which was peculiar to Panama, and that was what might be called the Culebra problem. This problem not only involved the excavation of fifty million to one hundred million cubic yards of material, depending upon the character of the canal, but it consisted in the transportation and disposal of that material over a distance of ten to twelve of fifteen miles away. The Culebra problem was the controlling factor to be considered both as to time, cost and difficulty. The time in which the Culebra cut can be excavated was the determining factor as to the time required for the construction of the canal.

After referring to the labor problem and the difficulties connected with it, Mr. Wallace spoke of the problem of sanitation and the care and health of the employees who were to be brought there for constructing the canal. This matter was in the hands of Dr. Gorgas, and he would like to say that the success of this work and the ability to bring men there would largely be due to his efforts and the support he received.

Sanitary Conditions as Encountered in Cuba and Panama, and What is Being Done to Render the Canal Zone Healthy.—This was the title of an address delivered by Dr. W. C. Gorgas, Chief Sanitary Officer of the Isthmian Canal Commission. He explained the sanitary conditions in Cuba, and stated that for two centuries the United States had been scourged with yellow fever often imported from Havana. When the United States occupied Cuba, there was a perfectly cast iron commercial quarantine against the West Indies, in all Gulf ports during every summer. Still worse was it if yellow fever broke out in the United States. To get rid of yellow fever in Havana meant that it would cease to menace the Southern States, so that the sanitation of the Republic of Cuba meant really the sanitation of Havana. For two years, therefore, Havana was cleaned industriously, for the reason it was thought that filth was the cause of yellow fever. Conditions changed, however, when the decision was reached that the *Stegomyia fasciata* was the cause of yellow fever. This theory was advocated by Dr. Carlos J. Finlay, of Havana, twenty years ago. The first practical effort to suppress yellow fever was made as inoculation tests and not as efforts to destroy the mosquito; but some fatal cases which occurred after inoculation stopped all enthusiasm in that direction, and then it was decided to attempt to destroy the mosquito. This met with unexpected and remarkable success. In less than a year Havana was entirely free from yellow fever, and since September, 1901, not a single case had occurred in that city. The United States came to Panama to build the canal and the work of the Sanitary Department was to preserve health while doing so. In all previous efforts the history of the canal had been darkened by great loss of life. Malaria and yellow fever were the canal's worst enemies. But the yellow fever problem here was really not so difficult as it was in Havana, and the result seemed equally as promising. Continuing, Dr. Gorgas said: "We know more about yellow fever now than we did at Havana; we are pretty certain to be able to eliminate that disease; but malaria is seen under very different conditions from what it was in Havana. Malaria in a big city is chiefly a disease of the suburbs; malaria along with yellow fever was eliminated from Havana by the destruction of the breeding-places of the mosquito, but on the isthmus conditions are different. Here there are twenty odd villages with 12,000 people scattered over nearly 50 miles; 70 per cent. of these

have been found to have the malarial organism in the blood; probably a larger percentage would be found, were the examinations to be extended over a greater period of time. Moreover, the parasite is not that of simple malarial fever, but the one which breeds the pernicious Chagres fever, of a much severer type, the estivo-autumnal parasite. The plan adopted along the canal is to eliminate the breeding places by superficial drainage. Much headway has already been made. For instance, at Ançon, the hospital is entirely free from the malarial mosquito. Dispensaries are being established, and all canal people are urged to use quinine. These are the two methods employed for destroying the malarial mosquito. Four-fifths of the money appropriated for sanitary matters now goes for the care of the sick, for the commission has determined to take care of those sick within the zone. There is now under way a hospital of 100 beds at Taboga; at Ançon, under Major La Garde, U.S.A., there will be hospital accommodations for about 500; at Miraflores there will be hospital accommodations for 100 chronic patients, including insane and lepers; at Colon, a hospital with 500 beds is expected. At Culebra, Gorgona, Bobia, small hospitals will be erected. At Ançon there is a good general laboratory in which are working Dr. Herrick and Dr. Kendall, both Johns Hopkins men.

Dr. Gorgas promised rapid advances, and he was sure that the expectations for complete control of conditions would soon be realized.

Earlier Conditions of the Canal.—Mr. Tracy Robinson delivered an address on this subject. He reverted to the opening of the Panama railroad on January 31, 1855. This, next to the discovery of the Pacific by Balboa, was the most important event that had occurred on Isthmian soil. In 1869 the overland connection from Omaha to San Francisco was completed, and the prosperity of the Pan-American route waned. He said the people of Panama expected great things from the influence of the medical profession on the new canal project. He believed that Panama under American government would some day be an object-lesson for the world. He joined his Panamian brethren in extending the hand of welcome to the members of the Congress. There had never been a real epidemic of yellow fever on the Isthmus for fifty years, although many had died of the fever. There had been 1,200 deaths in five years out of a total number of 6,000 men employed in the construction of the railroad. All the workers on the canal in the sanitary corps were up-to-date medical men—true missionaries. To them the people looked for health and strength. The trained physician led, and he would be the captain in the battle of scientific civilization against bigotry, ignorance, prejudice and their hosts of allies.

The Secretary-General of the Congress, Dr. José E. Calvo, extended to the members the hospitality of the city, and said that "if we have not the charm of large cities, we still take great pride in your visit, and hope that you will be rewarded for having come so far."

Mexico, Guatemala, United States of America, Honduras, Santo Domingo, Cuba, Peru, and Porto Rico sent official delegates, as well as the medical faculty of Costa Rica, the Academy of Sciences of Havana and other scientific bodies.

SECOND SESSION.—JANUARY 4TH.

There was an informal excursion in the morning to a suburb called Savanes, where the guests were received and entertained at luncheon by Dr. Icaza.

In the afternoon the scientific session was presided over by Dr. H. R. Carter.

ward too forcibly respiration would be arrested. A better way was to recall also the increased respiratory action caused by divulsion of the anus, and to call upon the accessory muscular apparatus to aid respiration. Surgical physiology of the circulation was more vital than that of the respiration. The control of the circulation often meant control of life itself. If by any reflex action the vasomotor system was disturbed, its function was impaired, and the blood pressure fell. If the surgeon remembered this he would guard against excessive manipulation, and he would try to support the circulation by such mechanical means as saline infusions, posture, or bandaging. It was known that a hard pulse and high blood pressure were characteristic of increased intracranial pressure. This might lead the surgeon into a false security. He should not push chloroform to full anesthesia, as by so doing the blood pressure is liable to fall and cause a sudden arrest of respiration and circulation. The heart might be inhibited from mechanical stimulation of the trunk of the superior laryngeal nerve in operations upon the larynx, and death might occur, although it should not. Furthermore, a blow upon the lower ribs or pit of the stomach did not cause collapse or death from disturbance of the solar plexus, but from inhibition of the heart. As to suspended animation, Dr. Crile stated that the different parts of the body had varying periods of suspended animation, and death fell unevenly to the different tissues and organs. He had been able to resuscitate a dog fifteen minutes after complete arrest of respiration and circulation. A decapitated dog was kept alive for twelve hours by a continuous slow infusion of one to fifteen thousand solution of adrenalin in salt solution. The lesson to be learned was that physiology must be studied carefully to benefit surgery.

Some Gynecological Superstitions.—Dr. Lucy Waite, of Chicago, said that these were hard to overthrow. One of the first superstitions was that the uterus had any normal position. It had not, but it might lie in any position. The second was that retrodeviation of the uterus was the cause of constipation. This was not so, as it could not be proved either by dissection or examination. She had 500 cases analyzed, but could not trace constipation to posture of the uterus alone. The uterus was found in anteroposition in 60 per cent., in retroposition in 40 per cent. Of the anteropositions, 52 per cent. gave a history of constipation, while 48 per cent. did not. Of the retropositions, 66 per cent. complained of chronic constipation, and 33 per cent. had normal bowel movements. The third was that backache was a symptom of retrodeviation. She regarded this as nonsense, as one thousand cases examined disproved that superstition. The fourth, that flexion or stenosis was the cause of dysmenorrhea. This was not so, nor was childbirth the only cure. Of 300 cases where the question was asked, "Have you had more or less pain since the birth of your children?" the answer of 135 was, "More pain," of 89 "Less pain," and of 76 "No difference." Some of these 76 had no pain before or since childbearing. Of the 135, some had no pain before childbearing. Many women had suffered worse after childbirth than before. She thought that the mania for operating ought to be checked on the death of these superstitions.

Dr. George W. Crile, of Cleveland, Ohio, asked the essayist whether all backaches were attributed to the uterus, and whether they were often accompanied by aches of the legs, to which Dr. Waite replied that not all backaches are traceable as referred pains to the uterus, but that there was usually some pelvic disturbance rather than any malposition of the uterus.

Extraction of Cataract.—Dr. S. D. Risley, of Philadelphia set forth the technic of extraction based upon certain complicating conditions, their relation to the opaque lens, and the extent to which the complications modified prognosis and rendered the removal of cataract difficult and dangerous. The cataractous eye was to be regarded as not free from disease. In studying cataracts, it would be found that early there were asthenopic symptoms, swollen and red caruncles, thickening of the retrotarsal folds and headache. As the cataract matured and reading was abandoned these diminished. There might also be encountered during the incipient stage anomalies of refraction and fundal changes, sometimes fluidity of the vitreous. There was an obvious relation between choroidal disease, eye strain and lens capacity; also between the lens and the gouty or rheumatic diathesis. The nutrition of the eyeball was largely dependent on the circulation of the uveal tract. Vitreous and lens were apt to suffer, as well as the posterior capsule; therefore, it was best not to operate in the immature stage, *i.e.*, until the disease changes had ceased. He never attempted operation with a dull gray or amber-colored lens that had ripened slowly or with one that was translucent. When the iris lacked luster and did not dilate easily, it was liable to traumatic iritis. It was best to treat such cases by iodide and bromide internally and by some mydriatic and to perform a preliminary iridectomy four to six weeks in advance, using cocaine if possible. If the lens was extracted in the capsule, Dr. Risley preferred a Kalt stitch through the cornea with a large corneal section; then a wire loop was introduced and the lens delivered by gentle traction. There was some but not unavoidable danger. In anterior capsulotomy, the danger was less and the corneal section might be smaller, but a secondary operation was usually necessary. For this he preferred two knives devised by himself introduced at the same time. He preferred a light firm bandage, with confinement in bed as short a time as possible.

THIRD SESSION.—JANUARY 5TH.

Coxa Vara and Differentiation Between It and Sthenic Inflammatory and Traumatic Affections of the Hip-Joint.—Dr. Nicholas Senn, of Chicago, stated that coxa vara was a disease of the femoral neck in adolescence, and hitherto had been rarely described in this country. Müller was the first, in 1888, to give it an earnest clinical study, and to prove that it was a disease entirely different from any other hitherto described. Hofmeister and Kocher, six years later, contributed to the study. A genuine coxa vara was characterized by a non-inflammatory softening of the neck of the femur. It was a self-limited disease, confined to the femoral neck, and characterized by anatomical changes. Dr. Senn reported two typical cases in young men, and a third in a man forty-two years old. The last case presented all the classical signs and the X-ray showed that there was no fracture of the femur, as had been suspected before the case came under his observation. There had been the usual pains in the hip-joints referred at times to the knee, coming on in paroxysms which would last for two weeks, followed by painless intervals of several days. There was no tenderness or impairment of joint motion. The pain was not aggravated by standing or walking. After two occasions in which the patient slipped and increased the pain, he noticed that the leg was shorter. When seen by the essayist he walked with a decided limp and complained only of muscular weakness. Any infection could be excluded, and there was certainly not a complete fracture. A spontaneous recovery, as well as the degree of

bending downward of the neck of the femur in its entire length, and the complete absence of neoplastic inflammatory products excluded absolutely the possibility of arthritis or senile coxitis. Very little was known with reference to the true nature of coxa vara. The softening of the neck of the femur was the most important element. Trauma, tuberculosis, or inflammatory affections must be excluded. Life itself was never threatened, as the disease was self-limited, and sooner or later ended in spontaneous recovery. The general treatment was unimportant. Local treatment should be directed toward relieving pain and limiting the bending of the neck of the femur. Both of these were secured by absolute rest in bed combined with extension. Operative treatment should be delayed as long as possible.

Sanitary Conditions in Cuba Since the Proclamation of the Republic.—Dr. Carlos J. Finlay, of Havana, Cuba, contributed a paper on this subject, which was read by Dr. Martinez, of Havana, in the absence of the author. The subject was divided into (1) special sanitation against yellow fever; (2) special sanitation against other infectious disease; (3) general sanitation for the preservation of public health. The author stated that there were many who did not yet acknowledge that the *Stegomyia fasciata* was the only means through which yellow fever could be propagated. The author claimed that this was the only method, and that to keep yellow fever patients from being bitten was the only means of subduing the disease itself. He referred in the highest terms to the noble work done by the late Major Walter Reed, Col. W. C. Gorgas, and others. He said that Dr. Gorgas, who was the chief sanitary officer of Cuba until May 20, 1902, first drove the infection from the island, and since his régime and up to the present date, December, 1904, notwithstanding the importation of 22 cases of yellow fever from foreign ports, not a single case of the disease had occurred in Havana, nor until two months ago in any other part of Cuban territory. The acute quarantinable diseases about which the Island of Cuba was particularly concerned were yellow fever, smallpox, cholera and plague. None of these diseases, except those cases mentioned, had occurred, with the exception of one case of smallpox, which was due to an accidental contagion which did not spread. Against smallpox they trusted to isolation and vaccination. Against diphtheria, isolation and anti-diphtheritic serum prepared in Havana had given excellent results. Cases of infectious diseases were isolated at home or in some special hospital.

Dr. Purnell, Acting Assistant Surgeon in the Marine Hospital Service at New Orleans, stated that although he accepted the mosquito theory, he did not do so absolutely, inasmuch as there were cases unexplained by this theory, and that measures of prevention besides the attack on the mosquito should be adopted. The great epidemic in Memphis, in 1879, occurred after a severe cold winter, but not until July 9, and if the mosquitoes alone were the cause the disease ought to have appeared in April. He had known of an outbreak in Jackson, Miss., among men working in buildings which ten years previously had been infected with the disease. Fomites had undoubtedly something to do with the spread of yellow fever.

Dr. H. R. Carter, of Panama, expressed himself as being positive that yellow fever was conveyed by the bite of a mosquito from sick to sick, and in this way he had assisted in stamping out epidemics by methods not necessarily directed against the mosquitoes alone, such as isolation and fumigation, but he knew that their efficacy had destroyed the mosquito incidentally. Sulphur was a good insecticide, but nothing else.

· Dr. Stern, of Jamaica and Panama, concurred in the remarks of Dr. Purnell in not accepting the mosquito as the only conveyer of yellow fever.

Dr. Chassaignac, of New Orleans, La., considered the mosquito theory beyond refutation. The Havana experiments had furnished positive proof of this, and he did not think there was any other means of transmitting or conveying the disease.

Dr. C. H. Hughes, of St. Louis, Mo., spoke of his experience with the disease during his early practice. He was not convinced that the mosquito was the only means of propagation and expressed himself as believing that flies might transmit the disease.

Dr. Carter referred to fomites, and said that there could be only two ways in which they could convey the infection. One was by direct contact, such as opening a trunk, and the other by environment. If either means was admitted, infection should take place anywhere.

Dr. W. C. Gorgas said he thought at one time fomites was the only cause of transmission of the disease. He then differed from Dr. Finlay, but Major Reed soon convinced him to the contrary. The harmlessness of baggage was observed in Havana, where people from the suburbs were constantly moving back and forth, but never brought infection with them.

Dr. Lewis Balch, in referring to fumigation, said that he relied upon two pounds of pyrethrum powder to 1,000 cubic feet, with two hours' exposure. This gave absolute results in killing the *Stegomyia fasciata*.

Dr. Thomas had used pyrethrum, but had found it without value, and said that sulphur was now used exclusively in Louisiana.

Dr. Echeverria, of Costa Rica, spoke in favor of the mosquito theory, and added that yellow fever had never been known to occur where the *Stegomyia* could not be found.

Dr. Martinez, in closing the discussion for Dr. Finlay, said that to explain isolated outbreaks, it was assumed that children preserved the organism in the blood, as they did malaria, and this offered a source of supply to the mosquito. The study of the development of the parasite in the mosquito showed that an intermediate host was necessary, just as it was in the tapeworm. The United States Army Commission had studied the question of fomites very thoroughly. In its report, one instance was cited where the blankets, clothing and bedding of patients ill or dead from yellow fever had been stored in a room, and used by two sets of non-immune fresh arrivals in Cuba, and yet no single instance of infection from this clothing had occurred.

Resolution.—Dr. Chas. Chassaignac, of New Orleans, offered the following resolution:

"*Resolved,* That owing to the suffering and to the serious danger to health and life for which the mosquito is known to be chiefly if not solely responsible, it is the imperative duty of all communities and governments to use all the means in their power for the destruction and gradual annihilation of the pestiferous insect in question." ·The resolution was seconded and unanimously carried.

Care and Cure of Epilepsy.—Dr. Chas. H. Hughes, of St. Louis, Mo., claimed that epilepsy should not in many cases be listed with the curable diseases. He reported ten cases that had been under observation for twenty-five years, in which there had been no recurrence. In treating epilepsy, he always demanded an agreement that the patient should be under control at least two years, during which time he would treat every function of the individual so as to keep his general health in the best possible condition. Of course, institutional

treatment was better in most cases than private treatment.

Report for the Delayed Passengers on the Athos.—Dr. A. E. MacDonald, of New York, stated that when the members accompanying him realized that they could not reach Panama on time, the delegates and members held meetings on board the Athos. Papers were read and discussed, of which records were kept, and he made a motion that such papers and discussions be allowed to be spread on the minutes of the Congress as a part of the regular proceedings. The resolution was adopted.

Permeability of Filters to the Protozoa of the Waters used in the City of Lima.—Dr. Hugo Biffi, of Lima, read a paper with this title, saying that the idea of the experiment was to see what filters were serviceable, not only to provide good drinking water to those using them, but to secure sterile water for laboratory purposes. They found that some amebæ and flagellate bacilli passed through all the filters. Most filters suffered from prolonged use. He considered the Berkefeld and Grandjean filters were the best.

Plague at Mazatlan, Mexico.—Dr. José Ramos, of Mexico, outlined the methods by which the Mexican government was able to suppress the outbreak of plague at Mazatlan in 1900. Complete isolation of plague patients was insisted on. Disinfection was thoroughly carried out; destruction of rats was attempted on a very large scale, and even houses were destroyed by fire to reach results. They had found the use of anti-plague serum very effective in suspected cases.

FIFTH SESSION.—JANUARY 7TH.

Trachoma in Mexico.—Dr. José Ramos, of Mexico, stated that this disease was gradually spreading in the Republic, and there were certain well-recognized areas where it was more frequently found, but there was no doubt that the elevation at which most of the people lived had a good influence on the disease, and that it was rather more benign than in other parts of the world. He urged that popular lectures for general practitioners be given throughout the country on the diagnosis and treatment of trachoma.

Dr. Calvo read by title all of the papers on the program, the authors of which were not present, or had no time to read them.

The delegates and members were warmly received and royally entertained.

The next place of meeting will be in Guatemala City, Guatemala, in 1908.

MEDICAL AND CHIRURGICAL FACULTY OF MARYLAND.

SECTION ON CLINICAL MEDICINE AND SURGERY.

Stated Meeting, held December 2, 1904.

Gastro-Enterostomy and Pyloroplasty.—This subject was reviewed by Dr. Finney and a report of his own operation with record of results to date was presented. At the time of the first published account of the Finney pyloroplasty five cases were reported. Since then 80 cases have been recorded in the literature and the results have been very satisfactory. The procedure was said to be really an anastomosis between stomach and duodenum with division of the intervening structures; and it should more properly be called a gastro-pyloro-duodenostomy. Dr. Finney had, he said, recently operated on his twenty-second case. In this series there had been two deaths: one in a diabetic, who died in coma, healing of the pyloroplasty being found to be perfect at autopsy; and the other, a death from intestinal volvulus. Five days after operation, the healing again being perfect. This case emphasized the fact that the so-called " vicious circle " so often occurring in anastomosis between stomach and intestine and characterized by persistent vomiting, may in reality be an intestinal obstruction. Dr. Finney said that his series warranted him in reporting progress, though the operation was only to be recommended in benign stenoses. He had, however, gradually extended the class of cases in which he performed pyloroplasty. Most often it was done for cicatricial obstruction. In two patients chronic indigestion without cause was the indication and both were relieved. It had also been efficacious for persistent uncontrollable vomiting. In two patients with active ulcer the operation was done successfully.

Objections to Finney Pyloroplasty.—The objections raised to the operation were said to be: (1) That it was difficult in cases where adhesions were present; Dr. Finney said this had not been the case in his series. (2) That it was not of use in the presence of active ulceration; two cases of those reported had, however, shown this condition and had done well. (3) That the operation did not give a low enough pyloric opening; but Dr. Finney said this could be made as low as desired.

Advantages of Pyloroplasty.—These, Dr. Finney said, were (1) absence of regurgitation of bile; (2) restoration of practically normal anatomical relations; (3) slight mutilation of tissue; (4) absence of opportunity for formation of peptic ulcer.

Gastro-Enterostomy.—The history of this operation was reviewed and the defects of each procedure noticed. Dr. Finney then described a method which he had recently used, similar to the procedure described by Scudder, of Boston. The portion of bowel chosen was at the junction of duodenum and jejunum. Here the intestine runs directly downward and anastomosis at this point provides direct passage for the food, allows for a posterior operation, uses the most dependent portion of the stomach and leaves a short intestinal loop, in this way diminishing the likelihood of peptic ulcer. The operation of gastro-enterostomy should, Dr. Finney said, be limited to cases of cancer in which a radical operation was out of the question.

Dr. Friedenwald reported the findings of stomach examinations made on patients operated on by the Finney pyloroplasty. Five cases were studied before and after operation. The gastric contents were collected one hour after an Ewald meal, five hours after a heavy dinner, and after a fast of ten hours. In all five cases the dilated stomach was shown to be restored to normal, the gastric secretion to be much improved and the retention of food in the stomach longer than normal to be abolished. Dr. Martin said that he had always done the Heineke-Mikulicz operation and had gotten fair results. He had had no deaths and knew of no objection to the operation. Von Hacker's gastro-enterostomy did theoretically allow of biliary regurgitation but practically the results were good after it. Dr. Friedenwald was asked if there were any signs in these patients of intestinal upsets due to the premature discharge of unprepared food from the stomach functioning without its sphincter. He answered that in the first three weeks following operation intestinal symptoms were present, but that these later disappeared.

Neglect of Eye Cases.—Dr. Theobald discussed this subject with particular reference to the occurrence of total blindness. There were, according to the eleventh census 50,000 totally blind persons in the United States or an average of one in 1,238 of population. Cohn and others have estimated that about 40 per cent. of the cases are avoidable; in other words, 20,000 totally blind persons in the United States are blind through somebody's fault. The percentage of total blindness is smaller among negroes than among whites, and in cities of over 50,000 population than elsewhere. It is high in Ireland and Russia and reaches a maximum of one case to every 3,300 of population in Iceland. In Holland, where average intelligence is high, education good and ophthalmology well practised, absolute blindness is less frequent than anywhere else in the world. The causes of this condition are said to be: (1) Congenital; a factor in only about four per cent. of the cases; (2) idiopathic eye conditions; (3) ophthalmia neonatorum. Nearly all of these cases could have been prevented—probably as many as 90 per cent. At Leipzig the introduction of Credé's prophylaxis reduced the occurrence of the condition from 10 to ¼ per cent. (4) Glaucoma (inflammatory.) This could almost always be checked by operation. (5) Diseases of the uveal tract. (6) Diseases of the cornea. Treatment ought to reduce immensely the frequency of blindness following this condition. (7) Sympathetic ophthalmia. This ought to occur only in those cases where the obstinacy of the patient prevented treatment. (8) High myopia. (9) General disease. In lues of the brain recogniton of the condition and prompt treatment will diminish the frequency of blindness. In diseases of the spinal cord there is often little to be done. Ulcers of the cornea in acute infectious diseases can usually be controlled by proper treatment. (10) Traumatism, stupidity and obstinacy on the part of patients and a disposition on the part of general practitioners to take the responsibility in cases really belonging to specialists. These were said to be the two main factors in avoidable blindness. Happily, in recent years, a decrease in the frequency of the condition has been noted among civilized peoples.

BOOK REVIEWS.

A TEXT-BOOK OF ALKALOIDAL THERAPEUTICS. By W. F. WAUGH, M.D., and W. C. ABBOTT, M.D., with the collaboration of E. M. EPSTEIN, M.D. The Clinic Publishing Co., Chicago.

FOR some time the authors have been propagating a new (sic) system of therapeutics, the prinicple of which is to employ active principles instead of crude drugs. This, to one outside the cult, would seem to be the general trend in medicine to-day, in so far as pharmacological research and success in isolating active principles on a commercial scale have kept pace with the demands of therapeutics. However, we have carefully scanned this exponent of the new (sic) system for something new, and have found that "alkaloidal therapeutics" embraces 146 remedies, of which only 36 are alkaloids and the rest such substances as iodoform, iron, mercury, nuclein, pepsin, podophyllin, salicylic acid, etc. Why the only "alkaloidal" potassium salts are the bichromate and permanganate, why butyl chloral hydrate is included and not chloral hydrate, the authors do not tell us. But they have a way of talking of morphine, strychnine, aconitine, etc., as if they really believe that it is a new idea for physicians to use morphine rather than opium, or strychnine rather than nux vomica. In fact, we wonder what is the object of the book, till we discover how careful the authors are to instil into the minds of the reader that these principles act best when in the form of "standard" granules, or so-and-so's (the name of some proprietary remedy), and we find that so-and-so and the maker of standard granules is always the manufacturing firm which bears the name of one of the authors. The book "Alkaloidal Therapeutics" would seem, therefore, to be an elaborate form of advertisment, well-written, and containing much valuable information.

A TEXT-BOOK OF HUMAN PHYSIOLOGY. By ALBERT P. BRUBAKER, A.M., M.D., Professor of Physiology and Hygiene in the Jefferson Medical College, Philadelphia. P. Blakiston's Son & Co., Philadelphia.

To ONE familiar with Brubaker's summaries of physiological research this work will be welcomed as fulfilling the promise given by the author's thoroughly practical outlook on current physiological progress.

To the student and practitioner in need of a short and well-digested physiology we can most cordially recommend this volume. It is succinct, authoritative and modern.

THE HUMAN STERNUM. By A. M. PATERSON, M.D., Derby Professor of Anatomy in the University of Liverpool; Hunterian Professor at the Royal College of Surgeons of England. The University Press, Liverpool, England.

THIS work consists of three lectures, which were delivered before the Royal College of Surgeons, England. The presentation of such a work of scientific anatomy has necessitated the collection and careful study of an enormous amount of material in all stages of development. The results of the writer's investigations are presented in comprehensive descriptions from embryological, comparative and morphological points of view. The commonly accepted view of the morphology of the sternum is not considered to be the correct one. The main object of the work consists in the presentation of evidence to show that the origin of the sternum is not from rib elements, its association with the costal cartilages being a secondary one, but that the primary condition is in association with the shoulder girdle. The scientific reader will find the book interesting and profitable.

TOXICOLOGY. A Manual for Students and Practitioners. By E. W. DWIGHT, M.D., Instructor in Legal Medicine, Harvard University. Lea Brothers & Company, Philadelphia and New York.

THIS is a brief account of the poisonous action of the more widely used drugs. It contains a large amount of matter compressed in brief compass, but is not always reliable.

We note a few important omissions: Acetanilid, antipyrine, salol, iodoform, trional, sulphonal and others, but this may perhaps be excused because of the author's wish to economize space.

THE PRACTICE OF OBSTETRICS. Designed for the Students and Practitioners of Medicine. By J. CLIFTON EDGAR, Professor of Obstetrics and Clinical Midwifery in the Cornell University Medical College. Second Edition. Revised. P. Blakiston's Son & Co., Philadelphia.

FOR richness of illustration and wealth of clinical material, as well as for practical value to the working obstetrician, we have not seen for a long time, a work which equals this volume by Dr. Edgar.

We desire to accord to it unstinted praise, as it deserves it in the very highest degree.

It is to be stated that the favorable judgment of the profession has been so unanimous that in four months after its appearance Dr. Edgar's book has been revised in a second edition. This second edition before us is even richer in illustrations than the first. The size is not much increased. We find, we believe, in this book a rare mingling of scientific findings, and beside practice, brought out in a highly satisfactory manner. We can confidently look forward to a third edition in the near future.

SURGICAL EMERGENCIES. The Surgery of the Abdomen, Part I. Appendicitis and other Diseases about the Appendix. By BAYARD HOLMES, B.S., M.D., Professor of Surgery in the University of Illinois; Professor of Clinical Surgery in the American Medical Missionary College, etc. D. Appleton, New York.

IT is with rare pleasure that one greets in this little volume a cheering appreciation and application of the classification of that great anatomist of Cornell, Bart Wilder. If, as is by no means the case, there were no other commending qualifications in the volume, this would be sufficient to secure its most cordial indorsement, for it is high time that general text-books of medicine and surgery break away from the medieval medical style and substitute a modern, rational, scientific nomenclature. In preparing his work, the author has taken skilful advantage of the fact that the perspective of the practising physician, of the consulting physician and of the surgeon is in each case very different.

For an unpretentiously made book, the illustrations are numerous and unusually good. Special attention is called to those portraying an ideal mannikin with luminosities showing the point of maximum pain and its radiations. These cannot fail to be of lasting value to the student.

THE PURIN BODIES OF FOODSTUFFS AND THE RÔLE OF URIC ACID IN HEALTH AND DISEASE. By I. WALKER HALL, M.D. Second Edition, Revised. P. Blakiston Sons & Co., Philadelphia.

THE purin bodies, including xanthin, hypoxanthins, caffeine, theobromine, uric acid and others, play an important part in the food, the therapeutics and the metabolism of the body. Unfortunately little is known of them. The author of this book has made estimations of the purin bodies in the more common foodstuffs, and studied their specific effects upon the metabolic processes in animals and man, taken into the body either subcutaneously or by mouth. Not only these, the exogenous purins, but also those derived from the cell changes necessary to the maintainance of bodily function are considered. The author reaches the conclusion that the circulation of purins is an important factor in the production of certain chronic pathological conditions. The book is an original contribution to a difficult, but promising subject, and is sure to stimulate further investigation.

INTERNATIONAL CLINICS. A Quarterly of Illustrated Clinical Lectures and Original Articles by leading members of the Medical Profession throughout the world. Edited by A. O. J. KELLY, M.D., Philadelphia.

THE present number of the International Clinics contains an especially good collection of special articles and clinical lessons on syphilis. Among those deserving of particular notice are articles by Dr. Wm. G. Spiller, of Philadelphia, on "Syphilis of the Nervous System," by Prof. Alfred Fournier, of the University of Paris, on "Syphilis and Suicide," and by Campbell Williams, of London, on "Uncertainty of Syphilitic Inoculation." Prof. Fournier's article calls attention to the danger that exists for persons of unstable mental health if they are bluntly told without proper preparation that they have syphilis. His experience includes some 18 cases of suicide associated with the disease.

In this number the Department of Treatment is especially suggestive.

THE HOUSEBOAT BOOK. The Log of a Cruise from Chicago to New Orleans. By Wm. F. WAUGH, M.D. The Clinic Publishing Co., Chicago, 1904.

DR. WAUGH gives a rather interesting account of his houseboat trip to New Orleans. Those contemplating a like trip will find in it many valuable hints. As a bit of physical therapeutics we could well imagine that such a trip might be just the thing for many an overworked physician. It would bring him back to Mother Nature for her curative potencies to have their effect.

FRIEDBERGER AND FRÖHNER'S VETERINARY PATHOLOGY. Translated and Edited by M. H. HAYES, F.R.C.V.S. Vol. I. W. T. Keener & Co., Chicago.

MEDICINE is so rapidly assuming its true biological character that works in veterinary pathology cannot fail to be of service even to the practising physician. In a sense, nearly every practitioner, particularly those in rural communities, are veterinarians, either for their own stock or for that of their neighbors, and this work will appeal, by reason of its essentially practical nature as well as scientific merit.

SERUMS, VACCINES AND TOXINES IN TREATMENT AND DIAGNOSIS. By W. CECIL BOSANQUET. W. T. Keener & Co., Chicago.

THIS is a little book of only 340 duodecimo pages, but is the best little book we have seen dealing with this important subject. One can slip it in the pocket and while traveling read it and be benefited, as it is thoroughly up-to-date, readable and withal practical. We most cordially commend it.

TRANSACTIONS OF THE FIFTH ANNUAL MEETING OF THE ROCKY MOUNTAIN INTER-STATE MEDICAL ASSOCIATION, held at Salt Lake City, 1903.

THE volume consists of the papers presented at the meeting. Some of these are Neuritis Due to Forward Dislocation of the Mandible, by G. A. Moleen, Intubation by F. E. Waxham, Surgical Anatomy of the Cervical Sympathetic, by H. D. Niles, Bilateral Excision of Middle and Superior Cervical Ganglia in Five Cases of Epilepsy, by S. D. Hopkins, and Elements in the Recovery of the Incipient and Acute Insane, by T. E. Courtney. There is also a very interesting report of the rare condition, volvulus of the stomach, by C. D. Spivak, and a review of the subject of Pyloric Obstruction, by A. C. Behle.

THE MODERN NURSING OF CONSUMPTION. By JANE H. WALKER, M.D., Medical Superintendent of the East Anglian Sanatorium. The Scientific Press, Ltd., London, 1904.

DR. WALKER'S little book contains many practical points for the care of the tuberculous. It is evidently the result of experience and is direct and judicious in its suggestions. Take but the one point that the rooms of tuberculous patients must always be dusted with a wet cloth—not a damp cloth, for this is almost sure not to collect all the dust and a good idea of how detailed the instructions are can be obtained. All those interested in the care of consumptives will find it useful.

BOOKS RECEIVED.

THE MEDICAL NEWS acknowledges the receipt of the following new publications. Reviews of those possessing special interest for the readers of the MEDICAL NEWS will shortly appear.

APPENDICITIS. By Dr. B. Holmes. 12mo, 350 pages. D. Appleton & Co., New York.

MULTIPLE PERSONALITY. By Drs. B. Sidis and Goodhart. 8vo, 462 pages. A. Appleton & Co., New York.

THE MODERN NURSING OF CONSUMPTION. By Dr. Jane Walker. 12mo, 48 pages. Scientific Press, London.

TOXICOLOGY. By Dr. E. W. Dwight. 12mo, 298 pages. Lea Brothers & Company, Philadelphia and New York.

THE HOUSEBOAT BOOK. By Dr. Wm. F. Waugh. 12mo, 211 pages. Illustrated. Clinic Publishing Co., Chicago.

DUALITY OF THOUGHT AND LANGUAGE. By Dr. E. Sutro. 12mo, 277 pages. The Physio-Psychic Society, New York.

PRACTICAL DIETETICS. By Dr. A. F. Pattie. Second edition. 12mo, 310 pages. Published by the author, New York.

MEDICAL LATIN. By Dr. W. T. Sinclair. Second edition. 12mo, 121 pages. P. Blakiston's Son & Co., Philadelphia.

THE ART OF COMPOUNDING. By Dr. W. L. Scoville. Third edition. 8vo, 338 pages. P. Blakiston's Son & Co., Philadelphia.

NEW METHODS OF TREATMENT. By Dr. Laumoiner. Translated by Dr. H. W. Syers. 12mo, 321 pages. W. T. Keener & Co., Chicago.

DISEASES OF THE NOSE, THROAT AND EAR. By Dr. S. S. Bishop. Third edition. 8vo, 563 pages. Illustrated. F. A. Davis Co., Philadelphia.

ACCIDENTS AND EMERGENCIES. By Dr. C. W. Dulles. Sixth edition. 12mo, 209 pages. Illustrated. P. Blakiston's Son & Co., Philadelphia.

OUTLINES OF PHYSIOLOGICAL CHEMISTRY. By Drs. S. P. Beebe and B. H. Buxton. 12mo, 195 pages. Illustrated. The Macmillan Co., New York.

MANUAL OF SERUM DIAGNOSIS. By Dr. A. Rostoki. Translated by Dr. Chas. Boldnan. 12mo, 86 pages. Illustrated. John Wiley & Sons, New York.

ESSENTIALS OF CHEMICAL PHYSIOLOGY. By Dr. W. D. Halliburton. Fifth edition. 8vo, 236 pages. Illustrated. Longmans, Green & Co., New York.

INTERNATIONAL CLINICS. By Dr. A. O. J. Kelly. Volume III. Fourteenth series. 8vo, 302 pages. Illustrated. J. B. Lippincott & Co., Philadelphia.

TRANSACTIONS OF THE AMERICAN CLIMATOLOGICAL SOCIETY FOR THE YEAR 1904. Volume XX. Guy Hinsdale, Secretary. 8vo, 291 pages. Philadelphia.

KIRK'S HANDBOOK OF PHYSIOLOGY. By Dr. W. D. Halliburton. Nineteenth edition. 8vo, 902 pages. Illustrated. P. Blakiston's Son & Co., Philadelphia.

DISEASES OF THE SKIN. By Dr. H. W. Stelwagon. Third edition. 8vo, 1,112 pages. Illustrated. W. B. Saunders & Co., New York, Philadelphia and London.

HANDBOOK OF THE ANATOMY AND DISEASES OF THE EYE AND EAR. By Drs. D. B. St. John Roosa and A. E. Davis. 12mo, 296 pages. F. A. Davis Co., Philadelphia.

A TEXT-BOOK OF PRACTICAL THERAPEUTICS. By Dr. II. A. Hare. Tenth edition. 8vo, 908 pages. Illustrated. Lea Brothers & Company, Philadelphia and New York.

A TEXT-BOOK OF PHYSIOLOGICAL CHEMISTRY. By Dr. O. Hammersten. Fourth edition. Translated by Dr. J. A. Mandel. 8vo, 701 pages. Illustrated. John Wiley & Sons, New York.

THE MEDICAL NEWS.
A WEEKLY JOURNAL OF MEDICAL SCIENCE.

VOL. 86.   NEW YORK, SATURDAY, FEBRUARY 11, 1905.   No. 6.

SPECIAL ARTICLE.

REPORT OF A SPORADIC OUTBREAK OF TYPHOID FEVER AT LAWRENCE, N. Y., DUE TO OYSTERS.

BY GEORGE A. SOPER, PH.D.,

OF NEW YORK.

To the Board of Health of the Village of Lawrence, N. Y.

GENTLEMEN :—I have the honor to present herewith my final report on the investigation of a sporadic outbreak of typhoid fever in Lawrence and its vicinity in the summer, fall and early winter of 1904.

The total number of cases of which I have knowledge was thirty-one. There were three deaths. Nearly eighty per cent. of the cases occurred outside the limits of the village of Lawrence. None were due to any insanitary condition within your village. More than two-thirds of the cases were traced directly or indirectly to shellfish taken from water polluted with sewage.

The investigation was made with more than usual care, partly because of the fact that public statements had recently been made by apparently competent authorities to the effect that oysters cannot transmit disease, and partly because other theories existed as to the cause of the outbreak.

Now that the investigation is concluded, it is probable that the results may offer a partial explanation of sporadic typhoid which has occurred elsewhere. It is said that at least two hundred times as many oysters and clams were shipped away as were eaten in your vicinity. If this is so, it is possible that thousands of cases of typhoid fever may have been caused among the people who ate these oysters. At first sight one might think that so much typhoid from a single cause would promptly lead to the discovery of that cause. Further thought, however, shows that this would not be likely. Several thousand cases of typhoid could easily occur without drawing suspicion to these oysters and clams. The shellfish from this source are shipped to widely separated points—some are said to go to Europe. Three or four thousand cases of typhoid scattered among so many people, over so large an area, at a season when typhoid is expected to be more or less prevalent, would scarcely attract attention.

The eating of polluted oysters is so common an occurrence, and the autumnal incidence of typhoid is so coincident with it, as to make it the duty of your Board of Health to take cognizance of the possible connection between the two for all time in the future. All public health authorities should be equally alive to the danger to which your attention has been called.

THE REASONS WHICH LED TO THIS INVESTIGATION.

The reasons which led to the investigation here described arose from a knowledge that about a half dozen cases of typhoid fever had appeared in the corporate limits of Lawrence and that a larger number of cases had broken out in adjacent districts. The exact number of cases was not known, for, as is usual in the United States, the physicians had not been in the habit of officially notifying the health authorities of their typhoid fever patients, and there were, consequently, no accurate records.

Acting on the principle that typhoid fever points to insanitary conditions somewhere, and believing that the future health and reputation of the village required that the defective conditions, wherever they might exist, should be brought to light and corrected, your Board engaged the writer to make a thorough investigation of the matter.

POLICY OF THE LAWRENCE BOARD OF HEALTH WITH RESPECT TO PUBLIC HEALTH WORK.

It was seen at once that the inquiry, if thorough, would need to be carried on as much in other villages as at Lawrence, and some question arose as to the authority required for such work. Fortunately, the policy of the Board with respect to work outside the strict limits of its legal jurisdiction was clearly defined. In a matter which so seriously affected the health, not only of the people of Lawrence but of the large district of which Lawrence is a part, it was decided that village boundaries should be forgotten and, so long as no objection was made, the investigation should be pursued wherever it might lead. This policy had been established by the Board in its excellent work of eliminating mosquitoes.

TOPOGRAPHY AND OTHER CHARACTERISTICS OF LAWRENCE AND VICINITY.

The village of Lawrence is, in reality, part of a practically continuous settlement which extends from Rockaway Beach to Hewletts, a distance of nine miles, and from the ocean, or its inlets, to Jamaica Bay, a distance of from one-quarter to one and one-half miles. This peninsula projects diagonally from the mainland of Long Island into the ocean, as shown in Fig. 1. It varies in elevation from two to more than twenty feet above high tide. It is narrowest and lowest along the ocean front at Rockaway Beach and Arverne, and widest and highest at Lawrence.

The soil is composed of sand and gravel, and is admirably adapted for drainage. Broad meadows and innumerable creeks and coves run up into the land from the ocean and bay. The average rise and fall of the tide is about six feet.

Notwithstanding the fact that the settlements on this long narrow strip are practically continuous, there are some similarities and differences among them which should be carefully noted. All are famous for their healthfulness. All are occupied the year round by a few residents and are particularly well patronized in summer. All are supplied with water by the Queens County Water Company.

Rockaway Beach, at the west end of the line, is chiefly a day pleasure resort, resembling Coney Island. It is said that as many as 300,000 people have visited it in one day.

east. It is one of the most beautiful and wealtl residential villages on Long Island. The hous are large and have, as a rule, several acres well-kept grounds about them. Lawrence has i public sewerage system. Most of the houses ha private systems of their own. The total popul tion of Lawrence is probably not over 500.

East of Lawrence lies Cedarhurst, partly o cupied by tradespepole and partly by well-to-i residents, Woodmere, a new and rapidly grov ing residential district, and Hewletts, an old settlement which is being transformed into summer colony.

Between Far Rockaway and Lawrence and the north of them, lies Inwood, an unpretentio

Fig. 1.

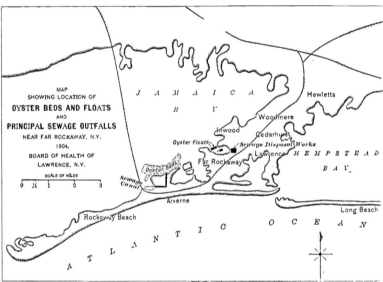

MAP
SHOWING LOCATION OF
OYSTER BEDS AND FLOATS
AND
PRINCIPAL SEWAGE OUTFALLS
NEAR FAR ROCKAWAY, N.Y.
1904.
BOARD OF HEALTH OF
LAWRENCE, N.Y.
SCALE OF MILES
0   ½   1   2   3

Arverne, close to Rockaway Beach, is a summer cottage colony of about 15,000 people. The houses are closely built; the streets are well paved and lighted. There is a sewerage system, the sewage flowing into what is known as the Amsdell Canal which carries it into Jamaica Bay.

Far Rockaway has a population of at least 15,000 in summer. It also sewers into Jamaica Bay, but its sewage is first conducted to a chemical purification plant which is intended to remove all of the dangerous and objectionable properties of the sewage. The communities thus far named lie within the corporate limits of New York City, in the Borough of Queens.

Lawrence lies next to Far Rockaway on the

village, many of whose inhabitants earn a liv from the oyster industries of Jamaica Bay. wood is the only community in this district wh receives little if any drinking water from water works of the Queens County Water C pany. Most of the drinking water at Inw comes from open wells situated in the bi yards of the houses. There is no sewer system. The village is closely built. One . tion is occupied by Italians and is extren squalid. A garbage burning plant and the sew disposal works of Far Rockaway lie close toget near the border between Far Rockaway and wood, as shown in Fig. 2. The immediate ritory about these works drains into the head a creek, popularly known as the "Cove," designated on the charts of the United States Hydrographic Office as Nigger Bar Channel. Inwood has 2,500 to 3,000 inhabitants.

PREVIOUS HISTORY OF TYPHOID FEVER IN THE VICINITY OF LAWRENCE.

In order to ascertain the location of every case of typhoid fever which had occurred in and about Lawrence in the six months preceding this investigation, as well as to gain a knowledge of the history of typhoid in this locality in past years, an invitation was sent by the Health

THE RECENT SPORADIC OUTBREAK.

From the physicians' statements and my own investigations I have found that the number of cases which occurred between Hewlett's and Far Rockaway from June 1 to December 1, 1904, was thirty-one.

Following is a table showing the dates upon which the beginning of the attack was marked; a chill or severe headache signalled the commencement of the disease.

Fig. 2.

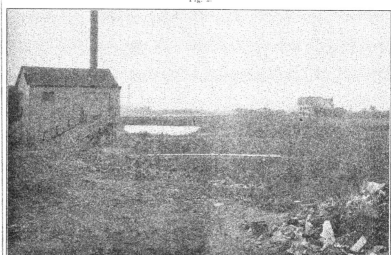

VIEW LOOKING TOWARD INWOOD FROM A POINT EAST OF SHERIDAN BOULEVARD.
The building in the near foreground is a garbage crematory. Beyond it is a pool of water adjoining the sewage disposal plant. All the drainage from this district passes into Inwood Cove.

Officer of Lawrence to every physician practising between Hewlett's and Far Rockaway to attend an informal meeting for the discussion of this subject. Eight accepted, one being compelled to remain away to attend a patient.

From the accounts of the physicians it appeared that typhoid fever was an unusual disease in the vicinity of Lawrence. The physicians ordinarily see no more than three or four cases in a year. Six or eight years ago, something like a prevalence of typhoid or malarial fever occurred at Far Rockaway. This outbreak was connected, in the minds of the physicians, with the construction of the public sewerage system, work upon which was hurried in anticipation of consolidation with New York City in 1898. In 1901 typhoid was less common; by 1902 it had disappeared.

TABLE No. 1.—*Dates upon which the patients were taken ill.*

Date 1904.	Number of People Attacked.	Date 1904.	Number of People Attacked.
June 10	2	Oct. 12	1
" 12	1	" 15	1
" 14	1	" 24	1
Aug. 7	1	" 26	3
" 18	1	" 28	1
Sept. 1	1	" 29	2
" 10	1	" 30	1
" 11	1	Nov. 1	1
" 15	1	" 6	1
" 25	1	" 9	1
Oct. 3	2	" 13	1
" 11	1	" 14	1
		" 18	2
		Total....31	

The cases were for the most part widely separated in point of distance. Among the four which occurred in June, no two lived nearer together than one half mile in a direct line. Later on, as will be seen beyond, several cases occurred in one house. Considering the period from June 1 to December 1, the distribution of cases is shown in the following table:

TABLE NO. 2.—*Showing Distribution of Cases.*

Locality.	Number of Cases.
Woodmere	1
Cedarhurst	3
Lawrence	7
Far Rockaway	8
Inwood	12
Total	31

It is practically certain that more cases than are here reported occurred at Far Rockaway during the summer. I have heard of several cases which were attended by physicians from New York City, whose addresses it has not been possible to ascertain. Cases are also known to have occurred at Arverne during the summer and several occurred at Rockaway Beach. Official confirmation of this statement can be found among the records of the New York City Department of Health at the Department headquarters in the Borough of Queens, Jamaica, L. I.

THE WATER, MILK AND FOOD SUPPLIES.

In the beginning of the investigation no single channel of infection seemed likely to prove common to all cases. Had the public water supply been infected a general epidemic would probably have resulted. Most of the attacks would have been among those who used the water. As it was, Inwood, where the use of the public water supply is not general, suffered more than any other district.

Still, for the sake of certainty, and in order to allay the fears of many persons, the public water supply was carefully examined. It was found that the Queens County Water Company supplied in the year ending January 1, 1904, a daily average of 1,904,812 gallons, the maximum being about 3,200,000 gallons, and the minimum about 800,000 gallons. There has always been enough water to supply the demand. No surface water has been used. The water is obtained from wells, many of them 160 feet deep, and driven through a thick layer of blue clay. The wells are situated in a practically uninhabited tract of land owned by the water company between Valley Stream and Hewlett's. The water, as it comes from the ground, contains a small amount of iron, and for this reason it is aerated and then filtered through what are known as natural, or gravity, filters. As some of the water is supplied to the people of New York City, it is analyzed every month by the chemists of the Department of Water Supply, Gas and Electricity. Through the courtesy of the Queens

County Water Company, I am enabled to presen the following results of analyses of the wate before and after treatment for the removal o iron. The chemical results are stated in part per million.

TABLE NO. 3.—*Results of Analyses of the Wate: of the Queens County Water Company Befor and After Filtration.*

Date of Collection Nov. 2, 1904.	Unfiltered.	Filtered.	Range since Regular Analyses were begun in 1898.
PHYSICAL EXAMINATION.			
Turbidity	5	0	....
Color	35	1	....
Odor	1	0	....
CHEMICAL EXAMINATION.			
Nitrogen as — Alb. Ammonia.	.018	.010	.002-.11
Free Ammonia	.020	.000	.000-.036
Nitrites	.001	.000	.000-.005
Nitrates	.05	.05	.000-.10
Total Solids	64.0	52.0	
Chlorine	5.0	5.4	.3-.4
Hardness	23.5	22.0	.8-.2:
Alkalinity	8.0	8.0	
Iron	.95	.00	
BACTERIOLOGICAL EXAMINATION.			
B. coli in — 0.1 c.c.	0	0	....
1.0 c.c.	0	0	....
10.0 c.c.	0	0	....
MICROSCOPICAL EXAMINATION.			
Standard units of microscopical matter per c.c. — Organisms	200	000	....
Amorphous matter	600	000	....

Two facts are evident from the foregoin results of analyses: First, the water has bee remarkably pure and satisfactory for a publi supply; and, second, it has suffered no deterior tion or alteration in quality from its usual hig standard.

In the begining it seemed possible that son of the cases of typhoid fever might be due milk which had become infected at its sour or in handling. Inspections were therefore ma of the dairies and bottling establishments determine whether any channels of infectic existed in this direction. None were found.

The sources of oysters and clams, as well of celery, lettuce and fruit, all of which a commonly eaten raw and may carry the infecti poison of typhoid fever, were too numerous warrant separate investigation in the absence any clue pointing toward them.

PLAN OF INVESTIGATION.

As the shortest and most feasible plan for d termining the cause of the outbreak, I decid to visit the home of each person who had be attacked by the fever and learn, if possible, to what channel of infection the patient had been exposed.

In this way I found that twenty-one of the patients had drunk the water of the Queens County Water Company; the rest had not tasted it. No milk supply was common to more than six. Two did not drink any milk or cream. Two drank waters which were not common to any other case. At least six patients had drunk no milk at all. Thirteen had eaten raw oysters within two weeks of their attack; one had eaten raw clams; one had handled fresh oyster shells; one had handled fresh clam shells. All the oysters and clams were from practically the same source. In addition to these sixteen cases, five cases could be explained on the ground of contact or comrade infection. Ten cases remain without an entirely satisfactory explanation; of these it is highly probable that three contracted their illness from oysters or clams and possible that one was made ill by bathing in the same water which infected the shellfish.

In addition to the thirteen whose typhoid is ascribed to oysters, it is important to note that three persons were taken with violent and continued diarrhea on three separate occasions following the eating of oysters from the source under suspicion. A fourth member of this same family, who also ate of the oysters became one of the typhoid fever victims already referred to.

These data can be conveniently arranged in the following manner:

TABLE No. 4.—*Cases of Typhoid Fever Ascribed to Various Causes.*

CAUSE.	No. of Cases.
Eating infected oysters...............	13
Eating infected clams...............	1
Handling infected oyster shells......	1
Handling infected clam shells.......	1
Due to comrade infection...........	5
Total cases satisfactorily explained	21
PROBABLE CAUSE.	
Eating or handling infected shellfish.	3
Bathing in infected water..........	1
Unknown	6
Total...................	31

Four of these six unknown cases occurred in June, five months before this investigation was begun, and were hence difficult to trace.

DETAILS OF EACH CASE ATTRIBUTED TO SHELLFISH.

An account of the most important items of evidence pointing to oysters and clams as the carriers of the contagium in the first sixteen cases, follows, the baymen being arbitrarily designated as A, B, C, etc.; the retail dealers as AA, BB, CC, etc.; and the milkmen by the Roman numerals I, II, III. etc.

Case No. 10.—Age thirty-seven years. Steam engineer in New York. Residence, Inwood. Taken ill September 11. Water from pump.

Milk from I. at Inwood. Went out on Jamaica Bay, September 1, and ate oysters taken from the grounds of A, about one-half mile east of trestle on both sides of Grass Hassock Channel.

Case No. 38.—Age forty years. Residence, Far Rockaway. Taken ill September 15. Water from Q. C. W. Co., and private well. Milk and cream from III., Far Rockaway. Ate raw oysters about September 3. Obtained oysters from AA. at Inwood. AA stole them from a float at Inwood.

Case No. 12.—Age twenty-five years. Residence, Far Rockaway. Taken ill September 25. Water from Q. C. W. Co. Milk from II., Far Rockaway. Ate raw oysters, on or about September 18. Obtained oysters from BB. He got them from the floats at Inwood.

Case No. 24.—Age eight years. Residence since September 20, Inwood. Previously lived one-half mile away, also in Inwood. Taken ill October 3. Water from pump. No milk or cream. No oysters or clams were eaten in this family. Played with clam shells thrown out from CC.'s grocery, next door to patient's previous home, September 18 to 20. CC., the grocer, got the clams from B., a bayman, about September 15. B. took them from Grass Hassock Channel, Jamaica Bay, in part payment for labor for cleaning up grounds of S. B. stored his oysters and clams on various floats at Inwood, borrowing the privilege.

Case No. 4.—Age twenty-nine years. Residence since September 25, Lawrence. Taken ill October 12. Water from Q. C. W. Co. Milk and cream from IV., at Woodmere, and VII., at Lawrence. Ate raw oysters October 5, supplied by DD., of Lawrence. On October 4 DD. had received a consignment of oysters from C, at Inwood. C. had obtained them from his bed in Grass Hassock Channel and had stored them in his float at Inwood.

Case No. 14.—Age thirty-five years. Residence, Inwood. Mechanic. Taken ill September 15. Water from pump. Milk from V., at Inwood. Started for trip to Coxsackie, N. Y., on a sloop from Inwood, October 3, taking several bushels of oysters obtained from D. D. got the oysters from his float at Inwood and originally obtained them from his bed in Grass Hassock Channel, Jamaica Bay.

Case No. 14.—Age thirty-five years. Residence, Inwood. Taken ill October 26. Water from well. Milk from I., at Inwood. Had oysters from EE. and G., of Inwood. Oysters taken from floats at Inwood and originally from Jamaica Bay.

Case No. 32.—Age eleven years. Residence, Cedarhurst. Taken ill October 26. Water from Q. C. W. Co. Milk from III., at Lawrence. No oysters. Ate raw clams from FF., Cedarhurst, on October 14 or 15. FF. gets his oysters and clams from C., at Inwood. They come from C.'s float at Inwood and originally from Grass Hassock Channel, Jamaica Bay.

Case No. 13.—Age thirty-eight years. Residence, Far Rockaway. Taken ill October 28. Water from Q. C. W. Co. No milk. Oysters obtained from AA., October 14, who stole them from a float at Inwood.

Case No. 9.—Age seventeen years. Residence, Inwood. Taken ill October 29. Water from Q. C. W. Co. Milk from V., at Inwood. Ate raw oysters October 15. Oysters supplied by E., from his float at Inwood. Oysters originally taken from Hassock Creek.

Case No. 5.—Age thirty-two years. Residence, Lawrence. Taken ill October 29. Water from Q. C. W. Co. Milk from VI., Lawrence. Ate raw oysters October 13, 20 and 27. Obtained

Case No. 31.—Age ten years. Residence, Far Rockaway. Taken ill October 30. Water from Q. C. W. Co. Milk and cream from VII., Far Rockaway. Raw oysters once a week from HH., Far Rockaway. Some oysters bought by HH. from JJ., Inwood. Some from KK., Inwood, about October 15. JJ. and KK. obtained their oysters from practically the same place, although JJ. probably stole theirs. KK. obtained his from D., his father. The father owns floats at Inwood and has a bed in Grass Hassock Channel.

Case No. 7.—Age thirty-four years. Residence, Woodmere. Taken ill November 1. Water from Q. C. W. Co. Does not drink milk. Ate raw oysters frequently from LL., Woodmere.

Fig. 3.

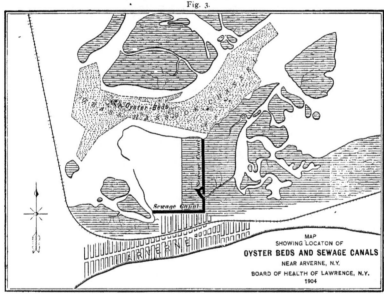

MAP
SHOWING LOCATON OF
OYSTER BEDS AND SEWAGE CANALS
NEAR ARVERNE, N.Y.
BOARD OF HEALTH OF LAWRENCE, N.Y.
1904

oysters from GG., a pedler. GG. obtained them from C., who supplied them from his float and took them originally from his bed in Grass Hassock Channel, Jamaica Bay.

Associated with this case are the three following cases of illness in the same family: 1. —, age seventy-six years, father-in-law of patient (*Case No. 5*); 2.—, age sixty-six years, mother-in-law of this patient; 3.—, age twenty-two years, wife of patient. All ate of the same lots of raw oysters on three successive Thursdays and each suffered for four to five days following with severe diarrhea and pain in the bowels. So convinced was this family that their illness was due to the oysters that they refused to buy any more from the peddler GG., who had formerly supplied them regularly.

LL. get their oysters from MM., Woodmere. MM. gets some from D., Inwood. These oysters came originally from D.'s bed near the trestle in Grass Hassock Channel, Jamaica Bay, and were floated in the cove at Inwood.

Case No. 15.—Age forty years. Residence Cedarhurst. Taken ill November 6. Water from Q. C. W. Co. Milk from VIII., Cedarhurst. Ate a dozen raw oysters about October 25. Obtained the oysters from JJ. Oysters originally from Jamaica Bay and Inwood floats.

Case No. 21.—Age five years. Residence, Inwood. Taken ill November 14. Water from a well. Never had milk or cream to drink. Never eats oysters or clams; played with oyster shell thrown out by F., about November 1. Oyster brought home by F. from his laying at Inwood.

Case No. 34.—Age twenty-five years. Residence, Far Rockaway. Taken ill November 18. Water from public water supply of the O. Co. W. Co. Milk from II., also IV., Far Rockaway. Ate raw oysters on October 29. Obtained oysters from HH., Far Rockaway. HH. gets some of his oysters from JJ., some from D., Inwood. Beds in Grass Hassock Channel, Jamaica Bay and floats at Inwood.

CHARACTER OF THE POLLUTION TO WHICH THE OYSTERS AND CLAMS WERE EXPOSED AT THE BEDS.

That the oyster beds which lie at the west end of Grass Hassock Channel are subject to sewage pollution is evident. The whole sewage of Ar-

water where it was formerly shut off. At the present time there exists a canal, deep and wide enough for a steam launch, and about half a mile long, between the sewers of Arverne and the oyster beds as shown in Fig. 3.

Oysters taken from the beds of C. and A. on November 22, were subjected in the bacteriological laboratory to what is known as the " presumptive test " for the *Bacillus coli communis.*

Results of Tests for the Presence of B. coli in Oysters from Grass Hassock Channel:

Sample No. 1.—In one-tenth cc. of the interior, negative; in one c.c., positive; in ten c.c., positive.

Sample No. 2.—In one-tenth c.c. of the interior,

Fig. 4.

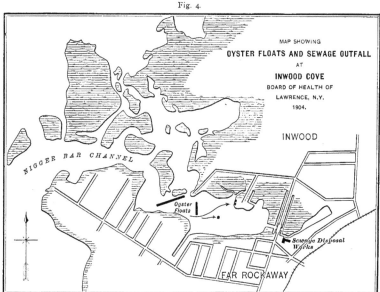

MAP SHOWING
OYSTER FLOATS AND SEWAGE OUTFALL
AT
INWOOD COVE
BOARD OF HEALTH OF
LAWRENCE, N.Y.
1904.

INWOOD

NIGGER BAR CHANNEL

Oyster Floats

Sewage Disposal Works

FAR ROCKAWAY

verne, which in summer has a population of about 15,000, debouches through two arms of a canal especially built to carry the sewage to the bay. The eastern arm of the canal was once cut off from the village sewer system by the construction of flood gates and an earth embankment, but these barriers are now out of repair and wholly ineffective. The water has worked its way around one of the abutments of the flood gates, and the gates themselves are wedged open with drift, so that the water runs either way through this former obstruction. Apparently to assist the draining of the meadows, a channel has deliberately been cut around the earth embankment, so that here, also, there is a free passage for the

negative; in one c.c., positive; in ten c.c., positive.

The western arm of the sewage canal empties into a natural channel of Jamaica Bay which flows in a direct line towards the beds of D., about three-quarters of a mile away. Given favorable conditions of tide and weather, it seems impossible to escape the conclusion that all of the oyster beds in this vicinity, and especially those of the planters whose layings are situated near the outlets of the canal, have been subject to pollution from the sewers of Arverne. Cases of typhoid occurred at Arverne through the summer, and as we know that typhoid stools are seldom if ever thoroughly disinfected where public sewerage systems exist, it seems probable that this sewage has been occasionally infected with typhoid fever germs. This probability is increased when we consider the likelihood that some convalescents from typhoid fever were among the 15,000 visitors to Arverne. Typhoid convalescents are as dangerous as patients in the active stages of the disease, for they may give off for weeks and months, enormous numbers of typhoid germs in their urine.

There seems no room to doubt that the oyster beds near the outfalls of the Arverne sewage canals have been from time to time infected, and that Case No. 10 contracted his typhoid fever through oysters which he obtained and ate in this locality on September 1.

water of this cove for from twenty-four hours to many days. It is probable that 100,000 to 200,000 bushels are brought to this point every year from the beds in Jamaica Bay and ultimately shipped away for sale. The local consumption of oysters is comparatively small. The nearby retail trade is supplied chiefly by C. and D.

At high tide the cove is perhaps an eighth of a mile wide. From the floats to the head of the cove the distance is about half a mile. At low tide the water leaves the bed of the cove exposed and at this time the oyster floats are out of water. Only a thin stream winds toward them from the eastern end of the cove, where the sewage disposal plant of Far Rockaway empties its effluent. The nearest float to the sewage works

Fig. 5.

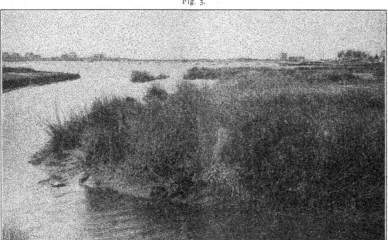

GENERAL VIEW OF INWOOD COVE FROM SHERIDAN BOULEVARD.
The effluent of the sewage disposal works empties into the creek in the immediate foreground. The oyster floats can be seen in the middle distance. On the extreme right is the dock where the oysters are landed.

POLLUTION OF SHELLFISH AFTER REMOVAL FROM THEIR BEDS.

The shellfish which came from Inwood were exposed to pollution at that place in an equally obvious manner. It is the custom among the oystermen to store the oysters which they bring from their Jamaica Bay beds in floats or cars which are located near the head of Nigger Bar Channel, otherwise known as the Cove, as appears from Figs. 4, 5 and 6. These floats are about 40 feet long, 15 feet wide, and one and a half feet deep. They are partly submerged, and are so built as to allow their contents to be covered by the water. The objects aimed at in putting the oysters in these floats need not be discussed here. It is sufficient for our present purpose to note that they are laid down in the

is that of C. For convenience, he has also a float-house on the shore, 100 yards away, as shown in Fig. 7. A little farther down the cove, is the float of D., one of a group of five. The remaining 12 floats, including those of E., lie about 500 feet to the west. Nearby is the laying of F.

THE FAR ROCKAWAY SEWAGE DISPOSAL PLANT.

Aside from the sewage disposal plant which I have described, the cove was polluted from other quarters. A few rods to the east of the sewage works is a garbage burning plant which drains into the creek. A settlement of several score of Italians lies close at hand. To the north of the sewage plant, and draining directly into the cove, is a pile of many hundred loads of manure and other filth. To the west, on the shore and easily reached by very high tides in the cove, are three loads of sewage sludge apparently taken from some cesspool.

The sewage disposal plant whose effluent empties into the water in which the oysters and clams are floated at Inwood is of comparatively recent construction, having been erected to purify the sewage collected by a sewerage system which was built at Far Rockaway in 1896 to '97. Theoretically the process is simple enough, but in practice considerable skill is required to operate it satisfactorily. The sewage is passed through a series of basins in which the impurities are supposed to be precipitated by the use of chemicals. The chemicals employed are chloride of iron and lime. They are added in solution, in small streams as the sewage enters the tanks and form hydrate of iron and chloride of lime. This is supposed to precipitate the impurities to the bottom of the tanks. The tanks are occasionally emptied and their accumulations dumped upon the meadows, after more or less disinfection.

TABLE No. 5.—*Analyses of the Affluent and Effluent of the Municipal Sewage Disposal Oyster Floats at Inwood, N. Y.*

Date and place of Collection of sample.	Nov. 30, 1904. Affluent.	Nov. 30, 1904. Effluent.
PHYSICAL EXAMINATION.		
Turbidity	89	75
Color	45	37.
Odor	4d	3d
CHEMICAL EXAMINATION.		
Alb. ammonia in suspension	1.600	.800
" " solution .	1.400	1.200
" " total	3.000	2.000
Free ammonia	13.000	17.400
Nitrites	.000	.000
Nitrates	.00	.00
Chlorine	90	104.
Hardness	75.	75.
Alkalinity	99.	99.
Iron	2.80	.75
Total solids	352.0	340.0
BACTERIOLOGICAL EXAMINATION.		
Number of bacteria per c.c. developed in forty-eight hours at 20° C.	5,240,000	7,320,000
In 0.10 c.c.	Positive	Positive
Bacillus coli { In 1.00 c.c.	"	"
In 10.00 c.c.	"	"
MICROSCOPICAL EXAMINATION.*		
Total microscopical organisms. ...	15,000	12,500
Amorphous matter	5,200	3,650
Important genera Mold Hyphae	1,200	1,000
Paramecium ..	3,750	2,500

* Number of standard units per c.c.

When I visited the plant on November 26, there was only a small stream of chloride of iron being added to the sewage. The lime solution was not being used. I was told that on Sundays

and holidays, lime was not employed because the chemist was away on those days. The efficiency of the plant under these circumstances being practically nil, it follows that on Sundays and on holidays crude sewage from the whole of Far Rockaway has been emptied into the cove at Inwood.

A second visit was made to this plant on November 30, for the purpose of taking samples of the sewage as it entered and left the plant. The process of purification was said to be in normal order. The chemical and biological analyses of these samples follow. The chemical results are stated in parts per million. (Table 5.)

TABLE No. 6.—*Analyses of Water Collected Near the Outlet of the Municipal Sewage Disposal Plant at Far Rockaway and Near the Oyster Floats at Inwood, N. Y.*

Date and place of Collection of sample.	Nov. 30, 1904. Near sewage Plant.	Nov. 30, 1904. Near Oyster Floats.
PHYSICAL EXAMINATION.		
Turbidity	12	3
Odor	13	11
Color	2d	1u
CHEMICAL EXAMINATION.		
Alb. ammonia in suspension	.200	.010
" " solution ..	1.000	.120
" " total	1.200	.130
Free ammonia	9.800	.140
Nitrites	.280	.006
Nitrates	1.45	.05
Chlorine	464.	15,750.
Hardness	207.	5,300.
Alkalinity	49.	97.
Iron	1.20	1.20
Total solids	1,033.	25,712.
BACTERIOLOGICAL EXAMINATION.		
Number of bacteria developed per c.c. after forty-eight hours at 20° C.	600,000	12,850
In 10.00 c.c.	Positive	Positive
Bacillus coli { In 1.00 c.c.	"	"
In 0.10 c.c.	"	"
MICROSCOPIC EXAMINATION.*		
Total microscopic organisms.....	395	50
Amorphous matter	2,500	250
Important genera Mold Hyphae	250	0
Paramecium..	75	0
Navicula	0	30

* Number of standard units per c.c.

The foregoing results show that while the chemical composition of the sewage was somewhat improved by passing through the disposal works, the number of bacteria were increased. This increase was nearly forty per cent. Colon bacilli were found as readily in the effluent as in the affluent. The odor of the sewage was reduced only 25 per cent., the color less than 18 per cent., and the turbidity less than 16 per cent. The amount of microscopic organisms of a much larger size than the bacteria were reduced sixteen per cent. The amorphous matter, as determined by the microscopical examination, was reduced 29 per cent. Taken as a whole, the results show that the improvement in the sewage was slight; the change was not greater than would have been produced, in all probability, had the sewage been allowed to pass through the settling basins without the addition of chemicals.

If the results of the analysis of the output of this plant is compared with the results of the analysis of the water of the Queens County Water Company, as given on page 244, it will be seen that the effluent of the sewage works was of a dangerous character. It is true that the sewage was diluted and purified to some extent after it was discharged into the cove, but the quantity of sewage was so large as compared to the quantity of the diluting water, particularly at low tide, and the distance to the oyster floats was so short, that the improvement must have been uncertain in amount.

RESULTS OF ANALYSES OF WATER AND OYSTERS AT THE FLOATS.

It seemed desirable to obtain information as to the quality of the water at the floats themselves, and to this end samples of water were taken at several points in the cove and carefully analyzed. To approach still closer to the point which it was desired ultimately to determine, specimens of oysters were taken from the floats at the same time. The oysters were collected from such of the 17 floats as would give a fair indication of the purity of them all. On the day when these samples were taken the conditions were unfavorable for finding evidence of sewage pollution. The winter population of Far Rockaway is much smaller than the population at the time when the oysters and the clams must have been infected and the quantity of sewage was correspondingly less. The tide was beginning to run up from the bay toward the sewage disposal plant. The chemical results are stated in parts per million. (Table 6.)

TABLE No. 7.—*Analyses of Specimens of Oysters Taken from the Floats at Inwood, on November 25 and 30, to Determine Their Condition. The Oysters Were Examined Inside and Outside for the Presence of Bacillus Coli.*

	Bacillus coli.					
Owner.	Inside the shell.			Outside of shell.		
	0.1 c c.	1.0 c c.	10.0 c.c.	0.1 c.c	1 c.c.	10.c.c.
D.	o	+	+	o	+	+
D.	+	+	+	+	+	+
C.	o	o	+	o	o	+
C.	o	+	+	o	o	+
G.	o	+	+	+	+	+
A.	o	+	+	+	+	+
I.	o	o	+	+	+	+
K.	+	+	+	+	+	+
L.	o	o	+	+	+	+
H.	o	o	+	+	+	+
F.*	—	—	—	o	o	+

.* Shells from the yard where Case No. 21, D., played. These shells had been exposed to the weather several weeks from the time they were thrown out to the time when they were examined.

These results show that the water near the sewage plant was grossly polluted; that it was markedly better near the oyster floats, but that even in this locality, under the favorable condition of an incoming tide, it bore unmistakable evidence of pollution. (Table 7.)

These results show that 20 per cent. of the oysters were certainly polluted on the inside, and 70 per cent. on the outside, according to the standards now generally adopted by sanitary experts. The evidence is conclusive on this point. In addition, the results of the examinations indicate that 60 per cent. were probably polluted on the inside and 80 per cent. on the outside.

SUMMARY.

Regarded as a whole, it would probably be difficult to find a more unsuitable spot in which to place oysters intended for consumption than the waters of Inwood Cove. The place is so obviously a catch-all for unwholesome drainage and miscellaneous filth, that it is surprising the oystermen themselves have not been alive to the dangers of the situation.

I believe the conditions found here and in the bay fully warrant the opinion that not only have the oysters and clams taken from these waters been unsafe to eat, but their shells have been dangerous to handle.

In my judgment, the pollution of Jamaica Bay by the sewage of Arverne, and of Inwood Cove by the sewage of Far Rockaway, and other unwholesome drainage, have caused, directly or indirectly, 21 of the 31 cases with which this investigation has been concerned.

DETAILS OF THE CASES OF TYPHOID WHICH WERE DUE TO OTHER CAUSES THAN SHELLFISH.

Although the investigation was closed before all of the remaining cases could be conclusively studied, there is reason for believing that the following patients were made ill in the manner now to be specified in each instance. The first five, it will be observed, are ascribed indirectly to shellfish.

DETAILS OF FIVE CASES OF CONTACT, OR COMRADE INFECTION.

Case No. 18.—Trained nurse. Residence, Lawrence. Taken ill August 18 and died. This woman had been in attendance upon Case No. 17, and undoubtedly contracted the fever from the infectious matter given off by this patient.

Case No. 21.—Age forty years. Laundress. Residence, Lawrence. Taken ill October 24. Washed bedding and linen from Case No. 1. Contracted the fever on this visit.

Case No. 25.—Age thirty-two years. Residence, Inwood. Taken ill November 9. Visited the house of Cases No. 24, No. 22 and No. 23, to carry food and help to this destitute family. Contracted the fever on this visit.

Case No. 22.—Age twenty-nine years. Residence, Inwood. Taken ill November 13. Mother of Case No. 24. Contracted the fever while nursing her daughter.

Case No. 23.—Age six years. Residence, Inwood. Taken ill November 18. Sister of Case No. 24. Contracted the fever from her sister.

DETAILS OF TEN CASES CONCERNING WHOSE ORIGIN THERE WAS DOUBT.

Case No. 27.—Age thirteen years. Residence, Inwood. Taken ill June 10. Water from pump. Milk from private cow. No oysters, clams or shells apparently associated with this case. On May 30, Decoration Day, took a bicycle ride to Lynbrook, visiting a cemetery and attending a large meeting at a race track.

Case No. 29.—Age fifty-two years. Residence, Inwood. Taken ill June 10. Water from Queens County Water Company. Milk from IX, Inwood. Had friends to dinner on May 30 and probably ate raw clams.

from V, Far Rockaway. One of a party of four at a clam bake about August 1. Clams bought from boys on the street who probably obtained them from Inwood.

Case No. 26.—Age fifteen years. Residence, Inwood. Taken ill Sept. 1. Water from well. No milk, cream, oysters or clams apparently associated with this case. Bathed in Inwood Cove.

Case No. 1.—Age thirty-five years. Residence, Cedarhurst. Taken ill September 10. Water from Queens County Water Company. Milk from IV, at Hewlett's. Visited Inwood, Lynwood, Far Rockaway and Rockaway Beach occasionally on his bicycle.

Case No. 3.—Age twenty-three years. Residence, Far Rockaway. Taken ill October 3. An intemperate man. Refused all information concerning his habits.

Fig. 6

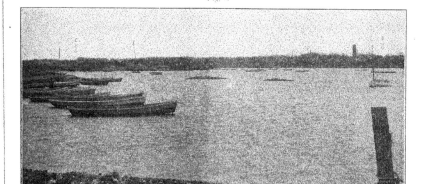

VIEW OF INWOOD COVE LOOKING TOWARD THE SEWAGE DISPOSAL WORKS.
The works occupy the long low building marked A; an oyster float belonging to C. is marked B; a float-house on shore belonging to C. is marked C.

Case No. 16.—Age sixteen years. Residence, Lawrence. Taken ill June 12. Water from Queens County Water Company. No milk, cream, oysters or clams apparently associated with this case. On May 30 took long walk on meadows with a dog, throwing the dog frequently into the water, thus possibly wetting hands with infected sewage.

Case No. 17.—Age forty-five years. Residence, Lawrence. Taken ill June 14. Water from the Queens County Water Company. No further information obtained concerning this case.

Case No. 19.—Age twenty-five years. Residence, Far Rockaway. Taken ill August 7. Water from Queens County Water Company. Milk

Case No. 11.—Age twenty-six years. Residence, Far Rockaway. Taken ill October 11. Water, at home, from Queens County Water Company. Milk from V, Far Rockaway. Cream from X, Far Rockaway. Does not eat oysters or clams. Takes luncheons at Jamaica, L. I., where typhoid fever was more than usually prevalent.

Case No. 6.—Age twenty-two years. Residence, Lawrence. Taken ill October 26. Water at home from Queens County Water Company. Milk from IV, Hewlett's. Had no oysters or clams at home. Luncheons taken in New York City. Went on hunting expedition to Eastport, N. Y., October 15 to 20.

RECOMMENDATIONS FOR THE PREVENTION OF TYPHOID IN THE FUTURE.

The history of Lawrence and its vicinity indicates that this region has been remarkably free from typhoid fever in the past and there seems reason to believe that, with ordinary care, it can be kept equally free from typhoid in future. The Rockaway peninsula is naturally healthful. The attention given by your Board to the recent sporadic outbreak should be taken by the people as an indication that sanitary questions are being carefully looked after and that public health in this vicinity will. for this added reason, be more than ordinarily secure.

At the same time, it must not be forgotten that typhoid fever is a disease which is more prevalent throughout the whole country than is

their returns. I think a better way, however, would be for your Board to request the physicians who practise between Hewlett's and Far Rockaway to keep you informed of their cases as a matter of courtesy and for the public good. In return for their trouble you could well afford to offer the doctors free examinations of such specimens of blood and urine as they would care to send you for the readier diagnosis of their doubtful cases of typhoid. Such laboratory examinations are of inestimable value and boards of health in many of the larger cities make them gratuitously for the physicians. An accurate reporting of all cases of infectious and contagious diseases lies at the foundation of all good work in public sanitation.

The Water Supply.—The water supply of the

Fig. 7.

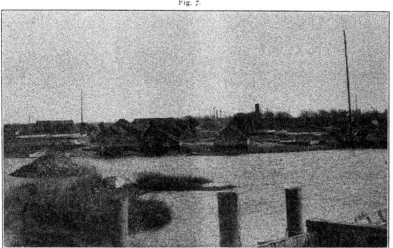

VIEW OF INWOOD OYSTER DOCK AND OYSTER HOUSES.
The sewage disposal plant is in the middle distance.

commonly understood. It is often very difficult to diagnose and is frequently called by names which do not suggest its infectious character. If any community wishes to exclude it absolutely, it will be necessary to exercise careful supervision over a number of matters which generally receive little or no attention.

The greatest security for the future can be obtained if you will secure a notification of the cases which occur in the villages in your vicinity and exercise a supervision over your supplies of water, milk and shellfish.

Notification of Cases.—Physicians can be required by law to report their cases of typhoid fever to the local board of health which has jurisdiction over the territory in which they practise, and in this manner you can learn of

Queens County Water Company is now of pure and satisfactory quality and will doubtless always be kept so. In order that you may keep informed of its quality, you are advised to arrange for a copy of the regular monthly analyses which are made of this water by the Department of Water, Gas and Electrictity of New York City and to request the company to inform you of any changes in the construction or operation of its plant which may, by any possibility, affect the quality of the water.

The Milk Supply.—The milk supply of your village, while not responsible for the recent cases of typhoid fever, has been found by inspection to be capable of improvement. It will not be possible to bring about ideal conditions at once, without severe hardship to the small producers and dealers, but a long stride toward the ultimate result can be made if the following simple requirements be insisted upon:

1. Require the milkmen to follow honestly the fifty dairy rules published by the Bureau of Animal Industries of the United States Department of Agriculture.

2. Do not allow the milkmen to bottle milk or wash, cool, air, or otherwise handle receptacles for milk in any dwelling house or barn, or within fifty feet of a dwelling or barn, privy or manure pile.

It is much better to have a separate building for the handling and bottling of milk and to have the water used for cleaning the receptacles brought from a distance in pipes. Wells situated in the back yards of houses or near stables should be analyzed, and if good, carefully protected against pollution.

3. Require the milkmen to sterilize by live steam or boiling water all bottles used for milk distribution.

4. Never allow a bottle or can of milk to be left at a house where there is a case of contagious or infectious disease. The milk should be emptied into a pitcher or other receptacle provided by the housekeeper.

5. Do not allow a case of infectious or contagious disease to remain in the house of a milkman. Either the patient should be removed from the premises or the milk business temporarily taken to another quarter.

Oysters and other Shellfish.—Your board has as much legal right to regulate the purity of shellfish as to regulate the purity of milk. One is quite as important as the other. It is, in fact, your duty to exclude from sale in the village over which you have jurisdiction, all oysters, clams and other shellfish which are liable to cause disease.

I positively believe you will find small difficulty in accomplishing this end if you will act with firmness, moderation and tact. It is to the interest of honest oystermen to afford you opportunities for inspecting their methods of cultivating and handling the shellfish and taking samples of the same for analysis.

In the event of your finding shellfish which are unsuitable for food in your territory, you have the legal right to forbid its sale, and if necessary, destroy it without any compensation to the owners.

Under the circumstances which exist at present, I think you would be justified in excluding from the village of Lawrence all oysters and other shellfish which have been taken from Jamaica Bay within the influence of the Arverne sewers or from the Cove at Inwood which receives the sewage of Far Rockaway.

Respectfully submitted,

GEORGE A. SOPER, Ph.D.,
Consulting Sanitary Engineer.

December 17, 1904.

ORIGINAL ARTICLES.

HEMATURIA AS A SYMPTOM OF HYDRONEPHROSIS. NEPHRECTOMY. CURE.

BY L. BOLTON BANGS, M.D.,
OF NEW YORK.

HAVING had considerable experience with hematuria due to various forms of renal disease, and never having met with a case similar to the one which I shall presently report, it seemed to me unusual and worthy of some study. This led me to search the literature for the experience of others with the result of finding that, with the exception of Israel, authors make very little mention of hematuria as a symptom of hydronephrosis, and Newman distinctly states that the latter "is not attended by hematuria." In this research I have had the assistance of Dr. Edward Preble (whose thoroughness and linguistic attainment I can recommend) and of the result of our combined labors, it may be stated, that "although pretty nearly every other condition of the kidney and pelvis is spoken of as a cause, common or exceptional, of hematuria, none of the systematic reference books on renal disease, nor any of the reviews in the special journals and in the *Index Medicus* mention hydronephrosis in this connection." In the past few years we have found 13 cases have been reported. Of these *nine* are by Israel, one by Morris, who quotes one by Allingham, one by Reclus and one by Albarran.

It would also appear from our combined research that hydronephrosis *per se* is a comparatively infrequent disease in this country, for nowhere in American literature do I find recorded any series of cases and no individual experience like that of . Israel, who reports forty cases, among them being the nine cases with hematuria as a symptom. It may therefore be inferred that either the better conditions under which our people live have prevented this form of renal disease or that American writers have not thought it worth while to publish their cases. The following case is presented as a contribution to this subject.

Case I.—Male, aged nineteen years, was brought to me with the following vague history: His father, who accompanied him, cannot remember that he had ever had any sickness until the present one, which began about a year previous. At that time he seemed to "run down;" complained of nausea and general malaise, and his mother noticed a sediment in his urine. Of this sediment no description is given. He was seen by a physician who said there was some slight "kidney trouble," and gave him some form of treatment. As he did not improve a distinguished Boston surgeon was consulted, who said there was blood in the urine, and that "the diagnosis was tuberculosis."

At present his symptoms are as follows: He

1 Read at the New York Academy of Medicine, Surgical Section, December 2, 1904.

is emaciated, but not markedly. He complains
of malaise and of an indefinite pain in both lumbar regions, described as of a dull character. He
has some burning when he voids his urine,
which is done at frequent intervals, and the
quantity is greatly increased; for, he says he
voids in the day about "five pints of urine," *i.e.,*
about 2,500 c.c. His urine, as voided in my
presence, is turbid, *alkaline,* and contains
shreds, flakes, and phosphates, but no perceptible blood. That the blood appears intermittently
and is variable in quantity is evident from a
statement made subsequently that he had noticed "that jolting increased the amount of
blood in his urine." He is chronically constipated, requiring daily use of cathartics, and this
is his chief complaint. Physical examination of
his sexual apparatus, including the prostate and
seminal vesicles, is negative. There are no nodules and no lesions to be discovered, and no increased sensibility. Bimanual palpation of the
left lumbar region shows a distinct fulness and
resistance in that region, but no definite or distinct outlines can be made out.

The following day the urine was separated
from the kidneys by means of the Harris separator and sent to a laboratory, with the following result:

Examination of urine of May 4; Harris separator. Right kidney: Small amount of blood;
no pus, no casts, no tubercle bacilli found.
Specific gravity, 1.008. Urea, 0.009 grms in 1
c.c. Functional capacity, 0.6. Left kidney: blood,
small amount; pus, moderate amount; casts,
small hyaline; no tubercle bacilli; specific gravity, 1.005; urea, 0.006; functional capacity, 0.25;
weight, 61.5 kilo.

Remarks.—Right kidney: The total absence
of renal elements with a functional capacity of
0.6, somewhat low but much better than the other
kidney, probably justifies the conclusion that
this kidney is normal. Left kidney: Lower gravity and lower relative amount of urea, larger
amount of albumin, numerous hyaline casts, together with a moderate amount of pus and
epithelium, presumably from the renal pelvis,
would, I believe, indicate some pyelitis, with,
probably, a more marked lesion of the parenchyma. The very low functional capacity (0.25), even
as compared with the other kidney, would cor-
roborate the suspicion of a more marked lesion
of the renal parenchyma.

It is evident that the left kidney is the seat of
his disease. He is given urotropin gr. v. four
times in the twenty-four hours and water copiously. Six days later it is recorded that he has
less backache and that his urine contains free
blood in moderate quantity. On this occasion a
soft catheter is passed into the bladder, which is
irrigated till the fluid returns clear. Bimanual
pressure is then made upon the left kidney and
instantly spurts of pale *bloody urine* follow in
characteristic and synchronous response to the
pressure. The bladder is again irrigated until

the fluid returns clear, and the same maneuver
being practised over the right kidney the result
is negative. Careful palpation of the left hypochondrium and loin shows that these regions
are occupied by a mass whose outlines, consistency and limits cannot be defined, but apparently
the left kidney is markedly enlarged and projects
laterally, as well as anteriorly. The left lumbar
region is flat on percussion, in strong contrast
to the other side where the percussion note is
distinctly tympanitic. The patient is given hygienic directions for the improvement of his general condition, to continue the water and urotropin and report in four weeks.

A month later he reported to me in better general condition, having increased in weight. He
had been relieved from pain, but blood in the
urine persisted. He has noticed that jolting, in
a wagon, for example, increases the amount of
blood in his urine. There is no change in the
renal tumor excepting that it is not so prominent
anteriorly. I was unable to make a positive diagnosis and advised an exploratory incision, which
was done a week later.

The kidney was reached without difficulty by
means of the Mayo Robson method, and after
the perirenal fat had been separated, a bilobed,
rounded tumor with thin walls presented. An
aspirating needle drew slightly clouded urinous
fluid. The tumor or sac walls was seized in two
places and incised. About a quart of fluid escaped,
some of which was preserved for examination.
Exploration of the sac showed that the kidney
was the seat of hydronephrosis and that comparatively little renal tissue was left, more being
at the extreme upper pole than elsewhere. There
was a moderately free hemorrhage from the interior of the sac, which was controlled by free
irrigation with very hot water, and the latter
also caused a marked contraction of the sac wall.
A small flexible bougie was passed through the
ureter to the bladder, as further proof that there
was no obstruction between the kidney and the
bladder.

The question of immediate nephrectomy was
considered, but it was thought advisable to give
him the benefit of drainage and perform a secondary nephrectomy, if necessary, under better
general conditions. The patient made a good
operative recovery and went to his home with a
drainage-tube in the left kidney, with instructions to remain under the observation of his physician and to return after a few months in order
that the question of nephrectomy might be considered. In the meantime his urine was to be
examined repeatedly, that from the bladder separately from that received from the drainage-tube.
The latter was dressed in such manner that the
urine was received in a rubber receptacle worn
beneath the clothing and without wetting the
latter.

At this time a comparison of the urine voided
from the bladder with the urinous fluid received
in the rubber receptacle showed that the left kid-

ney still excreted a large amount of fluid of a low specific gravity and containing a small percentage of urea._ Together they maintained the amount of excretion requisite for the patient's health.

The young man continued to improve steadily under the careful supervision of his family physician, who conferred with me by letter from time to time. The doctor, who is an instructor in the department of chemistry in the Tuft's College Medical School, made regular and systematic examinations of the urine. These showed a gradual improvement in the quality of the urine voided from the bladder, which was assumed to represent chiefly the urine of the right kidney. About eight months after the nephrotomy he wrote, " I have made a physical examination of the patient and find both his heart and lungs to be normal, while his general health is of the very best. I am inclined to the opinion that a gradual hypertrophy of the good kidney is taking place, and I believe that it is only a matter of time when it will properly perform the function of two kidneys. The presence of the diseased kidney in his body does not seem to be detrimental to his general health in the least, and I should, therefore, be conservative in any line of operative treatment until the compensatory hypertrophy is firmly established." With this view, so admirably stated by the physician, I fully agreed, and the young man was kept under observation for two months longer, when the urinary tests proving to be satisfactory and his general health remaining excellent, it was determined to remove the diseased and nearly useless kidney.

It is interesting to note here that the patient was kept for weeks continuously under the influence of urotropin. His physician wrote me that " under this treatment the condition of the bladder urine has greatly improved. Its acidity is normal for the first time in many months. The sinus urine, however, has shown little or no improvement, although by the bromine water test I have proven that the urotropin is being eliminated from both kidneys in the form of formaldehyde."

The operation was undertaken under ether anesthesia and the kidney sought for through the condensed tissues resulting from the previous operation. These had developed notably, especially along the line of the sinus, and made it difficult to separate the kidney from the surrounding tissues; consequently the manipulations necessary to accomplish this were prolonged, and during this time the sac bled freely from its interior. Supposing that a vessel had been ruptured in some way I opened the sac widely and unavailingly sought for a vessel. The hemorrhage continued free and uncontrollable till I folded the liberated parts of the sac on themselves, and, grasping the mass firmly in my left hand, compressed it as one would a sponge. The wound cavity then being cleared of blood and

clots, the remaining adhesions were seen or felt, easily separated and the pedicle reached, cleared and clamped.

When removed from the body the kidney presented the usual appearance of hydronephrosis, being converted into a large, thin-walled sac, with some kidney tissue spread out upon its inner surface, but whether the process had begun in the pelvis or not it was impossible to say. The amount of hemorrhage from the thin and expanded kidney tissue was surpising, and the young man lost enough blood before it could be controlled to cause a very serious condition of collapse, from which he was rallied after the operation by copious hot saline enemata, hypodermics of strychnine, etc.

Prior to the operation he had been voiding from 450 to 500 c.c. of urine from the bladder. Within the first twenty-four hours after the operation there was a gradual increase in the volume of urine, until on the second day, he voided over 3,600 c.c., showing that the one kidney responded to the stimulus of the salines, and that it was competent to excrete a very large quantity of urine. After this his progress toward recovery was uneventful and he returned to his home in about two weeks in excellent condition.

The diseased kidney was sent to the Carnegie Laboratory for examination. Their findings are as follows: It was the seat of hydronephrosis. Microscopical examination reveals a subacute pyelitis, with destruction of the epithelial lining of the renal pelvis in some places where a granulation tissue had developed. The pyramids were atrophic as a result of the hydronephrosis. Within the kidney the arteries showed a considerable endarteritis, leading in a few places to a great diminution of the lumina of the vessels affected and to an atrophy of the renal cortex. There were also a few areas of round-cell infiltration in the cortex, but no suppuration or *tuberculosis* could be found. The epithelium lining the convoluted tubules had undergone some parenchymatous and fatty degeneration. No bacteria appeared to be associated with the lesions found, although there were some bacilli and a few cocci near the surface of the organ. They were probably accidental.

Among the chief causes of hydronephrosis given by authors are mentioned: An obstruction to the overflow from the kidney due to something developed in the kidney itself, as, for example, calculus or new growths. Secondly, such changes in the position of the kidney as disturb the relation of ureter to the kidney; and, thirdly, obstruction in the course of the ureter. Israel considers changes in the position of the kidney to be the most frequent cause of hydronephrosis, and that it can take place as the result of either abnormal mobility, or of a congenitally low situation of the kidney. At the time of the nephrotomy I satisfied myself that there was no calculus either in the kidney or its pelvis, and that there was no obstruction in the course of the ureter; but, as to any misplacement of the kidney excepting that it was not in the bony pelvis, its magnitude had so changed its relations that I am unable to say. An enlargement of the operation wound might have made this point clearer, but the patient's condition did not warrant this. The report of the laboratory eliminates the question of neoplasm, but throws no light upon the etiology. Nor does any analysis of the clinical history make the causation clear. The patient had had unusually good health from his infancy up; there was no history of traumatism; there was no history of renal colic or of pain located in his left side; and prior to the onset of the nausea and general malaise there was no symptom indicating the begining of his malady. When the blood first appeared in the urine is also vague and indefinite, for its presence seems not to have been noticed till the fact was stated by the first consultant.

The obstinate constipation of which the patient complained and which appeared to be the cause of more misery to him than any other symptom, was no doubt due to pressure of the renal tumor upon the descending colon; for he did not suffer from this after the nephrotomy had reduced the size of the tumor; but its early stage, probably being regarded as a common functional affection, was not noted and it also affords no clue. Therefore how long the hydronephrosis had existed and the cause of the latter there is no means of knowing.

The character of the hematuria in this case is worthy of some study. The presence of blood in the urine was intermittent and variable in quantity; the latter being increased by slight trauma, such as has been mentioned, i.e., jolting in a wagon, and by the manipulations of the kidney necessary to a diagnosis. It was also suddenly increased by unknown causes, but at no time was there a serious amount of blood in the urine. After the nephrotomy the blood which appeared from time to time was found only in the urinous fluid received through the drainage-tube, and only once was this fluid of a bloody color. I have analyzed the examinations made for nine months of the urine from the bladder and the sinus respectively and at no time did blood, even microscopically, appear in the bladder urine. Parenthetically it may be noted that this fact lends additional doubt as to the accuracy of the Harris separator, for it will be remembered, blood was found in the urine segregated by that instrument from both kidneys. The ureters were not catheterized at the outset because the diagnosis of tuberculosis had been made by a man of such reputation that I preferred to make the diagnosis by other means rather than to take a risk (even minute) of extending the infection.

The degree of hemorrhage during the extirpation of the expanded and attenuated kidney seems to me under the circumstances noteworthy. In my experience, even when deliberately and freely incising a fairly normal kidney for different operative purposes, and even when the manipulation of the incised kidney was prolonged, there never has been any loss of blood in such proportion as to jeopardize the patient. In this case there seemed to be very little kidney tissue left where the incision was made and the blood appeared to come from the interior of the sac and not from its cut edges.

In conclusion, let me add a fact in regard to this case which, though but remotely pertinent to the postoperative history, may have some interest. The patient regained excellent health and about a year after the nephrectomy made an application for life insurance. In due time the medical department of a life insurance company wrote me for an opinion as to the young man's "longevity." I could reply only that I had no opinion as to the longevity of a person with one kidney, but that I knew of patients who were well and comfortable and apparently living out their time with one kidney doing all the work.

20 East Forty-sixth Street.

TWO CASES OF TRACHEAL STENOSIS FROM NEW GROWTH.

BY GEORGE EMERSON BREWER, M.D.,

OF NEW YORK;

PROFESSOR OF CLINICAL SURGERY, COLLEGE OF PHYSICIANS AND SURGEONS (COLUMBIA UNIVERSITY); JUNIOR SURGEON TO THE ROOSEVELT HOSPITAL.

THE following two cases of tracheal stenosis, necessitating grave operative procedures for their relief, are reported for the reason that, in the writer's opinion, the conditions are sufficiently rare to make them of general interest to the profession.

Case I. Papilloma of the Trachea, following Tracheotomy, for the Relief of Papillomatous Degeneration of the Laryngeal Mucous Membrane.—F. B., aged eleven years, was admitted to the Roosevelt Hospital in July last. When five years of age he suffered from extensive papillomatous disease of the larynx, which interfered considerably with respiration. After unsuccessful local treatment an operation was advised by those in attendance. This was declined by the parents, and the condition grew steadily worse until the dyspnea became so severe that an emergency tracheotomy was performed. The tube was worn continuously for a number of months, during which time local treatment was applied to the laryngeal mucous membrane. Several attempts were made to remove the tube, but in each instance marked difficulty in breathing followed, necessitating its immediate replacement.

After consulting a number of surgeons and laryngologists, he finally came under the care of Dr. Frank E. Miller, of this city, who by persistent local treatment succeeded in removing the greater portion of the laryngeal growth. This, while it left a sufficient opening in the glottis for ordinary respiration, afforded no relief; for as soon as the tube was removed the dyspnea was extreme. It was evident that an obstruction existed in the trachea immediately above the opening for the canula; and, from the length of time that the canula had been worn, it was deemed probable that the obstruction was of cicatricial nature.

The boy's condition was poor, he was anemic, had a chronic bronchitis and was exceedingly thin. Around the tracheal opening there was an extensive area of dermatitis.

Operation was advised, and on July 5, under chloroform anesthesia, an incision was made in the median line extending from the body of the hyoid to the sternum. The trachea was exposed with considerable difficulty below the original tracheotomy wound, incised, and a new tube inserted. The soft parts were then removed from the anterior surface of the larynx and upper segment of the trachea. After all hemorrhage had been arrested the patient was placed in the Trendelenburg position and the larynx and trachea freely opened by a median incision, extending from the thyrohyoid membrane to the original opening for the tube. A solution of cocaine and adrenalin chloride was immediately applied to the cut surfaces and to the laryngeal and tracheal mucous membrane. The tracheal wall was next retracted, exposing its entire mucous lining. Immediately above the old tracheal opening there was found a large papillomatous mass completely plugging its lumen and attached by a comparatively small pedicle to the left side of the trachea. The mass was about the size of a large blackberry. It was easily removed and its point of attachment touched with the actual cautery. Several papillomatous masses on and below the vocal chords were also removed. A large rubber tube was then placed within the trachea, extending from the lower tracheal opening upward through the larynx into the pharynx. This was secured by a thread passed from its upper extremity upward through the mouth and tied to the right ear. The trachea was closed over this by one or two catgut sutures, the cutaneous wound partly closed and dressing applied.

The operation was followed by moderate shock. The rubber tube was coughed out at the end of six hours. The tracheal canula was removed at the end of thirty-six hours. No embarrassment of respiration followed its removal, and his convalescence was uneventful. The patient has gained rapidly in flesh and strength, is able to go to school, and although the voice has not returned completely, it is constantly improving.

In this case the condition of the patient had become so deteriorated from chronic bronchitis, loss of sleep, bad nutrition and his inability to mingle with other boys and engage in their sports, that I regarded the prognosis as grave.

Recognizing that the operation would be a difficult as well as a protracted one, several precautionary measures were taken to avoid some of the dangers incident to such a procedure in a feeble and anemic subject.   ·

Chloroform was used for anesthesia to diminish the chances of increased tracheal irritation and pneumonia, as well as to avoid postoperative vomiting. To enable the anesthetist to use a minimum amount of the drug, a large dose of morphine was given hypodermatically fifteen minutes before the chloroform was started. As a result of these measures, only a very small quantity of chloroform was used, and although the patient was completely under its influence for nearly an hour and three-quarters, there was no postoperative vomiting and no increase in the bronchial irritation or secretion.

A large incision was employed laying open the entire larynx and cervical portion of the trachea. This enabled us to see the entire extent of the disease and to recognize at once its point of attachment.

The use of cocaine and adrenalin on the mucous membrane, served in the first place to avoid the rapid fall of blood pressure and consequent symptoms of grave shock, which almost invariably follow contact with the mucous membrane on the interior of the larynx; it also produced a marked anemia of the tissues preventing extensive oozing of blood, and more clearly defined the pathological changes in the mucous membrane, thus enabling us more rapidly to eradicate the disease.

The Trendelenburg posture kept the pharyngeal mucus out of the wound and rendered aspiration of blood less probable. It also rendered the use of chloroform safer.

Following the operation, the tracheal tube, which was allowed to remain in the lower tracheal opening for thirty-six hours, was kept constantly covered with gauze wet in hot boric acid solution. This filtered and moistened the inspired air and may have diminished the chance of postoperative pneumonia.

Case II. Adeno-Carcinoma of an Accessory Thyroid Gland causing Marked Tracheal Stenosis. —J. R. H., a physician, aged fifty-two years, consulted the writer in March, 1904. Three years ago on exertion he first noticed a slight difficulty in breathing. He attributed this to lack of exercise and progressively increasing body-weight. Some months later it was noticed that there occurred occasional attacks of rather pronounced dyspnea, always following some unusual exertion. Believing that the trouble was asthmatic in character, his treatment consisted of the usual remedies for this condition. During the six months preceding his first visit to the writer the difficulty in breathing had greatly increased, the dyspnea becoming almost continuous. At certain times it was intense and accompanied by cyanosis. This so interfered with his work that he at last consulted Dr. Francis J. Quinlan, of this city, who, on examination with the laryngoscope, readily detected a very decided encroachment upon the caliber of the trachea by an oval mass apparently springing from the right half of the tracheal wall. This tumor was smooth, oval, and covered, apparently, with healthy mucous membrane. It left a semilunar tracheal aperture about a quarter of an inch in diameter. The patient was also seen in consultation by Dr. Holbrook Curtis, who verified the diagnosis and referred him to the writer for treatment.

In addition to the above findings, the writer noticed a very slight bulging at the root of the neck, to the right and just above the sternoclavicular articulation. On deep palpation, a hard, oval mass was felt extending into the mediastinum. Moderate pressure on the mass caused an immediate increase in the dyspnea, and a greater degree of pressure produced absolute tracheal obstruction. From these findings, the diagnosis was made of an extratracheal tumor producing a marked indentation of the right wall of the trachea.

As a course of potassium iodide had already been tried without any improvement, an immediate operation was advised.

During the following four or five days, while the patient was arranging his affairs preparatory to entering the hospital, the dyspnea was markedly increased. He was unable to lie down, and on the night before entering the hospital his symptoms were so urgent that a brother physician passed the night in his house administering oxygen and stimulants freely. On the following afternoon he was again seen at the hospital by the writer, in consultation with Drs. Quinlan and Curtis. The symptoms were so urgent at that time that it was decided to operate immediately, as it was feared he would not survive until the following morning when an operation was planned.

In view of the alarming dyspnea and the difficulties of the operation, it was decided to entrust the anesthesia to Dr. Thomas L. Bennett, who promptly responded and administered chloroform. The patient at first took the anesthetic kindly, but as soon as the position of the head was changed to allow the performance of a preliminary tracheotomy, the dyspnea became extreme, an alarmingly and extreme degree of cyanosis developed.

An incision was made in the median line from the cricoid to the suprasternal notch, and thence continued downward toward the right in a curved direction for about three inches. The tissues overlying the trachea were rapidly divided and retracted, until the isthmus of the thyroid was exposed. This occupied practically the entire space between the cricoid and the sternum, and was exceedingly voluminous and highly vascular. Considerable delay was caused by the application of a number of mass ligatures, so that the thyroid tissues could be divided to expose the trachea. While this was in progress the patient ceased to breathe and the skin became livid. As the cut surface of the thyroid was bleeding profusely, it seemed unwise to make an attempt to open the trachea, which was pushed well to the

left by a large encapsulated tumor which lay beneath the thyroid gland, partly within and partly above the mediastinum. About a minute and a half was consumed in controlling the hemorrhage, during which time respiration was completely arrested. As soon as the hemorrhage was controlled the trachea was opened and an attempt made to introduce a tube. Owing to the narrowness of the lumen, only the smallest-sized infant tube could be introduced. Respiration was at once re-established, and the patient's color improved. The thyroid and other tissues were gradually dissected away from the tumor, which was found to be completely encapsulated, and to lie closely adherent to the trachea, the esophagus, the recurrent laryngeal nerve, the jugular and the innominate veins, and the innominate artery.

About one hour was consumed in dissecting the tumor free from these structures. The wound was then partly closed, a large gauze drain being left in its middle third, with the view to keeping the wound open and exposing the tracheal wall for subsequent X-ray treatment in case a histological examination revealed any signs of malignancy.

The patient's recovery was prompt, and, aside from a short period of idodoform poisoning, it was uneventful. Laryngoscopic examination showed a paralysis of the right vocal cord, but a great increase in the lumen of the trachea. The vocal paralysis was undoubtedly due to division of the recurrent laryngeal nerve. On examination, the tumor proved to be an adenoma, probably of an accessory thyroid, and it showed in places slight changes suggesting carcinomatous degeneration.

In this case the tracheotomy was by far the most difficult and hazardous part of the operation. As the patient was stout and had a short thick neck, as soon as the position of the head was changed to allow an exposure of the trachea, the tumor seemed to be forced against the tracheal wall and to produce complete obstruction. As the entire lower segment of the cervical portion of the trachea was covered by an exceedingly thick and vascular thyroid isthmus, this had to be divided between numerous ligatures before the trachea could be exposed low enough to allow the tube to pass the point of greatest obstruction.

As all of this had to be done after the patient had ceased to breathe, and as the cyanosis was extreme, it was difficult to resist the temptation to plunge at once into the trachea before the bleeding had been completely arrested. I am convinced, however, that had this been done before we had an absolutely dry wound, death would have immediately resulted, for had blood in any amount been drawn into the trachea it could not have been expelled by coughing through the small tube we were obliged to employ.

THE MANAGEMENT OF ACUTE GENERAL PERITONITIS.[1]

BY J. GARLAND SHERRILL, A.M., M.D.,
OF LOUISVILLE, KY.

Two forms of this affection are to be recognized clinically; the first, acute septic peritonitis, in which the poison is so intense that the patient dies from a profound toxemia before the local changes have progressed to the point of pus formation. Such cases follow perforating wounds of the intestines, perforation from typhoid ulcer, and ulcer of the stomach, gangrene and ulceration of the appendix, rupture of the urinary or the gall bladder, acute cholecystitis, ileus, puerperal infection, and less frequently disease of the ovary and tubes. The latter conditions are more often followed by a localized type of inflammation, as a result, perhaps, of a less virulent form of infection and because of the partial isolation of the pelvic structures from the other abdominal viscera.

The second type is general suppurative peritonitis in which pus is found free in the peritoneal cavity without any localization of the process, and the term should not be strictly limited to inflammation of the entire serous surface. This form may follow any of the causes mentioned above, but is especially prone to result from rupture of an appendicular or other abscess into the cavity. It would seem that these cases go on to suppuration because of a partial immunity which has developed during the time the causative abscess has been forming, which increases the local repsonse to the irritant and causes the disease to be prolonged sufficiently for pus formation to occur. Notwithstanding the possibility of such resistance to the infection these cases must always be considered as very grave. While they may not be so rapidly fatal, as the septic type, they are exceedingly likely to terminate in the same way.

To account for the difference in these two forms as regards toxemia, we must take into consideration the absorptive power of the peritoneal surface. This large lymph sac has great absorbing capacity, and when the more intense infections obtain entrance, the chemical products are very rapidly carried into the circulation, but when a local reaction is excited by the presence of a less virulent infection, the lymph channels become choked with leucocytes and just in proportion to this obstruction is absorption diminished. Finally, as suppuration occurs numbers of leucocytes, lymph, and serum appear on the membrane accompanied by an exfoliation of the epithelium, and it is possible that here again an absorbent surface is present. It would seem probable then that the suppurative cases are the more favorable ones for treatment. It has been claimed by very many competent observers, that septic peritonitis cases all die, and that post-operative cases are likewise always fatal, yet there are on record

a number of cases of recovery from operation done for the relief of these conditions, notably; Hintze reports two successful operations for postoperative peritonitis.

We are forced to admit that many cases, especially of the septic type, will die, no matter how soon they are seen, nor what plan of treatment is adopted. On the other hand, we may safely claim that there is a large proportion of cases which can be relieved by surgical interference, and some which can be conducted to a favorable issue by medical means alone. That the latter is successful in any large number of cases, we cannot admit, but when we consider that every case begins at a local point of infection, it is certainly true that medical measures are effective in some cases in keeping the process limited to a local inflammation. In offering this paper, I make no claim to present anything new, but do so with a desire to elicit from a discussion of this most interesting subject some ground upon which those who hold very widely different views can meet and formulate some reasonable plan of treatment which, with slight modification to suit individual cases, can be generally adopted by the profession. With the best authorities at variance upon a subject of this importance, the average practitioner is left quite at sea. The first question for consideration is, whether medical treatment or surgery offers most to these unfortunate individuals. Prior to 1843, when Volz advised the use of opium in these cases, the results were uniformly bad. This plan of treatment, first urged upon the profession of this country by Alonzo Clark, showed a considerably lower rate of mortality than the former methods in use, and was almost exclusively followed, until Tait urged the administration of salines to drain the inflamed peritoneum, and brought about another radical change in the treatment. The opium treatment is based upon the idea that by preventing peristalsis, adhesions form between the intestines, leakage is diminished, and tissue resistance can overcome the infection. The second plan is founded upon a radically different idea, namely, that in inflammation of the general peritoneum, salines remove offending material from the intestine and cause rapid removal of fluids from the blood, and an equally rapid elimination from the peritoneal cavity of the poison produced by the mycotic growth. More recently there has been a tendency to the rest treatment of inflammatory conditions within the abdomen, largely as the result of the stand taken by Ochsner in the treatment of appendicitis. He claims to get a quiet intestine, and the relief of pain by emptying the stomach, allowing nothing to be taken into its lumen, and avoiding the bad effects of opium. such as meteorism, constipation, and diminished kidney secretion. Others are using opium for the pain and salines to move the bowels, and are giving some food by the mouth. We find, therefore, three distinct plans of treatment, each of

[1] Read before the Southern Surgical and Gynecological Society.

which has been perhaps of benefit in some cases. As to which of these is best in cases where surgery is not indicated, or will not be permitted, it is difficult to determine. Ochsner's statistics seem to show the lowest mortality when the disease follows appendicitis.

I must confess that my cases have usually been considered surgical; therefore, I cannot deny his claims. I can see the advantage to be gained by relieving the stomach of the highly toxic fluids which are carried into it by reverse peristalsis, but I can more readily perceive the benefit to be obtained from a brisk purge in non-perforative cases and as well after a perforation has been closed by operation. It is generally admitted that this is a bacterial disease, frequently due to perforation of the alimentary canal, or to rupture of an abscess, various forms of organisms being found in different cases. The claim is justifiable that in the inception this is always a local infection, and in the large majority of cases its prompt recognition places it within the domain of surgery. Medical treatment is then indicated only in those cases where surgical aid is refused by the patient and in those in which the grave condition of the patient renders it likely that an operation will remove the slight chance remaining for recovery. In cases seen early, where operation is refused, it is exceedingly important before medical treatment is commenced, to determine if possible the causative lesion. In many cases this cannot be done, but careful attention to the history and symptomatology will in a majority of the cases enable the attendant to reach a conclusion upon which he may plan a logical course of treatment. In order to make clear this point, it will be necessary to distinguish not only between perforative and non-perforative cases, but also between perforations of the stomach and those of the intestine. We will therefore consider the form due to perforating ulcer of the stomach from a medical view point. The first importance should be given to absolute rest of the stomach, no lavage, no food, no medicine, no water nor anything else being allowed. An enema to unload the lower bowel and relieve meteorism should be used. Colon lavage can be safely employed, if necessary, followed by nutriment enemata as indicated. If there is reason to believe that the rupture is posterior, the hips and the shoulders as well can be raised, with a view to retain the process in the smaller sac of the peritoneum, as recommended by Lennander. The employment of heat or cold locally can be tried here as in all other varieties.

When the rupture is lower in the alimentary canal, and in cases of obstruction where there is danger or possibility of a rupture, gastric lavage can be safely employed, but purgation, and even large enemata are very dangerous. One case coming under my care with rupture from a blow was lost, probably because of injudicious efforts to cleanse the lower bowel, none of the fluid re-

turning. Absolutely nothing should enter the stomach after it has been thoroughly cleansed. Small enemata of concentrated solution of sulphate of magnesia with glycerin can be used to empty the rectum, and small nutriment enemata administered at proper intervals. If opium has any place in the treatment of peritonitis it is in a case of this kind, and it can be given quite fearlessly. The patient should be placed in a position of simply recumbency.

In cases following puerperal infection, surgical operation, the rupture of an abscess, and rupture of the appendix, a very different plan of treatment should be employed. Rupture of the appendix has been included under this division because the appendix which ruptures is in the vast majority of cases one whose lumen has become to a great extent isolated from the bowel, owing to the great swelling of the lymphoid tissue, or on account of torsion, or in some instances from cicatricial contraction. In favor of this view is the fact that one of the prominent factors in the production of inflammation of the appendix is an admitted inability of the organ to empty itself. Therefore, the danger following a ruptured appendix is not from fecal extravasation, but from the contained bacterial flora. There being little danger then of further increase in the dosage of the poison, I believe we are justified in the use of purgatives in this condition and in ruptured abscess and postoperative cases as well. It appears to me to be good practice to obtain a clean alimentary tract in cases of this character, because a prolific course of infection can be removed by elimination of the feces, also by causing a rapid osmosis from the peritoneal cavity without increased danger. My attention has been drawn to the acridity of the feces by some cases of large appendicular abscess of more than one week's standing in which a communication existed with the lumen of the cecum. After the abscess had been opened and its cavity cleansed, I have noted that the discharging feces was so poisonous that it produced marked sloughing of the wound margin. This sloughing only subsided when the alimentary canal had been thoroughly flushed by a brisk purge. The contention then seems reasonable that in cases where there is no leaking intestine, the treatment by gastric and rectal lavage and brisk saline catharsis is indicated. I do not mean to say that in all cases we can certainly exclude a leaking bowel, but when we can do so this should be our plan. I would especially urge that in the management of these cases, routine treatment should be eliminated as nearly as possible. It is extremely doubtful whether in any one of these forms of peritonitis topical applications, other than heat or cold, ever do any good. Leeching has some advocates and is perhaps worthy of a trial. In cases due to streptococcic infection, as shown by the presence of the organism in the blood, anti-streptococcic serum should be tried. Careful stimulation should be given for all.

In considering the surgical treatment of this subject, much stress should be placed upon operation as a measure for the prevention of general peritonitis. In the largest number of cases, prompt interference for the relief of any of the causative conditions before the serosa is soiled, or while the peritonitis is still confined to a limited portion of the membrane, offers the best chance of recovery.

Then, in all cases save where the two conditions already mentioned prevent operation, a section is indicated. The outcome of a given case will depend upon the following factors without reference to the special steps in the operation or the subsequent care, viz., (1) the virulence of the infection; (2) the quantity of the infecting medium, as extravasation from the bowel, or the amount of pus from a ruptured abscess; (3) the resistance of the patient, a factor never to be overlooked and rarely to be correctly estimated; (4) the activity of the organs of elimination, which in many instances can be fairly accurately determined and thus become an aid in prognosis; (5) the time at which the patient comes to operation after the poison enters the cavity; (6) the dexterity and thoroughness of the surgical procedure, no matter what is the special method of the operator in attempting to reach the desired end. Of all the factors mentioned only four come directly under the control of the surgeon. The amount of the poison may to some extent be lessened by early recognition and prompt interference. The time following infection then is of the greatest importance, and we can all agree that the sooner after the shock of a perforation is combatted, the operation is performed, the better the patient's chances, other things being equal. The power of elimination can be markedly stimulated and therefore is to some extent under the control of the surgeon. The sixth factor is also of great importance, and whatever the technic selected I should urge rapid but thorough work with the minimum amount of traumatism.

In the technic again we find a wide difference of opinion. How is it possible to reconcile the claims of the school, Finney and others, who do not believe in irrigating the abdominal cavity, but rely upon sponging to take up the infectious material, with those of another school who simply open and drain, doing nothing further, or with those of the third school, Deaver, Price, Blake and others, who advise the free use of hot saline solutions? These views are apparently so different that to reconcile them would seem impossible, yet the object of each is to free the patient of the noxious material and allow him to combat the poison already absorbed. By keeping this in mind, we can readily see that one operator reached success by carefully sponging loop after loop of intestines and also the spaces where fluids are so prone to collect, while the other uses water to remove the pus and bacteria, believing that in this way he can best accomplish

the end desired. Those who open the abdomen and drain without sponging or irrigation, are evidently of the opinion that any further surgery in cases where this plan is used would be immediately fatal and therefore hope to accomplish something from the incomplete surgery, thus making the best of a bad state of affairs.

It is scarcely my purpose to defend one plan of surgery and to decry another in these cases, believing that there are others who are specially equipped with facts to defend the positions which they have taken upon this subject. Yet I cannot refrain from commenting upon those who advocate sponging, and argue that irrigation tends to scatter the fluid containing the organisms and their toxins widely through the cavity, thus favoring further absorption; to some extent this criticism is just, especially when the irrigation is incompletely done. I believe also that the toxins are likely to be absorbed more rapidly when diluted with water; so that this danger should always be borne in mind to urge us to be most thorough in this flushing. On the other hand, those who irrigate claim that to obtain a perfect peritoneal toilet by sponging, it is necessary to subject the peritoneum to a great amount of trauma, thus adding greatly to the shock, and favoring the rapid passage into the blood not only of toxins, but of micro-organisms themselves.

These are matters of judgment to be decided by the individual operator. Personally, I feel that I can cleanse an abdomen, which is the seat of this form of inflammation, better by flushing than in any other way, and have found that my more recent results are better than former ones, simply because I do my work in a more thorough and systematic manner.

I am no longer content to flush only the pelvis, a very satisfactory procedure after the enucleation of a tubal or ovarian abscess, but irrigate in each loin and under the liver as well. Often surprise has been expressed at the amount of pus brought out after a large quantity of clear fluid had returned from pelvic irrigation. It appears to me that we must give more attention in these cases to the condition of the lesser peritoneal cavity, which in some cases will require flushing and drainage. After the irrigation, a large gauze sponge should be used to take up the fluid remaining in the abdomen, and this step may be repeated just before the wound is closed. Some operators fill the abdomen with saline solution, but I think this of little benefit when a drain is used. We cannot claim that either sponging or irrigation renders the cavity absolutely sterile, as experiments upon animals have shown this to be impossible. Yet the amount and virulence of the infection may be so diminished that many of these patients recover. Drainage is almost universally used, although Blake concludes it is often unnecessary. It can do very little harm and may save life in some instances. A number of gauze drains surrounded by rubber may be inserted in the pelvis and other portions of the abdomen where fluid tends to collect, and a posterior drain may also be used. Glass or ordinary fenestrated rubber tubes are preferred by some to the use of gauze. I have had recovery in some cases in which a single gauze drain allowed the removal of only a small quantity of serum, and am therefore convinced that the result depends more upon the thorough manner in which the toilet is made and the lesions repaired, than upon any special form or number of drains. Some operators inject solution of sulphated magnesia into the intestine during the operation and claim very beneficial results. The Fowler position will be found useful in many of these cases. The patient should have the usual treatment given all abdominal cases, should be carefully stimulated and should have no opiates unless demanded by great restlessness.

My individual experience has been that these patients fare as well with morphine as when it is not given. This impression may obtain because the more serious cases are the ones which demand morphine. If the patient ceases to vomit and the abdomen becomes flat, I do not hasten to administer a purge, and when vomiting and distention persist, purgation rarely relieves, although it deserves a trial. The convalescence may be interrupted by the formation of localized collections of pus which must be evacuated and the cases conducted in accordance with general surgical principles. Cases in which the pus shows streptococci should receive the serum. Very little mention has been made of the septic form of peritonitis (acute peritoneal sepsis of Mayo Robson) because it can only be suspected from the extreme toxemia and is usually positively recognized only after the death of the patient.

At its very onset, the pathology is identical with the suppurative form, and the only hope for the patient lies in the removal of the cause and the prevention of new infection by operation. The extreme gravity of such cases might tempt the surgeon to refuse operation, yet for the individual patient surgery is the only hope, and unless he is moribund should receive this chance.

In conclusion, these cases should be considered surgical with the two exceptions above mentioned. Operation should be done as a preventive measure before peritoneal infection and as soon after its occurrence as is possible, in some instances of prolonged shock before reaction is complete. The operation should be done as rapidly as is consistent with thoroughness, and above all things, we would urge that incomplete surgery be not done. Each surgeon must determine for himself how he can best free the peritoneum from infection, and he must realize that in the great majority of these cases the fate of the patient is determined when he leaves the table.

THE CLINICAL MANIFESTATIONS OF UTERINE FIBROIDS, AS INDICATIONS FOR EARLY OPERATIVE INTERVENTION.[1]

BY ARNOLD STURMDORF, M.D.,
OF NEW YORK.

IT is neither my object, nor within my time limit, to encumber this introductory discourse with anything approaching a complete and detailed enumeration of the various manifestations —immediate and remote—local and general—that constitute clinical indications for radical intervention in uterine fibroids: but rather to touch in a general way upon certain phases in this relation to the subject, on which our knowledge has been amplified and our conceptions cleared.

Modern research brings many demonstrated facts into striking contrast with older fancies, and in the study of uterine fibroids, has shed much light that has not as yet found diffusion in the general medical atmosphere. But long strides in our knowledge and mastery of this disease span a comparatively short time-interval, and the accumulated literature, though voluminous, is as yet so scattered that it is difficult, unless specially interested, to obtain a comprehensive view of the present status of this subject.

Barely two decades have elapsed, since a prohibitive mortality prompted Skene and others in this country, Keith, Schröder and Winckel abroad, to express themselves as follows:

" Uterine fibroids present a self-limited disease which rather torments than kills, in which every palliative means demands trial; and only when hemorrhage becomes uncontrollable, the progress rapid, with cystic or suppurative changes, health ruined or life endangered, can operation be justified."

Of every hundred women operated upon at that time eighty-five died, and Emmet, Sr., wrote: " Seeing the results of operation, no surgeon is justified in attempting to remove the uterus for the growth of a fibrous tumor, except as a forlorn hope."

To-day, the results of operative treatment for this condition constitute one of the most brilliant achievements of American surgery, and no woman, afflicted with uterine fibroids and subjected to modern operative technic, should lose her life—if operated at the proper time.

Unfortunately, however, the authoritative condemnation of operative intervention and the deplorable doctrines promulgated twenty years ago, continue to dominate a certain proportion of the medical mind, and this, notwithstanding that we have since learned, that these growths, while histologically benign, possess a clinical malignancy peculiarly their own; that they are not self-limited; that a climacteric millennium is a delusion and often indeed a snare; that they can kill as well torment, by inducing local and constitutional conditions hitherto unrecognized; and lastly that to the present time, all palliative ther-

[1] Being the introductory discourse in a Symposium on Uterine Fibroids held before the Medical Society of the County of New York at the New York Academy of Medicine, November 28, 1904.

would have lost their lives, had they not submitted to operation.

The actual list of death recorded from unoperated uterine fibroids, contrary to the general impression, is very long and instructive.

E. Stanmore Bishop, in a recent volume on this subject, published such a series of fatalities, carefully detailed from authentic accessible sources, presenting cases, in which death supervened as a direct result of the unoperated growth.

Gervis[1] published a case showing a large submucous fibroid, which had sloughed suddenly and completely, without obvious cause or premonitory symptoms.

There was double pyosalpinx and one tube had ruptured causing fatal peritonitis.

Lediard[2] reports patient with large abdominal tumor, causing dorsalgia, metrorrhagia and gastric disturbances accompanied by rise of temperature. Death after nine days of observation. Autopsy revealed miliary abscesses of recent development of both kidneys and infarcts of spleen.

Tait[3] reports patient aged thirty-four years, who died without operation. Post mortem revealed uterus as a black sloughing mass.

Lediard[4] reports fibrocystic myoma reaching $2\frac{1}{2}$ inches above uterus. After examination by sound, peritonitis; death on ninth day; autopsy: Both ovaries partly cystic, miliary abscesses in kidneys, spleen soft, enlarged, several recent infarcts, liver fatty, lungs edematous.

Edis[5] reports patient aged thirty-nine years. Amenorrhea for two months nine months ago, followed by flooding without warning. Soft and resilient tumor felt in posterior cul-de-sac; rigor, acute general peritonitis; death. Post mortem reveals general purulent peritonitis; both Fallopian tubes thickened and distended. Both ovaries contained small abscesses. The tumor in Douglas's pouch was a soft fibroid containing several small cysts.

Cotter[6] showed a subperitoneal fibroid removed after death. Patient aged forty-five years: diffuse suppurative peritonitis, much fetid pus, adherent intestines. Tumor attached to posterior surface of uterus by a short thick pedicle.

Favell[7] reports a case where the patient died from sudden profuse hemorrhage.

Bigonin[8] showed a uterine fibroid, involving the entire uterus. Patient aged thirty-eight years. Had noticed tumor for ten years. Two days before coming under observation she struck her hypogastrium against the edge of a table. On admission, violent pains and vomiting, abdominal distention; temperature 100° F.; death. Post mortem; Abdomen full of blood, from a large rent in the back of the tumor mass.

Lee Dickinson[9] reports patient aged forty-eight years, single. Growth noticed twelve

1 Trans. Obst. Soc., Lond. July 4, 1883.
2 British Medical Journal, 1883, Vol. 2, p. 941.
3 British Medical Journal, 1883, Vol. 2, p. 1076.
4 British Medical Journal, 1884, Vol. 2, p. 372.
5 British Medical Journal, 1888, Vol. 2, p. 940.
6 British Medical Journal, Vol. 1, p. 194.
7 British Medical Journal, Vol. 2, p. 1139.
8 Nouv. Arch. d'Obstet. et de Gynecol., April, 1892.
9 Lancet, London, Vol. I, p. 22.

months, grew rapidly during last twenty-seven days. Death from exhaustion due to hemorrhage and pressure symptoms. Post mortem: Tumor in anterior wall of uterus. Externally, both macro- and microscopical characteristics of a fibroid. Centrally soft and yellow.

This central portion had broken down into the cervical canal and through the posterior wall of uterus into the peritoneal cavity, forming a spouting hemorrhagic growth which filled the pelvis and extended upward into the left iliac fossa, surrounding and compressing the sigmoid flexure.

Sheard[1] reports a calcified subperitoneal tumor found after death from apoplexy.

Gouget[2] reports a broad ligament fibroid causing death by uraemia, hydronephrosis and atrophic interstitial nephritis.

Schletelig[3] reports death without operation from general chronic peritonitis. Pus under intestinal adhesions. Fibroma of broad ligament.

Cullingworth[4] reports widow, aged fifty-five years, with chronic constipation and attacks of severe abdominal pain. Menopause at fifty-three. Admitted to St. Thomas' Hospital October 8 for intestinal obstruction. Moribund on admission and died same evening. Post mortem: Rectum flattened and obstructed by uterine myoma; tumor adherent to pelvic wall and slightly to rectum. Entire colon distended; the cecal wall had given way and feces escaped into the abdomen. (St. Thomas' Hospital reports. 1895, p. 412): Woman admitted with large sloughing fibroid; septicemia; death.

Tarnier reports five pregnant women suffering from fibroids who died before delivery.

Kelly[5] reports case of woman, aged forty-five years, myoma of uterus with central necrosis; dilated ureters, pyelonephritis, emphysema of lungs, general marasmus; cardiac hypertrophy with hyaline fatty and calcareous degeneration. Death without operation.

Baldy mentions two deaths while undergoing treatment by ergot.

Thornley Stokes[6] mentions a case of a woman, aged thirty-four years, who died in syncope while waiting to be operated upon.

Henry Morris, quoted by Bishop, reports a case of uterine fibroid causing intermittent retention of urine. Double pyosalpinx and left ovarian abscess. Dilatation of ureters; acute double nephritis, purulent peritonitis; death.

Lombe Atthill[7] showed at a meeting of the Pathological Society, at Dublin, two large fibroids removed post mortem from a woman who died suddenly. Pus was found in the substance of the uterus and she lost her life from a resulting septic embolic pneumonia.

Hogan reports a case of pregnancy in a fibroid uterus. Rupture at the fourth month; death.

1 British Medical Journal, 1890, Vol. 1, p. 462.
2 Bull. Soc., Anal. d. Paris, 1892, p. 222.
3 Arch. für Gynec. u. Geb., Bd. 1, p. 425.
4 Trans. Obstet. Soc., Lond., 1897, Vol. 39.
5 Operative Gynecology, Vol. 2, p. 539.
6 British Medical Journal, 1881, Vol. 1, p. 195.
7 British Medical Journal, 1881, Vol. 2, p. 1058.

Finlay[1] reports patient, single, aged fifty-nine years. Had noticed an intra-abdominal tumor for fifteen years. It had caused no special trouble until quite recently, when it rapidly enlarged. She died of acute peritonitis shortly after coming under observation. At the necropsy, a smooth, encapsulated, globular tumor, the size of a fetal head at term, was found attached to the fundus uteri by a short narrow pedicle. Its summit was in a state of incipient disintegration. In this vicinity several coils of small intestines were adherent, one of which was perforated by a spur of the neoplasm. The adjacent part of the bladder was similarly affected. The rest of the tumor presented the appearance of a soft fibromyoma. An ordinary subperitoneal "fibroid," the size of a walnut, was attached to the right side of the uterus posteriorly. The cervical mucosa presented several small mucous polypi. Secondary nodules were found in the base of the right lung, in the wall of the left ventricle of the heart, in the left kidney and in the infraclavicular lymph glands on the left side. On histological examination the uterine tumor proved a myosarcoma, in which groups of round and spindle-shaped cells were interspersed with fibrous tracts containing unstriped muscle cells. The secondary growths were of similar structure, only the round-celled elements were more abundant.

Royal College of Surgeons' Museum—No. 4639. Woman aged thirty-six years. Twelve months before death noticed a hard lump in the right hypochondriac and lumbar regions. Owing to the length and flexibility of the pedicle, the tumor appeared during his life-time to be quite free from the uterus. The catamenia were normal till four months before death, which took place twelve hours after giving birth to a four months' fetus. The abortion was preceded by peritonitis and high temperature for several days. The tumor, a large one, was subperitoneal, springing from the back and left side of the fundus. Tumor measured ten by five inches, the pedicle was four inches long, 1½ inches broad, one-third inch thick.

No. 4642. Two calcified uterine fibromyomata. One large kidney-shaped mass, seven inches long by 3½ inches wide, composed of hard yellow earth substance deposited irregularly through a tough fibrous tissue; the external surface is minutely nodular and rough. It is invested with a thin capsule of fibro-cellular tissue, to which the adjacent abdominal organs are adherent. Several coils of intestines are attached, not by their free surfaces, but by their mesentery, and it would appear that any attempt to remove the tumor would have very injuriously interfered with the blood supply of these coils. The uterus was said to be ossified, probably because it has smaller tumors of the same kind in its walls. One such growth, closely attached to its wall, was connected by a strong band to the

1 British Medical Journal, 1883, Vol. 1, 459.

first tumor; a coil of intestine was acutely strangulated by this band, and was the immediate cause of death.

*St. George's Hospital Museum.—*No. 1411. Woman, aged forty-seven years, admitted in a dying state, and expired a few days afterward. She had suffered from symptoms of polypus uteri for eight years. No means had been taken to remove the tumor. Other fibrous tumors were embedded in the uterine walls. The vagina was considerably dilated, its lining membrane inflamed, and covered with mucopurulent secretion. The lower and anterior surface of the tumor was much ulcerated. The tumor itself lay in the vagina, and was attached above to the internal wall of the uterus by a long pedicle. Both ovaries were healthy. (Post mortem and Case Book, 1848, p. 5).

No. 14r. Case of death without operation from peritonitis resulting from an abscess between vagina and bladder. Woman, aged forty years. Two tumors, one the size of a tangerine in anterior wall, one the size of a cocoanut in posterior wall. The weight of the posterior tumor had caused introversion of uterus and the mass had pressed upon and caused serious obstruction of ureters. (Post mortem and Case Book, 1870, No. 342). Body fairly nourished and in good condition. Both pleuræ covered toward the bases with recent lymph and in the cavities was a considerable amount of fluid. No false passage leading from the urethra could be discovered. Pelves of kidneys and ureters were extremely dilated, surfaces granular and cysts existed in the cortices. Capsule very adherent.

14w. Uterus greatly distended by fibromyomata, enlarged to size of seven months' pregnancy. Jane S., aged thirty-five years, died in the hospital July 23, 1882. For six years menstruation had been profuse and painful and for three years the abdomen had been increasing in size. Three weeks before death, the patient was seized with severe burning pain in the sacral region, hips, and hypogastrium, and the discharge, which had simply been mucus, became brown and offensive (for six months a thick, yellow discharge). A soft mass was now discharged from the vagina. On examination a firm fleshy mass was seen protruding from between the labia; this filled up the vagina and could be traced into the os, where many more were felt. These were apparently loose, and were removed by the hand. They were blackish and horribly offensive. The patient suffered much from vomiting. Large masses of foul, sloughing organized matter were occasionally discharged from the vagina, and the patient sank. Post mortem: The abdominal cavity was found occupied by a large tumor reaching from liver to pubes, which proved to be the uterus altered as described. There were some flakes of recent lymph in the peritoneal cavity. All the other organs were natural. (Post mortem and Case Book, 1862, p. 200). Body corpulent, belly swollen, feet and ankles edematous. Heart flabby, valves natural. Lungs healthy. Ovaries and tubes healthy. Spleen rather large; contained a small fibrinous block. Intestines and folds of peritoneum were glued together by flakes of recent lymph. Death.

*St. Bartholomew's Hospital Museum.—*No. 1887. Cavity of uterus greatly enlarged and filled with retained blood. Anterior portion of tumor solid; forms about two-thirds of the whole mass. Left Fallopian tubes much thickened and dilated in its outer part. This was 12 inches long and contains blood. Anterior portion consisted of large tumor, measuring seven inches anteroposteriorly; was everywhere encapsulated by the wall of the uterus, except posteriorly where the cavity of the tumor opened into the cavity of the uterus by an oval aperture, five inches vertical by $3\frac{1}{2}$ inches transverse diameter. The wall of the uterus at this point was $2\frac{1}{2}$ inches thick below and $1\frac{1}{4}$ inches above. Immediately beneath the capsule is a layer of calcareous deposit. The whole of the central portion of the tumor is broken down, forming a large irregular cavity, filled with putty-like blood. Cause of hemorrhage was not discovered. Death without operation.

2960b. Woman, aged thirty-four years, admitted for difficulty in micturition and defecation of two years' duration. A rounded mass felt in the abdomen reaching to the level of umbilicus and continuous with a hard, thick, nodular tumor, which was discovered per vaginam to occupy the whole pelvic cavity and extend on to the perineum. Exploratory laparotomy. Patient died of peritonitis. Post mortem: Tumor found in condition of suppuration.

*Guy's Hospital Museum.—*2271.90. A large fibrous polypus distending the uterus. The tumor led to considerable hemorrhage. It projected through the os uteri, and the extremity of it was ligatured. The hemorrhage ceased but the patient eventually sank.

2275.80. Woman, aged forty-four years, in 1887, married, several children. Five years before was seized with severe hemorrhage. This continued at intervals, when in 1887 the attacks were more frequent. A profuse hemorrhage at last proved fatal. There was no other disease in the body (Guy's Hospital, Vol. 3, p. 143).

These are cases in which death supervened as a direct result of the unoperated growth. But *indirectly,* uterine fibroids are responsible for many more. Winckel's statistics show that in about 10 per cent. of *all* cases death ensues after a variable period.

These direct and indirect causes of death from unoperated uterine fibroids may, for convenience of illustration, be divided into five categories, whose order of frequency is as follows: (1) Pathological conditions induced in the adnexa; (2) structural changes or degenerations in the tumor; (3) compression or dislocation of adjacent viscera; (4) general metabolic, cardiovascular and renal changes *not* due to pressure, in fact, occurring frequently with tumors of insignificant dimensions; (5) pregnancy.

Pathological conditions of the adnexa, that is, salpingitis with or without ovaritis, eventuating in pyosalpinx or ovarian abscess, constitute one of the most frequent of fatal complications.

Twombly[1] estimated that 50 per cent. of interstitial fibroids were complicated with affected tubes. Meredith[2] states, that an analysis of Tait's cases showed 54 per cent. of tubal and 46 per cent. of ovarian disease. In this connection Bishop observes: " It has appeared to me to be more frequently seen, when previous treatment of a so-called palliative kind such as curettage was employed."

It is generally recognized, that even simple adnexal infections yield a grave ultimate prognosis.

Complicating uterine fibroids they furnish the largest contingent of fatalities in unoperated cases, while they dominate the immediate and remote prognosis in those operated upon.

Structural changes and degenerations within the tumor, are manifestations of an inherent tendency in some forms of these growths, and although second in order of frequency to adnexal complications, represent the most rapidly fatal incidents occurring in the course of uterine fibroids.

I will only allude to the cancerous, the edematous, the cystic and the telangiectatic degeneration with its thrombotic concomitants, to dwell with some emphasis on the marked vulnerability to necrobiotic changes displayed by these tumors, the result of their precarious circulatory conditions.

This circulatory arrangement in uterine fibroids presents an extremely meager arterial supply, abruptly drained by spacious venous channels devoid of valves; the resulting retardation of the scant blood current is further augmented by the suppression of the rhythmical uterine contractions which, under normal conditions, maintain its circulatory balance.

Peripheral inflammatory changes of the slightest degree, have proven sufficient to completely obstruct the circulation in these growths.

Thus, existing under such precarious nutritional conditions and in contiguity with infected adnexa or endometrium, a uterine fibroid may at any moment, and with a probability increasing with its size and weight, become converted into a sloughing infectious mass by agencies offering the slightest impediment to its blood supply.

The numerous reports of this fatality, as detailed above, emphasize one contributory factor in its production, upon which sufficient stress cannot be laid, namely, the employment of the curette and other mechanical intra-uterine manipulations, such as tamponade, cauterization, etc.

The closer the tumor to the endometrium, the more pronounced the symptoms, which, according to older conceptions, indicate the employment of such mechanical measures, but, unfortunately,

1 Boston Medical and Surgical Journal, May 20, 1897.
2 British Medical Journal, 1890, Vol. 1, p. 897.

this very proximity to the endometrium, enhances the liability of these growths to fatal traumatic infections from such manipulations. The gravity of this occurence is typically illustrated in the following case: A robust, married woman of the laboring class, forty-three years of age, who had never been pregnant and who presented neither menstrual nor other clinical antecedents of import, was suffering from an uncontrollable metrorrhagia of three weeks' standing, which had been preceded by five months of amenorrhea. The classic ergot, ice and tampon routine proving ineffectual, the attending physician resorted to curettage, which was promptly followed by severe rigors, high temperature and painful distention of the abdomen.

When the patient came under the writer's observation, twenty-four hours later, she presented the clinical evidences of a general septic peritonitis. The uterus was globular, soft, and reached a point midway between the pubes and umbilicus. Its os gave vent to foul solid sloughs and necrotic fibrous masses.

Death occurred within the day, and the autopsy revealed necrosis of the uterus, originating in a sloughing fibroid. There was a general septic peritonitis with thrombophlebitis of the iliac veins.

It is superfluous to dwell upon the immediate and remote effects of visceral compression and displacements exerted by uterine fibroids, inasmuch as these mechanical factors constitute the familiar chapter of their classic manifestations, and I simply allude to them, in passing to the enumeration of a vital group of pathological phenomena, of special interest and deepest significance to the internist as well as to the gynecologist.

The *nutritional,* the *cardiovascular* and the *renal* derangements, due to the presence of these tumors, but independent of their mechanical influences of visceral compression and displacements, often accompanying growths that are free and of insignificant dimensions, represent the last observed and least understood of fatal complications incidental to the development of uterine fibroids.

The occurrence of an anemia, *not* due to metrorrhagic depletion; a myocardial degeneration of characteristic and uniform type and a premature general end-arterial fibrosis with renal changes, compose this clinical triad, whose resemblance in symptomatic features to other and familiar forms of constitutional derangements, has produced much speculation and more diagnostic and therapeutic deflection.

The premature arteriosclerosis, evidenced by edema, embolic processes, hemiplegia and albuminuria, like its concomitant myocardial degeneration, have not received the general recognition —outside of the dead house—which their serious prognostic import would suggest.

In 1884, Hofmeier called attention to the frequency of cardiac diseases in cases of abdominal tumors, especially with fibromyomata. He collected 18 cases in which sudden death occurred from heart failure; three of these showed fatty degeneration and 15 brown atrophy of the myocardium.

Following this report, Fehling, Leopold, Strassman and Lehman, Fleck and many others, amplified our knowledge on this subject by the publication of numerous illustrative fatalities from this complication, and yet not a single textbook nor elaborate special treatise on cardiac pathology presents the barest allusion to these cardiovascular degenerations as accompanying uterine fibroids.

Bitter experience alone has taught many surgeons to dread the effect of anesthetic and operative shock on these hearts of patients with advanced uterine fibroids.

Volumes have been written upon these various phases, thus depicted in sketchy outline; yet these bare outlines sufficiently attest, that the prognosis in unoperated uterine fibroids involves incalculable and uncontrollable possibilities of the gravest nature, which nothing short of timely radical intervention can obviate.

Such timely resort to radical surgery is not only prompted by the fatal tendencies of the unmolested tumors and the happy results attending their early operative removal, but by the utter impotence of every other curative or palliative measure hitherto employed or suggested.

Meadows, quoted by Bishop (p. 128), expresses his sentiments in the following: "There is in truth no folly greater than to attempt the impossible and no worse treatment of conscience and character than the habitual practice of unreality . . . and I am firmly convinced that to persuade women for months and years to swallow medicines, mostly of a depressing and debilitating kind, in the vain hope that we can thereby bring about the absorption or expulsion of a hard fibroid tumor, is not only unscientific, but unreal and dishonest."

Our knowledge of the action of drugs and of the nature of these growths has greatly increased, and, the clearer our insight, the more completely does it dispose of the false reputation dishonestly acquired in this direction by the whole list of remedies from ancient ergot to modern organotherapy.

The same applies to the electrolytic treatment as elaborated by the late Apostoli.

It has been my privilege on various occasions, to present before the gynecological section of this Academy and elsewhere, a number of specimens and reports of cases, showing not only the utter uselessness, but the dangers attending the employment of this procedure. The reported results claimed for these therapeutic attempts, like the belief in a climacteric retrogression of uterine fibroids, reveal themselves to-day as dissipated myths: the menopause in numerous instances, as shown by Kleinwächter, inaugurating a period of renewed activity or pathological change in the growths.

Péan says: "J'ai operé plus de personnes arrivées à la menopause que de malades plus jeunes." Of his 250 operated cases 100 were between fifty and sixty years of age and 70 between forty and fifty years.

Herrman reported a case in which a tumor of this kind first appeared at the age of sixty-four years, thirteen years after the menopause.

Grinsdale has met with a similar case at sixty-seven; Champneys at sixty-nine, while Tait had to remove the whole uterus for a sloughing myoma at sixty-seven, twenty years after the menopause.

On the question of retrogression, spontaneous or otherwise, Roger Williams, in an elaborate treatise on uterine fibro-myomata, states: "With regard to the alleged disappearance of these tumors—or, indeed, of any true tumor—by absorption, I have never been able to convince myself of its reality. The weak point in the history of these cases of reputed absorption of myomata, is that which relates to the diagnosis of the growth . . . and . . . it is my belief, that in all such cases we have to do with inflammatory pseudoplasms."

The possible dangers of the curette have already found emphasis; its utter uselessness, however, in controlling uterine hemorrhage due to the presence of fibroid tumors, has recently been explained by the studies of Theilhaber and Hollinger.

As a result of these investigations, our conceptions as to the nature of metrorrhagic complications in general and in connection with uterine fibroids in particular, have undergone a radical change. The alleged endometrial changes have been proven an unfounded hypothesis, which has given place to the recognition of the demonstrated myopathic and vascular degenerations of the uterine body bearing these tumors; the resulting projectile and circulatory insufficiency and not endometrial disease are productive of hemorrhages which no amount of intra-uterine scratching can permanently control.

Thus, one of these misdirected therapeutic efforts after the other, down to the long-cherished curette, has foundered on the rock of experience, and the question to-day in the treatment of uterine fibroids simply resolves itself into a decision between early radical removal and a perilous inactivity—perilous not only in immediate and remote dangers, but in fostering those elements which add fatality to late operation, or lend disappointment from necessarily imperfect results.

At best it condemns the patient to invalidism more or less marked, during the years which should be the most useful and active of her existence. This is the very reverse of the usual optimistic view taken by those practitioners, who are inclined to regard the exceptional benign cases as embodying the rule and the usual result the exception."

It is within the memory of most, when appendicitis, gastro-intestinal perforations, gall-bladder disease, pancreatitis and adnexal abscess were treated by poultice and opium; when extra-uterine pregnancy was treated by morphine and electricity, and cures were reported. At the present time, to diagnose any of these conditions is to establish the indications for radical intervention.

Our knowledge of uterine fibroids places them in this same category; for just as in the conditions mentioned, treacherous calms will ultimately reveal themselves as incubation periods of serious potentialities, and a grave responsibility rests upon those who counsel delay, until what earlier would have been a safe operation of choice, has become, as a result of their counsel, a dangerous undertaking of necessity.

This responsibility is further enhanced by the fact that the immediate and remote operative results depend entirely upon the absence or presence of the complications which timely surgery alone can obviate, and against which every other therapeutic agent at present in our possession is powerless.

51 West Seventy-fourth Street.

LITERATURE UTILIZED.

Bishop, E. Stanmore. Uterine Fibromyomata.
Williams, W. Roger. Uterine Tumors, their Pathology and Treatment, 1901. Wm. Wood & Co.
Von Lorentz. Beitrag zur pathologischen Anatomie der chronischen Metritis. Arch. f. Gyn., Vol. 70, No. 2.
Fee. Myom und Herzerkrankung. Arch. f. Gyn., Vol. 71, No. 1 1k
Theilhaber and Hollinger. Die Ursachen der Blutungen bei Uterus Myomen. Arch. f. Gyn., Vol. 71, No. 2.
Strassman. Encyklopädie der Geburtshülfe und Gynecologie. Article Myom.
Noble. Am. Journal of Obstetrics. Vol. XLIV, No. 3.

MEDICAL PROGRESS.

PATHOLOGY AND BACTERIOLOGY.

Change in the Aorta in Syphilis.—The following changes were discovered in several carefully studied cases of syphilis of the aorta by S. ABRAMOW (*Virchow's Archiv*, Vol. 178, No. 3). In the first recent case, thickening of the intima, consisting chiefly of spindle-shaped cells, imbedded in homogeneous, intercellular substance, was marked. Portions of this thickened intima were made up of mucoid substance and the superficial layers consisted of thick, hyaline fibers. In the adventitia there was proliferation of capillaries, whose intima was thickened and adventitia infiltrated with round cells which extended into the media. Four more advanced cases showed cicatrized areas in the media where the muscle bundles were almost completely destroyed. The process in the adventitia no longer progressed and the fibers had become sclerotic. The thickened intima was also cicatrized and replaced by coarse connective-tissue fibres of hyaline appearance. The elastic elements of the aorta were more or less destroyed by breaking up into homogeneous flakes. The difference between syphilitic and ordinary aortitis is only quantitative. The diagnosis of syphilis can only be made, if distinct gummata have developed in the walls of the vessel.

Relationship of Splenic Anemia to Other Blood Diseases of Childhood.—The homopoietic organs of the infant up to the sixteenth year in health, the cavities of all bones contain red marrow in varying proportions mixed with fat. H. BATTY SHAW (*Lancet*, December 3, 1904) says truly that before attempting to answer any questions in this matter, it is necessary first of all to discuss the general conditions of the blood in healthy infants. At birth, the hemoglobin amounts to 100 or 104 per cent. This amount progressively falls to the third week, when it reaches 55 or 60 per cent. After this, it steadily rises until the color index is approximately one. At birth the leucocytes vary from 18,000 to 30,000. By the sixteenth day, they fall to 14,000, at the sixth month, 13,000. By the end of the first year, 10,000. At the sixth year from 7,500 to 9,000, a total of 30,000 leucocytes in a healthy child under three years of age after feeding is said to be far from rare. At about the twelfth day, the polymorphnuclear cells are 60 to 70 per cent. At the third year the mononuclear equal these. The conclusions of this paper are that there is no sharp line of demarcation between any of the pathological groups which have been dignified by special names. Clinical evidence, furthermore, fails to separate these maladies, and the same may be said of the blood examinations, except in the advanced forms of pernicious enemia and leucocythemia. A closer study of the lymphoid tissues throughout the body, and particularly of those elements lying within the reticulum of each tissue, is necessary. It is probable that in leucocythemia, the marrow is involved in every case; whether it be of a lymphocytic, myelocytic or of a mixed type. The spleen and lymphatic glands may or may not share in the hyperplasia of the lymphoid cells which normally occur there. By metaplasia, the lymphoid cells appear to give rise as in pernicious anemia to various forms of erythroblasts and erythrocytes. What provokes this hyperplasia is not known, nor is it understood why it should be more readily excited in the young than in adults. That this not infrequently occurs is vouched for by the occurrence of splenomegaly in the adult without profound blood changes, which condition is unknown in the infant. In view of the utter impossibility of reaching any definite conclusion which is based upon clinical evidence or laboratory findings, it is undoubtedly justifiable to hesitate to attempt to differentiate between lymphatic leucocythemia and the splenic anemia of infancy.

Experimental Production of Lymphocyte Exudates.—This question has been studied in animals by A. WOLFF and A. v. TORDAY (*Berl. klin. Woch.*, December 5, 1904). They found that the injection of tetanus and diphtheria toxin in mice and guinea-pigs brings on an exudate of lymphocytes, which continues for from one to twenty-four hours after the injections. The promptness with which this artificial production appears seems to dispose of the objection to accepting the theory that active lymphocytosis can take place. These objections were, that it is not possible to produce it experimentally and that the lymphocytes might come from connective cells. Lymphocytosis and leucocytosis varies with different species of animals. The mouse is inclined to show a lymphocytocis, and substances which set up merely a polynucleosis in guinea-pigs, bring about a lymphocytosis in mice.

The Path of Infection in Pulmonary Tuberculosis.—A method of infection which is declared by its author to be theoretically possible and clinically probable, is suggested by M. WASSERMANN (*Berl. klin. Woch.*, November 28, 1904). He cites a number of cases which seem to show that in many cases of pulmonary tuberculosis, the infection reaches the lung through the tonsils and pharynx through the cervical lymph nodes and the pleura. The pharyngeal mucous membrane allows the bacilli to pass through when there happens to be present some local inflammatory lesion in the latter. The cervical glands then become secondarily involved. The infection travels down the lymphatics to the pleura, where it sets up a localized pleuritis, with the formation of adhesions. The bacilli are then able to enter the lung itself. Adhesions form most readily at the apex because in this locality there is less amount of movement during respiration. The preliminary symptoms are usually not observed by the patient, but any involvement of the pleura is noted immediately, and this is very sensitive. The shooting pains in the shoulder are therefore the first thing complained of by the patient. Physical signs at the apex are absent, unless one is able to detect friction râles. The greater frequency of apical lesions on the right side may be accounted for by the greater activity of the right shoulder, which favors the lymphatic current on this side.

On Clinical Combination and Toxic Action as Exemplified in Hemolytic Sera.—A research the expenses of which were defrayed by a grant from the Carnegie Trustees was undertaken by R. MUIR and C. H. BROWNING (*Proc. Royal Soc.*, December 10, 1904), with the object of determining whether, where different complements differ in their action as shown by the dosage, both of complement and of immunebody required, this difference depends upon differences in their combining affinities or upon differences in their toxicity. The action of hemolytic serum depends upon two substances, namely, (a) the immunebody, which is developed as the result of the injection of the red corpuscles of an animal of different species, and (b) the complement, a labile substance which is present in the serum of the normal animal, and which is not increased as the result of such injections. Ehrlich has pointed out the similarity in the constitution of complements and of various toxins, and the author's own observations support his views. One may, in the study of hemolysis, consider the complement as a toxin, the red corpuscles treated with the appropriate immune body as the object in which the toxin is to act, and the hemolysis as the indication of the toxic action. Ehrlich regards the toxin as consisting of two chief atom-groups; the heptophore, or combining group, and the zymotoxic; but in speaking of the action of sera he does not always carry out this distinction completely. For example, the efficiency of different complements as tested by their hemolytic or bacteriolytic effects is often taken as evidence of the degree of chemical affinity between the complements and the immune-body. But it is manifest that theoretically a complement may combine perfectly through the medium of the immune-body and yet produce little hemolysis, owing to absence of sensitiveness to the zymotoxic groups—combination or "complementing" may occur and yet hemolysis be deficient or absent. The results of the authors' investigations show that in the action of the complement there are two distinct factors, viz., (a) power of chemical combination, and (b) toxic action, corresponding to the "haptophore" and the "zymotoxic" groups of Ehrlich; deficiency in the action of complement does not necessarily imply want of combining affinity, but may be entirely due to the non-sensitiveness of the tissue molecule to the zymotoxic group. In the case of the three hemolytic sera studied the outstanding fact is the large dose both of immune body and of complement necessary when one uses the complement of the same speecies of animal as that whose corpuscles are being tested. In all

three cases there is a relative non-sensitiveness of the corpuscles of the animal to the zymotoxic group of its own complement; hence a large dose of immune-body is necessary to bring into combination the amount of complement necessary for hemolysis. In one case (that of the ox) there is also a deficiency in the combining power of the complement with the receptors of the red corpuscles united to immune-body; from the two conditions acting together complete hemolysis cannot be obtained. No one has yet succeeded in producing an anti-substance or immune-body by injecting an animal with its own corpuscles or cells—such a body as with the aid of complement would produce destruction of these cells. This is manifestly a provision against self-poisoning and Ehrlich has applied to it the term autotoxicus horror. The resources which the authors have brought forward, if they were found to hold generally, would go to show that even if some substance should appear which acted as an immune body, there is a provision whereby the complement of an animal should produce comparatively little harmful effect.

PHYSIOLOGY.

The Molecular and Chemical Relationships of Transudates and Exudates.—The careful investigation of the physical chemistry of pathological fluids will probably furnish many valuable data from the standpoint of diagnosis and prognosis. A research in this field was conducted by K. BODIN (*Pflüger's Archiv*, September 30, 1904) with the following results: The molecular concentration phenomena of transudates and exudates are substantially the same. The osmotic concentration and the concentration of electrolytes in both exudates and transudates are approximately the same as those of normal blood serum. Just as in the latter, so in the former the concentration of the electrolytes presents slighter variations than the total concentration. It seems that the human serosa in both exudative and transudative processes always allow the inorganic salts to pass through in the same concentration, while the organic substances, according to the nature of the disease, are more or less held back. The content in ash is no reliable index of the content in electrolytes. From the standpoint of the NO-ions, transudates and exudates are neutral, like blood-serum, although like the latter, they both contain tritratable alkali. The author has not been able to discover any relation between the content in albumin and dry substance, on the one hand, and specific gravity on the other. There are no particular differences between the two groups of fluids as regards total proteids, serum-albumin, serum-globulins, ash and chlorides.

A New Method of Registering the Bodily Temperature.—The modern procedure of taking the rectal temperature at frequent intervals and regarding the highest temperature thus recorded as the maximal temperature for the day, is obviously imperfect, for it is possible that a still higher temperature may be reached in the intervals between the insertion of the thermometer. E. OERTMANN (*Pflüger's Archiv*, November 18, 1904) has devised a thermometer that will register the maximal temperature reached in any required period of time. The thermometer would necessarily have to be worn all this time in the patient's rectum; in order to render this possible and comfortable, the author devised an instrument similar to a hemorrhoidal pessary. It is shaped like a dumb-bell and is about 8 cm. long. One bulbous end is inserted in the rectum, the narrow part is firmly grasped by the sphincter ani, and the other bulbous end is outside the anus. A thermometer registering the maximal temperature is enclosed in this instrument in such a manner that the bulb of the thermometer is contained in the inner end of the pessary and the reading may be readily observed from the outside. The instrument may be worn as long as may be necessary.

The Reduction of Methylene Blue by Nervous Tissue.—The method discovered by Ehrlich and recently applied by Herter, of studying the varying reducing capacities of the tissues, has been utilized by H. T. RICKETTS (*Jour. Infect. Dis.*, November, 1904), in an investigation of the manner in which certain toxic substances affect the reducing power of nervous tissues. He used neurotoxic serum, that is, serum obtained by injecting extracts of nervous tissue from one animal into an animal of a different species. The blood serum of the latter then becomes highly toxic for the nervous tissues of the former animal. The author after intoxicating an animal with the foreign serum, injected methylene blue into its veins and then studied what effect the damaged nervous substance had in reducing the dye. He found that in this process of reduction the living cell is not essential, but that it may be brought about by emulsions of the tissue. The active reducing principles of these tissue emulsions consist of a thermolabile substance extracted by .85 per cent. NaCl, and a thermostabile substance closely associated with the solid tissue. Serum, old, fresh or heated at 70° F. for thirty minutes, may be substituted for the thermolabile substance as also may potassium hydrate. The reduction of methylene blue is accomplished by nascent hydrogen, which may have its source in fermentative processes, glycolytic or proteolytic. The action of KOH is referred to its catalytic properties. When serum is used as a reactivator, the reduction cannot be referred to ordinary ferments in view of the heat resistance of the substances contained. It may contain, in addition to ferments, some obscure catalyzing agents which act chemically.

PRESCRIPTION HINTS.

Fever and Sweats of Phthisis.—It is well known that consumptive patients support a high temperature without any apparent inconvenience. Frequently patients can be found amusing themselves having 102° F. of fever. In such cases, says Professor Tyonnel, it is not necessary to interfere. But in other cases, on the contrary, the fever is very high, fatiguing the patient, and treatment is necessary. Among the antipyretics at our disposal, antipyrine is the most innocent of all, and may be given with quinine:

    ℞ Hydrochlorate of quinine............grs. v
      Antipyrine. ....grs. x
    Two to four daily.

If the antipyrine is not well borne by the stomach, it should be given with Vichy water. Pyramidon, lowers the temperature very quickly, but it frequently excites profuse sweating. Preference might be given to the acid camphorate of pyramidon in wafers of grs. x; three or four daily.

Phenacetin is also a good remedy, and may be associated with quinine and pyramidon:

    ℞ Phenacetin ....grs. v
      Hydrochlorate of quinine...........∴.grs. iv
      Acid camphorate of pyramidon.......grs. vi
    For one wafer. Three or four in the twenty-four
    hours.

Sometimes simple rubbing with eau de cologne or lavender spirit every evening acts favorably and is inoffensive.

Atropine is without doubt the most active agent, although not without danger. Some patients complain of dryness of the throat from its use, and say that they can no longer expectorate, while others present cerebral trouble.

Camphoric acid, white agaric, and ergot of rye often succeed and may be combined as follows:

    ℞ Belladonna powder...................gr. ½
      White agaric powder.................grs. ii
      Ergot of rye.......................grs. iii
      Camphoric acid.....................grs. x
    For one wafer. Two to three in the course of the
    evening.

Hemoptysis.—Injections of 40 drops of a solution of adrenalin (1-1,000):

or

    Injections of gelatine, 1½ dram to 10 ozs.;

or

    ℞ Hydrochlorate of hydrastinin..........2 gr.
      Water ....5 ozs.
    A teaspoonful every hour;

or

    ℞ Hydrochlorate of hydrastinin..........½ gr.
      Hydrobromate of quinine.............. 1 gr.
      Ext: of balladonna...................⅛ gr.
    For one pill, two daily;

or

    ℞ Chloride of calcium................. 1 dram
      Laudanum ....30 min.
      Syrup of orange..................... 1 oz.
      Peppermint water................... 4 ozs.
    A tablespoonful every two hours.

Pruritus of the Vulva.—This obstinate affection i only too frequent and often resists treatment fo considerable periods of time. As is well known it is most troublesome at night. The following mix tures may be tried:

    ℞ Hydrarg. chlor. corrosiva } aa. 2 to 3 grs. (.10-.20
      Ammonii chlor. hydras. }
      Emulsion amygdalæ amaræ....qs. ℥vi (180.0)
    Robin and Dalché have reported considerable suc
    cess with a mixture of

    ℞ Orthoformi.......................... }
      Aristol............................. } aa. qs.
      Talcum.............................. }

or, if a pomade is desired,

    ℞ Menthol .... 1 gr. (.06)
      Guaiacol ....½ gr. (0.50)
      Zinci oxidi................... ℥iss (10.0)
      Vaselin....................... ℥i   (30.0)
    F. ung. Apply locally.

Asthma in Children.—

    ℞ Sodii arsenatis ....gr.⅓ (.002)
      Potassii Iodide...........}
      Potassii bromidi........} aa. gr.30 (2.0)
      Syr. aurantiæ flores...........℥ii (60.0)
    ℥ss t.i.d.

Nothing New Under the Sun.—Sir Henry ⸱ Blake, Governor of Ceylon, announced at a mee' ing of the Asiatic Society that Singalese medic: books of the sixth century described 67 varietie of mosquitoes and 424 kinds of malarial feve caused by mosquitoes.

THE MEDICAL NEWS.

A WEEKLY JOURNAL
OF MEDICAL SCIENCE.

COMMUNICATIONS in the form of Scientific Articles, Clinical Memoranda, Correspondence or News Items of interest to the profession are invited from all parts of the world. Reprints to the number of 250 of original articles contributed exclusively to the MEDICAL NEWS will be furnished without charge if the request therefor accompanies the manuscript. When necessary to elucidate the text, illustrations will be engraved from drawings or photographs furnished by the author. Manuscript should be typewritten.

SMITH ELY JELLIFFE, A.M., M.D., Ph.D., Editor,
No. 111 FIFTH AVENUE, NEW YORK.

Subscription Price, Including postage in U. S. and Canada.

PER ANNUM IN ADVANCE $4.00
SINGLE COPIES 10
WITH THE AMERICAN JOURNAL OF THE
MEDICAL SCIENCES, PER ANNUM . . 8.00

Subscriptions may begin at any date. The safest mode of remittance is by bank check or postal money order, drawn to the order of the undersigned. When neither is accessible, remittances may be made at the risk of the publishers, by forwarding in *registered* letters.

LEA BROTHERS & CO.,
No. 111 FIFTH AVENUE (corner of 18th St.), NEW YORK.

SATURDAY, FEBRUARY 11, 1905.

OYSTERS AND TYPHOID FEVER.

AT a time when the possibility that oysters may serve as a vehicle for the transmission of typhoid fever is a matter of doubt in the public mind, any new evidence on this point is of value.

The responsibility of the oyster, if established, is vast. Millions of bushels of these shellfish are annually grown and marketed on our coast and distributed through America and Europe without the least sanitary supervision. Many of the most celebrated varieties are sometimes bloated and bleached for market in streams which are in reality nothing less than open sewers. Is it possible that shellfish so treated occasionally become the carriers of disease? Are such sewage oysters at all responsible for the immense occurrence of sporadic typhoid fever which appears to be so baffling, not to say impossible to trace?

Dr. Daniel Lewis, Commissioner of Health of New York State, is on record as believing that typhoid fever is never caused by oysters. Recent U. S. Consular reports, widely quoted in the daily press, announce that a Commission, appointed by the Secretary of the Navy of France, has declared that oysters cannot transmit any disease to human beings. It is claimed that the oystermen themselves, who eat large quantities of shellfish, do not suffer to an unusual extent from typhoid.

But there is at least an equal weight of opinion on the other side of the question. We have the reports of Conn, Field and other capable observers in America, and of Houston, Klein, Bulstrode and many more in Europe, which go far to convince the reader of the guilt of the sewage oyster.

What shall we do about it? Shall we take the side of safety and advise our friends against raw oysters, or inform them that, before eating, their half shells should be analyzed? Because some oysters are little pockets of sewage, should we put a ban upon them all?

We do not want to produce a "scare." Oyster "scares" have occurred off and on for fifty years without producing any visible result beyond a temporary prostration of the business. But while we remain undecided, the oyster trade increases and typhoid fever multiplies.

The oyster business is a great and valuable asset to the people of this State, and as such, should be protected from the disastrous consequences of an unwarranted prejudice, but the public health comes first, and it is imperative that our oysters be kept absolutely pure.

For the protection of the public and the oystermen there is need of legislation based on a thorough sanitary investigation of the shellfish industry by persons of acknowledged and unprejudiced ability. We believe that the accompanying report (page 241 of MEDICAL NEWS), by Dr. George A. Soper, which we are enabled to publish through the courtesy of the Board of Health of Lawrence, offers an exceptionally strong argument in favor of this proposition.

THE ROENTGEN RAYS IN LEUCEMIA.

AT the December meeting of the New York State Medical Association, New York County Branch (see MEDICAL NEWS Society Proceedings, page 284, this week), Dr. Arthur Holding discussed the treatment of leucemia and pseudoleucemia by the X-rays. In *American Medicine* for December 24, 1904, there is an article by Dr. George Dock on the same subject. While the conclusions reached by these two writers are quite different, there is no doubt from the article of either that the Roentgen rays represent a very

interesting therapeutic factor in the treatment, especially of the conditions usually spoken of as
leucemic. Dr. Holding has been able to find altogether some 45 cases of leucemia and pseudoleucemia in the literature, and Dr. Dock has studied the original reports of 29 cases of genuine
leucemia, though he admits that there are probably others in the literature which have not been
clearly indicated by the title. It is perhaps the
best possible index of the rapidity with which
medical ideas are diffused at the present time and
the ready zeal with which experimental observations in therapeutics particularly are repeated,
that though one of the earliest cases of leucemia
treated by the X-rays was reported by Dr. Senn,
of Chicago, in April, 1903, there should be in the
short space of scarcely more than a year and a
half so many trials of his therapeutic suggestions.

Most of those who have used the X-rays in the
treatment of these serious blood conditions insist
that they must be employed very freely and without undue regard for possible evil results. Leucemia is a fatal affection and therefore justifies
heroic treatment. It not infrequently happens
that while a severe X-ray burn is healing, the
process of improvement in the blood condition
goes on almost uninterruptedly, though the exposures to the rays may have to be discontinued
for some time. As a rule, the whole person is exposed to the action of the X-rays except the head,
which may be protected by some form of flexible
metallic cover. There is no doubt that, at least
temporarily, beneficial results can be obtained in
most cases. Unfortunately as yet, time enough
has not passed to draw any definite conclusions
as to the absolute curative effect of this form of
treatment.

As to the contra-indications for the use of this
remedial measure there are as yet no definite
hints though some of its limitations are becoming
known. Unfortunately in a certain number of
cases toxic symptoms develop after a time and
then the general condition may suffer severely in
a way which may even resemble the state produced by acute sepsis. It is not uncommon to
have leucemic patients during the treatment die
suddenly or in a quasi-acute relapse of the disease, within a few days, after apparently progressive improvement has been going on for some
time. This is the most serious consideration in
the employment of this form of treatment. Even
when it does occur, however, there has usually
been a reasonably long period of improvement
and of great comfort to the patient. In all cases

there has been apparently some prolongation of
life. The thought cannot be suppressed that the
destruction of the superabundant white blood
cells brought about by exposure to the X-rays,
gives rise to toxalbuminous substances which
prove eventually fatal to the organism.

It is worth while to continue the experimentation with these methods of treatment in order to
determine the limitation of the benefits that may
be obtained from them. In this as in other reports with regard to the use of the X-ray, unfortunately there was an overzealous enthusiasm
on the part of those who reported some cases that
raised unwarranted hopes of an absolute cure
being possible. As Dr. Dock says, "In no case
has observation been carried out long enough to
speak of cure. The improvement must be considered functional and does not affect the original cause, nor in any permanent way the morbid
histology of the disease." It must not be forgotten at the same time that certain other forms of
treatment, and especially the employment of arsenic, has given some excellent results in leucemia at the hands of very conservative clinical
observers. Even where the X-rays are employed,
therefore, arsenic should not be neglected. The
most hopeful cases for any treatment are those of
beginning leucemia. If definite reports with regard to the effect of the X-rays in a certain number of these could be obtained, much more would
be learned and more satisfactorily than in any
other way. Here is an important field for investigation, open not only for those who are interested in X-ray work and who wish to add to our
knowledge of the value of an important therapeutic agent, but also to the general practitioner
of medicine to whom such cases come and who
may secure the cooperation of a colleague in order to test so promising a remedy for what have
hitherto been hopelessly fatal diseases.

INFLUENZA ONCE MORE.

THERE has been no doubt now for some years
that influenza has become endemic here in America ever since the great epidemic of the early
nineties, and that mild winters are likely to see it
rage with special virulence. The present winter
has proved no exception to this rule and in all
the large cities of this country a great many cases
of the disease, of rather severe type, have been
reported. The bulletin of the Health Department
of Chicago reported last week " that influenza is
more prevalent and more fatal in Chicago this

vinter than at any time since the epidemic year of 1891." In 1891 influenza was the chief agent in increasing the death rate of Chicago, more han one-fifth over that of the preceding year and numbers of the survivors have never since re-ained their former condition of mental and phyical health.

Undoubtedly the most prominent feature of he first great epidemic was the characteristically intense depression which followed even mild attacks of the disease. During the present winter this same feature for the disease has been brought to particular notice once more. There is no doubt in the minds of many physicians who remember the first great epidemic that some of the lasting after-effects were due to an unfortunate haste in the convalescence of patients from the disease. At that time, its after-effects were as yet unrealized and patients were often permitted to be up and about before such procedure was justified by their physical condition. At the present time the most important element in the therapeutics of the disease is insistence on the fact that patients must be kept in bed until their pulse and temperature has become absolutely normal and must not be allowed to go back to their occupation until they have thoroughly regained their strength. This will sometimes seem to a busy man a needless interference with his business life. The effects of imprudence in this matter are too serious for trifling, however, and this must be clearly represented to the patients in order to make them appreciate the dangerous possibilities of the disease.

With regard to the possible limitation of the spread of the affection, a very interesting and important field for observation lies invitingly open. The Board of Health in Chicago has emphasized the fact that no possible precaution should be neglected which may tend to limit the spread of the disease. As far as possible people should be advised to keep out of the way of contagion. Visiting by friends should be peremptorily discouraged, and in the case of delicate persons already under the care of a physician for other reasons, all visits to persons likely to be ill from influenza, even though the affection may be called bronchitis, or some other apparently harmless name, must be forbidden. Dosing with remedies supposed to prevent or abort influenza are not only of no avail, but are actually likely to lower resistive vitality and make persons more prone to the disease. At times of epidemics it must not be forgotten that crowded street cars probably

represent one of the most fruitful sources of the spread of contagious diseases, especially contagious respiratory diseases, in our large cities. Those who want to avoid the disease, should, as far as possible, keep out of the cars during the busy hours of the day and avoid attendance on crowded halls or assemblages in which there are likely to be many persons, some of them inevitably suffering from the prevailing affection.

In the present epidemic it has been noted, even more than almost any time in the last ten years, that the influenza does not confine itself to the respiratory mucous membrane, but that it is likely to work serious havoc on the mucous surfaces of the digestive tract. Under these circumstances, more than when the affection is only of the respiratory type, rest in bed and prolonged convalescence are necessary to prevent an unfortunate persistence of symptoms that may prove serious for the patient's subsequent health. In a word, the lessons learned in the past are that influenza must never be considered a trivial disease, and even when its symptoms are mildest, the depression that results is an index of how much the toxins of the disease have affected the central nervous system and how deep-seated has been an affection that otherwise seemed only a passing catarrh of mucous membranes. In this regard special stress must be laid on the fact that the reduction of temperature and the lessening of discomfort associated with the disease in the early stages by means of coal-tar products may easily tempt the patient to consider that the worst of the disease is over at a time when it is really only beginning to have its serious effect.

ECHOES AND NEWS.

NEW YORK.

Diphtheria Closes a School.—Dr. John T. Sprague, assistant superintendent of the Health Department in Richmond borough, has ordered the closing of Public School in Elm Park, because of the prevalence of diphtheria among the school children and other residents of that village. In the past two weeks forty-four cases of the disease have been reported to the Health Department.

In Memory of Dr. Thomas H. Manley.—In paying its tribute of profound respect to the memory of Dr. Thomas H. Manley, the Medical Board of the Harlem Hospital

RESOLVED, That by the death of Dr. Manley we have lost a highly esteemed and eminently proficient member of the Attending Staff. By his work at the hospital and his highly appreciated literary abilities, he has made his name known to the profession.

Resolved, That a copy of these resolutions be sent to the family of Dr. Manley, that it be published in the medical press, and that these words be entered upon our minutes.—Theodore Kuene, W. H. Luckett, *Committee.*

Record of State Hospital for Incipient Consumption.—The first report of the State Hospital for the treatment of incipient tuberculosis, which was established by an act of the legislature at Raybrook, in the Adirondacks, was presented to the New York State Medical Society by Superintendent John H. Pryor. Although the institution has been open only since July 1 indications point to complete success. Of the eighty-two patients admitted, eleven have been discharged as cured. Of the remainder five have not been in the hospital long enough to justify any conclusions; nineteen have apparently recovered; the disease of thirty-four has been arrested, and all the rest show improvement. "The law creating this institution and under which it has been in operation for a period of six months," says Superintendent Pryor, "seems to be eminently satisfactory."

That "Kinesipathy" Bill.—The *Times* asks the question "Are the Doctors Observing?" and makes the following comment: "Viewed from such a distance that only its surface can be seen by the unaided eye, Senator Sullivan's 'Kinesipathy' bill looks-like one to give a semblance of respectability and regularity to an assorted lot of rather dangerous quacks. For, if by some strange chance he should get it passed and signed, a multitude of 'professors' of rubbing and shaking would gain what is with the ignorant the enormous advantage of State recognition. Examined and certificated by a board chosen from among their own number and confirmed by the State Board of Regents, this whole great company of men and women who yearn to treat the sick—and get their fees—without taking the trouble to become doctors, would be safe from the occasional prosecution, which they are pleased to call persecution, and they would attain to a professional dignity that would be of enormous benefit to their business. It may be that Senator Sullivan has deeply studied the doings of the rubbers and the shakers, that he is competent to judge those doings, and that his introduction of the bill was the result of a warm and intelligent sympathy for suffering humanity. We hope so—we do, indeed. But we cannot help a doubt or two—little ones, which we are quite ready to abandon the moment a few real doctors give public expression to their approval of the measure. Till then we shall keep our little doubts and wonder how soon the medical societies are going to get—active."

Influence Brought to Bear on State Lunacy Board. —Strong influence is being brought to bear upon the Lunacy Commission by philanthropic persons to prevail upon that body not to complete the contract for the purchase of Isaac V. Baker's farm for a new insane asylum. If the Lunacy Commission refuses to entertain the appeal, those protesting against the acceptance of the Baker site will urge Gov. Higgins to interfere. The legislature of 1903 passed a special bill appropriating $50,000 for a site for the new hospital. When the Lunacy Commission, in the summer of 1903, directed experts to report on the different sites offered, it called specifically for information as to the water supply. The Commission last December voted to pay $42,000 for the Baker site, without any water supply, but with the understanding that an adequate water supply could be obtained for the site by an expenditure of at least $30,000 additional. The question, therefore, is, did the

Lunacy Board have any right to take action contemplating an expenditure of at least $72,000, when the legislature had appropriated only $50,000? It is contended that the Lunacy Board had no right to tie up the legislature to an additional expenditure for a water supply. While President Mabon of the Lunacy Board has declared that the proceedings for the buying of the site have gone so far that the Lunacy Board could not flop on the proposition if it wanted to, signs are not wanting that there is a possibility of the board dropping the site. It is suggested that some defect may be found in the searches. for the site or for the right of way that trails through the two miles of other people's farms to the proposed water supply. It is known that despite the fact that the Lunacy Commission voted to buy the land the latter part of December, neither the searches for the site nor the right of way are complete. In fact, no searches have yet been produced for the right of way.

Hospital Not Too Gorgeous.—Professor Orth, Virchow's successor in the chair of pathological anatomy at Berlin University, has been lecturing before the Berlin Medical College on his recent tour in the United States. He is reported to have said the most beautiful hospital he ever saw is Mount Sinai Hospital in New York. When he first sighted it he thought it was a magnificent hotel—such a profusion of marble, such gorgeous staircases, walls, etc. The professor says he never saw such luxury as in the rooms for patients, with their splendid furniture, electric lights and bathrooms. As far as poor patients are concerned, Professor Orth thinks that although comfort may play a large part in making a patient's life happy it is out of place on the scale of the Mount Sinai Hospital, where it can only result in unfitting such men to bear with the hardships of their home and in making them in future thoroughly dissatisfied with their lot in life.

Dr. S. S. Goldwater, superintendent of the hospital, makes the following reply:

To the Editor of the New York Times:

A cable dispatch published yesterday quotes a statement by Prof. Orth, of Berlin, concerning the alleged overindulgence of poor patients in the wards of Mount Sinai Hospital. It is not easy to believe that so enlightened a man as Virchow's successor in the Chair of Pathology at the Berlin University really sees any social danger in the provision of decent comforts for the sick poor.

Prof. Orth's views are reported as follows: "The professor says he never saw such luxury as in the rooms for patients at Mount Sinai Hospital, with their splendid furniture, electric lights, bathrooms, etc. Prof. Orth thinks that, although comfort may play a large part in making a patient's life happy, it is out of place on the scale of Mount Sinai Hospital, where it can only result in unfitting such men to bear with the hardships of their home life and in making them in the future thoroughly dissatisfied with their lot in life."

Now, what are the facts? For the well-to-do, Mount Sinai Hospital, in common with other institutions of the same class, provides such comforts as these patients are willing to pay for. For this no apology need be made, especially since the surplus revenue, if any, derived from this source can be utilized for the furtherance of the charitable work of the hospital; and so far as the poorer patients are concerned, what shall be said? Mount Sinai Hospital was established and is maintained for the purpose of rescuing those who have not the means to cope even for a short period with the heavy burden of an acute illness. For these the hospital provides clean beds, well-ventilated and well-lighted wards, expert voluntary medical attendance, wholesome food and good nursing. While in the hospital poor patients are protected from all the dangers and discomforts of overcrowding, of filth, of improper or insufficient food, and of ignorant or careless attendance.

In building and equipping a hospital, the sole aim is to furnish the means of fighting disease successfully, of putting the patient on his feet just as soon as possible, in order that he may resume his place in the social rank from which he springs. If a patient leaves the hospital with a new and higher appreciation of the value of air, sunlight, cleanliness, order, and decency, and with the determination to improve the conditions of his home, so that they may at least approximate decent standards, so much the better for the patient. Is not this the spirit which our social settlements are trying to engender, and may not the hospital properly take its place among the educational agencies making for social betterment?

No hospital in New York, so far as the writer is aware, is in a position to pamper its ward patients. If patients leave the hospital imbued with the sort of dissatisfaction of which Prof. Orth speaks, there is consolation in the fact that it is such dissatisfaction which has made our present civilization possible and which affords the promise of a higher plane of living for all humanity in the future.

PHILADELPHIA.

Bohemian Afternoon.—The Ladies' Auxiliary of the Jefferson Medical College gave a tea at the Horticulture Hall Saturday afternoon, the proceeds of which will be used to maintain and to supply books for the Library of the College.

To Lecture on the Care of Teeth.—According to the arrangements just completed Dr. J. Ashley Fraught will lecture to the public school children and their parents at the various schools during the month of March upon the care of teeth.

Professional Ethics.—In his address before the W. W. Keen Surgical Society, Dr. John H. Gibbon spoke to the members of this Society and the students of the Jefferson Medical College of professional ethics. After the address Dr. Gibbon was entertained at a banquet by the Society.

Epidemic of Smallpox.—This disease is again prevalent in York, Clearfield and Indiana counties. Dr. Benjamin Lee, secretary of the State Board of Health, attributes the outbreak to the activity of the smallpox contagion which was nurtured in the winter clothing packed away in closets and chests last spring.

New Hospital.—At 1234 North Fifty-fourth Street a new institution was opened which is to be known as the West Philadelphia General Homeopathic Hospital. It has ten free beds and a dispensary. W. E. Marbaker is president; Richard B. Morrel is vice-president; T. W. MacFarland is secretary, and Charles K. Hibbs is treasurer of the Board of Trustees. Dr. H. F. Williams is chief of the medical staff.

Meeting of the H. A. Hare Society of the Jefferson Medical College.—Prof. R. B. Preble, of the Northwestern University Medical School, Chicago, in his address before the Society and Members of the Faculty told how the pneumococcus by entering the blood stream produces constitutional effects without involving the lungs at all. By citing four cases he illustrated how utterly impossible it was to make the diagnosis until cultures were made from the blood. He laid great stress upon the sudden onset and the severity of pneumococcemia.

Wills' Hospital.—Realizing the importance of a society in which clinical workers in ophthalmology may be able to report their interesting daily cases and enjoy full and free individual discussion upon the same, and present theoretical and statistical papers upon ophthalmic subjects, Dr. Oliver, of Philadelphia, has recently organized the "Association of Clinical Assistants of Wills' Hospital." Membership by ballot is open to all those who have been or are connected with one or more of the clinical services in Wills' Hospital for a period of not less than three months' time. Meetings are held at the hospital at 8:30 P.M. on the first and third Wednesdays of each month. All who are eligible are invited to attend and join.

The Nathan Lewis Hatfield Prize for Original Research in Medicine Awarded by the College of Physicians in Philadelphia.—$500 will be awarded to the author of the best essay submitted in competition on or before March 1, 1906, subject: "The Clinical and Pathological Diagnosis of Sarcoma." Essays must be typewritten, designated by a motto or device, and accompanied by a sealed envelope bearing the same motto or device, and containing the name and address of the author. They must embody original observations and researches. The Committee reserve the right to make no award if none of the essays submitted is considered worthy of the prize. For further information address Francis R. Packard, M.D., Chairman, College of Physicians, 219 South Thirteenth Street, Philadelphia, Pa.

Meeting of the Eastern Section of the American Laryngological, Rhinological and Otological Society.—This meeting was held at the Jefferson Medical College with Dr. S. MacCuen Smith in the chair. During the morning session the following papers were read: "The Technic of the Radical Operation for Chronic Suppurative Otitis Media," by John D. Richards, M.D., of New York; "Report of a Case of Osteomyelitis of the Temporal Bone," by Charles W. Richardson, M.D., of Washington, D. C.; "Otitis Media Mucosa," by F. E. Sheppard, M.D., of Brooklyn, N. Y.; "Primary Epithelioma of the Auditory Canal," Joseph S. Gibbs, M.D., of Philadelphia; "A Case of Epithelioma of the Middle Ear," T. Passmore Berens, M.D., of New York; "Report of a Case of Mycosis of the Throat Treated with the X-ray," Lee Maidment Hurd, M.D., of New York. There were nine other papers read beside the last one mentioned during the afternoon session.

Regulations adopted.—At the last meeting of the Milk Exchange it was

Resolved, That the Philadelphia Milk Exchange urges upon its members and all engaged in producing and distributing the article, that no milk be purchased or sold unless conforming with the following rules: (1) Cows shall be healthy and free from disease. (2) Milk from any cow suspected of disease shall be discarded from the herd milk. (3) That the dairyman and his household are free from disease. (4) Pails used in milking should have a covered top, with small openings protected with a wire sieve or a cloth strainer. (5) All cans and dairy utensils shall be scrupulously clean before using. (6) No milk shall be sold from living rooms or rooms connected with the stable. (7) Absolute cleanliness of bottles and bottling apparatus. (8) There should be a clean room in which the bottles are filled. (9) Clean boxes for storage of the bottles or cans, and drains connected to avoid sewer gas. (10) Delivery wagons to be thoroughly cleaned both inside and outside.

Appointments—The Governor sent to the Senate the following names of the persons who are to be members of the board of Medical Examiners for three years: Dr. W. D. Hamaker, of Meadville, and Dr. M. P. Dickeson, of Glen Riddle, representing the Medical Society of Pennsylvania; Dr. J. C. Guernsey, of Philadelphia, and Dr. Edward Cranch, of Erie, to represent the Homeopathic Medical Society; Dr. William Rauch, of Johnstown, and Dr. J. M. Louther, of Somerset, to represent the Eclectic Medical Society. Dr. John H. Jopson has been elected a member to the surgical staff of the Presbyterian Hospital. Dr. W. W. Keen, Dr. J. William White, Dr. John B. Roberts, Dr. E. E. Montgomery, Dr. Orville Horwitz, Dr. John M. Baldy and Dr. Charles P. Noble have been appointed consulting surgeons to the Jewish Hospital. The consulting physicians appointed are, Drs. John H. Musser, James Tyson, J. C. Wilson, Roland G. Curtin, Alfred Stengel, J. M. Anders and Lawrence F. Flick. Dr. J. P. Crozer Griffith has been elected consulting pediatrist. Owing to the increasing number of patients in this hospital many additional surgeons and physicians were elected.

Meeting of the Academy of Surgery.—This meeting was held February 6. Dr. A. D. Whiting presented a paper on "Gangrene of the Scrotum." In none of his cases were the testes injured by the condition; he maintains that castration should not be performed unless these organs are extensively involved, and even then he is rather inclined to allow nature to get rid of them. In treating these cases incisions through the dartos should be made in the parts involved. Dr. Adinell Hewson showed "A Mulberry Calculus obtained from the dissecting room." He said that he was informed by the attending physician that the stone produced no symptoms during life. Owing to the absence of Dr. DeForest Willard, his paper was read by Dr. Hodge. This paper was entiled "Duodenal Ulcer; Gastro-enterostomy." The patient's gastric contents showed a hyperacidity and there was blood in the stools. From these facts the diagnosis of duodenal or gastric ulcer was made. The patient died soon after the operation, and at post mortem an ulcer was found in the duodenum which had perforated all the coats of the intestine, but by adhesions to the gall-bladder the contents of the organ did escape. Dr. A. B. Craig and Dr. A. G. Ellis read a paper entitled "An Experimental and Histological Study of Cargile Membrane." Dr. Craig found that the peritoneal fluids and the intestinal peristalsis dislodged the membrane so that it was necessary to fix it with sutures. He learned that when the Cargile membrane was either placed on denuded or on undenuded surfaces of the peritoneum adhesions formed just as in cases where no membrane was used. After removing the intestine upon which it had been allowed to remain for a certain length of time, the membrane could not be identified macroscopically. To determine whether the material was absorbed he placed a piece of chromicized and a piece of non-chromicized Cargile in separate glass tubes, which were then introduced into the peritoneal cavity of animals and allowed to remain for seven days; upon removal the unchromicized was dissolved but the chromicized was intact macroscopically. He then decided to determine whether the solvent action was due to the peritoneal fluids or whether it was due to the leucocytes, and accordingly placed the membrane in celloidin capsules, which fluids could permeate, but leucocytes could not. These capsules, after remaining in the peritoneal cavity, were found void of cells but contained a milky fluid; the chromicized membrane was almost dissolved. In concluding his part of the paper he said the Cargile may be of value to protect and prevent adhesions around wounded nerves, but it is of no value to prevent adhesion in the abdominal cavity. Dr. Ellis in the histological study of the tissue on which the Cargile was placed, found that it invariably produced an inflammation and that newly formed tissue was always present and in many instances invaded the Cargile. In one section he found a giant-cell between the Cargile and the nerve to which it was applied; the cells contained a fragment similar to Cargile. He believes the membrane is destroyed by lysins. In discussing this paper, Dr. Coplin reminded the Society that even non-vascularized bone from the same individual when introduced at any point in that body will act as an irritant, therefore Cargile could not possibly be put in the body without giving rise to irritation. Dr. Deaver told the Society he had used the Cargile extensively, but that all of his patients recovered, so that he was not able to see the changes it produced. Dr. W. W. Keen reported "A Case of Rupture in the Continuity of the Tendon of the Long Head of the Biceps." He overlapped the tendon and sutured with chromicized catgut. The injury was sustained in an effort to catch a hand-ball.

CHICAGO.

Contributions to Hospital Fund.—Up to the present writing the contributions for the Iroquois Memorial Association Hospital Fund amount to $11,959.

Report of Chief Lodging House Inspector.—The report of the Chief Lodging House Inspector informed the State Board of Health that there are no longer to be found in Chicago the disease-breeding spots that were designated as basement lodging houses, and other lodging houses that had double-deck and triple-deck beds, with small air space and poor ventilation.

Educational Campaign Against Disease.—An educational campaign against disease is to be started, through the high schools, by the department of pathology and bacteriology of the University of Chicago. It is hoped to arouse the students to take interest in practical work of a bacteriological nature, such as experimenting to demonstrate bacteria in air, water and milk.

Officers of State Board of Health.—Dr. George W. Webster, of Chicago, was recently re-elected president of the State Board of Health at its annual meeting. Other officers elected were: Dr. J. A. Egan, of Springfield, secretary; and treasurer, Dr. P. S. Wessel, of Moline. The Board mapped out aggressive plans to fight tuberculosis in every nook and corner of the State, giving its hearty approval to a bill recently introduced in the legislature that provides for the establishment of a State hospital for consumptives.

First Aid.—Dr. Nicholas Senn gave a lecture recently to the newly organized American White Cross First Aid Society. Among other things, Dr. Senn said that " Should you intercept a stray bullet, do not permit anyone, not even your wife, to wash the wound, but insist on the application of antiseptic absorbent cotton, which you or your companion is expected to have in an inside pocket." Several hundred persons attended the lecture, which was illustrated by the application of a bandage to a wound and the making of a sling for a fractured arm.

Bust of Dr. Fenger.—A memorial bust of Dr. Christian Fenger will be formally presented to the Chicago Medical Society soon by members. The bust is to be placed in the Cook County Hospital, where Dr. Fenger was a member of the surgical staff for twenty years. Dr. Ludwig Hektoen, Chairman of the Committee of Arrangements, states that there will be enough money left after paying the $3,000 for the bust to establish a Christian Fenger fellowship in one of the local medical colleges. It has not been decided which school is to be the recipient, as Dr. Fenger was a member of the faculty of three.

Plea for State Sanitarium.—In a lecture recently delivered at the Laflin Memorial Hall, Dr. George W. Webster made an eloquent plea for a State Sanitarium for consumptives. He said that unlimited funds would be at hand if the State expected an invasion of a force that would kill 8,000 people in a year; still it has made no move to establish a sanitarium for the care of sufferers from tuberculosis. After showing how heavy drinkers were quick victims to the disease, he dwelt at length on how tuberculosis could be prevented. He closed by asking that his hearers use their influence to secure a sanitarium for tuberculous patients.

Merit Bill for Medical Staff.—A bill placing the medical staff of the Cook County Hospital under civil service was introduced in the Illinois Senate by Senator Carl Müller, of Chicago. The measure is calculated to carry out the plan of President Brundage, of the County Board, of apportioning the members of the medical staff among the various recognized schools of medicine. It provides that "all such physicians and surgeons who serve without compensation shall be appointed only for a term of six years, and that the physicians and surgeons usually designated and known as irternes shall be appointed only for a term of eighteen months." It is further provided that the President of the County Board may appoint a consulting staff of physicians and surgeons. A medical staff under the present system is selected every two years.

CANADA.

Northwest Autonomy and the Canadian Medical Profession.—The Government of the Dominion of Canada is about to create two provinces out of what has to this date been denominated the Northwest Territories, and a writer in The Toronto Globe calls the attention of the Canadian medical profession to the matter, believing that same concerns them to a very great deal. This medical man argues that as the Northwest Territories were acquired by purchase from the Hudson Bay Company by the Dominion Government, that the medical profession throughout all of the older provinces of Canada have a great deal of concern in the creation of the two prospective provinces, and calls upon them to

see that power is not conferred upon the two new provinces by the federal authorities to exclude practitioners from entering therein after the autonomy has been granted. We do not think that many of the profession of medicine in the older provinces will take much notice of this appeal, but will rather prefer to let the profession in the Northwest have full control over all matters pertaining to the registration and practice of medicine in that important section of the Dominion of Canada.

Sacrilege in a Montreal Maternity Hospital.— Montreal medicine is a unit in denouncing the gross and brutal action of a high constable and his special assistant who, last week, with a warrant in their possession, invaded the Montreal Maternity Hospital, and in a most sacrilegious and unrighteous manner searched not only the public and private wards, but unceremoniously even stripped the coverings from the lying-in bed. It is monstrous that such a thing could have happened, or that the doctors and attendants of the institution, who had assured the two myrmidons of the law that no such person as they sought was present in the hospital, did not take it upon themselves to forcibly eject these brutes in human attire, who forcibly pursued their search, not even stopping at the apartments of the nurses or private patients. The editorial in the Montreal Medical Journal, which condemns their action, fairly boils over with righteous indignation and righteous wrath at the unmitigated scoundrelism exhibited by these minions of the law, and justly calls for their heads in an official envelope, which is certainly flat enough for the purpose. The authorities of the maternity immediately took the matter up with their solicitor, and will push it to the bitter end, being satisfied with nothing short of the dismissal of the two men in question. Pity 'tis that the private ward patients cannot get damages from those who issued such a warrant.

Canadian Medical Men and the British Medical Act (1858).—It was never brought so forcibly to the minds of the members of the Canadian medical profession that the British Medical Act was not all that it should be so far as Canadians were concerned, than at the time of the South African War. Then Canada furnished several contingents to help out British arms, but many Canadian medical men were refused commissions, and even a field hospital was refused on the ground that it was contrary to the British Medical Act of 1858. In 1903, and again in 1904, Lieutenant-General Laurie, a member of the Imperial House of Commons, who was formerly a member of the Canadian House of Commons, had a bill before the Imperial Parliament seeking to remove the disability whereby colonially trained physicians and surgeons could not receive appointments in his Majesty's army and navy. A copy of this bill has recently been sent to all of the local medical societies of Canada, so that, should Canadian physicians and surgeons desire to assist General Laurie when next he introduces this measure into the British Parliament, an expression of their opinion will be in the General's hands, who will have evidence to produce that the medical profession of the Dominion of Canada, desires that colonially trained physicians and surgeons should have admission to the army and navy of the empire same as those educated at home.

The Lepers of Canada.—Dr. Smith, the medical superintendent of the Leper Hospital at Tracadie,

N. B., has presented his annual report to the Dominion Government. According to this the Register of the Lazaretto shows that there are now fifteen inmates, ten males and five females. The number in the first stage of leprosy is six, in the second seven, and in the third one. The youngest patient is ten and the oldest patient is sixty-two years of age. There were four deaths during the past twelve months, and three new cases were admitted, one from without the province of New Brunswick. Of those on the Register, nine are of French origin, three Icelandic, and three of English origin. During the year Chaulmoogra oil, in combination, introduced two years ago, has been freely used by the inmates with beneficial success. Recently, Dr. Smith took a tour of investigation through adjoining parishes, and the doctor found one undoubted case of true leprosy. He also found three persons showing premonitory symptoms. Notwithstanding this he reports that leprosy is decreasing, but after careful investigation states that he fully believes in the communicability of the disease by contagion.

GENERAL.

Longevity.—A German statistician calls attention to the fact that the increased longevity in Europe within the last fifty years is more conspicuous in the case of women than of men.

Boston Societies.—Boston Medical Library in conjunction with the Suffolk District Branch of the Massachusetts Medical Society. The last meeting was held at the library February 1. Dr. F. B. Harrington was in the chair. The subject for discussion was "The Results of the Treatment of Cancer in and about the Mouth. Dr. Fred. C. Cobb spoke on the importance of early diagnosis. Dr. Farrar Cobb and Dr. Channing Simmons gave the results of cases operated on at the Massachusetts General Hospital from 1895 to 1900. Dr. Howard A. Lathrop and Dr. David D. Scannell gave the results at the Boston City Hospital. Dr. E. A. Codman spoke on the use of the X-ray in post-operative treatment.

International Congress.—The next international Congress of Medicine will be held at Lisbon, April 19 to 26, 1905. The national committee of the United States is constituted, according to the official bulletin, as follows: President, Dr. John H. Musser, of Philadelphia; secretary, Dr. Ramon Guiteras, of New York; members, Dr. Frank Billings, of Chicago; Dr. William Osler, of Baltimore; Dr. W. W. Keen, of Philadelphia; Dr. Frederick Shattuck, of Boston, and Dr. Abraham Jacobi, of New York. On the motion of Dr. Bergoinc, the executive committee has decided to make medical electricity a separate branch of Section IV. There is every prospect that the congress will be an eminently successful one. The number of promised communications at present amounts to 188.

Suicide.—The announcement of the Mutual Life Insurance Company that among its policyholders last year there were 162 suicides would seem surprising, writes the *Times*, if the latest available statistics did not warrant the conclusion that it was a relatively low rate in proportion to the number of those insured. Prof. Frederick L. Hoffman's investigations for the information of one of the large life insurance companies show that even in this country, where the conditions of life are a good deal easier than in many, suicide is a factor in the equa-

tion of human mortality which must be reckoned with, and is not so abnormal a happening that it does not admit of statistical classification in actuarial calculations. Moreover, it is progressive. In fifty of the principal American cities the suicide rate for the eleven years 1893 to 1903, inclusive, was 16.30 per 100,000 of inhabitants; in 1903 it was 18.39. During the period of 1892 to 1902, inclusive, New York (Manhattan and the Bronx) had a suicide rate of 21.6 per 100,000. In Hoboken, just across the river, it was 27.14; in St. Louis, 25.87; in Chicago, 23.64; in Milwaukee, 20.37; in Cincinnati, 18.75; in Newark, N. J., 18.25; in Brooklyn, 17.13. Nearly all other cities fell materially below the Brooklyn rate, except Oakland, Cal., with 23.35. It is popularly assumed that the suicidal tendency is stronger in France than elsewhere, but this does not seem to be borne out by statistics. The French suicide rate for ten years was 23.6, which is lower than that of Saxony, Denmark, and Schleswig-Holstein. The Paris rate is 42; but that of Dresden is 51, and that of Berlin 36. That the average of suicides in the United States is only about 3.5 per 100,000 is cause for congratulation, notwithstanding the fact that in Russia, Ireland and Spain it is still lower.

Health on the Isthmus.—Reports concerning conditions as to health on the Isthmus of Panama have been "cruelly exaggerated," according to a long cablegram received at the War Department February 4, from Governor George W. Davis at Panama. In the families of the Americans employed on the Isthmus, Governor Davis says, there have been three cases of yellow fever and only one case of death. Of the employees hired on the Isthmus, five have been stricken, but only one has succumbed to the disease. The total number of cases of Americans not employed on the Isthmus, including those of the cruiser Boston, where the disease broke out two weeks ago, have been nine cases and five deaths. Other cases originating on the Isthmus and reported elsewhere number seven, with two deaths. The total number of cases originating on the Isthmus is thirty-two, of which nine have proved fatal. Six cases are now convalescing. Since the American occupation, the dispatch says, two cases of smallpox have been reported, but none has originated there. There is no typhoid or plague. Of the 4,000 employees only three per cent. are ill of any disease. Governor Davis says that the sanitation of Panama is progressing as efficiently as in any city of the United States. Until the completion of the waterworks, in about three months, the water supply from the wells and springs will be used. Col. Gorgas, who was instrumental in dealing with the sanitation of Havana, is in charge of the work at Panama, and it is his opinion that the material and equipment now on hand are entirely sufficient for controlling the yellow fever. Col. Gorgas required about eight months to obliterate 5,000 cases of yellow fever in Havana, and it is believed that he can secure its complete eradication in Panama soon.

Medical Society of the Missouri Valley.—The seventeenth semi-annual meeting of this association will be held in Kansas City, March 23 and 24. An excellent program is being arranged for this occasion, and the profession, which is noted for its hospitality, will keep open house for the visitors upon this occasion. Dr. S. Grover Burnett, of Kansas City, is president of the society, and Dr. C. Lester Hall, chairman of the arrangement committee. Following is a list of the papers which have already been given a place upon the program: Paper, Geo. W. Cale, Springfield, Mo.; Surgical vs. X-Ray Treatment in Cases of Rodent Ulcer and Epitheliomata of the Face, with Demonstration of Operated Cases, C. O. Thienhaus, Milwaukee, Wis.; Transverse Ribbon-shaped Cornea Opacity, J. M. Sherer, Kansas City, Mo.; Rest in the Treatment of Select Cases of Mental Disease, F. P. Norbury, Jacksonville, Ill.; Paper, E. N. Wright, Olney, I. T.; Surgery of the Spine, C. E. Black, Jacksonville, Ill.; Synchronous Extra- and Intra-uterine Pregnancy, with report of case, D. C. Brockman, Ottumwa, Ia.; Remarks on the Surgery of Umbilical, Femoral and Inguinal Hernia, with reported cases, J. Young Brown, St. Louis; Case of Choroiditis, probably due to Necrosing Ethmoiditis, W. W. Bulette, Pueblo, Colo.; Pelvic Inflammation of Peri- and Parametritis, H. C. Crowell, Kansas City, Mo.; Renal Affections Simulating Abdominal and Pelvic Diseases, J. Block, Kansas City, Mo.; The New-Born Infant; Its Care and Management, A. D. Wilkinson, Lincoln, Neb.; Anesthetics, Dora Greene-Wilson, Kansas City, Mo.; Some Observations upon the Treatment of Inguinal Hernia, Prince E. Sawyer, Sioux City, Ia.; Functional Diagnosis of Kidney Diseases, A. C. Stokes, Omaha, Neb.; Hypertrophy of the Thyroid Gland, T. E. Potter, St. Joseph, Mo. A feature of the program will be a symposium on puerperal fever, opened by Dr. Robert T. Sloan, of Kansas City. A cordial invitation is extended to the profession and special rates will be granted by the railroads. Further information and copy of the complete program, which will be issued March 10, may be obtained by addressing the secretary, Dr. Chas. Wood Fassett, St. Joseph, Mo.

The Japanese Medical Corps.—The statistics which have been given out of the astonishingly low mortality in the Japanese army from disease since the present war began warrant the conclusion that the organization of the medical corps and its equipment are the best ever known in a military establishment. Since it took the field Gen. Oku's division has had only 40 deaths from disease. Of 20,642 cases of sickness treated, 18,500 recovered in the field. Only 5,609 had to be sent back home as more seriously sick than could be advantageously treated in field hospitals, and of these the total mortality is said to have been 40. Only 133 cases of typhoid fever have been reported, and 342 of dysentery. The sickness among the troops recruited for our little Spanish war reached enormous proportions, and the deaths were nearly 70 per cent. of the cases, warranting a grave prognosis when taken in hand. It is natural, perhaps, to conclude from such comparisons, and especially when the Japanese records are contrasted with the disgraceful zymotic statistics of the Boer war, that the Japanese are immeasurably ahead of us in their knowledge of camp hygiene and field medicine. Probably they are. But the differences in results cannot possibly be explained by attributing them to larger knowledge and greater skill and fidelity on the part of the surgeons of the Japanese army, as compared with those of our own and the British military establishments. This is an impossible supposition. That the Japanese organization is better we do not doubt, but such differences as are discoverable do not begin to explain why the percentage of enlisted men incapacitated by sickness is só low. The reason for this will probably be found in the willingness of the Japanese soldier to cooperate with the medical staff in doing what he

should to safeguard his own health. His diet is simple and well ordered; he is temperate; he prudently avoids a hundred dangers to which the American and British soldier is indifferent; he does not plunge headlong into vice the moment he gets outside his camp limits, and in his dainty way he comports himself at all times like a soldier and a gentleman. This is the difference. The Japanese is temperamentally an exponent of the simple life, and while apparently perfectly willing to die in the way of duty, he sets the American and the British volunteer an example of prudence and self-restraint which reduce the anxieties and responsibilities of the army surgeon to the least expression.

Ship Surgeons.—The dean of the surgeons of the Atlantic fleet, if not among the steamships of the world, is Dr. J. Fourness Brice, of the steamship Cymric of the Boston-Liverpool service of the White Star Line. Dr. Brice has practised his profession on shipboard since 1859. He was born in England in 1826, was graduated from the Royal College of Surgeons in London in 1850, and from the College of Physicians and Surgeons, New York, in 1858. His connection with the steamship service came about as the result of an accident. He had already come into extensive practice in South Yorkshire, having followed in the steps of a kinsman lately deceased. When one day on a foxhunt his mount fell, and the young physician received an injury that prevented his continuing in practice. He came to America, and, after an extended stay, returned as surgeon of the American steamship Congress. For two years Dr. Brice was an interne in a London hospital. Then he tried to reassume his Yorkshire practice, but his health was such that he could not go on, and he decided to look for a position as ship's surgeon. He secured an appointment to the Scotia of the Cunard Line, with which he continued for thirten years. In 1879 his allegiance was transferred to the White Star Line. After sailing on various vessels he was assigned to the steamship Germanic, on which he served for twenty-three years. Very recently he left that vessel and was transferred at his request to the steamship Cymric. Dr. Brice, in spite of his seventy-eight years, is an active, progressive physician. When he is ashore in America he spends most of his time in the hospitals in order to keep abreast of the times. When the ship is at Liverpool, however, he betakes himself to his Yorkshire home, where he enjoys the freedom of the moorlands and the society of his wife and two daughters. Dr. Brice has crossed the ocean nearly 900 times.

Another very well-known medical man at sea is Dr. R. Lloyd Parker, late past assistant surgeon in the United States Navy, who is now attached to the American liner St. Louis. Dr. Parker is a graduate of the University of Edinburgh in the class of 1879. As soon as he completed his hospital course he became a surgeon on a ship of the Allan Line for two trips, and then joined the staff of the American Line. During these years he has made nearly 600 transatlantic trips. Throughout the Spanish-American War Dr. Parker was a past assistant surgeon in the navy, attached to the United States steamship St. Louis. For his services in conveying the wounded of Admiral Cervera's fleet from Santiago to Portsmouth, N. H., Dr. Parker received the thanks of the Spanish Government.

Dr. O'Loughlin, of the Oceanic, a graduate of the Royal College of Surgeons and Physicians in Dubin New York, entered the White Star service in 1872 upon the conclusion of his hospital course. He has made more than 700 trips across the Western ocean. He has done a good deal of surgical work at sea, his last major operation being an amputation at the hip joint. Next to Dr. Brice, Dr. O'Loughlin has been longer at sea than any other transatlantic surgeon.

The ship surgeon, however he may devote some of his time to the amenities of civilized life, cannot be the social butterfly he is sometimes represented as being. Indeed, most surgeons see the passengers only at the table over which they preside, and occasionally on the promenade deck. The ship surgeon leads, in fact, practically the same kind of life as his confrère ashore. He is a busy man. The larger vessels seldom carry fewer than 500 people on each trip, and in the summer months 1,500 would be nearer an average number.

OBITUARY.

Dr. JAMES A. FREER, a well-known physician of Washington, D. C., was found dead last week outside of Washington. He was forty-six years old.

Dr. AUGUSTA SMITH, a widely known woman physician, died at her residence in St. Louis on February 4, as the result of being struck by a street car. Dr. Smith was seventy-three years old, and a graduate of the Bennett Medical College of Chicago. She was born at Fulton, N. Y.

Dr. WILLIAM H. RISK died at his home in Summit last week after a long illness. He had been president of the Board of Health of Summit for two years. He was born in 1842 and was educated in Lafayette College and at the University of Pennsylvania. He lived in Philadelphia many years and went to Summit in 1873. He was consulting physician to the Fresh Air and Convalescents' Home at Summit, also a member of the Morris County Medical Association and the New Jersey State Medical Society.

Dr. HOMER L. BARTLETT, one of Brooklyn's most prominent physicians, died February 2 in Thomasville, Ga., at the age of seventy-five years. Dr. Bartlett had been in poor health for some time, and four days ago he went to Thomasville, hoping that he would be benefited. He was born in Chittendon, Vt., in 1830, and was educated at the Bakerfield Academic Institute. He came to New York immediately and entered the College of Physicians and Surgeons under Dr. Willard Parker. In 1855 he took his medical degree, and the next year he made a name for himself by going into the town of New Utrecht, after all the physicians of the town had been killed by the cholera or had fled, and putting a stop to the plague by heroic work night and day. In 1857 he moved to the village of Flatbush, Brooklyn, and since that time was perhaps the foremost citizen of that part of Brooklyn. He organized the first health board Flatbush had, its original police board, the first village gas company, its water works and the Midwood Club. He was also the first trustee of the Erasmus Hall Academy, now a part of the city school system. Dr. Bartlett was vice-president of the Kings County Medical Association, a member of the American Medical Association, of the Association for the Advancement of Knowledge, of the State Charity Aid Association, and other associations, State and local. In late years Dr. Bartlett interested himself in compiling histories of the traditions and legends of Flatbush and Long Island. He is the author of a number of books.

SOCIETY PROCEEDINGS.

MEDICAL SOCIETY OF THE STATE OF NEW YORK.

Ninety-ninth Annual Meeting, held at Albany, January 31, February 1 and 2, 1905.

The President, Dr. Hamilton F. Wey, of Elmira, in the Chair.

SECOND DAY—FEBRUARY 1ST (*Continued*).

(Continued from Page 229.)

Railway Spine.—Dr. Edward B. Angell, of Rochester, N. Y., said that the use of this term, ever since Erichsen opened up this important chapter of accident neuroses for law and medicine, has not become any more definite than it was at the beginning. As a matter of fact Erichsen's classical article has been the guiding star of courts as well as of legal and medical experts and unfortunately very indefinite ideas as to true pathology have resulted. Much is said of concussion of the spine and of congestion of the spine, but little of the true morbid conditions that develop have been studied out. Dr. Angell then detailed some illustrative cases which served to show that as a rule these accident neuroses present manifestations out of all proportion to the injury which has been received. In most cases, it is a mental and not a bodily state that develops as the result of the accident. This is very clear from the shifting of tender points from the complaint of pains here and there throughout the body without any definite location of pathological conditions. Such symptoms are found even in cases in which there is no question of litigation for damages, and more than once they have been seen to persist long after settlement has been made.

Imperative Idea.—What develops in most cases is an imperative idea, a true delusion as to physical condition. The accident is often not the occasion of the symptoms, but the patient's opportunity. This imperative idea may be overcome sometimes by hypnosis and the curatively suggestive effect of money damages is well known. This by no means necessarily implies that the patients are only pretending as to their symptoms. The railway spine is unfortunate, for it is really a brain injury, though of course for this there may be a physical basis. What is needed is a more careful study of these cases and less theory with regard to them. On the other hand, medical experts should come to the realization of their duty to give testimony not for their patients as clients, but according to the reasons they are able to obtain for definite medical conclusions. One unfortunate effect of the abuse of medico-legal testimony is that at times the imperative idea in the patient's mind becomes a permanent obsession before the settlement of the case is reached and the after-life is prone to be that of a miserable neurotic wreck.

Dilatation of Spinal Capillaries.—Dr. Kinnear, of Albany, said that it does not seem so difficult to ascribe physical basis of railway spine as has sometimes been said. What happens when patients are profoundly shocked seems to be a profound anemia of the exterior body produced by tense contraction of cutaneous capillaries and consequently a forcing of blood into the interior organs and especially into the central nervous system. It is well known that when patients suffer from shock, they are cold all over, and this feeling of coldness is only an index of the fact that as when the skin is affected by cold, the blood is driven out of the cutaneous capillaries. The result of this state of affairs is a permanent dilatation of the blood vessels in the brain and cord. Hence the activity of the circulation is increased and the functional life of the sensory and motor cells is made more active. There is a constant sense of discomfort and a desire to be doing things with a sense of restlessness; this is the cause of the insomnia that so often follows such accidents. This pathological condition indeed serves to explain all of the abnormal manifestations of the so-called traumatic neuroses.

Classes of So-called Neuroses.—Dr. Flood said that there are four classes of patients who come under the physician's care as the result of railway accidents. In the first class are those who suffer from real organic injury in the central nervous system. In the second, there are the functional cases in which a true neurosis has developed after the accident. In the third class are the malingerers, who, having been in a real accident, pretend to have been injured or pretend to have been much more injured than is really the case. In the fourth class must be grouped a certain number of people who are robbers, who make it a business to go around the country looking for opportunities to have supposed accidents happen and collect damages for them. A number of these cases have been described in which men and women have gone from one State to another making a good living by the collection of damages for accidents that they themselves planned in such a way as to produce supposed traumatic neuroses, but without any serious bodily injury. In the great majority of cases of traumatic neurosis, no common changes have been found in the central nervous system of those who happen to die from some intercurrent disease during the course of their severe symptoms from the supposed nervous injury.

Hypnotism and Disappearance of Symptoms.— Dr. E. B. Angell, of Rochester, said that Dr. Kinnear's suggestion with regard to the permanent dilatation of the capillaries of the central nervous system would not be acceptable to any one who had found by actual observation that he could make supposedly severe symptoms of the traumatic neuroses disappear entirely during hypnotic suggestion. The hypnotic state has no direct influence on the permanently dilated capillaries, but only on the mental condition and imperative idea that is ruling the patient. Many of the symptoms that are observed in damage cases are pure simulation. It is unfortunate that physicians lend themselves to the exploiting of such cases and indeed sometimes suggest further symptoms than those which the patient already complains of as the result of persistent examination and interrogation.

Pelvic Conditions and Nervous Diseases.—Dr. A. L. Beahan, of Canandaigua, said that much more frequently than has been thought, various sclerotic conditions in the pelvis are responsible for nervous disorders in the female. This is true not only for sclerosis of the uterus and appendages, but also for such extrapelvic organs as the appendix. In many cases in the female, probably as the result of constipation that is so common in women, there is the sclerosis of the appendix. He has found in a number of cases that this bears a definite relation to certain menstrual disturbances. It is well known that there may be a vascular connection between the appendix in the female and the uterine appendages, and during the congested period incident to

menstruation, if there is any chronic obstruction to the flow of blood, the effect is apt to be noticed. Sclerosis of the reproductive organs themselves, however, is even more seriously and more frequently productive of various neurotic and menstrual manifestations. Low grade inflammations which bring about thickening of the ovarian capsule, yet without producing acute oophoritis are the commonest of these conditions.

Ovarian Manifestations.—Abortive ovulation probably due to some disturbance of blood supply incident to diversion of the circulation by cold or exposure to dampness may produce hematoma of the ovary or small cyst, and these are often productive of further pathological conditions. If they rupture into the abdominal cavity, the roughened surfaces that are left may produce adhesions fusing together portions of the reproductive organs or even occasionally of the small intestines. The development of such conditions produces a very definite effect upon the woman's nervous system and must always be considered whenever other and more obvious causes cannot be found. The means for restoration to health in these cases are sometimes palliative, but oftener surgical and careful consideration is needed in order that the woman may be given the benefit of proper remedial measures.

The Non-Sequitur in Medicine.—Dr. H. A. Fairbairn, of Brooklyn, said that unfortunately there has always been a tendency, which can be observed even at the present moment, to accept theory rather than observation as the basis of supposed medical progress. In the olden times metaphysical speculation invaded the domain of medicine, but even at the present time this has not been entirely superseded. It has been the rule to make assumptions from observations and base inferences thereon, and the consequence has been the disagreement of results and no real progress. Even carefully made observations, when followed by speculation, has nearly always led medicine astray rather than onward. The only thing that gives lasting advance in medicine is the observation of facts. Even if one generation should make false inferences from these, they will be useful for subsequent generations to enable them to establish true medical laws.

Poisoning by Potassium Bichromate.—Dr. Francis Eustace Fronczak, of Buffalo, said that the whole subject of the toxic influence of potassium bichromate is still in obscurity. Altogether less than six cases of poisoning are to be found in the medical and medicolegal literature so far at hand. As a consequence, the case which he has had the opportunity to study seems to make a valuable addition to the medical literature of jurisprudence which is otherwise very meager. He then gave details of the case in which an attempt had been made to kill a woman by mixing a large amount of potassium bichromate with a mixture of wine and alcohol. As a matter of fact the woman seems to have taken over 100 grains of the drug. The usual dosage given in books on the subject is from $\frac{1}{12}$ to $\frac{1}{2}$ a grain as quite sufficient to produce certain definite physiological effects. The toxic dose of bichromate is considered not to exceed at the most a few grains. Notwithstanding the fact that the woman took about 100 grains, she recovered without serious inconvenience. It would seem that the mixture of alcohol and wine proved sufficient to act as a neutralizing stimulant in preventing the toxic effects.

(To be Continued.)

JOHNS HOPKINS HOSPITAL MEDICAL SOCIETY.

Regular Meeting, held November 21, 1904.

Experimental Streptococcus Arthritis.—Dr. Rufus I. Cole reviewed this subject and reported some work he had done during the past year with the purpose of throwing light, if possible, on the nature of the arthritis of rheumatism. The tendency, he said, was nowadays to regard acute articular rheumatism as an acute infectious disease and the following four theories had been advanced to explain the condition: (1) Rheumatism is due to a specific organism as yet unknown. (2) It is due to a specific diploeoccus or streptococcus. (3) It is a mild pyemia resulting from infection with the ordinary streptococci or staphylococci. (4) It is due to an ordinary bacillus. Those who have argued for the specific nature of the disease have been able to isolate a diplococcus from the joints, the heart's blood and the exudates of many cases. Meier, noticing the close connection between angina and rheumatism, has been able to isolate from the throats of anginal patients streptococci which produced acute articular rheumatism in animals. Mentzer has held that the angina and the anginal rheumatism, in these cases, were due, not to a specific organism, but to the ordinary parasites of the mouth, most often to streptococci. Diplococci have, however, been isolated from many cases (most often from severe ones) the most recent report having been that of Lewis, of Philadelphia.

The Specificity of the Diplococcus of Rheumatism.—Dr. Cole said that those who claimed, for the organism isolated a specific nature based this claim chiefly on its morphology. A paired coccus, sometimes in chains, the pairing being most marked in recent cultures and the general features quite similar to those of the streptococcus—these were its main characters. Marmorek's test was said not to be reliable in classifying the organism; and the dark discoloration in growth on blood agar, at one time thought to be characteristic, was said to occur also with other organisms. By inoculation of the organism isolated the production of arthritis, of endocarditis and of chorea had been reported.

Experimental Arthritis.—Dr. Cole's own work was begun with a streptococcus isolated from the blood of a patient suffering with endocarditis, septicemia and joint pains. Inoculations were made into the ear-veins of several rabbits and an arthritis was produced in practically every case. Another series of experiments was then carried out in which streptococci were used for the inoculations taken from patients suffering with various non-rheumatic conditions and giving no rheumatic history. Six races of streptococci were thus used, no one of them being the streptococcus of rheumatism. In practically all of the rabbits so inoculated a typical arthritis was produced. The English technic was followed—an emulsion of the culture being injected into the ear veins. The rabbits first became somewhat languid and later became lame, first in one joint and then in another. At autopsy a thick, tenacious fluid was found in some joint of the body and here the cartilage was smooth but the synovial membrane injected. Smears from the exudate showed large numbers of diplococci with flattened sides. In two rabbits a typical endocarditis developed and two showed twitching, incoordinated, possibly choreic movements. In other words, with streptococci from seven different sources results followed inoculations identical with those following inoculations of the so-called diplococcus of rheumatism, and the latter is therefore not specific. Dr. Cole called attention to the fact that the cases reported in the literature as having furnished specific organisms have been usually the severe cases with pericarditis and other complications. This fact, together with the frequency of a secondary invasion of streptococci, argued, he thought, against the specificity of the organism obtained. Dr. Osler mentioned the specimens which Paynter had obtained in his experiments and called particular attention to the significant nature of the experimental subcutaneous fibroid nodules. He felt certain that the disease was an acute infection, but the organism, he thought, still undetermined. Dr. Cole said that Poynter and Paine had been able to get cultures from rheumatic joints but that the attempts made at the Johns Hopkins Hospital had never been successful. Philip, who has reported elaborately on the subject, has also never succeeded in growing organisms from rheumatic joints. Dr. Bloodgood said that it had recently been noticed that in cases in which no organisms could be found in arthritic exudates, the villi of the joint (particularly in gonorrheal cases) often contained bacteria.

The Mosquitoes of Maryland.—Dr. Kelly exhibited a case presented to him by Professor Smith, of Rutgers, in which the commoner varieties of mosquitoes—male, female and larval forms—were beautifully mounted. He asked that further work be done to find out what forms infested Baltimore and to eliminate the malarial bearers if possible. Dr. Thayer said that the work done thus far on the subject showed that three forms of *Anopheles* were common in Maryland; the *maculipennis* or *claviger*, the *punctipennis* and the *crucians*. The main source of the mosquitoes of Baltimore was said to be the drainage wells which very often go uncleaned for years.

Multiple Carcinomata of the Ileum.—Dr. Bunting showed the specimens from two cases of this condition. Primary malignant epithelial tumors of the small intestine were, he said, exceedingly rare. Only one has previously been seen in the Johns Hopkins Hospital and only thirty could be found by Lubarsch in the whole literature. The first patient reported was a negro who had died with cardiovascular symptoms. In the upper ileum six nodules were found which turned out, on section, to be carcinomata with alveoli consisting of small polymorphous cells and a firm fibrous stroma with hyaline degeneration here and there. The tumors, though they answered only two of Billroth's requirements, were probably all primary. These tumors, and the ones reported in the literature, have been similar—were small, occurred well along in the carcinoma age, grew slowly and were relatively benign. They resembled the small skin carcinomata seen on the scalp and arising from the Malpighian layer (the Basalzellen Karzinom of Krohnpeker). The second patient showed symptoms of obstruction and a palapable mass in the right iliac fossa. Inoperable carcinoma was found at operation and a colostomy was done. Autopsy showed multiple primary carcinomata of the small intestines with no peritoneal involvement. Dr. Bloodgood said that these skin carcinomata were more frequently seen than formerly—due in part to earlier diagnosis and in part to a realization by the laity that growths anywhere are not to be neglected. Clinically they were, he said, only slightly malignant and might almost be called benign epitheliomata.

Regular Meeting, held December 5, 1904.

DISCUSSION OF GASTRIC ULCER.

Etiology and Pathogenesis of Gastric Ulcer.—This phase was treated by Dr. Welch, who was, he said, struck with the fact that little of real importance had been added to our knowledge of the cause and development of round ulcer since the appearance of his own article on the subject, twenty years ago. The subject derived interest from the frequency of the condition and the great variety of complications and sequelæ; and it had been almost unique in having been treated so largely by the statistical method, the classical report being the publication of Brinton. The obvious fallacies of statistics were not, however, absent in this connection; and the frequency of round ulcer as determined by autopsy has varied largely with the care of search for it. It has been easy to overlook the scars of ulcers and to assume a round ulcer from a scar due to other causes. Large series of autopsies have shown either ulcers or the scars of them in about five per cent. of the cases. Clinically about one to two per cent. of adults in hospitals have shown the condition, though the incidence of the disease varies with locality.

Age and Sex Incidence of Gastric Ulcer.—The statistics published some years ago had shown round ulcer to be commonest in females from twenty to thirty years and in males from thirty to forty years. Recent statistics had, however, tended to restrict the enormous preponderance in females and in some instances to make the condition actually more frequent in males. Advanced life, also, has recently been shown to be less immune to round ulcer than was formely supposed to be the case.

Etiology of Round Ulcer.—Traumatism, recently emphasized in this connection, was said to be a possible cause more often than had previously been thought. Orth has recently advanced a theory which makes gastric ulcer analogous to cubitus, the condition having been seen in association with spinal curvature and with gall-stones and being thought of as an actual pressure slough. No good explanation for the disease has been given though there have been many hypotheses. It has been agreed that the presence of gastric juice is essential, for the ulcer occurs only in stomach, duodenum above the ampulla of Vater and, rarely, in the esophagus. No analogue to it has been found in the body, though some have thought it similar to the corroding ulcer of the uterine cervix. Whatever the ultimate explanation, local nutritional disturbance must be present; and circulatory changes (embolus, thrombosis, arterio-sclerosis, obliterative endarteritis) have, since Virchow's day, been thought of as causative. Such pathological changes have often been present near the ulcers but their causal relation to them has not been proven. Klebs has advanced a theory of spasm of the vascular wall as the cause of gastric ulcer; but the theory has not become anything more than pure hypothesis. Spasm of the muscle wall, followed by ischemia, has also been thought of in this connection, experimental ulcer having followed section of the vagi below the diaphragm in rabbits. This work, however, when repeated by Donati gave absolutely negative results. The probability is that gastric ulcer starts in many ways; the only prime requisite being a local nutritional disturbance. The real problem: Why an ulcer does not heal? has always remained unsolved; ane-

mia, hyperacidity and muscle-spasm having each been cited as the cause of the phenomenon, without good reason. Dr. Welch showed specimens of gastric ulcer illustrating various varieties and sequelæ of the condition.

Symptomatology of Gastric Ulcer.—Dr. Campbell Howard reviewed the manifestations of round ulcer as illustrated by the cases seen at the Johns Hopkins Hospital. Vomiting, pain and hematemesis had been the cardinal symptoms and had occurred in about the relative frequency usually reported. Pain was usually referred to the epigastrium, its site bore no relation to the site of the ulcer, and it varied from a discomfort to an acute colic. It was rarely continuous, was most marked after meals and was usually increased by pressure. In some patients it occurred independently of meals but most often it was greatest after the ingestion of food and the series exemplified the truth of Gerhard's maxim: "Those who refuse to eat because of pain have gastric ulcer." Vomiting was present in about 85 per cent. of the cases. It occurred at the height of digestion or just after the ingestion of food and varied noticeably with the severity of the pain. In some cases it was provoked for relief. The blood vomited was usually bright red but the coffee-ground vomitus was noted in two-thirds of the cases. In some cases fatal hemorrhage occurred without physical signs (of hemorrhage foudroyant of the French). Blood, Dr. Howard said, would be found in the stools more often if more carefully looked for. Nausea was usually absent. Dyspepsia due to hyperacidity, constipation and retention of appetite were usual. Loss of weight occurred in 54 of 82 cases—9 showing a loss of 40 lbs. Epigastric tenderness was often felt and sometimes tenderness or pressure over the back. A mass (due to abscess, perforation, exudate or scars) was present in twenty cases of the series. Only 27 per cent. of the cases showed hyperacidity and in nine hydrochloric acid was absent—seven of these showing the presence of lactic acid (due possibly to stagnation of food). The blood showed a chloranemia similar to that of carcinoma.

Complications of Gastric Ulcer.—Fatal hemorrhage occurred in 8.5 per cent. of the cases, perforation in 3.6 per cent. Obliteration of the liver dulness without ascites was said to mean perforation. Parotitis, tetany, perigastric adhesions and ulcus carcinomatosum were also seen.

Varieties of Gastric Ulcer.—The cases were divided into the acute and chronic types. Two classes of the former were distinguished—the primary (acute perforative) and the secondary (occurring in infectious diseases, heart disease, etc.). Five classes of the chronic type were recognized—the gastralgic, characterized chiefly by pain; the catarrhal, by vomiting; the hemorrhagic, by presence of blood; the cachectic, by wasting without gastric signs; and the dyspeptic, by the latent course.

Diagnosis of Gastric Ulcer.—This, said Dr. McCrae, is easy in the typical and difficult in the atypical cases. A large number of the cases are latent and cannot be diagnosed. Microscopical examination of the vomitus for blood should always be made. Similar conditions from which gastric ulcer must be differentiated are gastric neuroses (in which pain is not constant and gastric analyses negative), gallstone, gastric crises of locomotor ataxia, and all the acute abdominal conditions. In the chronic cases the diagnosis from cancer offers most difficulty. A constant hyperchlorhydria speaks for ulcer.

The Medical Treatment of Gastric Ulcer.—The case should, Dr. McCrae said, always be regarded as a possibly surgical one from the start and nurses and attendants warned to be on the watch for dangerous symptoms. Rest in bed for four weeks or longer, absence of irritation to the stomach and the provision of as good a blood supply as possible, were said to be the principles of treatment. All food should be stopped by mouth for from four to six days. Liquid nourishment, preferably whey or peptonized milk, should then be given for ten to fourteen days. One quart should be given per day and this should be diluted with alkalis. The diet should then be gradually increased, a soft solid diet being reached at the end of four weeks. Atropine, large quantities of alkali, bismuth, silver nitrate and olive oil were also said to be of use. Lavage, though not necessary as a routine, was said not to be contraindicated. The patient's diet should be carefully watched, even after he recovers. In chronic cases the treatment was said to be the same,—surgical interference being demanded when doubt exists as to the presence of malignancy and when repeated hemorrhages occur. For the pain, bromides, codeine and morphine should be used.

Surgical Treatment of Gastric Ulcer.—This subject was treated by Dr. Finney. He spoke first of the interest of gastric surgery and said that it was synonymous really with the surgery of the early and late features of gastric ulcer. It also illustrated the recent tendency of the internist and the surgeon to get together—the former realizing his limitations and the latter his possibilities. For the hemorrhage, the surgeon could not do much, on account of the inaccessibility of the bleeding point; and the early cases should be left to the physician. Later exploration was indicated, but little could be done beyond drainage. If hemorrhage was frequent, a jejunostomy and intestinal feeding were indicated. In perforation surgical treatment has been satisfactory when the cases have been seen early. Rapid cleansing, as slight insult to tissue as possible and closure without drain were the steps of procedure in early cases. For stenosis that operation was said to be best which disturbed relations as little as possible, and pyloroplasty was said to answer this requirement. For the remote conditions (dilation of stomach and the late train of neurotic symptoms) gastroenterostomy and pyloroplasty have proven useful. As a rule, the more found at operation the greater has been the relief the surgeon could give. Dr. Pancoast reported a case of perforating gastric ulcer who was jaundiced and showed bile in the urine. At operation a large amount of·free bile was found in the peritoneal cavity.

NEW YORK STATE MEDICAL ASSOCIATION, NEW YORK COUNTY BRANCH.

Regular Monthly Meeting, held December 19, 1904.

The President, Francis J. Quinlan, M.D., in the Chair.

The regular scientific business of the evening opened with an address by Dr. Constantine J. McGuire in memorial of the late Dr. William R. Pryor.

Dr. Pryor Memorial.—Dr. McGuire said that Dr. Pryor had been well above the average as a student and besides being distinguished in athletics at Princeton. He graduated from the College of Physicians and Surgeons in 1881. A few years later he became associated with the Polyclinic where he became a full professor of gynecology in 1895. While still a comparatively young man, he obtained a position at the Charity Hospital and was one of the moving spirits to bring about the needed reforms in that institution and to make the commisioners of health realize that more money must be spent on the medical and surgical department, if the poor were to be properly treated. He was an indefatigable worker for the City Hospital and often on cold wintry nights would sometimes go in a rowboat to see patients whom he had operated on during the day, not infrequently bringing with him delicacies for the sick not provided by the ordinary hospital dietary. The work for which Dr. Pryor will be known in gynecology consisted mainly of his development of the vaginal route as the principal avenue for the performance of most gynecological operations. He has done more to bring about the present favor in which vaginal operative gynecology is held than almost any other man. He will be long remembered for the introduction of the operation of bloodless hysterectomy, which he developed with wonderful technical skill and patient devotion to the problems involved. In recent years he had been occupied to no inconsiderable extent with the problem of puerperal sepsis and his suggestion of the employment of iodoform has borne more fruit in the saving of life in this awful disease than any other therapeutic method that has been suggested. He died, bravely facing the end, knowing that it was coming, realizing that that relentless foe to humanity, pernicious anemia, had a death-grip on him, containing his calmness and even his good spirits until the very end. Few men have been more worthy of their great profession than Dr. William R. Pryor.

Leucemia Treated by the X-rays.—Dr. Arthur Holding described a series of cases of leucemia treated by means of the X-rays. Altogether up to the present time 45 cases have been described in literature which have undergone this treatment, and while practically all of them have been improved, some have been cured. Cure is not considered to have taken place until the myelocytes have disappeared from the blood and the tumors have gone and not returned for several months. In only a few cases has the spleen decreased to normal. Many cases improved for some time and then after a relapse a fatal issue became inevitable. The general impression, however, that can scarcely fail to be gathered is that this method of treatment is not only well worth trying, but that it represents the most effective therapeutic measure at present at command for these otherwise inevitably progressive and fatal diseases.

Illustrative Cases, Case I.—The first case was one of splenomyelogenous leucemia in an Austrian male, aged thirty-five years. In 1903, this man noticed an enlargement of the glands under his axilla. Under the use of an ointment, these enlarged glands disappeared. Later, however, enlarged glands appeared above the clavicles. Then systemic symptoms began to develop. He suffered from nightsweats quite frequently and there was some cough, especially in the morning with white and frothy mucus. He began to lose in weight and especially the subcutaneous fat diminished. His postcervical glands now became enlarged, and the enlargement of his axillary glands recurred. His epitrochlear glands could now be felt, and it was very evident on examination that none of the glands involved an inflammatory condition, since they were all perfectly movable beneath the skin. After the use of tonics, cod liver oil and other means had failed, he was given X-rays on a number of occasions and the tumors disappeared. There was a corresponding improvement in his general condition and also in his blood condition.

Splenomyelogenous Leucemia, Case II.—This case occurred in a German woman whose first symptom was a sense of intense fulness in the abdomen shortly after eating. She suffered from malaria, but had never had either tuberculosis or syphilis. She noticed that starchy food or anything that produced gas in her stomach gave rise to great shortness of breath. There was a heavy weight bearing down upon her left side, and she feared the growth of a tumor. In February, 1903, physical examination showed an enormously enlarged spleen filling almost the entire left half of the abdomen. At this time the blood count showed somewhat over 3,000,-000 reds and 326,000 white blood corpuscles. The myelocytes represented 25 per cent. of this number. She was treated by cathartics and intestinal antiseptics, by hydrochloric acid and Fowler's solution and quinine, but without any effect until after the X-ray seances were begun. Almost at once improvement set in and the spleen became very much reduced in size. At the present time after some 30 treatments, the spleen has retired behind the border of the ribs and is not palpable, though it is still enlarged. Her blood condition has returned almost to normal. Indeed the red cells are in normal number and so is the amount of hemoglobin. There are still, however, some 30,000 white cells in each cubic millimeter. The differential count is much more encouraging now than it was before. At the present time the myelocytes number only six-tenths of one per cent.

X-ray Bath.—In opening the discussion Dr. E. B. Finch reported a case of splenomyelogenous leucemia in which the patient had been treated by complete exposure to the X-rays with the exception that head was covered with tinfoil. The result was a rapid reduction in the size of the tumor and an immediate general improvement in the patient's condition. With regard to the use of the X-rays for this condition, it is especially important to persist in its use and not to fear possible evil results. Sometimes it happens that while an X-ray burn is healing, the process of improvement in the blood condition seems to go on without interruption. In one case in which an enormous spleen was present, reaching far below the umbilicus, improvement was brought about by means of the X-ray treatment, though there had been copious hemorrhages and all hope was practically given up. The patient suffered from great pain, so that he had to be carried up. After the fifth X-rays exposure he was able to walk up. A year ago he left, very much improved in health and the improvement has continued ever since. In his case exposures had been made with the most powerful X-ray tubes for ten minutes in front, ten minutes at the back and ten minutes on the sides. High tension tubes were used, as a rule, because it was found that low tension tubes did not produce the desired result. It was found also that the low tubes produce burns quite as readily as the other. The X-rays must be used to their physiological limit. If the physician is to secure the best results, he must take a certain amount of risk in his treatment. After all, the disease is usually considered to be fatal and therefore risks are perfectly justifiable.

Reduction of All Enlarged Glands.—Dr. Finley R. Cook said that all enlarged glands responded to treatment by the X-rays, even in cases in which the enlargement was due to tuberculosis and already the glands had become soft and even where there was a mixed infection. .Enlargement of the thyroid glands were also favorably affected. Simple goiter, for instance, was made to disappear after six weeks' treatment consisting of three treatments per week. In Graves' disease, the thyroid gland became lessened in size and many of the nervous symptoms disappeared. Even when the enlargement of a spleen was due to malaria a reduction in its size followed exposure to the X-rays. Dr. Cook considered that the most fruitful aspect of the use of X-rays for enlarged glands must be as a preventive wherever a tendency to glandular hyperplasia was noted. In this way it seems not unlikely that glands might be kept from becoming malignant even though the original tumor was beginning to give off metastases.

X-ray and Hyperplasia.—Dr. Charles Warrenne Allen said that so much had recently been said against the X-rays that it was a pleasure to hear something favorable to them. In his own experience the X-rays had often proved a very valuable curative agent. As a result of their use in many affections, diseases formerly considered incurable were now known to be curable. He has been able not infrequently to cause tumors of the spleen to disappear and he has no doubt that further experience with the X-rays will show them to be of service in still further affections where their beneficial effects is as yet unsuspected.

Lymphatic Leucemia.—Dr. Grad said that he had recently had under his care a man nearly seventy years of age suffering from lymphatic leucemia of an acute type. This disease usually does not take long to bring the patient to a fatal issue. He was not able to save life, yet before death came, all the glands had been made to disappear and the spleen had become less in size. Forty-one exposures had been given in this case without producing any dermatitis. Systemic effects had been noticed and a high temperature had been noted as the result of the absorption of toxic material from the rapidly breaking down glands. In Hodgkin's disease, much better results may be expected and even a permanent cure is not out of the question.

In closing the discussion, Dr. Holding said that so far there are no reports of cases of cures of lymphatic leucemia. There is no doubt, however, that some benefit accrues from the use of the X-rays even in these cases. In splenomyelogenous leucemia and in Hodgkin's disease better results may be constantly looked for and indeed in some cases patients have remained entirely well for nearly two years after treatment.

Abuse of Water Drinking.—Dr. Morris Manges said that in recent years it has become the custom, almost on general principles, for physicians to recommend people who come to them for advice, to drink plentifully of water. It is supposed to flush out the system and is not likely to do any harm. Good authorities have protested recently against the possibility of serious danger from the taking of greater quantities of water than can be readily eliminated, especially in persons laboring from kidney and heart disease. In Von Leyden's text-book of the dietetic treatment of the disease and in Von Noorden's text-books on nutrition and metabolism especially with regard to nephritis, the dangers of overmuch water are pointed out. It is true that when more water is taken more is usually eliminated and a greater quantity of urea escapes from the system, but this is only for the moment, and later on, while the urine may remain abundant, it drops as regards its solid contents, and the consequence is that there is much elimination work without a corresponding removal of effete material.

Water as a Diuretic.—It is sometimes said that water is the best diuretic that we have. It must not be forgotten, however, that this is only true when water increases the blood pressure in the kidneys. On the other hand, the taking of an abundance of water leads to obesity because with an abundance of liquid, more food is likely to be taken and always more food is absorbed. In heart diseases an abundant supply of water may thoughtlessly increase the embarrassment of the heart by giving it much more fluid to drive through the circulation. It is only a popular delusion then that the more water a person drinks the better, though even by most physicians to doubt the advisability of kidney flushing is considered a rank heresy.

Method of Restriction.—When in the course of a chronic nephritis the heart has become incompetent, it is especially important to limit the amount of liquid taken. It has been suggested by German physicians that the patient should be carefully instructed not to take more than a quart of liquid at the most in a day. One day in a week, however, he may be allowed all he wants and this will serve the purpose of flushing out material that should be eliminated while not unduly increasing the work of the heart. In cases of contracted kidney, fluids must be restricted with special care, though of course in these cases, the occurrence of ascites is usually of itself a sufficient indication of a necessity for liquids. The value of a dry diet in heart disease can be readily recognized in most cases and should be considered to be a much more frequent indication than the abundant use of water. Especially is this true with regard to ice water.

Effects of Water.—Water in large quantities was supposed to have especial effect upon metabolism. It was thought even to help albuminous chemical processes within the body. This has been shown not to be true, and it has also been demonstrated that it neither decreases the amount of uric acid manufactured nor causes that material to disappear faster than would otherwise be the case. Minkowsky has shown that the old tests by which such advantages were claimed for water, did not give proper information when the urine was dilute. It seems clear therefore that small quantities of water, somewhat frequently repeated in order to allay thirst and prevent discomfort, are better for most kidney and heart patients than too free use of water.

Laying the Ghost of Flushing.—Dr. Simon Baruch said that Dr. Manges was to be congratulated on daring to lay the ghost of the flushing of the system by means of water. Water internally produces the same effect as water externally. Cold water externally applied will revive a fainting patient. If the person were very weak, however, and were put in a tub of cold water, collapse would almost surely follow. In the same way small quantities of cold water internally are similar. If about every two hours two to four ounces of ice water, that is water at about 40 degrees, be given, patients are distinctly

stimulated. This is especially true for the urinary secretions. The increased urination may go as high as 80 ounces per day. On the other hand it is dangerous to flush out whenever the heart is overburdened or when, as at the end of infectious diseases, it has suffered severely from the strain of the continued febrile processes in the body for several weeks. Of course when much water is leaving the body, as in cholera, then an abundant use of water is especially indicated. After hemorrhage also large quantities must be taken. In general, however, it must not be forgotten that water is not an entirely harmless agent and that it must be used according to the indications of each individual case.

Individualization.—Dr. Alfred Meyer said that even in health an excess of water may work harm,. but so also may an excess of anything else however good in itself. The present fad is for insisting on the eating of eggs in the early stages of consumption and he has seen not a few cases recently in which patients' digestions were hurt by an irrational use of so good an article of diet as eggs. With regard to the use of table waters, physicians need to warn patients who have suffered from angina pectoris, not to use much carbonated water, since during the course of the liberation of gas from such water mechanical interference with the heart's action may result. In general, for patients suffering from heart and kidney disease, it is important to note the effects of water drinking upon each of them. No general rule can be laid down. Each individual is a law unto himself. If an abundance of water seems to be helpful to the patient, as it often is, if there is costiveness present, or an insufficient amount of urine has been passed, then it may be continued. Its effect, however, must be constantly noted.

Water in Fevers.—Dr. Beverley Robinson said that in continued fevers, such as typhoid, he believes in the giving of water frely. Patients crave water very much and suffer much less discomfort if it is allowed them. He does not believe that the heart is injured in such cases and Debove's statistics of typhoid fever patients treated by large quantities internally show excellent results with this method. In acute nephritis, Dr. Robinson considers that the amount of fluid given should be very limited. In chronic nephritis, however, it is a matter entirely with the individual and more often than not, except where there is a tendency of anasarca, the use of water freely will be found to be beneficial rather than harmful.

Dr. Ransom said that no better stimulant to metabolism and chronic conditions can be found than the free use of water. He would not care to forego it, except where there were distinct contra-indications in a special case. It has been pointed out that it is of great use in all digestive processes, even in the saponification of fats in the intestines. Large quantities of it may be employed in many affections with gratifying results.

Chronic Nephritis.—Dr. Manges, in closing the discussion, said that the most important contra-indication to the use of water very freely is chronic nephritis. Undoubtedly there has been an abuse of it in this matter. Almost any patient who comes with the story of having suffered from chronic nephritis will be found to be using lithia or other table waters in large quantities by the prescription of his physician. In general it may be said that the important rule is to watch the quantity of urine passed and to see whether the water ingested is.

finding its way out of the system and is not being retained to increase the tension of the circulation and make the metabolic processes within the body more difficult than before. This is especially important in the continued fevers. Two-thirds of the water ingested should find its way out of the kidneys, and if it does not, it is accumulating within the system. If the water does not come out, the cause for such disturbance of elimination must be looked for and if possible removed. Of course it is important to treat the cases individually according to the indications in each case. Some patients are benefited by small amounts of cold water given frequently, some derive more benefit from even large quantities of water.

What Dr. Manges would protest against, however, is the inconsiderate giving of the advice to drink water freely in nearly all cases of kidney disease and in many other cases where it may be contra-indicated. It is not true that at least the water can do no harm. Large quantities of water may work serious harm in ailing persons. Here, as in everything else, the physician must use his intelligence and the knowledge gained from clinical observation in order to guide him in the use of this valuable remedy for various types of disease. There is no general rule for this any more than there is for anything else that is likely to do the patient good.

MANHATTAN DERMATOLOGICAL SOCIETY.

Regular Monthly Meeting, held December 2, 1904.

The President, I. P. Oberndorfer, M.D., in the Chair

Pruritus.—Dr. J. Sobel presented the following case: A woman, about fifty years old, complained of pruritus over the body at varying intervals for the past five years; since July last patient is taking occasional doses of cannabis indica and steadily 15-grain doses of natrium bromide t.i.d. Ten days ago patient noticed large papules and nodules along the tibiæ and on the feet; also a few nodular masses on the arms; the body is clear; the nodules involve subcutaneous tissue as well as the true skin. Owing to violaceous color and situation, Dr. Sobel at first thought he had to deal with an erythema nodosum; subsequently he changed his diagnosis to a bromoderma. There was no history of rheumatism, the joints are not involved and the urine is negative. Drs. Cocks, Kinch and Ochs said history favored diagnosis of bromine eruption; Dr. Gottheil inclined to call it erythema nodosum; Dr. C. W. Allen said it looked like an erythema nodosum, but there was a type of bromine eruption much resembling the eruption of an erythema nodosum. He thought this such a case; at least history favored such a diagnosis. Dr. Oberndorfer said the history in this case was suspicious of a possible connection between the eruption and the administration of bromine; he tends to side with Dr. Gottheil. Dr. Sobel, in concluding, quoted "Morrow" on a type of bromine eruption resembling and often mistaken for erythema nodosum.

Syphilis.—Dr. W. S. Gottheil presented two cases of tertiary and intractable syphilis, both exceedingly obstinate and rebellious to treatment. Case I was a gumma involving the upper lip and adjacent nasal structures; in spite of heroic treatment condition does not improve; patient states his body was never at any time perfectly clear since he contracted the disease, nearly twenty years ago. Case II was a large infiltrating gumma of the lower tibial region. Dr. Pisko spoke favorably of daily injections of bichloride. Dr. Kinch said tonic treatment must

also be given in these cases; he saw better results and Hg. and K. I. seemed to work better when tonic treatment with iron was inaugurated. Dr. Oberndorfer favored inunctions.

Chronic Onychia.—Dr. J. Sobel then showed a child with a chronic onychia, involving the finger nails, also, to a lesser extent, the toe nails; there was a history of thumb-sucking and nail-biting; the condition involved the nail-bed and surrounding cuticle.

Lupus Vulgaris.—Dr. Edward Pisko showed a case of lupus vulgaris; condition present for thirty years and treated abroad and here; treated with Koch's tuberculin with negative results, and under all and every kind of treatment likewise no result. Recently X-ray therapy was inaugurated; in all 45 exposures given since last May, with very gratifying results. Dr. Pisko exhibited photos of patient taken before X-ray exposures were begun; the results are very striking and encouraging.

Tuberculous Syphilide.—Dr. E. L. Cocks presented a young woman showing papular and nodular lesions on the face and neck. Patient does not deny exposure, but no lesions of a recent or remote infection can be made out; patient states she had a similar eruption on face about six months ago, which disappearing left small atrophic scars. The alæ nasi folds show fissures. The present eruption is of three weeks' duration. Dr. Cocks believes it to be specific. The members regard the eruption as a tuberculous syphilide.

Pityriasis Rosea.—Dr. B. F. Ochs showed a young woman with a typical eruption of pityriasis rosea on the body of ten days's duration; the mother lesion is well seen on the sternum; scalp shows slight seborrhea sicca. Dr. L. Weiss regards the eruption of pityriasis rosea as belonging to the erythematous diseases, non-parasitic and probably of internal origin, depending upon gastric disturbances or internal fermentation. He failed to find any micro-organism and therefore excludes it from the mycotic diseases; the clinical picture and course was totally different from true tinea circinatus et maculosum. Dr. Abrahams stated he was not yet convinced that pityriasis rosea was not of mycotic origin; failure to find microbe proves nothing. Dr. Allen still believes in its parasitic origin, although he cannot offer any new substantial proofs. It is distinct from ringworm; the latter is mycotic, the former may be; acute attacks occur over night, due to errors in diet, and he saw an alcoholic who was sure to get an acute outbreak whenever he stopped drinking. Dr. Oberndorfer said ringworm begins as a macule, spreads and heals in the center; pityriasis rosea as a primitive plague, with secondary squamous lesions; at one time both diseases were confounded and classified as the same disease.

Dr. Edward Pisko presented a young man showing squamous circinate lesions on the body of eleven days' duration and shown as the circinate type of pityriasis rosea. Drs. Weiss and Gottheil regard this case as tinea circinatus. Dr. Allen said it may be pityriasis rosea; the case will bear further investigation.

Dr. W. S. Gottheil then presented a girl of fourteen years, with so-called spontaneous outbreaks (consisting of scratch marks and excoriations) on the arms, legs and face; the first lesions were observed by the mother at the time of the girl's first menstruation. Dr. Gottheil is of the opinion that these lesions are self-induced by patient, and in this respect resembled a case presented to the society about one year ago.

Impetigo Circinatus.—Dr. Pisko showed a young man with eczematous lesions on little finger of right hand and left thumb, also an eczematous patch on right cheek; present about eight months and exceedingly rebellious to treatment; patient's occupation is that of a clerk. Dr. Gottheil said it resembled impetigo circinatus. Dr. Abrahams thought it was mycotic eczema. Dr. Kinch said it resembled the condition known as dermatitis repens. Dr. Allen said the fingers were eczematous, probably mycotic in origin; the face lesion may develop into a lupus subsequently. Dr. Oberndorfer expressed his opinion as being neuritic in origin.

Multiple Sarcoma.—Dr. Wachsman showed a case which he termed multiple sarcoma of the skin, basing diagnosis upon microscopical findings. This patient was presented by Dr. Pisko about a year ago. The consensus of opinion expressed was that this case was one of mycosis fungoides; an opinion shared when first presented by Dr. Pisko. Considerable discussion on the differential diagnosis and treatment followed. Dr. Gottheil reported a case of acute lead poisoning following local application of liq. Burrowi to a recent burn.

The following new officers were elected for the ensuing year: President, Dr. E. L. Cocks; vice-president, Dr. J. S. Sobel; secretary-treasurer, Dr. A. Bleiman.

BOOK REVIEWS.

LECTURES TO GENERAL PRACTITIONERS ON THE DISEASES OF THE STOMACH AND INTESTINES. By BOARDMAN REED, M.D., Professor of Diseases of the Gastro-Intestinal Tract, Hygiene, and Climatology in the Department of Medicine of Temple College, Philadelphia; Attending Physician to the Samaritan Hospital, etc., E. B. Treat & Company, New York.

THE author has endeavored in this single volume to meet the requirements of the general practitioner in the now extensive field of stomach and bowel disease. He does not follow the usual plan of considering all the diseases of the stomach and then those of the intestines, but, in a somewhat unique and instructive manner, groups stomach and bowels together as one tract. For example, he takes up in one group all their displacements, in another their different ulcers, in another their tumors, then their neuroses, etc. The cases of membranous catarrh he distinguishes as of two types, those strictly neurotic, and those accompanied by more or less enteritis; for their treatment he commends Von Noorden's detailed system of overfeeding and the administration of food which will leave much undigested residue. In discussing chronic gastritis, the writer differs from Cohnheim and some other foreigners, and agrees with Boas, Riegel, Einhorn, etc., that this disease may be manifested by hyperacid stomach contents as well as by subacid. On this basis he divides the cases into the sthenic and the asthenic types. Hyperchlorhydria he looks upon as either an indication of a beginning stage of gastritis, or a manifestation of Reichmann's diseases. In the chapter on Intestinal Parasites he wisely limits himself to the clinical findings, omitting the mass of biological details which are so easily found elsewhere. The section on diseases of the rectum and anus has been written by Dr. C. F. Martin. The following axiom is not without interest: "All fistulas in the neighborhood of the anus or rectum are the direct result of abscesses which have been either neglected or improperly treated." Diet, massage, electricity and gymnasium exercise are given ample consideration, diagnostic methods are detailed at length, and some useful tables of differential diagnosis, as under the headings of cancer and ulcer, are appended. "The Symptomatic Guide to Diagnosis," which the author

calls to our special attention, seems to us to have little if any value.

KIRKE'S HANDBOOK OF PHYSIOLOGY. By W. D. HALLIBURTON, M.D., F.R.S., Professor of Physiology, King's College, London. Nineteenth Edition, with nearly 700 illustrations including some colored plates. P. Blakiston's Son & Co., Philadelphia.

THE nineteenth edition of a text-book of physiology shows how well the book must be gotten up and how suitable it is for the purpose intended, that of a guide to the medical student. There is no doubt that for its size, Kirke's handbook is one of the best of the text-books on the subject we have. In its present form with 900 pages, it has somewhat outgrown the designation of handbook, but it has not suffered any loss in popularity by its growth in size. Dr. W. D. Halliburton is to be complimented on the thorough way in which successive revisions are done and the present edition is well up to date. There seems every reason to think that the future of the handbook is likely to be as successful as its past.

REFRACTION AND HOW TO REFRACT. Including Sections on Optics, Retinoscopy, the fitting of Spectacles and Eye-glasses, etc. By JAMES THORINGTON, A.M., M.D., Professor of Diseases of the Eye in the Philadelphia Polyclinic and College for Graduates in Medicine; Member of the American Ophthalmological Society. Third Edition. Two hundred and fifteen illustrations, thirteen of which are colored. Pp. xviii + 314. P. Blakiston's Son & Co., Philadelphia.

IT would be superfluous to review this book in detail; it is as widely and as favorably known as any book of its class, of which fact the appearance of the third edition is sufficient evidence.

This edition shows no important changes; it is still a book for beginners, and one regrets that the author, who is extremely well-fitted for the task, has not allowed the book to advance in the evolutionary scale. It is at present one of rather a large class of books, fairly easy to write and more remunerative than a completer treatise would be, but because it is a little better than most of its compeers, it should naturally advance until it takes precedence, as Donders and Landolt did in their day, and as Hess does to-day in Germany.

BOOKS RECEIVED.

PRACTICAL DIETETICS. By Dr. A. L. Benedict. 12mo, 380 pages. G. P. Englehardt & Co., Chicago.

NERVOUS AND MENTAL DISEASES. Epitome Series. By Dr. J. D. Nagle. 12mo, 276 pages. Illustrated. Lea Brothers & Company, Philadelphia and New York.

MANUAL OF PHYSIOLOGICAL AND CLINICAL CHEMISTRY. By Dr. E. H. Bartley. Second edition. 12mo, 188 pages. Illustrated. P. Blakiston's Son & Co., Philadelphia.

PATHOLOGICAL TECHNIQUE. By Drs. F. B. Mallory and Jas. H. Wright. Third Edition. 8vo, 469 pages. Illustrated. W. B. Saunders & Co., Philadelphia, New York and London.

ANNUAL REPORT OF THE SURGEON-GENERAL OF THE PUBLIC HEALTH AND MARINE HOSPITAL SERVICE OF THE UNITED STATES. 1903. 8vo, 572 pages. Illustrated. Government Press, Washington.

A TEXT-BOOK OF HUMAN PHYSIOLOGY. By Dr. L. Landois. Tenth revised edition. Edited by Dr. A. P. Brubaker. Translated by Dr. A. A. Eshner. 8vo, 1,025 pages. Illustrated. P. Blakiston's Son & Co., Philadelphia.

THE MEDICAL NEWS.

A WEEKLY JOURNAL OF MEDICAL SCIENCE.

VOL. 86.　　　NEW YORK, SATURDAY, FEBRUARY 18, 1905.　　　NO. 7.

ORIGINAL ARTICLES.

INTRAPLEURAL COMPLICATIONS IN PULMONARY TUBERCULOSIS.[1]

BY S. G. BONNEY, A.M., M.D.,

OF DENVER, COL.

FAIRLY close observation of over fifteen hundred cases of pulmonary tuberculosis in private work has demonstrated the frequent association of intrapleural complications, and their practical influence in determining final results. The object of this paper is to call attention to some of these more important conditions, to suggest briefly a few of their diagnostic considerations, to elaborate their prognostic import, and to emphasize their rational management. No attempt is here made to present new features of diagnosis or to introduce innovations of treatment, either in the manner of operation or mechanical appliances. Non-recognition of the existence of pleuritic complications is occasioned in the majority of instances, not because of any absence of readily available data for this purpose, but through failure to apply the established principles of diagnosis to the evidence presented. In like manner the unfortunate results of treatment frequently are not due so much to the lack of adequate therapeutic measures which could be employed, as to the misconception of their rational scope in individual instances. It may be said parenthetically, that, unlike many diseases of the lungs, the primary obstacles to success in the management of these complications may not be ascribed to delayed diagnosis. It is a humiliating reproach to state that not infrequently the interests of the patient would be better subserved if the condition remained entirely unrecognized. The justice of this direct reflection upon the management in the way of occasional meddlesome and unwarranted surgical interference will be explained later. While early diagnosis must be encouraged through actual thorough examinations of the chest and the accurate recognition of physical signs, yet the essential consideration for successful results consists in a correct interpretation of the prognostic significance and an intelligent appreciation of the rationale of remedial indications. It should be stated as a preliminary postulate that the existence of pulmonary tuberculosis in an individual, very materially modifies the consideration of those surgical methods which may be styled operations of expediency. At the same time the consumptive is entitled by virtue of every instinct of humanity, no matter how hopeless his condition, to

the fullest measure of surgical aid, in conditions involving so-called operations of necessity. My conclusions are derived from the mistakes as well as the successes incident to my personal experience. More of real benefit sometimes accrues from the opportunity to witness the deplorable results of mistaken judgment than from the elated observation of a successful issue following a fortunate but, perchance, snap choice of procedure. In support of views to be presented perhaps a few selected and illustrative cases properly should be introduced. A more or less comprehensive review of such cases will be permitted in another paper.

The intrapleural conditions in the course of pulmonary tuberculosis to be considered in this connection are: (1) Pleurisy with serous effusion; (2) empyema; (3) pneumothorax; (4) pneumopyothorax.

Pleurisy with Effusion.—That this condition is much more frequent than generally supposed is explained largely by the fact that it is often overlooked. Provided an effort is made to conduct a thorough painstaking chest examination, it is difficult to conceive how a moderate or large pleural effusion, presenting such classic physical signs as area of flatness with diminished intensity, or absence of voice or breath sounds conforming to the letter S curve, with dislocation of the organs, can remain unrecognized. That such is occasionally true even in typical cases must be regarded as due to faulty and superficial methods of examination. It is by far more often the small effusion that escapes detection, the area of flatness being confined to the lower posterior portion of the chest, sometimes without extending laterally as far as the posterior axillary line. Both friction rubs and respiratory sounds may be plainly heard in some instances. It is readily seen how such an effusion may be overlooked even by careful and experienced examiners. The only precautions necessary to prevent this mistake consists in percussing to the very base of each lung in the back, and outlining the lower borders of resonance for the sake of comparison.

Small and even moderate effusions have often existed among my cases entirely devoid of such rational symptoms to suggest their presence as fever, dyspnea, emaciation, malaise or loss of appetite, their recognition being incident only to the course of periodical examinations. It has been interesting to note that material general improvement has often taken place simultaneously with the development of these effusions. Several years before Murphy proclaimed his treatment of tuberculosis through compression of lung by the introduction of nitrogen gas in the

[1] Read at the Annual Meeting of the Colorado State Medical Society, October, 1904.

pleural cavity, it had been observed by several, myself included, that lung compression by pleural effusion sometimes produced a salutary effect upon the immediate course of tuberculosis, and that the removal of the effusion by aspiration was occasionally followed by an aggravation of some of the annoying symptoms. In my experience the fever attending the course of consumption is sometimes, although by no means always, diminished perceptibly after the development of a small effusion. At the same time is manifested perhaps an improvement in cough with marked lessening of the expectoration, absence of previous pleuritic pains and strangely a material gain in weight. A removal of the effusion, when practised under these conditions several years ago, was occasionally a precursor of an exacerbation of temperature, increase of cough and expectoration, loss of weight and renewed activity of the tuberculous process as shown by the physical signs. This would suggest the positive benefit sometimes derived from the intrapleural compression of lung for the time being, and such is my belief. It should be remembered, however, that this favorable influence of compression does not always obtain even in pleural effusions, that its benefits are usually but temporary, and that no artificial compression either by gas or external contrivances save in exceptional instances, and to fulfil special indications, is to be commended. In other words, it is not the treatment of the tuberculous lung, *per se*, that should constitute the rôle of the medical adviser, but rather the management of the tuberculous individual himself. Laudable as have been the efforts to secure a favorable influence upon the tuberculous process by direct mechanical compression, it must be stated that the clinical results have not been particularly gratifying. Experience has shown that in uncomplicated cases it is rather the dilatation of the air cells and the other physiological changes incident to moderate altitudes that constitutes the desideratum, rather than compression of lung. It is no detraction from the genius of Murphy to allude to the frequent impracticability of his method, and to disparage its adoption for general purposes. It does remain, however, for the practitioner to take cognizance of the practical truth emphasized by his work to the effect that an idiopathic compression from serous effusion may be of distinct value in some cases. The practical lesson relates to whether or not there exists special indications for its removal. Irrespective of the duration and sometimes of the extent of the effusion it is my custom not to resort to aspiration in the absence of fever and dyspnea or of such a degree of mechanical compression as threatens subsequently to seriously embarrass cardiac and respiratory functions. If these conditions exist, however, removal of the liquid becomes imperative and should brook of no delay regardless of all other considerations. The presence of fever in itself, without reference to other rational symptoms or

physical signs, does not afford a distinct and reliable indication either for or against aspiration. In conjunction with other clinical facts it may furnish a valuable and sufficient justification for its employment.

It is not my practice, as has been advocated by some, to delay aspiration until fever has ceased, on the ground that the rise of temperature indicates a continuance of inflammatory action, and that with this there must ensue a recurrence of the effusion. If such indications as relate to the pulse and respiration are perfectly clear, aspiration is employed regardless of fever. On the other hand, a persisting fever not previously present attending a moderate effusion without other clinical manifestations suggests the expediency of operation. Without the exhibition of such clearly defined data there is no excuse for resorting to the aspirating needle even to the extent of an exploratory puncture. Those who regard as a myth the danger of converting a serous effusion into a purulent one by the introduction of the needle, have certainly been most fortunate in their technic or have had but little experience. Permit me to state most emphatically that several times in my experience, after a scrupulous disinfection of skin and hands, the introduction of an irreproachable needle has been sufficient to convey an infection into the pleural cavity with the distressing sequelæ attending an empyema. The use of the exploratory needle for diagnostic purposes purely is entirely without any justification whatever in these cases. Given a case of pleural effusion of any nature and extent with any combination of rational symptoms, if the indications for its removal be sufficiently clear, let ordinary aspiration be employed, and with the additional information secured through the gross appearance and the bacteriological examination of the exudate, a subsequent course of procedure can be safely and intelligently conducted. If, however, the indications are not clear on the merits of the clinical symptoms to demand removal, why indulge in meddlesome and dangerous interference simply for the purpose of diagnosis which for the moment is relatively unimportant. Contrary to the opinion entertained by some that the character of the treatment is directly dependent upon the nature of the effusion, and hence the desirability of determining early its precise nature, let it be asserted that among consumptives the question of entering the pleural cavity in any way should be decided purely as previously stated, upon the combination of symptoms and physical signs. In all such cases these should furnish sufficient data to constitute a safe and satisfying working basis without recourse to that refinement of diagnosis which exalts the findings of the laboratory and the autopsy at the expense of the patient himself. In the event that the clinical manifestations warrant the performance of aspiration, or assuming that the pleural cavity has already been entered, it is readily conceded that the future course is subject to some extent to the character of the effusion, although not entirely so, as will be subsequently shown. The present contention is simply that among pulmonary invalids the precise determination of the nature of the liquid, whether serous or purulent, is entirely unnecessary as regards a future course of action, in view of the guidance and direction afforded by other means. The employment of the exploratory puncture for diagnostic purposes solely is, therefore, condemned. Not until the development of urgent or dangerous symptoms is it necessary to establish such a diagnosis as to involve or justify surgical measures. Ordinary aspiration, when once practised in accordance with authorized principles, should be repeated at intervals as long as the previous condition remains in force, and suspended whenever these conditions cease to exist. If the effusion is found at once to be purulent, or later becomes so, the discussion should be more properly embraced under the ensuing head, empyema.

Empyema.—Ten years ago, in 1894, in a paper entitled "Methods of Treatment of Empyema," read before this Society, it was my privilege to study and review the various measures (as advocated by men of authority), to compare their relative advantages and disadvantages, and to note the peculiar conditions in which each was applicable or contra-indicated.

At that time it was the general dictum of the medical profession that the treatment of all cases of empyema should be that of surgical interference, the only difference of opinion relating to the choice of the method. In the paper referred to the most important preliminary consideration was said to be the influence of the etiology upon the prognosis and treatment. It may be of interest to quote brief extracts from this paper, and ascertain to what extent one can indorse the views then entertained.

"The important practical thought to be emphasized in this connection is the recognition of the existence of several species of bacteria in the exudate, endowed with varying properties and possessing marked differences in their virulence; that the most benign of these characterize the empyemas of children and the metapneumonic pleurisies of adults, and thereby furnish to the physician a justification for not resorting immediately, in all instances, to the more radical and mutilative measures of treatment. The therapeutic indications are conceded to be, first, prompt and thorough evacuation of the pus; second, prevention of a re-accumulation by means of free and continuous drainage and by the maintenance of asepsis; and, finally, the obliteration of the pus secreting cavity through adequate provision for the expansion of the lung and the collapse of the chest wall. Save in extreme cases a general tuberculous infection never contra-indicates an operation from which satisfactory results are frequently obtained."

A single preliminary aspiration was advocated in children and possibly in the metapneumonic pleurisies of adults. "The choice of simple aspiration is not based upon any faith in its adequacy to effect a cure, but is made with an aim to afford temporary relief, and at the same time to establish a diagnosis, admitting that the purulent nature of the effusion, particularly in adults, almost invariably demands subsequent operative measures. Irrigation, as frequently performed, is not only incomplete but is usually superfluous, and is often attended with certain danger."

Then follows at length a review of the indications for the technic of the several methods, with especial mention of the syphon drainage as practised by Potain and Bulau.

Quoting again for a moment, "Immerman, an ardent advocate of syphon drainage, at the Ninth International Medical Congress, held in Vienna in 1890, reported 49 cases directly cured by this method out of a total of 57. Upon the same occasion, Curschman reported 63 excellent results out of 75 cases."

"The aim to be attained in all methods making use of this principle has been to secure the proper continuous drainage, without permitting the entrance of air to the pleural cavity. By this means it was designed to produce the fullest expansion of the lung, and favor the obliteration of the pus cavity by restoring the parts as fully and quickly as possible to their normal conditions. Its chief disadvantages are the occasional entrance of air around the tube, destroying at once the syphon action, the necessarily slow and imperfect drainage accomplished, on account of the weak aspirating force employed, and the liability of the occlusion of the tube by large masses of coagula. Even Immerman admits 'that this method gives good results only in recent empyemas, in which the pus is not too thick.' Pleurotomy consists in the free opening of the pleural cavity, and provides for the immediate and thorough evacuation of its contents. A complete exit is offered to the clots and organic débris and perfect facilities for a continuous discharge. It is my opinion that this method is indicated as an initial procedure in the treatment of all cases of empyema, excluding only the use of the single aspiration in children, previously alluded to. It is admitted that pleurotomy alone will not always suffice for the later treatment of old, protracted cases, owing to the existence of certain complicating conditions. Were this method, however, more frequently employed in the early stages of the disease, before an opportunity be given for the development of unfavorable conditions, there would result far less frequently the necessity for recourse to the severer procedures. The opening by incision into the pleural cavity may be accompanied in some instances, if necessary, by the resection of a small portion of a single rib. This should be distinguished from the multiple rib resection, which of itself constitutes a separate method, is subject to different principles and indicated by other conditions."

For several years following the writing of this paper the conclusions enunciated, derived from the experiences of others, were conscientiously applied to appropriate cases of tuberculosis with almost invariably unfortunate results. The essential principle was to perform pleurotomy upon the consumptive, provided his general condition was not materially impaired, regardless· of what is now accepted as vitally important consideration, i. e., fever, chills, sweats, emaciation, etc. The only consideration then was the presence of pus, which demanded prompt evacuation and drainage. If the condition of the patient in far advanced phthisis was desperate, it was thought more merciful to permit him to die without inflicting the added torture of an operation. In the light of a considerable experience, which has been educative if sad, it has become apparent to me that the above course is directly and radically wrong. Observation of numerous cases bear out what might be regarded as an assumption. Some of these cases will be reported at length in a future paper to sustain the position taken, and illustrate the perilous responsibility assumed in advocating the radical operation for those comparatively well, and in withholding such surgical aid from those in urgent need, though apparently beyond hope. The radical operation is necessarily followed either by a sudden expansion of the previously compressed lung, which affords opportunity for renewed activity of the tuberculous process, and usually results in very quick softening and cavity formation, or is attended by failure of the lung to expand and obliterate the pleural cavity, which means long continued pus formation and great danger of amyloid change. In the absence of such clinical indications as fever, sweats and chills, it seems exceedingly ill-considered, not to say foolhardy, to precipitate the patient into the midst of such peril. To witness the spectacle of a rapidly progressive or even long continued decline, with a fatal termination, in one who before operation was well nourished, devoid of fever, and to outward appearances in good condition, and to observe the astonishing recovery from an empyema in one who was at first refused operation by a surgeon as being already moribund, and to be privileged to note his condition improve through a period of two years to a complete arrest of the underlying tuberculous process, and to a permanent resumption of earning capacity, is sufficient to shake the faith in the tenability and wisdom of the previously accepted principles pertaining to a course of treatment to be accorded pulmonary invalids.

My present custom in the empyema of consumptives, particularly if not too far advanced, is to let it alone unless there is some good and sufficient cause for interference along the lines previously suggested. If removal is indicated, simple aspiration is first employed and repeated as frequently as demanded. If even temporary improvement does not attend such a measure, recourse should be had to the syphon drainage of Bulan, as was adopted and reported by Dr. Whitney a year ago. If for any reason the drainage is imperfect and the clinical results not of a satisfying nature, then, and not until then, is it justifiable to resort to the radical measures of opening the pleural cavity, with or without the rib resection in consumptives. The only exception to this relates to thoroughly septic cases with perhaps chills, fever, sweats, great prostration, with an advanced underlying tuberculous infection, and preferably with the empyema well circumscribed. Under such conditions no time should be lost through temporizing measures in securing free opening and thorough drainage.

It is unnecessary to describe in detail the distinctly surgical procedure of pleurotomy. It may be permissible, however, to call attention to one or two features that have repeatedly impressed me as of great importance. First, the opening should not be too low, on account of being later closed by the rising diaphragm as the cavity begins to become obliterated. The pus is not emptied from the thorax altogether through the force of gravity, but is pumped out to a large extent by the action of the lung in inspiration and expiration. Secondly, the opening should be maintained sufficiently patulous to permit free drainage. This does not refer strictly to the opening in the chest wall but to the tubes as well. I have frequently seen the fenestrated tubes so often used completely obliterated by the growth of granulation tissue from the opposite sides of the wall when the tube has been kept in position for some time. Third, the tube should be removed daily and cleansed and shortened from time to time. in order to avoid the violent paroxysms of coughing produced by irritation of the opposing and approaching pleura. Fourth, daily after removal of the tube, the patient should not merely be turned over on the side, but should also be subjected to a short series of pulmonary gymnastics in various positions, first with head and shoulders of affected side almost touching the floor, with the hips elevated on the side of the bed. Subsequently the hips should be lowered carefully to the floor with the shoulders elevated. This permits the fullest possible drainage from sacculated pouches that are not emptied by the ordinary turning of the patient. I have seen this demonstrated on my patients very many times after the cavity was supposed to be emptied. Gentle coughing is often sufficient at such a time, to either violently expel large masses of flocculent coaguli or at least cause them to present at the opening, and allow their subsequent removal by the forceps.

Pneumothorax.—The discussion of this somewhat frequent complication of consumption should include properly a separate consideration of the cases of acute onset, and the open, closed and valvular varieties. No mention will be here made of those cases with air and liquid combined in the pleural cavity. The diagnosis of acute pneumothorax, simple as it would appear, and with such cardinal clinical features as sudden onset, following a severe attack of coughing, pain in the side, collapse, cyanosis, exceedingly marked dyspnea or orthopnea, mental agony and the familiar air-hunger, to say nothing of such classic physical signs as tympanitic resonance, absence of voice or breath sounds, impaired mobility of affected side and dislocation of organs, is nevertheless very frequently overlooked. It has been my privilege to see several such cases in consultation, the nature of which had not been recognized, although hysteria and various cardiac and circulatory disturbances had been suspected. In the majority of cases that have come under my observation the pulse has been exceedingly good, usually slow and of good quality,, and the heart sounds, on superficial examination, normal, suggesting at once that the difficulty is not cardiac in character. A painstaking examination of the chest, which means its complete exploration, utilizing both auscultation and percussion, is always sufficient to establish a diagnosis. The real inability to do this usually, results from failure to make such an examination, which is sometimes difficult on account of the desperate condition of the patient, or from lack of a correct appreciation of the physical signs to be obtained. It seems to be often imagined that pneumothorax should invariably exhibit such typical text-book signs as bulging of rib spaces, complete immobility of side, resounding tympany, amphoric or cavernous respiration with possibly metallic tinkling, and should be ushered in by sudden severe pain following violent cough or violent exertion. As a matter of fact there have occurred among my patients numerous instances of acute pneumothorax without any assignable cause whatsoever, and many others of partial pneumothorax without so much as an initial symptom to suggest examination. Bulging of the rib spaces is by no means constant, nor any very marked immobility of the affected side, although both may be expected in severe cases. A perfectly defined tympany on percussion, so often looked for, is seldom observed. Amphoric or cavernous respiration can exist only in case of an open pneumothorax with air passing freely in and out with each respiration through an open communication with a bronchial tube. Metallic tinkling occurs only in case of liquid, as well as air, being present in the pleural cavity. In the absence of a suggestive history and the above physical signs, the diagnosis should be made by the diminished intensity of breath and voice sounds, complete absence of dullness and possibly displacement of heart. It may be noteworthy to mention in passing that I have seen one patient in whom the heart, instead of being pushed in the opposite direction, was found drawn toward the affected side by virtue of previously existing fibroid contracting change, and one patient in whom there was complete flatness over the affected side, suggesting pleural effusion, and in fact occasioning an error in diagnosis.

as shown when effort was made to remove the liquid. This flatness was undoubtedly caused by the very great degree of hyperdistention. Two other physicians seeing the case with me concurred in the diagnosis of large pleural effusion.

The prognosis of these acute cases must be regarded, first, from the standpoint of the immediate present, and, secondly, in case of a not quickly fatal result, from the basis of its chronic existence. It has been frequently observed by others as well as myself that patients surviving the first few hours and possibly day or two may linger for several years, according to the extent of their original tuberculous infection and subsequent management. In cases of open pneumothorax the indications for treatment consist solely in excessive stimulation for a few hours. In urgent cases, while stimulation is, of course, plainly indicated, the only relief that has been in any way satisfying to the patient, family, or to myself has resulted from aspiration of the air. This is only applicable to cases of the valvular type permitting the ingress of air with each inspiration, but preventing its exit upon expiration and occasioning a positive hyperdistention in the pleural cavity.

Most remarkable subjective and objective relief following the aspiration is immediately noticed. This is almost instantaneous with the first withdrawal of air. The relief is but temporary, possibly of but a few hours duration, and can only be secured again by a repetition of the aspiration. Two patients recently seen by me were repeatedly aspirated, with marked improvement following each aspiration, but a recurring relapse. Finally a trocar and canula were inserted in each instance, the canula being left in place. This procedure was instrumental in securing some relief from the distressing symptoms, and was attended with a marked egress of air from the chest, but in neither instance prolonging the life of the patient over a few days. It is, however, the treatment par excellence for such cases, and provided there is not already too much impairment of respiratory capacity of the lung of the other side through extensive tuberculous infection, will occasionally enable the patient to adapt himself to his radically changed respiratory conditions. Pending this happy accomplishment, free inhalations of oxygen are of immediate value as well as in the acute cases of the open variety.

The existence of closed pneumothorax implies the previous occurrence of a ruptured pleura either of sudden onset or associated with a gradual development, which tear has subsequently healed and effectually closed the opening. It is frequently impossible to distinguish this from the valvular variety save that in the latter the symptoms are more urgent, the suffering more intense, and the danger more imminent. There is also usually less immobility of the side and less bulging. Of course in such a case there would be great diminution or absence of respiratory sounds on auscultation. The prognostic influence of this type of pneumothorax upon pulmonary tuberculosis, if unassociated with liquid, is not necessarily unfavorable, in truth actual benefit may result from the compression. The danger lies in the opportunity afforded for infection and inflammatory action through the entrance of micro-organisms before healing of the rupture takes place, producing the formation of pus, and converting the condition into pneumopyothorax. Before this transformation takes place the treatment of the chronic pneumothorax consists in letting it alone.

Pneumopyothorax.—Save from a thorough and comprehensive chest examination this complication is very likely to be unrecognized. The condition is a chronic process, and often is lacking in rational symptoms to suggest its presence, although in case of a remaining open communication with a bronchus, close inquiry will elicit the periodical expectoration of large quantities of sputum, especially in the morning or upon change of position as leaning over, or turning upon the affected side in bed. While upon examination the presence of air may be detected, the existence of the liquid is not infrequently overlooked if occurring only in moderate amount. This is due partly to the fact that the liquid remains low in the pleural cavity, and is not molded around the lung as in the case of a pleural effusion. In pneumopyothorax, the upper level of the liquid conforms strictly to a horizontal plane, and being contained at the extreme base of the pleural cavity may readily escape notice if a searching examination be not made at this point. If attention is paid to this there should be no difficulty in recognizing the fluid on percussion, particularly in comparing the lower borders of percussion resonance on the two sides. This is made still easier by the usual development of emphysema on the well side, still further lowering its limit of resonance. A most striking corroborative physical sign is a very marked change in the level of flatness under the liquid with a corresponding change in the position of the patient. This, with the readily obtainable splashing sound and often the metallic tinkling, renders the diagnosis extremely easy when looked for.

The prognosis, aside from such considerations as the hyperdistention previously mentioned in cases of simple pneumothorax, is to a great degree dependent upon the degree of sepsis existing, if any. The treatment of pneumopyothorax, in the absence of marked intrathoracic distention occasioning cardiac or respiratory embarrassment, or of such a degree of sepsis as to produce fever, chills and sweating, consists in doing nothing as far as the complication is concerned, or, at the most, resorting to an occasional aspiration if indicated. If further measures are demanded by the existence of urgent symptoms, the syphon drainage, as used to meet somewhat similar indications in empyema, is the rational plan to be

adopted. If unfortunately this expedient is found impracticable or insufficient and the condition becomes progressively more alarming, recourse must be had to an operation, which to this class of cases is most serious of all, the permanent opening of the pleural cavity.

From my observation it would seem that for these unfortunates the old saying of Dante should be changed to " Abandon hope all ye who are entered here.'" The atelectatic lung thoroughly collapsed is usually bound down by firm adhesions precluding all prospect of its ever expanding to any extent. And now begins the long period of interminable suppuration and drainage, the cheerful prospect of repeated rib resections, an Estlander or a Schede, non-healing wounds, and finally amyloid change to end the ever-deferred hope. And still perhaps a few years of this is preferable to an earlier death, and surely affords a justification for the operation if the exigency exists.

OBSERVATIONS ON TWENTY-EIGHT CASES OF PROSTATECTOMY.

BY J. BENTLEY SQUIER, M.D.,

OF NEW YORK.

AMONG the vast amount of literature which has accumulated during the past ten years upon the operative treatment of prostatic hypertrophy, much has been said concerning the correct method of attacking the enlarged gland, the proper incision to expose it most freely and the manipulation by which it can be enucleated most easily. But surprising as it may seem, the subsequent details and events which occur in the course of the patient's convalescence have been referred to in a comparatively cursory manner, and it is the writer's opinion that a thorough understanding of postoperative conditions is of a greater importance than a knowledge of all the alphabetical incisions for the exposure of the gland, which have been offered by their many originators.

Suffice it to say that at present the most popular route to the prostate is through the perineum, the most popular incision is one which was first used two thousand years ago by Celsus, and the instrument upon which the urethra is opened was devised by Johannes de Romanes in 1555.

The operation of prostatectomy, either by suprapubic or perineal method, is not a difficult surgical feat. The danger lies in the fact that the condition of the patient for whom the operation is indicated is usually such as to make any surgical procedure a thing of gravity. The question of operative or non-operative interference depends on so many factors, social, physical and otherwise, that no general rule can be advanced. Each patient is a law unto himself. Operation can be offered with a clearer conscience, even though the risk be grave, to a poor derelict of humanity who has neither mentality nor means enough to launch himself upon a life of catheteri zation than to his more fortunate brother who is able to take advantage of all the measures which modern surgery has developed to make such a venture less perilous.

The expression " selection of cases " is a misleading one. It is too often a screen behind which many seek to hide a mortality rate. Can one select cases? Rather does one not have to meet the indication as it arises and select the operation or procedure which is most applicable to the case, the ability to do this wisely being the the goal toward which we should aim?

The choice between suprapubic and perineal operation, until recently, has been largely a personal equation with the individual surgeon, the operation advanced being that with which he had had the most experience, but now the pendulum of approval seems to swing toward perineal prostatectomy, this being the operation of election in the majority of cases on account of the advantages of the operation alone. These advantages, as summed up by Watson are, viz: (1) Low mortality; (2) completeness of result; (3) openness to visual dissection. In conversation with some of the advocates of the suprapubic operation, I have asked what were the main features of this method which have attracted them so forcibly. The answer has invariably been that if a calculus was found to be present it could be readily removed, and also that the middle lobe, if much enlarged, was so easy of access and of removal. These replies have not been convincing, because if one opens the urethra through a median perineal incision and after exploring the bladder with the finger, finds a stone present of too great size to be removed through the urethral incision without danger to the urethra, he still has recourse to the suprapubic method, the opening he has already made being used to drain the bladder after operation. In regard to the size of the median lobe making its removal through the perineal opening difficult or impossible, the writer is well aware that such cases may present themselves, but we believe this often to be largely a question of manual dexterity on the part of the operator. In the same manner one surgeon would do an abdominal hysterotomy when another would be able to remove a uterus of similar size through the vagina. In removal of the prostate one has the added advantage of being able to break up any one lobe into its component divisions before delivering it through the perineal incision.

Among the greatest number of patients suffering from the symptoms of prostatism, the discrepancy between the real amount of prostatic enlargement and the amount of discomfort the patient experiences is very marked. A comparatively small prostate often gives rise to disturbances out of all proportion to its size. These symptoms frequently develop before one is directed to the prostate as the seat of the trouble. By this is meant that the writer does not look upon prostatic hypertrophy as a senile condi-

tion, but as an interstitial change which has been insidious in its onset, first affecting the innervation of the gland and its enclosed urethra, giving rise through its close connection with the hypogastric plexus of the sympathetic, the lumbar plexus and spinal nerves to many reflex symptoms in the kidney and bladder, as well as those of a purely sexual character, and eventually, with the declining vigor of the patients' later years, becoming a mechanical obstruction to the outlet of an already overworked bladder. Five patients are at present under our observation, whose ages range from twenty-three to forty years, in all of whom the prostate is enlarged to twice the normal size or greater. They now suffer from symptoms due to faulty enervation of the organ only, but as they advance in years, and as the muscle of the bladder begins to partake of the general physical degeneration of old age, the added symptoms of obstruction will assert themselves.

That the time will come when such patients as these will be offered radical operation for relief before the symptom of obstruction has set in the writer firmly believes.

Since 1900 I have performed twenty-eight prostatectomies. Seven of these were removed by suprapubic incisions, with perineal drainage, and twenty-one by perineal incision only.

Of the patients operated upon by suprapubic method three died as result of operation, one from shock due to hemorrhage; two from uremia, one going into coma shortly after operation and the other living eighteen days.

One lived a year and a half after operation and died of pneumonia, the suprapubic wound in this case never being allowed to close. The patient experienced such relief from the suprapubic drainage that he refused to have the tube permanently removed. The only time he had any spontaneous urination was when the tube became plugged. The results in the other cases were brilliant, the patients being able to empty their bladders and control the act of micturition.

Of the twenty-one cases of perineal prostatectomy there have been two deaths. The first was a patient sixty-nine years of age, who succumbed to uremia three days after operation, the other, a patient of seventy-seven years, who lived but twenty four hours and died of suppression of the urine.

Both of the cases had advanced kidney lesions and severe cystitis. Operation was undertaken simply because their urinary difficulties were such as to make life unbearable.

The majority of the perineal operations have been performed upon almshouse inmates, who, almost without exception, have had, in addition to their prostatic hypertrophy, some pathological condition of their kidneys, lungs, or circulatory system, and it is extremely gratifying to see this class of patients come through operation with such a minimum of shock.

The incision which we prefer is the median

vertical. as the length of time for the healing of the wound after operation seems to be shorter when this incision is used. Horwitz claims that 95 per cent. of cases can be reached in this way. There is the objection to it that the chance of injuring the rectum is greater than with one of the more extensive incisions. The foregoing statement is based simply upon our own experience. Numerous observers state the reverse, including the possibility of rectal tearing as one of the objections to the horizontal incision or its modifications. They also place the moment of greatest danger to the rectum at the time of removal of the prostatic lobes. In the two cases in which this accident occurred to us, the injury took place during the separation of the rectum from the prostate.

In both instances the tear was immediately repaired and after operation a tube wrapped with iodoform gauze inserted into the rectum. In one case the accident did not materially affect the subsequent course of the patient's convalescence. The rectal tube was removed at the end of the fourth day, the perineal tube at the end of a week and the rectal tear caused no further complications, the patient making such an uninterrupted recovery. In the other case, however, a serious complication was left. The patient was sixty-four years of age, and in addition to his prostatism, had suffered for years from chronic constipation. At time of operation he was obliged to urinate every hour day and night. A soft catheter, at 9¾ inches drew eight ounces of residual urine. By rectum both lateral lobes were found enlarged to about three times the normal size and the rectum much dilated. The prostate was exposed by median incision and found to be hard and fibrous. While separating the rectum from the capsule of the prostate, the thin rectal wall was torn through.

The rent was repaired and a rectal tube inserted. The patient's convalescence was tedious. The perineal wound was over long in closing, the sutures sloughed in the rectal tear, and four months after operation the patient still had a permanent recto-urethral fistula. He has never passed urine through the penis. He has control over his bladder, but when he urinates the urine is expelled through the anus.

The diurnal frequency is normal. During the night he urinates once. Attempt has been made to heal this fistula by draining the bladder by means of an indwelling catheter. Unfortunately this attempt had to be discontinued, as the urethra would not tolerate the presence of a catheter. A secondary operation has been offered to the patient for the cure of this unusual condition, but has been deferred, the patient experiencing so great an amount of comfort since operation. Peculiar as it may seem the bladder has not become infected. The fistulous opening is in the membranous urethra.

Many cases have been reported in which the entire prostatic urethra has been removed with apparently no evil results. We have had one such experience, when in our enthusiasm to remove the whole of the gland the prostatic urethra was included.

While we deprecate such a procedure, this patient made an uneventful recovery, and has been seen a year after operation with a normal frequency of urination and an ability to empty the bladder completely, with no resulting contractures.

As to the possibility of removing the prostate gland, leaving the ejaculatory ducts patent, we feel that if such a thing happens it is more the result of good luck than good management. The anatomical relations of these ducts are too greatly disturbed by hypertrophical changes in the gland to make such a dissection probable. Sterility will be caused by occlusion of the ducts, but we are not prepared to believe that impotence will necessarily follow. The phenomenon of of erection is a complex process, depending upon proper innervation of the whole genital apparatus, and especially upon those nerves which affect the circulatory changes within the corpora cavernosa. If we were able to remove the prostate without damaging any of its delicate nerve supply, we might be reasonably sure of potency being present in the patient after such an operation had been performed, even though the ejaculatory ducts had been severed.

Unfortunately an elaborate dissection of this character seems to be only barely possible upon the cadaver.

Two patients under our observation have been able to cohabit satisfactorily since operation, in neither of whom was any attempt made to save the ducts from injury. On the contrary, the lateral lobes were removed in their entirety without trying to leave any "ejaculatory bridge." Most patients who have reached the stage of their disease where operation is undertaken for the relief of obstruction have already experienced such loss of sexual vigor as to make the question of postoperative virility one of but small moment to them.

The question, however, may arise especially with patients whose obstructive symptoms develop early, between fifty and sixty years of age, and may influence them to accept palliative treatment rather than operation, for at present we are in no position to state affirmatively whether or not the ability to perform the sexual act will remain after operation. This statement holds good for suprapubic as for perineal prostatectomy. In connection with injury to the ejaculatory ducts we desire to call attention to the frequency of postoperative epididymitis. It has occurred in seven of our cases. Two cases had both testicles involved, three cases the left testicle only, and two cases the right. In one case only did suppuration take place. Epididymitis has developed as early as the seventh day and as late as the fourteenth, usually on the ninth or tenth. In four of the cases the inflammation has been o an extremely acute character, the patients running a high temperature, with intense prostration. One patient ran a temperature between 103° and 105° F. for three days. Delirium was present, and the heart's action was so feeble and irregular that it seemed a question whether he would survive. At the end of a week the temperature dropped to normal and the patient recovered. This patient had both testicles, involved, and now, four months after operation, has had firm erections. He has not as yet tried to perform coitus.

The .epididymitis in these four cases cleared up from the fifth to the seventh day, and the temperature fell by crisis.

The case of suppurative epididymitis ran a subacute course, the patient being up and around the ward, the temperature never rising over 100° F. He did not call attention to the testicle until after suppuration had taken place and the abscess was almost ready to rupture. Questioning brought out the fact that the pain and swelling, which were slight, had developed about the seventh day after operation. It was, three weeks after operation when the abscess was opened. Two weeks later the sinus was healed and the subsequent course was uneventful.

Postoperative epididymitis takes place at "the time when granulation in the wound is well-established. These granulations, probably causing occlusion of the ducts, interfere with their drainage and dam up any existing infectious material. This may then travel back through the vasa, setting up inflammation in the testicles. .

We offer as a suggestion for the prevention of this complication, ligation of the vasa deferentia prior to performing prostatectomy. It is but the work of a moment and would not materially prolong the time of operation. When severe cystitis exists it may prove especially efficacious, as these are the cases in which epididymitis is most prone to occur.

Proust makes a point of isolating and ligating the ejaculatory ducts before the removal of the prostate. It no doubt acts the same as ligation of the vasa, but requires more time to do, as well as an elaborate dissection. We do not recommend that ligation of the vasa deferentia should be a routine procedure, but it may be found to be advantageous where the debility of the patient is so great that the possibility of testicular inflammation would gravely affect the prognosis.

One of our cases, of more than passing interest, presented the following history: He was sixty-seven years of age. He had been a sufferer from marked rheumatoid arthritis for years and was a "constant tippler." His urinary symptoms dated back seven years. Six years ago he had been operated upon for prostatic enlargement by the combined suprapubic and perineal method. The operation had given him practically no relief, and when he came under our observation he was dribbling urine continuously. Catheterization was only possible by use of a silver instrument, the

beak of which upon entering the bladder was deflected sharply to the left. He had six ounces of residual urine.

Rectal examination revealed a large mass in the situation of the right lobe of the prostate. This mass was firmly adherent to· scar tissue in the perineum. This patient begged to have something done, as his condition had become unbearable.

Perineal operation was decided upon, even though the rheumatoid arthritis had produced such an anchylosis in his hip-joints that it made it impossible to more than approximate the lithotomy position. The urethra, which was pushed way to the left, was opened by cutting down upon a silver .catheter. It was then found that the median and left lobes had been removed, their situations being occupied by scar tissue. The remaining lobe, which was in every way adherent to scar tissue, was enucleated with difficulty. Even though these dense adhesions made the operation tedious, the patient recovered from the immediate effects of it without incident. · The perineal tube was removed on the third day. The day following (four days after operation) a sharp hemorrhage took place from the perineal wound, and about eight ounces of blood were lost before it could be checked. Four days later a similar hemorrhage took place, but was readily controlled.

These postoperative hemorrhages have been the only ones which we have noticed in our whole series of cases. They were surprising, as the operation was remarkably free from bleeding on account of the extensive cicatricial tissue. No other complications have occurred in this patient's further convalescence. It is now a month since operation. He can control his urination, and though the perineal wound is not yet entirely healed, the major portion of the urine is passed through the penis, and he can empty the bladder completely. The hemorrhage in this case was doubtless due to the early removal of the tube and gauze drains. Nevertheless it is of prime importance, if quick healing of the wound is desired, to remove tubes and drains early. Our experience has shown that if the vertical perineal incision suffices to remove the gland, tube and gauze packing can be dispensed with much earlier than if one of the more extensive incisions is used. It is a recognized fact that elderly people do better if they are not confined to bed long after operation. Early removal of the tube is, therefore, to be desired. It has been our custom to remove the tube at the end of twenty-four or forty-eight hours, unless there exists such a grade of cystitis as to make a prolonged drainage necessary. Closure of the perineal wound will naturally take place at an earlier date if this is possible.

After the tube and drains have been removed from the wound, the bladder should be daily irrigated with a mild antiseptic solution. This is accomplished by introducing a catheter through the penis as, soon as the wound has closed sufficiently to make it possible. Some operators advise draining the bladder by means of an indwelling catheter after the removal of the perineal tube, leaving the catheter in until the wound is nearly healed. We have not found this procedure to be necessary in any of our cases. The earliest date in which the perineal wound has completely closed has been two weeks following operation. This occurred in one patient whose perineal tube was removed the day following operation, who was out of bed at the end of forty-eight hours and began passing water through the penis at the end of four days. It usually takes, however, from three to six weeks before the perineal sinus is completely healed. In none of our cases has there been any open sinus remaining after six weeks.

Three of our patients, prior to operation, suffered from a marked degree of pyelitis. With the removal of the obstruction to urination, the pyelitis was greatly improved. In one patient it disappeared entirely.

The ages of patients operated upon have been as follows: The youngest fifty-two, the oldest eighty-five years. Six patients were over eighty, eight between seventy and eighty years, and the remainder between fifty-two and seventy years. Age itself is apparently no contra-indication to operation.

The results of our series, taking three months after operation as the date of observation, have been very gratifying, but we have found that the majority of them have required a certain amount of treatment for some months following operation, directed toward curing up an old cystitis or increasing the muscular tone of the bladder. Although a patient may be able to empty the bladder completely after operation, in the majority of instances he never more than approximates a normal frequency of urination. This has been frequently due to the fact that a contracted bladder has existed before prostatectomy has been performed. Thus it will be necessary to keep many patients under observation and treatment for months in order to bring a diseased bladder back to its normal condition. This is where a knowledge of and skill in carrying out the details of bladder-treatment will greatly influence the final results. Passage of sounds has been a method of routine, but we have yet to see a case where there have been contractures serious enough materially to diminish the normal caliber of the membranous or prostatic urethra.

Many investigators have placed existing or non-existing renal insufficiency as the most important factor in determining for or against radical operation. Our experience has not borne this out. Seventy-five per cent. of those operated upon have more or less advanced renal lesions, and it has been frequently observed that kidneys which have been insufficient in their functions before operation, have been greatly improved by removing the urinary obstruction and giving them, as well as the bladder, free drainage. To our mind the effect of the anesthetic is of relatively greater danger to the kidneys than the effect of the operation, and the choice of the anesthetic of but small moment compared with the choice of the anesthetist.

THE OPIUM QUESTION IN THE PHILIPPINES.

BY JAMES A. LE ROY,

OF DURANGO, MEXICO.

WHEN the Philippine government proposed last year to establish a government monopoly of the sale of opium, both as the best means of preventing its being smuggled extensively and of so controlling its sale and use as to prevent, to the greatest possible extent, the spread of the habit among the natives of the islands, great opposition arose in the United States and in the islands themselves. The opposition that found expression in the United States, inducing the then Secretary of War to propose the postponement of the project under consideration until full examination could be made of the question, came from persons and associations, the latter mostly of a religious character, who opposed all connection of the government with the traffic in opium, on moral grounds. They preferred that absolute prohibition of the smoking of opium should be made the governmental policy. The opposition in the Philippines came to some extent from similar sources, but principally from the Chinese consumer and traffickers in opium, who, for the time being, joined hands with the missionary societies. They really preferred, or at least most of them did so, the maintainance of the *status quo*, getting their opium at the best price they could in consequence of the high tariff now placed upon it in the ports of the Philippines. Those of them who were engaged in the opium trade naturally wanted to see no monopoly established. It seemed quite evident, from their course of opposition, that they would rather see an attempt at absolute prohibition of the traffic, as the missionary societies desired, than have the government take in its own hands the regulation of the sale and smoking. In case of absolute prohibition there could still be the contraband trade; but, if the government should set up an elaborate inspection system, it would be better able to check smuggling.

The proposed law was at last definitely pigeonholed, and a committee of three was appointed to make investigations throughout the Orient and report with recommendations. The members of this committee were Major E. C. Carter, Chief Health Commissioner for the Philippines, Bishop W. P. Brent (head of the new Protestant Episcopal organization in the islands), and Dr. José Albert, a prominent Filipino physician of Manila and also president of the Federal Party. During the past fifteen months, the committee as a whole, or individual members of it, have made special investigations in Japan, Formosa, China, Hong-kong, Saigon, the Straits Settlements, Burma, Java and the Philippine Islands—meeting with opposition to their investigations only in Manila, on the part of the Chinese living there. Their report was submitted to the Philippine Commission several months since. It forms perhaps as comprehensive a survey of the opium traffic and the opium habit as has ever been made. Their findings are unanimous, and in general support the Philippine government in the proposition that the best method of regulating as well as of restricting the use of opium, in populations addicted to it, is by means of a government monopoly. They consider, however, that the conditions in the Philippines are, all in all, exceptionally favorable for wiping out the habit; and, while they propose a government monopoly as the best means of dealing with the traffic under the present conditions, they also propose that an early date be fixed for putting an end to the monopoly, after which time traffic in the drug and its use for any other than medicinal purposes shall be prohibited. In short, they advocate a system of "progressive prohibition," taking the form at the outset of a government monopoly.

After going at some length into the medical phases of the subject, they declare that only a superficial examination is sufficient to reveal the inadequacy of prohibition in places where the habit already obtains. In the first place, the irrepressible craving for the drug is so nearly impossible to resist that there may be said to be practically no cases of a spontaneous cure of the habit. Secondly, once begun, there is inevitably a gradual increase of the dosage. Though what may be called "opium intoxication" does not at first show itself, the person who resorts to the drug, very often on account of some ailment, finding that the symptoms of his disease disappear, and that generally the mental and reproductive functions are improved, yet inevitably, after a greater or less period of time, varying with the individual, these conditions change, first gradually, then rapidly, until at last the "end is reached in a physical, mental and moral degeneration."

The committee considered that there was no possibility of introducing the "local option" principle into the regulation of this traffic. As for the system of high license, or high tariff, they find that the use of opium has increased in the Philippines under the latter, and believe it would continue to do the same under a system of high license administered internally; under such a system also, a higher premium would be put on smuggling; and it is an unfortunate source of revenue, in any event. As for the system of "farming out" the sale of opium, now quite commonly in vogue in other Malay countries, the committee found it open to the same objections as that of high license, and added further: "The farmer endeavors to increase his profits by extending his business, and so the sale of opium

is increased; furthermore, it is hardly moral to delegate to an individual, not a representative of the people, such authority in the way of supervising, detecting and policing as the farmer usually exercises." As for immediate prohibition, they say: "The investigation of the committee leads it to believe that immediate prohibition is practicable only as a preventive measure in communities where opium-smoking has never obtained. In those communities where opium is used, and prohibition has been tried, it has been found to be a source of blackmail."

In general, a system of government monopoly is best where opium is already used, as government agents can thereby to a great extent regulate and restrict its use: the agents of its sale ought never to have any interests in profits from it; smuggling can be kept down at least as effectively under this system as under any other; and, by keeping the proceeds from the sale of opium at the point where they only meet the expenses of the system of regulation, it may be demonstrated that the latter is aimed only at control, repression and eventual abolition of the habit.

Their reasons for believing that no system of prohibition, abruptly introduced, would be of avail in the Philippines, and yet that the government can speedily shape conditions to that end, enforcing prohibition perhaps more effectually than is done in Japan, are as follows:

"In the Philippine Islands the practice of smoking opium is an exotic one, imported by the Chinese since time immemorial. The number of Chinese inhabitants in the Philippine Islands is about 70,000, distributed in varying numbers throughout all the provinces of the archipelago, the greater part being found in the larger towns, such as Manila, where there are about 40,000. From 1843 to 1898 the farming system was in vogue in the Philippines, its purpose being to raise revenue and to check the opium vice among the Filipinos, prohibition being considered an impossible utopia. Although this system prohibited the sale of opium to Filipinos and forbade their entering public smoking-shops, they were contaminated by the vice in all the provinces, though only to a small degree. From the statistics which we have secured and which accompany this report, it is clearly seen that the provinces in which the vice is most widely spread are Negros Oriental, Negros Occidental, Capiz, Surigoa. Cagayan and Isabela, there being many *pueblos* in which the vice is unknown to the natives, owing to the lack of social contact with the Chinese. The swallowing of pills is exceptional among those who abandon themselves to the vice, and hypodermic injections are unknown. The average number of smokers in the *pueblos* of the different provinces varies from a fraction of one to fifty. Filipino women rarely use opium, and the drug is never administered to children. As an exception to this rule may be mentioned the town of Tayasan in Negros Oriental, where the vice has taken hold of entire families."

From this analysis of the conditions affecting the use of opium in the Philippines, it is easy to see that absolute and immediate prohibition would not prohibit an opinion confirmed by its failure to do so in certain districts of Java where it is in effect.

". : . As we have already observed, the proportion of Filipino smokers to the entire population of the islands is insignificant, save in three or four *pueblos.* The danger, therefore. lies in the tendency of the vice to grow and spread, until the number of victims, now inconsiderable, may at some future time reach a point where it shall constitute an alarming evil. As long as the present Chinese exclusion act continues in force, there can be no influx of opium-smokers from without; and with a steady effort of the government to prevent an increase of the number of proselytes to the vice within, the habit will be confined to those who are already its slaves."

The committee recommends, therefore:

" That opium and the traffic therein be made a strict government monopoly immediately.'.

"That three years after that shall have been done, no opium shall be imported, brought or introduced into these islands, except by the government and for medical purposes only. The time necessary to enable one accustomed to the use of the drug to discontinue the habit has been estimated at from six months to twenty years. It has seemed necessary to the committee to state a definite period after which the use of opium shall be prohibited, because the force of any law or ordinance depends largely upon the exactness of the time at which it may be enforced. If a longer period than this were allowed, the time at which the *habitué* would begin to disaccustom himself to the use of the drug would be postponed indefinitely. Three years would seem to be a period of sufficient length. At the expiration of this time, the government will be in a position to determine what is wisest and best to be done."

Further recommendations designed to aid in this policy of "progressive prohibition," are: That the use of opium be prohibited to all inhabitants of the Philippines who are not males above twenty-one years of age; that those of the required status shall be allowed its use, obtaining the drug in prepared form from the agents established by the government. only on the presentation of a license, these licenses to be issued to such inhabitants (without distinction of race) only upon their written application, accompanied by the certificates of two trustworthy persons, one if practicable to be a physician, to the effect that the licensee is a "habitual user of opium and would be injured by being compelled to discontinue its use suddenly;" that habitual users of opium shall be disqualified to exercise the suffrage or to hold office; that for natives of the islands, violations of the laws regulating the use of opium shall be punished

twice by fine or imprisonment and the third time by disqualification for the franchise or for office, and that in the case of a third violation by a Chinese or other non-native inhabitants, the penalty shall be deportation; that no public smoking-places be allowed; that the cultivation of the poppy for the purpose of producing opium shall be declared illegal in the islands; that the government hospitals shall give free treatment to indigent opium-smokers entering for the purpose of ridding themselves of the' habit; and that a primer of hygiene be prepared for use in the public schools, in which the evil and debasing results of the opium habit shall be taught, this primer also being published in Chinese for distribution among the inhabitants of that race or reproduction in their newspapers. Other detailed recommendations are also made, such as are suggested by the experience obtained in other opium-smoking countries as best calculated to make the regulation on the part of the government the more effective.

Some such plan as this will now very soon be adopted in the Philippines. Considering the difficulties of instituting and maintaining the somewhat elaborate machinery for a government monopoly of the traffic, which should last but three years, Secretary of War Taft inclines to favoring a high-license system during the brief period within which the traffic shall be legal in the islands. In any event, whatever plan is adopted will look toward prohibition at an early date, probably within three years.

SOME SO-CALLED RHEUMATISMS.[1]

BY JAS. J. WALSH, M.D., PH.D., .
OF NEW YORK;
ADJUNCT PROFESSOR OF MEDICINE AT THE POLYCLINIC SCHOOL FOR
GRADUATES IN MEDICINE.

IN dispensary service and for office practice probably nothing comes more frequently for treatment to the physician than obscure pains of many kinds. usually worse on rainy days, and as a result of this, commonly called by the patients at least, and very frequently by their physicians also, rheumatic.

Chronic rheumatism is supposed to be one of the most frequent of diseases. The usually accepted explanation of it for about the last half century has been that the blood was too acid, and that as a consequence nerves were irritable and the circulation not so nutritious as it should be. Uric acid has been a slogan in medicine for a long time. We now have even a uric acid monthly. As for remedies that will cure the uric acid diathesis, their name is legion, and some of us suspect that they mean no more good for mankind than that other group of scripture fame whose name was said to be legion.

Fortunately a very decided reaction has taken place in the last five years, a reaction that had been foreshadowed ten years before by the work of physiological chemists, and at the present time

1 Read at the Annual Meeting of the New York State Medical Association, October 18, 1904.

there are very few serious scientific workers in medicine who consider that uric acid is of any etiological importance in the production of pathological conditions in the human economy. The cases that used to be called chronic rheumatism, however, still continue to come and must be treated. The question is, what are they? We have tried theory for half a century and it has failed us. It might seem well to go back and study the patients once more and see whether we would not find that there are grouped under this all embracing name " rheumatic " a number of conditions for which we can do much by recognizing their real cause in the habits and constitution of the individual. The present paper is meant only as a contribution to the clinical side of this important subject, diagnosis being considered rather than treatment, though once causation becomes clear, treatment is usually not a difficult matter and the indications stand out of themselves.

So-called rheumatic conditions in the upper arm and shoulder are not infrequent. I remember once having three of them present themselves at my dispensary service at the Polyclinic, all of them presumably suffering from rheumatism, all having been treated for this condition. One of them proved to be a motorman suffering from occupation pains that often come to those who use their arms overmuch, the pains seen so frequently, for instance, in baseball pitchers. These pains are always worse on rainy days. Why can one man pitch nearly every day all season and not suffer with his arm, while another man cannot? We can no more tell the reason for this difference than we can tell why one man is right-handed and another left-handed. One individual has a store of nervous energy that serves him very well. Another has a store of nervous energy that serves him well enough for his left hand but not for his right hand. The mystery would seem to be the original endowment of nerve force according to the individual's constitution. Your motorman who suffers severely from putting on the brake of the heavy car, will probably never be able to continue his occupation with comfort to himself unless his sore arm is due to some temporary condition, easily recognizable.

A second of my patients with rheumatism complained of his shoulder. He had been first easily fatigued, then it was painful when he moved much, most so on rainy days, and finally he had practically lost power in it entirely. His occupation was that of finisher in a molding works. He lifted a heavy hammer many hundreds of times a day with his right arm, striking quick short blows and using mainly his deltoid muscle in the lifting process. It was just his deltoid that was affected and the nerve supply had evidently given out. The third man complained not of his right hand, but of his left and of his forearm, not his shoulder, having lost power especially on the ulnar side of his hand.

He was a stonecutter, who held a chisel firmly in his left hand, grasping it mainly with the under or ulnar side of his hand, and consequently overusing his ulnar nerve.

There was just one feature in the history of all three that was the same. They did not drink alcohol to excess often, but they did take some whisky straight every day. The easiest explanation seemed to be that there was a neuritis set up in the nerves, which their occupations caused them to use so much, and that as a consequence, the low grade neuritis finally developed to such a condition as to make further use of the muscle supplied by the affected nerves practically impossible. Just why alcohol will select certain nerves and not others upon which to exercise its deteriorating influence and why lead usually affects an entirely different set we do not know. In the ordinary man of sedentary occupation who walks occasionally, as his only exercise, his most used nerve in his anterior peroneal. Those of us who are not used to walking much, know how soon this nerve complains of fatigue when we make some forced ambulatory effort. It is this nerve then that with most people is affected by alcohol. But any nerve that is overused will apparently be affected the same way, and as many outdoor workers take some whisky straight pretty regularly, it is not surprising to find that some of them have an idiosyncrasy and develop a low grade alcoholic neuritis.

Alcohol, however, is not the only substance that acts thus insidiously. I was once asked to treat a painter who was suffering from intense tired feelings in his right forearm. They were always worse on rainy days, and he had been treated for rheumatism without avail. He had no signs at all of wrist-drop, there were no suspicious signs on his gums and he had never suffered from constipation or anything like lead colic. It seemed far-fetched then to say that his muscles were fatigued mainly because of the irritating presence of lead in the nerves supplying his right forearm. He slipped on the ice, however, and sprained his wrist, and the next day turned up with a typical lead wrist-drop. This fact of having lead poison develop shortly after an accident is not unusual, just as a sprained ankle may sometimes be the signal for an outbreak of alcoholic neuritis in the lower leg which has been preparing for some time, the accident being partially at least accounted for in many cases by the awkwardness of muscles with insufficient nerve supply.

There is scarcely an occupation, however, in which movements are frequently repeated, or in which a particular position is maintained for a long time in which neuritis may not be seen. Lumbago is undoubtedly more frequent among tailors, especially those who sit on a table in the old fashioned way and bend their backs forcibly, than among any other class of men. The nervous effort required to maintain this bending position, most of the bend being in the lumbar region, is reflected back upon the lumbar plexus and vague pains in this region are quite common. Iron workers, puddlers, molders and the like, who stoop to lift and carry heavy objects also suffer from this affection very commonly. This is especially true if they are laboring under any toxic condition, lead, alcohol, diabetes, syphilis or the like, which exerts its influence upon the nutrition of the nerves.

Sciatica on the other hand is very common in those who actively bend the body at the hip, shovelers, for instance, who bend the right knee in going down to lift heavy shovelsful of material, are among workmen the most frequent sufferers from this disease. I have seen, however, a number of motormen accustomed to stand on their right foot and swing round the body on the right leg in putting on the brakes of heavy cars, who also suffered from it.

Those who have to stand on their feet much usually suffer in the lowest joint of the leg, at the ankle. There are very few waiters who do not suffer to some degree, at least, from flat foot. This affection is always worse on rainy days. I once pointed out as one of the reasons for this that on rainy days, people usually wear their old shoes, and old shoes do not support the foot as well as new ones. It is curious, however, how long flat foot may exist to a marked degree without giving any symptoms. Usually the symptoms develop rather suddenly. There is a story of the patient having done something quite unusual just before the trouble was first noticed. A man moves and has to hang up the pictures in his house, thus occupying an awkward position on the step-ladder, on his tip-toes, or otherwise, for several hours. A clerk, who has been handling goods on the counter, is asked to set them high up on shelves. The result is the giving way of the arch of the foot and a soreness that is usually called rheumatism, always worse on rainy days.

Just why sensitive nerves slightly irritated, or in a subinflammatory condition, should produce more discomfort on rainy days is not easy to say. Unfortunately it is usually considered that dampness and rheumatism are intimately associated, and consequently the word rheumatic is inserted in the description of the patient's condition. An affected tooth, however, often gives pain on a rainy day, a broken bone usually becomes sensitive just before a rain storm. The dislocated shoulder becomes an invaluable barometer, but one that most patients would dispense with very gladly. We do not call these conditions rheumatic, though they are associated quite as closely with dampness apparently, as the vague muscular pains. The fact of the matter seems to be that any drop in the barometer by making the pressure on the surface of the body less than it was before permits a dilatation of the capillaries at the periphery with a constant tendency to congestion, that makes nerves more sensitive than they were before, especially if they

have been affected by some low grade pathological condition. Even unaffected nerves, however, express their dislike of damp weather by making muscles much more easily fatigued than they were before; hence the depressed tired feeling of a day with low barometric pressure. The circulation is not so active, nutrition is not up to its proper standard, and fatigue comes sooner than it does on the cold, bracing day, which, by causing the capillaries to contract, raises blood pressure and causes rapid interchange in the metabolism of the muscles.

It must not be thought, however, that only workers, that is, manual laborers, are to be considered in this question of occupation pain. I have seen three cases now in writers, whose forearm bothered them some, whose shoulder bothered them much more, the conditions always being worse on rainy days so that they were considered to be rheumatic, though the pathological condition was really writer's cramp. Why some met get writer's cramp and others do not is another phase of the history that we have been discussing.

One thing, however, has been much impressed upon me, and that is that those who are normally left-handed and are taught to write with their right hand, suffer from writer's cramp much more readily than normally right-handed individuals. It would seem as though nature were taking her revenge for an interference with her original plan, for the man is right-brained and should not be compelled to use his right hand for a work requiring so much coordination as does writing.

A certain number of cases of sciatica will be found in those who sit in awkward positions or in unsuitable chairs while doing much writing or clerical work. I have seen an old woman, who was considered to be paralyzed, because she had lost all power in her feet and a certain amount of her sensation also below the knee, who yet got entirely well at once when she was taken out of a cushioned chair, which used to sink down in such a way as to allow the edge of the frame to press upon her sciatic nerves just at the place where these come closest to the surface. On the other hand I have had to treat a literary woman who sat much at her desk for pains that were considered to be rheumatic in the leg, but they did not get better until she had adopted another chair and another position for her writing, her former position bringing pressure to bear directly upon her right sciatic nerve. In a word, I think that much of the so-called uric acid diathesis with the consequent rheumatic pains is nothing more than neuritides of various kinds due to overexertion, pressure upon nerve trunks preventing proper nutrition, the presence of irritant substances in the blood, such as alcohol, lead and the blood disturbances of diabetes and to some inherited weakness of special sets of nerves.

CASE OF PRIMARY MALIGNANT TUMOR OF THE LUNG.

BY MAURICE PACKARD, A.M., M.D.,

OF NEW YORK [1]

LECTURER IN CLINICAL MEDICINE, NEW YORK POLYCLINIC HOSPITAL
AND MEDICAL SCHOOL; ATTENDING PHYSICIAN TO THE CLINIC
OF COMMUNICABLE PULMONARY DISEASES, DEPARTMENT
OF HEALTH.

ALTHOUGH many cases of neoplasms of the lung and pleura have been reported, still, since there are so many points in diagnosis and pathology in dispute, we are encouraged to believe that every new case may give some aid in the study of this interesting condition.

P. C., cigarmaker, fifty-five years old, presented himself at Prof. Adler's clinic and gave the following history: There was no trace of cancer or tuberculosis in the family and he denied ever having syphilis or any venereal disease. Five years ago, he became troubled with cough and pain, which was not accompanied by any expectoration. At first these symptoms seemed to disappear with appropriate treatment, but would soon return. In fact, his cough and pain never entirely left him. Two years ago his cough became more harassing and was accompanied with gradually increasing mucous expectoration, whereas until then there was only occasional shortness of breath on violent physical exertion; the dyspnea now became more intense and permanent, so that on the slightest movement he would have to stop in order "to catch his breath." Pain became more intense, sleep became disturbed, cough became more and more distressing, and during the last year expectoration was very frequently bloody. At times he expectorate pure blood; quantities varying from a few drops to a tablespoonful. On several occasions a genuine hemoptysis occurred with the expectoration of fully eight ounces or more of apparently pure blood. During all this time he maintained that his weight kept constant, and that he did not suffer from night-sweats or fever. His appetite remained good; there was no change of voice. Bowels were regular and micturition normal. Physical examination showed the following: Fairly well-nourished man, with average subcutaneous adipose tissue—five feet five inches in height and weighing about 130 pounds. Conjunctivæ rather pale, slight edema underneath eyes, complexion of face somewhat livid. No enlarged glands could be felt in the cervical, axillary, epitrochlear or inguinal regions. Both jugulars enormously dilated and tortuous. The superficial veins of the chest and upper portion of the abdomen, especially on right half of the trunk, were also greatly dilated and tortuous, standing out well above the surface of the skin and forming a huge "caput medusæ." A very slight superficial edema of the right chest was evident. The space above and below the clavicle was rather full. Respiratory motion was markedly reduced in right thorax. Careful measure-

1 Case presented at Clinical Society of New York Polyclinic, December, 1904, as a probable primary endothelioma of the lung.

ments of the thoracic arch showed no difference in diameter between right and left side. Apex beat of the heart was not visible, but faintly palpahle in normal position. Absolute flatness was found over nearly the whole right chest, extending from the axillary line forward and from the clavicle downward beyond the sternum and emerging over the superficial area of cardiac dulness. Over this area pectoral fremitus was completely absent. The voice was diminished. The breathing was faint, distant, and sub-bronchial in character. There were no râles. On the portion of the lung adjacent to the area of dulness expiration was harsh and prolonged. The right lung posteriorly and all of the left lung showed no essential changes. An aspirating needle introduced into the area of dulness, seemed to enter solid material. The heart sounds were rather feeble, but there were no murmurs. There was no accentuation of second pulmonary sound. Heart dulness did not extend beyond left mamillary line. Radical pulse was fairly soft and regular and of the same volume on both sides. Liver and spleen were not enlarged and no abnormalities could be detected in the abdomen. Reflexes were normal.

The examination of the stomach contents after a test meal showed free hydrochloric acid and the absence of lactic acid. The tube went down without difficulty.

Blood examination made a few days later showed. Hb., 62 per cent.; red cells, 3,989,000; white cells, 14,300.

Differential count gave polynuclears, 54 per cent.; lymphocytes, 34 per cent.; large mononuclears, $8\frac{1}{2}$ per cent.; eosinophiles, $3\frac{1}{2}$ per cent. Thus showing a preponderance of lymphocytes and a slight leucocytosis. Red cells stain evenly, but are not equal in size. Microcytes and pear-shaped cells are abundant, but there are no nucleated red cells, no poikilocytosis, and no stippling. The repeated examinations of the urine showed no noteworthy change. Temperature is normal, pulse about 80 per cent. and respiration at rest 28 per cent. Numerous and most searching examinations of the sputum were made. At no time could tubercle bacilli, elastic fibers or particles of tumor be found. Careful search for actinomyces, streptothrix and other abnormalities proved negative.

From the facts just stated, it seemed evident, that we had to deal with some form of neoplasm involving the right chest and the interior mediastinum, and compressing the large veins, most probably the superior cava. The fact that cough and pain in the right chest had been the first symptoms and had appeared five years ago, and the further fact that, according to the patient's repeated statements and assurances, the dilated veins and edema were of comparatively recent date, necessarily led to the assumption of a primary neoplasm of the right lung, that gradually involved in its growth the anterior mediastinum with its contents.

In view of the long duration of the affliction and the comparative state of good nutrition of the patient, the slight secondary anemia, the tardy involvement of lymph-nodes, we were inclined rather to exclude the more malignant form of sarcoma, and to consider a slow growing carcinoma or endothelioma of the lung as the most probable forms of neoplasm in this case.

The patient and his friends were advised of the unfavorable prognosis, and he was especially warned of a sudden hemorrhage at any time, endangering his life.

Patient remained under observation for two months, during which time the disease progressed with great rapidity.

Enlarged and hard lymph-nodes appeared first in the right axilla and then in the left, while the cervical and supraclavicular regions remained free. An area of slight dulness with harsh and prolonged respiration and diminished vocal fremitus appeared about the middle of right lung posteriorly, together with considerable pleuritic friction. Very soon thereafter, with increasing dyspnea and distressing pain and cough, fluid appeared in the right pleural cavity, which rapidly filled.

The chest was aspirated and twenty ounces of clear serous fluid removed. Almost immediately, the pleural sac began to fill up again, but the patient before he was ready for another aspiration, while in a carriage on his way to a meeting of a medical society, where he was to be demonstrated by Dr. Isaac Adler, was seized with a profuse hemorrhage, which ended his life.

Autopsy January 23, 1904, by Dr. Otto Shultze.—Macroscopical: A tumor mass was found involving lower end of trachea on right side, four rings above the bifurcation and on the left side just at the bifurcation. This tumor continues and involves right bronchus and posterior portion of left bronchus. Anteriorly the mass extends over the bronchus and reaches as high as two cm. above the origin of the innominate artery. Glands over the anterior portion on the right side of the dome of the pericardial sac are involved in the growth, and the upper lobe of the right lung is adherent to the sac. Growth extends directly through the anterior portion of the upper lobe of the right lung, following the larger branches of the bronchi to the costal pleura. Rest of the lobe toward apex is atelectatic and bronchi filled with pus. Middle lobe of right lung is the seat of hepatization, very light in color and slightly granular. Wherever the growth pierces the wall of the bronchus to the mucous membrane, the membrane presents an ulcerated and eroded appearance. Lower lobe partially atelectatic. Metastatic pleural surface of the diaphragm. Diaphragm contains a number of villi markedly injected. Left lung contains a few grayish white plaques (metastasis) ½ cm. in diameter on posterior surface of lower lobe, on the posterior margin of the base and also on the surface of the base. Embraced in the

mass and constricted by it is the superior vena cava, showing a distinctly puckered arrangement as viewed from right auricle. Right pulmonary artery shows longitudinal folds with a funnel-shaped narrowing down to the tumor where vessel is almost entirely compressed. Heart shows some brown atrophy, otherwise normal; peritoneum is perfectly free. Spleen is small and congested. Liver is normal in size—surface smooth—color pale. Stomach and intestines anemic, but otherwise normal. Patient had but one kidney, horseshoe in shape, and ureters passing anteriorly.

The microscopical examination showed a typcal flat-celled carcinoma in the primary growth, as well as in the metastatic deposits. Details of which will be published by Dr. Isaac Adler later.

160 West One Hundred and Twenty-first Street.

CALCULI IN BLANDIN'S AND SUBMAXILLARY GLANDS. REPORTS OF CASES.

BY HERMAN JARECKY, M.D.,
OF NEW YORK ;

VISITING OTOLOGIST, HARLEM HOSPITAL; EYE, EAR AND THROAT SURGEON, SYDENHAM HOSPITAL: ASSISTANT SURGEON, MANHATTAN EYE AND EAR HOSPITAL, ETC.

CALCULI are found in all of the salivary glands, although not very frequently, yet often enough to cause one to be on the lookout for their presence.

In 1896, Futterer[1] collected the reports of 160 and Roberg[2] in January, 1904, added 47; since then I have found in the literature mention of three ([a] to [5]), making the total, including my three, of 213 cases up to date.

They occur most frequently in the submaxillary gland or its duct known as Wharton's. This may be due to the secretion being more viscid from a larger proportion of mucin or perhaps to its situation. The openings of the ducts on each side of the frenum in the papillæ under the tip of the tongue are so situated that foreign bodies, as pieces of toothpicks, bristles from toothbrushes, micro-organisms can easily enter, and become nuclei for the concretions. The openings of the ducts may become obliterated or obstructed and lead to the formation of inspissated mucus in which the deposits of calcareous particles may take place. The calculi consist chiefly of calcium carbonate and phosphate, and usually assume the shape of the duct in which they lie. They vary in size from the smallest granule to those attaining a large size—as the one Puzey[6] reports—1½ inches in length and ½ inch in thickness, weighing 115 grains.

The diagnosis of the calculus in the Wharton's duct is easily made by passing one finger along the floor of the mouth, and another of the opposite hand below the jaw, so as to compress the duct between the fingers gradually throughout its entire length. Any hard concretion is bound to be felt. The calculus stops the flow of saliva and causes a distention of the duct and gland behind it, and a swelling under the angle of the jaw in the submaxillary, or by pressure, in the sublingual region. A fine probe can also be passed through the duct and the gritty feeling will reveal the nature of the obstruction.

These can easily be removed under local anesthesia. For operations around the ducts, I employ a fine-pointed canula with syringe and inject about one-half dram of a solution of adrenalin, 1 : 1000 and follow this by 5 to 20 drops of a 5 per cent. solution of cocaine directly into the canal. This makes the work absolutely bloodless and painless. Of course, general anesthesia can be employed when patients insist upon it, as was done in these cases which I herewith report.

Case I. Calculus in Blandin's Duct associated with one in Wharton's Duct.—This case is extremely interesting from its rarity. Blandin[7] in 1823 and Nuhn[8] in 1845 described underneath the tip of the tongue, on each side of the middle line, a gland the size and shape of an almond, having vessels and nerves but quite distinct from the sublingual.

If the tip of the tongue be curled up and the surface dried, pits marking the opening of the ducts, two or more on each side, may be seen.

In a general search through the literature, I find two cases reported of calculi in this situation. Gurlt[9] refers to Zacutus Lusitanus who mentions that a smooth hard stone the size of a hazel nut had been removed from the tip of the tongue.

Godlee[10] reports a case of a woman, twenty-four years old, with a tumor on the left side of the under-surface of the tongue near the tip. He passed in a trocar, and felt a hard substance which he removed. He then cut out the growth with a scissors. The wound healed readily and soundly. The examination of the mass revealed a calculus with an adeno-sarcoma surrounding it.

The patient of mine was Mr. M. S., aged thirty-four years, a German, referred by Dr. A. Sturm. He complained of a swelling extending from the tip of the tongue along the right side to beneath the jaw. It had been noticed three years prior as a small, soft swelling, which had gradually grown much larger and harder. The swollen part under the tip of the tongue caused excessive pain while eating. A diagnosis of calculi was made and an operation advised. As he objected to local anesthesia, a general anesthetic was given. Beneath the tip of the tongue, a small calculus was removed by a slight incision into a part of Blandin's gland and a larger one was found on opening Wharton's duct. Quite a large quantity of pus escaped. The calculus from Wharton's duct is pear-shaped, weighs four grains and is of a yellowish color, while the one from Blandin's is rod-shaped, weighs one-half grain and is of a reddish color. The parts healed nicely within a short time, a mild antiseptic wash being used.

Eight months later, the patient consulted me again, on account of a swelling on the same side, but this time limited to the side of the tongue.

The cut into Blandin's gland had thoroughly healed. Upon probing Wharton's duct, no calcareous particles were found, but quite a quantity of pus and saliva escaped. Since then, he has been perfectly well. It might be interesting to add that when he consulted me the first time, he had been informed that the swelling was in all probability malignant, and as a consequence, he had been exposed to the X-rays for their curative value, but naturally, without result. This is the only case on record of the association of a calculus in Blandin's gland with one of the submaxillary.

Case II. Calculus in Wharton's Duct attaining a large size without symptoms.—The patient, Abraham L., aged forty-three years, called at my office complaining of a swelling on the left side, of the tongue, and a small one under the jaw on the same side. Upon examining with a probe a calculus was discovered. A general anesthetic, ethyl chloride, as the patient absolutely insisted upon it, was administered by Dr. Milton Simon. Dr. B. M. Feldman, who referred the case, assisted during the operation. The calculus was removed from the anterior third of Wharton's duct and about two drams of thickish, yellowish pus accompanied it. The small swelling under the jaw was due to the pressure on the ducts of Rivinus of the sublingual gland. The calculus weighs six grains, having the general appearance of a large orange pit. The gentleman is one of the most prominent members of the criminal bar in New York City, and is constantly pleading in the courts; therefore, it was remarkable that the calculus should have attained such a size before it caused any annoying symptoms, as he had only noticed it about three weeks before he sought relief.

Case III. Small calculus with intermittent swelling of submaxillary gland.—Mr. I. S., aged thirty-seven years, of El Paso, Texas, complained of a swelling beneath the jaw, which would increase in size and then decrease again. The swelling was annoying and painful. Various applications, massage with camphorated oil, liniments, etc., had been employed unsuccessfully. He had been suffering from ethmoiditis, and nasal polypi, but these had been attended to.

Examination revealed a swelling below angle of the jaw, somewhat painful, but no fluctuation. Through the mouth at the beginning of Wharton's duct, a small hard substance was felt and a diagnosis of possible calculus was made. Under general anesthesia administered by Dr. M. Packard, the duct was opened and a calculus the size of a pea was found.

The reaction in this case was severe, the gland became swollen, and for a few days there was considerable difficulty in swallowing. This condition rapidly improved, the patient simply using a mild mouthwash. The duct was probed and found to be perfectly clear before the patient left for home a week after the operation. About one month later, I received a letter stating that the swelling of the gland had subsided in a few days, but that he felt something hard in the duct. Three months subsequently, I removed a small calculus from the opening of Wharton's duct under cocaine anesthesia. The second calculus must have been in the gland, and being so small worked its way out to the end of the duct. The first calculus must have acted as a valve at the beginning of the duct, causing obstruction and distention from time to time. There was no pus in this case.

Both these calculi are exceedingly small and rough. Their roughness is due perhaps to the fact that they were not in the duct long enough to be worn smooth by the action of the saliva and the muscles constricting the tube. The cause of the severe reaction must certainly have been due to the ethmoiditis, as during the operation quantities of muco-pus poured out, making the administration of the anesthetic quite difficult.

In concluding the paper, I would suggest in every case of swelling of doubtful diagnosis beneath or around the angle of the jaw, a routine examination of the floor of the mouth be made. A calculus would then be easily discovered, and the patient saved the annoyance of any unnecessary treatment or the worry of supposed malignancy.

115 West One Hundred and Twenty-first Street.

REFERENCES.

1. Futterer, G., Medicine, Detroit, 1896, II, p. 550.
2. Roberg, O., Annals of Surgery, Philadelphia, January, 1904, XXXIV, p. 669.
3. Roberts, W. O., Louisville Month. Jour. of Med. and Surg., June, 1904, II, p. 33.
4. Karpeles, S. R., Wash. Med. Annals, March, 1904, III, p. 14.
5. Lederman, M. D., Laryngoscope, May, 1904, p. 380.
6. Puzey, London Lancet, 1884, I, p. 424.
7. Butlin, Diseases of the Tongue, 1900, p. 9.
8. Nuhn, Ueber eine bis jetzt noch nicht näher beschriebene Drüse im Innern der Zungenspitze. Mannheim, F. Basserman, 1845.
9. Gurlt, Geschichte der Chirurgie, p. 438. Obs. 49.
10. Godlee. Transactions Pathological Society, London, 1887, XXXVIII, p. 346.

PROGNOSIS AND TREATMENT OF CHRONIC NEPHRITIS.[1]

BY A. C. MORGAN, M.D.,
OF PHILADELPHIA.

FROM our knowledge of the pathology of chronic nephritis we can see that the damage done to the kidney cannot be repaired; therefore, we must direct our treatment toward preventing or inhibiting advance of the pathologic process, and upon the results of this treatment the prognosis will largely depend.

So far as the existence of chronic nephritis alone is concerned, the patient is usually in no immediate danger, but it is the many pitfalls that line his path that modify the prognosis and determine the duration of the disease.

It is difficult to determine the actual duration in many cases, particularly in the interstitial form, because the disease is usually developed insidiously, and has existed for a greater or less period of time before manifesting symptoms, either primary or of its many complications.

"An absence of symptoms does not by any

1 Read before North Branch Philadelphia County Medical Society, October 8, 1904.

means exclude the existence of pathological changes, even in an advanced stage of disease" (Daland), and this is particularly true in this disease.

Much depends upon the causal factors in every case.

Dropsy occurring in the course of chronic nephritis is not necessarily of immediate bad omen, as malleolar dropsy may exist for years and the patient remain active, with but few other symptoms present.

When marked dropsy suddenly appears or previous dropsy becomes rapidly increased, it then becomes an active factor in the prognosis, as indicating either great structural change in the kidney, or heart failure, in either instance going on to a rapid end if treatment does not check its advance.

Chronic interstitial nephritis, barring complications, is a disease which may last for from five to thirty years, and offers a far better prognosis than the parenchymatous form, the latter often terminating within one year, five years being a wide limit of time in even the small white kidney to maintain functional activity.

The younger the patient and the earlier the appearance of symptoms, the graver the prognosis, as it is usually the parenchymatous form that is seen in persons under forty years, sclerotic changes belonging especially to advanced life.

Prognosis and Treatment of Chronic Nephritis.—Only a small proportion of patients suffering from chronic interstitial nephritis die from this cause alone, complications supervening to terminate the case in a majority of instances.

Chief among these are the pneumonias, especially bronchopneumonia, la grippe, cerebral hemorrhage, cardiac dilatation and inflammation of serous membranes, pericarditis being perhaps the gravest of the latter conditions.

Uremia, specially evidenced by convulsions, is a positive indication that failure of compensation of the kidney has occurred and the prognosis here is grave. Compensation may be restored one or more times, but the patient is badly crippled, and never regains his former degree of health but goes downward, finally, after a year or so, suffering his final attack of uremia or other complication, or dying of asthenia.

Treatment.—In the treatment of chronic nephritis much can be done by treating the patient and not the disease, endeavoring always at once to remove the cause, wherever known.

As chronic interstitial nephritis exists for years before its symptoms manifest themselves, or is accidentally discovered, proving that there is a long period of perfect compensation, diuretics should never be used until there is actual need for them. The same general rules as obtain in compensated heart murmurs should apply with equal force in this disease. Once the diagnosis is made the cardinal rule of "MODERATION" should govern us in considering the case in hand.

Some general rules as to hygiene are essential.

The patient should wear flannels the year round, that the skin action may be active and steady, and to protect him from marked changes of weather.

When possible, the winter should be passed in a warm, equable climate.

A country life, rather than seashore, is probably better for the patient as in the former environment there is less temptation and opportunity to indulge in the many dissipations of seashore life, such as social events, irregular hours of sleep and the like.

Bathing.—Cold baths are interdicted, as they throw too much work on the kidneys, but hot baths are serviceable as they enhance skin action, and thus relieve the kidneys. They may be warm packs, Turkish, vapor or hot-water baths.

Massage is particularly useful when the patient is confined to bed for any reason, aiding in elimination of effete products by the skin.

Rest in bed, when albumin is severe and persistent, or when the heart shows signs of weakness, is admirable in conserving the strength of the patient and should be insisted upon now and then. The patient should rest in bed for ten of every twenty-four hours to relieve heart action and diminish general activity.

Waters: An abundance of water is required to replace the excessive excretion of water and to keep the solids in solution. We must not go to excess with this line of treatment, however, as the tension may be increased by ingesting too much water and our efforts to aid would become reactive. Three liters of fluid daily is said to be a proper amount to be ingested (Anders). The carbonated waters are strongly indicated in order to counteract the high acidity of the urine which is usually present.

"An alkaline urine dissolves exudates" (Tyson).

Alcohol: "Malt liquors are bad; spirits are worse; the best are those which contain alcohol in from 5 to 8 per cent., such as acid wines" (Millard).

Diet: Nitrogenous foods must be decreased considerably as they increase the work of the kidney by favoring increased secretion of urea. We must not restrict the diet too much, as strength must always be maintained, and this adjustment will call for nice discrimination upon our part.

Coffee and tea should be partaken of sparingly, if at all. Milk, or articles of food prepared with milk should be given an important part in the dietary. Meats and meat gravies should be greatly reduced, though fish and oysters may be freely eaten. Patients should be abstemious in dining at social functions as the food there consumed is highly seasoned, and often washed down with the stronger alcoholic preparations.

Systematic Treatment.—Here our object is to inhibit or arrest the sclerotic and degenerative changes, and to overcome the ever-present and increasing anemia. For the first we have recourse to potassium iodide, hydriodic acid and

mercuric chloride; for the latter, to arsenic and iron.

Mr. Bright, in his first description of chronic nephritis, or Bright's disease, strongly urged the use of tannic acid for the albuminuria on account of its astringent effect, and a favorite treatment years ago was sodium tannic or gallic acid, in three to five grain doses, t.i.d.

Iron meets the dual requirement of an astringent and tonic, and is agreed upon by nearly all writers as being indicated, but must not be used in too large doses, as excessive doses lock up the secretions too much and cause danger of uremia.

Symptoms prominently occurring are best treated as follows:

High tension: As high tension is more or less essential in chronic nephritis with full compensation, we must carefully weigh the conditions present before we decide that the tension needs to be lowered, our guide being certain symptoms, as flushing of the face, congestive headaches, vertigo and epistaxis, while the danger of cerebral hemorrhage is always to be borne in mind.

If the heart is all right we may use veratrum viride or aconite over long periods, while glonoin is used if any cardiac weakness is manifest.

Low tension: this predisposes to serous effusions (transudates), and a decrease in the daily output of urine, thus increasing the tendency to uremia and must be combatted vigorously. Here digitalis, combined with glonoin is admirable, as the heart is weakened.

Effusions may be either transudates or exudates. In either case the indication is to get rid of the effusion as quickly as possible. If a transudate, increase the tension; if an exudate, absorptives or local applications are useful. If these measures fail we may tap the cavity and inject adrenal solution, which seems to have the happy effect of preventing further accumulation of fluid in serous sacs.

Salines, cathartics, by their osmotic action, play an important part in favoring absorption.

Counter-irritation: this is useful in the parenchymatous form, where there is so much congestion of the kidneys. Dry cups—better wet cups—are used over the kidney area, often relieving the congestion and immediately improving diuresis.

Drowsiness is to be met by decreasing and restricting the solid diet, by increase of liquids and free elimination by purging or sweating rather than by using diuretics too freely, holding this class of drugs for later use.

Dropsy: when edema is slight, massage, bandaging the limbs, rest in bed longer in the mornings, or a rest in the middle of the day may be sufficient to reduce or check it. When it increases and interferes with the function of any organ we must then rely upon diuretics and other eliminants to aid us. If the legs remain distended with fluid and the skin shining, pearly white, we may practise the "antiphlogistic touch of the therapeutic knife," as used by Pancoast, which consists in lightly puncturing the skin in many places with a fine lancet or scalpel, permitting the fluid to exude from the superficial tissues. Southey's tubes may also be used when above indications are present.

Many authors speak of the danger of erysipelas from these procedures, but it may be avoided by asepsis and common sense.

Diaphoretics: are useful from the very beginning of treatment as their use eliminates toxins and saves the kidneys much extra work, and they should be used regularly and systematically, relying upon baths,—water and hot air,—with occasional use of drugs, as sweet spirits of niter and spirits of Mindererus,—the latter in the well-known Basham's mixture, holding pilocarpine for occasional emergency use.

Diuretics should not be used when perfect compensation is present, but are indicated when there are scanty urine and much dropsy. When deficient heart action exists we use drugs which act on both heart and kidneys, such as caffeine, scoparius, digitalis and *Convallaria majalis*.

If dropsy is due to deficient kidney function and the heart is in good condition we may employ the potash salts, squills, sweet niter, diuretin and urotropin.

Asthma is a symptom of increasing intoxication and is often present for a considerable period of time before other marked symptoms of toxemia develop. Elimination, particularly by the accessory organs, must be practised thoroughly in order to overcome the condition. Chloral may be used. At times venesection will do good. Other cases do well on small doses of morphine hypodermatically, repeated only as needed.

Edema of glottis appears suddenly, is dangerous and needs prompt attention. Inhalation of steam, cocaine spray combined with adrenalin, scarification, counter-irritation or leeching may be practised, and, as a last resort, tracheotomy is to be done.

Epistaxis is due to high tension. The general indication is to lower blood tension. Locally, pressure of the non-elastic capillaries will do good.

Obstinate Vomiting or Diarrhea.—These are symptoms of great toxemia and must be promptly met. Vomiting is usually relieved by lavage; diarrhea by sweating, or diuretics. Do not check the diarrhea completely as it will cause retention of toxins and may precipitate uremia.

Pruritus is usually due to urea crystals irritating the skin. Hot bathing, followed by four per cent. carbolic acid solution, infusion of conium leaves, or chloral, may be useful.

Palpitation is met by the use of *Convallaria majalis* and, at times, morphine.

If the nephritis is dependent upon other diseases as a causal factor, the primary disease is to be treated and the condition of the blood pressure and urinary excretion are our guide to the treatment of the nephritis.

Uremia must be discussed, as the symptoms of chronic nephritis are often really those of mild degree minus convulsions.

When convulsions, unconsciousness, etc., appear we know that failure of compensation has occurred and that this point marks the beginning of the end.

Venesection should be done at once, whether tension is high or low, as it speedily eliminates toxins. This is to be followed by injection of normal saline solution, which dilutes the remaining portion of the blood and stimulates the various functions, guarding against raising the blood tension too much.

Spinal puncture has been resorted to recently upon the hypothesis that uremia is due to edema of the brain, but the results have not been conclusive thus far.

For the convulsions occurring in the parenchymatous form, morphine in good doses may be used, but in the interstitial form may be used sparingly. Chloroform, chloral and the bromides are also used to combat the convulsions.

The matter of using morphine in the uremia of chronic interstitial nephritis has been largely discussed, many authorities being found who take sides on the subject. Loomis, who first suggested it, Ziemsen, Osler, Stephen MacKenzie, Anders, Wilson, Delafield and Roberts Bartholow, all favored its use, while Tyson, Hirst, Waugh and others advise against it. While on duty under Dr. D. E. Hughes, at the Philadelphia Hospital some years ago, I saw him use it in many cases of uremic convulsions and cannot recall one case where any ill-effects were noted.

Personally I treated one case of chronic interstitial nephritis for over five years, during which time a pronounced bronchopneumonia and three attacks of uremia developed, using morphine hypodermatically for asthma that resisted other measures to combat, always with happy results. My usual routine was to give pilocarpine the morning following the hypodermic and I never saw any untoward effects of its use in this case.

Exacerbations are to be treated exactly the same as the ordinary acute attacks.

Edebohls' operation of stripping the kidney capsule in chronic nephritis seems to do good in nearly every case selected by him and other careful operators and is simply mentioned here as it is out of our domain in the limits of this paper.

MEDICAL PROGRESS.

SURGERY.

Volvulus of the Cecum.—This disorder is known to be one of the few conditions causing obstruction in the lower gut which present fulminating symptoms. E. M. CORNER and P. W. G. SARGENT (*Annals of Surgery*, January, 1905), of London, present their deductions from the study of 57 cases. Forty-two of these were males, 13 females, and in two the sex is not stated. Cecal volvulus is, therefore, three times as frequent in men as in women. It has occurred in every decade up to the eightieth year of age. A little over half the cases, however, are found between the ages of twenty and forty years. An analysis of this shows that although volvulus has always been described as one of the most acute forms of intestinal destruction, it is probable that the acute, subacute and chronic varieties exist. The total mortality was about 66 per cent., while the mortality after operation was 52 5-10 per cent. The cecum has been found in every region of the abdomen, even in the sac of in guinal herniæ. The left hypochondrium, however, is by far the most frequent situation. Here it is in relation with the spleen and stomach lying beneath the great omentum. The authors have attempted to make a classification of the different anatomical varieties. In the first, there is a mesentery common to the whole of the intestine, the cecum and varying length of the colon. The root of the mesentery is small, and its axis may be looked upon as that of the superior mesenteric vessels, it being around these that rotation occurs. The second variety is derived from the first, the root of the mesentery extending to a less degree than normal toward the right iliac fossa; thus the iliac mesentery is relatively shorter than that of the rest of the small gut or cecum, and offers a fixed point for the latter to rotate upon. In the first case, the rotation is in a segment of a circle; in the second, there being two fixed points, the curve is a segment of an ellipse. The third variety is a rotation of the cecum along its long axis. This form of axial rotation may be due to conditions either congenital or acquired.

The Matas Operation for Aneurism.—Every successful case reporting the application of this interesting technic is of the utmost value. HERMAN V. GESSNER (*Annals of Surgery*, January, 1905) cites the history of a negro, thirty-two years of age, who suffered from a syphilitic aneurism of the right popliteal artery. The tumor was five inches long by four and a quarter inches wide. He first noticed pain and swelling two months before admission. After constriction a median incision was made, and the internal popliteal nerves retracted inward. The sac was now opened and no clots were found. The lower opening was quite oblique, was easily found, and dark blood was escaping from it in small quantities. It was closed at once with No. 1 chromic catgut. The upper, or proximal, opening was found only after a prolonged search. It was one inch above the distal opening. No. 3 chromic catgut was used in a continuous Lembert stitch for closing this orifice. Removal of the Esmarch was followed by the escape of bright arterial blood, showing that the closure was defective or that some collateral existed. Hemostasis was effected by using a heavy Lembert stitch with an inch bite on either side of the sac. This further accomplished the firm approximation of the walls of the aneurism, so that no Neuberizing was necessary to do away with any dead space. At the close of the operation no pulsation could be felt in the dorsalis pedis. At the first dressing a moderate infection was found and the iodoform pack was replaced by a smaller one. The foot was warm, and pulsation was found where it had been absent in the dorsalis pedis. On August 15 the wound was entirely well. There was no pulsation whatever, although a slight tendency to edema was observed. On September 3d the patient appeared in excellent health. The circumference of the limb at the middle of the scar was 15⅜ inches against 14⅜ inches for opposite limb at same level. This difference was attributable to the scar and to the presence of the aneurismal sac. Pulsation is palpable in the dorsalis pedis. This case has, in the author's opinion, borne out one of the important claims made for the method, namely, non-interference with the collateral circulation. In spite of its early development, scarcely sufficient for the establishment of collateral circulation, the limb was supplied with blood after operation. Furthermore, the presence of a moderate degree of infection is shown by this case not to be incompatible with success.

PHYSIOLOGY.

The Physical Basis of Narcosis.—A subject that touches the borderlands of physiology, biology, pharmacology and clinical medicine, is that which attempts to explain the relative power of the various narcotics from the standpoint of physical chemistry. A new theory that seeks to show the mutual relationship of osmosis and narcosis and to discover the physical laws that underlie both, has been carefully worked out by J. TRAUBE (*Pflüger's Archiv*, December 1, 1904). Overton recently compared the various speeds with which different narcotics diffuse into protoplasm. He found that monatomic alcohol, aldehydes, ketones, etc., penetrate the cell wall more quickly than the diatomic alcohols and the amides of the monatomic acids, and then in decreasing order come glycerin, urea, etc., until are reached the salts of the strong inorganic and organic bases and acids, for which the cell-wall is wholly impermeable. The permeability is increased in homologous series by the substitution of hydrogen by methyl, and the latter by ethyl. He found that the narcotics pass through membranes the more quickly the more soluble they are in the lipoids such as fats, cholesterin, lecithin, etc. Overton and H. Meyer also pointed out that the good narcotics, anesthetics and antipyretics collectively belong to the substances that osmose quickly, and they proposed the theory that the efficiency of a good narcotic depends in the first instance on the degree of its solubility in lipoids. Overton assumes that the cell-wall, and if Quincke's theory be correct, that the walls of the foamy cell-contents contain lipoids, and the ease with which a substance penetrates these walls depends upon its solubility in these lipoids. Traube believes that there are grounds for denying that this is always the case. Instead of a foamy structure, he conceives of a membrane as a network of fine capillaries, without regard to whether it contains lipoids or not. Osmosis may be explained upon the principle of capillarity. Repeated investigations have shown that the greater the osmotic power of a water-soluble substance is, the more it lowers the capillary pressure of the water. Substances that are incapable of traversing membranes, increase the capillary pressure of the water in which they are dissolved. Diminution in capillarity and increased facility of osmosis run a parallel course. If two liquids are separated by a membrane, such that the surface tension of one is less than that of the other the former will osmose into the latter. Thus the difference in surface tension determines the direction and rapidity of osmosis. The force of osmosis is not osmotic pressure, but surface tension. In most, if not all instances in physiology, surface tension is to be put in the place of osmotic pressure in explaining dialysis. Whereas the number of molecules or ions determines the degree of osmotic pressure, it has no effect on surface tension; hence both forces must be considered distinct. In determining the various solubilities of different substances, the author found that those are the most soluble whose surface tension is the least. Solubility, solution tension and surface tension are therefore intimately related. The surface tension of solutions is determined by that of the dissolved substance. Solution tension and capillarity are more intimately connected than solubility and capillarity. Thus methyl and ethyl alcohol are both equally soluble in water, but the solution tension of the former is much greater than that of the latter. The author discovered the following law, namely, that substances of equal capillary activity belonging to homologous series (ordinary alcohols, fatty acids, esters, etc.), lower the rise of water in the capillary tube in the proportions of $1:3:3^2:3^3$ . . . . . The author believes that the rapidity with which the narcotics penetrate the walls of the ganglion cells of the brain, is not due to the fact that these substances are soluble in the lipoids of the cell-wall, but is to be attributed to the surface tension. When the narcotics have penetrated the interior of the cell, they then dissolve in the lipoids and unfold their narcotic power in proportion to this solubility. As pure non-toxic narcotics are to be regarded those that dissolve in the lipoids without causing any chemical reaction, either union with or decomposition of the proteids or other bodies of the cell. On the other hand there is a series of narcotics which have a decided toxic action; which is easily explained on the basis of their constitution, since they give use to accessory chemical reactions. As examples of the latter may be mentioned nicotin, ·llylalcohol, phenol, etc. Even the pure narcotics are not entirely non-toxic, since, while they are soluble in the lipoids, they in their turn dissolve some of the fatty substance. It is doubtful whether a really good narcotic will ever be found. Experiments show that in the pure narcotics there is a close relationship between surface tension and narcotic power. According to Overton, in homologous series the narcotic action increases with the increasing content of carbon, with the substitution of hydrogen by alcohol radicals, as well as from tertiary through iso—to normal compounds. The same holds true of the capillary activity of these substances. The substitution of hydrogen or amido groups in place of a hydrogen atom, lowers capillary activity as well as narcotic power. It is also found that the narcotic action of homologous substances (as alcohols, esters, etc.) with an increasing molecular weight, increases in the proportions of $1:3:3^2$.

Ferments of the Blood.—There can be little doubt that the property of blood to give off oxygen to the tissues, is due to a special ferment to which the name katalase has been applied. Some interesting researches upon this body are reported by A. JOLLES (*Münch. med. Woch.*, November 22, 1904). It is readily destroyed by heat and acids, but hardly affected by alkalies. The amount present in blood may be estimated as follows: 0,05 c.c. of blood are diluted up to 50 c.c. with physiological salt solution. 10 c.c. of this dilution are then mixed with 30 c.c. of accurately neutralized peroxide of hydrogen and allowed to stand for two hours. After acidifying, potassium iodide is added, and the amount of iodine set free by the peroxide still present, then titrated with thio-sulphate of sodium. Normally one cubic centimeter of blood will decompose 18 to 30 c.c. of peroxide. The amount of katalase seems to stand in relation with the percentage of hemoglobin; by

far the greater percentage is contained within the erythrocytes. Very low figures were occasionally obtained in tuberculosis, carcinoma, nephritis, jaundice and leucemia. The blood is also deficient in ferment in comatose conditions and it is possible that the symptoms here are in great part due to insufficient supply of oxygen in the nervous centers. There seems to be no fixed relation between the amount of katalase and oxydase (the ferment which converts hemoglobin into oxyhemoglobin) present.

Surface Tension and its Significance in the Organism.—Using as a test his own discovery that a solution of low surface tension will osmose through a membrane into a solution of higher surface tension, J. TRAUBE (*Pflünger's Archiv*, December 1, 1904) discuss the various manifestations of this force in the workings of the body. Since under normal conditions the blood does not pass into the stomach or intestines, one may conclude à priori that the surface tension of the contents of stomach and intestines is less than that of the blood. This is actually found to be the case. The author devised an instrument called the stalagmometer, which measures the number of drops in a given weight of fluid. By multiplying the result by a certain constant is obtained the number representing the capillarity of the liquid. The greater the number of drops the less is the surface tension of the solution. The blood has a very great surface tension. The significance of the formation of peptones depends upon a fact which has been experimentally established, namely: peptones reduce to a great degree the surface tension of the liquid in which they are dissolved, while proteids do not. As a result of this diminution of surface tension the peptones undergo dialysis. It has been found by Bernstein that only dilute solutions of peptone are found in the stomach and intestines, for peptones are mostly absorbed as quickly as they are formed. In digestive disorders in which the process of absorption is disturbed, there is a greater accumulation of peptones, with a resulting greater diminution of surface tension and hence a more active effort toward osmosis. In severe diseases, such as nephritis with gastric atony, ulcer of the stomach, and nervous anacidity, the surface tension of the gastric contents is much less than in the milder diseases. It is probable that this method of investigation will be of value from the standpoint of diagnosis. Indol and skatol are substances possessing a marked degree of capillary activity, that is, they strongly diminish the surface tension of the liquids in which they are dissolved. They thus have a marked influence upon intestinal absorption. It is found that a membrane which is semipermeable for a salt when it separates the pure aqueous salt solution from pure water, loses this semipermeability as soon as indol or skatol is added to the salt solution. The functions of bile are likewise partly dependent upon surface tension. Bile is a fluid of low surface tension. If this were not the case, it would not be capable of emulsifying fat, which has a low surface tension. Moreover this low surface tension enables the bile to moisten the wall of the intestine in order to hasten absorption. This same property explains how easily in icterus bile enters the blood and tissues during stasis in the biliary passages. In healthy kidneys the surface tension of the urine is much greater than that of the blood. In nephritis the surface tension of the urine is diminished, which explains the disturbances in the secretory activity of the kidneys. The urine can never have the low surface tension of bile or milk, and it is remarkable that the following law holds good, namely: capillary-active substances, which diminish surface tension, (such as phenol, indol, benzoic acid, etc.), on their passage into the urine are transformed into compounds (phenolsulphuric acid, indoxylsulphuric acid, hippuric acid, etc.), which are markedly capillary-inactive, maintaining the high surface tension of the urine. If substances like the former were allowed to enter the urine, the kidneys would soon cease to function. Unilateral stagalomometric investigation of the renal secretion, would be in order in cases of suspected disease of one kidney. Thus blood-pressure and osmotic pressure are not sufficient to explain renal activity. On the other hand, surface tension does not explain all the phenomena of osmosis. Thus blood pressure determines the flow of the nutritive elements of the blood in the direction of the lymph. Moreover the rapidity of osmosis depends in some degree upon the extent to which the opposing fluids are soluble in each other. Chemical forces must also be considered. The frictional coefficients of the osmosing fluids must also be borne in mind and above all the nature of the membrane itself. If a membrane contains fatty particles, the surface tension of the osmosing fluid is markedly diminished and the speed of osmosis is thereby increased. It is well known that alkaloids, antipyretics, diuretics, narcotics, excitants, etc., belong to the rapidly osmosing class of substances; they are also on the one hand soluble in lipoids, and on the other hand they diminish the surface tension of the liquids in which they are dissolved. This diminution is of great significance, for it explains the marked change in the surface tension of the circulating fluids, in certain conditions even reversing the direction of the exchanges of fluid and giving rise to the possibility of abnormal chemical changes in the organism. As an example, amyl alcohol contained in fusel oil lowers surface tension, and has the capacity of soaking well into vital membranes. Hence, if in the smallest quantities it moisten the walls of the biliary passages, the rapidity of the changes there would become an abnormal one. Ordinary alcohol also lowers surface tension and thereby its ingestion accelerates intestinal absorption, particularly that of fats; in this respect it has a certain therapeutic value. The author concludes that the action of many drugs is dependent not upon chemical changes, but upon such changes as have been indicated above. Even the smallest quantities of these substances may have a marked influence in this direction, not temporarily, but for a prolonged time. The fact that bacteria, ferments and colloids are in the first case agglutinated, and in the latter two precipitated by electrolytes, has been rightly attributed to surface tension. Each dissolved particle of salt may be compared to a small magnet, which by virtue of its high surface tension attracts to itself the colloidal particles, etc., and thereby causes precipitation. The author found that the surface tension of sodium and potassium salts increases with the number of sodium and potassim atoms in the molecule. The ameboid movements of white blood cells have been attributed by Quincke to changes of surface tension. This is possibly true also of the manifestations of chemotropism seen in the movements of the spermatozoon in the fertilization of the ovum. Bernstein worked out a theory of the muscular contraction as due to service tension. In the field of toxins, service ten-

sion may explain certain phenomena. Thus tetanus toxin travels to the brain by way of the fatty nerve-fibers, while antitoxin chooses the vascular path. The toxin also penetrates the cells while antitoxin does not. The toxin is dissolved in the lipoids of the brain tissue, while antitoxin is dissolved in the cerebrospinal fluid. The toxin dissolves red blood cells, while antitoxin does not; the toxin is found in the bile and milk and not in the urine, and it is just the opposite with the antitoxin. These facts indicate that tetanus toxin osmoses and dissolves in lipoids with ease, while antitoxin does not. These results suggest interesting developments in the domain of toxins. It would be useful to cultivate toxins in capillary-inactive media, and to add to antitoxins capillary-active substances, so as to increase their osmotic power and hence their usefulness.

PATHOLOGY AND BACTERIOLOGY.

Protozoa-like Structures in Syphilis.—A very interesting post-mortem finding in a fetus eight months old, bearing distinct signs of hereditary syphilis, is reported by D. JESIONEK and D. KIOLENE-MOGLOU (*Münch. med. Woch.*, October 25, 1904). In the kidneys, wherever the luetic changes were most pronounced, groups of 10 to 40 bodies were found which closely resembled certain protozoa in that they possessed a distinct capsule with homogenous protoplasm and well-defined nucleus. Similar bodies, but in less number, were found in the lungs and liver. Behavior toward dyes makes it improbable atht these structures were pre-formed tissue-elements. On the other hand, examination of syphilitic condylomata and of a second syphilitic fetus was absolutely negative, so that the real nature and significance of these elements could not be definitely decided.

Bacteriology of Noma.—A. HOFMAN and E. KÜSTER (*Münch. med. Woch.*, October 25, 1905) have succeeded in isolating a specific and hitherto undescribed bacteria from the tissues of a case of noma. If the necrotic tissues be examined a great variety of germs, including staphylococci, streptococci and diphtheria bacilli may be detected, but in the deeper structures, where inflammation is just beginning, only a short, slightly curved bacillus is found. This grows well on all culture media, but is not identical with other previously isolated in noma. The spirillum grows best in the presence of oxygen, is gramnegative and forms long chains. It may also be stained directly in the tissues, but here appears more like a bacillus.

Cause, Prevention and Diagnosis of Gastric and Intestinal Cancer.—The cells which make up malignant tumors are distinctly embryonal in character, but it is exceedingly improbable that they are human embryonel cells. G. KELLING (*Münch. med. Woch.*, October 25, 1904) is firmly convinced that all tumors of the intestinal tract result from the ingestion of fetal tissues derived from animals. Examples would be raw eggs, fetal cells from the uteri of the hog, etc. If macerated chicken embryos be injected into a mesenteric vein of a dog, distinct tumors will develop in the liver, and sometimes in the retroperitoneal structures after three to four months. The experiment is most often successful if old dogs are chosen, and the organs most susceptible to tumor formation are the liver and testicles. Proof that tumor-cells are really derived from other animals is to be found in the briochemical reaction. If a

rabbit be treated with an emulsion of tumor-cells its
serum will eventually precipitate human serum, but
also the serum of some other animal, usually chicken
or hog. If chicken or hog serum be injected, the
rabbit serum will in turn·precipitate the tumor extract. In a small percentage of cases no reaction
was obtained, probably because the embryonal cells
of some animal not tested was responsible for the
tumor. Possibly also the specific albumin may sometimes lose its characteristic properties. The precipitin reaction may also be used to test the blood of
suspected carcinoma cases. Every organism affected
with carcinoma will form a certain amount of precipitin against the parasitic cells, which can be
readily demonstrated by removing a few cubic centimeters of blood from the vein at the elbow, and
then mixing the serum obtained from this blood
with a dilute solution of albumin obtained from a
chicken or hog. In carcinoma a precipitate will appear in a few hours. Several cases with indefinite
symptoms of gastric cancer but positive serum reaction were operated and a tumor was found. Patients on whom the serum reaction is to be performed should not be fed on large amounts of raw
·eggs, since the albumin may pass into the blood and
give rise to the formation of precipitins, even if no
cancer is ·present.

**Pathology of Plants Compared with that of Ani-
mals.**—In an interesting article E. KÜSTER (*Münch.
med. Woch.*, November 15, 1904) discusses the various
pathological processes which have been observed in
vegetable tissue. While hypoplasia is occasionally
observed in different organs of the animal body, and
certain tissues even of the same organ may remain
behind in development, these processes are by far
more frequent in plants since these are more often
exposed to inhibitory influences. Even the vegetable reproductive organs are occasionally hypoplastic. Metaplasia, however, is less frequent and
limited only to abnormal development of the cell-
membrane and the contents of the cell. Changes in
form are especially rare, since the plant cell is usually surrounded by a firm membrane which fixes it to
its position. It follows that migration, inflammation
and infiltration are unknown in plant-pathology. Atrophy and necrosis do not occur; even the dead cell
retains its original shape. Hypertrophy of cells, on
the other hand, is, not rare; it may be due to absorption of water when the vegetable tissue is exposed
to excessive moisture, or an excess of nutritive material may be stored up when the conditions for
growth are exceptionally favorable. In the former
case the swelling is sometimes so marked that the
cell-membrane is ruptured and the cell contents deposit on the outside. The formation of giant-cells
is frequently induced by the presence of parasites;
they differ from the above only in that they have
multiple nuclei. Tumors often result from injury or
the action of parasites; they have no definite shape
or form; develop during a varying length of time,
and differ from the tumors of animal pathology in
that their growth is expansile and never infiltrating.
Their finer structure is extremely simple, yet some,
like the gall, are very complicated.

Toxin of Fatigue.—By means of a large number of
careful experiments, W. WEICHARDT (*Münch. med.
Woch.*, November 29, 1904) could prove that during
muscular exercise a toxin is formed in the muscles,
which can be easily separated from the other extractives by dialysis. If injected into fresh animals
this toxin will cause intense fatigue, fall of tem-

perature, stupor and death. It has the properties of
a true toxin, since it is not dialyzable, and gives rise
to the formation of an antitoxin if injected. The toxin
is saturated by the antitoxin both in the living body
and in the test-tube, according to the law of multi-
ples. Unlike the toxin, the antitoxin is readily
dialyzable and may be preserved for a long time.
If taken internally, the antitoxin seems to have a
remarkably stimulating action upon the muscle, so
that it may become a valuable therapeutic agent.

Streptococci of Lochia.—The lochial secretion of
the perfectly normal puerperal stage frequently contains a large number of streptococci. The explanation offered was ' that these were avirulent germs
which differed considerably from the ordinary pathogenic 'varieties. F. SCHENCK and A. SCHEIB (*Münch.
med. Woch.*, November 29, 1904) found the lochial secretion sterile in a large percentage of cases only
during the first few days after confinement; later,
streptococci were almost always present. These
germs were in every way identical with virulent
streptococci, since they were pathogenic to animals.
The serum of animals treated with lochial streptococci agglutinated streptococci of known virulency
as strongly as those which were injected. Cultures
of the two forms were alike in every way. It is,
therefore, probable that the granulating interior of
the womb is the only safeguard against general infection.

Microscopical Examination of Lochial Secretion.
—In every·case of temperature during the puerperium the lochial secretion should be examined most
carefully. The absence of streptococci, according to
A. LEO (*Münch. Woch.*, November 29, 1904) almost certainly excludes a severe affection of the genital tract. Fever, if present. may then be due to (1)
an extragenital cause; (2) simple retention of secretion; (3) a sapremic intoxication; (4) an infection
with gonococci, more rarely with colon, diphtheria
or tetanus bacilli. In the presence of streptococci,
the following facts must be kept in mind: (a) Chains
of four members are common during the normal
puerperium, and are thus of no significance. (b) Chains
of more·than four cocci in the vagina generally cause
fever or subfebrile temperature; if they occur in the
secretion of the uterus itself they are still more likely
to be responsible for the symptoms. The degree
of phagocystosis present gives a good idea of the
powers of resistance present. The time during which
streptococci are found is also of great importance;
if they occur late in the puerperium they are of less
significance than early.

Fate of Uric Acid Introduced into the System.—
Experiments conducted by W. EBSTEIN and E. BEN-
NIX (*Virchow's Archiv*, Vol. 178, No. 3) leave no doubt •
that uric acid, injected into the ear-vein of a rabbit
will deposit very soon in the epithelial cells of the convoluted tubules of the kidney in the form of spherical
crystals. If both kidneys are extirpated and even large
amounts of uric acid are then injected, no microscopical changes will be found in the liver or joints. Experiments conducted with unicellular organisms to determine which part of the cell has an affinity for the
acid, were negative, since these animal cells, unlike
vegetable cells, are extremely sensitive and rapidly die.
If xanthin, hypoxanthin or adenin is used instead of
uric acid, crystals will also be deposited in the cells and
lumen, but with guanin the distribution of crystals is
more uniform over the entire kidney.

Chorio-epithelioma of the Bladder.—It was formerly believed that a chorio-epithelioma could·only

develop from the placental site in the uterus, but since then several cases have been reported where tlie uterus was not the seat of the tumor. The following case of W. S. DJEWITZKI (*Virchow's Archiv*, Vol. 178, No. 3) is probably the first case of chorio-epithelioma developing from the bladder. The patient, an unmarried woman of seventy-five years, died shortly after a curettage for hemorrhage from fibroids. At autopsy, an ulcerated, reddish mass, occupied the greater part of the bladder. Numerous metastases were found in the lungs, intestines and spleen. Microscopical examination showed that the tumor and its metastases were made up of Langhans cells and syncytium. Two explanations are possible for the presence of this tumor in a woman who had never been pregnant. It may have developed from remains of the Wolffian duct which is normally placed in the posterior wall of the bladder during embryonal life, or it may have started from the epithelial lining of the bladder itself.

Arteriosclerosis of the Pulmonary Artery.—In studying the microscopical changes in arteriosclerosis. H. W. E. EHLERS (*Virchow's Archiv*, Vol. 178, No. 3) discovered that the structure of the normal pulmonary artery differs somewhat from that of other arteries in that the muscularis forms two distinct layers: an internal one with the elastic fibers arranged longitudinally and the external one, where the elastic fibers form a dense network. Frequently the two layers are separated by a membrane, resembling the internal elastic membrane. The small yellow areas of degeneration which are sometimes found at autopsies affect chiefly the longitudinal layer of the media. This layer is considerably thickened and converted into connective tissue or into a homogenous substance, poor in nuclei.

Arteriosclerosis in Nephritis.—The most important lesion of the smaller arteries in nephritis is a marked fatty degeneration. If the kidneys are stained with sudan, the arteries will appear as red rings, surrounded by a very narrow muscular coat. The process probably begins in the elastic lamellæ of the internal limiting membrane and all organs except the heart and the skeletal musculature seem to be affected. L. JORES (*Virchow's Archiv*, Vol. 178, No. 3) concludes that there are no characteristic vessel-changes for nephritis since the above lesions are common to arteriosclerosis as such. Not all cases of nephritis, however, are accompanied by these changes. The significance of arteriosclerosis in nephritis is not always the same: it may be the cause or the consequence of the renal affection or both lesions may result from a third, common etiological factor. Even extensive degeneration in the kidney is capable of being regulated so that we must deal with another factor to explain the formation of connective tissue. This the author thinks, is the gradual change in the vessel-walls, which will eventually render the glomeruli impassable and thus diminish the blood-supply necessary for the production of new parenchyma in the place of the old. In this sense every nephritis would be of the arteriosclerotic type and would merely be a symptom of the general arteriosclerotic changes.

Relation of Islands of Langerhans to Diabetes.—The much-disputed question of the relation of the so-called islands of Langerhans to diabetes has been answered by K. KARAKASCHEFF (*Deutsch. Archiv f. klin. Med.*, Vol. 82, Nos. 1 and 2) as follows: In most cases of diabetes, the islands are absolutely normal, in others they may even proliferate. Glands with seriously altered islands from cases who have never suffered from diabetes are not uncommon so that there cannot very well be any relation between the two. It is more likely that the metabolism of sugar is affected by lesion of the parenchyma of the gland. Injury or intoxication will affect both parts of the gland, but the islands, being more resistant than the parenchyma, will suffer less. Even if a certain amount of parenchyma is destroyed, the islands are able to form new acini, so that diabetes will not necessarily follow. Embryological studies will prove that the islands are not definite organs but earlier stages in the development of the acini, so that they may be regarded as reserve material which can replace destroyed parenchyma.

Parasites of Smallpox, Vaccinia and Varicella.—Nothing is more interesting in connection with medical progres than the records of efforts to prove the relation of ameboid bodies to certain acute infectious diseases. W. E. DeKORTE (*Lancet*, December 24, 1904) states that if human vaccine lymph be collected in capillary tubes on the ninth day of the disease, a considerable number of unicellular globes with refractile contents can be demonstrated. These bodies on the warm stage at 98° F. show considerable motility, the changes in shape being sometimes so rapid as almost to evade observation. Leucocytes in human blister fluid kept at the temperature of the body may remain intact for five days or more. But it has been shown that these cells disappear from the lymph spontaneously on or about the tenth day whether situated in the vesicle or stored in a capillary tube. For these reasons the author believes it conclusively proven that the bodies under consideration are certainly protozoan parasites. To what class they belong, however, he does not pretend to say. The parasite is found in secondary vaccination as well. In hunting for them it is well to centrifugalize the capillary tube. The protozoon of variola and vaccina is an ameboid organism measuring about one twenty-five hundredth of an inch. It has for the most part an oblate spheroidal shape, but encysted forms are found which may be four or five times as large. It consists essentially of cytoplasm, which in the encysted form is enclosed in the well-marked cell wall, and of a rounded or ovoid nucleus, which apparently has a definite membrane. This nucleus can be seen to possess a definite nucleolus. In the case of variola no definite pseudopsia has been seen. The author expects to publish a paper shortly on the method of cultivating the organisms.

Inoculation Carcinoma.—This much debated question is discussed in a very extensive and elaborate study of the subject by R. MILNER (*Archiv f. klin. Chir.*, Vol. 74, No. 4), who believes that from the data at hand the matter cannot by any means be decided conclusively. A large number of cases (over 200) have been collected, classified and studied. The conclusions of the author based on this study are as follows: The so-called inoculation carcinomata can only be considered to have been produced, according to the present state of knowledge, by the implantation of carcinomatous cells. The implantation of carcinoma cells on endothelium does occur, but not very commonly, and the advice of Hanau to conduct experimental inoculations on serous surfaces holds good even at the present day. The implantation of carcinomatous growths in fresh wounds experimentally has been repeatedly done, but has only succeeded in a very small proportion of the cases, and only when particular precautions were taken. The implantation of carcinoma cells on intact epithelium has never been accomplished experimentally, with the exception of that on the ovary. It is almost impossible to exclude the possibility of retrograde metastasis or primary multiplicity of the tumors. The unintentional transmission of cancer from one individual to another of the same species has never been positively observed. The fear of contagion by mere contact is therefore unfounded, but the accidental inoculation at operations cannot be so conclusively excluded, and' the precautions already formulated must be observed. Further studies are necessary, which will aid not merely in clearing up the general and special pathology of the carcinomata, but may also solve some time the question connected with other infectious diseases.

Bacteriological Examination of Blood.—The great importance of a bacteriological examination of the blood is again emphasized by G. Jochmann (*Zeitsch. f. klin. Med.*, Vol. 54, Nos. 5 and 6). If streptococci are found, the prognosis varies with primary and secondary conditions. Of nine cases of the former, as many as three recovered. The portal of entry may be the female genital tract, the skin, lungs, as well as the gastro-intestinal tract, urogenital tract, tonsils and middle ear. Secondary streptococcus infections, such as occur after scarlet fever, diphtheria, etc., are almost invariably fatal. The portal of entry in these cases is usually the tonsil. The identification of the germ is also of great value from a therapeutic point of view, for streptococcus infection will call for treatment with Tavel's or Aronson's serum, while no results can be expected from this if staphylococci are found. Staphylococcus infection is more hopeless, and not a single case observed by the author recovered. Metastatic foci are very common, and the clinical picture of what was formerly called pyemia is frequently seen. Pneumococci are also frequently encountered in the blood, and in the ordinary croupous pneumonia they occur in about 33 per cent. Two-thirds of these cases are fatal. Occasionally an empyema may form the starting point for a general infection. In general infection after gonorrhea, gonococci can usually be detected with ease upon the plated blood. In as many as 83 per cent of typhoid fever cases the author could grow typhoid germs from the blood. The period of continuous fever is the most favorable time for examination, but the results were frequently positive earlier, while the Widal was still negative, and also later, during the remittent stage. A large number of cases of articular rheumatism and sepsis were also examined, but the blood remained sterile in every instance unless the case was complicated by secondary infections.

Non-Fatal Rupture of Aortic Aneurism.—Although it is contrary to the general belief that rupture of the sac of an aortic aneurism must be fatal within a very few minutes, a few cases have been recorded in which life has been preserved not alone for hours, but actually for years after this lesion. Charles H. Melland (*Lancet*, November 19, 1904) recites the history of a laborer, fifty-six years of age, who was admitted to the Manchester Royal Infirmary, June 7. 1899. While at work, he had suddenly brought up a bucketful of blood. He was exsanguinated, with all the characteristic signs of that condition. As the hemorrhage had ceased, saline infusion was used, two pints being injected into his median basilic vein. He immediately rallied and improved. The history was then obtained, which showed that he had had a cough for eight months. During recent years, he had noticed a stabbing pain in the chest, which was made distinctly worse on exertion. At the hospital he improved very much for three weeks. The heart was somewhat hypertrophied. There was dulness in the second left interspace. There were tracheal tugging and inequality of the pupils. The pulses were markedly unequal, the right pulse being

of a water-hammer type. Three weeks later he had a severe hemorrhage. Two days after this it recurred, and he was again infused. An hour and a half after this, however, another hemorrhage proved fatal. At autopsy, the aorta was found to be so atheromatous that the orifices of the coronary aorta were practically occluded. The sacular aneurism arose from the convexity of the arch immediately beyond the left carotid, and was of about the size of a large hen's egg. The subclavian came off from the upper and outer part of the sac which was almost filled with laminated clot. Posteriorly, the aneurism had extended between the trachea and the esophagus. The trachea was thinned out and its mucous membrane softened. In this softened area there was a vertical slit, three-eighths of an inch long, through which the bleeding had occurred. As in the other reported cases, the limitation of the hemorrhage after free rupture must be attributed to the amount of clot in the sac, a portion of which had, no doubt, served as a valve to plug the opening. The value of saline injection in these cases is definitely proved, there being no doubt that the technic is indicated as soon as the hemorrhage is stopped.

PRESCRIPTION HINTS.

Treatment of Pruritus.—Various remedies employed in the modern treatment of pruritus are given by *La Quinzaine therapeutique, 10 janv., 1905.* Internally carbolic acid, in pills of 10 centigrams each, is preferred by many. Another school employs valerian as follows:

R Ammon. valerianate 0.5
Two to six pills daily.

Other remedies are the sulphate or valerianate of atropine (four granules of ¼ milligram daily), arsenious acid, cherry-laurel water, castoreum, musk, asafetida.

Locally, the following wash is recommended:

R Hydrocyanic acid 0.5-1.0
　Bichloride of mercury 0.5-1.0
　Sulphate of copper 1.0-5.0
　Carbolic acid 5.0-10.0
　Resorcin 5.0-20.0
　Chloral 5.0-25.0
　Bromide of potash 5.0-50.0
　Water 1000.0

Alcoholic solutions of menthol, resorcin, or sublimate are equally as efficacious. After washing, the parts may be powdered with the following:

R Powdered starch 100.0
　Subnitrate of bismuth 5-25.0
　Acid salicylic 1.0

For small surfaces, the following is good:

R Cocaine hydrochlor. 0.30
　Menthol 3.0
　Vaselin 30.0

Genito-perineal pruritus demands a search for fissures, excoriations, parasites, discharges, diabetes, albuminuria, etc.

In vaginal itching, a suppository of

R Cocaine chlor............. ⎫
　Morphine chlor. ...... ⎬ ....aa　0.02-0.03
　Cacao butter 3.0

is excellent.

Hydrotherapy, electrotherapy or surgical intervention may be indicated in any form.

THE MEDICAL NEWS.

A WEEKLY JOURNAL

OF MEDICAL SCIENCE.

COMMUNICATIONS in the form of Scientific Articles, Clinical Memoranda, Correspondence or News Items of interest to the profession are invited from all parts of the world. Reprints to the number of 250 of original articles contributed exclusively to the MEDICAL NEWS will be furnished without charge if the request therefor accompanies the manuscript. When necessary to elucidate the text, illustrations will be engraved from drawings or photographs furnished by the author. Manuscript should be typewritten.

SMITH ELY JELLIFFE, A.M., M.D., Ph.D., Editor,
No. 111 FIFTH AVENUE, NEW YORK.

Subscription Price, Including postage in U. S. and Canada.

PER ANNUM IN ADVANCE $4.00
SINGLE COPIES 10
WITH THE AMERICAN JOURNAL OF THE
MEDICAL SCIENCES, PER ANNUM . . 8.00

Subscriptions may begin at any date. The safest mode of remittance is by bank check or postal money order, drawn to the order of the undersigned. When neither is accessible, remittances may be made at the risk of the publishers, by forwarding in *registered* letters.

LEA BROTHERS & CO.,
No. 111 FIFTH AVENUE (corner of 18th St.), NEW YORK.

SATURDAY, FEBRUARY 18, 1905.

HOSPITAL CONSTRUCTION IN THE PRESENT AND FUTURE.

CINCINNATI is about to begin the construction of a hospital of some 800 beds. The committee having in charge the preparation of the plans of the new hospital are very proud of the manner in which their duty has been discharged; but their pride is not shared by all of their fellow-townsmen. A well-known Cincinnati physician is in despair over the outlook, and writes a truly pathetic appeal for light on the subject of hospital construction, the important landmarks of which, he declares, are shrouded in " Egyptian darkness." "On a high, rolling plateau," he writes, " 300 feet above the river we have twenty-four acres of land that is capable of being made anything the heart can wish. This beautiful site it is proposed to cover with an indefinite number of pavilions, that would make it look like an old Gothic camp, with a lot of tunnels that will be culture places for all that is vile. The estimated cost of this plan, for 800 beds, is from two to two-and-a-half million dollars; whereas a single large building of the same capacity, with all modern conveniences, would cost about half."

Our correspondent is evidently prepared to break with the tradition which for many years has dominated hospital architecture abroad—the tradition which has held up the pavilion system as the one permissible form of hospital construction. The followers of the pavilion idea, in their very laudable desire to avoid epidemics, to prevent overcrowding, to preserve good, natural ventilation, and to insure well-lighted wards, have held fast to the Hamburg-Eppendorf-Johns Hopkins models, and have erred in refusing to consider even the possibility of safeguarding patients' interests in hospital buildings of a radically different type.

In New York City the pavilion system, while never systematically attacked, has long been disregarded, for reasons chiefly economic. Hospitals must be easy of access to their patients, and on Manhattan Island accessible sites are so costly that a real pavilion hospital, consisting of widely separated one-story or at most two-story buildings, has not been thought of for many years. One may subdivide a huge pile like St. Luke's or Presbyterian into more or less disconnected units, and may call the units pavilions; but five-story or six-story buildings, housing superimposed wards, are not "pavilion hospitals" in the proper sense of the term. And yet, notwithstanding the absolute abandonment of the pavilion system (we refer, of course, to general and not to isolation hospitals) New York can boast of the possession of some of the finest hospitals in the world—hospitals affording to patients every comfort known to the inmates of the pavilion hospitals of Europe, and yielding, to their managers, the possibility of a much more convenient and economical administration. In the hospitals of New York overcrowding does not, or need not, find a place; natural ventilation is good and is supplemented, in some instances quite unnecessarily, by elaborate artificial aids; sunlight is not lacking; thanks to modern plumbing, filtered water, scrupulous cleanliness and efficient disinfection, epidemics are almost unknown; and even the pleasant garden breathing-spots which make so attractive the pavilion hospitals of Continental Europe, find a satisfactory substitute in such roof-gardens as one sees at the Lying-in Hospital, Mt. Sinai or in McKim, Mead & White's plans of the new Bellevue Hospital.

Ruppel, in his book on hospital construction (Anlage und Bau der Krankenhäuser nach hygienisch-technischen Grundsätzen, Jena, 1896), discusses the relative merits of two systems for the building of hospitals—the " corridor " system and the " pavilion " system. In the construction of a large hospital he recognizes no other alternative, and in considering the two systems named, he promptly condemns the corridor plan because of the possibility it offers for the conveyance of infection along the corridors from ward to ward. The book is written for a period or for a country in which the handling of individual cases, according to the highly developed practice of the best New York hospitals, is not known. We know of a children's hospital in this city, where so carefully are the patients and their hospital belongings (clothing, eating utensils, thermometers, etc.) individualized, that the appearance of a sporadic case of diphtheria, scarlet fever or measles, gives rise to scarcely any apprehension of an epidemic; for experience has shown that such methods as are here practised tend to prevent epidemics. New York affords many striking examples of the possibility of meeting all reasonable hygienic requirements in a tall, compact, modern, fireproof hospital building. Is it not advisable, then, in city construction, to avoid the magnificent distances, the costly ground-plan and the extremely difficult supervision which the pavilion hospital carries with it?

Without condemning the Cincinnati plans (for we have not had an opportunity to study them in detail), may we not with propriety suggest to the building committee the advisability of a careful study of the hospital architecture of New York, which, we venture to think, represents more nearly than does the "pavilion system," American hospital architecture of the future.

CAN THE ETHIOPIAN CHANGE HIS SKIN?

THE prophet Jeremiah certainly had no inkling of the tendencies or aspirations of modern science when he assumed that cutaneous pigmentation is a matter beyond human control. Recent discoveries in the biochemistry of the coloring matters of the integument impart a certain degree of plausibility to the hopes of the colored man. The science of physiology is passing through a sensational era. Even death hath lost its terrors. The heart that has lain frozen in the ice-box for seventy-two hours is made to beat under the magic hand of Kuliabko. The quest for the elixir of youth has not been relinquished, for no less a distinguished scientist than Metchnikoff is inclined to regard old age as a disease, the cure

of which is within the bounds of human possibility. A speculation of more modest scope is suggested by some of the recent work on the animal pigments.

In 1901, von Furth and Schneider isolated from the blood of insects a ferment tyrosinase, which acting upon tyrosin, one of the end-products of proteolytic digestion in the intestine, produces a melanin-like body. The beautiful colors of the butterfly's wings can thus be traced back to a lowly origin in the food-canal. Besides showing with what wise economy Nature sometimes utilizes the very wastes of the body, this discovery served as a forerunner of one of more immediate value. Florence M. Durham has reported to the Royal Society her discovery of the presence of tyrosinase in the skin of certain pigmented vertebrates, such as rabbits, rats, and guinea-pigs. In acting upon tyrosin, this ferment produces a pigment which corresponds in color with that of the animal from which the tyrosinase is obtained. This result suggests that for each color there is a specific tyrosinase. In all probability these ferments are present in the skin of human beings. Hence the natural color of the skin is to be attributed to pigments which have their source in the end-products of proteid digestion. As another instance of the extreme complexity of physiological processes, is the further discovery by Florence Durham that tyrosinase cannot bring about the transformation of tyrosin into pigment without the presence of an activating substance.

Tyrosinase is a ferment normally present in the skin. To what, then, are to be attributed the differences of color seen in the various races of mankind not to mention the innumerable gradations of complexion found in individuals of the same race? Three possibilities suggest themselves. First, the amount of tyrosinase may vary in different individuals. Second, the amount of tyrosinase may be constant but the activating substance may vary, or, owing to differences of environment, the ferment may unfold its activity to a varying degree. Third, the amounts of tyrosinase and activating substance may be constant, while the quantity of tyrosin produced in the organism, either in the intestinal tract or in the tissues, may vary within wide limits. The second possibility would seem best to serve as the basis of a working hypothesis, to explain the wide differences in cutaneous coloration.

In elaborating this hypothesis other factors

must be considered. The adaptive capacities of the organism and the influence of the sunlight have been determining factors in the evolution of the pigments of the skin. The colored and dusky races have had their origin under the hot sun of the tropics. It would seem as if the darkening of the skin from the accumulation of pigment is an adaptation by which the individual is protected against the ill-effects of excessive sunlight.

In this connection the experiments of R. C. Schiedt have an important bearing. This investigator deprived oysters of one of their shells and exposed them to pure light, with the result that the animals secreted pigment over the whole of their body. The chemical or blue rays produce the same pigment, but not so with the red rays, which, however, protect the animal against the pathological changes due to irritation. On placing the animal in darkness all pigment disappears.

These new experiments indicate that probably the deposition of pigment in the skin of higher animals is the result of a chemical process, initiated under the influence of the blue, or chemical rays, having for its object the protection of the organism from the irritating effects of the latter. From this viewpoint, the bronzing of the skin and the appearance of freckles in summer receive a rational explanation.

It may be that under certain conditions the organism may produce the pigment-forming ferment, which has been previously absent, or present at most in very small amount. Habitual exposure to strong sunlight, or in certain pathological conditions, the product of perverted metabolism, may initiate or stimulate the formation of tyrosinase, with the consequent deposition of pigment in the skin, or even in the internal organs. In the latter case, the presence of the pigment may be the starting-point of malignant newgrowths (melanosarcoma).

Besides being a normal, physiological manifestation of the organism, an adaptation for self-protection, cutaneous pigmentation occurs in a number of pathological conditions. Bronzing of the skin occurs in Addison's disease; in affections of the uterus (chloasma uterinum); in cystic degeneration of the ovaries; and, according to Withington, in scurvy; chronic tuberculosis, especially of the peritoneum; in cirrhosis, particularly in Hanot's hypertrophic cirrhosis with diabetes; in certain pancreatic affections, with or without diabetes; in old amyloid disease; in chronic splenic enlargement with or without malarial poisoning; in pellagra; in "vagabonds'" disease; in chronic rheumatoid arthritis; and in exophthalmic goiter. This wide range of the occurrence of cutaneous pigmentation, suggests that probably the latter is the result of some metabolic derangement.

In the light of what is now becoming known about the origin of the bodily pigments, one may assume that in severe wasting diseases there is a rapid destruction of the tissue proteids; tyrosin is produced in large amounts, and the organism seeks to get rid of this through the action of tyrosinase, which converting it into pigment, causes its deposition in the skin. Just as the body gets rid of a large excess of sulphur by causing its accumulation in the hair, under the form of keratin, so, possibly, the appearance of an undue amount of coloring matter in the skin is a manifestation of excretion. Schiedt found that pigments produced under pathological conditions are not permanent, and agrees with Loeb in believing that pigment granules are excretory products of protoplasm.

If one attempt to speculate further upon some of the hidden possibilities of continued investigations on this interesting theme, certain ludicrous results suggest themselves. Since the presence of pigment in the skin is the result of the action of tyrosinase, then, if one can obtain control over the latter, either regulate its action or destroy it altogether, one might change the complexion of an individual at will. Recent work on the antibodies has been extended to the production of antiferments. By injecting trypsin into the blood of an animal, the latter reacts with the formation of anti-trypsin. Why not inject tyrosin and obtain an anti-tyrosinase? Furthermore, since, according to Miss Durham, there is a specific tyrosinase corresponding to each color, one may also obtain specific anti-tyrosinases. If this should turn out to be the case, and there is nothing in it that is contrary to modern tendencies in physiology, then, with a broad variety of anti-tyrosinases before us, we may select the appropriate one, inject it into the individual desirous of changing his skin, and readily produce the result for which he has yearned. The race problem will have been solved. The brunette will no longer resort to notorious drugs for changing the color of her hair, but will find in anti-tyrosinase a scientific aid to her vanity.

THE LENGTH OF THE DENTAL CURRICULUM.

To all persons interested in dental education (except the few surviving advocates of a primeval art of "dental plumbing" as such), it is clear that dentistry is rightfully a medical specialty comparable for example to orthopedics or to what medical students universally term "G.-U." Argument in support of this proposition is not necessary. Every sapient individual appreciates, and the more fully every year, that an unwholesome mouth, befouled by carious teeth or rendered inefficient by the relative lack of teeth, is the widely inviting gateway for derangements and disease of the whole organism. This is the substantial basis on which rests the medical science of dentistry. The technic by which the complicated procedures of the dental practice of recent years are carried out is theoretically another matter. In practical fact, however, these aspects are indistinguishable in any notion of dental practice worthy any man's attention for an hour.

The problem which now confronts dental education in America, its home, is in some respects a serious one, for the official tendency is at the present time undoubtedly backward. Already most of the best dental colleges in the country had adopted a four-year course and had arranged an enlightened curriculum on a four-year basis. In most cases the first year's work was nearly or quite identical with that in the medical schools, the seemingly essential subjects, anatomy, chemistry, physiology, histology and the rest. This was working well, the more intelligent of the students appreciating thus much of the fundamental medical education, while their instructors were pleased and gratified to be able to provide them the substantial basis of a liberal knowledge not only of the mouth but of the whole organism which the mouth only serves. As was to be expected, the attendance at the larger schools showed conclusively that this advance in the dental profession was appreciated by those also, mostly dentists, who advise the new students what they should require in preparation for their life-work.

But meanwhile, many small schools, especially in the Western States, which found themselves somewhat discredited unless they, too, should adopt the enlarged four-year course, combined and quietly succeeded in passing in the American Association of Dental Faculties a vote dogmatically requiring its members to offer a three-year course. The meeting was held in a Western State last August. This requirement was to the numerous small schools originating it evidently a practical financial necessity, for their students would not pay readily for a four-year course in numbers sufficient to make possible the running of these schools. The result of the vote, however, has been to force nearly all the dental colleges of the country to adopt temporarily at least, and often under avowed protest, the three-year course in addition to the four-year curriculum already in running order.

Here a rather surprising thing appears: Offering both courses, the shorter is found to be by far the more popular! that is in any school it secures the large majority of the students. Why this disappointing fact is real it is not easy to decide. The alternatives presenting are these: Either most candidates for the dental profession look upon it far to narrowly as something more, but not much more, than an artisan's trade and consider that a year saved in hastily acquiring the needful skill is also so much money saved. Or else, in the opinion of most advisers of the student-youth, three years is actually long enough time for the learning of what the average dentist needs to know. Either supposition seems unfortunate to the medical mind aware of the complexities and of the intricate inter-relations of the human organism, certain, too, that the widest and the deepest knowledge in the long run of a dentist's practice is the most productive to him, is therefore cheapest in monetary and temporal values. It seems unlikely that a majority of experienced dentists would avow or admit the latter of these two alternatives. The problem then for the faculties of our dental colleges is how to correct the former supposition in the minds of those who are to send boys into the dental profession, for to most faculties it is obvious that four years is little enough in which to give a dentist the theory and practice he actually needs to become a *doctor* of dental medicine or surgery. In medicine at large the tendency distinctly is toward a lengthening of the course beyond four years; no one ever hears even a suggestion that the former two years or even three years are sufficient. Is dentistry, then, one of the most important of the branches of medicine, not developing and broadening, not keeping the pace of the times in the learned professions? And if not, why not?

Surely such a fear is baseless and as surely the present backward step in dental education will soon be made up,—and more. In this desirable result the practitioner of medicine as adviser to many a household, may take a part.

ECHOES AND NEWS.

NEW YORK.

Class Election at P. & S.—The fourth year class of the College of Physicians and Surgeons at a recent meeting elected the following officers: President, F. J. Barrett, of New York; Vice-President, R. Ottenberg, of New York; Secretary-Treasurer, R. M. Brown, of Missouri; Class Poets, J. Victor Haberman and J. C. Mabey, of New York.

New German Hospital Dispensary.—The German Hospital has sold its dispensary at One Hundred and Thirty-seventh Street and Second Avenue and will build a new one on the site near the hospital building at Park Avenue and Seventy-sixth Street. At the last meeting, recently, August Zinsser was elected president of the board of managers to succeed Theodore Killian, resigned. Mr. Killian had served as president for twenty years.

E. R. Squibb & Sons.—This well-known firm announces that their house has been reorganized for broader work and wider service. Mr. Theodore Weicker has been elected its president. Dr. Edward H. Squibb is Chairman of the Board of Directors, and Messrs. Charles F. Squibb, Lowell M. Palmer, Herman G. Weicker, William M. Spackman and Edward M. Shepard are directors. They will be able to meet hereafter the constantly growing demand for Squibb quality in a considerably larger line of products than they have been able to supply hitherto.

Montefiore Home's Report.—According to the annual report, recently received, of the Montefiore Home for Chronic Invalids and Consumptives the home has signalized the close of the first decade of its existence by obtaining 1,040 new contributors to its support. But though there are now more than 6,000 contributors, the total income of the home is only $100,000, as compared with $130,000, the annual expenditures. Altogether, the city institution and the sanitarium at Bedford Station have cared for 889 patients. Of this number all but 32 are free patients. The pressure of admission has throughout been very great, and there remained on the waiting list at the end of the year 65 persons, who had been admitted, but for whom room could not immediately be found; 1,266 applications were made for admission during the year, of which but 487 could be favorably acted upon. These constituted mostly urgent cases, to which class in every instance preference is being given by the executive committee. The care that has to be taken in making admissions, so that these shall become limited to applicants entirely deserving of the benefits of the institution is very great, and justice to this can only be done through much labor and through personal investigation on the part of the special committee charged with this duty. The institution has also given outdoor treatment, including medicated baths and therapeutic applications to a considerable number, who come from their own homes to the institution during the day. Including expenses of every nature, excepting only permanent additions to property. The average per capita cost has been $283.98, as compared with $302.76 during the preceding year, this covering both the city and country departments. Food account at the city institutions has shown an average of 18.84 cents per diem.

The Social Evil.—The American Society for Sanitary and Moral Prophylaxis was organized last week at a meeting of thirty well-known physicians, clergymen and men of public spirit at the New York Academy of Medicine, No. 17 West Forty-third Street. In genuine sincerity it is announced that the society pro-

poses to treat the social evil just as the community at present treats cholera, diphtheria or any other contagious diseases, which by its very presence menaces the health of large numbers. Dr. James Smith presided. Dr. Prince A. Morrow declared that the treatment of the social evil, as it is handled in this city, is nothing short of a crime. He denounced the interference of well-meaning reformers and faddists, who have dispersed this evil and by means of Raines law hotels and other institutions of the sort caused it to spread its blight all over the community. He declared it ought to be handled by the Health Department, just as they handle infectious and contagious diseases, and to treat it in any other way is a dangerous crime. Dr. Morrow wants to have literature distributed in colleges and schools where young men may get some idea of the extent of the peril to which many submit themselves. He suggested circulars and pamphlets and articles by competent authority in medical and lay journals. He expressed the belief that there is hardly a public woman in this city in normal health. Dr. Morrow's sentiments were accepted and indorsed without reserve by Prof. Felix Adler and Prof. Seligman, of Columbia, both of whom were present and made addresses. Dr. Ludwig Weiss and Edward T. Devine, of the Charities Organization Society, also discussed the subject. Bishop Potter and Dr. Lyman Abbott sent letters pledging their support to the society. Dr. Morrow said that $10,000 is practically pledged to start the work. Dr. Smith was authorized to draw up a constitution and by-laws, and at the next meeting officers will be chosen.

Dr. Farrand's Appointment.—Apropos of Prof. Livingston Farrand's appointment as secretary for the National Tuberculosis Movement, *Charities* writes: "Signal evidence of the draft which the greater social movements of the day are making upon the largest resources of the universities, is the announcement that Dr. Livingston Farrand, professor of anthropology at the Columbia University, has been appointed secretary of the National Association for the Study and Prevention of Tuberculosis. Within the year Dr. Samuel McCune Lindsley, professor of sociology at the University of Pennsylvania, has been named as secretary of the National Child Labor Committee. Both have offices in the United Charities Building, 105 East Twenty-second Street, New York. Of underlying significance is the fact that the tuberculosis association, which was inaugurated at a session of the American Medical Association, should enter upon a work which will grapple with the social, even more especially than the medical, problems of preventable disease, under the executive head of a man whose professional training and striking accomplishment have been in the field of natural science. Professor Farrand enters upon this new field, however, from one which could in no sense be called purely academic in its interests. His father was one of the founders of the Bureau of Charities in Newark, and following his own graduation from Princeton, he took a medical degree at the College of Physicians and Surgeons in New York, continuing thereafter an interest in both medical and humanitarian matters. He is a member of the Committee on Social Investigation of Greenwith House, New York, of which Professor Seligman is the chairman. It is in the field of psychology, ethnology and anthropology that Dr. Farrand has attained national reputation. Following studies at Cambridge and then at the German universities, he became a member of the faculty of Columbia University in 1893, and his new work will admit of his continuing in the chair of anthropology and the completing of certain researches now under way. Since

1896 Professor Farrand has been secretary of the American Psychological Association. He is recording secretary of the American Ethnological Society, member and president 1903) of the American Folklore Society, member of the American Society of Naturalists, the American Association for the Advancement of Science and the Washington Academy of Science, and fellow of the American Anthropological Association and the New York Academy of Science. His work as assistant curator of ethnology at the American Museum of Natural History has been notable. He was associated with Professor Boas in practically inaugurating that great series of expeditions among the Indians of the northwestern America and Eastern Asia, which will preserve lasting evidence of the life of the earliest Americans. Professor Farrand has taken part is no less than five expeditions, including the first Jesup North Pacific Expedition organized in 1897, and the Villard expedition among the Indian tribes of Washington, Idaho and Oregon. The art, social organization, religion and mythology of these people have been the subjects which have exacted the largest share of his time in working up the results of the undertakings. As a scientific investigator Professor Farrand has a reputation for uncompromising thoroughness and accuracy. In the words of a fellow scientist, " he unites executive ability, resource, and nerve"—all of them faculties upon which serious demand will be made by the large responsibility facing an anti-tuberculosis movement national in scope.

PHILADELPHIA.

Pottstown Hospital.—A new surgical ward is to be built to this hospital at a cost of $10,000. The sum named is to be taken out of the $25,000 appropriation expected.

Anti-Vaccinationists Active.—The Philadelphia Branch of the Antivaccination Society sent a delegation to Harrisburg to protest against the bill introduced by Representative Shearn, of Philadelphia. The bill in question makes vaccination compulsory in all first-class cities.

Orthopedic Graduates.—The Philadelphia Orthopedic Institute and School of Mechano-Therapy, 1566 Green Street, Philadelphia, has issued diplomas to thirty-four students in the scientific application of medical massage, Swedish movements and medical and orthopedic gymnastics; the same institution has issued diplomas to twenty-two students in electrotherapeutics.

Smallpox to be Curtailed.—The State Board of Health has ordered the officials of the town of Portage to obtain a pest house. If this order is not carried out the Board of Health threatens to quarantine the entire town and will call out the militia to enforce the order. All dogs running at large are ordered to be shot, for it is thought that they may be instrumental in spreading the disease.

Quarantine Raised.—The latter part of last week found the students at Gettysburg College a happy lot, for Dr. Welch of Philadelphia came to their rescue and pronounced the case which held them under quarantine chickenpox. When notified of their relief the students bombarded the wooden houses erected to shelter the guards. So intense was the fire of the students that the besieged had to find shelter behind trees.

Ether Ignites During Operation.—During an operation of tracheotomy it was found that the patient needed more anesthetic, and since the trachea had already been opened the ether had to be administered through the wound. Accordingly oxygen was passed through a bottle of ether and then given to the patient through the trachea. The etherized oxygen soon reached the gas jet burning above the operating table and ignited. Three of the assistants were burned, one badly, while the operator and the unconscious patient escaped. The accident occurred at the Samaritan Hospital.

Meeting of the Therapeutic Society.—The sixth annual meeting of the American Therapeutic Society will be held in this city on May 4, 5 and 6, 1905. The following men will read papers: Dr. Torald Solmann, of Cleveland, O.; Dr. Frederick Peterson, Dr. William J. Morton, Dr. Thomas E. Satterthwaite, Dr. Robert T. Morris, Dr. George B. Fowler, Dr. Wm. H. Porter, Dr. John B. White, Dr. Charles H. Knight and Dr. Carl Beck, of New York; Dr. Howard van Rensselaer, of Albany, N. Y.; Dr. George Butler, of Chicago; Dr. Howard H. Baker, Dr. Noble P. Barnes, Dr. H. W. Wiley, of Washington; Dr. S. Solis-Cohen, Dr. H. C. Wood, Dr. James M. Anders, and Dr. DeForest Willard, of Philadelphia. Dr. John V. Shoemaker is chairman on committee of arrangements. Headquarters will be at the Bellevue-Stratford.

Phipps Institute Report.—According to the first annual report of this institution 2,039 cases were treated. 1,130 were natives, 769 were foreigners and in 140 the nationality was not given. Of the whole number 6.5 per cent. were negroes. There was improvement in 537 cases, no improvement in 583, death occurred in 153, the results of the remaining cases are not recorded. In 656 cases the disease was present less than two years, in 485 from two to five years, in 171 from five to ten years, and in 148 not longer than ten years. Three hundred and sixty-five houseworkers and 101 laborers were affected with the disease. The longest stay of any patient in the hospital was 286 days. Although this was an advanced case the patient improved rapidly. The greatest gain in weight recorded in the dispensary service was 39¼ pounds.

A New Sanitarium for Consumptives.—Recently a charter has been obtained from Harrisburg incorporating the Reading Sanitarium for the Treatment of Tuberculosis. As a result of the activity of the Reading Medical Society many of the influential citizens of the place have been interested and they will personally and financially give aid to the project. The hospital will be established in one of the hills about Reading, but in the meantime a few beds will be isolated in the Reading Hospital until the special building is erected. The names of the directors under whose supervision the sanitarium will be erected are as follows: S. E. Ancona, the Rev. Robert Marshall Blachburn, the Rev. B. F. Callen, Dr. Israel Cleaver, Wm. W. Essick, Dr. F. W. Frankhauser, Dr. James R. Gerhard, Dr. Irvin H. Hartman, George M. Jones, Dr. J. W. Kauffman, Dr. Samuel L. Kutz, Wm. H. Luden, M. B. McKnight. John D. Mishler, Dr. John B. Raser, Dr. Howard S. Reeser, Dr. C. H. Shearer, Wm. D. Smith, P. R. Stetson, Dr. L. L. Thompson and O. M. Weand.

Wills' Hospital.—The first regular meeting of the Association of Clinical Assistants of Wills' Hospital was held at the hospital January 18, 1905. Dr. J. Hiland Dewey in the Chair. Dr. Stanley S. Smith read a report of a most interesting case of gumma of the iris and ciliary body occurring in the clinic of Dr. Charles A. Oliver. The case presented all the characteristic symptoms of the condition, and was fast becoming well. Dr. Smith stated that it was very instructive to note the secondary rapid diminution of vision produced by a haze in the media which had been probably caused by a deposition of the gummy infiltrates into the chambers of the eye. In the discussion, Dr. John T. Krall commented upon the comparative painlessness of specific cyclitis and the character of the infiltration into the aqueous and vitreous which was chiefly composed of round cell exudates. In support of the belief of others that gummata of the ciliary body usually occur on the upper border of the cornea, he had seen but one in which the swelling was situated to the lower side. The various methods of administering mercury were informally discussed, the consensus of opinion being in favor of the use of mercurial ointment by inunctions. Dr. Josephine W. Hildrup read a paper upon ten cases of interstitial keratitis, nine of which had been studied in the clinic of Dr. Oliver, and the remaining one in her own clinic at the Women's Hospital. The ages of the cases varied from six years to fifty-eight years. The dyscrasia had been very carefully studied in all. Females had been preponderant in the series. With but one or two exceptions, all of the cases had passed on to resolution. The discussion, which was quite informal, embraced the forms of treatment which were the mot prevalent among the surgeons in the Institution. Dr. James A. Kearney stated that he had seen much good from the use of inunctions of protiodide of mercury. Dr. Dewey spoke favorably of the use of dionin, claiming · that it had hastened resolution in a number of cases which he had seen. He had not had much experience with subconjunctival injections and had seen some unfortunate results, such as conjunctival ulceration, giving rise to disfigurement from their use. Dr. Kearney exhibited a case in which the right eye was being treated by the ordinary routine methods, supplementing these subconjunctival injections of common salt solution in the left eye; the latter organ (although the first involved) seeming to grow well much more rapidly than its fellow. Dr. Krall stated that he had learned to share the opinion of· others that if injections were made under the conjunctiva, their effects would be to produce a number of adhesions between the bulbar conjunctiva and Tenon's capsule; and stated that even though the injections were made into the capsule, their good results were but transitory as adhesions were sure to occur. In other words, he, with many other authorities, believed that such injections did more harm than good. Dr. Kearney presented a case of double pterygium from Dr. William Zentmeyer's clinic, in which one eye had been operated on by the von Arlt method and the other by the McReynolds'. He exhibited a case of entropion of the upper lid, taken from the same clinic, in which a Hotz operation had been performed with little or no improvement, followed ˌby a Jaesche-Arlt operation, which afforded a very satisfactory result. He also showed a case of entropion from the clinic of Dr. Frank Fisher in which the cilia had been transplanted and the tarsus removed, giving most excellent results. In the discussion, Dr. Krall was of the opinion that the McReynolds' operation had no advantage over the von Arlt. He believed that every case should be treated on its own merits, one method of operation not being applicable to all. Drs. Dewey, Milton A. Robinson, and Smith cited several cases in which different plans of treatment had been most successfully applied.

Philadelphia County Medical Society.—This meeting, which was held February 8, 1905, consisted of· a Symposium on Gastric Ulcer. Dr. Joseph McFarland discussed the etiology and pathology. He first considered the morbid anatomy, the location of the ulcer and discusses at length the theories advanced as possible causes of the condition but suggests nothing new.

He called attention to the experiments which have been performed to induce the lesions, some of which were successful. The serum of bacterial origin which when introduced into the stomachs of guinea-pigs produced ulcers, was also mentioned. He also spoke of the course of the disease and the complications. The next paper was read by Dr. A. P. Francine on the "Incidence in Philadelphia." He said that the disease is more common in the Northeast than in the South, except San Francisco. If the cases are 'chronic they are so from the start; the acute, he said, leave no scars and are often overlooked. The ulcers associated with tuberculosis and with nephritis are usually multiple. He believes more attention should be paid to the relation between nephritis and the stomach. In the 3,763 autopsies in Philadelphia, gastric ulcer was found in 51 of the cases, or 1.35 per cent. of the cases that came to autopsy. Dr. Campbell P. Howard, of Baltimore, by invitation, read a paper on "Symptomatology and Diagnosis." The symptoms are very obscure and misleading. The acute, he said, may be associated with other lesions. In 75 per cent. of the cases hemorrhage was the first symptom and perforation in three per cent. Of the Baltimore statistics 9 patients lost 40 pounds or over. In the next paper Dr. F. P. Henry discussed the "Medical Treatment." He informed the Society that gastric ulcer is a medical disease, and only when the case fails to improve after four or five weeks' of treatment should it go into the hands of the surgeon. In 75 per cent. of the cases medical treatment is successful. In speaking of the "Surgical Treatment" Dr. W. L. Rodman said that gastro-enterostomy and Finney's operation are the ones 'most favored. He is inclined to do incision when an indurated tumor is present arond the ulcer. He spoke of pylorectomy, the mortality of which, he said, is not much greater than that of gastro-enterostomy. Excision of the ulcer-bearing area in the majority of cases is not followed by a recurrence. In opening the discussion Dr. Alfred Stengel said it was absurd to say that 60 per cent. of all the cases of carcinomata of the stomach arose from the site of an old ulcer. He finds atropine a very useful drug in the treatment of the disease.

Pathological Society.—The meeting of this society was held February 9, 1905, with vice-president Ravenel in the chair. Dr. Coplin exhibited the specimens of three cases of hemorrhagic pancreatitis. The specimens of his first case were from a child with a syphilitic history; the pancreas in addition to the acute lesion show a sclerosis. The bile and pancreatic ducts were patulous. There were multiple hemorrhages in all the other organs. The child was jaundiced. Dr. A. O. J. Kelly exhibited a specimen showing acute hemorrhagic pancreatitis. Dr. J. H. Musser exhibited one specimen showing a carcinoma of the head of the pancreas and an interstitial pancreatitis; a second one showing a duodenal ulcer associated with cirrhosis of the liver; a third showing ulcerative endocarditis, and a fourth showing carcinoma of the stomach and peritonitis. Dr. John Funke read a paper entitled "Syphilis of the Liver—Sclero-Gummatous Type." He called the attention of the society to the fact that at postmortem he made the diagnosis of miliary tuberculosis of the liver, but that microscopic examination proved he had to deal with a sclero-gummatous lesion of the organ. He pointed out that the nodules which were mistaken for tubercles were really spherical masses of fibrous tisue. He laid stress upon the fact that the increase of intralobular fibrous tissue is in all probability an overgrowth of the already existing reticulum produced by the irritation of the syphilitic poison brought to the liver by the blood current. He tried to impress upon the society that the sclerosis did not necessarily originate at the periphery and extend into the lobules between the liver cells. In the sections several miliary gummata were found, which he believed were of recent origin, probably a result of a second infection. Dr. H. R. M. Landis read a paper entitled "Tuberculosis of the Liver." He pointed out that tuberculosis of the liver may occur as four types. The acute miliary; chronic caseous; the tubercular cirrhosis; that form involving the bile ducts. Of the fifty post mortems at the Phipps Institute in only two were microscopic evidence of the lesion, while in the 20 cases examined microscopically all but two showed tubercles. Dr. D. J. McCarthy exhibited as card specimens two cases of internal hydrocephalus due to a cerebellar tumor pressing upon the aqueduct of Sylvius. In the second case during an operation nearly one half of the cerebellum was removed which gave relief to the patient for a short period only. The symptoms recurred and then several operations were resorted to, during which so much of the cerebellum was removed that easy access to the brain stem was obtained. Dr. John Funke exhibited a card specimen showing ulcerative endocarditis not only involving the mitral leaflets but also involving the posterior wall of the left auricle.

CHICAGO.

St. Francis' Hospital.—During the year 1904 there were treated 212 cases at this institution in Evanston, 23 of which were cases of appendicitis.

Cocaine Sold as Medicine.—Legislation for the prohibition of the sale of medicines which contain too great a percentage of cocaine was recently proposed by Alderman Ryan at a meeting of a subcommittee of the License Committee of the City Council. Alderman Ryan declared that many of these medicines are merely a pretense for the sale of cocaine, and mentioned an article sold as a remedy for catarrh which is used almost exclusively by those addicted to the cocaine habit.

Modifications in Bill for State Sanatorium.—Honorable Edward J. Glacking, who is the father of a bill for the establishment of a State sanatorium for consumptives, recently had a conference with the Secretary of the State Board of Health, Dr. James A. Egan, during which changes were suggested in the bill, although its main provisions remain unchanged. The district and county medical societies of the State will be invited to cooperate in the movement, and will be asked to interest the representatives from their respective districts in this bill.

Removal of Tonsils in Schoolgirls.—Apropos of a recent cable dispatch from London, England, announcing Dr. Alice Neville Vowe Johnson as an advocate of the removal of tonsils of every one of the schoolgirls of that parish (Lambeth), the bulletin of the Health Department has this to say: "Dr. Johnson is a courageous woman and a wise physician. She knows, as every intelligent doctor knows, that the tonsil not only has no recognized useful function, but that it is the cause of more disease and death than the appendix itself. It is the nursery and hothouse for the propagation of every form of evil microbe, from that which causes ordinary 'quinsy sore throat' to the malignant septic organisms of diphtheria, pneumonia, tuberculosis, gangrene of the lungs, inflammation of the heart membranes and other fatal maladies. Even in conditions of health the tonsillar crypts are often filled with evil-smelling contents, consisting of disintegrating epithe-

lial cells, fibrinous débris, and various septic organisms, among which staphylococci, streptococci, pneumococci and leptothrix are abundant. If this disgusting category be not enough to secure the deep damnation and the taking off of every tonsil in the young throat, it may be added that it is the commonest cause of mouth-breathing, defective speech and hearing, and mental dullness among children. Honor to Dr. Johnson, of Lambeth. *A bas la tonsille.*"

CANADA.

Public Health in British Columbia.—An entire revision of the health regulations of the province of British Columbia will likely be made shortly. At present the health matters of the Pacific province are looked after by an official who consults with the Government of the province on all matters pertaining to the health thereof. It is proposed now to form and constitute a Board of Health composed of medical men, same as in some of the older provinces, and toward this end there has recently been held in Vancouver a conference of the Provincial Health Officer and representatives of the profession and representatives from the Dominion Health departments. The Government also proposes to hold a conference with the health officers of the leading five cities of British Columbia to see what is best to be done to put the health affairs of the province on the best possible footing.

The Medical Faculty of McGill will Seek Fuller Union with the University.—There was held last week a meeting of the corporation of McGill University, when a resolution was presented from the Medical Faculty to the effect that in the opinion of the Medical Faculty, and in the welfare and interests of medical education in Montreal, it would be well for the Medical Faculty to have full union with the University. The Committee from the Medical Faculty which conveyed this resolution to the Board of Governors consisting of Dean Roddick and Drs. Shepherd, Gardner, Ruttan, Adami and Armstrong. The deputation received a warm welcome from the Board of Governors, and expressed themselves with full satisfaction at the step the Medical Faculty desired to take. Another meeting will be held, at which the Special Committee will meet the Board of Governors to arrange for the desired end.

Reminiscences of the Toronto Hospital.—Appointments to the house staff of the Toronto General Hospital are only eligible to those who have been licensed to practise in the province of Ontario. The present medical superintendent, Dr. Charles O'Reilly, was appointed to office in 1876, and ever since he has ably filled his duties. During the time he has been associated with the hospital the maternity department has seen 4,000 births, and there have passed through his hands 220 house surgeons, many of whom are associated in the large hospitals and medical colleges of the United States and Great Britain. Among others who have been house surgeons at the Toronto General Hospital are Drs. L. F. Barker, Thomas Cullen, Thomas Futcher and Thomas McCrae, Baltimore, and Dr. Don Armour, London, England. Many prominent practitioners in Toronto have also been house surgeons at the General. The number of patients admitted annually to the wards have increased from 972 in 1876 to 3,811 in 1904.

Reminiscences of the Montreal General Hospital.—The Montreal General Hospital was opened for patients in 1822, and in the following year a document was sent to the Governor-in-Chief setting forth the need of a medical school, and showing the excellent facilities the hospital afforded for clinical training. Almost immediately the Montreal Medical Institute sprang into existence, its first teaching staff being composed of the doctors attending on the hospital. Six years later it became a part of McGill University. In 1854, Dr. Robert Craik, formerly Dean of the Medical Faculty of McGill University, was a house surgeon in the institution, when Montreal experienced its historic epidemic of Asiatic cholera The very first case brought into the hospital from a German emigrant ship scared away the six nurses and all the orderlies, and it fell to Dr. Craik and his only assistant, Dr. Chas. Ault, to admit these patients. From thirty to forty cases of cholera were always at the hospital that summer. Not a single case of infection occured in the hospital during the epidemic, and the two doctors had to depend upon convalescents for help in nursing. The training school for nurses was established at the Montreal General Hospital fourteen years ago, and since that time 241 nurses have been graduated. There are now 75 nurses in the hospital, including nurses-in-training and the graduates. In the jubilee year of the late Queen Victoria, a spacious home was erected for the nurses, and there is one room furnished by the Canadian Nurses' Association in memory of the late Dr. Kirkpatrick, a warm friend of the training school. Dr. F. G. Finley is the secretary of the medical staff.

GENERAL.

The Georgia Practician.—This new medical journal makes its initial bow this past week, and we offer it our hearty well wishes for a prosperous and useful career.

Infection from Books.—As bearing on the question frequently raised by timid people, as to whether our public libraries may not be factors in the spread of contagious diseases, *Public Libraries* for February prints the following letters, received from the librarians of the city libraries of Baltimore and Cleveland, respectively: " This library has been in existence now for about nineteen years, and during that time has had in its employ about 175 clerks of all ages, and among these clerks there has not been a case of any contagious disease, which I think is very good proof that there is very little danger. For the past eighteen years there has not been a single case of contagious disease of any kind in any of the public departments of the main library or its branches. As there are now more than 75 persons employed in these departments, and as each book is handled by not less than three people between the time of its return and re-issue, it seems probable that if contagion were readily carried by the books, the library employees would be affected."

New Hospital in Montclair.—Some years ago a woman walking in one of the streets of Montclair, N. J., saw a runaway team knock down a little girl. Hastening to her assistance, she saw it was a case where expert treatment would be needed, and that the child ought to be taken to a hospital. She found that there was none nearer than another town, many miles away—a long and painful ride for the little one, but which had to be endured. Going to her friends and acquaintances, this woman solicited subscriptions until she had enough to purchase a little plot of ground and erect a small one-story building of two or three rooms. This was the beginning of the Mountainside Hospital. As years went by, ground was added until it became a handsome property, and some serviceable, though far from ideal, buildings erected. About three years ago, however, the public interest in the hospital was so strong that the women and doctors connected with it determined to

erect a new, modern hospital building, especially for surgical treatment. The work was intrusted to Cady, Bergh & See, architects, of New York City, and it was opened last week. Its first floor is devoted to dispensary work, having a spacious waiting rom and examination rooms adjacent, and an accident ward opening directly on the ambulance way. There is also on this floor a museum furnished with a collection of models made by the late Dr. Ayers and given by his sons. The main floor of the building contains the offices of the managers, the physicians, the two wards for male and female patients, and the group of rooms embracing the operating pavilion and its associated rooms, the sterilizing, etherizing, washroom, and the surgeons' dressing room. The upper floor has eleven private rooms, beautifully furnished as memorials; also diet kitchen, linen rooms, etc. It is said that there is not a room or passage in which the sun does not shine at some time in the day. The surgical fittings and implements of the most modern type throughout are the gift of Dr. James Spencer Brown, one of the visiting surgeons. In the main corridor are placed tablets in memory of Dr. Pinkham, who made the first contribution to the Mountainside Hospital, and Dr. Love, whose influence greatly contributed to the growth of the enterprise.

Boston Societies.—Boston Medical Library Meetings, in conjunction with the Suffolk District Branch of the Massachusetts Medical Society. The last meeting was held February 11, at the library. The paper of the evening was by Prof. Russell H. Chittenden. of Yale University, on the subject, " Physiological Economy of Nutrition." Dr. George W. Gay was in the chair. Dr. W. T. Porter, of the Harvard Medical School introduced Prof. Chittenden. The reader first mentioned the various dietary experiments which had been held all over the world, and gave statistics based on these experiments of the average bodily need of the average workingman or laborer. The lowest of these figures, those of Germany, which are 118 gr. of nitrogenous food, 56 of fat and 500 of carbohydrates or twenty-four hours, have until recently been accepted as the minimum rate at which an ordinary man could live and yet do this work and preserve his nitrogenous equilibrium. Dr. Chittenden claimed that while these figures show on what the men on whom the experiments were performed actually lived, they do not really represent the needs of the body. The ideal diet, he says, is the smallest possible amount of nitrogenous food on which the body-weight and strength can be maintained. The dangers of an excess of the products of proteid katabolism in the body are coming to be realized more and more. and the less that is eaten above the actual required amount the better. Dr. Chittenden's experiments covered a period of from seven to eight months, and were done on three classes of people: (1) A group of five professors who took but very little physical exercise; (2) a group of U. S. army hospital corps assistants, men whose physical work was moderate, and who each day exercised in a gymnasium; (3) a group of university athletes, men in constant training and engaged all the time in a variety of athletic sports. These men gradually reduced their proteid ingesta from an average of 120 to 130 grams to about 40 to 30 grams; their nitrogen from 16 to 22 grams to 5 to 8 grams. The fats and carbohydrates were not limited. They lived under this régime for seven to eight months, and practically all, after an initial loss of weight due to the first cutting down, maintained their weight, and, furthermore, their strength, ability to work and to resist disease, and kept up their nitrogenous equilibrium— this on a diet of one-third of what had hitherto been considered the minimum—118 grams of proteids per twenty-four hours.

Prof. Lafayette B. Mendel, of Yale University, commented on these experiments from the point of view of one who at first thought them a dangerous procedure, but who had taken part in them and had been convinced of their value. He furthermore spoke of the ignorance on the part of the medical profession in general in regard to the weight and amount in grams or calories of the ordinary food consumed by patients.

Dr. Otto Folen, of the McLean Hospital at Waverley, described some experiments he had been performing on himself and a few others, in which a diet practically without nitrogenous food was taken in periods of from ten to fourteen days, and compared his results with those of Prof. Chittenden.

OBITUARY.

Dr. THOMAS H. SHERWOOD, a veteran of the Civil War, and for many years a medical examiner in the pension bureau at Washington, died at his home in that city on Thursday. He was a native of Delaware, was graduated in medicine at Philadelphia, and in 1851 was assistant surgeon of the Third Pennsylvania Cavalry. He also served as surgeon of the Twenty-seventh Pennsylvania Infantry, and was mustered out in 1865 with the brevet rank of captain for faithful and meritorious service during the war.

Dr. FRANK COWAN died February 12, at his home in Greensburgh, Pa., after an illness of several months. Dr. Cowan was born in Greensburgh, Pa., in December, 1844. He was the son of Edgar C. Cowan, who was a United States Senator, and after taking his medical degree became Secretary of the Senate Committee on Patents. Afterward he studied law, and in 1865 he was admitted to the bar. From that year until 1869 he was one of President Johnson's secretaries. Then he practised medicine, and then resumed the practice of the law.

Dr. PETER ROOSEVELT JOHNSON died at his home at Sag Harbor, L. I., last week, in his seventy-seventh year. He had not practised medicine for several years, but had interested himself in the study of Oriental religions. He owned large business property in Brooklyn, being a member of the corporation known as the "Johnson Estate." Dr. Johnson was a graduate of Columbia and of the College of Physicians and Surgeons in this city. He was one of a party of young adventurers who, in 1849, purchased a brig and sailed around Cape Horn to California in search of gold. The brig was wrecked and the party was stranded at Rio Janeiro for a long time.

CORRESPONDENCE.

OUR LONDON LETTER.

(From our Special Correspondent.)

LONDON, February 4.

A ROYAL PRINCESS OPERATED ON FOR APPENDICITIS—SIR FREDERICK TREVES ON PROFESSIONAL · SUCCESS—TWO TYPES OF PHYSICIAN—HYGIENIC MATRIMONY—VITAL STATISTICS OF LONDON—THE PREVENTION OF LIVE BURIAL—CREMATION IN GREAT BRITAIN—DEATH OF A NONAGENARIAN DOCTOR.

SIR ·FREDERICK TREVES's enemies—if he has any—will be driven to think that the stars in their courses fight for him. As if fate had not been sufficiently kind to him in giving him the sacrosanct person of His Most Gracious Majesty to flesh his knife upon, it has now delivered the King's daughter into his surgical hands.

Appendicitis seems to have a special predilection for our royal family, for besides the monarch himself and the Princess Victoria, his niece, another Princess Victoria (of Schleswig-Holstein) had to undergo an operation not long ago. The Princess Victoria of England is in her thirty-seventh year, and the fact that she is unmarried has led to a general belief that she suffers from some constitutional delicacy. However, this may be, her health has been unsatisfactory for a considerable time past, making sea voyages and periods of rest and seclusion at various places necessary. The appendiceal crisis seems to have been precipitated by an attack of influenza in the early part of January. At present all the omens are said to be propitious, and the distinguished surgeon will be able to add another successful case to his long list. It is related that at the Congress of Vienna, when Lord Castlereagh appeared in a black coat amid the crowd of diplomats arrayed in gorgeous uniforms and blazing with decorations, Talleyrand said, *Ma foi, milord, c'est très distingué!* Treves would be still more *distingué* if he presented himself at Court wearing a ribbon made of aristocratic appendices like an Indian brave with his belt of scalps. Many of his professional brethren doubtless envy him the glory shed upon his head by the sunshine of royal favor, but there is nothing else to excite their jealousy. His fame can scarcely be greater than it is, but his retirement makes it impossible for him to take fees. His services to the King brought him more honor than profit; for his attendance on the Princess he will get nothing except perhaps an additional decoration. It is believed by many that he will be made a peer, and probably he could have a peerage or anything else he wished—except money—for the asking. It may be wondered at that exalted persons should think it no indignity to accept without payment professional services, which given gratuitously to ordinary mortals would stamp upon them the brand of pauperism. Royalty, however, finds it convenient to believe that the mere honor of rendering it service is in itself sufficient reward.

The mention of Treves's name recalls the fact that he has been confiding to the Rev. R. J. Campbell, a Nonconformist preacher of what Byron might have called "forty-parson power," and editor of a periodical called *The Young Man*, his views on success in practice. He says that as a student he was "signally undistinguished." He suffered a good deal by the advice tendered to him to mend his ways. One of the most encouraging counsellors at the commencement of his career was a consulting surgeon of the London Hospital where he was a student. Referring to a surgeon then enjoying great fame the Mentor said: "I don't see why you should not do as well as he has done, because at your age he was a perfect fool." This naturally made Treves extremely happy. Speaking of the complaint often made by unsuccessful men that they have no luck, Treves said that as far as the medical profession was concerned, there was no such thing as luck. "Luck meant that a man was ready for a certain chance when it came along." Again, some students complained that they had no genius. As to this, Treves says that "genius is some sort of neurosis—an uncalculated nervous disease." He added that the few men of genius he had met were exceedingly impossible persons. Such people are, he thinks, entirely out of place in the medical profession, where even cleverness is not to be encouraged. "Indeed, of all desperately dangerous persons, the brilliant surgeon is the most lamentable. Cleverness finds its proper place not in the operating theatre but in the Egyptian Hall," the home of conjuring and legerdemain. In regard to lack of influence Treves declares that "no person succeeds better than the man who stands entirely upon his own feet, depending on no one to assist his progress." He goes on to say: "The absence of means is another ground of lamentation; but the men who have succeeded most conspicuously are the men who started on nothing. The things that made for progress are difficult to define. Hard work comes first. Then there must be close observation. Of course, too, a man must know his profession. As Sir William Jenner put it, 'He must be in a position to be dogmatic.' There are two classes of dogmatic persons—those who knew everything and those who knew nothing of a subject. Again, a man must be kind. It is not kind to blurt out to a lady the news that she has a malignant disease. The last quality to a successful medical man is honesty, and it cannot too emphatically be laid stress upon. The late Sir Andrew Clark was a man who had no knowledge of dulness, and an infinite capacity for work. He was a particularly shrewd observer, amusing in his dogmatism, a man than whom none had a kinder heart, and almost pedantically honest. Sir Andrew started without money, friends, or influence, and he rose to the highest position in his profession." Treves's account of himself and his repudiation of luck as a factor of success must be taken with the proverbial grain of salt. His student days were, indeed, it is said, marked by a certain amount of Bob-Sawyerism; but he was a hard worker from the first, and his rise was exceptionally rapid owing partly to his own merits, but largely to that "luck" which he now somewhat ungratefuly scorns. Had it been his fate to serve, as John Abernethy and other distinguished men had to do, for a quarter of a century in a subordinate position he would assuredly not have been able to retire from practice at the age of fifty. His way was not blocked by veterans lagging superfluous on the stage. Of course, as Treves points out, a man must be able to take advantage of the chance when it comes to him, or it will profit him nothing. Nevertheless, it is true that many men never come within touch of the tide in the affairs of men which, taken at the flood, leads on to fortune. In expressing contempt for brilliancy, again Treves speaks just a little *pro domo sua*, for his most ardent admirers will not claim for him the possession of that quality. He is not a surgical artist, but a strenuous man who knows what he means to do, and drives straight through all obstacles at the object he has in view.

As Treves mentions William Jenner and Andrew Clark, I may be allowed to tell a story which illustrates an interesting difference of type in great physicians. Jenner was called to see a case which, after careful examination—and he could handle the abdominal organs almost as easily as if they had been on a plate before him—he pronounced to be one of cancer of the liver. Declaring, with the brusqueness of manner characteristic of him, that there was nothing to be done, he took his fee and his departure. The friends then invited Clark to see the patient. He told them that there was certainly a swelling "not of a benignant character," but added that the resources of medicine could do much to mitigate the lot of the sufferer during the few and evil days before him. The patient lived some three months, during which Clark visited him daily. If the patient did not live longer than he otherwise would have done, he doubtless died comfortably, while the physician was all the richer. Treves's statement that Andrew Clark rose without friends or influence is not strictly accurate. He made

little way until the cholera of 1886 brought Mrs. Gladstone to, visit the sick in the London Hospital. She was impressed by Clark's *copia fundi*, which equalled even that of her distinguished husband, of whose health she at once made the struggling physician the keeper. She sang the praises of her Scotch doctor in Society, and Clark soon exchanged a small dingy house in the East End for a palatial establishment in Cavendish Square. The bracketing together of the two men is rather grotesque. Jenner was one of the greatest clinicians and teachers that ever lived, whereas Clark's name, as far as the history of medical science is concerned, may truly be said to have been "writ in water."

The cry about the physical deterioration of the British people, which has been praised by prophets of various kinds, has lately found an echo in the pulpit. The Rev. Dr. Watson, better known to the lovers of the "Kailyard" school of literature as "Ian Maclaren," preaching at Liverpool, insisted that no young man should think of getting married without first being accepted as a first class life by an insurance office of unquestionable standing. Interviewed on the subject, the preacher said he would include women as well as men in the application of the rule. He explained that he did not mean that a delicate person should not marry, because many such people are constitutionally sound. The reason for insisting on a certificate from a good insurance company was that a person gets the benefit of an unprejudiced and independent examination. Dr. Watson expressed a hope that the time would come when the State would not sanction marriage unless both contracting parties could qualify for such a health certificate. His views will doubtless commend themselves to the insurance companies. But it may safely be predicted that the British people will need a very long course of education in the higher social hygiene before they surrender the right of marrying and giving in marriage as they please.

The report of the Public Health Committee of the London County Council for the year 1903, which was issued recently, shows the lowest death rate ever recorded, namely, 15.2 per 1,000, as against 17.2 in 1902, and a 62 years average of 22.3. On the other hand the report also shows the lowest birth-rate recorded since the regular tabulation of these statistics—28.4 per 1,000. How consistently and steadily the birthrate has fallen is shown in the subjoined table:

1861-70	35.4	1895	30.6
1881-90	33.2	1898	29.7
1891	31.9	1902	28.5
Total births, 1903		130,906	
Total deaths		69,737	

Excess of births	61,169

As the struggle of the public health authorities against the specific epidemic diseases first began to assert its supremacy in 1879, it is necessary to seek other causes to account for the declining birth-rate. One cause is to be found in the decline of marriage, the rate for 1903 standing at 17.4 as against 20.3 in the ten years from 1861 to 1870. The reduction in the marriage rate, however, is not in any degree commensurate with the fall in the birthrate, and to the decline in marriages must, therefore, be added as the chief cause of the reduction the growing dislike of motherhood. Even as it is, motherhood does not appear to be very successful for the rate of infant mortality is terribly high. During 1903 the total number of infantile deaths was 16,978, or 130 in every 1,000 births. It is true that this is the lowest rate on record since 1891, when the rate was 153 per 1,000, but when it is noted that it means that forty-six infants die in every twenty-four hours, it is not surprising to learn that the Public Health Committee are giving the matter their "anxious consideration." Looking at the specific causes of mortality, it is to be noted that the figures for consumption, cancer, diarrhœa, and measles are all alarmingly high, though all, except cancer, show a decline as compared with 1902, while smallpox has shown a remarkable falling off. In regard to the milk supply of London, a further attempt is to be made by the Council in the next session of Parliament to obtain greater powers for ensuring purity—"which," the Public Health Committee add, "we think are urgently needed in the interests of the London public."

From time to time some gruesome story of live burial causes a scare in the public mind. Three cases of cataleptic trance, with alleged narrow escapes from too previous interment, have lately been reported, with sensational details, in the newspapers, and the Association for the Prevention of Premature Burial is naturally making the most of them. At the annual meeting of that body, held the other day, Dr. W. R. Hadwen, ·of Gloucester, said the recent case at Accrington should give pause to any skeptic who denied the danger of premature burial. Thousands of death certificates were given without a doctor having seen the body. In 1903 the Home Secretary had to admit that during the previous five years no fewer than 53,000 certificates were given without the cause of death being shown. He proceeded to say that an old woman who was formerly caretaker at the Cholera Hospital in Gloucester had told of the haste made to dispose of the bodies ·of patients who died from cholera. "Sometimes," she said, "we used to hear them kicking after the lid was screwed down, but we never opened it again, because we knew they had got to die anyhow." Hadwen is the doctor who carried out the testamentary injunction of the late Miss Frances Power Cobbe that her throat should be cut after death to "mak' sikker," as Kirkpatrick said to Robert Bruce, when he said he thought he had killed the Red Comyn. He is a leader in the Israel of anti-ism, anti-vaccinist, antivivisectionist, etc., etc. In the eyes of the medical profession he is a nonentity, but he doubtless comforts himself for this lack of appreciation by saying with Falstaff that wisdom calls out in the street and no man regards it. It must, however, be admitted that it is true that doctors often give certificates without seeing the body or taking any particular trouble to verify the fact of death. This evil the association above referred to is endeavoring to remedy. With that object it has drafted a Bill to be submitted to Parliament, which contains the following provisions: (1) No burial shall take place without a medical certificate of death. (2) No certificate shall be given without a personal examination of the body, and the certificate shall state the signs from which death is inferred. (3) The appointment by the Home Office of death verifiers in every district of England and Wales, who shall give their whole time to the duties. (4) The municipal authorities shall have power to establish waiting mortuaries, in which bodies shall remain until putrefactive decomposition sets in. The enforcement of some safeguards of this kind would certainly remove a hideous fear that lurks at the bottom of many people's minds. It is extremely doubtful, however, whether the bill will become law, for the medical profession is disposed to pooh-pooh the whole subject, and the association by which it is promoted consists of the most part of rabid cranks of one kind or another,

who are sure to spoil their case by wild statements like those made by Hadwen.

Probably the fear of live burial makes some people seek post-mortem safety in cremation. That method of disposing of the dead makes steady but somewhat slow progress in this country. There are ten crematories in existence in the following places: London (2), Woking, Manchester, Glasgow, Liverpool, Hull, Birmingham, Leicester and Darlington; and two more will be opened in the course of the present year at Leeds and Bradford. The total number of cremations carried out since 1885, when the first crematory (Woking) was opened, is 4,407. The religious, or rather theological, objection is disappearing, but the requirements of the Cremation Society as to death certificates are much more stringent than those for ordinary burial, and afflicted families therefore have the remains of their defunct members incinerated only when they are compelled to do so.

The recent death of Dr. William Williams Morgan of Newport in Wales, at the age of ninety-six, recalls the fact that in this country, too, soldiers fired on people clamoring for their rights as human beings. At the time of the Chartist riots in 1839, he had not long begun to practise at Newport. Hearing firing from the direction of the principal square of the town, he went thither on an errand of mercy. He found the square empty of all save the dead and wounded, though frightened people were peering round the corners. From the windows of an adjacent hotel the muzzles of the soldiers' muskets protruded. He approached the nearest wounded man, holding up his hand as a signal of peace, but before anything could be done the man died. Dr. Morgan afterward learned that the soldiers were only prevented from firing on him by the town constable, who knew him as a doctor. Another wounded man whom doctor Morgan found professed to have been shot at while going to the post office, but he had a sword down the leg of his trousers. Eleven persons were killed during the riots. Dr. Morgan, who was a pupil of Sir Astley Cooper at Guy's Hospital, became a member of the medical profession in 1835.

SOCIETY PROCEEDINGS.

MEDICAL SOCIETY OF THE STATE OF NEW YORK.

Ninety-ninth Annual Meeting, held at Albany, January 31, February 1 and 2, 1905.

The President, Dr. Hamilton F. Wey, of Elmira, in the Chair.

SECOND DAY—FEBRUARY 1ST (*Continued*).

(Continued from Page 281.)

SYMPOSIUM ON DISEASES OF THE PROSTATE.

Etiology of Prostatic Hypertrophy.—The symposium was opened by Dr. L. Bolton Bangs, of New York, who said that when modern pathology took its rise the enlargement of the prostate that was found to occur in old men, was at first set down as inflammatory. Virchow in his work on tumors said that it was due to chronic inflammation which started in the glandular substance of the prostate. This view did not attract much attention, however. On the contrary for many years the French opinion that a certain amount of enlargement of the prostate was, a usual senile process and that precocious enlargement of the prostate was due to presenility, occupied the attention of the medical world. This has now been practically disproved. Lately has come the opinion once more that the enlargement observed is due to a chronic inflammatory process which usually has been in progress for many years. It is to this latter view that Dr. Bangs gives his adhesion.

Insidious Chronic Inflammation.—Dr. Bangs considers that the process by which the enlargement of the prostate takes place, remains latent for many years, though it would be readily detected if opportunities for observation occurred. This inflammation starts in the prostatic urethra, near the veru montanum. It may be due to many causes, but is practically always the result of excessive irritation of the genito-urinary tract because of overfunction, or some wrong form of function. Ordinary excesses sexual are almost sure to result this way, but such abuses as masturbation or coitus reservatus may produce it. This region is subject to violent engorgement and unless this engorgement is properly relieved by a period of absolute rest, the tendency to low grade chronic inflammation soon develops.

Developmental Relations.— The development of the prostate depends to a great extent on the development of the testis. Its condition in after-life depends to a great extent to the condition of the testis. Hence it is easy to understand how overfunction in one gland is followed by congestion and enlargement in the other. There may be years of prodromal symptoms, that have not been recognized as pointing to an affection of the prostate.

Unphysiological Sexuality.—Dr. Bangs has carefully investigated over 300 cases of the origin of enlargement of the prostate. In over 85 per cent. of the cases, unphysiological sexuality was found in the history. In younger men a state of sexual erethism is developed as the result of abuse which may make the prostate extremely tender on examination. In such cases speedy marriage may produce a cessation of symptoms. It must be remembered, however, that there may be abuses in the marriage state that will keep up the conditions of congestion, and so there will be no abatement of symptoms, especially is this true in regard to the practice of coitus reservatus. The irritation thus set up is only a step to inflammation and is not inflammation itself, but it predisposes the prostatic tissues to be affected by micro-organisms of any kind that may pass in the urethra or may find their way there through the blood stream. To Dr. Bangs it is evident that prostatic hypertrophy is not due to gonorrhea alone, since in certain cases in which there is frank confession of other sexual abuses and without any good reason to deny gonorrhea, no gonorrhea is in the history.

Perineal Prostatectomy.—Dr. George R. Fowler, of Brooklyn, said that the perineal route for the removal of the prostate is the most suitable for the majority of cases of enlarged prostate. Through the suprapubic route, the total removal of a large prostate is possible, but the ejaculatory ducts cannot well be spared. As the present tendency in surgery is more and more toward earlier operations, so as to prevent the serious symptoms that often make the eventual operation dangerous, this question of the preservaion of the sex functions becomes important. More manipulative skill is needed for the perineal route, but it is a more satisfactory operation in many ways. It may be done under general anesthesia, or under spinal anesthesia, and Tinker has done it under intraneural injections into the pudendal nerves.

Technic.—The resection of the prostate is perfectly possible from the perineum and the bleeding in these cases is not as severe or as difficult to control as might be expected. Ordinarily the prostate can be shelled out without any difficulty. If there is bleeding, the wound may be packed, but drainage tubes should be avoided. One secret of success is frequent change of dressing. If a drainage tube has to be employed, then it should be removed not later than forty-eight hours after the operation. Absolutely the most important bit of postoperative technic is to get the patient out of bed as soon as possible. This facilitates the drainage, prevents difficulties from infiltration of urine and by encouraging the patient, greatly shortens convalescence.

Methods in Prostatic Surgery.—Dr. Willy Meyer, of New York, said that no one operation is suitable for all forms of prostatic enlargement. In some cases the perineal route is undoubtedly the best. In cases where there is great enlargement of the prostate, the suprapubic route gives the most satisfaction. It is possible, with care, to preserve the sexual power by either route, since the ejaculatory ducts are not involved in the portion of the prostate that is usually most enlarged. As the operation is done earlier, the question of sex-power preservation becomes more important. In some cases, the knife is absolutely refused. Then the operator should be ready to suggest Bottini's method and employ it if it is permitted. Only if all these methods of treatment are refused, should the patient be introduced to the use of the catheter. This should not be entrusted to the patient, however, unless he is in such a station in life that he can be expected to take the precautions necessary to avoid infection. In a word, physicians should be expected to familiarize themselves with all methods of operation and select the method which is most suitable for the individual patient.

Prostatism Without Prostatic Enlargement.—Dr. Charles A. Chetwood, of New York, said that the train of symptoms usually considered to be connected with enlarged prostate may develop without enlargement of the prostate. There may be urgency and frequency of urination with pain during and after the act and even with some residual urine. This has sometimes been spoken of as due to contracture of the neck of the bladder. The pathological basis of the condition seems to be a fibroid stenosis of the vesival orifice. It is not due, as is sometimes said, to spasm, not to a fold of mucous membrane, but to the deposit of inflammatory exudate. This may or may not be due to gonorrheal origin, though it usually is due to the gonococcus. Enlarged prostate may be present without symptoms unless this contracture of the vesical neck exists. The blocking of the urinary passages may eventually lead to pyelonephritis.

Suprapubic Prostatectomy.—Dr. Howard Lilienthal, of New York, reported 31 cases of removal of the prostate by the suprapubic route without a death. In all of these there has been perfect recovery of function except in two patients. If the patient is uremic, the operation may be done in two stages without any difficulty and with very satisfactory results. With regard to the sexual power, it has been lost in no cases in which the patients were potent before. In many of the cases it has been found to have increased after the operation. Most of Dr. Lilienthal's operations were done on feeble subjects in advanced years. Two of them were suffering from diabetes and one from tabes. In several cases the operation followed a failure of relief of symptoms by the Bottini method. In

Dr. Lilienthal's opinion, this method of surgical removal of the prostate is preferable to all others.

Points in Technic.—For two days before the operation the patient is prepared for it by emptying the bladder with the catheter every three hours day and night. The urine is made antiseptic by salol administered in five-grain doses. Urotropin is given after the operation. The incision is two to two and a half inches long through the abdominal wall and then the bladder is inflated so as to push up the peritoneal fold. The bladder itself is then punctured, the puncture being stretched sufficiently by digital irritation so as to remove any stones that may be present in the bladder and also the prostate itself. The enucleation of the prostrate is usually rather easy, especially when the organ is pushed up by the finger of an assistant in the rectum. Care is taken not to tear the prostatic mucous membrane. If there should be abundant hemorrhage, which is rare, then strips of gauze are placed in the bladder to encourage clotting, but not to pack the viscus. By careful siphonage the patient is kept dry and comfortable. He is out of bed on the second or third day and the siphon may be removed before two weeks. The average length of time in the hospital is 4½ weeks.

Advantages of the Operation.—The advantages of operation through the suprapubic incision are the having the field of operation directly under the eye of the surgeon so that the cause of the obstruction may be observed. There is total absence of shock and this is of decided advantage in weak cases. Where there has been infection of the upper genito-urinary tract, the operation may be performed in two stages. Speed in surgery for the aged is important and this is the quickest method of operation with least loss of blood. Besides impotency rarely supervenes.

Perineal Prostatectomy.—Dr. Hugh H. Young, of Baltimore, detailed the results of two years' experience of removal of the prostate through the perineum. He considers that no one method is adapted to all cases and his experience has not been confined to the perineal route. He first did prostatectomy by the suprapubic method and it seemed ideal. After having three deaths in 30 cases, however, and finding how tedious convalescence was, he looked around for another method. He found that Bottini's method gave wonderful results and the millennium in prostatic surgery seemed to have come. There were some inexplicable failures, however, besides in 85 cases there were six deaths and some of them in subjects that were strong and with regard to whom no good reason for the fatal issue could be found. Then he tried the perineal route.

Technic of Operation.—The skin incision is made in the shape of an inverted V, though this incision is carried no farther than the skin. The prostatic gland is then reached by the ordinary lithotomy incision and as much of it removed as is deemed advisable. In 75 cases thus operated, he has had no deaths and in only two cases is there any residual urine. He is careful as a rule to save that portion of the prostatic gland in which the ejaculatory ducts are contained and by so doing has avoided the epididymitis due to inflammatory closure or infection of the spermatic duct for which Albarran sometimes ties the spermatic duct in the groin. Where the prostatic urethra is preserved, the fistula in the perineum closes rapidly. The advantages of the perineal route are many. The prostate is nearest to the surface here and the procedures necessary are more

under control. Convalescence is shorter than by the suprapubic route. Besides there is an absence of any tendency to hernia or any possibility of it, and when care is exercised, there is a preservation of sexual power.

Urinary Incontinence After Prostatectomy.—Dr. E. Wood Ruggles, of Rochester, said that in a certain number of cases there is incontinence of urine after prostatectomy. The course of the case is rather interesting in certain respects. Incontinence is apt to follow the operation for some time. Then for a period there may be good control. Afterward, control may be lost again. It would seem as though the scar in the prostatic region was first soft and incapable of enabling the bladder to retain the urine. Afterward by contraction it became harder and enabled the bladder to control the stream of urine. Later on, however, as the result of infection or over-irritation, the scar softened again with consequent incontinence. It is now known that it is not the removal of a portion of the bladder that causes the incontinence, for cases have been reported in which a slough of the bladder has occurred involving one-third of that viscus without bringing on incontinence.

Real Sphincter.—The real agent for the control of the urine in Dr. Ruggles' mind seems to be the external sphincter, the so-called compressor urethra. It is the partial or complete paralysis of this muscle that gives rise to the anomalous set of events which have been described in the postoperative course or certain cases of prostatectomy. It seems especially important then that care should be taken to avoid wounding the muscle in making the necessary incisions for prostatectomy. It is not, as has been thought by some, that the prostatic urethra is injured that is responsible for the continence. Freyer and Moynihan, in England, make it a rule to remove the prostatic urethra in their cases, yet their patients do not suffer from incontinence. Hence the advisability of paying more attention than has been the custom to the nerve supply of the compressor or urethra.

First American Operator.—Dr. Francis S. Watson, of Boston, said that a better state of mind is developing among American surgeons with regard to prostatectomy. They are especially to be congratulated in that it is no longer considered quite the thing to have a pet operation. Individual patients must be operated upon according to the necessity of their case. Very large prostates are better removed through the suprapubic incision. Most prostates, however, should be removed through the median perineal incision. Dr. Watson said that American surgeons should remember gratefully the work of Gouley in this regard. He stands between Mercier, the French surgeon, and American surgery as the bridge that leads up to the modern evolution of prostatic surgery. Undoubtedly he must be considered as the originator of perineal prostatectomy. It was from him that Dr. Watson first learned the rapid method of enucleating the prostate with the finger. He pointed out the planes of cleavage in the prostatic tissues out of which the large gland could readily be shaved. This is the operation now used more than any other and destined to supersede all others, except for special cases.

Sexual Power in Prostatics.—Dr. Watson said that he is rather surprised to find how much stress is being laid upon the necessity of preservation of sexual power in patients operated upon for the relief of prostatic symptoms. Perhaps the greater delicacy of feeling on the part of surgery in this respect is due to the difference of patients in a more southerly climate. In the more ascetic atmosphere of northern Boston, patients suffering from severe prostatism have no interest in sexual matters. If, however, the prostatic urethra be saved, then the ejaculatory ducts remain uninjured and all that is possible to do for the preservation of sexual power is accomplished.

Differing Enlargements of the Prostate.—By a series of lantern slides Dr. Watson then showed the varying forms of pathological prostates and the methods of operating upon them. He emphasized the necessity for care in shelling-out the prostate and the thinness of the capsule in many cases that made it easy to lose the way. Where all three of the lobes of the prostate are enlarged, all of them should be removed, and this is indeed the essence of Freyer's so-called new operation, which is, however, not really different from the operations that preceded it. With regard to the operation of choice in any given case, the surgeon's judgment must be used. Where any one method is used to the exclusion of others, the results are not so favorable. With the suprapubic route, as compared to the perineal route, even in the best hands there will always be ten per cent. more of mortality than with the perineal route in good hands.

Importance of Diagnosis.—Dr. Albert Vanderveer, of Albany, said that the mere occurrence of symptoms of prostatism does not necessarily imply the existence of an enlarged prostate. The surgeon must be sure of the actual existence of some enlargement. In certain cases Dr. Vanderveer believes that the use of the catheter may be encouraged for a time. It seems especially fortunate that more conservative methods are now the custom. The old operation of the removal of the testicles was an example of an extreme fad in surgery. In operating by the perineal route, Dr. Vanderveer considers that gentleness so as not to tear the prostatic urethra is important. In postoperative technic, the most important thing is to get patients out of bed early, since this restores their confidence and gives them courage for convalescence.

Development of Prostatectomy.—Dr. Samuel Alexander said that the revulsion of feeling against such operations as the removal of the testicles had proved excellent for the evolution of prostatectomy. The hit or miss operations of the days before that time had been replaced by operations done with full knowledge of the anatomy of the part. Gouley had undoubtedly done good work, but his operation always left a portion of the prostate behind the urethra and thus often failed to afford relief.

Dr. Willis McDonald, of Albany, said that he had gone through all the phases from Gouley to Bottini and the suprapubic route. He still believed that some old men can be left to a catheter life under special circumstances. He does not think that in order to get into a house, when the front door is at hand, that he should have to climb up on the roof, and so he prefers the perineal route.

Dr. Parker Syms, of New York, said that prostatic surgery owed most to American surgeons. While Gouley had accomplished much, undoubtedly Alexander's work had been of great significance, coming particularly as it did when direct operations upon the prostate were not in favor. The perineal route is undoubtedly the method of choice for most cases.

The Blood in Epilepsy.—Dr. B. Onuf read a paper on the subject which had been prepared by himself and Dr. Horace LoGrasso, of the Craig Colony, at Sonyea. Dr. Onuf said that so far the use of the bromides in epilepsy has not been found to produce any material deterioration of the blood. Epilepsy itself has, according to most observers, had no definite effect. There is no difference in the red blood cells and no constant variation of the white blood cells. There has been some diminution noted in the number of eosinophiles. The attacks themselves of epilepsy seem to have some effect on the red blood cells making them more spherical in shape and smaller in some cases and the blood plates become more frequent. The leucocytes sometimes drop in number just before a seizure takes place and do not come back to normal for some time. The first increase is noted in the lymphocytes which increase after an hour. The eosinophiles, however, may not return to normal for ten hours. In their experience at Sonyea, there seems to be a definite curve of reduction in the number of white cells whenever there are a series of seizures.

Fluctuations of Leucocytes.—In a number of cases, carefully observed, it was found that epileptics seemed to have a special tendency to fluctuation in the number of leucocytes and this physiological or pathological peculiarity seems to have a definite connection with their effection. There is always a tendency to a higher leucocytosis whenever the attacks become more frequent. Much more study is needed, however, to determine absolutely what the relationship of these changes is to epilepsy.

Extensive Carcinoma of Tongue and Neck.—Dr. William Seaman Bainbridge, of New York, presented a patient from whom he had removed the entire tongue and the large part of the floor of the mouth, with both sublingual and submaxillary glands, and all the lymphatic glands along the great vessels from the base of the skull to the dome of both pleural cavities. The patient not only recovered, but now, at the end of ten months, he is able to eat, talk and taste readily. His talking, and the fact that he tastes well are especially interesting, since apparently all organs necessary for these functions have been removed. The patient is a theatrical man, forty-eight years of age, whose mother died of cancer at the age of seventy-four years. He had smoked cigars for twenty years, often as many as twenty cigars a day and always on the left side of his mouth. Some years ago he noticed a pimple on his tongue, which proved refractory to treatment, but which disappeared on giving up smoking. When he took up smoking again, it recurred and now proved more obstinate than ever, becoming an open ulcer that would not heal.

Constitutional Symptoms.—The patient lost flesh, became sallow in color and generally cachectic. The ulcer continued to spread on the anterior portion of the tongue and in spite of the advice from several surgeons that an operation was necessary, the patient refused. He was treated with the X-rays for nine weeks but grew steadily worse. Portions of the tongue were removed and two pathologists independently declared the new growth to be very vascular epithelioma. At the end of the X-ray treatment, the tumor had extended across the tongue and the cervical glands on both sides were enlarged. Finally he consented to operation.

toid on the other side. Besides this branch incisions were made along the anterior surface of the sterno-cleidomastoid down to the clavicle. Care was taken during the course of the operation in the removal of the cancerously affected tissues that healthy structures should not be bathed in cancer cells. All the sheaths of the vessels were removed and the whole tongue was removed. Shellac was then applied over the wound. The patient had reduced in weight to 139 pounds. He gained 10 pounds in the hospital after the operation and now weighs 160 pounds. He can masticate any food, can talk very intelligibly and tastes well. He has no difficulty in swallowing any kind of liquid except water. This is his own story.

At the end of his discussion of the case Dr. Bainbridge said that no case of inoperable cancer had ever been cured by X-rays or by any other form of radiation. At most, a temporary improvement takes place and, in the most virulent forms of cancer, even this alleviation is not noticed.

Failure of X-ray.—Joseph D. Bryant, of New York, said that he believed that special emphasis should be laid on the fact that the X-rays are not curative in any of the severer forms of malignant disease and no delay in operation should be permitted when the chances are slight of being able to make a complete operation. Idiosyncrasy plays a large rôle in the matter of recurrence of cancer. In some patients what seems to the surgeon complete removal of all cancerous tissues recurrence is rapidly followed. In other cases, contrary to all expectation, recurrence is delayed or even may not take place at all.

Prophylaxis in Pregnancy.—Dr. T. Avery Rogers, of Plattsburg, N. Y., said that the most important part of prophylaxis during pregnancy consists in the care of the kidney and the skin. The accident most to be feared is cancer. This seems to be growing more frequent in recent years and seems to occur much oftener than ought to be expected in certain parts of the country. The statistics ordinarily count one case of eclampsia out of 500 labors. In and around Plattsburg, however, out of 75 births, 11 cases of eclampsia have occurred. Indeed the affection seems to be quite common and there is possibility of an infectious origin. The question whether it is climatic or microbic in origin is interesting and is open for further study. The queston of diet in these cases is also important. It is said that in Vienna, where many of the population drink wine containing the tartrates of sodium and potassium, there is less eclampsia than in other parts of the world. There is, however, insufficient urinary examination made with care to foresee the possibility of eclampsia and thus avoid it most effectually. It is not when nervous symptoms are already beginning that the patient should come under treatment, but a considerable period before this, when only the urine gives any warning of the approach of the danger.

Hackley Bequests.—The will of Charles H. Hackley, the Muskegon philanthropist, which was filed February 15, makes large bequests in addition to provisions for relatives and friends. To the Hackley Manual Training School of Muskegon $250,000 is given, which, added to $360,000 already given by Mr. Hackley, makes the school's total endowment $610,000; as an endowment for the Hackley Hospital, $300,000, less any sums given in Mr. Hackley's lifetime for this purpose; for the maintenance of the Hackley Public Library, $200,000; for the purchase of pictures for this library, $150,000.

NEW YORK ACADEMY OF MEDICINE.
SECTION ON GENITO-URINARY DISEASES.
Stated Meeting, held November 16, 1904.

The President, James Pedersen, M.D., in the Chair.

Tuberculosis of the Bladder.—Dr. Eugene Fuller reported the case of a man, twenty-five years old, who presented himself with symptoms of one week's duration. Although he had lost flesh he considered himself perfectly well until one week previous, when he began to have frequent and urgent urination. There was some blood at the end of the urination. By rectal examination nothing could be felt, and he never had any gonorrhea. It seemed to Dr. Fuller as though the case might be one of tumor of the bladder. On passing a searcher a hard inflammatory mass was detected. The patient was taken to the hospital and placed in bed. Examination of the urine revealed a very few tubercle bacilli. Although there was danger of stirring up trouble by further instrumentation, nevertheless it was done with the utmost care and under profound anesthesia and there was found a tuberculous excrescence involving quite a large area extending back around the lumen of the left ureter. This instrumentation did no damage. One of the interesting points of the case was that the examination being conducted without causing trauma was not succeeded by any inflammatory reaction.

A second case, which occurred in a woman thirty-five years old, who was brought to him for incontinence of urine. The bladder really had no capacity, the patient soiling herself all the time. She gave the history that two years before she had frequency in micturition without any assignable cause. A careful examination was made microscopically but no gonococci found. Tubercle bacilli could not then be found. She was supposed to have a tumor of the bladder and expected to be operated on for this condition. On rectal examination the whole bladder seemed to be involved. The uterus was bound down. She was placed in the hospital. The bladder could not be distended at all, even under complete anesthesia. The bladder was thickened and collapsed. This viscus was inflated with air and scraped; these scrapings showed an abundance of tubercle bacilli. The woman left the hospital without much relief and her outlook was bad. Dr. Fuller doubted if the bladder would ever gain its elasticity because of the pericystitis and because of the damage done by washing the bladder for two years with various strong solutions. The trauma produced by such washings would naturally stir up the tuberculous condition and tend to provoke it to invade the muscular and the perivesical tissues, the result being the existing pericystitis.

Prostatectomy.—Dr. Martin W. Ware presented a specimen of an enlarged prostrate removed from a patient, sixty-five years old, who was admitted to the Mt. Sinai Hospital on July 22. His trouble dated back five or six years when he began to urinate frequently and got up for this purpose three times during the night. The first alarming symptom that caused him to consult a physician was severe pain in the suprapubic region associated with marked hemorrhages during micturition. He was then catheterized and received some relief. During last May he had another severe hemorrhage lasting three or four days, and he had to be catheterized quite frequently for retention associated with the

Technic of Operation.—An incision was made from the tip of the mastoid to the tip of the mas-

hemorrhage. At the time he presented himself for admission to the hospital he was being catheterized during the day as often as six or seven times, and he had complete retention when admitted. He appeared to be a well-nourished man and had a moderate degree of fever, 99° to 100° F., pulse in good condition. His bladder was found to extend to the umbilicus and he was unable to pass a single drop of water. He was immediately catheterized and 60 ounces of urine, bad smelling, cloudy and turbid was removed. There were no evidences of nephritis notwithstanding the large quantity of cloudy urine passed. He was placed in bed and watched for a few days. Examination per rectum revealed a mass, not very large; a cystoscope was introduced and there some bleeding was seen to arise from the prostate which jutted into the bladder; there was a moderate enlargement of both lobes of the prostate. No untoward results followed the introduction of the cystoscope. He was given the option of operation and accepted. A perineal prostatectomy was performed, the perineal route being selected because the prostate was within reach of the finger; although the suprapubic route might have been as easily performed the perineal route was selected because of anatomical reasons. Nitrous oxide gas was used and the prostate was removed with ease in fifteen minutes. A perineal drainage tube was introduced. Within forty-eight hours the man was in perfect condition and wanted to get up and stand; he was allowed to do so. On the third day he got into a chair, and before a week was up he walked 'about the ward. At the end of three or four weeks the sinus in the perineum closed and then he had the same absolute retention that he had on admission. There had been no leakage. The cystoscope revealed at the neck of the bladder a condition frequently found in females especially, i.e., edema of the bullosum vesicæ tissues. Faradization of the bladder both by urethra and by rectum was of no avail, and he went away but to return again. Then the cystoscope revealed the edema had entirely disappeared. The endoscope showed a prominence at the site of the verruca montana which might have been sufficient to cause the obstruction. It was cauterized with actual cautery and later Bottini's operation was performed. All treatment applied was of no avail. It was then decided to do a suprapubic cystotomy but nothing was found. The bladder was so atonic that a portion of the bladder wall apparently fell against the urethral orifice. This case showed that the contention of Sir Henry Thompson and Guyon was not absolutely wrong. Such bladders may gain their tone.

Dr. Ware presented a second specimen that he had removed from a patient seventy years old. The symptoms prior to his admission to the hospital were typical of enlarged prostate. He had frequent micturitions associated with hematuria and quite a temperature; had had to be catheterized five or six times a day; occasionally he had retention. The rectal examination showed an enlargement of the prostate. The cystoscope showed that no stone was present. The residual urine amounted to four ounces. There was a marked cystitis. There were some hemorrhagic patches on the bladder wall. January 27 he entered the hospital because of retention. On July 8 he was operated upon under nitrous oxide anesthesia; the suprapubic operation was performed in twenty minutes. The suprapubic wound did not close until August 20. Then the condition

of the patient was such that he had only one ounce of residual urine. The cystitis had not been markedly benefited. At the end of six weeks he still had residual urine. He was then discharged. The physician who had him in charge said that he had not been markedly improved and he still had to use the catheter.

These two cases reported by Dr. Ware were intended to show that all patients on whom a prostatectomy technically successfully performed were not markedly relieved at once.

Dr. Howard Lilienthal, in the discussion, asked Dr. Ware if, in his first case, it would not have been better to have done the suprapubic operation in the first place. Was the bladder drained?

Dr. Ware replied that it was drained.

Dr. Lilienthal did not think it possible for prolonged drainage in itself to cause a shrinkage of the bladder. The function of urination would come back after the removal of an obstruction unless there had been something more than mere overdistention of the bladder walls. If the trouble had been due to central nervous disease, operation might not cure. It seemed to him that if the suprapubic operation had been done in the first place it would have saved this patient considerable trouble.

Dr. John Van der Poel said he had had a somewhat similar case of perineal prostatectomy with comparatively little result, where it was difficult for him to make out the middle lobe. The patient was relieved of his retention after operation, but since then he had had frequent urination, almost as often as prior to operation. He has now two or three ounces of residual urine, and it is suspected that there is a bar or middle lobe, which had not been detected at the time of the operation. The results in these operations were not always gratifying. With reference to Dr. Fuller's case, he said he had introduced the cystoscope in patients with frequent urination, in order to exclude any bladder lesion, where the instrumentation seemed to give relief in much the same way as passing a sound seemed to do in such cases. He believed that most of the cases of tuberculosis of the bladder got along far better without local treatment, relying upon hygienic and other measures. Dr. Cabot, of Boston, illustrated this fact in the reports of several cases he has published, where complete recovery had been reported.

Dr. Thomas H. Manley referred to a patient, an old man who had entered his service at Harlem Hospital a year ago, who came there for relief of urinary retention. He stated that his prostate had been removed at the New York Hospital, two years before, but without relief. He bore a transverse scar in the perineum; and examined for rectum, showed no trace of prostate. Dr. Manley said that in the bladder of those beyond middle life, there were often senile, with organic changes in their walls. In these cases an enlarged prostate was but one factor in urinary obstruction.

Dr. Franz J. A. Torek said that the report of Dr. Ware's first case reminded him strongly of spinal cord disease. He had once a case presenting similar symptoms with retention of urine, the condition existing twenty-eight years. He did a Bottini operation for hypertrophy of the prostate with absolutely no good following. A suprapubic fistula was made at a later operation, and this relieved him considerably.

Dr. Joseph Wiener said that one should bear in mind that every case of retention occurring in old men who happened to have an enlarged prostate could not be cured by prostatectomy. Of course where there was an enlarged prostrate which caused retention of urine the removal of that prostate would always relieve the condition.

Dr. Parker Syms said that when one operates for obstruction to urination the successful removal of the cause of obstruction, as an enlarged prostate, does not necessarily cure the results of this obstruction; in other words the bladder often requires careful treatment after operation. In this regard some of Dr. Syms early cases of prostatectomy were more favorable than some of his later ones; that is to say many of his later cases have required very careful after-treatment to cure cystitis and other damage which had been produced before operation. Dr. Syms spoke of two patients now in Lebanon Hospital who had been operated upon in other hospitals by the suprapubic route. One is a hopeless invalid, and Dr. Syms thinks that this is on account of the route chosen. The operation wound had not healed at the end of two years, during which time his bladder had become contracted and seriously damaged by infection. The other patient is not in so serious a condition, but his bladder is contracted because the wound was many months in healing. However, his bladder is now being dilated, and it is hoped that he may make a fair recovery.

The Chairman asked Dr. Ware if the atonic condition of the bladder in the first case he reported was recognized before the prostatectomy was performed, which was answered in the affirmative. Continuing, the Chairman said that the discussion pointed out quite clearly the necessity for careful discrimination before deciding whether perineal or suprapubic prostatectomy should be performed in a given case. Dr. Ware's case under discussion reminded him of an experience he had last summer with a patient upon whom he performed perineal prostatectomy in whom a suprapubic prostatectomy, as it turned out, would probably have yielded better results. The intravesical portion was so large and was situated so high that it was impossible to remove it all through the perineum. Prolonged drainage of the bladder failing to accomplish the desired result, he incised the intravesical portion of the prostate with the Bottini instrument by way of the perineum, as practised by Chetwood. It was feared that the patient would not stand a suprapubic prostatectomy as a secondary operation. At a subsequent meeting he hoped to give the net result in this case. He agreed with Dr. Van der Poel's experience regarding the effect that sometimes follows an exploratory instrumentation of a tuberculous bladder; but he called attention to the fact that this temporary improvement does not follow subsequent, repeated instrumentation. He thought it was now generally agreed that vesical tuberculosis should be treated hygienically, as Dr. Van der Poel had said.

Dr. Ware closed the discussion. The specimens were not presented in order to exploit any particular method of operation and he did not intend to convey the impression that prostatectomy was the panacea in all cases of urinary retention. It was nothing of the sort. All cases could not be cured. Watson and other men whose statistics could be relied upon had stated this fact. Socin in *Deutsche Chirurgie* states among 77 cases of suprapubic prostatectomy, 31 per cent. were completely cured; the mortality rate was 20 per cent. The public should not be told that these operations were not attended with any risks at all.

Regarding the possibility of any nervous lesion to account for the retention referred to by Dr. Toroli, he answered by saying that there was absolutely no such lesion; the patient had been examined by a neurologist and no lesion was demonstrable. The mucous membrane of the bladder was rather smooth and the muscular walls had quite an appreciable thickness. After prostatectomy was performed and the catheter left in the bladder he seemed to have quite a good deal of expulsive force. How the bladder could regain its tone after being out of work for long periods of time he failed to see.

Calculi Removed by Litholapaxy.—Dr. James Pedersen presented two cases:

Case I.—The patient is a well-developed boy, fourteen years old. Painful urination began when he was two years old. Medical treatment gave temporary relief until his sixth year. Since then the symptoms have been progressive and have become especially severe within the past two years. Without anesthesia a small bougie-à-boule introduced into the bladder, at once encountered a calculus. After the usual preparatory treatment of the bladder its capacity was found to be five ounces. The operation was performed under general anesthesia. The meatus, which measured 22 F., was divided to 28 F. The calculus was extremely hard; as the crushing progressed some sections of it were found to be much harder than others. The fragments were evacuated through a 28 F. evacuating tube. The patient left the hospital on the fifth day. Since the operation (October 24) patient has been entirely free from pain; but some vesical irritability persists. He is being treated for this by his physician who brought him to Pedersen. As is his custom, he had the patient report at his office two weeks after the operation and searched the bladder for any stray fragments or small particles that had escaped evacuation at the time of operation. Evacuating tube 24 F. was used and proved the bladder entirely clear of fragments.

Case II.—The patient is fifty-two years of age. No bladder symptoms up to a year ago when intense burning during micturition developed extending along the length of the urethra. Frequency, urgency and slight hematuria followed. On July 12, 1904, cystoscopy was performed, without anesthesia. The tolerance of the bladder admitted five ounces. Two calculi was discovered; one the size of a hazelnut the other twice that size, lying together in the postprostatic pouch. With a slender lithotrite the smaller was seized and the larger was moved about to prove that is was free in the bladder. Operation July 15, 1904, under general anesthesia. The patient was out of bed on the third day and returned home on the fourth day. He reported at my office on the sixth day that nocturnal urination had ceased and that he was able to retain urine at will during the day; but that a trifling sensation during urination remained. Six days later all symptoms had disappeared and the urine was normal. Two weeks after the operation cystoscopy revealed two small grains at the base of the bladder. These were evacuated in the usual way.

Observations on Twenty-eight Cases of Prostatectomy.—Dr. J. Bentley Squier, Jr., read this paper. It will be found on page 294 of this issue of the MEDICAL NEWS.

Dr. L. Bolton Bangs, in the discussion, said he was much interested in the progress that had taken place in prostatic work during recent years. It certainly is encouraging and he wished to congratulate the reader of the paper for the frank manner in which he had presented his experience. He said he had been particularly interested lately in reading the papers on this subject; many were very instructive and many were very dogmatic and made one wonder if we were yet living in the dark ages and what the object of the paper was. He thought it would be more creditable if surgeons who wrote so many articles should pay more attention to the question of diagnosis; it seemed that the question how to operate was of less importance than the question of whether operation was indicated or not. The details of diagnosis seemed to be overlooked, again the after results had not been reported as fully as he would like to see them. The operation of prostatectomy had not met all his expectations and had not given the same satisfaction that he had been led to hope for from the reports of the experiences of his colleagues. He did not believe it was necessary to say that because a man had some residual urine and a certain amount of prostatic hypertrophy he must be subjected to operation; there were many cases notwithstanding the presence of residual urine which did not need this operation, or any operation whatever. Nor would they necessarily be placed upon catheter life. There were cases also whose postoperative condition was not improved. Neither of Dr. Ware's cases was improved and Dr. Bangs had had somewhat the same experience in dealing with younger men whose bladder were infected and who required long continued drainage. Similarly he found that prostatics with prolonged obstruction causing secondary changes in the bladder, even after the prostatic obstruction was removed, were not appreciably relieved of their symptoms. The conditions that existed prior to operation should be more carefully inquired into. The reader of the paper had called attention to a point which, he confessed, he had not paid sufficient attention to, and that was the question of the discrimination of the patients. Not long ago Dr. Bangs attended a meeting of medical and surgical men at which a paper was read by a distinguished member of the profession who stated that he did not attach much value to the opinions of hospital surgeons, because their opinions were based upon experience with the class of cases met with in hospitals whose social conditions required radical measures, and therefore the surgeon's judgment often was biased when considering the needs of the better classes. Therefore, it seemed to Dr. Bangs that we should discriminate more carefully. For example you will meet with individuals in the higher walks of life who have entered catheter life and who go on for years in excellent health. Admitting that a bladder with residual urine is a culture chamber, always liable to infection, many of these cases that come under our supervision if given proper and judicous care will not require operation. Catheter life should not always be despised in certain individuals. Hygiene has its place as a preventer of infection. Judicious, thoughtful, refined catheter life was not necessarily dangerous, but we must also discriminate between individuals. With regard to technic he said that many believed that the suprapubic operation was the only operation, while others believed that the perineal was the only correct method. Dr. Bangs believed that only a careful anti-operative diagnosis would enable us to determine just which operation was the proper one. In his opinion the perineal operation would meet all the indications in the majority of cases. There was no

difficulty encountered, as a rule, in removing stone by the perineal route and there should not be much difficulty in attacking the prostate by this method. With regard to leaving the so-called " sexual-bridge " according to the technic of Young, of Baltimore, he agreed with the writer of the paper that its possibility was doubtful and made no real difference. Regarding postoperative epididymitis he had seen patients suffering more vital depression from this than from the whole operative procedure. As to following the suggestion made of ligating the vas deferens, he dissented and would not do this as a stock procedure. The question of the difficulty of doing either the suprapubic or the perineal operation did not concern us. He had had more difficulty and experienced more surgical thrill in doing some of the operations of general surgery—for example in dissecting out a tumor of the base of the neck, than in any prostate operation which he had yet encountered. The important question seemed to be, is an operation indicated; if so, what operation?

Dr. Eugene Fuller believed that many people were operated for prostatic senile hypertrophy when none existed at all and when the cause of trouble was to be found simply in inflammatory conditions following gonorrhea, for instance. In such inflammatory cases there would of course be found nothing to enucleate. Cases of developing prostatic obstructions should be more considered. For instance, take a man in the late fifties with beginning prostatic obstruction; it did not seem to him that, in such cases, provided the general condition of the patient was good, it was worth while to procrastinate about operation. If such a man wished to live but a short time, all right; but if he wished to live a long time then it was best to operate and remove the prostate which otherwise would go on developing. Regarding the question how such an operation would leave these patients in 99 per cent. of the cases they should be left in a satisfactory condition. Such men who refuse operation cannot get well, and if they should wish to go away, as to the woods hunting or fishing, they must take catheters and be prepared for accidents which may happen; anyway they run a risk which they would not run of they submitted to operative procedures. It was like trifling with an inflamed appendix. But, if a man develops an obstruction while he is in his seventies, this then is another class to consider; the surgeon here should be more conservative and more inclined to operate only when the catheter should be found to fail. Dr. Fuller said the prostate could be removed either by way of the perineum or suprapubically. He had done the perineal operation of prostatectomy about 75 times and the suprapubic one about three times as many times. Many believed the perineal operation to be the one of choice in certain instances. Other questions besides getting the prostate out must be always considered in selecting the route. Dr. Fuller here related the history of one of his cases showing the point that one could not rely entirely upon one route; it was necessary to individualize in such operations as in many others. If a bladder was found to be absolutely atonic the perineal operation was not the one of choice; but if the bladder was strong and hypertrophied and had sufficient expulsion power, then the perineal operation was, as a rule, the proper one. The question of the sexual function in connection with prostatectomy had of late received considerable attention. In the speaker's experience prostatectomy was more apt to improve that function than injure it. If one exercised sufficient care it was not necessary to damage the sexual apparatus at all. In many cases with large hypertrophies of the prostate, the glands pressed upon the ejaculatory ducts, and after prostatectomies in such instances the sacs regained their tone and the sexual function correspondingly improved. In the performance of the perineal operation Dr. Fuller used a small incision and divulsed the tissues much as Dr. Syms did, although he did not think it was necessary to use the balloon. He condemned the use of sharp-clawed instruments employed as tractors. Dr. Fuller said that as far as he was personally concerned the operation of prostatectomy was way beyond its experimental stage. He felt that with him it was no more of an experiment than was the removal of the appendix with the general surgeon.

Dr. Parker Syms agreed with Dr. Fuller's statement that prostatectomy was beyond the experimental stage inasmuch we have still a great deal to learn. Regarding indications for operation he is inclined to be rather more conservative than some of the other speakers, for he believes we should wait until the bladder, urinary apparatus, or general health of the patient shows that damage is being done by the prostatic obstruction. A moderate amount of residual urine is no indication for prostatectomy, and he does not think we should operate in anticipation of bad results, simply because of the gradual enlargement of this gland. One should wait until there is evidence of injury present and then operate.

In regard to catheter life he thought that a patient in the hands of one as skilful as Dr. Bangs might perhaps go along very safely, but that does not represent the criterion of catheter life. Dr. Syms feels that for a patient about to enter catheter life it would be far safer to operate than to allow him to take up the use of the catheter. Some months ago he roughly estimated the mortality in those of his patients who had declined operation and continued the use of the catheter; about 50 per cent. of these patients had died within a year and a half to two years. He had expressed himself so many times before on the technic of the operation that he hesitated to say much more. He believes the perineal route to be the only one of choice for anatomical as well as surgical reasons, but the reports of some of the gentlemen would show that good results might be obtained by the suprapubic operation. The operation should be performed with as much speed as possible and the lower route is the quicker. The suprapubic operation may be easier, but he preferred to work by the peritoneum. The after-effects of the suprapubic operation were more serious than those of perineal prostatectomy. If he expected to cope with hemorrhage he preferred to operate by the perineal route. As he operates, the bladder is not injured except by the introduction of the finger, and if there is any liability to hemorrhage it can be easily controlled because the blood cannot pass into the bladder if the tube fits properly and one has only to pack the space from which the prostate came. It is also true that the prostatic wound does not come in contact with the urine until after the drainage tube is removed. In perineal prostatectomy there is but little damage to surrounding tissues and there should be no damage to the bladder. He opens the prostatic sheath and enucleates the prostate without tearing or lacerating the lobes. In a properly performed perineal prostatectomy there should be no hemorrhage. He never expects to lose more than

an ounce or two of blood. He lays stress on the median incision in the perineum. He believes that it is far better than the dissecting operation of the French which has been presented to us by Young. He paid tribute to the work of Goodfellow, of San Francisco, who antedates us all in perineal prostatectomy. His work was first published in 1892; he uses no retractor, but enucleates the prostate through a small incision made in the perineum. Goodfellow reports over seventy cases without a death. Dr. Syms operates through a small median incision. The membranous urethra is opened and the tissues are pushed back and on to one side until the prostatic sheath is exposed. This is opened by a vertical incision on the left side and through this incision the left lobe is removed. Sometimes the entire prostate is removed through this incision, and sometimes he makes a second vertical incision on the right side through which he removes the right lobe. Goodfellow has shown that it is not necessary to use a retractor. Syms finds his rubber retractor of great use. It pulls down the neck of the bladder and holds the prostate steady, aiding the enucleation. As each lobe of the prostate is removed the space is closed by pressure of the retractor and oozing is checked. With regard to conserving the sexual function as emphasized by Young, of Baltimore, he believes the idea is rather a phantom. In many cases sexual function which has been lost will be restored, and in other cases sexual function will be lost as the result of the operation, and in other cases it will not be affected. The fact that epididymitis is a very frequent complication after operation shows that the ducts are not closed or destroyed, or the friction could not take place. With regard to final results he will only speak in a general way, for he hopes ere long to report his cases in detail. He will only say that his final results have been very satisfactory. His patients have done so well that he is convinced that the operation is a truly scientific and commendable one.

Dr. Martin W. Ware believed that one essential in the right direction was in appreciating the patient's condition by means of the cystoscope prior to operation and he said the consensus of opinion was in favor of doing this. One of the conditions which would lead us toward a rational suprapubic or perineal operation would be one of stone in the bladder; in such cases one would not hesitate to introduce a searcher to find if a stone was present. Therefore, why should one hesitate to introduce a cystoscope and learn the position of the stone? It depended upon the situation of the stone, and its nature, whether the perineal or suprapubic operation was to be preferred. The cystoscope enabled us to choose between these two routes not only in doing lithotomy but also in performing prostatectomies.

Dr. Howard Lilienthal said that taking everything into consideration regarding the time to operate it had been stated once and for all by Paul Thorndike, of Boston, that "when catheter fails to give relief that is the time to operate." Regarding the choice of operation he preferred to do the suprapubic one. He was glad that Dr. Syms changed his opinion expressed some time ago; then he said that it was about as sensible to attack the prostate suprapubically as to attack a tonsil through the back of the head. And yet not every tonsil could be removed through the mouth and incisions in the sphenomaxillary region might be necessary. Epididymitis was more or less common after these operations; it was also a common complication in prostatism without operation. Dr. Lilienthal thought that a long time would elapse before the final word was spoken regarding the merits of either the suprapubic or perineal operation and he did not believe one should be too quick in deciding any questions regarding them. With regard to the use of the cystoscope, if one had decided upon the suprapubic operation its use would be absolutely unnecessary; but if one had not decided upon this upper route, and wished to gain further information regarding the bladder conditions, then the cystoscope might be a very valuable aid.

Dr. Joseph Wiener said that his personal experience with this operation was the same as Dr. Howard Lilienthal's and he preferred the suprapubic route for operating because of the good results obtained. The series of good results Dr. Lilienthal had obtained caused him two years ago to adopt it in his work, and this route had always given him satisfaction. His cases had all been done under nitrous oxide anesthesia. The element of time he considered to be of extreme importance, and he usually consumed ten minutes, from the time the knife was used until the packing was in the bladder. He did not believe that any surgeon experienced in this work would tear a hole into the rectum; he did not know of a single case of suprapubic prostatectomy in which this accident occurred. It did occur during the perineal operation. The question of stone in the bladder was an important one and Dr. Bangs had stated that every one could be removed by way of the perineum. He had operated on one case where the stone could not have been removed through a perineal incision. He was surprised to hear Dr. Squier say that in the perineal operation one could break up the lobe of the prostate and remove it. By the suprapubic route one can remove the gland in its entirety which was a decided advantage. In this upper operation there is less hemorrhage; there is the absolute certainty of removing the gland entire and in one piece; one can save a great deal of time by shelling out the gland in one piece. The cystoscope he considered a dangerous instrument in the presence of marked hypertrophy of the prostate. In his early operation he had a few cases of epididymitis; he then passed a sound. In his last four or five cases he placed a catheter in the urethra and closed the bladder wound two days after operation, did not use any sound, and had not had a trace of epididymitis. The perineal operation was one of decided disadvantage in that it required frequent sounding. Dr. Wiener recapitulated as follows: In the suprapubic operation one did more rapid work; a stone could be more readily removed; the rectum was not damaged; the cystoscope was not employed; epididymitis was not common. Other factors that contributed to the success of the operation were, no instrumentation prior to operation; nitrous oxide anesthesia, rapid work.

Dr. John Van der Poel said that, in pulling down the prostate in perineal prostatectomy, his personal preference was for the retractor of Dr. Young, of Baltimore, which was almost precisely the same as that devised in France. Where this retractor was often combined with the finger of the assistant in the rectum there was, as a rule, no difficulty in getting at the organ and, at the same time, the assistant's finger in the rectum often gave timely warning as to the proximity of the rectal wall. He believed that Dr.

Young's operation, in saving the sexual bridge, was practically unnecessary in the majority of cases, who were beyond the age of sexual life and, in many cases, time being a very important factor, the general condition of the patients not being of the best, it not being the shortest method of operation, too much time was required for the dissection; as it was preferable to operate quickly, the sooner the patients were off the table the better; hence he did not think the dissecting operation advisable.

BOOK REVIEWS.

A HISTORY OF SCIENCE. BY HENRY SMITH WILLIAMS, M.D., LL.D., assisted by EDWARD H. WILLIAMS, M.D. In Five Volumes. Illustrated. Volume I—The Beginnings of Science. Volume II—The Beginnings of Modern Science. Volume III—Modern Development of the Physical Sciences. Volume IV—Modern Development of the Chemical and Biological Sciences. Volume V—Aspects of Recent Science. Harper & Brothers, New York and London.

IT is both flattering and surprising to the medical man to note the great number of physicians who have been pioneers in scientific discoveries. Thus Dr. Julius Robert Mayer (Vol. III, p. 259) discovered the "Conservation of Energy;" Dr. William Gilbert (Vol. II, p. 111) is known as the "Father of Electricity;" Dr. Thomas Young (Vol. III, pp. 215-225) discovered the wave-theory of light; Dr. Joseph Black (Vol. IV, p. 12) discovered carbonic acid and is considered to have been one of the founders of modern chemistry.

Notwithstanding this, physicians as a class are often prone to lose sight of the fact that medicine rests almost entirely upon the application of the principles and methods of other sciences; we know natural science is the foundation upon which medical facts are largely based. The frequency with which chemical and physical laws are daily requisitioned in medical practice is of common experience. What would the opthalmologist do without applied optics, the internist without acoustic laws? It is not inaptly said that medicine is an applied science which receives its sustenance and growth in greater part from the primary sciences—chemistry, physics, geometry and the like.

The value to the medical student of a preliminary education in these sciences needs but little more emphasis than the necessity of the physician's continued interest in these subjects after graduation. Researches in pure science are not often permitted to the practising physician, such as these undertaken by Mayer and Gilbert, but a practical working knowledge of the history of science, its epoch-making discoveries and their portent in advancing our concepts of modern medicine is free to all. This data properly arranged is now at hand in the work before us—The History of Science. The historical digest embodied in the work, its orientation of the scientific trend of thought in the past and present is altogether admirable. It should be a matter of professional pride to us that this excellent science series is from the hands of medical colleagues, Dr. Henry Smith Williams and his brother, Dr. Edward H. Williams, of this city.

The fascination of the science-story is irresistible; its literary charm is co-extensive with the lucid and careful statements of facts in the work. The comprehensiveness of the contents, arrangement and the general book-making are most praiseworthy. The History of Science should form a part of every physician's library, and we believe the professional and lay reader will find equal delight in these volumes. The work is unique, as there is nothing like it in the English language.

HANDBOOK OF THE ANATOMY AND DISEASES OF THE EYE AND EAR. For Students and Practitioners. By D. B. ST. JOHN ROOSA, M.D., LL.D., Professor of Diseases of the Eye and Ear in the New York Post-graduate Medical School; formerly President of the New York Academy of Medicine, Etc., and A. EDWARD DAVIS, A.M., M.D., Professor of Diseases of the Eye in the New York Post-graduate Medical School; Fellow of the New York Academy of Medicine. 300 pages. F. A. Davis Company, Philadelphia.

THIS is an excellent little book. It contains very briefly and clearly what a student should know and does not confuse the untrained mind with needless descriptions and pictures of what must be learned by clinical observation, nor does it offer the usual assortment of remedies for diseases, the knowledge of which can be acquired only through actual experience.

Exception may be taken to certain views, and the statement that no inconvenience is felt unless astigmatism=0.75 D. or 1. D. is one that might mislead.

The book is well printed, is of convenient size, and is supplied with an elaborate index.

MODERN OPHTHALMOLOGY. A Practical Treatise on the Anatomy, Physiology, and Diseases of the Eye. By JAMES MOORE BALL, M.D., Professor of Ophthalmology in the St. Louis College of Physicians and Surgeons. With 417 illustrations in the text and numerous figures on 21 colored plates. Pp. xxii+820. F. A. Davis Company, Philadelphia.

THIS elaborate and rather ponderous work may be commended for many reasons, and it is an ungrateful task to criticize a book to which the best of intentions and much energy has been directed.

The text shows an extensive acquaintance with the best authorities, and when a personal attitude is apparent, it is of a conservative nature. The treatment of glaucoma may be considered an exception, as undue stress is laid upon removal of the sympathetic ganglion. Sympatheticectomy is the rather clumsy name given the operation by the author. The pictures relating to this subject are not convincing, especially those of the microscopical appearances from which one might infer that there are changes in the ganglia in glaucoma which are characteristic of this disease, which have not been demonstrated by other observers.

The colored plates are good, especially those of the fundus by the practised hand of Miss Washington. The author has had the collaboration of several well-known men in important subjects, and the work has been well done, if somewhat unevenly.

The book is well printed, on good, slightly glazed paper, and contains a very complete index.

THE PATHOLOGY OF THE EYE. By J. HERBERT PARSONS, B.S., D.S.(Lond.), F.R.C.S.(Eng.), Assistant Ophthalmic Surgeon, University College Hospital; Curator and Pathologist, Royal London (Moorfields) Ophthalmic Hospital; Lecturer on Physiological Optics, University College, London. Volume 1. Histology. Part 1. Pp. xiii+388. G. P. Putnam's Sons, New York. Hodder and Stoughton, London.

IT is a matter of sincere congratulation that a work of such importance has appeared in the English language. If the succeeding volumes shall show the scholarly qualities evident in the volume at hand, we have no hesitation in saying that it will stand as a monument of thoroughness and precision, unsurpassed by similar works

in any language. It is apparent to anyone who is familiar with our current ophthalmological literature, that a sounder basis of pathological knowledge has been urgently needed. The chief sources of information have been in journals, for the most part German, and have been spread over such an arid space, that familiarity with them is impossible except to those with Teutonic patience and the time to devote to research.

The author disarms criticism, if such were possible, by disclaiming dogmatism and finality, and by assuming in questions where decision is impossible, an admirably judicial tone. He says " It must be admitted with regret that few of the problems before us have been solved. I shall therefore endeavor to set forth the facts which have been discovered. . . . The various theories based upon these facts will be reviewed and weighed, with the object of determining their relative value, and of arriving at the best working hypothesis for directing future research."

The work will be divided into four volumes, the first two dealing with the Pathological Histology of the Eye, the last two with the General Pathology of the Eye.

In Volumes I and II the parts of the eye and its annexes will be taken seriatim and the histology of the various morbid conditions described. In Volumes III and IV the diseases which affect the eye as a whole will be discussed, and an endeavor will be made to trace them to their ultimate causes. This will therefore include such conditions as glaucoma, sympathetic ophthalmia, congenital malformations, etc.

From this statement of the author's purpose, it will be seen that the book is indispensable to all who are interested in ophthalmology, and it is evident from the first volume that the author is exceptionally fitted to undertake this great work.

The illustrations, 267 in number, form an important feature. Most of them are from photographs which have not been touched up, reproduced in half tone; they gain in precision what, in some instances, they may lose in clearness. Comment in detail may be postponed until the completion of the work, which, it is to be hoped, will not be long deferred.

The work of the publishers cannot be too highly commended.

PRACTICAL DIETICS, with Reference to Diet in Disease. By ALIDA FRANCES PATTEE. Second Edition. Published by the author, New York.

THIS book was originally written as a simple manual and text-book for nurses in the classroom or in outside practice, and the recognition accorded to the first edition, has prompted the preparation of a second edition within a year after the appearance of the first. The object of food, food values and their classification, and general rules for feeding the sick, form an introduction to the work, the body of which is made up of a classified list of recipes adapted to various diseases. In addition there are chapters on diet in disease and dietaries, and numerous practical suggestions for adding to the comfort of the patient. Reference to certain proprietary articles in the text might as well have been omitted without affecting the usefulness of the book.

BOOKS RECEIVED.

LABORATORY GUIDE IN ELEMENTARY BACTERIOLOGY. By Dr. W. D. Frost. 8vo, 395 pages. Illustrated. The Macmillan Co., New York.

CLINICAL DIAGNOSIS. By Dr. L. N. Boston. 8vo, 549 pages. Illustrated. W. B. Saunders & Co., New York, Philadelphia and London.

THE MEDICAL NEWS.
A WEEKLY JOURNAL OF MEDICAL SCIENCE.

VOL. 86.   NEW YORK, SATURDAY, FEBRUARY 25, 1905.   NO. 8.

ORIGINAL ARTICLES.

THE EXPECTANT TREATMENT OF APPENDICITIS. AN EXCURSION INTO THE FIELD BETWEEN SURGERY AND MEDICINE.

BY A. C. BERNAYS, M.D.,

OF ST. LOUIS, MO.

I FEEL that I have a call to say a few words in order to give the results of a long experience and some reflections on this subject. My views are exactly contrary to some that have recently been very extensively circulated by papers read at medical societies, and by their publication in many medical journals and also in lay journals. Most of these papers emanate from my friend, A. J. Ochsner, of Chicago, and are intended to influence the general practitioner in his method of treatment of appendicitis cases which are not deemed suitable for operation.

The operative treatment of appendicitis is regarded the world over as an American surgical achievement. On a recent trip to Europe and a more recent one to Japan I find that everywhere America is given much credit, or most of the credit, for having developed this department of surgery. But nowhere do they seem to know exactly who the men are that did the important work. And I must confess that I, who have followed American and foreign surgical literature very closely, would find it a difficult task to assign the credit to any one or to any ten or twenty men, among my coworkers in this country. A great many have contributed to the work of building up the almost complete structure as we have it now. The German, French, English, Swiss and Italian authors and contributors to surgical literature do not always give credit where it belongs. I for one feel that I am given too much credit by some European authors and not enough by others for the contributions I have made in this most important field of operative surgery. But in the last edition of Kocher's Text-book on Operative Surgery, published in Jena, in 1902, and now translated into English by Mr. Harold J. Stiles, F.R.C.S.Ed., of England, published by Adam and Charles Black, of London, in 1903, and in America by the Macmillan Co., we Americans are fairly treated. This volume is really not a text-book, but is a volume full of original suggestions and methods. Its author is the grand master of surgery, who, although a Swiss, was elected President of the German Society of Surgeons at Berlin, in 1902 This book is by far the most valuable memoir on surgery ever written by one man in the world's history. There is nothing so belittling as a priority dispute among scientific men, and men like the great foreign masters of surgery have no in-

clination to take from us Americans what we have fairly earned, on the contrary, I find them more than fair—they are generous.

The idea, that by the expectant treatment, cases of acute appendicitis may be tided over the febrile stage and the appendix removed later on during the afebrile stage, is gaining ground among general practitioners. Many physicians have been misled into trying expectant treatment as a regular routine measure. I do not think that Ochsner ever intended to advocate this method to the exclusion of the primary operation early in the attack, and I know of no surgeon of experience who does not always operate if called early enough. The expectant treatment is only to be thought of in cases that are seen after the best time for operation has been allowed to pass.

This secondary operation has been called the interval operation, because it is believed by some that if the appendix is not removed it may give rise to a second attack, hence the operation being performed between two attacks is called interval operation.

It is assumed that a first attack will be followed by a second one, a second by a third, and so on. How much truth there is in this assumption I do not know. I am conscious that I have done good in many of the hundreds of "interval" cases that I have done. I am sure that I have never seen a death follow an interval operation. I am also sure that some interval operations are not easy, providing that the object,—that is, the removal of the appendix and of adhesions and other lesions that may have been left behind by the attack,—is completely and thoroughly fulfilled. It is a fact that in many so-called interval operations the appendix is found "shamefully normal" or only slight, innocuous changes are found in or about the much-sought-for little rudimentary organ. I confess that in some of these cases the good to the patient was exclusively due to the psychical effect brought to bear. In some of the cases this psychical effect was such as to completely cure the patient of his *perityphlitophobia*. (God save the mark!) Could it be that some colleague, untainted by philology, would prefer appendo-phobia?

While I am making confessions, perhaps unwisely, but with a sort of satisfaction, I will add that I cannot throw off a feeling of embarrassment when I pull up a perfectly normal appendix before a corona of students or distinguished visitors. This embarrassment must be quite serious when a normal appendix is removed in six or eight cases in one day, as recently happened in a well-known hospital. Fortunately the histologist will always find infiltration of "small round cells" in the mucosa and submucosa. The friendly pathologist does not mention that the mucosa of the appendix is always richly supplied with lymph-follicles. hence the copious infiltration of leucocytes will always be present, no matter how normal an appendix may be. After all is said, each case will still be left to the judgment of the physician and the surgeon. I would gently insinuate that the interval operation is not always necessary, and when it is remembered that a first attack is not always followed by a second attack, nor a second by a third, we will all agree that an interval operation may sometimes be unnecessary though it be harmless.[1]

About thirty years ago, at the time when I began the practice of medicine, after having finished a university course of, five years, one of the important things I had learned was the treatment of peritonitis.[2] The method in vogue then at Heidelberg, Vienna, Paris, in fact at all the universities which I attended during the years 1872 to and including 1876, was as follows: Very scant, liquid diet, amounting to starvation in some clinics, frequent copious enemata, rectal feeding, opium, initial doses of calomel, castor oil, etc., the régime varying but little in different clinics. In England and in America the "opium splint" was thoroughly introduced. In the service of Spencer Wells, opium was given after all abdominal sections in order to prevent peritonitis. His lowest mortality in one hundred cases of ovariotomy was 13 per cent.; his average was 16 per cent. Then came Lawson Tait, who, even before Bouchard, arrived at a crude auto-intoxication theory and, acting upon it, changed the opium method, which he had tried for years, into the purgation and cathartic treatment.

At one stroke he reduced the mortality of abdominal section from 15 per cent. to less than five per cent. This feat of Lawson Tait's should be counted among the greatest therapeutic triumphs, coming before the auto-intoxication experiments of the French scientific experimenters. —as it did. Lawson Tait, in his empirical, unscientific way, said that purgation with salts etc., not only flushed and cleansed the sewers of the organism of their toxic contents. but he claimed that the lymphatics of the intestines and mesentery, being loaded with used-up toxic material, were drained by active catharsis. His empirical teachings have now been sustained by experiment. and the opium treatment relegated to the records, where many therapeutic mistakes are put away.

It is proper to mention here that Spencer Wells was more thorough in his antisepsis and cleanliness than was Lawson Tait. In my opinion the difference between their results is largely due to the abandonment of opium and the free use of purgation by Tait. In America fortunately the Tait system was rapidly introduced by the many pupils who followed his methods. and the opium treatment of peritonitis was crowded out after a severe struggle on the part of the conservative mossbacks, a rare specimen of which tribe I occasionally run across even at the present time.

In order to most drastically observe the difference between the effects of treatment by the "opium splint" method and the cathartic purgative method, it is sometimes possible to make a comparison in a large general hospital where cases of peritonitis are often admitted in late stages of the disease.

For instance: A physician of the old school has treated a case of peritonitis caused by appendicitis by the expectant method. We will say the opium splint has been well applied to the poor man's belly. He had also, had lavage. gastric and colonic, he has a temperature of 103.5° F. at night, pulse is 118 to 120 per minute, abdomen tympanitic, no appetite, in short, he is "getting well" under the expectant method of treatment. He has been sick two weeks and it is believed he will get well, and probably he may, but he is a very sick man. He is very properly being treated by all the approved and most careful liquid nourishment per mouth and per rectum methods. His money gives out and he is taken to the City Hospital.

At the City Hospital there is a young man at the top, say a pupil of mine or a pupil of some other surgeon, who has done many abdominal sections, say, over one thousand. When the patient is seen by the Superintendent, or. if it were in my service at the Lutheran Hospital. my assistant or even the head nurse would have given an enema. a large enema with warm water and a roaring big dose of salts immediately on admission. I would have ordered this treatment continued after I had seen the case, most certainly if I saw a narrow pupil indicating that the patient had had opium or morphine. Need I say that in twelve hours there would be a different picture, the temperature will have fallen, the patient's abdomen will be flat, he will have an appetite, his pulse will be lower, he will fall into a healthy sleep and it will soon be plain to all concerned that a rapid recovery is to be expected. A case of peritonitis caused by appendicitis being treated just like the other. only substituting daily use of salts for the opium would probably never get into the miserable condition in which the above-quoted case was found on admission—simply because in the one case the used up and toxic matter, instead of being flushed out of the sewers. is confined in the intestinal tract and its lymphatics.

Now in order to clearly show what I am polemicizing, let me quote one of Ochsner's sentences which he offers with a view of reducing the mortality:

[1] The harmlessness depends to a great extent upon the technic. The length or method of closing the incision being most important.
[2] It will be admitted by all that nearly 95 per cent. of cases treated as peritonitis in those days were pure cases of appendicitis. These figures being nearly correct when speaking of male wards. in female wards the figures are slightly different. not referring to gall-bladder. stomach and other rarer conditions.

" Thesis 4.—In all cases of acute appendicitis, without regard to the treatment contemplated, the administration of food and cathartics by mouth should be absolutely prohibited and large enemata should never be given."

To this thesis or proposition I would offer the following amendment, or, rather, substitute:

In all cases of acute appendicitis the administration of food should be very scant, but cathartics and large enemata of warm water should be regularly given. In order to make a more perfect antithesis, I might add the phrase " without regard to the treatment contemplated," because even though an early operation be intended the purgation and the enema would greatly favor the patient, besides greatly facilitating the surgeon's work.

By contrasting the two sentences of advice the reader at once sees the difference and can decide which method he will follow in his practice. From the standpoint of a surgeon my experiences leave no room for doubt, the results will be vastly better when operating upon a case that has been regularly purged, than in those cases that have not been flushed out by cathartics and enemata. Acting upon this conviction I recommend my substitute to the general practitioner who may decide in favor of an expectant treatment of appendicitis.

For fear of being misunderstood, I will add that the ideal method of treament is the operative method, carried out in the beginning of the attack. If for some cause this time has been allowed to pass, then I also agree that the expectant treatment may come into consideration and will often give better results than the operation in late cases. The best time for operation having passed, the purgation treatment will give the best results and not the method which has by some been called the Ochsner method. This latter method looks like turning backward the hands of the clock in its progress, and ignoring the advances recently made in the art of medical practice, returning to a time now over twenty years past.

This is not the place to discuss the long-settled question of the possibility of purging a patient by means of cathartics into his own peritoneal cavity or cœloma. I rather think that the warning against cathartics and enemata is based upon a fear of rupturing an existing walled-off abscess into the cœloma or peritoneal cavity. But this danger seems to me quite as imaginary as the first mentioned and not really based upon well authenticated autopsies. But a discussion of these questions would lead us into experimental pathology and pathological anatomy.

I have seen many perforated appendices and the escaped fluid was always limited to the fluid contained in the appendix before the perforation. In 350 cases operated on during the last few years I have notes bearing on this question. In all of these cases cathartics had been given

before the operation and if they had not been given, I ordered them to be given, as well as enemata before making the operation. In no case did I ever see escape of intestinal contents, caused by the cathartic, either into the abscess cavity or the peritoneal cavity. Of course, the fluid, pus or at least purulent material had a fecal odor, in fact fecal concretions, coproliths and similar substances having fecal odor were often found. Only rarely would manual pressure upon the exposed cecum press out fecal contents and I am sure that cathartics would never expel contents of the intestine through a perforation as long as the abdomen is closed. The contents will always follow along the line of least resistance, which nature has wisely placed along the lumen of the intestine. Were it not for this provision of nature our efforts in abdominal surgery would amount to but little, for no kind of suture, ligature or union would hold against internal intestinal pressure.

Several other theses besides No. 4 are erroneous, notably No. 9, which says: " All practitioners of medicine and surgery as well as the general public, should be impressed with the importance of prohibiting the use of cathartics and food by mouth as well as the use of large enemata in cases suffering from acute appendicitis." In the interest of reducing the mortality this thesis should read: *All practitioners of medicine, and the public, if you like, should know that the proper treatment of acute appendicitis is by the regular use of cathartics and copious warm enemata and the restriction of food by mouth, to a minimum of liquid nourishment, and rest in bed with large, moist, warm, antiseptic poultices over the belly.*

Ochsner's thesis No. 2 is also misleading. I will quote it *in toto:* " No. 2.—Patients suffering from acute appendicitis should be operated on as soon as the diagnosis is made provided they come under treatment while infectious material is still confined to the appendix if a competent surgeon is available."

According to my observation, on opening the abdomen the infection will be found to have spread beyond the outer coat of the appendix and to have involved the adjacent intestines and their peritoneum in at least nine hundred and ninety cases out of any thousand cases. It may be that in ten of the cases the disease will be limited to the inside of the appendix in acute cases, in which the diagnosis is made by a competent man. In cases in which the infectious material is confined to the appendix there should be no postoperative mortality. I have not been so lucky as to find ten cases confined to the appendix in my entire life and I have seen over 1,700 appendices through an abdominal section. I do not agree that the diagnosis can be made with regularity and certainty as long as the infection is confined to the mucous or inner coat of the appendix, where it nearly always—I may say, where it always—starts.

This thesis No. 2 must be dropped because it deals with a condition that is rarely diagnosed. The other theses may pass, they deal with subjects that are well understood and I may say that I only wish to do away with the theses that oppose the use of cathartics, because I believe their regular use will very materially decrease the mortality of acute appendicitis, no matter by what other methods they are treated. My strong views against the use of opium are sufficiently well known, having been published and read before important societies, for instance the Oregon State as well as the Iowa R. R. Surgeons' Society as long ago as 1896 or even earlier.

A few words about statistics. I believe Ochsner's to be more true than most others, but I am constrained to say that but very little can be proven by statistics, because different men mean different things although they be talking or writing about the same thing. Just compare what I have said about thesis No. 2. Ochsner evidently does not mean to limit the operation to cases in which the infection is confined to the appendix. He would not see five acute cases of that variety per year, even though he has a wonderfully large material to select from. I do not wish to disparage the publication of statistics, but I merely wish to say that they cannot be used without much danger of error, no matter how truthful and careful the compilers may be, for the reason above given. The old saying that anything can be proven by statistics is still true and always will be true, as long as men compile them with the object of proving theories or results. I will therefore leave the test of the two opposing methods to the army of hard-working physicians, who will have to choose the method that seems to them most plausible. That good results will follow both methods is probably correct, but the purgation method, in my judgment, is the most preferable and will get better results than the method which I have been combating. How many per cent. the purgation method will cure I cannot state, because I do not believe in statistics. I could easily produce perfectly truthful statistics of cases treated by the expectant purgative method showing a very low mortality, but they would justly be regarded by others as I regard theirs. Let us remember that statistics are, after all is said and done, only ex parte evidence, be they "as true as gospel or even truer than that," as the great Christian Fenger once said to me.

American Bacteriologists.—According to *Science*, at the meeting of the Society of American Bacteriologists, held in Philadelphia on December 28, 1904, the following officers were elected: President, Prof. E. O. Jordan; Vice-President, Prof. S. C. Prescott; Secretary and Treasurer, Prof. E. P. Gorham; Council, Prof. F. G. Novy, Dr. Erwin F. Smith, Prof. F. D. Chester, Dr. J. J. Kinyoun; delegate to the council of the American Association for the Advancement of Science, Prof W. H. Welch.

OBSERVATIONS UPON THE MORPHOLOGY AND CLASSIFICATION OF THE MYCOBACTERIUM (Bacillus) TUBERCULOSIS.[1]

BY CHAS. F. CRAIG, M.D.,

OF SAN FRANCISCO, CAL.;

FIRST LIEUTENANT, ASSISTANT SURGEON, U. S. A., PATHOLOGIST AND BACTERIOLOGIST TO THE UNITED STATES ARMY GENERAL HOSPITAL, PRESIDIO OF SAN FRANCISCO, CALIFORNIA.

THE very radical changes which have occurred during recent years in our conception ot the position of the organism causing tuberculosis makes it of importance to put upon record any observations which assist in placing the organism upon a definite basis as regards classification. Until within a very recent date the organism concerned in the etiology of tuberculous disease was considered a typical example of a bacillus, but the researches of many investigators has definitely proven that it can no longer be classed as belonging to the group of bacilli, but is in all probability an *Actinomyces*.

In 1898, I described in the *Journal of Experimental Medicine*[1] the occurrence of branching in the tubercle bacillus. Previous to this time, in 1897,[2] I had described certain other variations in in the morphology of this organism, and since that time have been especially interested during the routine examination of specimens of tuberculosis sputum, in observing the great number of departures from the classical description of this organism as given in text-books upon bacteriology. During my service in this laboratory I have preserved 509 specimens of sputum from as many cases of tuberculosis, with special reference to a careful study of the morphology of the organism. I have been very greatly impressed with the effect which a tropical climate seems to have upon the growth of this organism, as evidenced by its structure. Almost all the specimens which I have examined have been obtained from soldiers returning from the Philippine Islands, at least 480 of the specimens being from that number of cases of tuberculosis which have been invalided home from Manila. The study of this question is of importance both from a scientific and a practical standpoint. From a scientific standpoint, the great variations which occur in the morphology of the parasite would seem to indicate that it does not belong to the group of organisms known as bacilli, but rather to some higher group, and from a practical standpoint the study is valuable because a large number of the specimens showed organisms which depart so radically from the descriptions given that unless one is prepared to accept them, they would hardly be diagnosed as tubercle bacilli. The study of this question is also of importance because of the attention which is being given just at this time to the variations between the tuberculous organisms of man and animals, as the variations observed in the organism occurring in the human sputum, so far as the morphology is con-

[1] Published with permission of the Surgeon-General of the United States Army. From the Annual Report of the United States Army General Hospital Presidio, San Francisco, Cal., 1904.

cerned, are greater even than those observed in the mammalian and human organisms.

As generally described, the tubercle bacillus consists of a slender, straight or slightly curved rod, one-half to two-thirds as long as the diameter of the red blood corpuscle. As a rule, it stains readily with special stains used for this purpose, but here and there unstained areas are observed within it, which by some authorities have been regarded as spores, but that they are spores is not accepted by the best observers. This classical description of the organism certainly applies in a great majority of instances to those observed in sputum of patients contracting the disease in temperate regions, although even in these regions very great departures from the classical description are by no means rare. In my experience, however, with the organism as it occurs in the sputum of patients returning from the tropics, this description is very inadequate, as in almost all specimens organisms are seen which differ so radically from it that it has often seemed as though other organisms were being observed. It is this effect of the tropics upon the growth of the organism, as shown by its morphology, that I would especially call attention to. It would seem that the greater moisture and heat of such regions enables the organisms to grow very luxuriously, and in forms which are not usually met with in the sputum of patients in temperate climates. It is a well-known fact that cases of tuberculosis in the tropics run a rapidly fatal course. This must, of course, be due to the greater multiplication of the organisms, their greater virulence and size; and, if anything can be told from the morphological appearance of an organism as to its virulence, certainly the organisms seen in the sputum of these cases bear out the well-known clinical facts.

Variations in Length.—The greatest variations occur in the length of the organisms, some being so short as to be almost like cocci, but the majority much longer than those usually found. Long filamentous forms are very common, at least 75 per cent. of the sputums which have been examined showing them. This form is not uncommon in old cultures, but is rare in sputum in cases occurring in this country. These long filamentous forms stain well, but often present a beaded appearance due to unstained intervals within them. They are generally slightly curved and often are curved in opposite directions two or three times in their course. I have seen these organisms so long that if they had been stained alone, without others of more typical appearance surrounding them, a diagnosis of tubercle bacilli would not have been made. A very common appearance observed in the long form is a deeply staining dot at one end somewhat broader than the organism itself, thus giving it a slightly clubbed appearance.

Very short organisms are often present and these are generally much thicker than the long ones. This difference in thickness is very marked

in some instances. It is not due to the opposition of one or two organisms, because the most careful focusing fails to reveal any distinction, the organism staining solidly throughout. Many organisms are seen of the typical length, and it should be understood that no one specimen presents organisms of one length, but in almost every specimen will be found long filamentous forms, the very short forms, and those of ordinary length.

Variations in Breadth.—One of the most notable variations occurring in tubercle bacilli in the sputum of patients from the tropics has been increase of breadth. As ordinarily seen the tubercle bacillus is remarkable for its delicacy, the breadth being in many cases very slight. In the majority of specimens, however, in patients from the tropics, the organism is quite thick, certainly three or four times as thick as those observed in the sputum of cases in this country. These thickened organisms stain very deeply and do not, as a rule, show the unstained areas which are so noticeable in many specimens.

Variations in Contour.—Beside the classical bacilli which answer to the description given in the text-books, specimens of sputum from these cases show very great variation in the contour of the organism. Very many specimens show organisms which present in some portion of their length a well-marked knob. Others are swollen at the end or toward the center, while many are completely bent, forming a letter U or S. Curved forms are very common, the curves generally being very well marked.

Variations in Staining Power.—Most of the organisms observed in these cases stain very intensely and retain the stain under the most severe acid treatment. There are numerous instances in which the stain is interrupted, leaving unstained areas irregular in shape, and often distinct interruptions are observed extending entirely across the organism, thus giving it the appearance of a chain of cocci. Very deeply staining areas are often observed, especially at the ends of the long forms. These areas are generally greater in diameter than the rest of the organism.

A brief description will here be given of the most common departures from the classical type, as observed in the sputum from the class of cases mentioned:

1. *The Streptococcic Form.*—I have applied this name to this type of the organism because in the stained specimens it resembles a chain of streptococci. This appearance is due to an interruption of the stain, the result being a chain of deeply stained areas alternating with unstained intervals. If such forms occurred alone in the sputum and the decolorizing agent was not used to differentiate them, they would invariably be taken for streptococci, but as numerous other organisms are always present which are more typical in structure, this mistake will not readily be made. These unstained intervals in the para-

site have been regarded by some authorities as spores, but a careful examination will show that these intervals are not spore-shaped, and that no method used for the demonstration of spores will stain them. This form of the organism is much more difficult to differentiate than the form which shows slight unstained intervals, but with a narrow stained band connecting the stained portion. This band or enveloping material in such instances retains the stain, but in the streptococci form it does not. The length of this form of the organism varies considerably, sometimes being very short and sometimes almost filamentous. In the latter case the resemblance to a chain of streptococci is still more marked.

2. *The Clubbed Form.*—As I have already mentioned, numerous instances are seen in which the end of the bacillus is enlarged and takes the stain very deeply. Such organisms resemble very much the clubbed form of the diphtheria bacillus and also certain forms of actinomycetes. Very often these clubbed organisms will be seen collected in masses. Careful focusing will demonstrate that many of them are branched and interlaced. These organisms generally stain very well throughout their entire length, but there are unstained intervals, minute in size, scattered along them. The clubbed extremity always stains much more intensely than the remainder of the organism.

3. *Budding Forms.*—In at least two-thirds of the sputums examined. this form of the organism has been found if it was looked for long enough. It consists of a rather long rod at one or more portions of which there occurs a distinct enlargement or knob. projecting laterally. This enlargement stains deeply and is rounded in appearance. The enlargements occur most frequently in the filamentous forms. sometimes three or more being seen in one organism. This budding. as I have termed it. is undoubtedly the first stage of branching which has occurred so frequently in the organisms found in patients returning from the tropics, and which will now be described.

4. *Branching Forms.*—In 1898[3] I described true branching tubercle bacilli occurring in the sputum, which was the first description. I believe. of this form of the organism occurring in this country. Previous to my description a considerable amount of attention had been paid to this form of the parasite by Coppen Jones and Fischel. At that time I considered branching as an exceedingly rare occurrence, and that it was probably due to diminished virulence of the organisms, as such forms are not very uncommon in old cultures. Since then I have paid especial attention to this form of the organism and have been impressed with the great frequency with which it occurs in the sputum of tuberculous cases which have originated in the tropics. In over 80 per cent. of the cases which I have examined branching forms of the tubercle bacillus have been demonstrated in the sputum. They occur

with such frequency that I believe them to be a normal development of the organism under certain conditions, being most often present in cases occurring in a tropical climate. I have been able to trace in very many specimens the entire stage of growth of the branching form from the budding forms to the fully developed filamentous branch. The first stage of the process is the budding form which has already been described. The next stage consists in an outgrowth of the bud into a short branch. The number of branches present vary, some organisms showing but one, others two or three, or even more, growing at an angle from the parent organism. In this early stage they are generally shorter than the parent body and stain uniformly throughout, although the parent organism may show unstained areas. The organisms showing branching are always longer than those surrounding them, and it may be said that branching only occurs in the long filamentous forms. They resist decolorizing solutions much more effectively than do the unbranching parasites.

From this young branching form to the fully developed branching organism is simply a question of growth, the branch extending in length until it finally, in many instances. becomes longer than the parent body, and itself sends off other branches, so that in many instances an interlacing network is formed, due to the luxuriant branching of the organism. Of these fully developed branch forms there are many variations. Sometimes only one long branch is given off, sometimes two or more. Very often one or more long branches will be seen accompanied by several bodies. indicating the commencement of other branches. The fully developed branches often show unstained intervals similar to those in the parent organism. Where this branching has occured in two or more organisms which lie near one another, a mass of organisms is formed in which the branches interlace and produce the appearance of an actinomycotic growth. Many specimens of sputum show these large masses of bacilli, and the appearance presented is so entirely diverse from what one would expect to see in tuberculous sputum that if other organisms were not present which were more typical in appearance, one would believe that the patient was affected with actinomycosis. In my observations, it has been possible to trace in the sputum the entire process of branching from the knobbed forms to the formation of mycelial groups. The organism which is destined to present this change becomes longer than usual and presents at some portion one or more knob-like outgrowths. These outgrowths gradually lengthen, and at last become true branches, and they in turn are capable of budding and giving off other branches.

This process should be carefully distinguished from the false branching which is often present. due to the apposition of the end of one bacillus to some portion of the length of another. This, at first sight, gives the appearance of true branching, but careful focusing will always demonstrate that there are two separate organisms concerned instead of one.

Significance of Variations in Morphology.— The question now arises, What do these peculiar forms of the organism of tuberculosis indicate? From this very short description of the variations in morphology of this parasite it will be seen that it is not a morphological unit, but that during its growth it is capable of assuming many forms, some of which are not those which are common to organisms classed as bacilli. In the first place, the occurrence in a class of cases where the conditions are most favorable as regards the growth of bacteria, would seem to indicate that these changes are not degenerative in character, but that instead they indicate a very free and luxuriant development. The view that they are degenerative in character is advocated by A. Fischer,[4] who believes that they are involution forms, but there are several objections to this view, the most important being that they are not limited to old cultures which have undergone loss of virulence, but are present in rapidly advancing cases of the disease in the sputum, and that in their staining reactions they do not differ from the typical appearing organisms. From my observations I am convinced that the occurrence of these forms necessitates some change in our views as to the classification of this parasite. Klein[5] believes that the branching is a reversion to an ancestral type which presented mycelial growth. Fischel[6] has pointed out the analogy between these forms and the actinomyces, and both he and Coppen Jones,[7] who have studied these forms very extensively, believe that they belong to the same group of organisms. Bruns[8] regards them as involution forms when observed under parasitic conditions. He says: "They pertain to the saprophytic growth form of a higher organism, which as a parasite in the animal body appears in the form of rods." The only objection to his theory is that these forms occur so frequently in the sputum of human beings, in my experience, that they can hardly be regarded as abnormal, and that they depend for their occurrence upon certain favorable circumstances which are not present as a rule in the human body. The description in recent years of certain lung infections due to the *Streptothricæ* has led several authors to express the opinion that the tubercle bacillus is very closely allied to this organism. Kruse[9] is inclined to believe that they should be placed under it, and Johan-Olsan[10] distinctly places the tubercle bacillus under the *Streptothricæ*. This group is especially characterized by branched filamentous forms or organisms, and is placed between the bacteria proper and hyphomycetes. Lehmann and Neumann[11] in their "Principles of Bacteriology," have classed the tubercle bacillus under the actinomyces and have given it the name *Mycobacterium tuberculosis*. From my observations, I am inclined to agree with this

classification, as I do not believe, in the light of our present knowledge, that the organism can any longer be considered as a bacillus. It answers in every way to the description of the actinomyces, as it presents true branching, the club formation and mycelial formation. In sections of tissue Friedrich[12] found collections of this organism forming dense. radiating groups, which answer in every way to those which I have observed in the sputum. In view of the fact that these forms occur so often and are so entirely different in their morphology from bacilli, it would seem that the retention of the name of bacillus for this organism, except because it is so well known and recognized, is not scientific, for the parasite undoubtedly belongs to the group of actinomyces, and the name given it by Lehmann and Neumann is much more correct from the botanical standpoint. The science of bacteriology is hampered by unscientific classifications, and any observations which will enable us to make these classifications more correct botanically are of the greatest service. It is of little practical importance whether the tubercle bacillus shall be known by that name or by some other, but it is of great importance from a scientific standpoint. An organism which presents such great variations in its morphology should no longer be classed among the simple bacilli, as such a classification gives an entirely erroneous idea of its appearance. The forms which I have described should be known, as their occurrence in small numbers and unaccompanied by the typical organism as described in the text-books would, without doubt, lead to an erroneous diagnosis and great injustice to the patient. For this reason I have called attention briefly to the variations which the organism presents, especially in the sputum of cases contracting the disease in the tropics, and I believe that futher observation will only prove that this organism is very pleomorphous and should no longer be classed as a bacillus. In a future report I shall describe more at length the various forms which I have mentioned, together with observations on the virulence of sputum containing such forms.

BIBLIOGRAPHY.

1. Journal of Experimental Medicine, Vol. III, No. 3, 1898.
2. Medicine, June, 1897.
3. Journal of Experimental Medicine, Vol. III, No. 3, 1898.
4. Vorlesungen über Bakterien, Jena, 1897, p. 25.
5. Annual Report of Local Government Board, 1889, p. 203.
6. Untersuchungen über Morphologie u. Biologie d. Tuberculoseerregers. Wien, 1893.
7. Centralblatt für Bact., XIII (1893), XVII (1895), XX (1896).
8. Centralblatt für Bakt., XVII (1895).
9. Flügges. Die Micro-organismen. 2. Th., Leipzig, 1806.
10. Centralblatt für Bakt., Abth. II, 111 (1897).
11. Principles of Bacteriology. Saunders & Co., 1903.
12. Deutsche med. Wochenschrift, 1897.

Winnipeg General Hospital.—Dr. A. M. Campbell was appointed medical superintendent of the Winnipeg General Hospital at the last regular monthly meeting of the Board of Governors. The number of patients treated in January, 1905, was 593, as against 483 for the same month in 1904. The number of deaths amounted to 40, as against 19 for the same month in the previous year.

CLINICAL STUDIES IN URETERIC MEATOSCOPY.[12]

BY WALTER C. KLOTZ, M.D.,

OF NEW YORK.

THE importance of ureteral catheterization in determining the functional activity of the healthy kidney, and as an aid to diagnosis in renal disease has been generally recognized. At the same time this method possesses some disadvantages and certain limitations. While in most cases it can readily be carried out, it may be very difficult and tedious, and in some instances it is quite impossible. It has also been found that the information in regard to lesions of the kidney, obtained by means of the ureter catheter is occasionally disappointing. Thus a chemical and physical examination of the separated urines, offers a valuable means of determining the source of pus, blood or bacteria present in the urine,—but in some cases of renal disease, the urine is negative, and under such circumstances, a differentiation of the urine is obviously useless. Again, if the ureter is wholly or partially obstructed, the complete absence of or a marked relative diminution in the quantity of the urine from one side, may be a valuable sign, but care must be taken to ascertain that the catheter is not occluded with pus or mucus, and it must be borne in mind, that even in health both kidneys do not always secrete the same amount of urine in the same time. Used as a probe the catheter may detect an obstruction of the ureter, but it is not always possible to decide by this means whether such an obstruction is due to stricture, a calculus, or a kinking of the ureter. The ureteral catheter may pass a calculus in the ureter, without meeting with any obstruction, especially if the ureter is dilated or sacculated, while a calculus in the pelvis, of the kidney, can very rarely be detected by palpation with a ureter probe, particularly when a male cystoscope is employed.

On the other hand, valuable information can often be obtained, by the simple cystoscopic inspection of the ureteric orifices. It is possible in this way not only to note the escape of pus or blood from one or the other ureter and whether one or both kidneys are secreting urine, but it has also been observed, that in cases of renal disease, the ureteric orifice on the same side presents an appearance, differing distinctly from that of the normal. While these changes have been regarded as characteristic of certain conditions in the kidney, their exact clinical significance has remained undetermined. The subject seemed of sufficient surgical interest to demand further investigation, for if reliable data could be obtained without catheterizing the ureters, it would be a distinct advantage. With a view of determining how far these changes could be relied upon as a means of diagnosis in diseases of the kidney, and encouraged by Fenwicks' recent work along the same lines I have during the last year more carefully noted the cystoscopic findings in cases referred to me for ureteral catheterization, on account of suspected renal disease. At the same time I have endeavored to compare the value of both methods under similar conditions. At present only a small number of cases have been subjected to critical study, and in this preliminary report, no attempt will be made to draw any positive conclusions or to set up any fixed rules for the interpretation of the changes in the ureteric orifices, described more fully in connection with the clinical histories reported below.

In the following cases, most of which occurred in my service as cystoscopist to Roosevelt Hospital, I shall present only the bare facts, and in order to make these reports as brief as possible, I have included only such features as have a direct bearing on the cystoscopic examination. I am indebted to the gentleman referred to under each case for the use of clinical data and the reports of operations.

The first group comprises 12 cases of nephrolithiasis. This condition was the one most frequently encountered, and at the same time it is one in which the diagnosis is often most difficult.

Case I. M. W., female, aged thirty-five years; private patient of Dr. N. W. Green. History of partial suppression and pain in region of kidney on right side. Urine contains few red blood cells, but no pus, symptoms improved under general treatment. Cystoscopy, January 30, 1904, bladder normal, left ureteric orifice normal, secreting clear urine, right ureteric area occupied by a circumscribed swelling of reddened and edematous mucous membrane, almost obliterating the ureteric orifice situated at the summit of the tumor, no efflux or urine noted. Diagnosis: Renal calculus. Operation report: Small calculus in pelvis of right kidney.

Case II.—M. S., male, aged thirty years; patient on Dr. Brewer's service, Roosevelt Hospital. History of renal colic right side, X-ray shows shadow over lower third of right ureter. Cystoscopy, March 1, 1904, bladder normal, left ureteric orifice normal, secreting clear urine, right ureteric orifice shows redness and edema of surrounding mucous membrane, lips of orifice swollen, almost obliterating the actual orifice, efflux of urine cloudy, left ureter catheterized but catheter obstructed about 1 cm. in the ureter, right ureter could not be entered by catheter. Diagnosis: Calculus in kidney or ureter. Operation report, large mulberry calculus in lower third of right ureter.

Case III.—M. R., male; aged fifty-six years; patient on Dr. Brewer's service, Roosevelt Hospital. History of renal colic left side, urine contains pus and granular sediment. Cystoscopy, August 11, 1904; bladder normal, few calculous fragments, right ureteric orifice normal, secreting clear urine, left ureteric orifice shows a distinct elevation of mucous membrane, the lips everted and edematous, and the surrounding surface of the interureteric fold red and congested;

[1] From the Out-Patient Department, Roosevelt Hospital, New York.
[2] Read before the Surgical Section of the New York Academy of Medicine, January 6, 1905.

no efflux noted (Fig. 1). Left ureter catheterized, and catheter passed up 14 inches, no urine obtained after waiting one hour. Diagnosis: Calculus, impacted in pelvis or upper end of ureter. Operation report: Small kidney, calculus in pelvis of kidney, complete stricture of ureter about two inches below pelvis.

Case IV.—M. M., male; aged forty-six years; patient on Dr. Brewer's service, Roosevelt Hospital. History of renal colic on right side; X-ray shows shadow over right kidney, urine contains pus. Cystoscopy: August 12, 1904; trigone of bladder red and congested, right ureteric orifice lips elevated swollen and edematous, margins of orifice eroded, no efflux of urine noted, left ureteric orifice, also shows some eversion, edema and slight redness, but no erosion. Both ureters catheterized, on both sides the catheters could be passed to pelves of kidney. The urine from the left side was clear and of

velt Hospital. History of attacks of pain over the course of the left ureter for several years. X-ray shows small shadow over lower third of left ureter, urine negative. Cystoscopy, December 16, 1904: Bladder shows trabeculation of posterior wall, both ureteric orifices normal, both ureters catheterized, on right side the catheter could be passed up the usual distance of 15 inches, on the left side the catheter was passed the full length or 20 inches without meeting with any resistance, the urine from the right side was clear and of good quantity, considerably less urine was secreted from the left side. Diagnosis: Dilatation of left ureter, no signs of calculus. Operation report: Small stone adjacent to, but outside the wall of the ureter in its lower third, stricture of ureter, chronic ureteritis.

It is probable, that in this case the ureter catheter on the side of the lesion was doubled up by the stricture of the ureter, and in this

Fig. 1.

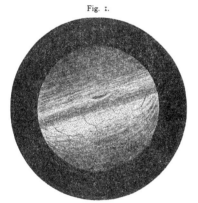

Normal Right Ureteric Orifice (Case III).

Fig. 2.

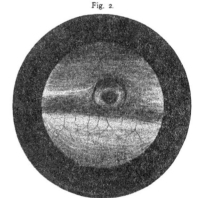

Left Ureteric Orifice, Everted and Edematous, Renal Calculus (Case VII).

good quantity,· the urine from the right side was scanty, and contained much pus. Diagnosis: Calculus of right kidney. Left kidney normal. Operation report: Large branching calculus in pelvis of right kidney. Further history and subsequent operation disclosed calculus imbedded in cortical abscess in left kidney.

Case V.—M. B., female; age thirty years; private patient of Dr. Brewer. History of repeated attacks of renal colic on the right side, X-ray shows constant shadow over right ureter, urine clear, no pus, no red blood cells. Cystoscopy, October 19, 1904: Bladder normal, both ureteric orifices normal, but somewhat large and open, both kidneys secreting clear urine, both ureters catheterized, urine from both sides clear, and of good quality. Diagnosis negative. No operation.·

Case VI.—M. D., male; aged forty-three years; patient of Dr. Brewer's service, Roose-

way the apparent great length of the ureter might be explained.

Case VII.—H. M., female; aged twenty-six years; patient on Dr. Blake's service, Roosevelt Hospital. History of renal colic on left side accompanied be dark color of urine, symptoms subsided under general treatment, at time of examination urine was clear and contained no pus and no red blood cells. Cystoscopy, October 27, 1904: Both ureteric orifices normal, typical in form (Fig. 2), both ureters catheterized, and catheters passed to pelvis of kidneys, urine from both sides clear and good quality, otherwise negative. No operation.

Case · VIII.—M. T., male; age thirty-seven years; private patient of Dr. N. W. Green. History of renal calculus, perinephritic abscess and nephrotomy four years ago, since then has pyuria and occasional attacks of dull pain in lumbar region. 'Cystoscopy, February 12, 1904: Mucous membrane of trigone and base of bladder red and congested, areas of congestion on posterior wall, no ulceration, no calculus, urine very cloudy, pus and bacteria, no casts. Right ureteric orifice normal but small, no efflux of urine noted, left ureteric orifice normal, secreting clear urine. Right ureter catheterized, catheter passed up 15 inches, no urine obtained after waiting one hour. Diagnosis: Chronic cystitis following old calculous pyelitis; right kidney not functionating. No operation, irrigations of bladder, urinary antiseptics, slow improvement.

Case. IX.—V. S., female; aged twenty-eight years; patient on Dr. Blake's service, Roosevelt Hospital. History of pain over left kidney, X-ray shows doubtful shadow over left kidney, urine clear, no pus, no blood cells. Cystoscopy, November 13, 1904: Bladder normal except region of trigone on the left side which presents a stippled red appearance, like multiple, punctate, submucous hemorrhages, the lips of the left ureteric orifice were somewhat edematous, but not characteristically elevated or everted, the right ureteric orifice was normal, but very small, efflux of clear urine. Right ureter catheterized, urine clear and good quantity, attempts to catheterize left ureter abandoned on account of pain to patient. Diagnosis: Irritation of left renal pelvis, probably due to stone. Operation report negative; no calculus in pelvis or ureter, kidney healthy.

In this case as well as in the following, it is possible that a small calculus was passed before the operation, as in both cases there were typical clinical symptoms of renal calculus.

Case X.—M. B., male; aged twenty-eight years, patient on Dr. Brewer's service, Roosevelt Hospital. History of typical attacks of severe renal colic. X-ray negative. Urine clear, a little pus, and a few red blood cells. Cystoscopy, December 19, 1904: Right ureteric orifice normal, secreting clear urine, left ureteric orifice shows very marked circumscribed swelling of mucous membrane with intense edema, orifice almost completely obliterated, in attempting to catheterize the ureter, the catheter could be engaged in the orifice, but resisted all attempts to push it into the ureter. Right ureter readily catheterized, good quantity of urine collected. Diagnosis: Calculus in lower extremity of ureter. Operation report no stone found in kidney or ureter.

Case XI.—M. S., male; aged forty-four years; patient Dr. Brewer's service, Roosevelt Hospital. History of renal colic on left side, and of having passed stones, urine contains pus and red blood cells. Cystoscopy, January 2, 1905: Few calculous fragments in bladder, left ureteric orifice, large open, elliptical, lips everted and edematous, efflux purulent. Right ureteric orifice normal, secreting clear urine. Urethra too small to admit catheterizing instrument. Diagnosis: Renal calculus, and pyelitis left side. Operation de-

ferred. (Operation, since reading of paper, showed extensive pyonephrosis.)

Case XII.—M. S., male; aged thirty-five years; patient on Dr. Brewer's service, Roosevelt Hospital. History of renal pain, and attacks of colic, has frequently passed stones, urine very purulent and contains granular sediment. Cystoscopy, January 2, 1905: Left ureteric orifice, normal but somewhat open and rounder than usual, right ureteric orifice normal, somewhat longer than left. Both ureters catheterized, Urine from right sde clear, urine from left side very turbid and cloudy, contains much pus. Diagnosis: Pyelitis left side. Operation deferred.

Similar changes were noted in the ureteric orifice in cases of renal tuberculosis and pyonephrosis as shown in the following histories.

Case XIII.—W. W., male; aged sixteen years; private patient of Dr. Brewer. History of fre-

Fig. 3.

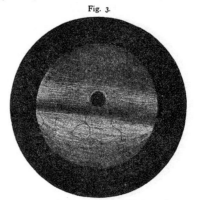

Left Ureteric Orifice, "Golf-Holed," Renal Tuberculosis (Case XIV).

quency of micturition, tubercle bacilli found in the urine, pain on right side. Cystoscopy, August 1, 1904.: Mucous membrane of trigone red and congested, right ureteric orifice swollen and distinctly reddened, margins ulcerated. Left ureteric orifice normal, left ureter catheterized, urine clear, contains no tubercle bacilli. Diagnosis: Tuberculosis, right kidney. Operation report: Scattered tubercles in right kidney.

Case XIV.—M. O. B., male; aged twenty-eight years, patient on Dr. Brewer's service, Roosevelt Hospital. History: Frequency of micturition on right side, urine contains pus and tubercle bacilli. Cystoscopy, October 28, 1904: Prostate swollen and congested, bladder normal, right ureteric orifice appears as a normal slit, the mucous membrane immediately external to it is deeply congested and thrown into market folds (Fig. 3), giving it a papillomatous appearance. The left ureteric orifice appears as an open round hole without any eversion or pouting of the lips (golf-hole type) the surrounding mucous membrane is normal (Fig. 4). Both ureters catheterized, the urine from the right side was negative the urine from the left side contained tubercle bacilli. Diagnosis: Tuberculosis of left kidney, possibly also of right. No operation.

In this case the appearance of the mucous membrane in the vicinity of the right ureteric orifice, while the orifice itself was normal and the urine from that side contained no tubercle bacilli, might be explained by the jets of tuberculous urine from the left kidney, being thrown against the mucous membrane of the opposite side and in thus producing an infection of this region of the bladder.

Case XV.—K. K., female; aged thirty-three years; patient on Dr. Blake's service, Roosevelt Hospital. History of renal pain on the right

Fig. 4.

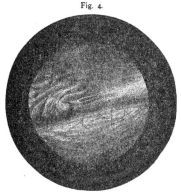

Right Ureteric Orifice Surrounded by Tuberculous Inflammation (Case XIV).

side, urine is cloudy and contains pus, no tubercle bacilli. X-ray negative. Cystoscopy, December 30, 1904: Bladder shows evidence of former cystitis, right ureter surrounded by a group of small, rounded, nodular tumors, a further group of similar tumors extends from the ureteric orifice toward the center of the trigone. The left ureteric orifice is normal. The whole trigone is markedly swollen and congested. Both ureters catheterized, no urine collected from right side, urine from left side clear and good quantity. Diagnosis: Pyelonephritis right side. Operation report: Pyonephrosis. (Probably tuberculosis.)

Case XVI.—M. D., female; aged about forty years; patient on Dr. Brewer's service, Roosevelt Hospital. History of a previous operation for abdominal and pelvic abscess, general sepsis, pyuria. Cystoscopy, September 1, 1904: Bladder normal, both ureteric orifices normal, both ureters catheterized, urine from left side clear

and good quantity, urine from right side very scanty and purulent. Diagnosis: Pyelonephritis. Operation report: Pyonephritis, right kidney.

Case XVII.—M. G., male; aged thirty-five years; patient Dr. Brewer's service, Roosevelt Hospital. History of typical attacks of renal colic right side, congenital pinhole meatus of urethra. Urine contains some pus. Cystoscopy, October 13, 1904: Prostate enlarged and congested, bladder much dilated, posterior wall trabeculated. Right ureteric orifice appears as an elongated elliptical opening with rigid thickened edges, no efflux noted. Left ureteric orifice normal. Right ureter shows obstruction to further passage of catheter, about one centimeter from vesical end, no urine collected, left ureter catheterized, urine clear and good quantity. Diagnosis: dilatation of bladder, ureter and pelvis, stricture of ureter, near vesical end, right kidney probably diseased from back pressure. Operation report: Kidney normal, pelvis not dilated, complete stricture of ureter 14 inches below pelvis.

Case XVIII.—M. N., male; aged twenty-five years; personal, O. P. D. Roosevelt Hospital. History of frequent micturition, no urethritis, no cystitis, pain in right lumbar region, urine clear, no tubercle bacilli. Cystoscopy, November 12, 1904: Bladder normal, left ureteric orifice normal, right ureteric orifice large, open, oval in shape, lips thickened, both kidneys secreting clear urine. Diagnosis: Probable dilatation of pelvis, cause unknown. No operation—further observation.

Case XIX.—M. H. male; aged forty-one years; personal O. P. D. Roosevelt Hospital. Frequency of micturition, four times at night, some cough, has had urethritis urine clear, no pus, no blood, no tubercle bacilli. Cystoscopy, December 3, 1904: Trigone and left interureteric fold red and congested, left ureteric orifice shows distinct, rounded, conical elevation, orifice itself small and round, secreting clear urine; right ureteric orifice normal, secreting clear urine. Diagnosis: No positive opinion; some affection of left kidney. No operation—further observation.

Case XX.—M. B., male; aged thirty-four years; personal O. P. D. Roosevelt Hospital. History: Pain in lumbar region, has had urethritis and stricture, urine contains some pus. Cystoscopy, December 15, 1904: Bladder normal except for some redness and congestion in region of trigone; prostate moderately enlarged and congested; both ureteric orifices normal; both ureters catheterized; urine from both sides abundant and clear. Diagnosis: Prostatitis. No operation; local treatment.

Taking up the results obtained in the above series of cases, and considering only the eleven cases in which lesions of the kidney were found at operation, it will be found that in four out of five cases of nephrolithiasis changes were noted in the ureteric orifice on the diseased side. In the case in which no change was noted in the ureteric orifice, the calculus was found outside the wall of the ureter and had probably existed in this situation for some time. In the two cases of suspected nephrolithiasis (Cases IX and X) in which changes were noted in the ureteric orifices and in which no stone was found at operation, it is possible that a stone was passed either just before cystoscopy, or between the time of cystoscopy and operation. In the remaining six confirmed cases of renal disease, changes were found in the ureteric orifice in five. In the case in which ureteric meatoscopy was negative, ureteral catheterization was of distinct service. ,

While these figures cannot be accepted as a basis for any conclusions, the results so far would show that even if ureteric meatoscopy cannot replace ureteral catheterization in all cases, it may frequently furnish additional information and be of great service in those cases where ureteral catheterization cannot be carried out. It is to be expected also that with increased observation, it will be possible to make finer distinctions as to the appearance of the ureteric orifices and to more confidently draw inferences, as to their clinical significance. But before ureteric meatoscopy can be placed upon an absolutely safe clinical basis it will be necessary to definitely settle the following questions: What constitutes a normal and an abnormal ureteric orifice? What are the causes of any pathological changes, whether in a given case these causes exist in the kidney, the pelvis or the ureter? And, finally, whether the absence of change in the ureteric orifice is of any value in making a negative diagnosis? For the present these questions must remain unanswered.

SPRAINS OF THE KNEE AND ANKLE-JOINTS.[1]

BY J. T. WILSON, M.D.,

OF SHERMAN, TEXAS.

THE frequency of these injuries, the acute suffering produced and the occasional bad results following, suggested the subject of this paper and serve as an apology for it.

In the treatment nothing original or new is presented, but the management which has seemed productive of the greatest relief, which has given most satisfaction and been generally adopted is emphasized. These sprains are produced in a variety of ways and of every degree, the lesions involving for the most part the ligaments by which the joints are held together. In treating sprains of the knee and ankle-joints it is necessary to have in view at least the general outlines, of the anatomy of these joints for their more comprehensive and intelligent management. Both are complex joints of the ginglymoid variety. The knee is composed of the condyles of the femur, head of the tibia and patella whose articular surfaces are covered with cartilage, and it

1 Read before the North Texas Medical Association, December 13, 1904.

will be remembered that these are held together by fourteen ligaments all firmly attached, which make it one of the strongest joints. The synovial membrane is the largest and most extensive of any joint in the body, is a serous membrane and when injured liable to serious pathological changes. The joint is well supplied with blood vessels and nerves; tendons of the muscles of the thigh are distributed about the articulation and four of them inserted into the patella. Its chief movements are flexion and extension with slight rotary. The ligamentum patella is the only ligament put upon the stretch during flexion, all the others are relaxed. Owing to the great amount of flexion of the leg upon the thigh, the two being brought in actual contact with ease, it is much more difficult to injure this ligament; on the other hand since in extension the ligamentum patella is relaxed and all the others are stretched, extension being limited to a certain extent, it will be readily seen that in this position serious injury can be inflicted with a moderate amount of force. Usually these injuries are caused by extensive violence, but occasionally we meet with one of considerable severity the result of an apparently insignificant twist. In slight sprains there may be only stretching of one or more ligaments, in severe sprains there is more or less laceration of the ligaments and bruising of the parts, rupture of some of the small arterial branches and nerves or nerve filaments, followed by more or less effusion, occasionally there is displacement of a ligament, or a scale of bone may be torn off; some of the cases may be complicated with dislocation or fracture and it is always important when there is much swelling and deformity to examine carefully for these complications. It may be necessary to use an anesthetic to make the diagnosis certain, but it is entirely justifiable. A correct knowledge of the condition will guide us in the management and upon it also may depend the results. A failure to arrive at a correct diagnosis has been the cause of improper treatment, leaving permanent injury and deformity. When the swelling and tenderness is extensive a correct diagnosis is often difficult, but these should be reduced and the diagnosis made as soon as practicable. A bad sprain is more difficult to recover from and takes a longer time, frequently, than a simple fracture.

Any serious trouble with a joint is liable to involve the bone and its periosteal covering. There is also the possibility of infection which would render the complication a grave one.

The immediate effect of a sprain of the knee is considerable pain, sometimes of a sickening character, an effusion, possibly part hemorrhage, and swelling progressing rapidly, rupture of one or more ligaments possibly including the capsular ligament. If the synovial membrane is involved to a considerable extent it renders recovery more tedious. "If a joint unsupported is painful when used, but painless when properly supported it is an indication of laceration or severe stretching of supporting ligaments."[1] It is difficult to estimate how much damage is done to a joint in severe sprains, but it varies and depends largely upon the direction of the force, if it is applied to the knee in a state of extension, the damage will be greater in proportion to the degree of violence, and here in addition to stretching and laceration there may be displacement or a detachment of an articular cartilage. It is of great importance to know if there is a bone lesion to complicate the case.

The more promptly treatment is commenced after the accident the better the results obtained. I have found that if the patient is seen early, immersion of the part in very hot water will bring speedy relief from the pain. As it is very inconvenient to immerse the knee, flannel cloths saturated with water as hot as can be borne with which the knee is enveloped and covered with a dry cloth, oil cloth or rubber tissue, form an excellent substitute. This can be kept up by having two cloths; as fast as one begins to get a little cool it is replaced by the other, the water in which they are dipped being kept almost at the boiling point, and the application continued for from forty minutes to an hour. If not only relieves pain but retards swelling. If there is a simple contusion, a stretching of the tissues without laceration, a gentle massage for ten or fifteen minutes, followed by the Cotterell dressing, e.g., strapping the joints with strips of adhesive plaster firmly applied longitudinally, beginning six or eight inches above and extending as far below the knee, overlapping each other and surrounded by a well-fitting roller bandage, is the most effective and satisfactory treatment. The patient can with the aid of a crutch or cane walk around to a limited degree with but little discomfort. With a more extensive injury the rubber plaster can be applied both in a circular and longitudinal direction, the popliteal space being properly protected. This is not an immovable dressing, and while it supports the parts very nicely it admits of a limited amount of motion which is desirable in this character of sprain. The patient is advised not to bear too much weight upon the limb and is restricted in the amount of walking. This dressing can be removed in five or six days in order that the parts may be bathed, massaged and passive motion instituted, when it can be reapplied; after this time the joint should receive a daily treatment of massage and movements, which can be done, though very imperfectly, over the rubber strips, yet sufficiently to be of considerable benefit. The dressings, however, can be removed every second or third day for this treatment and reapplied. If the skin should become irritated as it sometimes does, a tight stocking leg, as advocated by Hoffman, can be drawn over the knee and the strips applied over this.

When the sprain is more severe, the ligaments and tissues lacerated, the swelling, heat and effusion considerable, a different procedure is required. The hot water is applied as before, the effusion aspirated under strictly aseptic precautions and the joint put at absolute rest by a fixed dressing. I have had the best results follow the application of a firm roller enveloping the entire leg, beginning at and including the foot over which is applied a well-fitting plaster-of-Paris dressing, the popliteal space being properly protected, this plaster dressing extending from the ankle to the upper third of the thigh, the patient put to bed, limb elevated and placed in as comfortable position as possible. It is very important that this fixed dressing should not remain undisturbed long, as changes are liable to take place leaving a permanent injury. As the swelling recedes the bandages are liable to become loosened and the parts deprived of the proper support, a condition which will probably occur within three or four days. The dressing should then be removed, the plaster cut from top to bottom, preferably on one side, with a slice cut out so that the shape will not be affected, the joint massaged and gentle passive motion very cautiously instituted. The amount of massage and movement will depend upon the condition. If there is much heat, swelling and tenderness this procedure is omitted or practised very gently and to a limited degree. A second aspiration is justifiable if effusion has reaccumulated. If not removed it will cause much distention, retard healing and may cause permanent injury. The effusion in a joint is absorbed, as a rule, rather slowly. The dressing is now reapplied, the plaster tightened and held in place by an outside roller. These dressings should be applied in such a manner that the pressure may be equable, and should now be removed every day to admit of massage and passive motion, both of which must be performed with care and judgment and increased in degree as the tenderness gives way and the joint grows stronger. After a rest of about ten days or two weeks, if there is no pain of moment, the patient will be required to walk some each day. As soon as this fixation dressing can be dispensed with a nicely molded leather case may be applied, firmly laced, with advantage, or a steel bar apparatus which admits of slight motion of the joint and gives good support, and should be worn as long as there is any pain or much weakness. Some pain should not be a bar to the institution of motion. If this should be neglected and there should unfortunately follow ankylosis in any degree, if there is no heat or swelling the adhesions should be forcibly broken up under an anesthetic.

The ankle-joint is also classed as a hinge joint, yet has some lateral motion, the bones of which it is composed are the tibia, fibula and the upper convex surface of the astragalus. It is invested with stout ligaments, blood-vessels and nerves, is a very strong joint and connected by important structures. A severe sprain will sometimes involve not only one or more of the ligaments which immediately connect it, but the tendons of

---
[1] J. C. Bloodgood in Progressive Medicine.

the muscles which pass through them, the synovial membrane, and may tear the annular ligament, or displace some of the tendons. Of all joints it is the one that is probably most frequently sprained. In severe sprain with considerable swelling it is often difficult to decide if it is complicated by fracture or dislocation. It is not an easy matter sometimes to make a satisfactory examination because of the intense pain and swelling; to accomplish this it may be necessary to use an anesthetic. It is important to know the extent of the damage and what structures are involved. In some obscure cases an X-ray examination might reveal the lesions.

In most cases the lateral ligaments are involved and as in the knee when the injury is extensive, it may implicate the synovial membrane, rupture some of the vessels and nerves. The pain is often severe and the slightest movement increases it, motion is suspended, if lifted up the foot drops, in such cases it is probable that there is extensive laceration of the structures involved and there is generally a good deal of effusion quickly following the swelling which may be slow to disappear. Manipulation of the foot and putting the ligaments on the stretch will often indicate what structures are torn. It is important in the treatment of sprains of the ankle joint to know if possible what tissues are implicated. If the injury is slight or only moderately severe the foot and ankle is immersed in water as hot as can be borne and the temperature kept up to the point of toleration for thirty-five to fifty minutes when the pain will be greatly mitigated and the swelling in a measure retarded; then the treatment advocated by Gibney will give the best results of any that I have used.

He employs the Cotterell dressing as follows: "Employ massage for five or ten minutes with the foot well elevated. Next apply strips of rubber plaster about an inch in width and from twelve to eighteen inches in length over the part sprained beginning back of the injury. Aim to leave the part of the foot not affected as well uncovered as possible, but reinforce well as the strips are applied under the malleolus or malleoli. The first strip for a sprain of the external malleolus is applied beginning just above the ankle on the unaffected side of the foot, and ending on the affected side, about half way up the calf. This strip is usually along side the tendo achilles and makes firm support under the heel. The second strip starts on the inner side of the unaffected part of the foot, near the ball of the toe, comes round over the back of the heel, and ends about the base of the little toe. It crosses the first one just above the border of the heel. The third strip overlaps the first half way, the fourth the second, and so on until the part sprained is fully covered by this crisscross strapping. A cheesecloth bandage is applied, more with the idea of securing close adhesion of the plaster, and is removed within twenty-four hours. As soon as the dressing is completed the stocking and boot should be applied. The patient is now ready to begin walking, and this should be insisted upon in the presence of the surgeon. Direct him to walk about the room for eight or ten times, by the time this task is completed there will be very little lameness or disability. While it is undesirable to insist on too much walking for the next few days it is essential that the patient should walk as much as it is necessary for him to walk and attend to any duties that require a moderate amount of walking. At the end of the week it is well to remove the strips and reapply in the same manner as above. Two or three such dressings will complete the cure.[1]

For such cases as these, if treatment is well carried out, I doubt if any other plan can be devised that will give better results. The patient should be cautioned against another accident which might again twist the joint, while it is weak, and put the ligaments on the stretch. The amount of walking should be prescribed by the surgeon and the patient kept under his control. If the sprain is severe with extensive laceration of the tissues, the pain, swelling and effusion will be greater and a different method of treatment is required. The best results in these injuries are obtained by differentiating the various degrees and applying appropriate treatment for each. Beginning by the application of hot water in these cases is also of great benefit, then the patient should be put to bed, the foot elevated and put in the most comfortable position, so that it will be properly supported and at rest, with the application of soothing or hot evaporating lotions. In twenty-four or at most thirty-six hours if the effusion is found to be excessive it is aspirated with a small, clean needle, gentle massage, the application of a smooth, firm roller over which is applied a fixed dressing that will control motion and give proper support. Usually plaster of Paris answers well, which, except the heel and toes, should cover the foot and ankle extending half way to the knee. The foot is now placed in an elevated comfortable position. If there is not pain enough to annoy the patient this dressing can remain undisturbed for five or six days, when it is removed and a treatment of gentle massage is given. It is rather too early to begin passive motion of the joint, but the massage should be now practised every day and in three or four days if the swelling, heat and tenderness has diminished, the foot is moved cautiously by flexion and extension only, and is continued every day. If, however, the joint resents this interference by a relighting of inflammatory symptoms, it must be put at rest again undisturbed for a short period, and another attempt made with the same treatment and the effects watched. The amount of heat, swelling and pain should guide us in these manipulations. In the intervals the joint should be kept in the fixed dressing. Probably in two weeks a lighter plaster dressing can be applied but of sufficient firm-

---

[1] Dennis' Surgery.

ness to give support and as soon as dry the patient required to walk with a crutch and cane, bearing some weight on the affected foot, but it must be removed daily for massage and passive motion. The temperature, swelling and sensibility of the joint are important guides to active measures. As soon as the patient can walk with but little discomfort the plaster dressing is discontinued and a suitable, well-fitting leather case ordered, or a steel-barred apparatus with hinge joint. The wounded joint may be tender and weak for several months during which time the supporting apparatus is to be worn. While it is all important in these bad cases that in the beginning the injured member should be at absolute rest and all motion prohibited, this mode of dressing has its limits and if left too long is liable to cause damage that might be permanent. It is important during the entire treatment of a sprain to watch the general health. A suitable diet is prescribed, the bowels and kidneys kept acting and rest at night secured. Attention to these details will hasten the cure.

It requires great vigilance on the part of the surgeon to prevent the too free use of opiates, both for the present and future welfare of the patient who should be kept under observation until all pathological lesions have disappeared and the joint has resumed its normal function.

SYPHILIS OF THE LUNG SIMULATING PHTHISIS.[1]

BY WILLIAM E. HUGHES, M.D.,

AND

ROBERT N. WILLSON, M.D.,

OF PHILADELPHIA.

AS EARLY as 1858, Virchow described a pulmonary condition which he called " white hepatization " and which he noted especially in the lungs of syphilitic newly born infants. He also noted a brown induration and a collection of brown pigment in the lungs of a number of adults accompanying a similar congenital " white hepatization." This pigmentation he considered due to an impediment to the blood stream in its passage through the pulmonary tissue, consequent upon the filling of the alveoli by round cells. Virchow apparently did not feel, however, like committing himself to the statement that these hepatized areas were undoubtedly syphilitic processes. Wagner in 1863, Pavlinoff in 1879, Schnitzler in 1879, Hiller in 1884, Heller in 1888, and more recently many others including Councilman, Greenfield, Kidd, Perry, Rolleston, Weber, Wilks, Aufrecht, and Stengel, have also reported cases of apparent syphilitic pulmonary involvement. The question is often asked: " In cases that do not come to autopsy can we be sure that the process has not yet been of a simple bronchopneumonic character¦ or even of a tubercular nature; especially since tuberculosis is a frequent accompaniment of syphilis? "

When such pathologists as Virchow fail posi-

[1] Read before the Philadelphia County Medical Society, November 23, 1904.

tively to diagnose the condition under the microscope, how indeed are we to assure ourselves of the clinical condition in a doubtful case of pulmonary involvement in a syphilitic patient? And still more difficult, how shall we make the diagnosis in the presence of a doubtful pulmonary lesion in a case supposedly not, but actually, syphilitic? These are not only interesting queries, but practical issues as the instance reported in this paper will demonstrate.

Case.—H. H., white, aged thirty-two years, born in Russia; an ironworker. His father, mother, two brothers and two sisters living and well. Patient has had measles and smallpox. Has been repeatedly exposed to venereal infection, but denies having suffered from venereal disease of any description. Claims never to have had a chancre or other sore upon his penis, or elsewhere on his body. Has experienced no sore throat, no alopecia and no eruption. Has always been engaged in hard labor, for years as a sailor and recently as an ironworker. Six weeks prior to admission to the Philadelphia General Hospital, on December 31, 1903, he contracted a " a severe cold " which persisted about a month. He then became stronger and better physically, but the cough continued, as did also the expectoration which had been profuse from the outset. About December 15, 1903, he began to expectorate blood. At first this appeared in occasional small streaks in the sputum, but has gradually increased in quantity, until at the time of admission it appeared in quantity with every coughing attack. The patient then appeared well nourished, of large muscular frame, his skin of good color and, except for his cough, he said he felt perfectly well. He was also frightened at the continual loss of blood. The physical examination found his mouth and throat normal in appearance, the glands of the postcervical and sternomastoid regions not palpable, the pulse rapid and small and not easily compressible. The pupils were equal and reacted promptly to light and distance. The patient was right-handed, but on inspection the right chest seemed more prominent than normal, especially over the lower portion. The expansion was relatively impaired over this area, though still remarkably free. The circumference of the right chest from midsternum to the spine at the level of the eleventh spinous process was 20 inches (50 cm.); that of the left side at a corresponding level was 18 inches (45 cm.); at the height of the scapular spine the right chest measured 20⅝ inches (50.9 cm.) and the left side 19⅝ inches (49 cm.). The expansion over the pulmonary bases was, on the right side three-quarters of an inch, and one-half inch on the left. Percussion resonance was also impaired over the entire right lower lobe, especially posteriorly. Tactile fremitus was slightly increased. On deep inspiration, over a space as large as the palm of the hand, just below the upper border of the right lower lobe, fine crackling râles and a scraping friction sound were heard. Percussion over this area also gave distinct dulness, not amounting to flatness. Above and to the outside of of this area Skodaic tympany was easily obtained.

The middle and upper lobes on the right side showed prolonged inspiratory' and expiratory sounds, also rather harsh, but no other abnormality. The apex was negative anteriorly and posteriorly. The left lung appeared to be altogether normal, except for a rather poor expansion. The abdominal examination was negative. There was no eruption on any portion of the body, and no scar nor induration was discoverable on the penis. The glands were enlarged only in the inguinal region, where both the deep and superficial chains were palpable on both sides. From December 31, 1903, to the date of his discharge, January 14, 1904, temperature which was 100° F. on admission, varied between this point and 97° F., where it was disposed to remain during the last days of his stay in the hospital. The pulse was 110 on admission, and averaged 90 during the subsequent period. The respirations gradually fell from 30 to normal. The blood showed a slight reduction of hemoglobin; the urine was normal.

The patient experienced little or no discomfort on the right side, but had a constant hacking cough, and brought up enormous quantities (two or more sputum-cupsful) of sanguinopurulent matter daily. The expectoration was very profuse in the morning, shortly after rising. There were no nightsweats, there was little or no loss of weight, the appetite was good, and the genreal impression given was that of a man with a strictly localized pulmonary lesion, and a general economy that was still amply competent to combat the advance.

On the presumption that the latter was tuberculous, the sputum was examined repeatedly, but on no occasion could tubercle bacilli be detected. Pneumococci were present in numbers. January 6, 1904, there was no cessation on the part of the pulmonary bleeding, which had now become so free that there was no more blood than mucopus in the sputum. The latter invariably showed, however, a thorough admixture with the blood, assuming rather a prune-juice than a bright red color. The patient was demonstrated on this day in Hughes' clinic, and an exploratory puncture made in the eighth interspace in the midscapular line. The first puncture yielded no fluid, probably owing to a faulty mechanism of the apparatus. The second insertion of the needle, however, to our surprise gave a syringeful of dark red blood, floating in which were large flakes of lymph, evidently from the surface of the pleura. The wound was sealed, and the patient returned to the ward in good condition, but still expectorating blood and mucopus as before.

In the doubt as to the diagnosis three condi-

tions seemed possible, with the probability in the following order of mention; incipient pulmonary malignant disease, tubercular phthisis, and syphilis. It seemed to be very improbable that the lesion was parasitic (actinomyces, hydatid, etc.), since no evidence pointing to such an origin could be discovered in the sputum. Calcium chloride and gelatin were employed, together with prolonged, absolute rest in bed, but without effect upon the pulmonary bleeding, which appeared to be on the increase. This fact, together with the absence of constitutional involvement, and the circumstance that the patient appeared to be otherwise in excellent physical condition, seemed to render tuberculosis unlikely, though still of course possible. Syphilis was also considered, though deemed unlikely in the light of the entire absence of a history of primary, secondary or tertiary lesions. Moreover pulmonary syphilis is by no means a frequent occurrence in medical literature.

The most probable condition, therefore, appeared to be an early malignant, in all likelihood sarcomatous, involvement of the lung and pleura and the tentative diagnosis of sarcoma was accordingly made. Microscopical examination of the flakes of lymph, obtained in the fluid drawn by puncture, it should be stated, gave no clue as to the nature of the pathologic process.

More as a matter of interest and empiricism than with the expectation of alleviating the symptoms, the patient was placed on January 7, 1904, upon large doses of potassium iodide (one dram three times a day), with the idea that harm could be done only in the unlikely event that the condition was tuberculous. To our astonishment and satisfaction within twenty-four hours the expectoration diminished in quantity and the patient stated that he was bringing up less blood. The treatment was persisted in, and after three days the sputum, while still free in quantity, contained no blood, the cough had largely disappeared, and the patient insisted on leaving the hospital in the belief that he was cured. He was persuaded to remain four days longer and on January 14, 1904, could no longer be detained, and was lost sight of. When discharged he was free from cough, his sputum was mucopurulent, but in slight quantity, and he himself felt perfectly well. The respiratory sounds over the area of former consolidation were still rough, and moist râles could be heard; the percussion note was almost similar in like positions on the right and left sides.

In looking back upon this case, it is natural at once to suggest that the condition was one of bronchopneumonia, with delayed resolution, the latter taking place finally at a time coincident with the administration of potassium iodide. This appeared to us so unlikely, however, that we excluded it in favor of less unlikely conditions. The duration for at least twelve weeks without seriously affecting the general condition of the patient, the free expectorating of prune juice fluid, beginning with the eleventh week of the disease, and the prompt, and seemingly almost complete recovery from active symptoms within a week of the first administration of potassium iodide, all seemed to point to a condition other than that of a simple bronchopneumonic consolidation.

Malignant disease it certainly was not in the light of the result of treatment. Equally certain is the fact that we must now exclude tuberculosis, which, though sometimes remaining stationary under the influence of potassium iodide, is usually urged on into an acute exacerbation, and is never really benefited by any combination of the iodides.

We have remaining but one probable condition, pulmonary syphilis; and our diagnosis rests simply and solely up to the present moment upon exclusion and upon the therapeutic grounds. In speaking of this case to a genitourinary specialist, we were received with the comment: "So, this is what the internist calls syphilis!"

We would reply: "If not syphilis, what else?" There are many discoveries made by so-called chance, and by so-called experiment, and some of our most valuable items of knowledge have been obtained by reasoning backward, as it were; this method being the only one that offered a purchase from which to reason and observe in the right direction.

Even in the absence of the classical eruption, and the evidence of a primary sore, and even lacking a general glandular enlargement (none of which we believe to be indispensable accompaniments of latent syphilis) we feel compelled to look upon this case as one of pulmonary syphilis, at first latent, and then manifesting itself by the symptoms of a localized pulmonary lesion. Until our friends, who have up to this time spent their lives in a vain quest for the causal germ of syphilis, proclaim the success of their pursuit, we shall consider it our duty from the double standpoint of the patient and the clinician to regard such conditions as respond promptly to treatment by potassium iodide or mercury, and to no other, as luetic, provided, of course, that we find no evidence suggesting another condition as more probable.

It is interesting from the pathologic standpoint, and in view of Virchow's comment upon the occurrence of brown induration and pigment and its histogenesis, that so many of these cases present hemoptysis as a prominent clinical feature. Aufrecht's case is especially noteworthy in comparison with our own, in that the autopsy showed the presence of a tumor of coagulated blood, arching over the left bronchus, and pressing upon the tracheal wall. The tumor was formed "by an almost globe-like dilatation of the aorta, as large as a plum," communicating with the lumen of the arch by an opening one centimeter in diameter. The result of puncture in our case might well have been consequent upon the insertion of the needle into some such aneurismal clot, or equally well into a circumscribed extravasation, due, as suggested by Virchow, to an impediment to the blood stream. In the latter event the stage of the disease when observed by us must have been one antecedent to that of brown induration and its attendant pigmentation.

Stengel gives the post-mortem findings in one case of undoubted pulmonary syphilis, of which the clinical history was lacking. He also submits the clinical history of another case, first looked upon and treated as an instance of pulmonary tuberculosis, but recovering after six months of treatment with potassium iodide. The latter case is open to the objection, of course, that the improvement was so slow as to admit of question whether is was not a case of phthisis after all, recovering in spite of the use of potassium iodide.

Many cases of well recognized incipient phthisis do indeed recover within an even shorter period. In other words the improvement may or may not have been due to the antispecific treatment. Certainly, however, the iodide had no deleterious effect. Stengel also quotes the interesting case of Brambilla, of a supposedly tuberculous patient being given the mercurial inunction intended for a syphilitic in the adjoining bed, followed by the prompt recovery from all his symptoms. The clinical histories of such cases must have at least one important influence, in the direction of proving that a certain few cases, apparently tuberculous, will improve and convalesce symptomatically under antisyphilitic treatment. This once determined, the question as to whether we can rightfully call them instances of pulmonary syphilis, assumes secondary importance.

The probability approaches a certainty more nearly with each new case, and in due time a sufficient number of post-mortem records will have been obtained in cases that have shown just such a clinical history and the doubt will be dispelled. In the meantime the uncertainty will cause some hesitation in the positive diagnosis of incipient tuberculosis in subjects known to have or suspected to have a syphilitic taint.

REFERENCES.

Hiller. Charité Annalen, Berlin, 1884, S. 184.
Pavlinoff. Virchow's Archiv, 1879, S. 162.
Rollet. Wiener med. Presse, 1875, S. 1101.
Schnitzler. Wiener med. Presse, 1879 u. 1883.
Virchow. Archiv f. path. Anatomie, 1858, S. 310.
Wagner. Archiv der Heilkunde, 1863.
Aufrecht. Amer. Edit. Nothnagel's Encyclopedia of Practical Medicine.
Councilman. Johns Hopkins Hosp. Bulletin, Vol. II. 1891.
Greenfield. London Path. Soc. Transactions, XXVIII, p. 248.
Heller. Deutsch. Archiv f. klin. Med., XLIVI, S. 149.
Kidd. Lancet, 1890, and Lond. Path. Soc. Trans., XXXVII, p. 111.
Pefry. London Path. Transactions, XIII, p. 53.
Rolleston. London Path. Soc. Trans., XLII, p. 50.
Weber. London Path. Soc. Transactions, XVII, p. 152.
Stengel. University of Penna. Med. Bulletin, May, 1903.

MEDICAL PROGRESS.

SURGERY.

Decapsulation of the Kidney.—The effect of decapsulation of the kidney on animals has been studied very carefully by G. HERXHEIMER and J. W. HALL (*Virchow's Archiv*, Vol. 179, No. 1). Most animals stand the operation well and albumin does not appear in the urine. A new capsule forms very rapidly; after twenty days it is very evident and usually thicker and more irregular than the original capsule. A moderate number of small vessels were encountered, but in no place did these vessels penetrate into the interior of the kidney and form anastomoses with the renal vessels. A number of rabbits were treated with chrome alum before the operation in order to set up a nephritis and study the effects of decapsulation upon this. The operation was also tolerated well but the amount of albumen excreted was just as high as in the animals which were not operated. It required an equally long time for both sets of animals to recuperate, so that, at least in this form of nephritis, no good effects can be expected from decapsulation.

Intestinal Anastomosis by the Connell Suture.—H. H. SINCLAIR (*Med. Rec.*, February 4, 1905) describes three cases in which he performed intestinal anastomosis by the Connell method. The patients all made good recoveries and the author suggests that perhaps the lack of a simple method of doing an intestinal anastomosis has been one of the causes of mortality in strangulated hernia and volvulus.

Intermuscular Hemorrhage from Muscular Action.—A. H. SMITH (*Med. Rec.*, February 4, 1905) says that a sharp distinction is to be drawn between those cases in which the escape of blood within the intact sheath of a muscle is the important factor, and those in which laceration of muscle and sheath plays the principal part. Contrary to what might be expected, the former sort of cases may give rise to greater immediate suffering and more lasting impairment of function than the latter. While almost any muscle may be the seat of rupture, those that act through the tendon Achilles are especially liable to the accident. The strain on this structure in walking is at certain moments equal to three times the weight of the body, and if it is brought to bear suddenly, the tendon may be ruptured, or some of the muscular structures which act through it may give way. Incoordination of the fibers of a muscle also may cause some of them to rupture, and this irregular contraction probably is the cause of the lesion in those cases in which there is no conscious muscular effect at the moment of the accident. The author describes two cases of hemorrhage into the calf muscles due to muscular action, and two other cases, affecting the gastrocnémius and the sternomastoid muscles respectively, in which there was a demonstrable rent in muscle and sheath. In the former two cases the effusion of a moderate amount of blood into the confined space afforded by the intact sheath caused much pain and protracted disability, whereas in the latter the suffering was comparatively slight, and recovery was relatively prompt.

The Infection of Physicians by Syphilis.—The seriousness of this condition is ably discussed by A. BLASCHKO (*Berl. klin. Woch.*, December 26, 1904), who had twelve physicians as patients with this disease, acquired during their work. In most of them the primary lesion was on the finger, and not fully recognized at first. Three conditions must be differentiated from chancre in this region, herpes, anatomical tubercle and the soft chancre. Herpes in most instances may be

readily enough distinguished, but more difficulty is encountered in the presence of the other two. In some cases the primary lesion may be small, causes little disturbance and heals rapidly without forming a scar. In these cases the development of general symptoms or an indolent bubo first calls attention to the disease. In one case there was absolutely no evidence of external infection, and the writer thinks that this may be one of a class where the primary lesion is never developed and where it is possible that the infection took place through an insect sting. The chief source of infection seems to be wounds, either accidental and unnoticed, or made by the puncture of instruments used on syphilitic patients. Hang-nails are a frequent source of infection when making gynecological or other examinations, or when attending syphilitic women during an abortion. Blaschko thinks that there is no absolute way of preventing infection. The vigorous scrubbing which is indulged in before operation is a frequent source of wound production, and where the skin of the hands is very tender it should be avoided and washing with marble soap without a brush be deemed sufficient. Moreover, it is better to avoid carrying virulent germs about on the hands, by a thorough cleansing after operation on an infectious case. The use of rubber gloves is also warmly recommended. Small wounds should be carefully cleansed and painted with a two to three per cent. solution of nitrate of silver. Suspected punctured wounds may be treated with tincture of iodine. The writer does not agree with the generally accepted theory that extragenital syphilis is more severe than the other type, and none of his patients developed any complications. Treatment should never be instituted on mere suspicion, but the appearance of characteristic signs should always be awaited. The question of stopping his practice is a most important one, but if the proper precautions are observed there is no reason why an infected physician need cease to work. Otherwise he must observe the same restrictions as are incumbent upon other individuals.

Cauterization by Zinc Chloride.—The action of this drug on wounds as a protective against infection has been studied by L. BROSE (*Deut. med. Woch.*, December 22, 1904). His experiments were conducted on rabbits and on the bacteria themselves. The author finds that even in concentrated solutions the zinc chloride is devoid of antiseptic properties, but that the eschar which results when brought into contact with aseptic wound surfaces prevents subsequent infection. The penetrating powers of this substance are so marked that it protects the wound even when applied a full minute after the application of the infectious agent. The slough produced is not a culture medium, for bacteria and other pathogenic organisms cannot be recovered from it for two or three days after they have been applied.

Marked Mental Improvement Following Operation for Depressed Fracture of the Skull.—B. VAN D. HEDGES (*Med. Rec.*, January 28, 1905) describes the case of a boy of eight years, who four years previously had been struck on the head by a brick, which had caused a marked depression in the bone at the seat of the injury. From this time there was evidence of a change in his mental and moral make-up. Intellectually he was at a standstill and all moral sense appeared to be lost. Over a year ago the author removed the area of depressed bone, and since that time the boy's mental and moral condition has become normal. The depression was about one inch in diameter, one-quarter inch in depth and situated in the median line, along the course of the sagittal suture, the center of the depression being one inch and a half anterior to the vertical point and four and one-half inches from the glabellar point.

Trendelenburg's Operation.—A critical study of of the use and abuse of this most excellent and widely used technic for the treatment of varicose veins is of the utmost value. VIANNAY (*Revue de Chirurgie*, January, 1905) presents an exhaustive treatise on the subject. Not the least interesting of his chapters is that which is devoted to a consideration of the condition of the operative intervention before the time of Trendelenburg. He concludes that in France, direct intervention was practised by means of ligating the internal saphenous vein either with or without resection of the vessel. Gagnebe in 1830, Velpeau in 1838 and Ricord in 1839 were among the French operators who worked on this technic. Shede, Riesel, in Germany, Steel, Colley, Anandale, in England, also practised the same operation. Viannay concludes that when one has decided to interrupt the continuity of the internal saphenous vein, in the case of a varix, which shows the presence of valvular insufficiency, all intervention directed upon a single point in the vein is insufficient and illusionary, with the single exception of resection high in Scarpas triangle. Although in many cases this intervention may suffice, it is usually better to interrupt the internal saphenous in a series of sections, or as the author states by a veritable luxury of precautions, to exsect it entirely. These conclusions are corroborated by operative results. Not having had a sufficient number of cases from which to deduce conclusions to present practical results, no figures are given by the author. The monograph is full of interest and the conclusions not based on personal observations are the direct results of careful study of the statistics of others.

Enlargement of the Spleen Simulating a Pelvic Growth.—Splenomegaly is ordinarily not easily confounded with pelvic growths, but the following case, as recorded by A. J. STURMER (*Brit. Jour. of Obst.*, October, 1904) shows that such a mistake is possible. Elsie E., aged twenty-five years, multipara, native of India, was admitted to the Government Maternity Hospital, Madras, June 30, 1904, complaining of a painless swelling of the abdomen, which had existed for sixteen months. She had not menstruated in two years and four months. Micturition was normal. She had gradually lost flesh. There had been fever off and on for a year previous to her marriage, and occasionally afterward. Malarial fever was very prevalent in the woman's home. At the time of admission to the hospital the patient was well-nourished, not anemic; bowels regular. Pulse 108, temperature normal. The abdomen presented considerable enlargement; a large irregular mass was found to occupy the right iliac and lumbar regions encroaching upon the left side, extending from the pubes to three fingers-breadth below the ribs. It filled more of the right side of the abdomen than the left. The tumor was hard and freely movable, especially toward the right side. A distinct fluid thrill could be elicited in both flanks. It could not be determined whether this was in the tumor or free in the peritoneal cavity. There was dulness all over the tumor, but the flanks were tympanitic. The hand could easily be passed under the ribs over the top of the tumor, and could be made to pass underneath it, therefore it was decided that it did not take its origin from above. Vaginal examination was practically negative. On opening the peritoneal cavity some fluid came away, and a bluish-red mass presented. On passing the hand into the right iliac fossa the splenic notch could be made out, as it rested upon the right ilium. Above the spleen did not pass under the ribs; incision was therefore enlarged, and finally the spleen was delivered. The pedicle was long. The splenic artery was about the size of a goose-quill, divided into two branches before entering the spleen, and these two branches were first tied, and then the main vessel ligatured. Finally the spleen was cut away. The appendix was found to contain a round worm—not an uncommon experience; it was cut across and the outer portion of the worm removed. The spleen weighed four pounds three ounces, and was remarkable for the number of notches,—three or four deep cuts at its edge,—near the usual notch. On leaving the hospital the patient was strong and able to walk about, to all intents in good health and had gained considerably in weight.

Surgical Treatment of Chronic Dyspepsia.—The progress made in the treatment of a rather typical form of gastric dyspepsia has been marked by continued growth during the last few years. JOHN G. SHELDON (*Annals of Surgery*, January, 1905) states that it is generally admitted that from fatigue of the gastric muscle followed by gastric atony and elongation of the gastric muscle fibers, enlargement of the cavity does occur. When this condition is of but temporary duration, special attention has been given to derangements of the secretory functions of the organ. Treatment by various disgestive ferments often affords relief in these cases, especially if they are seconded by antacids. Mayo says that it is the mechanics of the stomach that are usually at fault and not its chemics. Einhorn has shown that even achylia gastrica can occur and produce no symptoms if the motor function of the stomach is not impaired. The succession of changes which take place in these long-standing cases of chronic dyspepsia, due to muscular atony, seem to the author to be as follows: There is deficient drainage, resulting either from pouch formation or from lack of muscular force to expel the contents. The retained material undergoes chemical changes which produce products having a local effect on the gastric mucosa. These are absorbed and are capable of producing more or less marked general changes. As time goes on the inflammation of the mucosa becomes chronic, or, in other words, chronic gastritis develops. It has long been recognized that severe cases of tetany may be due to gastric toxemia. The author believes that many nervous symptoms, less severe than tetany, but due to disturbances of a like quantity but of a less quantity are often manifested in cases suffering from dilatation. This covers that great field of debilitated individuals who are known as neurasthenics. It has been believed for too long that the nervous symptoms are primary and that the dyspepsia is secondary, although it must be admitted that gastric symptoms may very definitely and certainly be produced by primary nervous disturbances. Regarding the experiments which have been carried out to show the effect of nerve section in animals, all of which have tended to show conflicting conclusions by their authors, Ewald says all these experimental stimulations have had an indefinite and uncertain value. We have many examples of tetany being relieved by drainage of the stomach and also of the disappearance of nervous symptoms following drainage in cases of obstructed pylorus. As to the cause of the chronic constipation, which is almost always associated with neurasthenia, it has been claimed that the small amount of solid material which these patients pass into their gut, is responsible for the condition. Lohrisch has shown that the absence of sufficient dry residue in the intestines inhibits the growth of the intestinal flora and diminishes the production of indol, skatol, etc. The author, however, believes that the constipation is the direct result of defective drainage of the stomach and is not due to secondary causes. From a series of cases and from a study of those of many other surgeons he concludes that any case of severe and long-standing dyspepsia, that has resisted the usual methods of treatment and that has shown no permanent improvement after the stomach has been rested for two weeks by rectal feeding, should be subjected to gastro-enterostomy.

An Operation for Inguinal Hernia.—Multiplication of technics intended to simplify the treatment of characteristic lesions shows that the ideal has not yet been reached. CHARLES J. SCUDDER (*Annals of Surgery*, January, 1905) gives his interpretation of the essential details of Bassini's operation. He has never yet found it necessary or advisable to excise the veins of the cord. He considers the transplantation of the cord of little importance, although he is more and more inclined not to transplant it. He keeps his patient in bed for two weeks, on a bed-rest for the third week and advises a bandage for one month simply for the comfort of the patient. He exposes the region by the usual incision, incises the external oblique, in the usual way and frees it for about two fingers' breadth around the cut edges. The cremaster is split parallel to its fibers and separated from the sac and cord. The sac is developed by blunt dissection. It is then opened, emptied and divided transversely down through the cord and its vessels. The proximal part of the sac is isolated from the cord and from the abdominal muscles. He considers that the purse-string suture may slip. He consequently sews the sac across its cut end over and over. The distal portion of the sac, namely the scrotal part, he has ordinarily disregarded, except to gently curette its inner surface. It is unnecessary to remove it in most cases. Downward traction upon the proximal portion of the sac facilitates the suturing of the peritoneum. The cord and distal portion of the sac are now lifted from their bed if it is decided to transplant them. The sutures are then placed and it has been the author's custom always to put one or two external to the spot where the cord pierces the peritoneum. The external oblique fascia is closed over the cord by a continuous chromic catgut suture, taken with a loop or hemstitch. This overlaps the two layers of fascia as satisfactorily as is done by the mattress suture of Halstead. The skin is closed by silkworm gut, which is covered with sterile gauze. Silver foil, ointments, paste and powder have no advantage over this dressing. Absolute hemostasis, ample cutaneous incision and minimum of trauma to the cord are essentials to success.

Treatment of Fracture of the Lower Jaw.—Although this bone is known to heal more kindly than any other in the body, its treatment after fracture has been the source of many vexatious discussions. RUDOLPH MATAS (*Annals of Surgery*, January, 1905) states that the ideals aimed at are ac-

curate reduction combined with suitable provision for the gygiene of the mouth. The meeting of these conditions should not interfere with the oral and maxillary functions. He further states that this problem has taxed the originality and resources both of the practical surgeon and of the dental specialist. No less than 15 articles on fractured lower jaws have appeared in journals from January to September, 1904. Celsius wired the adjoining teeth. Angle and Lohers perfected this method by the use of clamps and bars to lock the teeth together. Moulded dental splints, which accurately fit over the crowns of the teeth cast on molds of the teeth made from plaster-of-Paris impression usually give far better results than the wiring method. The difficulty, however, with these types of splints is that they require a specialist for their preparation. The technic of the author is devised particularly to meet the want of the majority of people who enter a large hospital service. The majority of these patients have in general hospitals to be treated by men of ordinary experience and without the necessary training to prepare a dental splint. Ninety per cent. of these fractures occur in adult males. The splint is described as follows: It is constructed on the principle of a clamp which holds the entire projecting arch of the jaw from the chin to the angles firmly in the grip of a flexible mouthpiece, which fits like a gutter over the entire dental arch, and of an external plate or chin cup, which extends from the symphysis to the angle. The mouthpiece and chin plate are both detachable. The chin cup is made adjustable to various degrees of prognathism by a sliding-joint fixed by a pin and thrumb screw. The mouthpiece is horseshoe in shape. It is hollowed in three planes to fit loosely over the crowns of the teeth. The softness and flexibility of which the splint is made allows the operator to adjust the splint accurately to the lower dental arch. This splint is made in three different sizes. The chin piece is made of perforated aluminum and is shaped to fit the contour of the jaw. It has a sliding-joint upon which it moves backward and forward. The clamp which holds the two pieces together is made of soft steel and consists of an upper and lower limb screwed together in front of the mouth. The upper limb projects from the middle of the mouth and is so arranged that dribbling is prevented and that eating and drinking is made possible. The pressure required to hold the jaw in the grasp of the two pieces is obtained by a screw attached by a swivel-joint to the upper limb of the clamp. When the splint is applied, the contour of the dental arch should be restored when the fracture is reduced and while the bone is held in place by combined internal and external manipulation; one of the metallic dental gutters is selected, depending on the age of the patient, and fitted on the arch of the teeth. It can be molded with the fingers. It may be necessary, in the case of destroyed teeth to fill the gutter with a modeling wax, such as is used by dentists. The outside clamp is then adjusted and padded and the clamp is tightened. The patient is then taught to irrigate his mouth, which should be done every hour or so. If the contusion of the soft parts has been extensive, care should be taken to relax the pressure of the screw; otherwise injury may be done by the unyielding splints. In this case, until the swelling has subsided, a Barton-Gibson, or sling-bandage, may be used to reinforce the splint. This article is illustrated very fully.

Hepatic Wounds.—With the rapid evolution of abdominal surgery, the question of recognition and treatment of hepatic injuries has received increasing attention. BENJAMIN T. TILTON (*Annals of Surgery*, January, 1905) states that the liver is injured with greater frequency than any other abdominal viscus. Of 365 cases of subcutaneous injuries of solid viscera the liver was injured in 189. The spleen, kidney, and pancreas combined in but 179. The factors which favor a high percentage of injury are (1) that it lies wedged between the ribs and vertebral column and (2) that it is very heavy and elastic and only slightly movable. It is nine times as heavy as the spleen and ten times as heavy as the kidney. Furthermore, the physiological function of digestion renders it more liable to injury, since the gland is engorged with blood. Again the organ is particularly liable to disease. Alcoholism, tuberculosis, malarial lesions, new growths and the production of fibrous tissue rendering it even more friable than in its normal condition. Chiari has reported a case of carcinomatous liver occurring when the patient was simply turned over in bed. The author reports a number of cases of traumatisms to the liver which were treated surgically in his service at Bellevue, and from a study of these he deduces the following data as to symptoms: Escape of venous blood with or without bile, particularly in scab wounds over the region of the liver is a very important sign. Hepatic injuries usually cause pain to radiate to the right shoulder. Inasmuch as there is also local pain on respiration, the chest does not move as much on the right as on the left. This may lead to a misconstruction of the diagnosis, for it suggests to the casual observer thoracic injury. The blood gravitates into the right iliac fossa and may give well-marked dulness. Disappearance of liver dulness is due to beginning tympanitis and is therefore not of great diagnostic importance. Jaundice is occasionally present, but usually does not appear until the second or fourth day. Ludwig found it 24 times in 267 cases. Its presence usually signifies injuries of the bile duct. In very severe cases the prognosis is exceedingly grave. no matter how early intervention may have been practised. Hemorrhage was the cause of death in 69 out of 162 fatal cases. Abscess and peritonitis are of course responsible for many deaths. In all probabiliy, in the opinion of the author, there are many mild cases of liver laceration which go on to entire recovery without ever having been diagnosed. Of 25 cases of hepatic injury occurring in the last ten years in the New York hospitals, which were uncomplicated by serious lesions of other abdominal organs, 12 were ruptures, 9 gunshot wounds, 4 stab wounds. Eleven deaths resulted, being a mortality of 44 per cent. The modern tendency is toward early laparotomy. The very important and never-failing rigidity of the abdominal muscles is probably the most important indication for laparotomy. It may be that operation must be performed simply for the control of hemorrhage, the extent of which is indicated by the increasing dulness of the iliac fossa. Sutures or gauze packing control bleeding well. The thermocautery is of very little value. The author concludes that the prognosis of the severe cases of wounds of the liver alone has improved under early operative treatment. This is inaugurated for the control of hemorrhage, for thorough examination and for prevention of infection. Mild cases without symptoms of collapse or internal hemorrhage should be treated expectantly. The mortality of hepatic injuries will probably diminish very considerably as early operation is more generally resorted to.

Ureteral Catheterization for Therapeutic Measures.—It is conceded by all that the segregation of the urine by this method has a far-reaching value for diagnostic purposes. Few people have, however, employed it as yet as a therapeutic measure. G. v. ILLYES (*Deut. Zeitsch. f. Chir.*, January, 1905) reports seven cases from the clinic of Dollinger in whom very marked improvement had been noted as a result of ureteral irrigations. In one case the results were astonishing, the procedure having to all appearance cured the individual of a pyelitis. In the remaining six there was a perceptible although a less-marked improvement. The author concludes that this method of treatment is more than justifiable as a means of preparing patients who are in a profoundly septic condition, for operation, since by washing out these pus capities, their system can in a slight measure rehabilitate itself and establish fresh resisting powers which may be sufficient to determine between life and death after operation. He considers the danger of the technic as trifling and believes that in proper hands its simplicity and ease of execution is so great as to warrant its more general employment.

MEDICINE.

Albuminuria after Palpating the Kidney.—An interesting observation is recorded by J. SCHREIBER (*Zeitsch. f. klin. Med.*, Vol. 55). If a floating kidney be palpated in the usual manner, albumin will almost always appear in the urine, even where only a small portion of the kidney can be grasped between the fingers. The color of the urine, voided after palpation, is generally somewhat paler, and microscopical examination shows an abundance of epithelial cells from the pelvis, ureter and bladder, cylindroids, red and white blood cells, but hardly ever casts. The albuminuria is probably caused by the passage of serum from the capillaries into the tubules. Probably some lymph also reaches the latter since there frequently is no relation between the degree of pressure exerted and the amount of albumin. The observation is of great clinical value, since a doubtul organ in the abdomen may be safely diagnosed as kidney, if albuminuria follows after palpation.

Complications of Acromegaly.—Several cases of acromegaly, which may throw some light upon the pathogenesis of this peculiar disorder, are described by E. STADELMANN (*Zeitsch. f. klin Med.*, Vol. 55). In one marked polyuria and glycosuria were concomitant symptoms. The patient died of diabetic coma but no changes could be found in the pancreas at autopsy. The pituitary body was converted into a large tumor which proved to be a malignant adenoma on section. A second case was complicated by hypertrophy and dilatation of the heart, intra- and extrathoracic struma, protrusion of the eyeballs and moderate arteriosclerosis. A benign adenoma of the hypophysis and a marked interstitial pancreatis were found at autopsy, yet the patient had never passed any sugar with his urine. These two cases make the relation between pancreas and diabetes more doubtful than ever. Both cases presented the typical symptoms of acromegaly, but the fact that the bones were more hypertrophic in one and the soft parts in the other, make it desirable to speak of two types of this disease.

Struma and Cataract.—Turbidity of the lens of the eye is often associated with diabetes, but it is less commonly known than a number of other affections, notably hypertrophy of the thyroid, also play an etiological rôle. A. VOSSIUS (*Zeitsch. f. klin. Med.*, Vol. 55) believes this is due to some toxin secreted by the gland. All patients observed were of the female sex and the goiter was large and complicated by stridor and compression of the trachea. As a rule, the cataract affected only the nucleus and the perinuclear zones so that the peripher remained clear.

Polycythemia and Splenic Tumor.—All the recorded cases of polycythemia, more commonly known in this country as Osell's disease, have been tabulated by W. WEINTRAUB (*Zeitsch. f. klin. Med.*, Vol. 55). The majority of patients were males, usually in middle life. An etiological factor could not be discovered and it is almost certain that alcohol, syphilis or malaria play no rôle. The subjective symptoms may be divided into those due to deficient blood-supply of the brain (attacks of unconsciousness, headache, vertigo, tinnites, vomiting and general depression) and into those caused by the enlargement of the spleen (pressure in the left hypochondrium, pains, due to perisplenitis, gastric and intestinal disturbances). The most prominent objective sign is the cyanosis. The color of the skin is not, however, blue but more of a violet, and suggests pronounced hyperemia. The mucous membranes of the lips, tongue, gums and vocal cords are usually of a dark cherry-red. The spleen is often so large that a leucemia is first suspected. In the few cases with autopsy notes only a simple hyperplesia of the spleen could be detected but in one instance tuberculous changes were found in this organ. It is extremely doubtful, however, that this has any bearing on the condition, for many similar lesions are reported without blood changes. The liver is often enlarged and of soft consistency. The most characteristic change in the blood is a marked increase in the number of red cells and the percentage of hemoglobin. The highest figures recorded are 12 million for the former and 200 per cent. for the latter. The red cells rarely show morphological changes and the leucocytes are frequently increased, yet a differential count does not vary much from the normal. The specific gravity and dry residue usually fall within the normal limits while the amount of albumin may even be subnormal. Symptoms appearing later in the course of the disease are dyspnea, hydrops and albuminuria of unknown cause since albumin is only present in traces, with at most a few hyaline casts. The blood-pressure was found increased by some, normal by others. A coincident uratic diathesis (gout, renal stones) is not rare, but probably due to the continuous leucocytosis with its increased breaking-down of nuclein bases. A rational therapy does not exist, but good results frequently follow repeated venesections. Polycythemia may also occur without splenic tumor, but is then usually due to intoxication, with carbon monoxide or phosphorus, to congenital heart-lesions or to high altitudes. The true cause of polycythemia is not known, but probably the destruction of red cells does not go on as rapidly as in normal blood.

Relation of Tuberculosis to Pseudoleucemia.—H. FALKENHEIM (*Zeitsch. f. klin. Med.*, Vol. 55) reviews the literature upon the connection between tuberculosis and pseudoleucemia and finds that upon first sight intimate relations seem to exist between the two conditions. A number of cases are on record where even the pathologist believed the glands were typical of pseudoleucemia, yet where tubercle bacilli were found in the tissues. The belief is gaining more and more ground that at least a certain percentage of cases of lymphadeny, running with intermittent fever, are tuberculous affections. Sternberg has recently described changes in the lymphnode, supposed to be characteristic of tuberculosis. The lymph-spaces are dilated, the endothelial cells proliferated and within the stroma there are found, besides the usual lymphoid cells, groups of large, uni- or multinuclear cells with abundant protoplasm and round or indented, intensely staining nucleus containing nucleoli or karyokinetic figures. In ten out of fifteen cases, unmistakable signs of tuberculosis were present in other organs and tubercle bacilli were occasionally found in the glands. Although many writers have confirmed the observations of Sternberg, the author does not believe that the evidence is conclusive. In most cases, the tuberculous changes were more recent than the lymphatic hyperplasia, and there is no reason why one may not assume that the tubercle bacilli have been passively transported into the glands by way of the lymph-channels. Reed has injected glands with typical changes into guinea-pigs and has given the patients tuberculin injections, always with negative results. Finally, the cells of Sternberg have also been found in lymphosarcomata. It need not surprise that a body weakened by a malignant disease should occasionally be invaded by tuberculosis, but it is wrong to attribute the former to the latter for this reason.

Fever in Syphilis of Liver.—An important fact to remember in cases of fever of unknown cause, is that syphilis of the liver may be responsible for the rise. F. KLEMPERER (*Zeitsch. f. klin Med.*, Vol. 55) states that the fever is intermittent or remittent in type and frequently accompanied with chills or chilliness, but does not have the regularity of malarial fever. Attacks of profuse nocturnal perspiration frequently molest the patients. The liver is enlarged, but not necessarily irregular, and some tenderness may be present, so a diagnosis of liver abscess or suppurative cholecystitis is made. Other cases are treated a long time for malaria, tuberculosis or sepsis without improvement. The effects of mercury and iodide of potash are indeed remarkable, for a fever which has lasted for months may disappear in a few days. Similar symptoms may occur with syphilis of the lungs, which is usually treated for tuberculosis and with cerebrospinal syphilis. The pathological findings are generally gummata, which give rise to fever as they break down.

Theory of Infection by Tuberculosis in Children.—It has been claimed by v. Behring within recent years that in adults, infection with the tubercle bacillus does not necessarily produce phthisis. He believes that sometime during early life there has been a tuberculous infection, which may have been latent or not given any outward signs of its presence, and that this is what predisposes to the invasion of the organism later in life by the same disease. The same infantile infection may also on the other hand bring about a condition of immunity against later infection. H. BEITZKE (*Berl. klin. Woch.*, January 9, 1905) claims that v. Behring's theory remains unsubstantiated by facts and rests purely on a speculative basis. The writer undertook to demonstrate this latent form of tuberculosis in infancy by a search for the tubercle bacilli in the blood of infants which had died from other disease without any gross evidences of tuberculous lesions. As the bacilli are believed to reach the blood through the intestinal tract, it seemed probable that they would be found in the venous blood mixed with the lymph, or in the right heart. The blood was accordingly abstracted under proper precautions from the right ventricle and injected into guinea pigs. Of 98 cases which were available, only 48 proved of any value for the purposes of the investigation. Control tests with cases which had died of tuberculosis, all gave positive results. In one animal which died spontaneously in four weeks after injection, no changes were found at the site of inoculation or in the regional glands, but the liver and spleen contained a large number of miliary nodules, and the lungs showed fine punctate hemorrhages. No bacilli were found. The case can only be looked upon as doubtful because the child from whom the blood was taken was only two days old at the time of death. In the other 47 cases the results were entirely negative in both animal experiments or by Jousset's methods of inoscopy. The writer thinks that the proofs of v. Behring's theories are in no way conclusive and until they can be made so, the theory formulated by this investigator cannot be accepted.

Graves' Disease and Adenoids.—That adenoid vegetations may be the cause of this condition, as well as of epilepsy and chorea, is the belief of B. HOLZ (*Berl. klin. Woch.*, January 23, 1905), who reports a number of cases to substantiate his statements. In two children with marked adenoid hypertrophy he found a well-developed exophthalmos and other signs of Graves' disease, but no cardiac symptoms or enlargement of the thyroid. In both, clearing out of the adenoids was followed within two weeks by a disappearance of the exophthalmos. In one child there was a recurrence of the adenoids within two years and also a reappearance of the exophthalmos, which also disappeared after the adenoid vegetations were removed for the second time. In another case, a marked case of chorea was likewise benefited. The author concludes that exophthalmos, if not merely a protrusion of the bulb due to mechanical reasons, may be considered as establishing the diagnosis, even if no other well marked signs of Graves' disease are present. This disease furthermore is essentially a toxemia of the central nervous system brought about by an abnormal internal secretion. It seems very likely that the disease can be produced by hypertrophy of the adenoid, and that this same factor may bring about epilepsy or chorea. Furthermore by the removal of these offending growths, all these conditions may be cured.

Fever in Cholelithiasis.—There can be little doubt at the present day that the fever accompanying gallstones is due to bacterial action, for trauma to the mucous membranes, experimentally induced in animals, is never followed by reaction. The most common germs found in the gall-bladder are the colon and the typhoid bacilli, but staphylococci, streptococci and even sarcinæ have been encountered. The pneumococcus, on the other hand, does not find conditions favorable for growth in the bile. There are about twenty cases on record where the bile itself proved sterile, but the interior of stones contained in the gall-bladder harbored germs. The different layers of the same stone were even found to contain different germs, thus proving that two different infections had occurred. Microörganisms may reach the interior of the gall-bladder in two different ways: they may descend from the radicals to the chief biliary ducts or else may travel from the papilla of Vater upward against the stream. The

former is more common with infection with one germ; the latter with mixed infections. In almost all cases that were operated during the fever the bile was strongly infected; in the few cases reported with sterile contents the fever was usually due to some other lesion. According to H. EHRET (*Zeit. f. klin. Med.,* Vol. 55) even the normal bile contains a small number or germs; aerobic germs seem to predominate in the lower, larger branches, and anaerobic ones in the upper, smaller ones. Even in the case of streptococci, they are not pathogenic. Specific germs, such as the typhoid bacillus, have not been encountered in health. The presence of bacteria alone is not responsible for the fever, for many cases have been operated with distinct lesions in the gall-bladder and many pathogenic germs, yet perfectly normal temperature. This corresponds with the finding of pneumococci in healthy lungs and of diphtheria bacilli on healthy tonsils. Probably the body is already immunized in such cases or the germs are prevented from entering the system. It has been proven by animal experiment that germs injected into the gall-bladder disappear rapidly, even if the biliary ducts are ligated, so that there can be no doubt that the body is able to cope with a certain amount of infection. The degree of resistance offered by the body is therefore just as important in bringing about fever as the infection itself. The following experiments speak for an active immunization: (1) If colon or other germs be injected into the ear-vein of dogs it will be more difficult to set up a cholecystitis three or four weeks later and the animals will react with only very slight fever. (2) Animals which have gone through an experimental cholecystitis will hardly react to injections of coli, etc. (3) If new germs of the biliary system are affected after a cholecystitis has existed for some time, the subsequent symptoms are less severe. (4) If streptococci are injected where colon bacilli are already present, a new rise of temperature will generally be noticed. Typhoid injected into a gallbladder containing colon bacilli is, however, often without effect. (5) The animals experimented upon usually survive the operation, unless operated during the attack. Many facts important in diagnosis may be adduced from the above observations. Thus, the presence of fever in the absence of other complications, invariably means an infection. Normal temperature does not exclude infection, but if it is certain that fever has never existed at a previous date, one may safely conclude that active processes are not going on in the biliary passages. The presence of fever or its height does not permit one to diagnose the exact lesions present since the highet temperatures often go with very slight changes and little or no temperature with advanced lesion. The following laws may, however, be laid down: (1) In doubtful cases a rise from the normal to a high temperature within a few days will argue against cholangitis or cholecystitis. (2) The prognosis is more favorable if the fever appears late in the course of the disease, but unfavorable if very chronic cases run with very high fever. Frequently repeated attacks of high temperature speak for chronic obstruction of the choledochus. (3) High continuous fever is not an unfavorable sign by itself. (4) If the fever stops by crisis the infected area has probably become sterile, while if it ends by lysis the biliary passages may remain infected for a long time. If the fever is complicated with icterus, the infection involves the finer ducts or at least extends into them; in the absence of jaundice, these ducts are probably free. The simultaneous appearance of fever and jaundice may also point to a chronic obstruction of the choledochus, especially if the attacks are sudden, regular and intense. Three stages may be recognized in almost every case of cholelithiasis: a prefebrile, febrile and postfebrile stage. A spontaneous cure is possible in the latter stage. As a rule it is not safe to operate during the fever since the body has not become sufficiently immunized to withstand contamination of the peritoneum or general infection.

Value of Ficker's Diagnosticum.—Ficker's diagnosticum, an emulsion of dead and broken-up typhoid germs, is recommended from many sides in the place of a living culture, for Widal tests, since it is permanent and will thus enable every physician to test for agglutination. Most reports are favorable, yet H. SELTER (*Münch. med. Woch.*, January 17, 1905) has tested quite a few blood-specimens where the Ficker test was negative, yet that with the living culture positive. During the height of the disease, both tests were generally positive, but in early and late cases the living bacilli are certainly to be preferred. In most cases it is better if a physician sends his blood-specimens to a laboratory, since here tests with the paratyphoid germs can also be made.

Typhoid Agglutination with Allied Germs.—An interesting contribution to the already extensive literature on typhoid agglutination is furnished by A. GRÜNBERG and P. JOLLY (*Münch. med. Woch.*, January 17, 1905). These authors found that the agglutination of the blood from different cases of typhoid varies considerably and stands in no definite relation to the severity of the disease so that it is well possible that a mild case will agglutinate strongly and a severe one moderately only. Even the number of typhoid bacilli found in the blood after blood cultures will not give an idea of the patient's condition. The blood of positive typhoid cases was also tested with paratyphoid germs and positive agglutination was obtained in as high as 70 per cent. In some of these, the paratyphoid agglutination was much higher than the typhoid agglutination even though it was positively proven by blood-culture that the disease was typhoid. In 55 per cent. the colon bacillus was strongly clumped, and in 22 per cent. the bacillus enteriditis of Gärtner. It follows that the Widal reaction is not absolutely specific, and that only a blood-culture will positively determine the germ which causes the disease.

X-Ray Treatment of Leucemia.—Nicholas Senn, in 1903, reported a case of leucemia successfully treated with the rays. In 1904, Bryant and Crane reported two cases of leucemia with recovery. These were also subjected to the X-ray. J. C. G. LEDINGHAM and R. G. McKERRON (*Lancet*, January 14, 1905) report the results of a similar treatment of splenomedullary leucemia occurring in a boy eleven years of age. The splenic enlargement was enormous and the blood picture was absolutely typical. The abdominal distention was marked, the lower border of the spleen reaching to within a finger's breadth of the pubes. There were 3,570 red cells per cubic millimeter, 2,304 white cells, hemoglobin 80 per cent. The temperature was elevated when the boy was admitted to the hospital, but after staying in bed for a day or so, it became normal. It was noticed that this occurred every time that the patient was allowed to get out of bed. Arsenic was badly borne and had to be given up. For the one and a half years previous to the time that he was in the hospital wards, there had been but little change in the boy's general condition except for the fact that the spleen had grown larger. During the six months prior to X-ray treatment, the blood showed the following average

count: White cells 200,000, with variations of 40,000 on either side; red cells 3,300,000. The ratio remained at the fairly constant figure of one to 15. Hemoglobin percentage taken by Haldan's instrument remained fairly constant at about 55 per cent. The result of the differential counts are given in the paper in the minutest detail. Following Senn's methods, the rays were applied over the spleen and the lower epiphysis of the femora. The exposures lasted ten to fifteen minutes every other day. Through three months of treatment, no constitutional effects at all were noted aside from a slight prickling sensation. This condition was in marked contrast with those produced in the cases of Senn and Bryant. The curves presented show that the leucocytes came down in six weeks to 23,000. The red cells during June, July and August averaged 4,500,000. The hemoglobin, however, remained stationery. It must not be forgotten that arsenical treatment may produce similar changes. Extraordinary as the results of the rays were upon the blood picture, they were even more so in their action upon the general condition of the patient. From having been bedridden, he was within a month able to go up and down stairs. At the beginning of the treatment, his maximum girth was 32 inches. On September 24 it was 26½ inches. There was a corresponding gain in weight. The following theories have been suggested to explain the mode of action of radiotherapy in leucemia. Senn believed that his results were due to antiparasitic action, and if Lowit's views on the etiology of leucemia are correct, this may seem plausible. Mosse and Milchner, working with rabbits found alterations in the lymphoid and myeloid elements of the marrow under the X-ray. The experiments of Joachim and others would seem to show that all the bone-marrow in the body would have to be exposed to the rays in order to produce results. Finally, Lepine and Boulay have shown that enzymes can be influenced by the rays, and since Ehrlich holds that an enzymes may be responsible for the condition, it is possible that its destruction prevents the further influx of leucocytes into the system.

PATHOLOGY AND BACTERIOLOGY.

Vital Examination of Leucocytes.—If a moist blood-film be examined over a hanging-drop chamber, so as to retard drying, the ameboid motions of both multi- and uninuclear leucocytes may be demonstrated for hours, sometimes even for days. A drop of water placed in the bottom of the chamber will cause the leucocytes to swell up, and will impart very rapid oscillating motion to the granules. The same may be seen in the pus cells of cystitis or gonorrhea, and is a sign that the cells are losing their vitality. A new method of staining the elements of the blood has been discovered by D. ROSEN and E. BIBERGEIL (*Virchow's Archiv*, Vol. 178, No. 3). A solution of the dye employed is simply spread out in a thin film upon a cover-slip; over this the blood is spread and the specimen then examined in the hanging-drop, before the blood has dried. If a mixture of pyronin and methyl-green is employed, the nuclei will first appear red, later green. Even in the later stages, a delicate red network arranged like the spokes of a wheel, will appear within the nucleus. The blood-platelets also show a red and a green substance. All dyes have a deleterious action upon the leucocytes, but the acid ones are more injurious than the basic. If eosin be employed, it will first dissolve in the serum, so that the cells appear to float in a pink fluid. Soon the leucocytes will swell up and appear rounded and the granules in their interior will become very active. The lymphocytes never show this phenomenon since their protoplasm does not contain true granules. The same applies to the lymphocytes and myelocytes of the lymph-nodes and bone marrow. The granules generally take up the dye soon after the cell has lost its vitality. Basic dyes first tinge the protoplasm, then the nucleus, but the latter will retain more of the dye. Neutral dyes are split up into their component parts before the nucleus is stained. The protoplasm is first tinged slightly with the mixed dye, then the nucleus takes up the basic dye. The neutrophile granules become decolorized later, so that they appear as if only the basic dye had been employed.

Organic Phosphorus in the Urine in Pathological Conditions.—The determination of the inorganic P_2O_5 cannot be regarded as a true index of phosphorus metabolism, according to D. SYMMERS (Jour. of Pathol. and Bacteriol., January, 1905), since an appreciable and important amount of P_2O_5 in organic combination is excreted in the urine in various pathological conditions, so that frequently 25 or 50 per cent., and in occasional instances, almost all the P_2O_5 appears in the organic state. The excretion of organic P_2O_5 is to an extent rhythmical, periods of excessive excretion alternating with what may be either retention or diminished production, so that in cases in which an average output is to be established frequent determination must be made. The excretion of organic phosphorus is pronounced in lymphatic leucemia, where there is a marked change in the ratios of nitrogen to organic phosphorus as well as an absolute increase in the percentage of organic P_2O_5 in the total P_2O_5, while the ratio of nitrogen to total P_2O_5, and so the inorganic P_2O_5 shows little if any departure from the normal. In nervous diseases of the degenerative type the absolute amounts of organic P_2O_5 as well as their percentage to the total P_2O_5, are increased, sometimes to an enormous extent. It seems impossible that such amounts could be derived directly from the obstruction of nervous tissues. In this connection the question of tropic influence assumes importance. It seems unlikely that the increased excretion of P_2O_5 could be derived from bone. The confirmation of this statement is seen in the fact that in osteomalacia the output of P_2O_5 has not been found increased. There is weight in the assumption that the increased phosphorus output depends upon general metabolic causes, probably in the waste of phosphorized endogenous compounds. The abnormal increase of organic P_2O_5 may be an increase in the production of phosphorized endogenous metabolic compounds, or an expression of lessened oxidation, with the inorganic phosphates as the end-product.

The Pathology of Pernicious Anemia.—A histological study of seventeen cases of pernicious anemia was made by G. L. GULLAND and A. GOODALL (Jour. of Path. and Bact., January, 1905), from which the authors draw the following conclusions: The essential feature of the disease and the criterion in its diagnosis is, that it is a megaloblastic anemia. The widespread evidences of blood destruction occurring in liver, spleen, leucolymph glands and marrow, indicate abnormal vulnerability in the blood cells rather than a pathologically excessive leucolytic action on the part of so many diverse tissues. The accumulation of iron in the liver is due partly to the disintegration of weakened or weakly blood corpuscles by endothelial cells and leucocytes and partly (and to a much greater extent) to storage of iron, which is the product of red blood corpuscles which have been disintegrated by phagocytes elsewhere. This accumulation of iron in the liver is not peculiar to pernicious anemia, and is the normal result of the abnormal amount of blood destruction. There is no direct evidence of special disease of the intestine, and the intestine need not be the primary seat of toxin production, though in certain cases, and notably in bothricephalus anemia, it probably is. In some part of the body a toxin is produced which acts directly on the bone marrow, interfering with normoblastic blood formation, leading to megaloblastic formation, and acting with negative chemiotaxis upon leucocytes, especially of the neutrophile variety. The large old blood corpuscles produced by such a marrow, perhaps as much from their size as from inherent weakness, fall a ready prey to endothelial cells and leucocytes in the hemolytic organs, notably hemolymph gland, spleen and marrow. It is quite possible that certain individuals, from congenital defect in the marrow, may be specially prone to the disease, as there is little doubt that the megaloblastic degeneration represents a reversion to the fetal type.

The Plurality of Cytolysins in Snake Venom.— Of considerable importance from the standpoint of cellular intoxications are the result of the researches on the mechanism of the cytolytic activities of snake venom, conducted by S. FLEXNER and H. NOGUCHI (Jour. of Path. and Bact., January, 1905). They find that venom contains solvents for the parenchymatous cells of several animals, and that considerable differences in activity in this respect occur, according to the source of the venom. The solvent action of venoms upon various kinds of animal cells is shown to be due, not to the presence of a single solvent, but to a number of solvents which are distinct one from another. The solvents for any given organic cell of one animal may be abstracted from venom by absorption without removing the solvents for the same kind of cells belonging to another animal species. Cytolysis is brought about through the interaction of amboceptors (of the venom) and complements of the respective animals. That the solution of cells is not the result of enzyme action is shown by the fact that the amboceptors for liver and testicular cells resist heat.

Dog-Tongued Elongation of Left Hepatic Lobe.— The variations of the size of the left lobe of the liver, sufficient to cause symptoms, have been recognized and reported in but one case, that of LANGENBUCH (Annals of Surgery, January, 1905). In this case the liver is described as a short corset organ in which in addition to the right lobe being pressed upward into the diaphragmatic space, the left lobe is pushed across in the left hypochondrium, where it spreads over the fundus of the stomach and over the spleen. The woman had had pain for eight years; she was nirty years old. While lying on her back the pain was almost intolerable. The treatment of this case consisted in resection of the left lobe. Ascites existed for a short time after operation. Hammond's subject was a girl, sixteen years of age. She had had a painless swelling of the epigastrium for nine years. She had never had any evidence of hepatic disease, but had suffered from palpitation of the heart, dyspnea and feeling of gastric distention. She was free from these symptoms when in an upright position and when the stomach was empty. Examination showed what appeared to be immensely distended stomach. The mass appeared to be influenced by respiration. The right hepatic lobe could be felt just below the costal margin. The heart apex was heard best in the fourth interspace. The condition had been diagnosed as gastroptosis colon distention, hydatid cyst and malignant hepatic disease. The author considered it probably a cyst of the pancreas. The temperature and blood count were normal. The pulse in the sitting posture was 78 and in the recumbent 126. On abdominal section the left lobe was found to extend entirely across the lesser curvature of the stomach, into the left hypochondrium, where it was flattened out over the spleen. There were no adhesions. It could be lifted from its position easily. It was thin. The capsule seemed normal. There were no nodules or any evidence of pathologic change. The right lobe appeared normal, as were the other organs in the neighborhood. On attempting to replace this lobe, the respiration immediately became markedly embarrassed. The entire lobe was accordingly sutured to the abdominal wall. The results were perfect. The length of the lobar from the free margin of the liver to its apex was 6¼ inches, width 1¾ inches. Inasmuch as it has been shown by both Pronfick and Von Meister that resection of a part of the liver will be followed by regeneration, nothing could be gained by such operation, and ventrosuspension seemed the only practical course to take. While in this case the history shows that the deformity had existed from early childhood and had perhaps been congenital, there is no doubt that a gradual extension of this tongue from the main body of the liver had taken place quite rapidly in the last two years. The patient's occupation, that of a laundress, had caused sufficient trauma to encourage growth. It has been shown at autopsy that when the left lobe is deformed, it is usually folded upon itself and more or less incurved.

Morphology and Biology of Tubercle Bacillus.— The best medium for growing tubercle bacilli is coagulated blood-serum, according to E. LEVY (*Zeitsch f. klin. Med.*, Vol. 55). A pure culture can easily be obtained, if infected material is injected into guinea-pigs and the organs of the tuberculous animals are then transplanted on the serum. A new tube is inoculated every four weeks and the fifth or sixth generation will then grow luxuriantly upon agar, which should contain no more than two per cent of glycerin. The so-called spores, the author believes, are not really spores, but may be compared to similar structures better studied in actinomyces. Portions of the filament here have lost their contents by diffusion through the membrane or by retraction. What remains within the capsule of the tubercle bacillus is still capable of reproduction, even though the process is so slow that it cannot be observed under the microscope in the hanging drop. The occurrence of branching and of club-shaped ends makes it very possible that the tubercle bacillus is closely allied to the group of ray-fungi.

Para-Urethritis.—Associated with the urethra are often to be found a series of gland-like structures which may become of pathological significance in the presence of an infection. They are more frequently seen with hypospadias than in the normal penis, or when hypospadias is not present, on the lips of the meatus. They vary in extent from slight depressions to long ducts and may be independent of the urethra or connected with its lumen. J. W. CHURCHMAN (*Jour. Am. Med. Ass'n.* January 14, 1905) reports two cases of urethral infection which show that gonorrheal disease of these ducts may occur in the male and that it may manifest itself either during the course of an ordinary urethritis or before urethral symptoms have appeared. Paraurethritis in its early stages may simulate inflammatory lesions of the surface of the glans, notably beginning chancroid, chancre or herpes. Paraurethral infection, once it has become established, can be destroyed only with great difficulty, the organisms appearing in abundance even after cauterization of the duct. The author thinks that the infection can be overcome without surgical interference by persisting in conservative treatment and the continual existence of a neighboring focus of infection does not necessarily mean a bad urethral invasion if careful prophylactic measures are taken.

PEDIATRICS.

The Metabolism of an Artificially Fed Infant.—A careful study of the exchanges of matter and energy in his own artificially fed infant was made by F. TANGL (*Pflüger's Archiv*, September 30, 1904). Although born at term, the child was considerably below the normal weight, but was otherwise healthy. It was fed upon modified cow's milk prepared after the method of Székely and Kovács. The principle of this method depends upon the fact that by means of carbon dioxide, cow's milk under great pressure will precipitate its casein. Skimmed milk is warmed to 60° C. and then put under a pressure of 20 to 25 atmospheres, when with the aid of CO_2 the casein is thrown down. Two parts of the whey are then mixed with one part of cream and then 1½ parts of equal parts of milk and cane-sugar is added. This mixture is then pasteurized in bottles. The virtues of this preparation are supposed to lie in the removal of the superfluous casein without the addition of any foreign agent, the CO_2 producing no change in the milk, and being itself easily removed. This preparation has the following composition: Water, 87.2 per cent.; fat, 3.7 per cent.; casein, 1.5 per cent.; albumin, .9 per cent.; sugar, 6.3 per cent., and ash, .7 per cent. The author found that this food was well assimilated by his infant, which, although delicate, was nourished as well as a normal child and, with the exception of the inorganic constituents, as well as a breastfed infant. The absorption and utilization of the proteids was excellent. Of the total energyvalue of the modified milk, 89.2 per cent. was utilized by the infant, which, although delicate, got the same proportion of energy from its food as the strong, healthy infant gets from ordinary cow's milk. Moreover, the bodily growth, the taking-on of flesh, and the deposition of mineral salts, followed the same course as in a strong infant fed on cow's milk.

Pyloric Stenosis in Infancy.—This condition, since attention has been called to the clinical features, is no longer a medical curiosity; but the following case is of interest because of its successful termination after surgical interference. An infant of eleven months was apparently well until the sixth month, when it began to vomit after nursing. It also developed an attack of bronchopneumonia followed by empyema, which was aspirated. At the time of admission to the hospital at eleven months, the child was greatly emaciated. A rubber drainage tube was inserted into the empyema sinus and the pulmonary symptoms cleared up. The vomiting persisted in spite of measures of treatment applied. A diagnosis of stenosis of the pylorus was based on the vomiting, dilated stomach, constipation, absence of bile in the vomited matter and loss of weight. At the operation of the pylorus was found decidedly thickened, but no evidences of inflammation were present. A gastro-enterostomy was done after Kocher's method and a few days after the child was able to retain milk. The stools also became normal, and the patient gained in weight rapidly and remained well. H. L. K. SHAW and A. W. ELTING (*Albany Med. Annals,* January, 1905), who report this case, have collected reports of forty operations upon infants with pyloric stenosis, of which nineteen were gastro-enterostomies, with a mortality of 63 per cent., the remainder pyloroplasties and Loretta's operation. The writers believe that pyloric stenosis in the infant is of much more frequent occurrence than is commonly supposed; that medical treatment in these cases has proved uncertain and unsatisfactory; that surgical interference should be practised before the strength and vitality of the patient have become seriously reduced, and that pyloroplasty and anterior gastro-enterostomy are the operations of choice.

~ **Infantile Syphilis.**—This term is confessedly much to be preferred to the rather frequently used "inherited" or "congenital' forms of syphilis. GEORGE F. STILL (*Lancet,* November 19, 1904) states that some writers would apply the term "inherited" in such cases only in which the syphilis rates from the time of conception, reserving the term of "congenital" for those in which it was transmitted at some later period of intra-uterine life. Speaking of the transmission of syphilis to the offspring, the writer said that one of the most striking features in the family history of syphilitic children is the frequent absence of any syphilitic history in the mother. This demonstrates the truth of what is embodied in Cole's, that a mother who has shown no symptoms of syphilis may nurse a congenitally syphilitic child without fear of infection. Coutts has suggested that this immunity is derived from the syphilitic fetus, who imparts is own antitoxin to the mother. The order and frequency of the symptoms are considered by the author under the following headings: *Marasmus.* —All in all, this is probably the most noticeable as well as the most frequently observed symptom. In its gravest forms it frequently dates almost from the birth. Snuffles occur almost always within the first three months. The author found it present in 70 per cent. of his cases. The lesion may be very severe, or it may amount simply to an inconsiderable nasal obstruction. The discharge is, however, occasionally blood-stained. On account of the disability in breathing, the child cannot nurse. The depression of the bridge of the nose may be produced very rapidly. *Skin eruptions.*—These generally appear soon after the snuffles, almost always within the first three months. They are very uncommon after six months. The author found a characteristic eruption in 69 per cent. of his cases. Macular patches predominated with erythematous, desquamative, fissural, bullous and condylomatous following in order of frequency. Two very important symptoms are characteristic of inherited syphilis. One is the extraordinary growth of hair which is usually developed at birth, the other being, within a few months, an exactly opposite condition, viz., extreme thinning of the hair. Another very characteristic lesion is onchyia. Enlargement of the spleen,—the statistics on this point are variable, averages having been made as low as 10 per cent. and as high as 58 per cent. Forty-five per cent. of the author's cases showed enlargement. Orchitis is a rare condition, having been

present in only five out of 64. Ten per cent. of the author's cases, up to the age of twelve, showed cerebral affection of one kind or another. In considering the contagiousnes of inherited syphilis, the author has said that it was hardly possible to overemphasize the importance of Colles's law. Coutts says, "I have personally never known an instance where syphilis was contracted from an infant with the inherited complaint. L. D. Buckley, however, states that "hundreds and thousands of cases of innocent syphilis have had their origin in innocent babies, and too great care can hardly be exercised." delivery. None of these three children showed evidence of spontaneous improvement, although the eldest was kept under observation several months before operation. Four years ago the eldest child was operated on, and the depression was elevated., It proved extremely elastic, however, and nothing but a fracture of the part in several segments sufficed to overcome the deformity. Although four years have elapsed the region is not yet covered in and still pulsates freely. In the two younger children the method employed was inversion of the depressed area. Circular parallel trephines armed with rim-flange guards were used to cut out discs. These in each case measured 3½ inches in diameter. The steps of the operation are briefly: (1) Exposure of the scalp; (2) removal of the depressed area; (3) inversion of this bone in a sterile towel, and the reduction by thumb pressure of the bend as far as may seem to correspond with the natural curve of the skull; (4) replace it, still inverted, on the dura; (5) close the scalp suture. The author concludes that depressed greenstick fractures do not recover spontaneously. This should not be expected of greenstick parturition fractures any more than of similar fractures elsewhere. This is true of cases over one month of age, and in which Kerr's method has been found inadequate. Inversion is unquestionably the best technic yet offered, and infinitely preferable to elevation.

Lobar Pneumonia in Infancy.—JOHN LOVETT MORSE (*Am. Med.,* January 28, 1905) believes pneumonia is far more common during the first two years of life than is generally supposed. Its course and prognosis differ materially from the descriptions given in many of the older as well as in some of the newer textbooks. The onset is less stormy than is usually described. A chill practically never occurs; convulsions are very unusual. Cough rarely amounts to much in the beginning. High fever usually develops rapidly and is generally accompanied by drowsiness and apathy. The most common period of pyrexia is seven days. A shorter duration is more common in infancy than later. The average duration is longer in the fatal cases. Remissions of even as much as three or five degrees are not uncommon. Crisis is less common than later. Lysis is especially common in cases of long duration. Collapse during the crisis is less frequent than is usually taught. The usual pulse-rate is between 150 and 170, being over 150 in 75 per cent. The usual respiratory rate is between 55 and 80. It is more often above 80 than below 55. The rate of respiration is always increased out of proportion to that of the pulse. This change in the pulse-respiration ratio is most important in diagnosis. Cough is seldom a prominent symptom. Gastro-intestinal symptoms are very common and very important. Marked anorexia is the rule. Vomiting is not very common. Diarrhea is more common than constipation. Distention of the abdomen is frequent, difficult to relieve and often hastens the fatal termination.

The urine often shows the evidences of acute degeneration and occasionally of acute inflammation of the kidneys. The usual mental condition is one of drowsiness or apathy. Cerebral symptoms are usually functional in origin and are frequently associated with a high temperature. The nervous symptoms are often due to a complicating inflammation of the middle ear. The diminution of the respiratory sound on the affected side is often the earliest sign and is of great importance in diagnosis. The order of frequency of involvement of the lobes is left lower, right upper, right lower and left upper. There is no relation between the mortality and the part of the lung involved. The mortality varies directly with the amount of lung involved. Acute inflammation of the middle ear is the most common complication. The pneumonia mortality in The Infants' Hospital series was 25 per cent. This is higher than that in private practice. The younger the infant, the worse the prognosis. The prognosis varies with the amount and not with the part of lung involved. Fever lasting more than nine days is of serious import. The prognosis is good when the temperature is not over 103° F. It is serious when over 106° F. Variations between these two points are unimportant. The prognosis is good when the pulse is not over 140 or the respiration over 55. The amount of the increase above these limits is of little importance. The gastrointestinal are the most dangerous of the more common complications. The treatment is hygienic and supportive rather than medicinal. Far more harm can be done by overmedication than by undermedication. The infant should not be disturbed. It must have the greatest possible amount of fresh, cool air The diet must be regulated to suit the weakened digestion and food forced if necessary. Stimulation should be used when indicated, and not as a routine measure. Strychnine is most useful, alcohol next. The fever should not be treated unless it causes marked nervous symptoms or depression. It should then be treated by cold externally and not by antipyretics internally. Cold must be used cautiously, as infants bear it badly. Fan baths and cold packs are best borne. Local applications should be used only for pain; oxygen for cyanosis. Creosote, the various serums and other "specifics" have no effect on the course of the disease.

NEUROLOGY AND PSYCHIATRY.

Hypochondriasis.—As the result of extended observations, A. SCHOTT (*Berl. klin. Woch.*, December 19, 1904) believes that this condition is not a nosological entity, but rather that it is an indication of degeneration. Hypochondriasis is a very frequent accompaniment of neurasthenia and hysteria, and may appear in all forms of insanity. In dementia præcox, hypochondriacal states demand particularly careful analysis and observation on account of the danger of confusing it with simple neurasthenia or hysteria. In the presence of very marked hypochondriacal conditions, the tendency to suicide or self-destruction must always be reckoned with, and where it becomes an insanity the danger to the patient's surroundings must be taken into account. In every case of hypochondriasis a careful bodily examination is indicated, and all peripheral sources of nerve irritation are to be removed as far as possible. The treatment must be directed to the underlying sources of illness, and the use of drugs should be restricted.

Fecal Vomiting and Reversed Peristalsis in Functional Nervous Disease.—The importance of fecal vomiting as a diagnostic feature of intestinal obstruction is such that the possibility of the occurrence of the symptom in other less grave conditions

is overlooked. In the case reported by F. P. WEBER (*Brain*, Summer, 1904) three successive laparotomies had been performed in a patient in whom fecal vomiting and reversed peristalsis were merely hysterical manifestations. This, as well as the study of similar cases in the literature, lead the author to conclude that functional nervous vomiting, like the hemi-anesthesia, palsies and spasms of hysteria, must be regarded as due to an abnormal state of the cerebral cortex, and is just as much a symptom of functional brain disease as the vomiting in cases of cerebral tumor is of organic brain disease. Fecal vomiting of functional nervous origin is merely a rare and extremely exaggerated form of ordinary hysterical vomiting. The vomiting in functional brain disease may sometimes be more violent and severe than it ever is in organic cerebral disease, since fecal vomiting is scarcely known to occur in cases of cerebral tumor. Some light is thrown on this point by the fact that a delusion is apt to be more stable and better "organized" in a monomaniac, whose brain, could it be examined, would probably show no obvious change, than in a general paralytic, whose brain is the site of grave organic disease. For the occurrence of fecal vomiting of functional nervous origin active intestinal antiperistalsis is absolutely necessary. But it is not certain that antiperistalsis necessarily always plays a part in the fecal vomiting known to surgeons as a symptom of organic intestinal obstruction. The fecal vomiting in organic obstruction of the bowels is seldom, if ever, more than "feculent," that is to say, having the odor of feces without containing obvious (visible) fecal particles or masses. Vomiting of formed feces, in the absence of malingering and gastrocolic fistula, practically only occurs in functional nervous cases. This may partly be accounted for by remembering that antiperistalsis, if it occurs at all, is likely to be more forcible when the muscular walls of the gut have not been previously weakened by overdistention or gross organic disease. Hysterical malingering is, of course, apt to develop in the same class of patients in whom fecal vomiting occurs, also the possibility of genuine fecal vomiting occurring side by side with simulation must be borne in mind.

Erotomania.—LEONARD CORNING (*Am. Med.*, January 21, 1905) adverts to the great confusion existing among writers in the use of this term, and more particularly to the frequent confounding of the disorder with nymphomania and satyriasis. Erotomania he finds to be a delirious amorous obsession, pathologic, essentially psychic and devoid of carnal appetite. Erotomania, in the first instance then, is a hypertrophy, so to speak, of the ideal. Later, if thwarted in his pursuits, the erotomaniac may disclose mortification, chagrin, profound depression, even to the point of suicide; or exasperation against the subjects of his obsession or her natural protectors. Under the sway of this emotion he may commit murder. In the interesting and unique case detailed by the author, both the persecutory and depressive stages were successively in evidence. From an exhaustive study of cases coming under his observation, Corning concludes: (1) Erotomania, like other manifestations of paranoia, is due to degeneration. (2) Erotomania may occur in either men or women, but is more common in the former. (3) Broadly, it is an affection of the imagination, a morbid extravagance of the ideal. (4) In its individual manifestations, it presents the characters of a love,

over, of carnal appetite. (5) There is nearly always, though not invariably, a tendency to personification; the subject foists his ideality upon a living person, or upon an inanimate object (statue, picture). In the latter case, his apostrophes and gestures disclose the personifying propensity. (6) The delirious idea of the erotomaniac, like others of the same class traceable to degeneracy, is impulsive, obsessional, irresistibly compelling. Though his intelligence may show him the consequence of yielding to his obsession, he is powerless to resist it. He should, therefore, not be held to a legal responsibility for his acts, but should be restrained, and, if necessary, committed to a hospital for the insane. (7) Erotomania may occasionally coexist with nymphomania or some other form of sexual aberration, or with mysticism. (8) The obsession of the erotomaniac is usually for an individual of the opposite sex. (9) While erotomania may disclose itself in youth, it is really a disease of adult life, coming on after puberty and ending usually in dementia.

Psychiatry in its Relation to Other Sciences.— CHARLES L. DANA (*Am. Med.*, January 21, 1905) shows the relations of psychiatry to its nearest allied sciences,—economics, psychology, physics, neurology, and internal medicine, pathology and physiological chemistry, criminology, forensic or legal medicine, and anthropology. He indicates the lines along which work can be carried with mutual help to all, and especially to the advancement of a sounder knowledge of that capstone of all medical sciences, the pathology of the mind.

Gluttony as a Cause of Symptomatic Epileptic Convulsions.— W. P. SPRATLING (*Med. Rec.*, January 28, 1905) describes a type of epilepsy due to errors of diet which is fairly common and is generally amenable to treatment. The patients are usually middle-aged men of plethoric physique, leading inactive lives, and eating and drinking to excess. The primary cause of the convulsive attacks in these cases seems to lie, first in a weak stomach and second in some obscure disorder of metabolism. The type of convulsion induced is usually of the grand mal variety, though petit mal seizures are also observed. The treatment is that of the toxic state induced by the faulty metabolism, and is mainly dietetic and hygienic.

THERAPEUTICS.

X-ray Treatment of Urethral Caruncle.— The X-ray is now so well established as a remedial measure that one is hardly surprised to hear that it has been successfully used in some hitherto refractory conditions. G. H. STOVER (*Den. Med. Times*, October, 1904) reports two cases of urethral caruncle successfully removed by means of the X-ray, which he considers the first cases to have been recorded. The first case had appeared originally fifteen years ago and had recurred after two operations. Twenty-five X-ray treatments were given, using a tube of medium low vacuum, at a distance of five inches, the seances lasting ten minutes. The size of the growth diminished after the fourth or fifth exposure, and the pain became gradually less. In the second case the growth had been removed some six years before but had returned. Six exposures were given with a low tube at a distance of six inches, with ten-minute seances during a period of about three weeks. After the fourth exposure the patient stated that she had no more pain or soreness.

Large Fibro-Sarcoma Treated by Roentgen Radiation.— Many medical practitioners are skeptical as to the utility of the Roentgen rays in deep-seated malig-

nant conditions and as a matter of fact the failures are more numerous than the successes. Occasionally, however, clinical manifestations are observed, of a nature to draw attention to the curative power of this agent. CLARENCE E. SKINNER (*Arch. of Elec. and Rad.*, October, 1904) reports a case of inoperable spindle-celled sarcoma, ten by five by eight inches in dimensions, producing lethal symptoms in the patient, and which had resisted all measures applied for its relief, which was entirely removed and the patient restored to unimpaired usefulness and health, by 136 applications of the X-ray of high penetration from a tube excited by a static machine, the treatment having extended over a period of 849 days, being an average of one application every 6.2 days. The case demonstrates that sometimes the rays effect a complete cure; that the lack of satisfactory results in many cases is probably not due to mere size in the tumor or thickness of intervening tissue, but to some undetermined factors which it is not unlikely we shall know more of later; that there is in all probability some connection between systemic toxemia and reduction of the growth, as in this case there were periodic recurrences of toxemia with invariable shrinkings in the size of the tumor; and that in inoperable cases the Roentgen-ray treatment should be persisted in as long as possible, even when there is no observable result.

Inoperable and Recurrent Sarcoma Successfully Treated by Roentgen Ray.— It is now widely held that the greatest value of the Roentgen radiation in connection with malignant growths is in postoperative cases to lessen the danger of the recurrence, and in inoperable cases to diminish suffering and perhaps prolong life. The number of complete cures in the latter type of cases is necessarily small, and the three cases reported by GEO. C. JOHNSTON (*Jour. of Adv. Therap.*, November, 1904) are of interest. *Case I* was in a man fifty-six years of age, suffering from a growth, the nature of which the author does not state which involved the abdominal muscles, the peritoneum and the omentum. Much of the growth and incidentally the abdominal wall were removed, still leaving a considerable portion of the tumor. Treatment was given daily for two months, bi-weekly for three months and once or twice each week for another month. The pain had disappeared, the abdominal wall softened and the patient had gained thirty pounds. Examination fails to reveal any evidence of the existence of tumor. *Case II*, a recurrent sarcoma of the vulva in an unmarried woman of forty-two years, had been apparently removed in its entirety by operation, but recurred in the scar at the end of six months, when it was again removed. At the end of several months the growth again recurred, this time involving the skin, subcutaneous tissues and the periosteum. Ten-minute treatments were given daily for three weeks. The pain had disappeared and a recess of ten days was given the patient. Treatment was resumed with the same technic every other day for the next six weeks. Treatments were then given with a high tube twice each week for two months. Six treatments were then given with a softer tube, resulting in a dermatitis necessitating a discontinuance of the treatment. Upon recovering from the dermatitis, it was found that the last trace of the sarcomatous deposit had disappeared. *Case III* presented involvement of the entire upper chest, the suprasternal notch and the left triangle of the neck. There had been three operations. The treatment was given every day for three weeks with a low tube. The author does not mention the duration of the balance of the treatment, but states that though two years have elapsed, the patient is apparently well. There were no evidences of toxemia in any of those cases and when any of them was burned, the reaction was prompt. The author concludes from these cases that we are justified in believing that in this agent, when promptly and intelligently applied, the profession has a curative that is entitled to the respectful attention of the medical world, and that its indications should be carefully studied.

Hodgkin's Disease.—Although the prognosis in Hodgkin's disease has been generally considered practically hopeless, the undoubted benefit derived in some cases from applications to the X-ray justifies us in hoping that we have, if not a permanent, at least a temporary relief at our disposal in this obscure and severe condition. JOHN V. SHOEMAKER (*N. Y. Med. Jour. and Phila. Med. Jour.*, November 12, 1904) reports a case in a physician, fifty-two years of age, who was treated while in the last stages of the disease by the X-rays. The patient died, but the changes in his condition were remarkable and worthy of record. Daily exposures were given for ten minutes during sixteen days. The entire body was exposed to a high vacuum tube placed alternately over the abdomen, left side and back. The size of the glands began to diminish by the end of the first week and were one-third the original size at the end of sixteen days. The spleen decreased gradually. These results obtained in sixteen days in a moribund patient warrant our hoping for some success in the early stages of the disease. The dangers to be confronted are: That there may not be time to produce an effect; that the rapid disintegration of the morbid tissues may cause toxemia; and burn.

Surgical Use of the X-ray.—The liability of making a false diagnosis by too hasty interpretation of X-ray results, and the dangerous possibilities lurking therein, is cause for unending vigilance on the part of the skiagrapher. A. L. GRAY (*Mobile Med. and Surg. Jour.*, November 4, 1904) reports a case in point. The patient, a small child, had swallowed a safety pin, which, resisting all efforts at removal, remained lodged in the alimentary tract, and gave rise to severe pain and an enterocolitis. The child was examined with the fluoroscope because of objections to anesthetics on the part of the parents. A small mass which might have been the head of the pin was located in the hepatic flexure of the colon. Operation was deferred on account of the position of the obstacle which apparently rendered natural passage possible. After several days, the child growing steadily worse, another examination by fluoroscope was made and a similar spot located in the hypogastric region, the original spot having disappeared. The child was then anesthetized and a radiograph made, which plainly showed the pin in the esophagus. The stomach being opened, a probe was passed through the mouth and the pin pushed downward and removed. It was subsequently ascertained that the child had been given large doses of subnitrate of bismuth for the bowel trouble, and it is presumed that the latter was responsible for the errors in the fluoroscopic examinations.

Movements Produced in the Stomach and Bowels by Electricity.—G. G. MARSHALL (*Med. Rec.*, January 7, 1905) conducted a series of experiments on animals in order to determine the degree of reaction caused by the application of the electric current to the stomach and intestines. The faradic, galvanic, and faradogalvanic currents were used in different degrees of intensity, and the method of applying the electrodes was also varied in many ways. While the pyloric end of the stomach feebly contracted, and the intestines contracted uniformly under the immediate application of a small metal electrode, no reaction followed when a thin layer of wet cotton was placed over the metal. The contraction produced in the intestine had no semblance to peristaltic movements, only the circular fibers being constricted. Hence the conclusion is drawn that electricity as generally administered, either percutaneously or directly, never causes contractions or increased peristalsis of these viscera, and the author shows how contractions of the thoracic muscles may simulate a gastric reaction, and so deceive physician and patient. Experiments are also described which demonstrate that the gastric mucosa offers no unusual resistance to the passage of electric currents, and that the failure to produce contractions in the organ is in no way due to a non-conductive character of its mucous membrane.

Roentgen Rays in Cancer.—Since 1896, when Despeigne first utilized the X-rays in a case of cancer of the stomach without any results, this therapeutic agent has been used the world over with varying success. DIEMIL PASHA (*Revue de Chirurgie*, January, 1905) states that within the last six months Dumur and Lamoine have published the histories of a number of cases cured by this means. One of these was cited as a case of cancerous stomach cured by radiotherapy. Side by side with these favorable reports, the same authors have published a long series of distressing failures as well as some more encouraging, in which there was a cessation of the functional disturbances without permanent cure. The author recites the history of the treatment in seven subjects. In the case of the three which he reports as cured, the cancers were superficial and primary. Three were ameliorated and one was treated without success. The author admits that we know comparatively nothing of the action of the rays on cancer whether it has to do, as Perthe has contended, by retarding epithelial growth, or whether the process consists in an electro-chemical inflammation of specific local origin as Jacinski has suggested—nobody knows. The author tends to the conclusion that the action is probably an antiparasitic one. He further concludes that radiotherapy may have a very favorable action on malignant tumors in general; that it yields absolute cures in cases where the lesion is superficial, primary and only slightly advanced; that it is a most excellent palliative treatment for deep-seated, advanced growths and exercises an influence upon cachexia.

PRESCRIPTION HINTS.

Chronic Bronchitis.—The following combination is recommended by E. Fletcher Ingals to relieve the cough in chronic bronchitis when opiates are not contra-indicated:

R Morph. sulph.........................gr. 1
  Ammon. carb.....................gr. 30-40
  Syr. pruni virg.............)
  Mist. glycerrhizae comp..... ∫ ...aa. oz.   4

M. Sig. One teaspoonful in water to relieve the cough;
or,

R Terpin hydratis....................gr. 2
  Ext. cannabis ind.................gr. 1-20
  Codeinæ ....gr. ⅛
  Ol. menth. pip....................gtt. ½
  Sacchari albi.......................gr. 3

M. Ft. capsulæ No. 1. Sig. One every four hours until the cough is relieved.

THE MEDICAL NEWS.

A WEEKLY JOURNAL
OF MEDICAL SCIENCE.

COMMUNICATIONS in the form of Scientific Articles, Clinical Memoranda, Correspondence or News Items of interest to the profession are invited from all parts of the world. Reprints to the number of 250 of original articles contributed exclusively to the MEDICAL NEWS will be furnished without charge if the request therefor accompanies the manuscript. When necessary to elucidate the text, illustrations will be engraved from drawings or photographs furnished by the author. Manuscript should be typewritten.

SMITH ELY JELLIFFE, A.M., M.D., Ph.D., Editor,
No. 111 FIFTH AVENUE, NEW YORK.

Subscription Price, Including postage in U. S. and Canada.

PER ANNUM IN ADVANCE	. . . .	$4.00
SINGLE COPIES	. . . . .	.10
WITH THE AMERICAN JOURNAL OF THE MEDICAL SCIENCES, PER ANNUM	. .	8.00

Subscriptions may begin at any date. The safest mode of remittance is by bank check or postal money order, drawn to the order of the undersigned. When neither is accessible, remittances may be made at the risk of the publishers, by forwarding in *registered* letters.

LEA BROTHERS & CO.,
No. 111 FIFTH AVENUE (corner of 18th St.), NEW YORK.

SATURDAY, FEBRUARY 25, 1905.

THE DRYNESS OF INDOOR AIR.

THE supply of fresh air, that is of oxygen-laden air, has for many years now received from physiologists, physicians, and nurses as well as from the more knowing of the public, no little attention,—not nearly enough, to be sure, but still an encouraging degree of effective notice. Even architects and builders have given a half-hearted sort of attention to ventilation, so that nowadays in some of the finest and most carefully built buildings it is possible often to find the carbon-dioxide percentage almost down to the hygienic maximum of six-hundredths. The anti-tuberculosis crusade is helping this matter greatly, and it is likely that the Americans now being born will look back with something of the same sort of horror on our present closed windows and "bundling up" as that we now feel toward surgery before the days of anesthetics or toward city milk-service of a quarter century ago. Oxygen, purveyor of long life, the world is learning at last to appreciate, and the mean life-span lengthens correspondingly.

But there is another aspect of the atmosphere we breathe which gets relatively no fraction of the attention that it deserves to receive. Nearly everybody ignores the highly important demand on the part of the respiratory passages and of the skin in general for moisture in the air about us in our offices, factories, shops and dwellings. When the atmosphere out of doors is very dry or very humid most persons realize it, and incontinently curse the " weather man," but they nearly all quite neglect to maledict the much more responsible authors of the harmful dryness of the air they live in inside of buildings. But slow always is the advancement of learning among the mass of men,—and truly testudinal where ancient habit and factors of trouble and of some expense of money hold it back, and with it the promised benefit.

In buildings heated by direct radiation and without forced drafts of air immediately from outdoors, tests with the wet-bulb thermometer often show a relative humidity of from twenty to thirty per cent., while the average in the open air of temperate climates is approximately seventy per cent. In dwellings heated by tight stoves this percentage of twenty or thirty is much reduced, often to the degree that the air feels "burned" even to the average individual. Apartments heated by indirect radiation or by furnaces usually show more moisture in their air because of the strong draft required from out-of-doors and usually from near the ground. Even in buildings provided with elaborate ventilating arrangements, the air's humidity is seldom adequate, for it unfortunately must be admitted that the very large majority of ventilating systems, which do not include power for forcing currents of air in and out, are failures, and plants with such power, steam or electric, are of course still relatively few. This failure of most air-supplying systems is at once obvious to any one who has made numerous tests of the proportion of carbon dioxide in the air of public and private buildings. The reason lies largely in the expense but in part surely too in the purely perfunctory way in which most architects plan the air-supply of their structures. But even were the allowance of air in the average building adequate, this would only in small part supply the needful moisture in the winter-time indoors.

Now this almost universal deficiency of watery vapor, suffered month after month and year after year, is a more serious matter for its victims, (and they are millions), than even most of us realize. The throat specialists can tell one how great the injury, so widespread, is, and they are unanimous with the hygienists and physiologists in preaching improvement. Many persons do not appreciate how large a surface of mucous membrane is exposed to the inflowing tidal air between the nostrils and the alveoli. Abnormally dry air passing so frequently over this large area of sensitive membrane dries it and soon begins to irritate it. The result in a few months is nasal catarrh, a "hacking" perpetual pharyngitis, and various affections of the mouth, the Eustachian tubes, the pharynx, larynx, trachea and bronchi. Defect in the vigor of these exposed membranes makes various infections more easy by lessening the membrane's power of resistance and thereby the way is open to secondary evils worse than the unpleasant and harmful primary inflammation. But again moist air feels warmer than does dry air of a similar temperature. A room at 65° F., if the air be properly moist, seems warmer and far more comfortable than a dry room at 72° or 74° F. Here is a saving in heat, which means not only a saving of money, but also the prevention of no small amount of harm and trouble to the organism.

In a large telephone building in an eastern city, the numerous young women were formerly much troubled and incapacitated from work by the dryness of the air they breathed. An apparatus was recently put in which evaporates daily sixty-six gallons of water and distributes it about the building. The effect was immediately apparent in the decrease of illness among the employees, not to mention their increased comfort. The watery vapor required in a room is greater in amount than might be expected in advance. A pan of water on a radiator or on a stove, unless actually boiling continually, is of no account in supplying the moisture deficiency even in a single room. The large pan constructed in most furnaces must be kept supplied with water to be of any service whatever! Steam escaping from a radiator-vent is adequate for that room, but impracticable owing to the noise.

The problem then is a hard one with our present habits of heating the rooms in which we pass our days. One solution, for certain times and places, lies in open windows and in ventilating systems which really supply fresh air in amount to satisfy the ever-hungry blood. Another solution is in makeshifts to keep the air moist by hook or by crook. The best, real solution, for promulgation among men at large, and for adoption as fast as the pressing need becomes known among us, is the construction, with the houses of various sorts, of some sort of air-moistening device. Meanwhile it behooves medical men to keep in mind this crying need of our modern civilization,

so unphysiologic in so many different ways. Of all these this need of moisture in the air we breathe is by no means least.

NEUROFIBRILS AND THEIR FUNCTION.

No better illustration of the advancement of biological learning is at hand than the histology of the nervous system in the last ten years affords. To-day the unprophetic physiologist knows not what to suppose and can ' only stand and wait," hopeful that ere long the secret of the nerves will be revealed.

In the neurone theory the physiologist, as well as the histological embryologist, had something definite, and though puzzled by the uniqueness of its supposed mode of action, he hailed it as an added hope in the solution of the great neural mystery. What a storm, then, a priori, met the drawings and descriptions of Apáthy and of Bethé, showing fibrillar continuity between the neurones! And this despite the fact that men as trustworthy as Dogiel, Schultz, Lugaro, Golgi, Nissl and Mann more or less promptly corroborated the findings of the discoverers. Nissl's conversion to the belief is especially significant because there is little doubt that study of his chromatophile bodies retarded somewhat the general seeing of the intracellular fibrils and their continuity with those of the neuraxes and dendrites.

At the present time the majority of workers familiar with the new staining methods and with the research reports of the last two years, are nearly ready to accept many things opposite in tenor from the demands of the neurone theory, especially such (though these are yet but few) as have seen the books of Bethe and of Nissl. Looked at broadly, the present views are but the settling back of the pendulum set moving at least ten years ago by the observations which led up to the neurone theory, so named by Waldeyer, and whose climax was found in the comprehensive book of Barker. From the old-fashioned notion of nerve-cell and fibers the trend distinctly now is round toward the same point of view again, save that a wealth of detail has been added to both cell and fiber, and that the trophic function of the cell has meanwhile been exalted— possibly too far.

Were we to roughly describe a plate at the end of Nissl's book (which he expressly declares is nothing more than a suggestion, "not even an hypothesis"), showing perhaps how neural things tend, we should quickly see the nature of the anti-neuronal drift. Imagine, then, that the gray matter of the nervous system (save the "gray" fibers, which are ill-called so because they appear darker than the highly refractive medullated fibers with their covering of fatty myelin), that the gray matter is pervaded everywhere with the finest of fine networks, the diameters of whose threads and of whose meshes are both exceeding small. This is the "neural gray." Here and there this reticulum gives off a most delicate fiber and several of these threads combine to form one of the "primitive" fibrillæ which in turn combine in hundreds to form a nerve fiber (the neuraxis of a neuron, the axis cylinder of the nerves). Around the nerve fibrils is a closely fitting reticulum known already as Golgi's net, and where this fibril ends in the gray matter it comes into connection with the neural gray network, than which it is coarser and much more conspicuous, especially to Golgi. By threads as yet unseen this Golgi's net connects everywhere with the ends of the fibrils, which in turn combine into fibers. Between these fibrils and the ultimate meshes of the neural gray there are then two modes of connection,—one by the mediation of still smaller direct fibrillilæ (if we may make the word) and the other by means of the widespread connections of Golgi's net surrounding the ends of the fibrils.

But around the nerve-cells, too, extends everywhere both Golgi's net and, outside that, the "neural gray." Through the cell extend numberless fibrillæ, some of which go far in the projections of the cell, but many of which also, by the mediation of Golgi's net, are in direct connection with the universal basal reticulum of the neural protoplasm, which this "neural gray" essentially is. Thus the conducting paths of the nerves, the fibrils of the fibers, are in constant and intimate connection with the very substance of the gray matter's protoplasm and conduct its impulses and those from active tissue protoplasm, doubtless, of other sorts.

Functionally this suggestion if proven substantially true would mean much. That it will be so proven no one at the present time would dare to prophesy, but should it be, we should have at length an hypothesis adequate to account for phenomena under the neurone theory blind and with only a semblance of satisfaction in their explanation. Thus in the first place observe that the gross fiber of the nerves is wholly inadequate to convey the messages which seemingly should pass through it, say from the end-organs of a portion of an eye-muscle, if the fiber conducts as an unit a single message. Still more striking may be the deficiency in the organ of Corti of the ear. This consideration makes it in general probable that the fibril rather than the fiber is the neural path. Again, nothing which adequately represents any connection between these fibrils and the essential parts of the nerve cell, namely, the nucleus, and Nissl's bodies, has ever been pointed out. On the other hand, the neural gray and Golgi's net do suggest the possibility of a means of connecting the nervous impulse in the fibril with a sufficient source of metabolic energy. In this suggestion, if nowhere else, the nerve fibril runs continuously into the very heart and being of neural protoplasm where it could receive all that the vastly complex katabolism of lecithin and "phosphines" and nucleoproteids could give it. As for the use of the nerve cells, it is not too hard to conceive that they might modify by their metabolism, perhaps anabolic, the messages as they pass, and support the nutrition of the fibrils or of the neuroplasm around them. The pigment granules found in many nerve cells indicate the presence of most delicate metabolism of some sort.

But idle, nearly, are the wanderings of the imagination when let loose from the editorial fibrils—that is to say, neurones—into the realms of the details of the nervous system, ænigma magna of the day.

ABDOMINAL PREGNANCY IN ANIMALS AND WOMEN.

IN the *Archiv für Geburtshülfe und Gynäkologie,* 1896, Band LII, S. 376, Leopold published the history of a remarkable case. A woman four months pregnant fell down stairs and injured herself in the abdomen. At the termination of the period of gestation an examination led to the diagnosis of extra-uterine pregnancy. The abdomen was opened and a fetus of about the fourth month of gestation enveloped in a thin sac was found to occupy the abdomen. The umbilical cord passed through an opening in the posterior wall of the uterus. This organ, in which was also located the placenta, was removed. The evident conclusion from these pathological data is that the uterus was injured when the woman fell and the fetus in its amnion was intruded into the abdomen through a rent in the posterior uterine wall. This condition has been termed "utero-abdominal" pregnancy.

In the *Lancet,* December 10, 1904, John Bland-

Sutton states that the chief interest of Leopold's case lies in the fact that, although this form of pregnancy is extremely rare in women, it is the commonest form of extra-uterine pregnancy in mammals with long two-horned uteri. The author is satisfied that tubal pregnancy in these mammals is exceedingly rare, he having failed to discover a single convincing record or specimen. There are, however, undoubtedly many cases correctly recorded of puppies and kittens enclosed in tightly fitting sacs which have been found adherent to the omentum and the intestines. Some observers have been led to the conclusion that these abnormalities represent examples of primary abdominal pregnancy.

That this is a purely unverified speculation continues to be Sutton's opinion. Thirteen years ago he advanced the belief that in mammals possessing bicornate uteri, the horns of which are of some length and frequently containing several fetuses, the uterus not uncommonly ruptures, because of its violent efforts to expel a contents which has grown proportionately too large for the maternal parts. In the vast majority of cases this accident is fatal to the mother. Occasionally, however, she survives and the extruded fetuses become adherent to the omentum, the uterine rent cicatrizes, the amniotic fluid is absorbed, the placenta disappears; the amnion shrinks and compresses the fetus tightly. Occasionally these sacs remain free in the abdominal cavity.

The phenomenon of so-called "abdominal pregnancy" in mammals has recently been stimulated by the observations of Pembrey and Kamann. These observers have experimented with rabbits. A doe was killed within a week of the last littering. On opening the abdomen five white discoidal bodies were found. They showed no attachment to the abdominal organs, and in all but the smallest the head, body and limbs of a fetus could be felt. Pembrey found a scar on the front of the uterus just below the junction of the cornua. A further description of his findings is to be had in the Transactions of the Obstetrical Society of London, Vol. XLVI, p. 283, 1904.

Kamann (*Monatsschrift für Geburtshülfe und Gynäkologie*, 1903, Band XVII, p. 588, Berlin) from a study of similar conditions concludes that in the case under his observation the embryos were discharged into the abdomen after primary rupture of the uterus.

In his book on the Surgical Diseases of the Ovaries and Fallopian Tubes, second edition, 1896, Sutton refers to the literature of the reported cases in which the cornu has undergone axial rotation. This is not uncommon in the mammals under consideration, namely, those having two-horned uteri. Pozzi, Martin and others have recorded cases of axial rotation in gravid Fallopian tubes in women.

In women utero-abdominal pregnancy is rare, for the simple reason that rupture of the uterus almost invariably is followed by death, but the case of Leopold furnishes conclusive proof that, occasionally at least, the human being may survive it. It is instructive to note that these conclusions are given added weight from comparative observations in animals by Sutton. Primary abdominal pregnancy is probably a myth of the past.

ECHOES AND NEWS.

NEW YORK.

Medical Library and Historical Journal.—Owing to the almost total destruction by fire of the establishment of its printers on February 13, it begs the kind indulgence of its subscribers and advertisers for delayed publication of the January, 1905, number. Fortunately, duplicate copies of all important MSS. were made before sending them to the printer, so the heavy loss incurred by the *Journal* will not be shared by its contributors or readers. The Editor desires to announce that immediate steps have been taken for the making of new plates and duplicating the entire number, which was in press, and that this issue will be published at the earliest possible date.

Denuding the Forests of the Empire State.—The destruction of the forests of the State of New York seems to be going on, but few people know how rapidly this work is progressing. Some computations on this subject have recenly been made and the figures are startling in the extreme. For instance, it is estimated by men who have looked carefully into the matter, and have taken actual results for a considerable period of time as the basis for their calculations, and it is stated as a positive fact that it takes thirty-five acres of pulp wood land per day to furnish the paper stock for the Hearst papers alone. in New York, Boston and Chicago. Here is the basis for the statement: Newspaper is made of 20 per cent. of sulphite pulp and 80 per cent. of ground wood pulp. One cord of wood produces 1,200 pounds of sulphite pulp. One cord of wood produces 1,800 pounds of ground wood pulp. The average lumber land in certain sections of the State produces ten cords of pulp wood per acre. Therefore, the ten cords produced for newspaper use, 16,800 pounds of stock, and the 300 tons divided by this equals thirty-five acres per day. Think of it, thirty-five acres of land being denuded for the pulp to furnish one newspaper in New York, Boston and Chicago, for one day. But the effect on the State water supply is something that cannot yet be estimated. A few centuries of this and the Adirondacks will be as barren as the Desert of Sahara.

Manhattan Maternity.—The Manhattan Maternity Hospital and Dispensary, at 327 East Sixtieth Street, was opened last week. The new institution is a model of its kind, containing every known improvement for the field it is to fill. It will include a training school for nurses and eight student-physicians can be accommodated in the building. There will be a large outdoor department, connected with the dispensary, which will cover practically the whole of the upper east side. The building has been put up and partially endowed by Henry A. C. Taylor. On the Board of Directors are Moses Taylor, President; Frank L. Polk, Secretary and Treasurer; Daniel Lamont, Percy R. Pyne, William Sloan, H. R. Taylor, H. S. Thompson, and Cornelius Vanderbilt. The building is square, of five stories and basement, and built of brick with a white enamel finish that it may be kept perfectly clean. On the main floor are the dispensary, the examining and admitting rooms, an office and Superintendent's reception room, with the students' dormitory and dining room. On the floor above are the wards, accommodating eighteen patients, and the nurseries for both the ward and private patient babies. There are tiny single cribs in the latter, and in the former little three-baby cribs with a couple of single ones for isolating the children when that is necessary. The ward patients' dining-room is also on this floor. All the rooms are bright and light, there being windows on all sides of the building. On the third are the private rooms. On the fourth floor at one side is the operating room and amphitheatre, with seats extending up into the top story.

Two Dangerous Bills.—To the Doctors of New York State: There are two bills now before the legislature of this State which we believe the medical profession should express itself as uncompromisingly opposed to. They are Senate Bill No. 261, introduced by Senator Fitzgerald, of New York City, entitled An Act to regulate the practice of Kinesipathy in the State of New York, and Senate Bill No. 298, introduced by Senator Davis, of Buffalo. Senate Bill No. 261 is somewhat vague in its provisions, but aims to include under the term "Kinesipathists" all massage operators. It might be made to serve a good purpose, possibly, if a clause was inserted providing that "in no case shall the practise of Kinesipathy be employed for the treatment of any disease or injury of the human body except under the advice and guidance of a licensed practitioner of medicine." If this is not inserted the bill might be construed as giving masseurs the right to treat diseases and injuries of the human body by means of the method known as Kinesipathy, in which case the bill would be worse than the Osteopathic Bill. The second bill, Senate Bill No. 298, entitled An Act regulating the practice of Osteopathy in the State of New York, provides for the creation of a Board of Examiners in Osteopathy, to appear before which one has to show evidence of attendance for three years at a regularly conducted school of "Osteopathy." Where such schools are located or what constitutes a regularly conducted school of "Osteopathy" I do not know. The secret of the bill is contained in a clause which provides that the Regents may accept, as the equivalent of this course of study, five or more years of practice. Section 11 of the bill provides that "Osteopathists" when duly licensed and registered in accordance with this act shall have all the rights and privileges and be subject to the rules and regulations that govern other physicians or medical practitioners in matters

pertaining to public health, but they shall not be authorized to prescribe drugs or to perform surgery." From this it will be seen that the enactment of this law will give to every person who has been practising the system known as "Osteopathy" for five years the right to register and obtain all the rights and privileges now possessed by physicians who have studied medicine for four years and who have complied with all the conditions of our medical laws, except that they cannot prescribe drugs. The fact that there is a law now on the Statute Book regulating the practice of the healing art and that these people who call themselves "Osteopathists" have been practising that art without complying with the law, is evidence enough, at least so it would seem, that they are lawbreakers; and yet, notwithstanding this, they have the assurance to go to the legislature and ask that special legislation be enacted for their protection. They cannot even plead that "Osteopathy" is prohibited in this State, for there are no restrictions placed on the person who qualifies under our present medical law. The regularly licensed physician can practise what is called 'Osteopathy' or any other peculiar system of healing, and doubtless does when there seems to be any particular reason for so doing. The fact is that "Osteopathy," as a distinct and separate method of treating disease, is not only a humbug and a fraud, but is positively dangerous in the hand of any but educated physicians. Will not the doctors of New York interest themselves in this matter and write their representative in the legislature exposing this fraud? Try and get the doctors in your county to do the same. When possible have your medical societies pass resolutions opposing the bill. The matter is now in the hands of the Senate Judiciary Committee, of which Hon. Edgar T. Brackett is Chairman. A list of members of the Senate Judiciary Committee is here added. Please send in protests at once. There will be a hearing on the Osteopathic Bill before the Senate Judiciary Committee Wednesday, March 1, at two o'clock P.M., in the Judiciary Room in the Capitol Building, at Albany. Will you try to attend personally and if possible have a delegation from your County appear in opposition to the bill? The Osteopathic Bill has since been introduced in the Assembly and referred to the Committee on Public Health. The hearing on March 1 will be a joint one before the Senate Judiciary and the Assembly Public Health. Below are the names of members of these two committees. If any of them are from your County please get all the doctors in their districts to write them to vote against the bill. *Assembly Committee on Public Health:* Hon. James C. Sheldon, *Chairman,* Cattaraugus; George H. Whitney, Saratoga; James K. Apgar, Westchester; Richard C. Perry, Kings; Frank L. Stevens, Rensselaer; Ezra P. Prentice, New York; Matthew Hurd, Rockland, Leonidas D. West, Yates; Edward Rosenstein, New York; John Wolf, Kings, John W. Gurnett, Schuyler.

Senate Judiciary Committee: Hon. Edgar T. Brackett, *Chairman,* Saratoga; George A. Davis, Erie; Nathaniel A. Elsberg, New York; William W. Armstrong, Monroe; Jotham P. Allds, Chenango; Spencer K. Warnick, Montgomery; Merton E. Lewis, Monroe; George H. Cobb, Jefferson; Alferd R. Page, New York; John Raines, Ontario; Patrick H. McCarren, Kings; Jacob Marks and Thomas F. Grady, New York.

FRANK VAN FLEET, M.D.,
Chairman of the Committee on Legislation.

PHILADELPHIA.

Appointed.—Dr. E. Harris Scatchard, of Germantown, has been elected superintendent of St. Luke's Homeopathic Hospital to succeed Dr. Carl Vischer, who has resigned because of the increased demand of his private practice.

Resigned.—Owing to the fact that he has accepted the position of assistant professor of surgery at the Jefferson Medical College, Dr. John H. Gibbon has resigned from the Medical Board of Examiners of the Civil Service Bureau.

Prize Award.—The essay on "The Biology of the Micro-organisms of Actinomycosis," written by Dr. James Homer Wright, of Boston, Mass., captured the Samuel D. Gross prize for the Academy of Surgery, for the year 1905.

Bequests.—The will of Isaac Rosskam bequeathed $18,500 to charitable institutions, of which $5,000 was given to the Jewish Hospital Association to maintain a Rosskam bed, $2,000 to the National Jewish Hospital for Consumptives, Denver, Col., and $1,000 to the Free Hospital for Poor Consumptives, White Haven, Pa.

Association of Infectious Diseases.—Dr. Edward Martin placed the authorities of the Municipal Hospital in a peculiar position by sending them a patient who was suffering with diphtheria, measles, chickenpox and scarlet fever. After some consideration the child was given a special ward with two nurses to take care of her.

Pneumonia Causing Alarm.—Of the 104 patients in the Germantown Hospital last week 21 were cases of pneumonia; of the 77 patients in the Samaritan Hospital 12 were afflicted with this malady; in the German Hospital six of the 85 medical cases were suffering with this disease; in the Hahnemann Hospital two thirds of the medical cases this winter have been pneumonia. Of the 509 deaths last week 102 were due to pneumonia.

The Associated Health Authorities and Sanitarians of Pennsylvania.—The twelfth annual convention of this body assembled at Harrisburg, February 13 and 14, 1905, and there unanimously indorsed the following bills now before the State legislature pending action: (1) The Establishment of a Bureau for the Registration of Vital Statistics. (2) The protection of the Inland Water Supplies of the State. (3) The Establishment of a State Department of Health. Dr. John S. Fulton, Secretary of the State Board of Health of Maryland, who delivered the annual address, stated that in many respects Pennsylvania in greatness was second in the list, but in a matter of vital statistics comes next to Oklahoma. In opening the symposium on Tuberculosis by the members of the medical staff of the Phipps Institute, of Philadelphia, Dr. Charles J. Hatfield, who spoke on "The Modes of Infection," maintained that there is little danger of infection through the ingestion of meat, but that sanitary inspection of milk, the sources from which it is derived, and the handlers of the product is of the greatest importance. He regards the dust from houses in which tuberculous patients are kept as extremely dangerous while the street dust he does not fear. Dr. Wm. B. Stanton read a paper on "The Importance of Popular Education in Regard to Tuberculosis." Although, he said, isolation of all cases is impossible and segregation impracticable, the consumptive can be taught to take care of his sputum and the healthy man his body; if those measures are adopted, prevention will be greatly enhanced. In his paper on "The Necessity for Early

Diagnosis in Tuberculosis," Dr. Joseph Walsh maintained there were two reasons for doing so: (a) It will give the patient the best possible chance for life. (b) It will prevent the patient from infecting other people. In discussing the free antitoxin question at the close of the session, Dr. A. H. Stewart, of the Philadelphia Board of Health, said the time had come when the State of Pennsylvania should furnish antitoxin free to rich and poor alike in all cases of diphtheria. Dr. Hugh Hamilton, of Philadelphia, in speaking of pollution of the water supply, maintained that, the complexities and intricacies of the pure water supply in this State were made more complicated by the reckless artificial pollution of the streams through several industries. Dr. A. H. Stewart, in discussing the "Disinfection for Communicable Diseases," stated that he found the best way to kill germs in an infected room was to apply the solution containing the gas directly to every portion of the room, walls and floors. The following officers were elected: President *ex officio,* Gov. Pennypacker; First Vice-President, Dr. T. M. McKee, of Kittanning; Second Vice-President, Dr. R. S. Maison, of Chester; Treasurer, Dr. Jesse Green, of West Chester; Secretary, Dr. W. R. Batt, of Philadelphia.

Section on General Medicine of the College of Physicians.—This meeting was held February 13, 1905. Dr. O. J. Kelly showed a patient who had recovered from "Pyopneumothorax after Evacuation through a Bronchus, Subsequent Resection of a Rib." When he saw the patient there were feeble signs of pleural effusion; about fourteen days later the patient expectorated pus, after which time the displacement of the organs was less marked; a little later, however, the symptoms of pyopneumothorax were distinct. At operation 30 ounces of pus were found. Dr. Eshner showed a case of aortic regurgitation. The murmur could be heard when the ear was placed from 2.5 to 4 cm. from the chest wall. Dr. Eshner then read a paper entitled "Universal Congenital Atrichia." The patient tells him that hair have never been present at any point upon his body. Eshner found atrophic changes in the nails and teeth. The patient scarcely ever perspires; he has retinitis albicans. Drs. Sailer, Geisler and Welty then read a paper entitled "Polycythemia and Chronic Cyanosis, with a Report of Three Cases." Upon their first cases they performed an autopsy but found no communications between the various cavities of the heart; the ductus arteriosus was not patulous. The red blood cells were and remained about 8,000,000 until the patient developed a lumbar abscess, when they fell. The hemoglobin could not be estimated. The second case had 8,000,000 red blood cells and hemoglobin 110 per cent. In their differential counts they found an occasional myelocyte, few normoblasts and basophiles and few basophilic red blood cells. The third case had as high as 9,240,000 red blood cells, and 120 per cent. hemoglobin. They studied a number of cases of advanced emphysema, but in none could an increase in the erythrocytes be determined nor were any of them cyanotic. Dr. Robinson showed a case of polycythemia. Dr. Sailer, in the discussion of his paper, noted Ehrlich pointed out that an iron-free diet brought about an improvement in the condition of the patient. Dr. J. Norman Henry read a paper entitled "Paratyphoid Fever with a Report of Six Cases." He maintains that there are two forms of the paratyphoid bacillus, one known as the paratyphoid A and the other as B. They can be differentiated from the colon bacillus by the fact that the paratyphoids do not ferment saccharose and do not coagulate milk. They are found in the blood, urine' and rose spots. He stated that the symptoms are identical with those of typhoid except the Widal reaction is negative when *Bacillus typhosus* is used to carry out the test, but there is clumping and cessation of motility when the paratyphoid bacillus is employed. Then, too, the duration of the disease is shorter than in typhoid fever and the paratyphoid may end by crisis. This disease may be complicated with typhoid fever. At post mortem he did not find involvement of the Pyer's patches ŋor the solitary follicles.

CHICAGO.

Open Willard Hospital.—The Frances E. Willard National Temperance Hospital was recently dedicated to the memory of the temperance worker. The hospital will accommodate seventy patients. It is the only institution of its kind in the country that eliminates alcohol 'in the treatment of patients.

New Hospital Law.—An ordinance to compel hospitals to operate morgues for the care of those who die in their charge until relatives have been notified was recently recommended by the Health Committee of the Council. Bodies must not be removed from hospitals for twenty-four hours after death unless permission is given by the relatives. The removal of bodies in any vehicle which may be afterward used to carry the living is prohibited.

Dr. Dudley threatens Suit to Enjoin a Publication.—An injunction suit to restrain the Globe Educational Society from using his name in connection with *Practical Home Treatment*, a publication of the Society, is to be filed by Dr. E. C. Dudley. Dr. Dudley declares he never saw a copy of the book of which he is advertised as one of thirty-two "eminent specialists," whose medical advice it contains until a prospectus of the work was brought to him recently by a canvasser employed by the concern. The people who got up the book have used his name as that of one of the authors of the book without his knowledge, and they have published also the names of several physicians who, are dead, among them Dr. Christian Fenger.

Unions to Fight Tuberculosis. — Tuberculosis farms to be established in different sections of the United States by labor organizations for the treatment of union workers afflicted with consumption were recently advocated by President George W. Perkins, of the Cigarmakers' International Union. The Cigarmakers' Union has had under consideration for a month or more the establishment of such an institution for the benefit of that organization. A new plan, now in preparation, probably will be adopted. The new scheme is broadened to include other international unions. According to the plan, farms will be located in North Carolina, the Adirondack Mountains, in the Middle West, and on the Pacific Coast. On account of the inroads of the disease into the ranks of the cigarmakers that union is interested particularly in the project. Since 1888 the per cent. of mortality among 47,000 members of the organization had 'been reduced from 51 to 24. Mr. Perkins contended there was room for still greater reduction in deaths. To combat the disease successfully, however, requires special advantages in the way of tuberculosis farms. Mr. Perkins heartily favors the project, and expects

within a month or two to see other labor organizations co-operating.

Court Rules Surgeon Must Get Patient's Consent Before Major Operation.—Any surgeon who performs a major surgical operation on a patient, without the consent of the patient, is, under the law, guilty of malice, and' is liable to punitive damages. Even the consent of the nearest relative to such operation, provided the patient be of sound mind, does not relieve the surgeon of liability. This principle has just been enunciated by the Appellate Court in a decision affirming Judge Tuley's finding of $3,000 damages against Dr. E. H. Pratt, who, it is said, in 1897 operated ón a Mrs. Davis without her consent and against her wishes. As a result of the operation, it is claimed, she became insane, and is now an inmate of the Kankakee Asylum. The Appellate Court's opinion, written by Judge E. O. Brown, holds that the surgeon deliberately deceived the patient regarding his intentions to perform an operation, and declares that the performing of a major operation without consulting and obtaining the consent of the patient, except in a case of emergency, amounts in law to malice and the surgeon is responsible for damages. Dr. Pratt, in his defense, asserted that the husband had given him *carte blanche* at the first interview to perform whatever operation he considered necessary, but admitted that this agreement was not made in the hearing of Mrs. Davis.

Dr. Senn on Brilliance and Genius.—It seems that an American daily recently published a short extract of an address of Sir Frederick Treves, which appeared under the head "Brilliant Surgeons not Wanted." Among other things, Treves is reported to have said: "Genius is some sort of neurosis, an uncalculated nervous disease. The few men of genius I have met were exceedingly impossible persons. They are certainly entirely out of place in the medical profession, where even cleverness is not to be encouraged. Indeed, of all desperately dangerous persons the brilliant surgeon is the most lamentable." The source from which this quotation emanated attracted Dr. Senn's attention. Further, he states that "for many years the medical profession has regarded Sir Frederick as a genius for good and substantial reasons. A genius in the sense in which this term is used in the quotation consists in a distinguished mental superiority; uncommon intellectual power; especially superior power of invention or origination of any kind, or of forming new combinations, or making new applications. Is Frederick such an enviable distinction in its own ranks? I think not. If it had not been for a liberal amount of inborn genius he never would have attained the worldwide reputation he so well deserves. The man who speaks so disparagingly of the brilliant surgeon and genius as an attribute of medical men is an indefatigable investigator, a skilful anatotions of existing principles or facts. Has the medimist, a prolific author, a pathfinder in the unknown fields of surgical patholoyy and operative technic, and certainly a clever operator.

CANADA.

A Union Banquet in Montreal.—On the evening of February 21 the profession of Montreal, both English and French, sat down to a love feast, and the hatchet was buried forever. The occasion was a joint banquet of the Medico-Chirurgical Society cal profession made a mistake in according Sir and La Société Médicale, and was significant in that it will tend to draw these two portions of the profession in that city into bonds of closer union.

Analysis of Montreal's Water.—A special commission is conducting day by day an analysis of the water of the city of Montreal. Frequent microscopical examinations have been made, and Dr. George Charlton, now of the Regina bacteriological station, has stated that he has found upward of forty varieties of organisms in Montreal's water. So far the examinations have not revealed the presence of any typhoid bacilli.

Vancouver General Hospital.—The annual meeting of the Trustees of the Vancouver (B. C.) General Hospital was held in that city on February 8. Dr. A. M. Robertson, the medical superintendent, submitted the following report: During 1904 the total number of patients admitted to the wards was 851, and 785 were discharged. The deaths numbered 63, and there were left in the hospital on January 1, 1905, 61 patients. The number of patients' days treatment during the year was 20,206, being an average of 55.2 patients per diem. The average cost per capita was 1.56. There were treated 307 cases of medical disease, 400 surgical cases, 28 eye cases, 40 cases of diseases of women, while 272 operations were performed, 23 being for appendicitis.

Actinomycosis Before the Montreal Medico-Chirurgical Society.—At a recent meeting of the Montreal Medico-Chirurgical Society, the subject of actinomycosis received considerable attention. It was introduced by Dr. James Bell, who reported nine cases, in which the diagnosis had been confirmed in all by bacteriological methods. Professor Adami discussed certain points in connection with he development of our knowledge of this disease and its causation. Dr. W. W. Chapman dealth with the clinical aspect of actinomycosis. From the medical aspect the subject was dealth with by Dr. W. F. Hamilton. Dr. A. G. Nichols had in charge the subject of bacteriology of the disease. All the papers are published in the February issue of the Montreal Medical Journal.

Fighting Tuberculosis in Montreal.—An important report has recently been made to the Hygienic Committee of the City of Montreal. Last June Dr. de Martigny, of Montreal, was apointed a special commissioner by the Montreal Hygienic Committee to proceed to Paris and investigate the Marmorek system of treating consumption. On his return to Montreal a short time ago, after having spent some months in Paris, Dr. de Martigny submitted his report. He is thoroughly convinced from his observations and experiments that Marmorek's serum possesses wonderful efficacy, and feels satisfied that if it were employed in the treatment of all of the tuberculous of Montreal, that tuberculosis would soon, or in ten years at least, be as scarce as smallpox. Dr. de Martigny concludes his report by strongly recommending the employment of Marmorek's serum in the treatment of tuberculosis, stating that the treatment in itself is harmless.

Personals.—Dr. Breffney O'Reilly, only son of Dr. Charles O'Reilly, medical superintendent of the Toronto General Hospital, has gone to Baltimore on special invitation from Dr. Osler to attend the last lectures of that noted clinician before he takes his departure to England. Two graduates of McGill University, Dr. McConnell, son of Dr. J. B. McConnell, of Montreal, and Dr. Wolferstan Thomas, of the same city, have been appointed by the Liverpool School of Tropical Medicine to study tropical diseases, the former to proceed to the west coast of Africa and the latter to South America, on the Amazone.

* Dr. Robert Allan Pyne, Toronto, Registrar of the College of Physicians and Surgeons of Ontario, has entered the cabinet of the Hon. Mr. Whitney, having been assigned the portfolio of Minister of Education. Two other doctors are also in the new cabinet, viz., Dr. Reaume, of Windsor, and Dr. Willoughby, of Durham.

Prof. J. George Adami, of McGill University, Montreal, will deliver an address at the annual meeting of the Canadian Association for the Prevention of Tuberculosis, which meets at Ottawa on March 15.

Dr. George A. Charlton, late Governor's Fellow of Pathology at McGill University, and late Fellow of the Rockefeller Institute, has been appointed pathologist and bacteriologist to the Government of the Northwest Territories.

Dr. Oscar Klotz, the Governor's Fellow in pathology at McGill University, which was instituted in 1899, has resigned. This fellowship is open to graduates in medicine, is tenable for two years, and has attached to it a salary of $500 per annum.

Senator Fulford, of Brockville, Ont., has donated the sum of $10,000 toward a nurses' home for the hospital at that place.

Dr. Frank Wesbrook, professor of bacteriology in the State University of Minnesota, and who was recently elected President of the American Public Health Association, has been paying a visit to his old home in Winnipeg.

Dr. James B. Huntington, of Boston, Mass., was in Victoria, B. C., the other day on his way to Japan. Dr. Huntington has been summoned to Japan by the Japanese Government to take charge of the military hospital at Nagasaki.

Dr. Bracken, secretary of the Minnesota State Board of Health, has been in Winnipeg during the past week gathering information regarding the typhoid outbreak there and other health matters in connection with Winnipeg.

GENERAL.

German Congress of Orthopedics.—The Fourth Congress of the German Association for Orthopedic Surgery will open its proceedings April 25, 1905, in Breslau.

No Yellow Fever at Colon.—The Isthmian Canal Commission has received a report from Health Officer Spratling, at Cristobol, Canal Zone, saying positively that it has not been shown that yellow fever does exist or has existed at Colon since he assumed the duties of health officer of Colon, on July 9, 1904. This report is in reply to statements that yellow fever exists at Colon and is concealed or unrecognized.

Compulsory Vaccination Legal.—Justice Harlan, of the Supreme Court of the United States, February 20, delivered the opinion in the case of Jacobson vs. the United States, involving the validity of the Massachusetts State law, giving authority to the health authorities of cities and towns in the State to impose compulsory vaccination regulations. He held the law to be constitutional on the ground that the protection of the health of a community may be exercised by the State as a police regulation.

Boston Medical Library Meetings.—The last meeting was held at the Library February 15. Dr. Geo. Seaes was in the chair. Prof. Gary Calkins, of Columbia University, spoke on the Protozoa in the Etiology of Infectious Diseases. So far, he said, there was only one disease definitely known to be used by a protozoa. Instead of speaking on this already widely known subject he confined himself to describing, by means of lantern slides, certain morphological changes in the life cycle and reproductive phenomena of various protozoa and their relation to higher organisms and to phenomena seen in disease.

Dr. E. E. Tyzzer, of the Pathological Department of the Harvard Medical School, spoke on some medical studies in the Philippines. Dr. Tyzzer, along with Dr. Brinckerhoff, had been sent by the Pathological Department to continue the study of smallpox in the Philippines, where conditions were more favorable than in this country. In his remarks he did not speak on smallpox, as the material and data collected were not yet entirely worked up,' but confined himself to general consideration on the hygienic conditions and the diseases prevalent in those islands. Forty-one per cent. of all deaths were in children under one year, this was largely due to the lack of proper food, there being no fresh milk, all the cattle having been carried off by rinderpest. Amebic dysentery was the one disease of importance to which Americans were subject, and only by careful boiling all water could it be escaped. There were about 6,000 lepers on the islands, with only 500 segregated. Plague appeared in 1899 but has now died out; cholera, in 1902, 157,-000 cases and 102,000 deaths! The last case appeared in February, 1904. Dengue fever and beri-beri crop up occasionally; typhoid is rare. Rinderpest appeared shortly before the American occupation and killed off 90 to 95 per cent. of all cattle; cattle now are inoculated against the disease, and only 3 per cent. die. He spoke enthusiastically of the excellent laboratory facilities in Manila, and of the good work in all branches of medicine done by the Americans.

American Physiological Society.—The following eminent foreign physiologists have been elected honorary members of the American Physiological Society: Th. W. Engelmann, professor of physiology in the University of Berlin; A. Dastre, professor of physiology at the Sorbonne, Paris; J. N. Langley, professor of physiology, Cambridge University; C. S. Sherrington, professor of physiology, University of Liverpool; Fr. Hofmeister, professor of physiological chemistry at the University of Strasburg; J. P. Pawlow, director of the Physiological Laboratory at the Imperial Institute for Experimental Medicine, St. Petersburg.—(*Science*.)

An Excellent Scheme.—We learn from the *British Medical Journal* that the Danish government has issued a stamp bearing the head of the late Prof. Finsen with the object of placing within reach of the poorer classes a means of subscribing to the national monument by which it is proposed to commemorate the work of the Danish investigator. On the occasion of the Christmas and New Year holidays the Danish Postmaster-General also issued four million illustrated postcards. The profits on the sale of these postcards are to form the basis of a fund for the erection of a sanatorium for indigent consumptives.

An Antiquackery Congress in France.—A congress "for the repression of illegal medical practice," writes the *British Medical Journal*, is to be held in Paris in May next under the presidency of Professor Brouardel. Among the questions to be debated the Organizing Committee has decided that special prominence shall be given to illegal practice by non-medical persons, lay or clerical, with a charitable purpose or under pretext of charity. A report on the subject will be presented by Maitre Bruno-Dubron, Doctor of Law, Advocate of the Court of Paris, and sometime secretary of the Conference of Advocates. He will deal with the illegal practice of medicine by ministers of religion, teachers, benevolent associations, etc. He will consider the measures of repression that can be employed against them, and the measures that can be adopted for the prevention of such abuses, notably the regulation of medical assistance given in educational establishments and in factories, and the legal sanctions to be enforced in case of failure to apply the law. Communications relative to the congress should be addressed to M. le Secrétaire Général du Congrès pour la répression de l'exercice illégal de la Médicine, Hotel des Sociétés Savantes, rue Serpente 28, Paris.

Army Medical Corps Examinations.—Preliminary examinations for appointment of assistant surgeons in the army will be held on May 1 and August 1, 1905, at several points to be hereafter designated. Permission to appear for examination can be obtained upon application to the Surgeon-General U. S. Army, Washington, D. C., and from whom full information concerning the examination can be procured. The essential requirements to securing an invitation are that the applicant shall be a citizen of the United States, shall be between twenty-two and thirty years of age, a graduate of a medical school legally authorized to confer the degree of doctor of medicine, shall be of good moral character and habits, and shall have had at least one year's hospital training or its equivalent in practice. The examination will be held concurrently throughout the country at points where boards can be convened. Due consideration will be given to the localities from which applications are received, in order to lessen the travelling expenses of applicants as much as possible. In order to perfect all necessary arrangements for the examinations of May 1, applications must be complete and in the possession of the Surgeon-General on or before April 1, and for the examination of August 1, on or before July 1. Early attention is, therefore, enjoined upon all intended applicants. There are at present twenty vacancies in the Medical Corps of the army.

Early Diagnosis of Tuberculosis.—The State Board of Health of Illinois has just issued for distribution to the physicians of the State, a circular on "The Early Diagnosis of Tuberculosis," which will bring to the physician in concise and systematic form, all of the information on the diagnosis of the disease to be obtained from a most exhaustive review of American or foreign medical literature, and which might be an example to other State Health Boards to follow in the fight with tuberculosis. The great interest in consumption, manifested during the past few years, has resulted in extensive scientific investigation, and the importance of early diagnosis both in saving the life of the patient, and protecting those with whom he comes in contact, has directed much of this investigation to the earliest reliable signs of the existence of the disease. Attention of the medical men of the State is directed to the laboratory of the State Board of Health at Springfield, and it is announced that examination of sputum of patients supposed to be tuberculous will be made without cost at any time. The establishment of container stations, for the distribution of

mailing cases for specimens, one in each county of
the State, is also announced, and special attention is
drawn to the fact that, wherever consumption is
found by physicians to exist in unusual numbers, inspectors will be sent to assist in the investigation of
the cause, and in taking necessary steps to check its
spread.

Manuel Garcia.—The *British Medical Journal* gives
further details in regard to the celebration of the
hundredth birthday of Señor Manuel Garcia, which
occurs on March 17. The anniversary is to be made
the occasion of a great demonstration in his honor
by laryngologists of every nationality, who will at
the same time celebrate the jubilee of their specialty.
The program, as far as at present arranged, is
as follows: At midday a ceremonial meeting will
be held at the rooms of the Royal Medico-Chirurgical Society, Hanover Square. The Spanish am-
bassador will attend to congratulate the illustrious
centenarian in the name of the Government of his
native country, and addresses will be presented by
the Royal Society, before which Señor Garcia read
his paper entitled "Physiological Observations on
the Human Voice" just fifty years ago; by delegates
of the Berlin, South German, French, Dutch and
Belgian Laryngological Societies; by musical societies and by old pupils of the famous maestro. In
order not to overtax the strength of Señor Garcia,
the addresses will for the most part be only formally
presented, and the whole duration of the proceedings will not exceed one hour. The meeting will
conclude with the presentation. to Señor Garcia
of his portrait painted by Mr. John Sargent, R. A.,
at the request of admirers throughout the world,
together with an album containing the names of the
subscribers. In the afternoon a scientific meeting
will be held in the same place for the purpose of
giving foreign specialists an opportunity of seeing
the methods of work and results of their British
brethren. In the evening there will be a dinner,
probably at the Hotel Cecil, at which ladies will
be present, and it is expected that Señor Garcia will
make a speech. Notwithstanding his great age, he
is still fairly vigorous in body, and he was able to
attend the annual dinner of the Laryngological Society on January 13. His mental powers are absolutely undimmed by age.

Hall of Fame.—The editor of the *Western Medical
Review* desires to nominate five physicians, all of
whom well deserve the honor which such an election
confers. (1) Benjamin Rush, of whom at the time
of his death it was said, "the name of Dr. Rush
gave a splendor to the American character and
greatly added to its reputation throughout the republic of letters. His works are read coextensively
with the language in which they are written. He
has been one of the most prominent pillars on which
his country's claim to be ranked with the learned
nations has pre-eminently rested ever since Dr.
Franklin was no more. Few or none of his contemporary fellow laborers can prefer superior or even
equal claims as reformers and improvers of the
theoy and practice of medicine." As a signer of the
Declaration of Independence he gave public mark
to his patriotism, shown already in a thousand other
ways. (2) David Ramsay, physician, historian, pa-
triot—of him as a graduate from college Dr. Rush
said: "He is far superior to any person we ever
graduated at our college. His abilities are not only
good but great. His talents and knowledge are universal. I never saw so much strength of memory
and imagination united to so fine a judgment." His

historical writings were as successful as his practice
of medicine, which is saying much, and by every
effort he contributed to securing the independence
of our country. (3) John Collins Warren, First
professor of anatomy and surgery in the Harvard
Medical School, patron of the first administration
of ether for surgical purposes, and founder of the
Boston Medical and Surgical Journal, one of the first
medical publications of the present day. (4) J.,
Marion Sims, who revolutionized the practice of
the surgical treatment of the diseases of women.
He enjoyed a greater reputation than any other
American surgeon, operating with brilliant success
in all the capitals of Europe. He founded in 1855
the great Woman's Hospital in New York City, and
the methods which he devised and perfected are
among the richest gifts any member of the profession has ever given to humanity. (5) Oliver Wendell Holmes, physician, medical teacher, poet, remembered by thousands not more lovingly for his
books than by many others, physicians who by lecture or by printed page have been his pupils. He
rendered a great service to the medical profession
by first calling attention to the contagiousness of
puerperal fever, and his poems and prose writings
will be read with delight as long as the language
endures.

Dr. Osler on the Race in Canada.—In an address recently delivered to the Canadian Club, Professor Osler
spoke of the "incessant dribbling" of their young
men into the United States. A million Canadians,
he said, were in the States, many in prominent positions in finance and in the professions, particularly
medicine and theology. There they have been successful by reason of industry and thoroughness, "the
only qualities worth anything in the make-up of a
young man." It is not only the young men, however, that are being drained away; what Professor
Osler regards as a more serious loss is that of the
young women. He had as a patient once a neurasthenic man of thirty or thereabouts whom he asked
why he did not get married. "Because," was the
reply, "all the girls I wanted have gone to the
States." It appears that of 651 women in six of the
great eastern hospitals in the States 196, or almost
a third, are Canadians. To check this migration
of possible mothers, Professor Osler suggested a
tax on bachelors over twenty-five or twenty-six, or,
as an alternative, an export tax of £20 on every girl
leaving Canada. He admitted that she was worth
more than that, a statement which was received with
approval by his audience, who seemed to agree with
him that she was worth £200, and it would pay to give
her family that amount to keep her at home. He went
on to say that it was sane and reasonable of Canadians to think of themselves as a strong race; they
are satisfactorily situated for the development of
one strong in body. Rarely has a strong nation
appeared elsewhere than in the north. The cold
and rigor of winter are much to their advantage, and
will produce a stronger type than any other on the
continent. Waxing prophetic, Professor Osler fore-
tells that in our generation by far the most virile
nation will dwell north of the Great Lakes. The
amalgamation and commingling of the heterogenous
elements of English, Irish and Scotch is, in his
opinion, the best mixture the world had ever seen.
If he had his way he would have an act of parliament
passed that every fourth Upper Canadian should
marry a French-Canadian girl, because in that way
the future of the race would be assured. To grow
a strong race mentally, elementary education should

be fostered by well equipped schools and teachers. It is not good for boys to be brought up under women; the Canadian people must pay better salaries, and make their teachers feel that they are doing useful and honorable work for their country, with a prospect of provision for age and for their families. Prof. Osler holds that the most important thing is to grow a strong race morally, and that is the hardest of all. He does not think Canada immoral. Homicides are less frequent than in certain other countries, and drunkenness not so prevalent, though some of them with Scotch fathers might have a little tissue thirst. Illegitimacy is rare, and divorce is not common. Morally, the country has made a good start, but there is, he thinks, far too much evil speaking, lying, and slandering in connection with political life. This is entirely superfluous and unnecessary. Young men in this atmosphere of slander and hostility toward opponents suffer great harm. Dr. Osler regards it as an infinitely worse vice than drunkenness. The only way to meet it is to deal with political opponents in an everyday Christian spirit, or, if not in the character of St. Paul's noble Christian, at least in that of Aristotle's true gentleman.—(*British Medical Journal.*)

OBITUARY.

Dr. MORTIMER WRIGHT SHAW, a practising physician, of Cedar Street, New York, died at Middletown, N. Y., on February 22, of pneumonia. He was thirty-seven years old. Dr. Shaw was graduated at the Long Island College Hospital in 1892.

Dr. ELIHU RUSSELL HOUGHTON died last Sunday at his home, No. 167 West Ninety-first Street, New York. He was graduated from Amherst in 1885, and entered Bellevue Medical College. He had served in the United States Navy and in the Immigration and Marine Hospital Service.

Dr. JAMES E. CRISFIELD, of Dansville, N. Y., died February 21, at Jacksonville, Fla. He was the oldest practising physician in Livingston County, N. Y., and prominent in Democratic politics of his section of the State, and for a time served as a member of the New York State Democratic Committee.

Dr. SPENCER VAN DALSEN died at his residence, in Paterson, N. J., on February 17, of bronchial pneumonia. He was born in that city fifty-two years ago. Dr. Van Dalsen was a member of the Passaic County Medical Society, becoming identified with that association in 1876, the same year he was graduated from the College of Physicians and Surgeons in New York.

SOCIETY PROCEEDINGS.

BOSTON MEDICAL LIBRARY MEETINGS IN CONJUNCTION WITH THE SUFFOLK DISTRICT BRANCH OF THE MASSACHUSETTS MEDICAL SOCIETY.

Stated Meeting, held December 21, 1904.

The President, George Sears, M.D., in the Chair.

Nephritis.—The subject of the evening was nephritis. Dr. Franz Pfaff first spoke of the medical treatment. In past years attempts had been made to treat the signs of nephritis, the albuminaria and casts. Drugs such as tannic acid, potassium chlorate were given for this purpose. Sometimes disinfectants as methylene blue were used. At present with regard to inflammatory conditions of the kidneys at least, the object in view is to fulfil the physiological

action of the kidneys, whether by the so-called rest treatment, sparing the kidneys and getting other organs and systems to act vicariously for it, as the reins and the intestinal tract, or by stimulating the kidneys directly by means of drugs which affect the renal epithelium, or by stimulating the heart and thereby increasing the flow of blood to the kidneys. Whether to use one method or the other depends on the individual case and its symptoms, the general condition of the patient and the special condition of the heart, kidneys and urine.

In regard to the latter, a single specimen is of no use. Repeated examinations of the mixed twenty-four-hour urine must be made in order to get any accurate results; very often the morning urine will be quite normal, free from casts, albumin, etc., while a specimen of mixed urine may show quite a nephritis.

Rest and Stimulating Methods.—The primary object of both the rest and the stimulating methods of treatment is to get rid of the waste products of the blood. Usually, in all acute inflammatory and acute exacerbations of chronic processes, the kidneys should be spared work. This is done by reducing the ingestion of food, especially the proteids, so as to reduce proteid metabolism. In the course of a year the kidneys excrete seventy to eighty pounds of inorganic salts and about six hundred quarts of urine. This amount of work can, for a short time at least, be very greatly diminished. Next comes the question as to how far we can go in reducing the proteids, and what proteid shall we use. In infants milk works very well, but in adults there is more residue and much less absorption. One hundred grams a day of proteid material is necessary for the healthy person. During a limited period, two, three, or four weeks, this can be reduced 40 to 50 per cent. by increasing the carbohydrates and fats, the loss can be made good and the body equilibrium maintained. Rice is by all means the best carbohydrate to use; macaroni and white bread stand next in order. As regards the ingestion of water, in some cases large amounts are to be taken and in others it is to be reduced. Van Noorden advises, in all cases of nephritis, acute and chronic, to cut down greatly on the amount of water.

Dr. Pfaff considers this view very unsafe, and from experience is sure that in nine out of ten cases treated in this way albumin and the numbers of casts will increase. A normal or slightly increased amount of urine should be passed, and water in amounts sufficient to do this given. If the edema and ascites is present, reduce the water ingestion. Certain patients normally drink too much water, and this should be considered in treatment. The intestine is the chief means of carrying on the vicarious functions of the kidneys; the skin in a lesser degree can be used by hot baths. Salts and vegetable purgatives, such as aloes and gamboge, are the best cathartics to use. If all these means of treatment fail then, and not till then, should the kidney be stimulated. The salts of caffeine and theobromine act directly on the renal epithelium. If by their use the urine shows more albumin and casts they should be discontinued. In chronic kidney disease a milk diet is not practicable for any length of time; meat, red or white, it matters not, must be given in amounts at least 20 per cent. less than normal, and the difference made up by carbohydrates. Animal broths should be avoided as well as alcohol in any form. Under such a diet weight can be gained, but no attempt should be made to put it on, as it means increased metabolism.

Surgical Treatment of Nephritis.—Dr. Paul Thorndyke spoke on this condition. During the last few years a marked change has come into view as regards nephritis. This was stated by a paper by Reginald Harrison, who in the *London Lancet* of January 4. 1896, spoke of the beneficial effects of operation on certain cases of albuminuria, whereby he was obliged to cut and slash the kidney parenchyma. The operations were not done for the nephritis, but for pain and hematuria. Edebohls, of New York, was the first to operate directly to benefit nephritis itself. The speaker carefully described Dr. Edebohls' technic, and gave statistics showing his results. Seventy-five per cent. of cases of chronic diffuse nephritis dies very soon, showing that this class was particularly unfavorable for operation. By a series of animal experiments, done by L. C. Gifford, of Boston, it was shown that after stripping off the capsule a new one, rather thicker than the first, was formed within thirty days, and that relief could thus be only temporary as far as the capsule itself was concerned. There was a possibility that the blood supply might be increased. On the whole, the speaker considered the question well worthy of further study, and a very valuable field for further investigation.

The Progress of Nephritis from the Standpoint of Insurance.—Dr. Frank Wells dilated on this phase of the disease.—He said that all applicants whose urine showed albumin by either of the ordinary tests were refused, or at least held for further investigation, but that the great expense made it very hard to follow the after life of such refused applicants, and, therefore, statistics on which to base a prognosis were scarce. He went on to speak of the great number of deaths every year from Bright's disease, especially in the large cities, where pressure of living is high, and worry and consequent alcohol consumption is very great.

Uremia and Nephritis Following Scarlet Fever.—Dr. J. W. Elliott mentioned two cases he had operated on for nephritis; one a chronic diffuse case in uremia at the time of the operation, and the other a young adult with a nephritis following scarlet fever. The former case died in three months, and on autopsy an apparently normal capsule was found. The other case is now alive and well. He thinks that the operation has some value, but is not at all sure that the operation as done by Edebohls is to be the one of the future.

Dr. Edward Reynolds considered the operation to be still *sub judice*. He thught that an operation in early cases. without uremia, might be of value; he did not advise decapsulation, but liberal slashing of the kidney substance.

Bilateral Decapsulation.—Dr. J. B. Blake advised strongly. if anything surgical was to be done, the bilateral decapsulation of the two kidneys at once by two surgeons and their assistants. Improvement in the cases at the Boston City Hospital was variable in degree and amount, but that in young people, after medical treatment had failed and they were still getting worse, the operation was advisable and gave the best chance of doing good.

Dr. Henry Jackson, speaking on diet in nephritis, emphasized the fact that each case must be studied and individualized until a suitable diet was found. Animal broths were, in his opinion, very good.

Dr. E. G. Cutler, on the subject of operating, said that if medical means, properly carried out over a

long enough time, were of no avail, an operation should be considered.

Treatment of Nephritis in Children.—This was the topic of Dr. John L. Morse, who said that the same lines should be followed as in treating adults. What harms the kidneys is urea, creatinin and phosphoric acid. Too much milk is very apt to be given. For a boy of four years 15 grams of proteids equaling 12 ounces of milk per 24° was enough for a few days. Meat extractives in broths should be avoided because of the large amount of creatinin. Phosphoric acid was contained in the yolks of eggs, and could be neutralized by calcium carbonate and thus given in milk. As regards drugs, no stimulant like digitalis or creatinin should be given in the acute stage. There are three classes of nephritis; one with much edema and uremia and very little urine, to be treated with the lowest possible diet, a little water, cathartics, and hot packs; second, with slight edema, no uremia. These should be given more milk with cream and cereals, and water varied according to the edema. Third, convalescent stage, when starches and fats were added to the milk and all the water wanted was given.

MEDICAL SOCIETY OF THE STATE OF NEW YORK.

Ninety-ninth Annual Meeting, held at Albany, January 31, February 1 and 2, 1905.

The President, Dr. Hamilton F. Wey, of Elmira, in the Chair.

(Continued from page 330.)

The Public Health Laboratory.—Dr. Herbert D. Pease, of Albany, said that the laboratories that have been established by public funds have more than repaid the public by the discoveries that have been made in them, and by the usefulness which they have developed. At the present time they are doing good work in the recognition of diphtheria by bacteriological diagnosis, by the discovery of the tubercle bacillus, by the Widal test, by the examination of feces, especially for the existence of parasites, by the determination of the potability of water, and by the examination of samples of milk so as to decide whether they are fit for use or not. In very recent years they have become still further useful by the examination for the presence of adulterants in foods by the determination of the power of disinfectants, by acting as a criterion for antitoxin as regards its strength and purity, as also for vaccine material, and finally by the fact that examinations for rabies and material for the treatment of this dread disease are provided.

Unsettled Problems.—Of course, it may well be said that many of the problems of laboratory work are as yet unsettled. The laboratories themselves are, however. doing the most that is possible for the settlement of problems of disease. How much more is now known of the diphtheria bacillus, of its form and various simulants. of its existence in healthy throats, and of its distribution, than before the establishment of laboratories. With regard to the tubercle bacillus. there are not a few problems that laboratory workers have been busily engaged at and new light is being shed on them every day. What is needed in order that laboratory knowledge may become more definite is more laboratory investigation. In order to make our medical progress assured one of the best elements is to further encourage the laboratory workers. The study of virulence, its increase and decrease under varying circumstances, and the future of disease and of immunity, these are all in the lap of the future laboratory work.

Opening of the Skull.—Dr. Charles H. Frazier, of Philadelphia, said that the failure of many operations for tumors of the brain were due to the fact that the opening made in the skull was too small to discover the lesion. It is impossible, as a rule, to determine the site of the lesion with sufficient exactness to guide the surgeon for a small opening. There is no more risk in the large opening than in the small, and, as a matter of fact, the mistake has been in making the opening too small rather than too large. He exhibited a skull on which osteoplastic flaps had been raised, some of them four inches in length, illustrating the method which he employs for intracranial investigation. The large flap in the prefrontal region is raised whenever there are psychic symptoms; in the posterior parietal region the flap is raised for such symptoms as astereognosis; in the occipital region for hemianopsia and other similar symptoms. The flap over the motor area is so raised that two-thirds of the region uncovered shall be in front of the central fissure rather than exactly over it, as used to be the case. In making the incision into the scalp a larger flap is made than of the bone. After the bone flap is turned upward the edges of the scalp may be tucked in around it, thus keeping up the vitality of the bone and preventing its separation from the pericranium from which it derives its nourishment, and separation might mean necrosis. The portions of the flap are covered with gauze so as to protect them from any possible injury during the course of the operation. A flap corresponding in size to that of the bone is made in the dura mater. The incision to this issue heals very kindly and very thoroughly. At subsequent operations, even a few months after the first operation, no signs of the opening in the dura could be found.

Postoperative Dressings.—The main purpose to be kept in view in putting on the dressings is that adequate drainage shall be supplied. For this purpose the flap incision itself in the scalp is not used, but special incisions are made somewhat beyond these. Rubber tissue is conducted from the bone out through these openings. A certain amount of oozing is sure to occur from the bone and also from the dura, sometimes even for the brain itself. If provision is not made for its conduction outward a clot will form, and this may become organized giving subsequent trouble by pressure upon the brain. The absence of a direct communication between the outer air, because of the indirect path along which the rubber tissue runs, saves the patient many risks of infection.

Making the Bone Flap.—In Dr. Frazier's experience the best instrument for this is Crile's spiral drill. This is run by means of an electric engine. The end of the drill is protected by a flange, which fits beneath the bone and keeps the dura out of the way. When the trephine opening is first made through which the drill is passed a director is used to separate the dura from the skull in case there should be adhesions. By means of this drill it takes but a few minutes, from five to seven, to make a large bony flap. Time is a very precious thing in these operations, and there is no instrument that is as useful as the spiral osteotome.

Other Instruments.—Stelwagon, of Philadelphia, invented an extremely ingenious circular saw which can be used with excellent effect whenever an elec-

tric engine is not available. This, however, necessitates the cutting of a semicircular or circular flap of bone, while the spiral osteotome will make any sort of a flap, no matter how irregular its lines. Doyen's circular saw is a useful instrument, but cuts only in straight lines and requires several trephine openings. The ordinary chain saw has the same objection, and besides is rather slow, necessitating operations in two stages, often. With Crile's instrument the operation in two stages is never necessitated.

Blood Pressure.—As to the condition of the patient, Dr. Frazier has found that the most important element indicative of his condition is the blood pressure. This is of itself quite sufficient to enable the surgeon to know the exact state of his patient as regards shock. Its more frequent use would undoubtedly reduce mortality, especially in operations upon the central nervous system. The ordinary blood-pressure apparatus is not difficult of adjustment, and after the operator has become familiar with it it is rather easy to keep in touch with.

Palliative Trephining.—This procedure, which the French sometimes call decompressive trephining, will be found useful in very many cases. In brain tumors that are beyond the reach of surgical intervention, intracranial pressure becomes the most fruitful source of symptoms. Patients suffer from vomiting, from choked disc, from intense headache, for which no relief can be afforded, and finally from blindness. Practically all of these symptoms are relieved at once by the relief of increased intracranial pressure through a trephine opening, and the raising of the bone flap. For this purpose the region of choice is the parietal region. The reasons are obvious. Against the frontal region there are cosmetic objections. In the occipital region hernia of the brain is much more likely to occur. Perhaps the most striking benefit conferred by this palliative operation is the saving of vision. At times, unfortunately, patients have come under Dr. Frazier's care whose vision was already too far gone for relief of pressure to be of avail in saving of it. Experience shows, however, how much good is accomplished, and more and more of these operations will be done as time goes on.

Opening the Skull.—Dr. Farquhar Curtis, of New York, said that the instruments and technical methods presented by Dr. Frazier are of service not alone in operations for brain tumor, but for all cases where opening of the skull is necessary. Up to this time he has used the wire saw. There is always some difficulty in fastening this from one trephine opening to the other. Crile's instrument is undoubtedly the best for the purpose. The secret of successful brain surgery is the making of large flaps. There is no more danger in a flap that is four inches across than in one that is two inches. The oblique drainage is an important element in the after-treatment. Dr. Curtis, however, has found rubber cloth better than rubber tissue. Portions of this latter are likely to be left in the wound, because it is rather friable. The development of the technic of operations upon the cranium will undoubtedly lead to the relief of many patients who have hitherto suffered from almost obstinate symptoms from intracranial pressure, and because more tumors will actually be removed and depressed bone raised than has been the case in the past.

Two-Stage Operations.—Dr. Frazier, in closing the discussion, said that his experience with these is very limited. He has found so little shock when the opening into the brain is made rapidly that he has never had to wait for the recovery of the patient before proceeding to complete the operation. In a number of observations carefully made he has found that the removal of the growth does not add to the gravity of the patient's condition, and so he now always proceeds with the operation. In this matter a revolution has been worked by the newer method. For such men as Von Bergmann the two-stage operation seemed to be absolutely necessary.

Vasomotor Disturbance from Sunlight.—Dr. Samuel B. Ward, of Albany, reported a case in which erythema and urticaria developed whenever the patient was exposed to the sunlight. A number of observations under varying circumstances were made in order to discover just how and why the skin lesions occurred. When the patient was exposed to direct sunlight the temperature of the skin being normal just before the exposure at about 87 degrees and the general temperature being normal, within ten minutes the temperature of the skin was raised nearly ten degrees, though the general temperature remained the same. The arms and shoulders were exposed, and they became of a brilliant scarlet color. Besides this erythema there were white, round wheals of urticaria, which were very itchy and irritable. After a time swelling set in, and this became so marked as not to allow bending at the elbow. The redness went down in fifteen minutes, but the swelling remained for some time. While the erythema was present the sensation was tested. and was found to be normal for heat and the tactile sense.

Experimental Observations.—A portion of the skin surface was exposed to the X-rays for some time, but no untoward effect was found. Ordinary heat rays produced no bad effect, for the patient can sit before the fire without discomfort. Evidently the element that has an injurious action is in the sunlight, for she is unable to go out more than one day of twenty without having these lesions recur. In order to determine what portion of the sunlight produced the effect, portions of the arm were covered with red and yellow glass. Beneath the yellow glass there was some slight change in the skin appearance produced. Beneath the red glass there was no change. though the sunlight produced its usual effect where no glass intervened between it and the skin. It is evident that actinic rays of the sun, those which produce photographic effects, are responsible for the changes noticed.

Sensitiveness to Cold.—A certain number of cases of sensitiveness to cold in various parts of the skin somewhat corresponding to this case have been reported as a consequence of freezing. These cases are interesting by contrast. It seems probable that the vasomotor nerves are so affected by the pathological conditions of freezing that they refuse to act whenever exposed to cold again. Some trouble with the vasomotors seems to be present in Dr. Ward's case. The patient cannot take one-two-hundredth of a grain of nitroglycerin without lying down because of the rush of blood to the head which it occasions.

Similar Case.—Dr. Ruggles, of Buffalo. reported a case in which the patient. a young woman of twenty, suffering somewhat from constipation and menstrual irregularity, had her face frost-bitten, and had since suffered from urticaria whenever exposed to cold. In this case the lesions occur only on the face, never on the hands. They are absolutely symmetrical, though true urticaria is said never to occur symmetrically. The trouble would seem to be in the peripheral nerves. and to be due to a vasomotor neurosis.

Central Neurosis.—Dr. Kinnear said that such cases would seem to be due to a central neurosis. and he believes that the application of cold over the spine will benefit them to a great extent. As the result of the shock or some nervous disturbance the nerve centers assume a tendency to become hyperemic. As a consequence the peripheral vasomotor apparatus is no longer properly under control, and peripheral hyperemia with even the leakage of serum into the skin, which is the basis of urticaria, may occur.

Idiosyncrasies.—Dr. Frederick Curtis, of Albany, said that patients have these curious but inexplicable idiosyncrasies. He has had under observation one who suffered from urticaria whenever clean sheets were placed on the bed. The only thing to do for these patients is to teach them to avoid the cause of their disturbed cutaneous condition.

CHICAGO SURGICAL SOCIETY.

Regular Meeting, held December 5, 1904.

The President, L. L. McArthur, M.D., in the Chair.

Actinomycosis.—Dr. Arthur Dean Bevan, in a paper on this subject, referred, first, to the early history of this disease, saying that von Langenbeck first noticed the sulphur-green-like bodies of actinomycosis as early as 1845; and that Bollinger recognized the ray fungus in lumpy jaw in cattle. Israel, in 1878, recognized the ray fungus as the cause of the disease in man. Belfield first recognized the ray fungus. in lumpy jaw in cattle in this city, and Murphy reported the first case of actinomycosis in man in this country in 1883. Clinically, the disease appears in four different forms, with four different groups of infection: (1) The head and neck actinomycosis, with infection from the mouth and pharynx; (2) actinomycosis of the chest through the respiratory tract; (3) abdominal actinomycosis, with infection probably always through the alimentary canal; possibly, however, in rare instances through the female genital organs; (4) actinomycosis of the skin. The lymphatic glands are seldom involved, but he reported one case in his group of cases in which there was invasion of the lymphatics.

Enormous Infiltration.—Dr. John B. Murphy said that an important feature brought out was the demonstration of lymphatic involvement. In none of the cases that came under his observation was it shown that the lymphatic glands became involved, or that the infection was transmitted through the lymphatic chain and arrested in the lymphatic glands. Another point was the enormous infiltration that occurred around a small focus of suppuration. This is one of the first things that attracted Dr. Murphy's attention in the first case of actinomycosis he saw in 1883. This was a typical case of actinomycosis of the jaw, in which the infiltration extended down to and involved the neck to the extent of an inch or more on each side. There was apparently a small fluctuating focus. When the involved area was opened, a number of yellow bodies escaped. These appeared molded. They were not round or oval. The infiltration described by Dr. Bevan in his case of actinomycosis of the pelvis was one of the classical conditions of the disease in the peritoneum. While the disease affects bones. muscles, and destroys the tissues with which it comes in contact, it elects fatty tissue, and passes by preference along the fatty tissue tracts. involving skin, muscle or bone, lifting its periosteum, attacking the periosteum, or sometimes attacking the fatty tissue close to the periosteum without attacking bone. As to treatment, Dr. Murphy's first, second and third cases recovered, but the forth one terminated fatally, which was one of peritoneal actinomycosis, where the micro-organisms escaped either through the stomach wall or transverse colon. There was no perforation of the stomach wall nor of the large intestine. There was infiltration of the fatty tissue on both sides, the micro-organism having passed up into the diaphragm and beneath the surface of the liver. Relative to actinomycosis of the appendix, he has seen two cases, one of his own and another he saw in consultation with Dr. Lee. In the first the actinomycotic process was confined practically within the appendix. The appendix was extirpated, followed by recovery. The case of Dr. Lee pursued an entirely different course.

Dr. E. Wyllys Andrews said one cannot help noticing the large percentage of recoveries which had been referred to, which was quite contrary to his own experience in the rather limited number or cases he has observed in the last few years. Most of the cases he has seen have either died or, if they were living, there is an increasing actinomycotic mass in other parts of the body. He recalls one man who has a mass in his chest, and who, he thinks, is going to die. These cases ought to be worked up with exceeding care. If one analyzes all the cases of actinomycosis of the alimentary canal, he would scarcely find one involving the stomach, and the probabilities are that the acidity of the stomach prevents the active generation of the germs there. A comparatively small number are found in the upper intestine. In nearly one-half of all cases reported the actynomyces are found in the cecum and in the appendix. He has not seen a case of actinomycosis involving the rectal region.

Hematogenous Infection.—Dr. M. L. Harris has seen during the past year three cases of actynomycosis, which apparently were hematogenous infections. The first case was in a country boy, who was admitted to the hospital with a slowly developing swelling in the prevesical space. It had the characteristic hardness. He opened the mass and obtained a small amount of pus. Inoculations from the pus gave a pure culture of *Staphylococcus pyogenes albus.* In the first pus which was evacuated no granules were recognized, but on the dressings a few days after the characteristic granules were at once recognized, and when submitted to the microscope demonstrated to be actinomycosis. The case progressed, the exudate spread, sinuses and fistulæ were formed about the abdominal wall into the lateral wall of the pelvis. The boy was operated on several times; these tracts thoroughly cleared out, and during the operations the abdominal cavity was opened, because the speaker was suspicious of a primary intestinal origin. The abscess did not originate in the appendix, nor could he find any point of the intestinal tract that was involved, so he was unable to explain how the infection reached the prevesical space, except through the blood. The patient was subjected to all the recognized treatments for actinomycosis. Iodide of potash was given internally, continually and interruptedly. He was given X-ray treatment very thoroughly, but, in spite of all treatment, he progressed from bad to worse, and after a period of several months died. A peculiarity in this case was the

very marked reduction of hemoglobin. The red cells were not reduced in number, but the hemoglobin was reduced to a low point before death. Dr. Harris detailed at considerable length the other two cases that have come under his observation, and said, that the three of them seemed to be instances of hematogenous infection, the organisms having been carried in through the blood, as there was no local point of infection, so far as he could determine.

Dr. A. J. Ochsner said there are a great many cases of actinomycosis in Chicago and its vicinity, although most of them had not been accurately diagnosed. He was almost never without a case of actinomycosis. He has one at the present time under treatment. He recalls half a dozen cases in which the face and neck were involved, one in which the larynx was affected, in a number the abdomen was involved, in one the eighth rib, and in others the appendix. He has had two or three cases of actinomycosis of the lungs. As to treatment, he believes surgeons should follow the method of veterinary surgeons, if they wish to succeed in treating this disease. In late cases of actinomycosis in cattle the veterinary surgeon has the animal killed. He never tries to cure a late case of this disease in cattle. In the early cases, however, an effort is made to remove the entire mass by thorough curettage, followed by the administration of large quantity of iodide of potash. Veterinary surgeons give a large quantity of iodide of potash for several days in succession and then they interrupt its use, giving the spores time to develop into ray fungi, after which they repeat the dose for a day or two, then withdraw it for a day or two again, repeat it again, and so on, and in cases where the actinomycotic process is localized the cattle recover. Actinomycosis in the human being should be treated on the same principles. About eight or nine years ago the speaker followed the method of giving iodide of potash in increasingly large doses, but in several cases in succession there was apparently no effect upon the disease until he reached the dose of a dram three times a day, and then the progress of the disease became arrested. He remembers the first case in which he was impressed with the importance of large doses of iodide of potash and this was an instance in which he operated a dozen times. It was a case of actinomycosis of the scalp. The disease burrowed and burrowed, and every week or so he found it necessary to scrape the scalp and apply every remedy he could think of, without much improvement. However, when he reached 60 grains of iodide of potash three times a day the disease was arrested. The next case he had acted in a similar manner, and since then he has made it a rule to give 90 grains of iodide of potash in a half pint of hot milk at two in the morning, two in the afternoon and ten at night, for as many days as the patient can stand it. If the patient can bear it for a week, then it is withdrawn for some days, after which it is repeated for three or four days, withdrawn again, and later repeated once a month. The reason why he repeats odide of potash once a month is this, that in one of his fatal cases he did this for a time, and the patient was apparently well, but two years later the patient had a recurrence and died of the disease. A circumscribed encysted abscess was found at autopsy in the lower end of the right pleura.

Actinomycosis of the Alveolar Process.—Dr. L. L. McArthur reported the case of a young woman, very fond of golf, who frequently was rebuked by her husband for dragging at hay and chewing it while playing golf. She developed actinomycosis of the alveolar process, which required three or four months' treatment by a dentist before it healed. Nine or ten months later, while playing golf in the South, she began to have pain in the right iliac region, and this pain being of a rather colicky character, on her return home she consulted her family physician, Dr. Carey, who, feeling a mass there, and noticing she had elevation of temperature, sent her to the speaker's service at St. Luke's Hospital, believing it to be a probable appendical abscess. Dr. MacArthur concurred in this diagnosis and advised operative measures. On opening the abdomen, a tumor was found in the ileocecal region, involving the appendix, ileum and cecum, for a distance of four of five inches on the cecum. The tumor in its clinical aspect, although having no miliary bodies in it, seemed to him to be a hypertrophic tuberculosis, and on that basis, with the consent of the family physician, he made a resection of the entire ileocecal region, implanting in the side of the hepatic flexure of the colon the resected ileum. On lifting up from the iliac fossa this mass, a few drops of pus were seen on the fascia covering the iliac muscles. This was mopped up, drainage provided for, and the wound closed. The wound healed after a few weeks, the patient left the hospital, and for three months was quite well, when she began to have a cough and high temperature, with chills and night sweats, and during his absence from the city she was seen by his assistant, Dr. Hollister, who considered the case—although he was unable to demonstrate tubercle bacilli in the sputum—one of acute tuberculous trouble. the patient having lived in the house of a patient who had died a few months before of tuberculosis, and many of her living things still being in the house, such as bedding, clothing, etc. On Dr. McArthur's return, the patient being extremely ill, he saw her and found a tender area, with an enlargement in the neighborhood of Reidel's lobe of the liver, and considered the condition one of hepatic abscess with burrowing through the diaphragm. He urged operative interference. The husband refused to have any operation performed until she had become extremely run down and had a temperature varying from 103° to 106° F. for three or four weeks. Then, at his urgent solicitation, the patient was brought to the hospital, he made an incision over this area, and found an abscess which had perforated the posterior sheath of the rectus muscle, and in which were then to be seen for the first time the typical granules, and the nature of the case became clear. The patient lingered along for about two weeks, and finally died. A careful post-mortem examination was made by Dr. Hektoen, and a very thorough report of the case was made. In the sputum there were found the typical leptothrix-like threads, but never any suspicion was had of granules. In the stomach abscess opened there were typical granules to be found, and from them cultures were made which proved typically characteristic, so that here was a person in the habit of chewing grain and hay, who had disease of the jaw, who had a hypertrophic actinomycotic infection, which often is indistinguishable from tuberculosis, who recovered from that and later developed hepatic abscesses, with perforation of the diaphragm. Post-mortem examination showed multiple stomach abscesses burrowing into the diaphragm.

NEW YORK OBSTETRICAL SOCIETY.

Stated Meeting, held November 16, 1904.

The President, J. Riddle Goffe, M.D., in the Chair.

Tubo-Abdominal Gestation.—Dr. E. B. Cragin presented a photograph and the specimen of this condition occurring in a primipara thirty-four years of age, who had been dilated and curetted for sterility seven years previously. Vomiting and pain had been present at intervals throughout the pregnancy. A diagnosis of full term ectopic pregnancy with dead fetus was confirmed by the operation. The sac was found adherent to the abdominal wall and floor of the pelvis, and roofed over by coils of adherent intestine. The entire sac containing the placenta was enucleated from the adherent surroundings until it was only attached by the upper portion of the broad ligament, which, forming a pedicle like an ovarian cyst, was ligated and the entire sac removed. No denudation of the peritoneum had occurred so that the abdominal wound was entirely closed and the patient made an uneventful recovery. Further examination of the sac showed the amnion and chorion to be covered by the expanded tube on the proximal side, while the distal portion had been reinforced by the adherent coils of intestine and panital peritoneum. He therefore considers this case to be one of tubo-abdominal gestation, in contrast to the three cases reported by him in 1900 to the American Gynecological Society, and to the one subsequently reported in the same year to the New York Obstetrical Society, all of which were of the intraligamentous variety.

Retrorectal Dermoid of the Pelvic Connective Tissue.—Dr. Hiram N. Vineberg presented a dermoid cyst that he had removed from a patient, thirty-five years of age, who presented herself with a complete prolapse, rectocele and cystocele one year subsequent to an instrumental delivery. There was also to be felt behind the rectocele an elastic tumor extending to the left and behind the rectal wall. A probable diagnosis of a dermoid of the subperitoneal connective tissue was made. but an operation for the uterine prolapse was only done at this time, leaving the rectocele and tumor. One year later the patient returned with rectocele larger and the tumor of double its previous size. After failing to remove the tumor through the vaginal wall, it was enucleated through an incision extending from the coccyx to the anal margin. The rectocele was then repaired.

Full-term Extra-Uterine Pregnancy.—Dr. Hiram N. Vineberg presented such a specimen that he had removed from a patient twenty-eight years of age, who had suffered from abdominal pains at irregular intervals throughout the pregnancy. The loss of flesh had been so marked that a diagnosis of a malignant growth was possible. Although there was considerable hemorrhage and difficulty in removing the sac, it was all enucleated except a small piece which was sewed into the abdominal wound. Recovery and closure of the fistula in five weeks.

Simultaneous Extra- and Intra-Uterine Pregnancy.—Dr. Hiram N. Vineberg related the history of a patient to whom he was called on account of an attack of pain in the right side of the abdomen, which resembled both appendicitis and gall-stone colic From the history and examination, however, he suspected an ectopic pregnancy. A distinct tumor behind the uterus disappeared during an examination under anasthesia, and while performing a curettage by which the material of a four to five weeks' preg nancy was removed, the patient collapsed. An incision in the posterior fornix revealed free blood, and an immediate laparotomy without the ordinary preparations or instruments revealed a ruptured tubal pregnancy. Microscopical examination showed chorionic villi in the tube and in the material removed from the uterus.

Dr. E. B. Cragin, in the discussion, referred to a case depicted in the American Text-book of Gynecology, upon which he operated one night for ectopic pregnancy, and the next day a fetus with its membranes was passed from the uterus.

Dr. H. N. Vineberg recalled two cases of intra- and extra-uterine pregnancy. In one the diagnosis was not made until labor began, when the tubal rupture occurred.

Toxemia of Pregnancy.—Dr. James Ewing (guest) gave a lantern demonstration and read a paper, entitled, "The Pathological Anatomy and Pathogenesis of the Toxemia of Pregnancy." He first demonstrated and described the different pathological varieties as they occurred under the two clinical forms, eclampsia and hyperemesis. Under the cases of eclampsia, so-called clinically, because of the presence at some time in the course of the disease of convulsions, were included the following pathological varieties: (1) Hemorrhagic hepatitis; constituting the lesion of 95 per cent. of all such cases, in which the liver was of normal size, but of reduced consistence. Hemorrhagic foci were seen on both the surface and sections. Microscopically, there was a uniform and intense degeneration of the liver cells, showing a disintegration of protoplasm and abolition of liver function. There were also minute hemorrhages, usually in relation to focal necrosis. (2) Acute yellow atrophy; clinically, intermediate between eclampsia and acute yellow atrophy, in which the convulsions are less prominent, but toxic symptoms are more marked and not limited to the last month of pregnancy. The liver is slightly reduced in size and reduced in consistence. It is mottled red and yellow. There is hydropic and fatty degeneration of the inner two-thirds of the lobules; an intermediate zone of necrosis and a peripheral zone of slight granular and fatty degeneration. (3) Minimal hepatic lesions: The liver may appear normal, showing only a reduced consistence, and indications of slight congestion and cloudy swelling. Microscopically, there is a moderate diffuse granular and fatty degeneration with foci of partial necrosis, showing autolysis of liver cells, and alteration of function.

Hyperemesis.—The lesions were given of three fatal cases, in which no convulsions occurred, but which were clinically diagnosed as pernicious vomiting of pregnancy. In two of these, the liver presented the same lesions as appear in eclampsia, in one the liver was distinctly atrophic. There may be the same necrotic process, but it may not be reduced in size, and may have less marked degeneration, and changes which might be overlooked, but which indicate extensive autolysis and profound disturbance of function.

Dr. Ewing also demonstrated acute degeneration in the liver of a rabbit dying immediately after giving birth to young. He also mentions a similar lesion occurring in a rabbit after injection into it of the blood of one of his fatal cases of toxemia. After referring to the relation of toxemia to postgestational acute yellow atrophy, he spoke of the frequent occurrence of leucemia shortly after pregnancy, and the presence of leucin and tyrosin in the urine of both

leucemia and toxemia, and the similarity of the hepatic lesions in both diseases. Brief reference was also made to the possible relation of toxemia to postpartum anemia and sepsis.

Pathogenesis.—The disturbance of nitrogenous metabolism, which is responsible for the clinical manifestations of the toxemia of pregnancy, is due to a failure of oxidizing capacity on the part of the liver. The proteid derivatives, chiefly amido-acids and ammonia, also those containing sulphur, are not combined into urea, but circulate in the blood in poisonous forms, and are excreted to some extent by the kidneys. The complex nature of the sources of these poisons renders less obscure the fact that the clinical manifestations may vary from mild vomiting to acute yellow atrophy. Although the mild and fatal cases of eclampsia are admitted to be identical in nature, a mild form of acute atrophy is not generally recognized. Mild vomiting is considered physiological and severe vomiting is thought to be an exaggerated form of the other without a definite pathological basis. Ewing, however, believes that acute atrophy is frequently followed by recovery. He thinks, too, there is no reason for separating either clinically or pathologically the mild and severe forms of vomiting, which seldom is the only symptom of the disease. Disturbance of nitrogenous metabolism is present in cases of non-fatal vomiting, and unoxidized proteid derivatives as leucin appears in the urine. The hypobromite test he considers unreliable, as leucin, tyrosin and ammonia are all estimated with the urea. The absence of jaundice in fatal cases of vomiting means that the bile-producing function of the liver is inhibited. The present view of the nature of the toxemia classes it as a functional disturbance of the liver, usually attended by severe anatomical lesions, and secondarily with a functional disturbance and anatomical lesions of the kidneys and other organs. It is primary in the liver, as the synthesis of urea is exclusively a function of the liver. Disturbances of the kidneys doubtless exist from the first, but only become pronounced when the poisons resulting from the failure of liver oxidation cause degeneration and exudative inflammation of those organs. As the morbid process is originally a functional disturbance of the liver, its intensity is not entirely dependent upon any anatomical changes, so that fatal cases occur with minimal lesions. Various factors are present in this disturbance of nitrogenous metabolism—the retention of principles ordinarily thrown off at menstruation, increased metabolism from the growth of the fetus, the thyroid gland. The presence of a large amount of unabsorbed saline solution in the intestinal tract in severe cases, and the marked concentration of the blood, leads Ewing to suggest the more frequent and early intravenous infusion of some saline solution like Ringer's.

Some Causes for Puerperal Morbidity Antedating Delivery.—This was the title of the paper read by Dr. J. Clinton Edgar.

The Fetal Manifestations in the Toxemia of Pregnancy.—Dr. W. S. Stone read this paper.

Dr. E. B. Cragin, in the discussion, stated he was more impressed with the fact that the three complications of pregnancy—pernicious vomiting, acute yellow atrophy and eclampsia, all belong to the same group and are due to toxemia. He recalled several cases diagnosed as eclampsia, which the pathologist reported as having the lesion of acute yellow atrophy.

Dr. G. L. Brodhead thought that cases of pregnancy could not be observed too closely from the time of the first skipping of the menstruation until full term is reached.

Dr. H. N. Vineberg thought that to say, as Dr. Edgar did, that patients who had had a severe toxemia should not be allowed to conceive was too strong a statement, as in his own experience he had seen several cases go through subsequent pregnancies without any toxemic symptoms.

Dr. J. Milton Mabbott asked if the closure of the os by the mucous plug could be responsible for the toxemia, as thus the relief of some of these cases after dilatation could be explained. He regarded post-partum acute yellow atrophy a virulent variety of sepsis.

BOOK REVIEWS.

THE PHYSIOLOGICAL FEEDING OF INFANTS. By ERIC PRITCHARD, M.A., M.D.(Oxon.), M.R.C.P.(Lond.). Second edition, greatly enlarged and entirely rewritten. Chicago, W. T. Keener & Co.

THE term "physiological" as used in this title would seem to include conditions of both health and disease, and does not fully indicate the scope of the work. A glance at the chapter-headings will show that it is more comprehensive than one might suppose. In Part I they are: Breast Feeding, Method of Percentage Feeding, Milk Modification, in accordance with the physiological requirements and with the infant's symptoms (such as vomiting, colic, diarrhea, constipation), modification of food in difficult cases and in special conditions. Part II is devoted to the Development and Physiology of Infancy, and here the author discourses upon the skeleton, the muscular system, the digestive system, etc.

Among other things he says: "The normal stimulus to the secretion of pepsin is necessary for the proper development of the stomach, therefore it is far more satisfactory at the commencement of life to feed an infant on milk which contains a low proteid percentage, than to supply him with a large percentage of proteids which have been previously digested."

An appendix includes recipes for various liquid foods, percentage tables of the composition of various kinds of milk, cream, condensed milk and patent foods, and methods for subsidiary feeding including the feeding of premature infants. It is a concise and instructive treatise.

EXAMINATION OF THE URINE. By G. A. DE SANTOS SAXE, M.D., Pathologist to the Columbus Hospital, New York City. 12mo volume of 391 pages, fully illustrated, including 8 colored plates. W. B. Saunders & Company, Philadelphia, New York, London.

Dr. SAXE, already known to the medical profession as the inventor of an excellent little instrument for determining the specific gravity of small quantities of urine, has made a very successful attempt in presenting the subject of Urinology in a concise and practical way. The physiology of the kidneys serves as introduction, after which the physical and chemical tests are fully discussed. Some of the obsolete and also some of the more recent tests for albumin and sugar could have been omitted without affecting the value of the book, while a few more reliable methods of estimating uric acid would have been in place, for the uricometer, like the purinometer, is hardly to be relied upon for any degree of accuracy. We also miss tests for pentose and alkapton, which certainly are of more importance at present than the determination of electrical

conductivity, to which two full pages are devoted. In the part on bacteriology, no mention is made of the importance of looking for the typhoid bacillus in doubtful cases, and of its methods of identification. All in all, the book will form a valuable guide to the uranologist, and a number of questions appended to each chapter, will greatly facilitate the task of students.

MEDICAL LABORATORY METHODS AND TESTS. By HERBERT FRENCH, M.A., M.R.C.P. (Lond.), Medical Registar, Guy's Hospital, Gillson Scholar, Society of Apothecaries of London; Radcliffe Traveling Fellow, Oxford University. W. T. Keener & Co., Chicago.

THIS volume is intended as a small handbook for the medical laboratory and has been written in response to repeated complaints that there is no really small book dealing with the chemical and microscopical tests most useful to medical men. The text is divided into nine chapters, dealing with examination of the urine, blood, sputum, pus, gastric contents, feces, skin and exudates and the tests for common poisons. The descriptions are necessarily concise and to the point, but the illustrations are frequently too crude for a clear interpretation. As a handy reference book to be used in the laboratory, the volume will undoubtedly serve its purpose.

CLINICAL URINOLOGY. By ALFRED C. CROFTON, Professor of Medicine, Chicago Post-Graduate Medical College and Hospital, Physician-in-Chief to St Mary's Hospital, Pathologist to St. Luke's Hospital. Illustrated. William Wood & Company, New York.

THIS book is a novel departure from the usual treatise, since it is not merely a laboratory guide to the analysis of urine, for a purely clinical disquisition on the disorders that produce urinary abnormalities, but is intended as a description of the borderland which lies between the laboratory and the clinic. Many subjects are presented from an entirely new point of view and many tests are cited which are not usually found in treatises of this kind. The text is exceptionally readable, but the illustrations somewhat scant. Everything of practical value is included, but certain subjects which have not so far vindicated their claim to recognition as valuable adjuncts to urinary diagnosis, have been omitted. Why the Ehrlich diazo-reaction has been included among the latter is not quite evident, for this test is certainly of the greatest value in the diagnosis of typhoid and miliary tuberculosis.

BOOKS RECEIVED.

THE MEDICAL NEWS.

A WEEKLY JOURNAL OF MEDICAL SCIENCE.

VOL. 86.   NEW YORK, SATURDAY, MARCH 4, 1905.   NO. 9.

ORIGINAL ARTICLES.

THE EQUILIBRIUM BETWEEN INFECTION AND IMMUNITY AS ILLUSTRATED IN THE TONSILLAR CRYPT.[1]

BY JONATHAN WRIGHT, M.D.,

OF NEW YORK.

[From the Throat Department of the Pathological Laboratory of the Manhattan Eye, Ear and Throat Hospital.]

IN a recent publication[2] I have again drawn attention to the object lesson, the illustration, which nature affords us of the conflicts of the animal organism with its environment in the faucial tonsil. Its crypts may be accepted as the counterpart of the laboratory test tube, holding as it does a mixed bacterial culture. Its epithelial lining pervious to dust particles, but impervious under conditions of health to the same-sized bacterial particles is hardly analogous to the vitreous wall of the test-tube, because we must suppose that the bacteria are kept out of the tissues not altogether by mechanical means, but by being annihilated and dissolved as soon as they enter the epithelial layers. How far purely mechanical agents act as protectors to the animal organism it is impossible to say. It is probable they act chiefly in diminishing the dose and retarding the action both of pathogenic bacteria and of their toxins. On various occasions I have attempted to emphasize their importance, but in doing this, care must be taken not to exaggerate it. From the experiments of Goodale and others with colored granules, from my own observations of dust particles passing the epithelial layer in health, and of bacteria passing the epithelial layer in disease, it is evident enough that there must be something beyond mechanical obstruction which, under ordinary conditions of health, keeps the tissue beneath the epithelium free of bacterial life which swarms in some of the crypts on the outer side of the epithelial cells. As I have just intimated, in addition to the epithelial hedge which retards ingress, the various forces which keep the bacteria on the move, the act of deglutition, the excretion of fluids from the surface by osmosis, gravitation itself, all combine to lessen the numbers of germs which remain within the open-mouthed crypts. Yet in sparse numbers they may be seen even on the surface of the tonsils. When we come to study sections falling through the plugged crypts of the tonsil, the sealed flasks of nature's laboratory, then indeed we must realize that all these accessory protective influences are

[1] Read before the Section of Laryngology of the New York Academy of Medicine, February, I, 1905.
[2] Actinomycosis of the Tonsils, with some remarks on the portals of Infection. The American Journal of the Medical Sciences, July, 1904.

no longer in play, but we have only the mechanical resistance offered by the epithelium.

When we study the epithelium around tuberculous or syphilitic ulcers, when we note that the ephitelium of the tonsillar crypt which contains actinomyces, or even other fungus forms, acts in a peculiar way—becomes granular and proliferates in festoons, we suspect this is the answer to the stimulus of a specific poison. Such is the histological evidence.

Clinically, we know individuals with chronic lacunar tonsillitis, ragged tonsils and plugged crypts, are prone to various indispositions, traceable to this tonsillar condition, but yet it is much more evident they do not all die or even perceptibly influence mortality statistics. After diphtheria the tonsils are still more ragged, and diphtheria bacilli are regularly for prolonged periods denizens of the pharynx. It is said they are found in about one out of ten fairly healthy people. Pyogenic cocci and streptococci are found in larger proportions. It is even known that non-tuberculous people occasionally have tubercle bacilli in the pharynx. I need not repeat more of the clinical side of the problem. It has been too readily accepted as probable, that this malaise and discomfort is due to the absorption of bacteria in the crypts. Yet this cannot be demonstrated histologically until an acute attack of diphtheria or quinsy supervenes, for in quiescent conditions dust particles pass and bacteria do not. When we remember that streptococci are perhaps the most constant, among pathogenic forms of the crypt dwellers, and when from recent researches we gather that their endotoxin is especially active, we may infer whence arises disturbance both local and constitutional in chronic tonsillar diseases. Presumably the ill health of patients with ragged tonsils is due to the absorption, therefore, not of pyogenic cocci, but of their endotoxin, which we may believe has been set free during the process of bacteriolysis within the crypt.

Plainly, as I have said, we are in the presence of some wonderful mechanism of nature, evolved through eons of time and established at the portals of infection by which harmless atoms glide through the stomata of cells or their interstices which are impassable to microphytes. From what follows we may understand how the parasites inimical to the animal perish, but it is not entirely clear why the saprophytes, the harmless bacteria, are not seen passing with the dust particles.

Hitherto the revelations of the antitoxic power of the blood-sera have been insufficient to explain the problem the terms of which I have tried to make plain by what has preceded. That explains the nullification of the toxic power of the pathogenic germ, after it passes within the tissues, but it does not explain immunity from infection—to translate literally—the freedom from the carrying in of the germ; that is an entirely distinct thing. It in no way explains the efficiency in conditions of health of the epithelial barrier of the crypts. Without an explanation of that the whole modern theory of immunity is incomplete and unsatisfactory. Even with that it is neither entirely complete nor thoroughly satisfactory. In the title of this paper I have used the word *Immunity* in apposition to *Infection*. As differentiation advances the term immunity is becoming shadowy and ill-defined, but it still possesses enough significance to allow of its use here without obscuring my meaning.

At the forks where the foodway and breathway meet we have a local problem, a local phenomenon which puzzles the clinician and the microscopist, and if it leaves the laboratory bacteriologist complacent it is only because of his limitations. Yet it is from bacteriological research that we receive a hint which renders us hopeful of still further enlightenment.

Recently Pfeiffer in Germany and Bordet in France and their co-workers[1] have more definitely laid down the difference between a bacterial toxin and an endotoxin, pointing out that the former term should be more carefully reserved for use in designating such general phenomena as are exhibited by the diphtheria and the tetanus bacillus in the animal body. Endotoxin on the other hand is the term to apply to that property of pathogenic bacteria, which does not cause the appearance in the animal organism of an anti-endotoxin to counteract its poisonous effects, but does cause the manufacture of a bacteriolysin which dissolves the invading organism. Unfortunately at present workers at these problems are so interested in the beauties of symbols for phenomena they do not understand, that much of the effect of Ehrlich's splendid work is being compromised by the terms of his theory. The receptor and the amboceptor and the haptophore and the complement, a Gothic phantasmagoria with a classic nomenclature, it is to be hoped is a passing madness which will cease when we really know more of the phenomena which it is thought these words explain.

In further distinction to the toxin the endotoxin is a property which it is difficult but not impossible to separate from the bacterial bodies. Now in close juxtaposition to an epithelial cell,[2] as I showed in some recent observations on a case of tonsillar actinomycosis, such as habitually occurs with more common forms in a

tonsillar crypt, it exerts a destructive or at least an inimical effect on the vitality of the cell. But at the same time it must, in accord with the researches to which I have referred, produce in the cell a lysin which tends to dissolve the germ. This, while to some extent destructive to the bacterium as it lies within the crypt, must be still more effective when it enters the epithelial hedge. How much influence we must ascribe to autolysis of the bacterium, the crumbling of its protoplasm from old are, the struggle for existence with its antagonists and its congeners, is uncertain.

We see, therefore, how in the throat this bacteriolysis is the most important of adjuvants to the antitoxin of diphtheria, for it is exerted on the bacterium before it enters the circulatory system, while it is still on the surface, and it is probably much more efficient when beneath the epithelial line.

After a recovery from diphtheria, whether through the use of an antitoxin manufactured within the body or without, as Wolff declares: " It is left to the bacteriolytic power of the body to make an end of the infection." Usually, for a longer or shorter time, so far as the tonsillar crypt is concerned, it does not succeed. Sometimes the diphtheria bacillus becomes a permanent dweller in the tonsillar crypt. A truce has been struck, an equilibrium established between the endotoxin and the bacteriolysin. If this is so for the Klebs-Löffler bacillus, which stimulates the animal organism to the production of an antitoxin, how much more important must be that power of the endotoxin which calls forth from adjacent cells, epithelium or leucocytes, a bacteriolysin for the protection of the animal organism against other poisonous parasites in the tonsillar crypts.

The staphylococcus and the streptococcus are more frequent and numerous in the tonsillar crypt than the diphtheria bacillus, and the tubercle bacillus is less frequent but much more deadly. There is no satisfactory proof that the system manufactures an antitoxin to combat these germs when introduced. When they exist in the tonsillar crypt and the host suffers no harm, when it is impossible to detect them passing through the epithelium in health, when, in other words, a general peace reigns between the animal cell and its enemies, we must picture to ourselves that so far as pathogenic germs are concerned an equilibrium exists between infection and immunity, and this tendency to the establishment of an equilibrium is a cardinal doctrine of Spencerian philosophy. Of course this end is not so simply attained as here foreshadowed. It is still too early to speak otherwise than vaguely of it. The virulence of the germ, the fighting powers of the cell decline *pari passu* until something occurs to help one or the other, and then the germ is exterminated or the organism suffers, according to which one has received reinforcements.

---

1 In the Centralblatt fur Bakteriologie, etc. (I, Abth. Originale, Band 37, Heft 2, 1904) the weary reader will find that Wolff has summarized and to some extent added to and elucidated the work of others.
2 I fell into the error of calling the influence which produced the morbid state of the epithelium a toxin, a more distinctive term and more in accord with recent work would have been an endotoxin.

We must realize that the same principle is to be applied to all situations in the animal economy where germs may lodge for a time—the intestinal canal and its adnexa; nay, the apex of the lung and the lymph-nodes as well as the folds of the pharynx.

Since modern research has begun to travel this road we have long since come in full view of the close of the era of exclusive bacterial etiology of disease, and again looms up the importance of that unknown factor which upsets the equilibrium. It may be a freshly virulent germ, or an auxiliary germ, but the presumptive evidence is that it is usually a change of the intrinsic rather than of the specific extrinsic factor.

Returning from the realm of speculation to the concrete problem presented by the tonsillar crypt, the observer familiar with its flora will realize that there is still a very serious element of doubt as to whether it is indeed the bacteriolysin or the mechanical obstruction offered by the epithelium which shields the tissue beneath from invasion. In the previous work to which I have referred, I have suggested that it is some sensitive mechanical arrangement which closes the stomata and interstices of cells to the ingress of bacteria and allows the inorganic particles to pass through, but perhaps this does not help the matter very much. We are indebted to the labors of the workers on the problem of immunity for an explanation why the pathogenic bacteria do not float into the lymph-spaces with the dust, but what of the saprophytes? Does their endotoxin bring forth its response in a bacteriolysin? If so, why? Evolutionary doctrine points out how the hurtful germ came to be kept out, but why are the harmless organisms halted? We have here apparently a break in our chain of circumstantial evidence.

It seems probable from experimentation with various forms of protoplasm, that the animal organism evolves defensive properties to destroy by lysis even comparatively harmless protoplasmic particles, when the system through lack of sufficient excretory power becomes embarrassed by their presence. Thus the constant presence of the protoplasm of so-called harmless bacteria in the tonsillar crypt may evolve a resisting power in the adjacent epithelium, which we may suppose is the equivalent of a bacteriolysis. We are warranted in supposing this is so by the results obtained from injecting into the animal organism repeated doses of the organs, or the leucocytes or erythrocytes of other animals. It is said after one or two injections dissolution of the injected cells takes place, not only within the phagocytes of the host but outside of them, in the plasma of the blood or the lymph.

Wolff's conclusion is "that the bacterial endotoxins form no separate class of poisons with laws especially applying to them, but that the endotoxins are simply albumen of foreign origin, and therefore poisonous like every other foreign albumen." We thus understand how the bacterial protoplasm may excite bacteriolytic ferments in the epithelial cells, irrespective of their specific effect on the animal organism.

There have been some investigations of late which directly support this conclusion. The injection of the *Bacillus prodigiosus*, a harmless parasite, for instance[1] at first produced no effect in animals. Repetitions, however, quickly brought about a condition of the system which, if persisted in, resulted in the death of the animal. Now this is the way the animal organism reacts experimentally to the introduction of foreign protoplasm in general. We may suppose then that the same law applies, in the bacteriolytic process, to pathogenic and non-pathogenic germs in the tonsillar crypt.

In what cells of the human organism this chemicobiological process really does go on, remains uncertain. I have assumed that it may proceed in the epithelium or in fact in any of the cells of the body, but if we are limited to Metchnikoff's idea that it is confined to the leucocytes, the subepithelial tonsillar tissue would be *par excellence* the site of such activity, but, as I have said, there are certain phenomena in the behavior of the epithelium, exposed to the bacterial influences of the tonsillar crypt, which influence me strongly in supposing that there also the process is going on. Indeed on reflection that it is the epithelium everywhere which is exposed primarily to the noxious influence of the animal's environment, it would seem the place where we should expect reactions most pronounced in many cases.

As I bring this disquisition to an end, Dr. Theobald Smith's lucid essay[2] comes to hand. The prominence which he gives to the idea of equilibrium falls in so well with the trend of what I have written above and is a so much broader exposé of the standpoint of modern biology in medicine, that I can only refer to it with admiration, without, however, entirely subscribing even to his very modest and cautious estimation of the value of the chemicobiological solution.

MULTIPLE NEURITIS IN WOOD ALCOHOL POISONING.

BY SMITH ELY JELLIFFE, M.D.,

OF NEW YORK;

VISITING NEUROLOGIST, CITY HOSPITAL, NEW YORK; INSTRUCTOR IN PHARMACOLOGY AND THERAPEUTICS, COLUMBIA UNIVERSITY.

IN view of the recent bringing to light of the fact that many deaths have been caused by the use of methyl alcohol, and further, by reason of the renewed interest taken in the subject of methyl alcohol optic neuritis as evidenced by the more recent work of Buller and Wood,[3] it

---

[1] Bertarelli, Centralblatt f. Bakt. XXXVII. Bd., Heft 6.
[2] Some Problems in the Life History of Pathogenic Organisms. Science. December 16, 1904.
[3] Introduction to a discussion held at the New York Academy of Medicine. January 17, 1905.

has seemed pertinent to inquire if types of neuritis other than that affecting the optic nerve may be caused by the use of methyl alcohol taken internally, either as a liquid or as a vapor.

It is well known that ethyl alcohol—ordinary grain alcohol—produces as a result of long use not only optic neuritis (first brought into prominence by Eichorst in 1876), but also the familiar type of peripheral multiple neuritis, first described in this country by James Jackson,[2] of Boston, as far back as 1822 as " A Peculiar Disease Resulting from the Use of Ardent Spirits."

Up to the present time, however, I have been unable to find any record of multiple neuritis induced by methyl alcohol. My search through literature has been extensive but not exhaustive, and at first sight it would seem highly improbable that attention had not been called to this condition, but it appears to have been overlooked, or I have overlooked it.

Inasmuch as the optic neuritis of wood alcohol poisoning has been thoroughly covered by some scores of investigators. Ward Holden,[3] Birch-Hirschfield,[4] Rymowitzsch,[5] de Schweinitz,[6] among them, I have limited the present note to some personal observations on peripheral neuritis resulting from the use of wood alcohol.

Of this affection per se three patients have come under my observation. By reason of the time limitations for this discussion their histories are presented very briefly.

The first patient was seen in 1898. He was a business man, thirty-four years old, and a moderately constant drinker. Sprees were not frequent but he drank small quantities, particularly at night before going to bed. During business hours he rarely indulged. He drank a special brand of whisky which was sold to him by an enterprising druggist, a friend of his, for 25 cents a quart or a dollar a gallon. His friend told him that it was tax-free whisky (moonshine whisky), that he bought on the quiet from some friends in the country. As a matter of fact it was a 35 per cent. Columbian spirits whisky with suitable flavors to make a " richly blended article." He was proud of his ability to " get next " to such a bonanza.

My notes made at the time do not cover the question of the length of time of his indulgence, but he had been drinking this whisky, and other whiskies also, the latter, however, in comparatively small quantities, for at least three months, if not six.

He began to suffer from severe gastric irritability and marked hyperesthesia in the upper extremities, particularly in both arms and hands. This was followed by incomplete paralysis of the extensors and typical drop-wrist. He also had a mild grade of ptosis.

I saw him while in the early stage of paralysis and also found that he had a partial amblyopia. It was very restricted. The patient recovered after four months of treatment, but he still complained of some blurring of vision. Since that time I have lost sight of him.

My notes are not extensive in this case but they are sufficiently explicit to enable me to exclude practically all other causes of neuritis. He was not a beer drinker. Arsenic may be eliminated. Other metal toxemias were excluded, as were also the posttoxic affections of the infectious diseases, malaria, grippe, typhoid, diphtheria, etc. The dyscrasiæ were also excluded. It is true that he occasionally drank good whisky, but most of his drinking was done in the evening at his own home from his own private special stock. I have always felt that this was a distinct example of neuritis from wood alcohol. The neuritis did not differ in any particular from neuritis due to ethyl alcohol.

Two other cases may be of interest in this connection, as showing a much lighter grade of affection and a different mode of ingress of the poison.

Both of these patients were painters, particularly varnishers. They did nothing but shellac work, on desks, furniture, etc., and they worked long hours and in comparatively small rooms.

The shellacs that they used were for the most part dissolved in wood alcohol and they were exposed to the evaporating fumes. They were comparatively unaware of any distinct action of the alcohol. As for one of them I never could make up my mind that he did not use the diluted alcohol to drink. Indeed, instances of drinking the wood alcohol washings from shellac barrels are not unknown. One of the patients reported on by Buller and Wood indulged in this manner.

Both of these patients suffered from the hyperesthesic form of the disease. The involvement was also of the upper extremities alone. There were the familiar paresthesiæ, numbing, pricking and shooting pains in the back of the hands and forearms. The pains were at times severe and there was intense pain upon pressure over the nerve trunks. The joints were involved to a slight extent only. There was also a certain amount of edema or puffiness.

These were instances, I believe, of beginning peripheral neuritis due to breathing the fumes of wood alcohol. It might be recalled that de Schweinitz[7] and others have described typical optic neuritis and blindness as a result of breathing the fumes of wood alcohol.

Both of these patients were intelligent men and noting similar symptoms they were led to seek medical aid before serious consequence arose. It is true that the involvement was slight only, but it seemed at one time in the disease particularly in one of the patients, that paralysis might develop. There was distinct motor weakness in both instances, and it might be added that they seemed more anxious about the impairment of their muscular power than they were about the sensory symptoms.

In so far as this whole question of wood alcohol poisoning is of comparatively recent development it might prove of service, particularly opening a discussion, to recapitulate, in a stricted sense, somewhat concerning our knowledge of the comparative toxicity of the different alcohols, particularly the peculiar characteristics of wood alcohol.

The alcohols that interest us are hydroxides of the marsh gas series: Methyl, CH_3OH; Ethyl, C_2H_5OH; Propyl, C_3H_7OH; Butyl, C_4H_9OH; Amyl, $C_5H_{11}OH$. Wood alcohol, grain alcohol, and amyl alcohol or fusel oil represent the most familiar.

Pharmacologists are in practical accord that from the lowest to the highest of the series there is for acute poisoning a gradual increase in the toxic action of these alcohols, and the early figures of Joffroy and Serveaux[8] have been practically confirmed by a large series of experiments with various animals. In general it may be said that the comparative toxicity in acute poisoning is: Methyl, .5 to .7; ethyl, 1; propyl, 2 to 3; butyl, 3 to 5; amyl, 5 to 8. These figures are not absolute for all species, but they represent a mean of the results of many investigations.

Thus Dujardin-Beaumetz and Audigé,[10] almost the earliest observers, working with dogs, showed that the toxic doses in grams per kilo of animal were arranged as follows: Wood alcohol (ordinary), 5 to 6; pure wood alcohol, 7; ethyl, 7.75; propyl, 3.75; butyl, 1.85; amyl, 1.50. Joffroy and Serveaux's[8] figures for the equivalents in toxic power for rabbits were as follows: Methyl alcohol, 25.25; ethyl alcohol, 11.70; propyl alcohol, 3.40; butyl alcohol, 1.45; amyl alcohol, .63; furfurol, .24, and Bär's experiments on guinea-pigs to control the figures of the earlier French writers showed practically the same results. Poisoning increased with the boiling point of the alcohol. He would arrange them as follows: Methyl, .8; ethyl, 1.0; propyl, 2; butyl, 3; amyl, 4. Less than one per cent. of higher alcohols added to ethyl alcohol does not seriously modify its toxicity, but four per cent. causes a distinct rise in toxic power. One to two per cent. of furfurol also increases the poisonous action of ethyl alcohol.

Reid Hunt's[11] more recent and exhaustive work on dogs shows somewhat similar results. He raises the question, however, that the results as observed in acute intoxication of the lower animals may not be applicable to man.

It may thus be seen that, dose for dose, for lower animals, including monkeys, and possibly also for man, although there are reasons why this may not be true, methyl alcohol is slightly less toxic than ordinary alcohol.

But the matter is distinctly different when repeated dosage is concerned. Here experimentation with the lower animals has shown that wood alcohol differs in its action from other alcohols. It is markedly cumulative in its action while the others are not or distinctly less so. The action of a single toxic dose, moreover, is much more prolonged than for any of the other alcohols, for Pohl and others have shown that the maximum output of decomposition products following wood alco-

hol doses does not occur until the third or fourth day. Thus lower animals may take ethyl alcohol or the higher alcohols for considerable periods of time, weeks, months or even years, and if the doses are not too large there is soon established a balance between absorption and elimination, and the animal continues to live and develops slowly the characteristic tissue changes of alcoholic degeneration. This is also true for fusel oil and for furfurol, two of the most poisonous ingredients of many intoxicating drinks.

Under methy alcohol, however, even if the doses given are not distinctly toxic, after a comparatively short time, two or three weeks, the animal dies, usually of coma, inanition, fatty degeneration of the liver, and almost invariably develops changes in the nervous tissues of the eye. It is thus very evident that the type of poisoning is different with methyl alcohol, and that probably the products of decomposition of methyl alcohol in the body are different from those of the higher alcohols.

Just what the exact steps are in the oxidations, more particularly of ethyl alcohol and wood alcohol, we are not yet in a position to state positively. Pohl[12] has shown that the probable course of the oxidation of ethyl alcohol is into ethyl aldeyde, to ethyl acetate, acetic acid, carbon dioxide and water; thus in the urine, beyond the small amount of unchanged alcohol, there are no traces of the decomposition products. For wood alcohol the oxidations are probably into formic aldehyde and then to formic acid, and the latter acid has been found in considerable quantities in the urine by Pohl, by Reid Hunt and others who have worked on this side of the problem. Pohl failed to find any increase of formic acid in the blood or tissues, however.

Pohl, Hunt and others have concluded then that in view of the prolonged action of methyl alcohol and the high toxic action when given in small repeated doses, it is probably very slowly oxidized and hence probably remains, first as methyl alcohol in contact with the tissues for a long time, and that probaly formaldehyde and formic acid play some part in the poisoning. Hunt has said that formic acid is probably six times as toxic as wood alcohol.

It is not therefore necessary to say that it is because of the impurities in wood alcohol, furfurol, acetone, etc., that this body is toxic: it is because of its very slow oxidation processes, and its own characteristic decomposition compounds.

Before wood alcohol was put upon the market as an odorless substitute for grain alcohol, as it was about 1896, under the name of Columbian Spirits, its very penetrating odor prevented, in large part, its use for adulterating whiskies and other alcoholic preparations, tinctures, essences, colognes, flavoring extracts, etc., but at the present time, if we are to take the statements of many competent analytical chemists that a large percentage of all these preparations is adulterated, and that largely by wood alcohol, the situation is not reassuring. The Board of Pharmacy in this city at one time found an extensive use of wood alcohol in the manufacture of the tinctures of official preparations, to be used in serious illness, and, be it accorded to their credit, they have been indefatigable in their efforts to stop such highly reprehensible practices—and with success.

Why then do we not find a number of patients suffering from methyl alcohol peripheral neuritis, and why are there not more reported cases in literature?

There are a number of reasons why! One is that death occurs so promptly in many instances that there is not enough time to develop the lesion in the peripheral nerves; or because of the greater susceptibility of the ganglion cells of the retina, partial or complete blindness appears so promptly that the methyl alcohol mixtures are not taken for a greater length of time.

As for the reasons for this relatively greater susceptibility of the retinal ganglionic structures it can be accepted at the present time only as a fact, bearing in mind that the alcohols as a class affect the more complex nervous elements of the cerebrum and highly differentiated special senses more rapidly than the comparatively more primary spinal neurons of the peripheral nervous system.

Peripheral neuritis from wood alcohol does not seem to have been observed in any of the animals experimented on. Here again the early death precludes the development of the lesion, and, moreover, most of the investigators had in mind solely the effects to be observed in the retina and optic nerves. The more general subject of experimental wood alcohol peripheral neuritis is therefore in need of investigation.

64 West Fifty-sixth Street.

LITERATURE.

1. Buller and Wood. Journal, A. M. A., October 1, 1904, et seq. (Extensive study of poisoning and optic neuritis.)
2. Jackson. New England Journal of Medicine and Surgery, 11, 1822, p. 351.
3. Ward Holden. Archiv für Augenheilkunde, Vol. 40, p. 351.
4. Birch-Hirschfeld. Archiv für Ophthalmologie, 54, 1902, p. 68, (With bibliography for Optic Neuritis).
5. Rymowitzsch. St. Petersburg Dissertation, 1896.
6. de Schweinitz. Toxic Amblyopias.
7. de Schweinitz. Ophthalmic Record, June, 1901, p. 289.
8. Joffroy et Serveaux. Arch. de Méd. expérimentales, Vol. 4, p. 473.
9. Bär. Archiv für Anatomie und Physiologie, (Phys. Abth.) 1898, 304, p. 283.
10. Dujardin-Beaumetz et Audigé. Comptes rendus, 83, 1876, p. 80.
11. Reid Hunt. Johns Hopkins Hospital Bulletin, 13, 1902, p. 213.
12. Pohl. Arch. f. d. exp. Path. u. Pharmakologie, 31, 1893, p. 281.

No College Affiliation Yet.—At a recent meeting of the Board of Trustees of the University of Illinois, no action was taken relative to a closer affiliation between the university and the Chicago College of Physicians and Surgeons. At present the university and the medical school work under an agreement made in 1900. Recently, it is said, an offer was made by two philanthropists to endow the school as soon as it came into the possession of the University. President James and the Board of Trustees may take steps hortly to bring this about.

APPENDICITIS, AS A VISCERAL MANIFESTATION OF ERYTHEMA EXUDATIVUM MULTIFORME.

BY JAMES S. CHENOWETH, M.D.,
OF LOUISVILLE, KY.

ERYTHEMA exudativum multiforme, as its name would indicate, is an affection characterized by polymorphic skin lesions of an erythematous type. It may occur in the course of some general disease or in an apparently idiopathic manner.

The eruption may be the first and only manifestation of the disease; frequently, however, its appearance is preceded for several hours or days by prodromal symptoms, consisting of general malaise, headache, backache, gastric disturbances and fever.

Visceral lesions, which have been noted in a large percentage of cases, may precede or follow the eruption and may cause a fatal termination. In certain cases the lungs, brain, kidneys, stomach, and intestines have been pathologically affected. These visceral lesions are not uncommonly attended by intense colic, high fever, nose bleed, hematuria, hematemesis and intestinal hemorrhage, one or all of which may be present in any given case.

In a paper read before the Louisville Surgical Society, November 23, 1896,[1] I reported two cases of appendicitis, occurring in connection with erythema exudativum multiforme, calling attention, I believe, for the first time to the possibility of such a causation of certain cases of this disease.

The importance of these vasomotor circulatory disturbances as affecting the appendix has not, in my opinion, been sufficiently recognized, as more extended experience leads me to believe that these cases are by no means rare. The matter of diagnosis is one of grave importance. In the first place these attacks of colic, the so-called abdominal crisis of exudative erythema, may easily lead the inexperienced to make a diagnosis of appendicitis, when no lesion of that organ exists, on the other hand the more serious mistake may be made of overlooking the co-existing appendix trouble, unless it be recognized that these vasomotor circulatory disturbances do at times result in congestion of and even hemorrhage into the appendix, with the result that we may have bacterial infection and inflammation or actual gangrene of this organ. The peculiar anatomical arrangement of the appendix, the abundant lymphoid tissue enclosed by a dense fibromuscular sheath, and the possession of a terminal circulation, make it particularly liable to serious circulatory disturbances What would in other portions of the intestine be a simple and temporary edema, may here result in a most serious condition.

The diagnosis of appendicitis in these case must rest upon the classical signs, pain (localize or general in character), tenderness over the ap pendix, and localized muscular rigidity. In m experience the abdominal crises of exudative ery

1 Mathew's Quarterly Journal, January, 1897.

thema have not been attended by muscular rigidity, and localized tenderness except in those cases in which the appendix has been involved, as demonstrated by operation in four cases.

Two of these cases are quite typical. The first was that of a boy, aged fifteen years, operated upon January 7, 1895. His mother had rheumatism and tonsillitis; one aunt had rheumatism, a second, exudative erythema; his father had rheumatism and died of endocarditis; a sister was under my care with erythema nodosum.

This boy came under my observation in the fall of 1890, suffering from tonsillitis and nose-bleed. From that time until the spring of 1894 I attended him at various times with tonsillitis, nosebleed, colic and urticaria.

In May, 1894, after a horse-back ride, he had a severe attack of colic attended by vomiting. His pain was general over the abdomen, and unattended by local tenderness or muscular rigidity. His temperature was slightly elevated. The August following he had a second attack accompanied by fever, pain and vomiting, which subsided in a few days.

On November 23 following, he started on a hunt in Indiana. The first day out the weather turned very cold and he slipped on the frozen ground and cut a deep gash in his hand, which necessitated a return that night. Next day he had an attack of asthma with nose-bleed. This lasted with intermissions until December 6. On January 6, one month later, I was hurriedly called to find him suffering from colic and vomiting. He was quite nervous and tossing about the bed. Temperature 99.2° F., pulse 100, abdomen not distended; pain was most intense under the border of ribs on *left* side, and over the appendix. There was now present local rigidity and tenderness over the appendix. Enema of glycerin and water brought away only a little gas. Calomel grs. 1½ was retained. Five hours later he began to cough and his nose bled. Urine was scanty and contained some blood. Twenty-two hours after the commencement of the attack his temperature was 100.6° F., pulse 105. He had vomited several times and bowels had not moved.

An increasing tenderness in the region of appendix warned me against further delay, and notwithstanding many misgivings as to his general condition his abdomen was opened. The appendix immediately presented. There were no adhesions or signs of previous inflammation. The appendix was three inches long, the meso-appendix extending half its length. It was tensely distended, containing some mucopurulent fluid, and a good-sized blood clot. Hemorrhage had taken place into the walls of the appendix and mesentery, which were almost black in color.

The case went on without incident until the eighth day when the stitches were removed, union being perfect. On the ninth day, his stomach became deranged through some error of diet. This was followed by severe abdominal pains chiefly on the left side. On the next day an ery-

thematous eruption appeared on the abdomen. During the next few weeks he showed nearly every possible phase of exudative erythema, pain and edema in the muscles and joints, urticarial lesions of all styles, bleeding from the nose, hematemesis, hematuria, and hemorrhage from the intestine, always preceded by intense colic. Purpuric spots appeared in the legs.

He finally recovered and has remained in good health with the exception of an occasional attack of erythema, sometimes accompanied by colic, and hematuria of short duration. I saw him in one attack during the past month.

The second case was that of a boy, aged fourteen years, taken sick in May, 1895. His family history is interesting. His father I operated upon for a large appendical abscess. A sister, twenty-four years of age, suffered from dysmenorrhea and tonsillitis. Several times I was called to see her, and found her suffering with violent colicky pain, usually located in left hypochondrium, and for which I could assign no cause. On one occasion this was attended by vomiting and an outbreak of urticaria. A second sister had rheumatism and tonsillitis, and finally developed appendicitis.

I first saw the boy about twelve o'clock in the day. He had been employed in a milk depot for a week, and the day before my visit had done a hard day's work for a boy of his age, handling the heavy cans, etc., and while overheated, drank a large quantity of ice cold milk before leaving the dairy. The next morning the awoke and at once complained of nausea and sore throat. A little later a number of large erythematous wheals appeared over the body and simultaneously he complained of intense abdominal pain, most intense over the region of appendix but generalized.

His temperature was 100.2° F., pulse 90; localized tenderness and marked rigidity of muscles over appendix. A diagnosis of erythema exudativum with appendicitis was made and the boy removed to Norton Infirmary, and operated upon at 9 P.M. of the same day.

On opening the abdomen the appendix was found pointing downward, and overlapped by the cecum; its walls were hyperplastic, and quite hard from the dense infiltration of its walls. The mesentery was thickened and extended almost to the tip of the organ. The distal third of the appendix and corresponding portion of the mesentery presented a dark, mottled appearance from the extravasation of blood into this hyperplastic tissue. The lumen of the appendix was pervious, and contained only a little mucoid material with fecal odor. Recovery in this case was rapid, the erythema subsiding in the course of a week.

The clinical as well as microscopical study of these cases seemed to demonstrate the fact that the pathological condition in the appendix was primarily and essentially the same as that taking place in the skin. That the erythema was not secondary to the appendicitis, is clear from the fact that previous attacks of erythema had occurred in both cases and have occurred at intervals since the removal of the appendix.

The occurrence of appendicitis in these cases is of course not to be regarded as due to the erythematous eruption on the skin, but rather, as the title of this paper would indicate, as one of the visceral manifestations of that condition, of which the presence of such an eruption is the most common and easily recognized sign.

Just how often such circulatory disturbances occur in the appendix of sufficient severity to damage its integrity, and permit of bacterial invasion is a matter of conjecture. It would seem to me. however, that too much stress has been laid upon bacteria as the primary agents in the production of appendicitis, to the exclusion of all constitutional conditions. Certainly, if we would do anything toward the prevention of this disease it must be through the recognition of those general conditions which at least strongly predispose to its development.

SHORT AND EASY METHODS OF ARRIVING AT GOOD RESULTS IN DISEASES OF THE EAR AND UPPER AIR TRACT, ILLUSTRATED BY RECENT CASES.[1]

BY W. SOHIER BRYANT, M.D.,
OF NEW YORK.

Anditory Delusions.—Miss A. K., age twenty-seven years, January 13, 1904. She complains of voices and sounds. The voices talk about the thoughts that are in her mind. They say bad things about her. She has a slight "chronic middle-ear catarrh." I treat her with catheter, Siegel, and nitrate of silver. January 21.—Patient looks well. She does not hear the voices as clearly. The tinnitus is mostly in the right ear. The voices are heard in whichever ear is down on the pillow at night. March 10.—Hearing slightly improved. The voices have ceased. No recurrence three weeks later.

A very important case showing the connection between tinnitus and insane delusions, the tinnitus in a psychopathic patient taking the form of voices.

Caries of Tympanum; Radical Operation.—Miss M., aged twenty-four years. A year ago she lost a sister after a radical operation, who had the same aural complications as herself. September 14. 1904, when I first examined the patient, the tympanum had been curetted for the otorrhea some time previous, but otorrhea continues and there is a large carious surface on upper and inner wall of tympanum and antrum. Tenderness on pressure over antrum. Temperature 99° F. Slight, very fetid discharge. I performed the radical operation. Owing to the anatomical irregularities, the sigmoid sinus impinging against the posterior wall of the auditory canal, with only 1 mm. of bone intervening. the posterior cranial fossa had to

1 In the Fourth Pan-American Medical Congress, Panama.

be opened, exposing the greater part of the sigmoid sinus. The carious condition of the tegumen necessitated opening the middle cranial fossa and exposing a considerable area of dura. All diseased tissues were removed. The meatus was split and stitched back into the wound, which was closed and packed from the meatus, leaving only a pencil drain from the exposed dura. Temperature did not rise above 100.5° F. Drain removed September 18. Patient went home on September 28, with wound healed by first intention. Epidermitization progressed favorably. On October 26, the tympanum was all covered with skin except at mouth of Eustachian tube. November 11, the ear was dry and sound. November 25, watch nine inches. Patient has gained twelve pounds since the operation. Last seen December 17, in perfect condition. Shows satisfactory healing of tympanic cavity in eight weeks without skin grafting more than the plastic with the meatal flap. Mastoid wound entirely healed in thirteen days.

Epidural Abscess; Operation; Rapid Recovery.—Mr. G. T., aged twenty-one years. Patient of Dr. Michelis. (Shown at the 1904 meeting of the American Otological Society). Three months ago grippe and earache. Two months ago severe headache commenced. The first time I saw him, patient had seropurulent non-fetid discharge and not very marked tenderness behind ear. No superficial redness nor swelling. Tympanum filled with sensitive tissue. Marked tenderness over base of mastoid, extending posteriorly. Continuous severe headache. Constant seropurulent discharge. Temperature 100°. F., pulse 88. On June 19 I performed my usual mastoid operation, using the front bent gouge. The mastoid cells and the whole process are filled with granulations and are removed. Posteriorly there is an area of bare dura about as big as a silver dollar, covered with pus and granulations. All the diseased bone is removed. Wound irrigated with saline solution and closed. Dry treatment for the tympanum. Temperature did not rise above 100° F. July 4, tympanum perfectly healed, acoumeter 13 inches. July 10, wound healed solid. Hearing very good. Patient still continues well. Shows the advantage of closing a comparatively clean cranial wound for union by first intention, and dry treatment of the tympanum. Tympanum completely healed in fourteen days. Wound healed solid in twenty days.

Severe Aural Symptoms Cured with Expectant Treatment.—Mrs. X., aged thirty-two years, daughter of one of the few rich men of New York. Left ear discharged many years. Head symptoms commenced, May, 1903, became violent in the summer and a mastoid operation was done with transient relief. March 15, 1904. on account of vertigo with epileptiform exacerbations, extreme tenderness in scar and over bone of mastoid and occiput, and swelling and tenderness down the neck. Headache, temperature

99° F. A radical operation was done by Dr. Crockett, of Boston. I assisted and had subsequent charge of the convalescence. Patient much relieved by operation, wound healed by first intention. Maximum temperature 99+° F. A facial paralysis appeared the day after the operation. March 22, meatus and bone behind ear very tender, shooting pains; April 2, very annoying vertigo, convergent strabismus, more or less constant pain and tenderness behind, below, in ear and down neck, and in right occipital region, and paralysis worse. Cleaning the canal and tympanum seemed to relieve the condition. Exacerbation on April 12, 23 and May 5. A third operation was not advised on account of the prominent position of the patient. Pharyngitis was associated with these exacerbations. May 20, felt difficulty in moving left leg and arm. June 16, no dizziness. June 21, a relapse, walking difficult, on account of vertigo, tenderness. June 24, ear discharge increased with relief of symptoms. July 25, ear dry, hearing good, symptoms very mild. November 12, tenderness gone; November 18, bad attacks, pharynx involved, but ear remains dry and healed, no redness of canal. December 14, another similar attack. It appears that the submerged tonsil is chiefly to blame for these attacks. Cleaning the tympanum and nitrate of silver rapidly relieved the attacks. The facial paralysis very much improved with strychnine, massage and electricity.

An alarming group of symptoms due partly to the ear and partly to the throat, but apparently without any immediate danger.

Epithelioma of Concha.—Mr. S., aged sixty years. October 31, 1903, has an ulceration of the concha as large as a five-cent piece, behind posterior edge of right meatus. He says ear has discharged for six years. No glandular enlargement noted. I removed a specimen for histological examination. It was pronounced epithelioma by Dr. Dixon. March 24, 1904, ulceration has slightly extended. After three weeks, with four X-ray exposures per week, by Dr. Morton, the ulceration has entirely cicatrized and disappeared. No recurrence. This justifies a good prognosis for epithelioma of the auricle before involvement of the glands.

Facial Paralysis.—Mrs. X., aged twenty-eight years. October 25, 1904, left facial paralysis four days' standing. Cause not known. The eye can be three-quarters closed, paralysis most marked about mouth. Ear normal. Tenderness below and in front of the ear extends onto mastoid process. Valsalvan inflations easy. Hearing slightly defective by air conduction. Left side of pharynx red and somewhat swollen, has been painful for two weeks. Pain in the throat in the posterior and inferior mandibular region. Could not eat for pain in ear. Could not shut mouth for a few days. Treatment strychnine and heat; silver applications to the pharynx. Patient improved rapidly. In ten days

could whistle slightly. Shows an unusually rapid recovery in spite of the neglect of electricity.

Absence of Liquefied Contents; Obstinate Fetid Otorrhœa from Attic and Antrum. Hearing Improved by Dressings.—Miss N., aged twenty-seven years. Referred to me by Dr. Joseph A. Kenefick, October 7, 1904. She has had a running ear for more than five years, and much treatment, including ossiculectomy four years ago. Tympanum is devoid of all structures except stapes. There is scanty, very fetid discharge. The epitympanic space very extensive and filled with decomposing material. I cleansed the ear with H_2O_2, alcohol, and boric acid, and nitrate of silver solution. The vault and tegumen are extremely sensitive. October 7, nearly dry but fetid; October 29, clean, damp, but no smell; November 12, less tenderness; November 28, very little tenderness; December 5, dry and not sensitive; December 14, ear in fine condition. Hearing by watch 3.5 inches; after insertion of cotton tack it is eight inches, and with paper dressing nine inches. Fetid discharge from vault of attic and mastoid antrum cured in eight weeks.

Fetid Otorrhœa of Very Long Duration from the Antrum through a Small Perforation.—Mr. T. C. J., merchant, aged thirty-nine years, December 1, 1903. Scanty, thin, fetid, purulent discharge from left ear, which has lasted for many years in spite of prolonged treatment by others. There is a perforation occupying the upper posterior quadrant, leading up into the antrum. The anterior part of tympanum is shut off by a cicatrix. I syringe the ear with Blake canula and solutions of boric acid and nitrate of silver. After five treatments on alternate days the ear has ceased discharging and is healed. December 21, 1904, hearing fair. Patient has gained much strength. Constant fetid discharge from mastoid antrum cured in eight days.

Caries of the Malleus and Perforation of Shrapnel's Membrane.—Capt. D., U.S.A., aged thirty-four years. Referred by Dr. Clarence J. Blake, of Boston, who made the diagnosis of perforation of Shrapnel's membrane with caries of the neck of the malleus. Purulent discharge came on in right ear during service in Cuba, 1898. Ear has discharged more or less ever since, in spite of varied treatment. It was much aggravated by recent service in the Philippines. Capt. D.'s application to the Surgeon General for allowance for special medical treatment being granted, I commenced treatment, February 27, 1904. I find a perforation in Shrapnel's membrane and a slight amount of mucopurulent discharge. I syringed with boric acid solution, nitrate of silver, and alcohol. On March 3, hears acoumeter five feet. On March 9, discharge has ceased. Acoumeter 7½ feet. Discharge soon reappeared, but was brought under control once more. March 27, acoumeter 15 feet. Again the discharge reappears, and again was stopped. May 3, the ear became permanently dry, and treatment discontinued. May 17, hearing was 35 feet with acoumeter. Patient last seen November 28. Ear has not bothered him any more.

Purulent discharge through Shrapnel's membrane lasting for over six years, permanently stopped 9½ weeks of treatment.

Chronic Purulent Otitis Media with Pinhole Perforation of Membrane.—Mr. K., aged twenty-three years, first seen May 20, 1904. Has had for four years purulent discharge from right ear, on account of which he is not now serving in Austrian army. He has had much treatment in Europe. I found mucopurulent discharge oozing through a small pin-hole perforation behind the tip of the malleus. Membrane opaque slightly red and very thick. Thick mucopurulent discharge in vault of pharynx. Acoumeter three feet. I enlarged the perforation in membrane by a horizontal incision, and treat by syringe of boric acid, nitrate of silver and alcohol for the ear; alkalol spray for the nose. July 23, hearing acoumeter 15 feet. August 22, hearing acoumeter 30 feet. Discharge stopped. Perforation shows no tendency to close up. September 14, patient still in good condition. A very obstinate purulent inflammation of the middle ear is healed in 13½ weeks.

Acute Salpingitis and Epitympanitis.—Miss J. A., aged twenty-six years, referred by Dr. Van Loan, December 13, 1904. Has had cold in the head a month. Deafness two weeks. Lost weight, pain in left ear and ringing sounds, discomfort in right. Watch, left ear, 4 inches; after treatment 17 inches. Right ear, 18 inches; after treatment 48 inches. Left Shrapnel membrane red and bulging. Right ear partly filled with fluid. Catheter and saline sprays. December 15, no pain or noise. Right ear, watch 96 inches, left ear, watch, 24 inches. Rapid recovery of an acute condition in forty-eight hours. Hearing, watch right, 4 inches, increased to 24 inches, and in left ear from 18 inches to 96 inches.

Mechanical Assistance for Defective Hearing in Loss Due to Suppurative Process. Cured by Nasal Treatment.—Mr. F. B., aged twenty-five years. June 15, 1904. Has had purulent ears for many years. Left ear discharging now, right cicatrized. I found hypertrophied lower turbinates and thick mucopurulent discharge. Acoumeter, right ear, 2 inches; left ear, zero. After inflation, left, 2 inches; right, 4 inches. I improved the nasal condition with operative and palliative treatment and the ears dry up. July 3, both ears cicatrized. August 14, with cotton dressing, hearing for right ear, acoumeter, 7 inches, left ear 14 inches. August 31, without cotton, 4 inches in right ear and 2 inches in left ear. With cotton replaced, hearing 18 inches in the left ear. September 6, right ear, acoumeter 48 inches with cotton; left ear, 2 inches without and 9 with. October 24, right ear, without cotton, 23 inches; left ear 10 inches

with paper dressing in ear, 12 inches with cotton dressing. Patient thinks he hears well enough for ordinary business purposes. Otorrhea, stopped in seventeen days. Hearing brought up from acoumeter, right 2 inches, by use of dressings, to over 48 inches in three weeks, then without the dressing to 23 inches in ten weeks. From acoumeter left 0 inch, by use of dressings, to 12 inches in ten weeks.

Grave Tinnitus.—Mr. J. M., aged forty years, referred to me by Dr. Alfred Michaelis, February 14, 1904. Patient neurotic and haggard in appearance. Says he has an unbearable tinnitus in his left ear, preventing sleep and attention to business. Conversation and appearance suggest lack of mental balance. The ear began to run thirty-six or thirty-seven years ago. The tinnitus began twelve years ago. In September, 1903, underwent the radical mastoid operation for tinnitus, without any effect on the tinnitus. The ear shows a large epidermatized tympanic cavity; no discharge. Told the patient that it is possible to remove the auditory nerve and thereby stop the tinnitus, but milder measures had to be tried first. Give hygienic suggestions. February 27, 1904, patient attempted to end his troubles by taking poison. June 24, general condition improved, sleeps better, has been practically free from tinnitus a few days. December, 1904. Hygiene has improved his physical condition and restored his mental balance. He says he is getting used to the tinnitus. After ten months the patient's mental attitude is much improved.

Commencing Stapes Fixation.—Mr. F. L., aged twenty-eight years, referred to me by Dr. C. A. Crockett, of Boston, October, 21, 1904, with diagnosis of commencing stapes fixation of right ear. The right drum membrane is dark-colored and of normal transparency, nasal mucous membrane dark red. Tinnitus, like a sea-shell, crackling and musical notes. I used catheter, iodine vapor instillations, and nitrate of silver to the pharynx. Ear feels and looks much better after the treatment. December 12th, acoumeter, 96 inches. The shell-sound tinnitus remains but is much lower and intermittent. Valsalva possible but slow. Strychnine sulphate seven-sixtieth grains per day. In 7½ weeks the stapes fixation has been materially improved.

Adhesive Middle-Ear Catarrh.—Mrs. P., referred to me by Dr. Potter, of New York. Aged seventy-one years. Gouty tendency. December 2, 1904, itching of canals, ears feel thick. Nasal mucosa dark red. Acoumeter, left 27 inches, right 10 feet. Adrenal powder, silver nitrate to tubes and lanolin to canal. December 14, subjective symptoms stopped. Left ear acoumeter, 42 inches; right ear, 15 feet. Rapid improvement of hearing in adhesive processes in the patient; from right acoumeter, 120 inches, left, 27 inches; to right acoumeter, 180 inches, left, 42 inches, in eleven days.

Very Obstinate Case of the Atrophic Form of Chronic Catarrhal Otitis Media with Deafness and Tinnitus.—Seen at the New York Eye and Ear Infirmary, February 4, 1904. Mrs. G. G., aged twenty-nine years, complains of tinnitus, simultaneous or alternating in the ears. High and low bells ringing. She says she has had the sounds in her right ear for two years and in left ear six. Right drum membrane has a large calcified area in anterior half. Hearing by air conduction very bad in left ear, good in right. Air passes by catheter and Valsalva, best into left tympanum. Fork lateralized in left ear. Nasal mucous membrane dark red and thickened. I treated her with the catheter, iodine vapor and applications of nitrate of silver to the nasopharynx. Negative results continue for a long time. August 9, 1904. Has been better of late, and now hears well. August 18, 1904: Tinnitus stopped in right ear, and nasal mucous membrane is light pink and clean. Finally tinnitus stopped, and hearing very good. A short relapse in November, easily controlled. Mucous membrane good color; all right again December 4. In twenty-eight weeks the atrophic condition has been overcome. Result entirely satisfactory to the patient.

Deafness Due to Adhesive Processes, Defect and Relaxations in the Sound-Conducting Mechanism.—Mrs. S., a society woman, aged forty-three years; referred to me February 8, 1904, by Dr. Clarence J. Blake, of Boston, for continuance of treatment he had commenced. Right ear has a dry perforation which is being treated by paper dressing to induce proper adhesions. Left ear: Drum membrane relaxed, being treated with collodion dressing. The acoumeter heard at a distance of four inches by the left and 12 inches by the right ear. I continued the treatment of paper and collodion dressings. On March 22, the perforation is healed and the hearing in the right ear is, acoumeter, 96 inches and in the left, 72 inches, in spite of the patient's being quite exhausted from the season in New York. In six weeks the hearing has improved from acoumeter, 12 inches right and 4 inches left, to ninety-six inches right and seventy-two inches left.

Subacute Closure of Eustachian Tube.—Mr. H. D. H., aged thirty-eight years; referred to me by Dr. Joseph Collins, December 1, 1904. Has had a cold in the head since November 12. Ears began to feel full November 20. Has had various kinds of treatment from others. He hears, acoumeter, 14 inches in right and 48 inches in left; after Politzerization, right, 54 inches, left, 96 inches. Insufflation of powdered suprarenal gland. Apply a solution of nitrate of silver in the red and swollen nasal fossæ, and gave a menthol-eucalyptol spray for home use. December 3, acoumeter, left 12 feet, right 8 feet. After Politzerization acoumeter heard over 20 feet by each ear. December 8, acoumeter in right over 15 feet and watch 3 feet. After

Politzerization, watch 6 feet. December 18, watch right, 7 feet, left, 5 feet. Patient was more than satisfied. In forty-eight hours the hearing improved from 14 and 48 inches for acoumeter, to over 240 inches for each ear. This improvement increased 50 per cent. more on the seventh day of treatment.

Stricture of Eustachian Tube with Adhesive Catarrhal Processes in the Tympanum.—Miss D., referred to me by Dr. Clarence J. Blake, of Boston, September 10, 1904. When a child she had a discharge from the right ear, and recently an acute attack of streptococcic infection in the attic. Nasal mucous membrane is dark red, nose clear, no air enters tympanum by Valsalva. The patient had closure of the right Eustachian tube and occasional tinnitus. I treated her with the catheter. The air entered tympanum with difficulty. Then applications of nitrate of silver in the nasopharynx, and alkalol spray. After the third treatment she hears watch, left 9 inches, right 6 inches. Air goes into left tympanum by Valsalva. On October 21, Valsalva easy; patient feels much better. No abnormal sensations in ears. Drum membranes look very nearly normal. Watch, right ear, 40 inches, left, 54 inches. October 28, no unpleasant symptoms. Patient satisfied to stop treatment. The stricture was cured in six weeks with relief of the adhesive condition.

Loss of Acoustic Balance with Tubal Stricture.—The Rev. Mr. J., twenty-six years old. October 25, 1904, complains of impaired hearing in left ear. Tuning fork lateralized to the left with much increased bone-conduction, slight ringing tinnitus. Valsalva not free. Membrane good color, slightly relaxed. Apply solution of nitrate of silver to the nares. November 1, Valsalva easier. On the fifth visit, November 11, hears watch 72 inches in right ear and is well pleased with improvement. Treatment: catheter, strychnine, suprarenal powder and nitrate of silver. December 7, watch 7 feet; fork still lateralized in the left. Apply thin collodion dressing to left ear. Watch heard 10 feet. December 9, watch heard 15 feet by left ear. Valsalva very easy, and ready return. Application of collodion. Hears watch twice as far in left ear as in right. Left ear, 30 feet, equivalent to $^{30}/_{10}$. Right ear, 15 feet, equivalent to $^{15}/_{10}$. Stricture cured in six weeks. Acoustic balance restored in forty-eight hours, and deafness exchanged for hyperacoustic.

Valvular Occlusion of the External Auditory Meatus by a New Growth, Causing Grave Reflex Symptoms (Reported before the American Otological Society, 1903).—Seen at the Massachusetts Charitable Eye and Ear Infirmary, through the kindness of Dr. Z. L. Jack, April 14, 1903. Mrs. E. W., a well-nourished, neurotic woman with a haggard expression, aged thirty-one years. Declares that she can no longer endure her distress, which she is unable to describe. Complains bitterly of indescribable misery and discomfort in her head, sleeplessness due to the oppression in left ear, and severe headache, deafness and inability to do any work, read, sew or fix her attention, without extreme effort, inability to sleep and consequent irritability, nervous exhaustion and mental confusion. She said that she was helpless, no use to herself or any one else, and that she wished to die if she could not be cured. She locates the source of her trouble in her left ear, which has been treated by many " specialists," but her condition has steadily grown worse. Nose is occluded by engorged turbinals. She has a slight strabismus. Appearance and hearing of right ear normal; left ear, $^3/_{20}$, conversation voice. Inspection shows a normal meatus, except that at the orifice the upper wall sags sufficiently to be in contact with the lower for a distance inward of about half an inch, and closes the meatus like a valve. Drum membrane appears normal. On questioning the patient it appears that the meatus becomes hermetically occluded and that the vacuum forming on outer surface of the drum causes her unpleasant symptoms by drawing out the drum membrane. I removed a small free subcutaneous fibroid of the keloid type under nitrous oxide anesthesia. Wound healed in three days. Left drum membrane and hearing normal. The patient said that as soon as she had quite gained her mental equilibrium after the anesthetic, she found complete relief from her disagreeable symptoms, and that she now has perfect nasal breathing, a condition which she can scarcely remember to have enjoyed before. November 1, 1903, she still has occasional headaches, but none of the same symptoms she formerly had.

Foreign Body in Meatus.—Seen through the kindness of Dr. Gorham Bacon, February 18, 1904. Mr. M. C., aged twenty-two years, complains of tinnitus in left ear. Inspection shows a piece of cerumenous-looking substance resting against the drum membrane. This I readily removed with a syringe. It proved to be a bean. Patient declares that the bean has been in his ear since his seventh year. After drying the canal, all symptoms have disappeared, and the membrane appears normal. The canal was large and had a spacious posterior pocket. There was very little cerumen and epithelium removed with the bean. The skin was separate from the bean, which was brown, like a baked bean.

Vertigo from Impacted Cerumen.—Seen through the kindness of Dr. Albert II. Buck, November 2, 1903. Mr. J. B., aged forty-two years, complains of " swinging " vertigo for the last four months. Says he " drops right in his tracks. Feels it coming from the legs up." He says his left ear has been stopped for three or four years. Inspection discloses impacted cerumen in left meatus. Hearing in the other ear good. I removed the cerumen with the syringe, and all sensations and symptoms of vertigo disappear on the instant.

Deafness of Twenty Years Cured by Removing Cerumen.—Seen at the Vanderbilt Clinic of the College of Physicians and Surgeons, through the kindness of Dr. Robert Lewis, Jr., October 18, 1903. Mr. A. B., aged twenty-seven years, complains of increasing deafness in his left ear. Cerumen is seen packed in both meati. First I syringed the cerumen out of the right ear. Immediately the patient was wonder-struck, declaring that he hears in the right ear for the first time. He admitted later·that in childhood he had heard with both ears. The membrane appeared in fair condition. The hearing in the left ear was also restored by syringing out the other plug of cerumen.

Empyema of All the Sinuses of the Nose.—Seen through the kindness of Dr. John L. Adams. Mr. N. S., twenty years of age, paper-box maker. History of case dates back a year and a half. Now complains of occluded nares and profuse purulent discharge. Inspection of the nares showed purulent discharge coming from the vault and from between the middle and lower turbinates on both sides. Transillumination shows the frontal and maxillary sinuses opaque. I removed part of both lower turbinates; later on, part of the middle turbinates, at several sittings. Opened up and drained the frontal sinuses through the nose. I partially removed the ethmoidal cells with the curette and Myles' punch. The sphenoid sinuses found discharging;· and I opened both with the curette. Opened the right maxillary sinus through the middle meatus. At frequent intervals cleansing and curetting. August 27, 1904, after neglect of treatment, patient returns for the first time, with frontal pain and tenderness, which is relieved by curetting and opening up the sinuses for free drainage. Patient pale and appetite poor. December 12, patient well, with good color. Nasal secretion not yet perfectly clear.

Complicated Nasal Obstruction, Causing Serious Aural and Reflex Disturbances.—Seen at St. Bartholomew's Clinic. Mr. R. S., aged twenty-three years. Complains of severe frontal parietal and occipital headache, trifacial neuralgia, difficulty in reading and in fixing the attention for any length of time, sneezing fits, severe nose-bleeds commencing spontaneously at four years of age, tinnitus, dizziness, and discharging ears. Inspection shows nose absolutely occluded by an S-shaped deflection of the septum, combined with extensive bilateral spurs. I performed a modified Asche operation under ether. After convalescence I removed the spurs on both sides, and later on part of lower turbinates. Nasal breathing is established and all symptoms gradually improved; headaches cease, mental condition improves, eyesight acute, and later on (December 28) the ears, without special treatment, cease discharging entirely and cicatrize. Tinnitus ceases August 13, 1904. The hearing is improved and remains good in one ear and fair in the other. All unpleasant symptoms disappeared. Last seen, December, 1904. Patient in the same good condition.

Mouth-Breathing from Chronic Engorgement of the Turbinates.—Seen at the Presbyterian Hospital, October 10, 1904; Mr. J. P., aged twenty-three years, a cigar manufacturer. Trouble for five years with constant nasal occlusion. Inspection: Nares occluded by enormously engorged lower turbinates, mucous membrane fairly good color. I insufflated powdered suprarenal gland. The turbinates shrink, leaving free nasal fossæ, and disclosing a small spur. I then apply a solution of nitrate of silver, and instruct the patient to spray his nose with Dobell's solution twice daily. A week later patient is seen again. There has been no recurrence of nasal obstruction. Nares normal. All treatment stopped. The cure will probably be permanent if the patient changes his occupation. Chronically engorged turbinals restored to normal function after one treatment.

THE DIAGNOSIS OF MALARIA BY THE FINDING OF PIGMENTED WHITE CORPUSCLES IN UNSTAINED BLOOD FILMS.

BY J. R. CLEMENS, M.D.,

OF ST. LOUIS, MO.

SOME twenty months ago I came across an article by Patrick Manson in C. G. Gibson's Text-book of Medicine. The article in question was on malaria, and it was under the heading of diagnosis that my attention was arrested by the following: " The finding of pigmented white corpuscles is absolutely pathognomonic and a diagnosis may be made on that finding alone." Since the reading of that statement I have examined over 500 unstained blood films in which pigmented whites were found and I have never had occasion to regret the diagnosis I made in each case—malaria. The advantage of diagnosing malaria in unstained specimens by the presence of pigmented whites over the diagnosis of malaria by staining and looking for the inconstant *Plasmodia* will be brought out clearly, I think, by a comparison of the parallel columns below, which will also accentuate the simplicity and infallibility of Manson's method over that of the school who still cling to the staining method and search (often in vain) for the elusive *Plasmodia*.

Diagnosis by Pigmented Whites in Unstained Specimens.	Diagnosis by *Plasmodia* in Stained Specimens.
A *constant* index, found always, irrespective of the time of sporulation or the action of quinine. (Within certain limits.)	Often absent; influenced by quinine and the time at which the blood is taken.

The examination of unstained specimens possesses the further advantages of celerity and simplicity of technic which anybody can master in one demonstration and the recognition of unstained pigmented whites is infinitely more easy than that of the *Plasmodia* in stained specimens. Besides, the most elaborate and skilful staining is often made in vain, for the good reason that there are no *Plasmodia* to stain and, therefore, a diagnosis by this method must often remain in doubt. There can be no doubt to the follower of Manson, for a pigmented white can only mean (with two rare exceptions) malaria, and if there be malaria present there will always be pigmented whites.

I have found the pigmented whites trusty guides in all manner of irregular malarial attacks masquerading under the guise of typhoid, rheumatism, appendicitis, acute diarrheas, gastric crisis, vomiting, periodic vertiginous attacks, etc., and relying on them have told the patients they had malaria and further proved it within a few hours by the effects of quinine. If such a degree of accuracy is given by unstained pigmented whites, why, I ask, go to the trouble of waiting at the bedside for a paroxysm or staining. The Manson method is open to all, the staining method to but few, hedged in as it is by so many provisos and exceptions.

PSAMMOMA OF THE MAXILLARY SINUS.[1]

BY JOHN C. MUNRO, M.D.,

OF BOSTON, MASS.;

SURGEON-IN-CHIEF CARNEY HOSPITAL; LECTURER IN SURGERY, HARVARD MEDICAL SCHOOL.

THE formation of sand bodies may take place frequently in various portions of the central nervous system, such as the inner surface of the dura, the arachnoid, the pineal body, etc., without going on to the formation of a definite tumor. Virchow limits the term psammoma to tumors located in the central nervous system and its coverings, although the same type of sand bodies may be found in tumors of various sorts, such as fibroma, papilloma, carcinoma, sarcoma, etc. Ziegler describes the psammoma as " sarcoma or fibrosarcoma of the dura, inner meninges or pineal gland, which contain concretions of lime in greater or less abundance. Some of these concretions are similar in structure to the normal brain sand, the basis of their formation being a concentric mass of cells which have undergone hyaline degeneration. They usually form round nodules and may be of multiple occurrence." When, however, the sand bodies are found in tumors, the type of the latter must be determined partly from the sand bodies but essentially according to the constituent type of tissue (Virchow). Consonant with Virchow's theory of the origin of tumors he ascribes them to irritation or chronic inflammation. He has separated, moreover, from his great class of sarcomata this form of tumor under the name of psammoma as it belongs, with respect to its histological construction in general, to the connective tissue type of growth (Steudener). Biegel has limited the term psammoma to tumors in which there is slow

[1] Read by invitation before the Rocky Mountain Interstate Medical Association, September, 1904.

growth with scarcely any tendency to multiply, and standing between the fibromata and the solid spindle-cell sarcomata, a sharp line of differentiation, however, being difficult of demonstration. In the carcinomata, including as well endotheliomata, we may not infrequently find deposits of lime salts, mainly as concretion-like masses, just as we find them in psammoma. " These concretions may form either from the cells or in the connective tissue. They occur particularly in the papillary adenomata of the ovary and in cancer of the mammary glands " (Ziegler). The psammo-carcinomata, furthermore, form metastases of a type corresponding to that of the original growth, so that the secondary growths are found in organs of most varying types—in short, where a carcinoma may grow a psammo-carcinoma may also be found (Marben). The majority of these psammomata have been described as originating in the ovary, with metastases, involving practically any of the intra-abdominal organs, but in addition to these there are a few psammo-carcinomata reported as primary in the liver, bones, skin, etc. (Marben). The case reported to-day apparently belongs to a similar type as found in the central nervous system and occasionally in distant organs such as the submaxillary glands, etc. As a careful examination of the literature has failed to unearth an analogous case, it has been deemed worth while to place this one on record.

Case.—Delia C., about twenty years old, servant girl, first consulted Dr. Allen Greenwood, who has kindly given me the following history: "Delia C., called at my office in December, 1902. Seven years prior to this she noticed that the left eye was a little more prominent than the right. Year by year this had become more marked, until at the time of her visit it had become so prominent that it was a source of annoyance on account of the resulting disfigurement. At no time had there been any pain and the vision of the eye had not been interfered with. She had never noticed diplopia.

"Examination showed the following condition: The left eye was markedly proptosed so that the lids could be closed with difficulty. The apex of the cornea was on a plane 2 cm. anterior to that of the other eye. The eye could be moved freely in all directions but the extent of the motion was limited about 50 degrees less than normal, so that a diplopia could be produced by directing the vision as far from the line of central fixation as possible in any direction. The fundus was normal and the V. $= {}^{20}/_{20}$. The eye could not be pushed directly backward, but could be pushed a little upward and backward. Palpation revealed a smooth rounded mass in the lower part of the orbit beginning at the infra-orbital ridge and running upward and backward as far as the eye would allow the finger to go. How much farther it extended could not be ascertained with the finger, but it appeared from the feeling that the bulk of the mass was back of the equator of the globe. There was a sulcus between the mass and the ridge of the orbital floor which admitted the finger-nail, showing that while the mass might be connected with the infra-orbital plate the ridge was not involved. Laterally the mass could be felt to extend out to the side walls of the orbit at the level of the canthi.

" The slow development of the growth would count against its being malignant and delay was advised as I thought it might be an exostosis arising from the infra-orbital plate.

" I saw her again in May, 1903, when it appeared that the proptosis had slightly increased and I advised an exploratory Krönlein's operation; sending her to Dr. J. C. Munro for that purpose."

When the patient came to me in May, 1903, I found the condition as described by Dr. Greenwood and advised operation, supposing that we should find an infra-orbital bony growth. Under ether a modified Krönlein's operation for exposing the orbit was carried out. A curved incision at right angles to the line of the external canthus was made and the outer wall of the orbit was chiseled out in the form of a spherical triangle without stripping the periosteum. The edges of the bone were beveled so that when replaced the fragment rested in practically normal position. The bony, together with the undisturbed soft tissues overlying it, was turned backward on a hinge of periosteum, skin, etc. A slightly fluctuating tumor was found lying behind, below and to the outer side of the globe, on chiseling the outer edges of the wall, which proved to be soft bone of the thickness of blotting paper, a large cyst-like tumor was encountered, full of reddish granular material, feeling like a mixture of sand and putty. This was curetted out in large quantity and lay for the most part below and behind the globe, evidently having pushed upward from the antrum, the bony plate felt behind the orbital ridge before operation, proving to be the orbital floor forced upward like a trap-door by the invading growth. A further opening was then made through the mouth into the antrum. At first about a dram of puriform mucus escaped, but above this, filling the antrum, was the same gritty material that had been found in the orbit. This was thoroughly curetted out, the inner surface of the walls feeling rough but not nodular. There was considerable venous oozing while the curetting was going on, but it was easily controlled by packing. The orbital floor was then pushed back into place and the antrum packed with iodoform gauze. In replacing the bone-flap of the orbit the deep fascia was sutured with catgut and the skin closed with buried silkworm gut. No shock followed the operation.

For some time following operation there was marked edema and ecchymosis of the lids and conjunctiva as well as ecchymosis of the lids of the right eye. Some relief to the edema followed removal of the packing, and under irrigation and iced cloths no injury to the cornea followed. Convalescence was not as satisfactory as had been anticipated. The pulse and temperature kept steadily above normal and in spite of persistent irrigation a foul discharge kept up and the exophthalmos did not subside satisfactorily. The patient had a poor appetite and was in bed most of the time. The temporal wound healed per primam and left no deformity. The patient finally consented to a second operation with a view to removal of the upper jaw if necessary, as it did not seem unlikely that the growth was becoming malignant if it had not been so from the first.

Two months after the first operation the patient was again etherized. The left common carotid was closed with a Crile clamp, and the opening in the antrum enlarged for exploration. The latter, however, was found free of growth. As, on examination with the finger, fulness posterior to the upper jaw, was found, an incision was made along the side of the nose and through the upper lip, in order to turn the cheek back. The anterior wall of the upper jaw was removed up to the infra-orbital foramen. A hard tumor could be felt in the roof of the pharynx pushing the mucous membrane downward, apparently having taken its origin from the antrum. This tumor proved to be psammomatous, exactly similar to that found at the first operation. On removing the pharyngeal portion more growth was found, so far as could be determined, in the sphenoidal and ethmoidal cells of both sides and surrounding the left lateral wall of the nasal cavity, which was removed. The vomer had been pushed far to the right but was not involved in the growth. The tumor lay also on the upper surface of the palate, but the latter itself appeared normal and did not require to be removed. Above, the growth extended to but did not involve the frontal sinuses. So far as could be told all of the tumor was removed. Exploration into the cavity of the orbit showed no sign of recurrence in any region. The resulting extensive cavity was packed with gauze and the wound closed with silkworm gut and horsehair. Very little bleeding followed removal of the carotid compression and there was only a moderate degree of shock at the close of the operation.

The patient rapidly convalesced and was discharged in good condition at the end of a few weeks.

Examination of the growth removed at the first operation was made by Dr. J. H. Pratt and is as follows: Tumor of orbit and antrum of Highmore. Macroscopic examination.—The specimen consists of a mass about 15 c.c. in bulk. In appearance it does not look unlike fine sand soaked with blood. When a small portion of this substance was placed in a test tube and hydrochloric acid added, there was some effervescence, but the granules did not entirely dissolve. These sand-like particles were readily separated from one another.

Microscopical examination.—Some of the material was decalcified in sulphuric acid and embedded in celloidin. It was found that the calcareous bodies were separated by tissue consisting of very closely packed, long, spindle cells with little or no intracellular fibrillar substance. The nodules varied in shape, averaging 50 to 70 mm. in size, and some had a more or less concentric structure. They were in such close contact that the areas of tissue between them were very narrow.

Diagnosis—Psammoma of peculiar type. which possibly should be classed as sarcoma.

Before the first operation there was no suspicion of any growth involving the respiratory tract and no examination was made of the throat as everything pointed to a localized orbital lesion. After operation, however, although it was supposed that all the growth was removed, a poor general condition seemed to indicate that the tumor might be a malignant one, as examination of the throat did not suggest anything so extensive as was found at the second operation. Later, when operation was urged, consent was not obtained until it was apparent that something more radical must be undertaken. As to the origin taking place definitely in the maxillary sinus rather than in one of the deeper sinuses, an accurate determination could not be made. The invasion into the orbit must have been from below and must have dated back for seven or more years. The position and condition of the orbital floor seems to establish that definitely. The absence of nasal or throat symptoms would point to a slow growing tumor of the maxillary sinus, gradually filling the cavity and pushing the lateral wall of the nose inward, invading the sinuses of the ethmoid and sphenoid later and possibly rapidly at the time of operation or thereabouts. Had the growth started originally in the ethmoid or sphenoid it hardly seems possible that it could have filled the antrum, and then the orbit, without causing more nasal and throat symptoms. Origin from the dura was considered, but there were no indications of a basal fissure or other structural deformity.

The prognosis was doubtful, but, considering the cellular structure of the tumor, it seemed very possible that recurrence might take place at some time, even though the original course of the disease had been very slow.

Examination of the patient in September, 1904, sixteen months after the first operation, showed a barely visible scar except for a slight notch at the mucous border of the lip. The anterior wall of the upper jaw had reformed so that this part of the face appeared normal; both nares were free, and the septum was back nearly in its normal position. The sulcus between the alveolus and the cheek was firmly healed without any sinus. There was slight varicosity of the lower lid, and along the infra-orbital ridge could be felt a slight, irregular thickening. Just above the inner canthus a small bony prominence could be felt but not seen. There was no pouching of the palate. The voice had only a faint trace of the hollow sound that follows removal of the upper jaw. The tears flowed normally through the duct instead of over the cheek as was the case before operation. The eye was still prominent and turned outward, but the globe was normally covered by the lids on pressure. It could not be turned inward beyond the median line. Apparently sight was normal, although the right eye was commonly made use of. The patient had been entirely relieved of the headaches that harassed her before operation, and she had been working steadily and gaining weight for several months. During the winter she felt the cold very much in the left side of the face. There was no evidence of return of the growth, but the result in restoration of the globe to its normal position was a disappointment.

MEDICAL PROGRESS.

MEDICINE.

Meningismus Typhosus and Meningotyphoid.—Three interesting cases of typhoid, accompanied by symptoms of meningitis, have been observed by C. STRÄUBLI (*Deutsch. Arch. f. klin. Med.,* Vol. 82, Nos. 1 and 2). The first case was noteworthy in that the lumbar puncture was negative and a suppurative mediastinitis was found at autopsy. The second case was accompanied by signs of cortical aphasia. Owing to the fact that the meningitic symptoms disappeared rapidly without leaving anatomical changes, the condition must be called typhoid meningismus, probably due to functional disturbances, induced by bacterial toxins. The third case was very evidently a meningotyphoid, since typhoid bacilli were found in the purulent cerebrospinal fluid. The distinction between typhoid meningismus and meningotyphoid is of great prognostic importance, since the former may be followed by recovery, while the latter is generally fatal.

Pneumonia and Pregnancy.—ROBERT C. RANSDELL (*Am. Med.,* February 11, 1905) reports two cases. In the first case, pregnancy was complicated by pneumonia and measles. The patient was delivered of a stillborn child on the third day of pneumonia and died on the sixth. In the second case pregnancy was complicated by pneumonia and the presence of a large uterine fibroid. The patient was delivered of a healthy full-term child on the third day of pneumonia and died on the eleventh day. From a careful study of his own cases and those from the literature the author concludes the death rate is appreciably higher in the pregnant woman than in the ordinary patient. Abortion takes place in more than half the cases. The mortality is much higher in the last three months of pregnancy than in the first six. The causes of death can be attributed to (*a*) diminution in hemoglobins, (*b*) degenerative changes in heart muscle, (*c*) overloading of the right heart and pulmonary circulation after birth. The large percentage of abortions is due to accumulation of carbonic acid in blood.

Pathogenesis of Banti's Disease.—Owing to the fact that several cases of Banti's disease, observed by F. UMBER (*Zeitsch. f. klin. Med.,* Vol. 55) were perfectly cured by splenectomy, this author firmly believes in a toxic cause for this disease. In one case, the extirpated spleen showed a deposit of pigment and an enormous overfilling of the sinuses and capillaries with blood, while the arterioles gave evidences of hyaline degenera-

tion. In a piece of the liver which had also been removed, the periportal connective tissue was rich in lymphocytes. The chief clinical symptoms were enormous splenic tumor, hypertrophy of the liver, moderate jaundice and anemia with morphological changes in the erythrocytes. The number and relative proportion of leucocytes was normal. After removal of the spleen each symptom disappeared rapidly, so that the toxic agency was undoubtedly present in this organ. The second case coincided in every way with the first.

Simultaneous Occurrence of Syphilis and Tabes.—From a large number of cases on record, C. ADRIAN (*Zeitsch. f. klin. Med.,* Vol. 55) concludes that with pronounced tabes, the syphilitic virus may still continue active within the body, so that a combination of manifest syphilis of the skin or internal organs with typical tabes is not of such rare occurrence. It seems that syphilitic spinal meningitis is particularly common. With late occurrence of tabetic symptoms, active syphilis is less common; the combination is more frequent in the male sex, since syphilis is here more frequently encountered and the disposition to posterior degeneration is greater. Since tabes appears later in the majority of cases than tertiary lues, a somewhat more favorable prognosis may be made where both conditions are combined, since the process may often be arrested by active antisyphilitic treatment.

Relation of Trauma to Diabetes.—After carefully reviewing the entire literature of diabetes supposed to be caused directly by trauma, W. KAUSCH (*Zeitsch. f. klin. Med.,* Vol. 55) comes to the conclusion that no relation exists between the two. Many alleged cases belong to the so-called "diabetes decipiens," or diabetes without symptoms other than glycosuria, and the presence of sugar was here only detected when the urine was accidentally examined after the trauma. It is true without doubt, however, that different forms of glycosuria, from alimentary glycosuria up to the severest diabetes are observed after injury. The mildest forms are seen most frequently and are especially common after injuries to the skull. Since the sugar generally disappears rapidly, such cases cannot be called diabetics. Where the glycosuria is paramount, it is likely that the condition has already persisted for some time, but has become aggravated by trauma.

Change in Size of Heart on Change of Position.—On skiagraphing the heart, F. MORITZ (*Deutsch. f. klin. Med.,* Vol. 82, Nos. 1 and 2) has repeatedly observed that the shadow is considerably smaller if the patient stands, than when he lies down. The effect is not a purely optical one since the heart descends in the upright position of the body and shortens somewhat in the transverse and sagittal diameter. Even though the long axis lengthens slightly, the entire anterior surface will be smaller. The correctness of this observation on the human being has been proven without doubt by animal experiments. The change in size and volume is partially due to descent of the diaphragm, with the traction it exerts upon the pericardium, partially to the hydrostatic action of the upright position. The inspiratory narrowing of the orthodiagraphic shadow is also due to real diminution in size. It follows that every exposure should be made with the patient in the horizontal posture. Other advantages of the latter are: The respiratory movements are less extensive and the heart is more regular, the diaphragm occupies a median position and is not affected by the liver and intestines, the abdominal wall is relaxed, and weak individuals are less fatigued by long exposures.

Intermittent Polyuria in Addison's Disease.—During the twelve months that a patient with Addison's disease, in the practice of E. BENDIX (*Deutsch. Arch. f. klin. Med.,* Vol. 82. Nos 1 and 2) was under careful observation, the course of his illness varied considerably. At times, the adynamic condition was so pronounced that he could not get up or eat without assistance; at the same time loss of body-weight and psychical depression made their appearance. From time to time, the patient suffered seriously from gastro-intestinal crisis, marked by tenderness and tension of the abdomen, combined with vomiting and singultus. The most peculiar symptom was an intermittent polyuria, for which no cause could be detected. At autopsy, both suprarenal glands were in a state of complete caseation.

Intravital Stimulation of Autolytic Processes in the Body.—According to D. HEILE (*Zeitsch. f. klin. Med.*, Vol. 55), the action of iodoform on tuberculous abscesses and of the Roentgen rays on diseased tissues in general, is best explained by an increased autolysis. Ordinary pus from a cold abscess will not digest a flake of fibrin or give the biuret reaction, but pus from other sources or tuberculous pus from a cavity which has been treated for some time with iodoform emulsion, will readily dissolve fibrin and give a positive biuret, since there is sufficient ferment present to disintegrate the albuminous principles. This ferment is derived from the nuclei of the leucocytes. since the amount of purin bases in ordinary pus and in tuberculous pus after treatment, is much higher than in tuberculous pus before treatment. It follows that the chief beneficial action of iodoform is a chemotactic one. The Roentgen rays also stimulates autolysis. If the spleen of a rabbit whose abdomen has been exposed to the rays for half an hour be examined after twenty-four hours, it will be found that autolysis has advanced much further than in a control spleen. The urine of patients exposed to the Roentgen ray contains more uric acid and more purin bases than before the treatment. The cause of this phenomenon is an increased breaking-down of body cells combined with chemotoxis and destruction of the emigrated leucocytes.

Perforating Ulcer of the Foot.—ADRIAN (*Gazz. deg. Osped.*, January 24, 1905) makes a study of 445 cases of perforating ulcer. The course is as follows: (1) Formation of a callosity. In consequence of a slight traumatism, such as a prolonged walk, a hemorrhage takes place under the corn, and a thinning of the horny layer appears until it gradually passes into the second stage of the formation of an ulcer. (2) The ulcer forms a sinus to the bone. Other clinical manifestations are alteration of sensibility within the ulcer, later hyperproduction of epidermis; alleviation of the secretion of sweat, inflammation of the bone and joints. These ulcers are rare in children. The etiological factors are as follows: (1) Mechanical theory, compression of the foot by shoe in some one place. (2) Change in the blood-vessels of the toe. (3) Nervous causes. It is often difficult to deny an association of a perforating ulcer with a peripheral neuritis. A large number of cases show some long-standing lesion of the sciatic nerve or its branches, in which case an anesthesia of the sole of the foot may persist. Fracture or dislocation in the leg above may cause this. Rheumatism, arthritis deformans or flatfoot may cause a perforating ulcer. Disease of the central nervous system. especially tabes dorsalis, syringomyelia, general paralysis and tumor of the spinal cord will produce perforating ulcer. In tabes it often appears in the pre-ataxic period. Unlike the ulceration occurring in diabetes, there is no tendency to spread on the surface. The prognosis should always be reserved.

Prognostic Factor in Pneumonia.— In the course of his investigations into the nature of the sputum septicemia in animals A. Fränkel showed many years ago that the rabbits which were used in his experiments exhibited a varying degree of susceptibility when injected with the sputa of pneumonic patients. Of twenty animals which were thus treated with the sputa from as many different individuals ten died, presenting the typical picture of sputum septicemia, while ten others remained either unaffected or died from other causes. Similar results have since been obtained by other observers. No systematic examinations, however, were made regarding the virulence of pneumonic sputa at different stages of the disease, until quite recently, when STÜRTZ (*Zeitschift f. klin. Med.,*) was prompted to take the matter up after noting that mice which had been inoculated with the sputa of clinically severe cases of pneumonia succumbed more rapidly than those which had been injected with material from lighter cases. The results which he obtained are very interesting and suggest the possibility of determining the prognosis in a given case by animal inoculation. The technic employed is very simple: The patients are instructed to repeatedly rinse the mouth with water, when the sputum masses which are next expectorated are received in sterilized spit cups. A white mouse is then subcutaneously inoculated with 1 c.c. and kept under observation. Following this procedure Stürtz ascertained the important fact that the virulence of the sputum as measured by its effect upon the mouse, in the course of an individual case, is directly proportionate to the intensity of the morbid process in the corresponding patient. The result obtained in the mouse may therefore be regarded as an approximate index of the virulence of the pneumonic process in a concrete case. It was thus found that in especially severe or fatal cases the sputum virulence was high, resulting in the death of the mouse in from eight to ten hours. Cases of moderate severity. on the other hand show an initial virulence of from eleven to twenty hours, while in light cases the animals only succumb after from twenty to forty-five hours. Exacerbations of the pneumonic process are associated with corresponding exacerbations of the sputum virulence, and it is important to note that the occurrence of such changes is demonstrable by the animal experiment earlier than by the physical signs; this seems to be especially the case in very severe and highly virulent cases. Bearing in mind how often it occurs that a patient with pneumonia who has just passed the climax of hepatisation in one lobe, and whose heart is already profoundly enfeebled, is unexpectedly brought to a most tension of the process, even though it only be lobular in kind, the value of such a method, as suggested by Stürtz is self-apparent. In severe cases it would indeed be well to inoculate the mouse every morning and every evening, so as to be warned by the extension of the morbid process in time. Stürtz's conclusions regarding the value of the method from the prognostic standpoint are based upon an investigation of twenty cases only. But this work has been carefully done and deserves credit.

OBSTETRICS AND GYNECOLOGY.

Rupture of the Uterus During Delivery.—After a most thorough review of this subject N. IVANOFF (*Annal. de Gyn. et d'Obstet.*, October, 1904) gives the following as his conclusions: (1) The majority of ruptures in placenta previa are due to violence on the part of the accoucheur; (2) This is also true in cases of transverse presentation; (3) If in transverse presentations, tentative maneuvers are employed to deliver. when version is finally attempted, there is a predisposition to rupture. (4) Braun's hook for decapitation, a most imperfect instrument, should not be used where rupture has taken place. (5) A large proportion of the ruptures begin on one or the other side of the cervix; they have a tendency to spread longitudinally and to extend into the cellular tissue of the broad ligaments. (6) In the case of hydrocephalia, besides the distention and wounding of the uterine walls, rupture often takes place because the condition is not recognized until it is too late to prevent its occurrence. (7) In cases where there is a constriction of the body of the uterus, a rupture may occur because of the distention of the lower part of the uterine wall and because of the increased pressure produced against the fundus in the directions where there is present an abnormally reduced cavity, so that even an abnormal convexity is present, making more or less violence in the concavity of the fundus. (8) A contracted pelvis predisposes, naturally, the uterine walls to rupture. (9) Spontaneous ruptures in flat pelvis are almost always produced in the supravaginal portion of the cervix and transversely. The time elapsing from the beginning of labor and the rupture is ordinarily very short. (10) The so-called cases of "colporrhexis," in the majority of cases, are only transverse ruptures of the supravaginal portion of the cervix. (11) In contracted pelves, if there have been many difficult and operative deliveries, the treatment along conservative lines presents dangers especially if palpation establishes beforehand the existence of scars in the supravaginal portion of the cervix. (12) One of the predisposing factors to uterine ruptures, other than modifications of the uterine wall produced by the cicatrices already mentioned, and by malignant tumors and by insufficient development of the organ, etc., is inflammatory cellular infiltration. (13) All the modifications of a pathologic nature involving the elastic tissue of the uterus, by which some authors wish to explain the production of rupture, are in reality physiological modifications which supervene during pregnancy, delivery, and during the puerperium. No one has ever found true pathological changes in the elastic tissue of a ruptured uterus. (14) The conservative method of treatment of rupture of the uterus gives a result twice as favorable as that from surgical intervention. (15) The treatment of every rupture during delivery should be operative, for that method alone gives us the possibility of checking hemorrhage, definitely (to ward against secondary hemorrhage) and to ascertain the cause of the condition.

An Acephalic Monster.—A number of these cases have been reported, most of them of three main types: Acephalus monobrachius, paracephalus and myacephalus. ANNIE C. GOWDEY (*Brit. Jour of Obst.*, November, 1904) presents the following case which is unique in that it possessed both upper limbs though in a more or less immature state. In this case the mother was delivered of a full term fetus at the same confinement with the monster, the former being born first but at an easier delivery. There was but one placenta with two umbilical cords and only one chorion. The monster was absolutely without any semblance of a head. At the upper end there was a circular line of hair with a central depression. The forearm was absent in the right upper limb, the hand, which possessed only three digits, being in contact with the lower end of the humerus. The left upper limb consisted of a very short humerus. a forearm, and hand with five digits.

Talipes varus was present and marked in both feet. There were five toes on the right foot—all webbed; the left foot had only three toes. The mother was highly nervous and but twenty-one years old. She had had one previous child by another husband. which was five years old, strong and healthy. There was nothing of note in the mother's family history. on the father's side there was a suspicion of tuberculosis. The sex of the monster, like the majority of others of its kind, was female. According to Ballantyne, fetal malformations are associated with tubercle in the parents; it is interesting to note that the father's history in this case was suspicious.

Cancer of the Body of the Uterus.—The female sex is much more often affected by malignant disease than the male, and of all the organs of the body, says THOMAS WILSON (*Brit. Jour. of Obstet.*, October, 1904) by far the most frequently attacked is the uterus. The report in the *Birmingham Medical Review*, published May to July, 1900, shows that 4,972 persons died of cancer in ten years in a population of 750,000. 60.8 per cent. of the deaths from cancer occurred in females. From the figures in the report it would seem that one out of every four deaths from malignant diseases in women is due to involvement of the uterus. It would seem that carcinoma chiefly affects women who have passed the menopause, and that the age at which the menses cease often departs from the normal but not in any definite direction. Cancer of the body of the uterus is usually described as beginning in one of two ways, either from the glands of the uterus or from the squamous epithelium. The growths in the body of the uterus may be either diffuse or localized. They may also be classified according to the characteristics of the surface of the tumor, which may be smooth and nodular, coarsely papular, or closely set with fine filiform villous projections. None of these forms corresponds to a distinct histological variety of tumor. The exact origin and, especially the nature of the tumor germ or matrix, which presumably gives rise to the tumor, is therefore entirely a matter of inference. There can be distinguished local and remote paths of extension of cancer. The local invasion takes place (1) by simple continuity, alveoli spreading out along the lines of least resistance, in the case of the uterus, in the intersection between' the connective tissue and muscular fibers, and in the lymph spaces; or (2) by some more extensive form of local spreading which takes place along the blood and lymphatic vessels that remain in the uterus itself. The remote paths are the lymphatic and blood-vessels which drain the uterus, either of which convey emboli from the original growth. Recurrence after operation may be understood by a reference to the modes of spread just described; thus the recurrence may be local; (1) at the site of the original growth or (2) at a little distance from the former site but still within the limits of the organ; (3) recurrences may take place at any part along the course of the lymphatics leading from the organ, or in the lymphatic glands. (4) remote metastases may occur from emboli from the primary growth having been carried out by the blood stream and lodged in some of the remote organs or tissues. When fibroids are present in a uterus. if the menses have been stopped for a time and then begun again, or if the bleeding increases, or if a profuse serous, mucous or colored discharge makes its appearance, especially at the climacteric, the cavity of the uterus should be explored without delay, and in case of doubt the uterus should be removed. It is important to recognize that expert knowledge is necessary both in the use of a curette in these cases and in the examinations of the curettings afterward, and it is to be desired that suspected instances of the disease shall be investigated by competent observers at the earliest possible moment. In this way only can the best results of treatment be obtained. The occurrence of true cancer in the body of the uterus in women under forty-five years appears to be comparatively rare.

A Lithopedion Forty-one Years in the Abdominal Cavity.—Though many similar cases have been recorded, F. W. N. HAULTAIN (*Brit. Jour. of Obstet.*, October, 1904) has only been able to find nine cases in the literature where the tumor has been present in the abdominal cavity over forty years. A tenth case is reported by this author with the following history: The patient, aged seventy-one years, became pregnant when thirty years of age, and when at full term went into labor without tangible result. The abdominal swelling remained, and for some time gradually diminished in size. In February, 1904, the patient died somewhat suddenly of cardiac disease. On post-mortem examination a large lithopedion, placed behind the uterus, and densely adherent to the intestines, was found. The fetus was disposed with the head downward, but no true relation could be determined. The patient was well aware of the presence of the fetus all her life, but aside from occasional attacks of abdominal pain she enjoyed good health and performed her duties until shortly before her death. Menstruation returned a few months after her spurious labor and continued to the age of forty-five years. There had been no subsequent pregnancies. The fetus had preserved to a remarkable degree its normal configuration. Flexion still existed; the limbs to the finest digits were in absolute preservation, and the nails projected over the finger-tips. The tissues were contracted and calcarious over the limbs, but on the back scalp and breech, they seemed of normal thickness. There was no sac. In the majority of cases of advanced ectopic pregnancy decomposition results with subsequent disintegration and passage of the fetal membranes through the hollow viscera; and it is difficult to discover the reasons which in one case tend toward calcification and in the other to disintegration. Prolonged retention of the fetus in a normal uterus with resulting lithopedion has not as yet been conclusively proven, but Pearson reports a case where one remained in a rudimentary horn of a double uterus for twenty-six years.

Rupture of the Uterus.—The observation of NIKONOFF (*Roussky Vrach*, No. 46, 1904) is based on five cases of rupture of the uterus occurring during labor, from which the following conclusions are drawn: (1) Besides the two well-established varieties of rupture of the uterus that take place during labor, namely, spontaneous and traumatic, there is also a class of cases where the rupture extends from the anterior wall, from a purely traumatic forcible origin. (2) In some exceptional cases one rupture takes place slowly and gradually, and is not accompanied either by any very prominent reaction or profuse hemorrhage; in such cases the diagnosis presents some difficulties; thus, in the author's first case, that of an old multipara, labor continued for thirty hours before the symptoms became sufficiently distinct, nor were there any cessation of pains or the ap-

pearance of acute pains that usually signalize the beginning of rupture of the uterus; in fact, the woman was able to sleep quietly for some six hours with part of the fetus in the peritoneal cavity. (3) The diagnosis of a complete rupture of the uterus with the escape of the fetus into the peritoneal cavity presents usually no difficulty and can be made with the aid of ordinary palpation; the anamnesis and accompanying phenomena but tend to verify same. (4) Internal examination often fails to supply us with exact data (before the extraction of the fetus), so that in certain cases is may be omitted altogether, especially when there exist serious objections thereto, such as the possibility of infecting the deeper portions of the sexual apparatus. (5) The prognosis of rupture of the uterus depends on many conditions which must be considered in every individual case; it may be stated in a general way that it is somewhat more favorable at present than it was some time ago; the mortality should not be above 40 or 50 per cent., and under favorable conditions it may even be lower. (6) The extraction of the fetus per vias naturales should be avoided until the patient be placed under conditions that admit of a capital operation, if it is at all possible. (7) If operative interference is inadmissible, the fetus should be extracted, and the tear either sewed up or at least tamponed per vaginam. (8) Having prepared for the operation extract the fetus: (a) if it be found in the uterine cavity, or if its extraction through the abdominal wound present any difficulty (as, for instance, hydrocephalus), an attempt should be made to extract per vias naturales, and then either tampon, sew up or remove the uterus per vaginam or by abdominal section, in accord with the necessities of the individual case. In case of hydrocephalus it is first necessary to perform perforation of the head and then either extract per vias naturales or make ready for a Cæsarean section; (b) if the fetus be found in the abdominal cavity, a laparotomy should at once be resorted to without any preliminary attempt at extraction through the natural paths. (9) In the majority of cases it will become necessary to remove the uterus either wholly or partially; in some exceptional cases it may be closed with sutures. (10) After the operation extreme asepsis is absolutely required as regards the abdominal cavity, the best being a copious and frequent flushing with sterilized physiological salt solution. If the uterus is removed or only partially so, a very wide drainage tube should be inserted with its end through the vagina. (11) In the event of a threatened postoperative paralysis of the intestine, large doses of atropine, subcutaneously, should be tried. (12) If there be observed after operation any symptoms of sepsis, the exudate should be investigated bacteriologically, and, if necessary, resort should be had to specific sera.

Infantile Intestinal Diverticula.—The diverticulum ilei may take origin in almost any portion of the ileum, but the majority appear at or about the junction of the jejunum and ileum. J. W. HYDE (*Am. Jour. Obstet.*, December, 1904), having made a study of this condition, states that the diverticula may end in a blind pouch which may be attached to some portion of the interior abdominal wall. In other instances there may be a fistulous exit at the umbilicus as well as above or below this point. It is not clear why diverticula have been found more frequently in males. The accoucheur should always examine the cord carefully before and after separation, and when the character of a fistulous exit indicates the presence of a diverticulum, the best plan of treatment is the radical operation at as early a date as conditions will permit.

Dangerous Hemorrhage from the Urinary Tract During Pregnancy.—Hemorrhage from sources other than the genital tract during pregnancy are rare, the most frequent cause being a rupture of varicosites. PAUL V. KUBINYI (*Centralbl. f. Gyn.*, No. 48, 1904) relates the history of a patient, who in the eighth month of her pregnancy, after lifting a heavy weight, suffered from a severe hematuria with subsequent retention of urine. Catheterization for three days only brought away a few blood clots, the patient had headache, general malaise and vomited a few times. Diagnosis of rupture and tumor of the bladder had been successively made by different physicians. Digital examination confirmed the writer's diagnosis of retention from the formation of a blood clot at the neck of the bladder, the urethra having been previously dilated by Hegar's dilators up to No. 17. After removing half a liter of foul-smelling blood clot, several liters of urine came away. A few days later cystoscopic examination showed the presence of a large blood vessel running transversely across the neck of the bladder. In considering the cause of the rupture, changes in the vessel walls and a sudden increase of blood pressure were thought to be the important factors. The possibility of the kidney as the source of the blood was excluded because of the presence of the large clots and the absence of other signs of nephritis.

Transmission of Toxins from Mother to Fetus.—The manner in which toxins during pregnancy exert their effects on the fetus, has been studied by C. SCHMIDLECHNER (*Zeitschr. f. Geb. u. Gyn.*, Vol. 52, No. 3). For the purpose of determining whether in case the mother becomes ill, the toxin produced is transmitted to the fetus and what are the changes resulting in the organs of the latter, he injected diphtheria toxin in pregnant guinea-pigs. The results of nineteen experiments are reported as follows,—intoxication of the mother is followed by a transference of the toxin into the blood of the fetus and produces in the organs of the latter the same changes as in those of the mother. The intensity of the changes depends on the amount of toxin which has entered the body of the mother. The effects of the toxin are developed more rapidly in the fetus than in the mother and to a higher degree. The transmission of toxins can take place only through the medium of the placenta and requires very little time. The surplus toxin which finds its way into the fetal circulation, remains unchanged for a time. If some of this fetal blood is injected into another animal, it produces the same changes in the organism of the latter as in that of the original animal and its young.

Spinal Analgesia in Gynecological and Obstetrical Practice.—This method of anesthesia with tropocaine has been used by M. STOLZ (*Archiv f. Gyn.*, Vol. 73, No. 3) in 155 gynecological and 25 obstetrical cases with very satisfactory results. The conclusions arrived at in his very complete article are as follows. (1) Spinal analgesia with 0.05 to 0.08 of tropacocaine dissolved in the cerebrospinal fluid, is not dangerous and only in exceptional instances is followed by any unpleasant after-effects. Larger doses increase the effect both in length of time and intensity; larger amounts of fluid the extent of the area of analgesia. Therefore as many centigrams of cerebrospinal fluid are to be employed for the solution as the number of centigrams of tropocaine it is intended to inject. (2) For oper-

ations around the anus and external genitalia which do not consume longer than forty-five minutes, an injection of 0.05 of tropacocaine will be sufficient. For longer operations, from 0.07 to 0.08 may be necessary. Abdominal section could be done without disturbance in 56.3 per cent of the cases. In 30.9 per cent general narcosis was found necessary in addition and 12.7 per cent spinal analgesia was found insufficient from the outset. Inhalation anesthesia as a supplement to the spinal form is very satisfactory, and only a very small quantity of the anesthetic is necessary. (3) Lumbar puncture is accomplished with more difficulty in pregnant, than in non-pregnant women, because it requires special attention to antisepsis and special skill in its application, which is not usually possible outside of the hospital. It is therefore less practical than the inhalation anesthesia. The injection of 0.05 tropocaine during labor produces analgesia of the external genitals for an hour afterward. The labor pains are much affected but the abdominal pressure is absent and only is brought into action by voluntary effort. In two cases of eclampsia, no effect was observed on the convulsions.

Use and Abuse of Curettage of the Uterus.—E. A. BROWD (*Med. Rec.*, January 28, 1905) says that the apparent simplicity and security of the operation has led to the frequent performance of curettage of the uterus in cases in which the procedure is not only of no service, but may even be directly contra-indicated. It is useful in cases of endometritis not associated with pelvic inflammations, exudates, or diseased adnexa, in subinvolution of the uterus or retained secundines, in endocervicitis as a prophylactic against carcinoma, in mole pregnancies and in all cases of endometritis of so-called hyperplastic nature. In post-partum infections there is room for much judgment, for while saprophytic cases with refained membranes, etc., are benefited by curettage, the measure is distinctly contra-indicated if the infection is of the septic type. Curettage should not be regarded as a routine treatment for sterility, for it may aggravate existing pathological conditions, while the danger of perforation is very great in curetting for syphilitic, tuberculous, sarcomatous or cancerous degeneration of the endometrium. It should never be performed without an anesthetic, owing to the danger of perforation due to sudden movements of the patient, or in dirty surroundings that cannot be rendered aseptic. A number of cases are cited in which disregard of these rules was followed by serious consequences.

THERAPEUTICS.

Value of Hetol in Tuberculosis.—Very many contradictory articles in literature upon the value of betol in arresting a tuberculous process, show that the question is not yet definitely decided. O. PRYM (*Münch. med. Woch.*, November 1, 1904) has noticed decided improvement in only five out of 22 cases. Yet the tubercle bacilli never disappeared from the sputum, and the objective symptoms remained stationary. As many as eight cases became decidedly worse and reacted toward injections with high fever. The tolerance seems to vary within very wide limits and the most advanced cases are not always the ones that show the most intense reaction. The author concludes by stating that great care should be exercised in selecting the cases and that constant supervision should be practised. The reports of F. Schrage, contained in the came number are however more favorable. In a third article, H. Frey speaks well of the antituberculous serum of Marmoreck. General toxic symptoms were never observed, the only reaction ever complained of being a local or general urticaria. The results obtained, while not amounting to real cures, justify an extensive trial of this serum.

Sulphate of Copper Alone, and in Combination with Lime, for the Destruction of Mosquito Larvæ, as a Deodorant, and as a Disinfectant.—A. H. Doty (*Med. Rec.*, January 21, 1905) reports on the results of a series of experimental tests undertaken to determine the question indicated by the title. It was found that a solution containing one pound of sulphate of copper and one pound of unslacked or rock lime (calcium oxide) in ten gallons of water was promptly effectual in causing the death of mosquito larvæ when added in the proportions of one gallon of solution to fifty gallons of the infected water. Solutions of copper or of lime alone were less satisfactory. The result is not due to a toxic action of either of the chemicals, but to the fact that a precipitate is formed which rapidly removes from the water the organic matter upon which the larvæ depend for nourishment and life. This method is applicable only in collections of stagnant and offensive water, where it not only destroys the larvæ, but also deodorizes the fluid, but in swamps or bodies of water covering large areas, other measures are preferable. As a deodorant, the mixture of copper and lime in the proportions stated is the most valuable and practical agent we possess for the purpose. Its action is rapid and permanent, it is practically harmless, is cheap and easily made, and can be employed equally well for deodorizing solids or fluids. The experiments on the germicidal properties of copper sulphate show that it has possibilities as a disinfectant, but no definite statements can as yet be made.

Painful Affections of the Feet; Diagnosis and Treatment.—C. Ogilvy (*Med. Rec.*, January 21, 1903) discusses the commoner causes of foot pain, with the appropriate treatment. The diagnosis of "rheumatism of the feet" is often made, but is usually incorrect, the symptoms in most cases being due to some deformity, such as eversion, or flatfoot. In eversion, or what is commonly called "weak ankle," the foot is everted, the internal malleolus projects very prominently, the toes point outward and the line of strain falls to the inner side of the foot, throwing excessive weight in the inner half of the longitudinal arch. This leads to loss of elasticity of the arch, the foot breaks down and flat foot results. Flatfoot in its first stages is not diagnosed correctly in 50 per cent. of the cases, yet an early diagnosis is of the greatest importance, for it is a difficult matter to transform an everted painful foot with a broken-down arch into one which is capable of performing all its functions without pain or discomfort. The treatment may require the use of the Thomas heel, the Whitman plate, the plaster bandage, operation, exercise and massage, singly or in combination, according to the nature of the case. Metatarsophalangeal pain is due to weakness of the anterior arch and is treated by the application of a felt pad and adhesive plaster. Bursitis of the heel is less frequently met with and is treated by hollowing out the heel of the shoe or by dissecting out the bursa. The subject of proper footwear is also considered and the essential points of a well fitting shoe are enumerated.

The Trend of Modern Prescription Writing.—An *Ass'n*, January 7, 1905) on this subject is based on interesting paper by M. C. Thrush (*Jour. Am. Med.* the examination of 500 prescriptions received in each of two leading drug stores in Philadelphia, the results showing the importance of proper training in this branch and the evidence of apparent neglect. The following conclusions seem warranted: That the trend of modern prescription writing is in favor of proprietary preparations. That the use of polypharmaceutical preparations is diminishing to a great extent and their use is chiefly confined to the older practitioners. That the number of incompatibles observed is greater than it should be. That the metric system is but little employed at the present time in prescription writing, a condition to be greatly deplored. That over one-third of the prescriptions are incorrectly written, and this is especially noticeable among the younger practitioners. That certain non-official preparations are quite popular and that some of these deserve admission to the U. S. Pharmacopœia. That the more educated the physician, the greater the use of pharmacopœial preparations, and the greater the tendency to simple instead of complex, non-scientific, polypharmaceutic and proprietary preparations.

Treatment of Phthisis by Iodoform Infusion.—This is not the first communication presented on this very important subject. Thomas W. Dewar (*Brit. Med. Jour.*, January 14, 1905) made a preliminary report in the same journal November 21, 1903. In a continued communication, he cites nine cases from which he concludes as follows: They were under no restraint and the diet and hygiene used was that most suitable to each particular one. Five consecutive patients were remarkably improved, and by this the author means that there has been the usual gain in weight and a freedom from tubercle bacilli which in every instance had been plentiful in the sputa. It may, as he says, have been coincident, but if so, it was a remarkable one. In the sixth and seventh cases the advance was certainly retarded. The author believes that the contention in his first paper that the continuous injection of an etheral solution of iodoform was followed by improvement, that it was innocuous in moderate doses and powerful to arrest pulmonary tuberculosis, was correct.

Treatment of Leucemia with Roentgen Ray.—The experience of several authors on the use of the Roentgen rays in leucemia, is contained in the *Münch. Med. Woch.*, January 24, 1905. In both cases of E. Meyer and O. Eisenreich the general condition improved wonderfully after a total exposure of about 500 minutes and with it, the body-weight, percentage of hemoglobin and number of red cells increased so that the patients could again earn their living. The number of leucocytes dropped from several hundred thousand to near normal, but the spleen diminished in size appreciably in only one. In the patient of W. Wendel, marked improvement was observed only when the sternum and the epiphyses of the long bones were exposed. It is doubtful if a permanent cure can be obtained even with the Roentgen rays, but there can hardly be any question that the disease will be kept effectually under control. Good results in four out of five cases are also reported by D. Schieffer.

NEUROLOGY AND PSYCHIATRY.

Multiple Sclerosis.—It seems that among individuals living in the country, the most common organic disease of the nervous system is multiple sclerosis, while the inhabitants of cities are more frequently affected with tabes. The classical type of multiple sclerosis as described by Charcot is rare. Thus, P. Morawitz (*Deutsch. Arch. f. klin. Med.*, Vol. 82, Nos. 1 and 2) found scanning speech in only 12 per cent., nystagmus and tremor in about 50 per cent. As opposed to hysteria, eye-disturbances are rather frequent, thus, atrophy of the optic nerve was seen in about 40 per cent. Extensive disturbances of sensibility are, however, rare; usually only a hyperesthesia is found which involves only the distal portions of the extremities. The abdominal reflexes are often exaggerated in hysteria, but lost in about 50 per cent. in sclerosis. In the latter condition, the Babinski reflex is often positive, showing that an organic affection of the nervous system is present. Bladder disturbances in sclerosis are usually transient, but recurrent difficulty in urination or moderate incontinence, while in hysteria one often sees ischuria, developing acutely and intensely after a psychical trauma.

Cryoscopy in Epidemic Cerebrospinal Meningitis. —J. H. BAILEY (*Med. Rec.*, February 11, 1905) made a cryoscopic study of sixty-nine specimens of cerebrospinal fluid, and though the results are not yet available for practical purposes they have scientific value. Using T as a symbol for the total freezing point of the cerebrospinal fluid, some of the conclusions reached are as follows: Upper limit of T is -.815; lower limit, -.50; a variation of -.315. The vast majority of cases, however, 79 per cent., ranged from -.52 to -.64, a variation of only -.12. Average T is -.575, very close to the normal freezing point of blood. T oscillates much less than the freezing point of urine. The greater part of T is due to the sodium chloride content. T varies not only in specimens from different cases, but, also, in specimens from the same case at different times. T is not of any prognostic significance; some of the patients that recovered showed a high T, others a low T; while the same is true of several cases that terminated fatally.

Hysteria in Surgery.—There is no disease that simulates or "mimics" so many other diseases as hysteria, which may throw off his diagnostic balance even the most experienced clinician. N. A. VELYAMINOFF (*Prakt. Vrach*, Nos. 47, 48, 1904) presents a highly instructive account of his experience with hysteria as met with in a surgical practice based on observation extending over many years. Hysterical phenomena in the gastro-intestinal sphere are encountered throughout the entire length of the tract beginning with hysterical dysphagia down to disturbances of the anal opening. Hysterical spasm of the pylorus is a condition by no means unknown, which may tax the ingenuity of the most skilful diagnostician, as gastro-enterostomy has been performed more than once under the impression of organic disease of the pylorus. The author describes a case of a young woman who presented an abdominal tumor in the lower right abdomen the size of a fist with the symptoms of intestinal stricture accompanied by increased peristalsis of the part above the constriction. During the examination, however, the patient "removed" the swelling to another part of the abdomen; this was then a case of hysterical spasm of the intestine brought on, as was shown later, by some unpleasant sensation, as, in this instance, by the sight of a lemon. A somewhat similar case was that of coccygodynia, which was mistaken for anal fissure for which appropriate treatment proved unavailing. Nevertheless in differentiating hysterical affections that may simulate organic surgical disease we must keep in mind the following points: The hysterical symptoms are much less prominent and distinct; they are not constant but are changeable as to intensity; the degree of intensity is variable, while the entire picture of the disease is easily and frequently changeable, in-asmuch as evidently important symptoms disappear, or become exaggerated under some mental strain or in connection with the sexual functions. Moreover, a hysterical patient always presents various hysterical stigmata in addition to the symptoms of the given affection which assist greatly in differential diagnosis. The author describes at some length a few interesting cases of hysterical spinal disease simulating spondylitis and scoliosis. The French have long since established the existence of what they call "rachialgie hysterique," which is practically identical with spinal irritation of the old authors and traumatic neurosis and railway spine of the English and American authors. In one of the author's cases, that of a girl of twenty-six years, burdened with tuberculous heredity, though living under the most favorable circumstances, the question of a tuberculous spondylitis could only be excluded after a most thorough examination and observation extending over some time (for particulars of this most interesting case the reader must be referred to the original), while in the other case, also that of a woman, of twenty-five years, repeated examinations and close and unremitting observation in the hospital established eventually the positive diagnosis of a hysterical kypho-scoliosis. The author considers the pseudo-kyphotic curvature of the spine or rather the swelling of the vertebræ that simulates in these cases curvature as due to hysterical angioneurotic edema of the soft parts surrounding the vertebræ and possibly to edema of the periosteum. To the same class belong cases of hysterical scoliosis, as observed by Albert and Hoffa, and two of which are reported by the author in his article. Of equal interest and importance are the cases of hysterical swellings of the breast, what the French call "sein hystérique," of which the author observed 63 cases during the last twenty years. Of these he distinguished tumors that invade but a few lobules, and those that attack the entire mammary gland, the latter rather less frequent. The former may be of various sizes and consistency, though this may change quite often. They are usually smooth, but at times also lobulated. As distinguished from real neoplasms these tumors pass gradually into the healthy tissue, and are usually very movable; besides the tumor there are also found other smaller lobes in the breast. The patients frequently complain of pain of a neuralgic character (mastodynia) spreading along the intercostal nerves and to the corresponding upper extremity. The author distinguishes four types of patients in whom this condition is encountered: (1) Girls between twenty and thirty years of age, of strong sexual tendencies, in whom marriage and pregnancy usually causes the disappearance of the tumor. (2) "Psychopathic" girls between twenty-five to thirty-five, undoubted hysterical subjects with degenerative stigmata, dissatisfied with their maiden state, constantly dwelling on sexual matters. (3) Married women of unfortunate family life, constantly excited by old and impotent husbands, the so-called Balzac woman suffering from chronic inflammatory conditions of the sexual sphere and, finally, (4) old hysterical women, addicted to the reading of medical works of a doubtful character, and having seen cases among friends and relatives. Therapeutically, it is of the highest importance to abstain from operative interference, the more so, as, strange to say, trauma predisposes to the development of malignant growths, as the author observed in four cases;

still extreme circumspection should be exercised, especially when dealing with women in the "cancer" age.

The Epileptic Criminal; with Report of Two Cases. —T. H. EVANS (*Med. Rec.*, February 4, 1905.) gives the histories of an epileptic who, in a period of depression, committed a murder, and of a woman belonging to the borderland epileptic type who, in an access of jealousy, attempted to kill her lover. Taking these instances as a text the author concludes that: (1) The essence of crime is in the intention, and the ability not so to intend. (2) No punishment is adequate to any crime; restraint not only after a crime has been committed, but efforts to hinder any such deed, is preferable always. (3) The victims of epileptics ought to have legal ground for suit against the community as well as those in charge of the epileptic. (4) Reservations ought to be established, in which degenerates and the normally irresponsible could oe colonized and treated, allowing all possible freedom of initiative for useful and safe pursuits therein. (5) Marriage of neurotics should be regulated. We can afford to lose the few sane descendants if we could also cut out their degenerate progeny. Democratic principles encourage, in this as in other matters, the average, and discourage the exceptional or abnormal—great or small. (6) All epileptics are to be viewed with suspicion. Many cases of psychic erraticism, cranks, and mistaken reformers, are to be taken as examples of epileptic psychic equivalents. The major forms of epilepsy may not prove so dangerous to the community as these veiled manifestations.

PHYSIOLOGY.

On the Presence of Tyrosinase in the Skin.— The relation of pigment to the development of certain malignant neoplasms, particularly melanosarcoma, has been partly illuminated by recent discoveries on the origin of animal pigments. In 1901, v. Fürth and Schneider showed that a tyrosinase could be obtained from the blood of certain insects. This tyrosinase acted upon a chromogen present in the blood, and converted it into a melanin-like substance. When a solution of tyrosin in water was treated with the ferment a melanin-like body was also obtained. FLORENCE M. DURHAM (*Proc. Royal Soc.*, December 10, 1904) in further investigations in this field, finds that an extract can be made from the skins of certain pigmented vertebrates (rabbits, rats, guinea-pigs, chickens), which will act upon tyrosin and produce a pigmented substance. This action suggests the presence of a tyrosinase in the skins of these animals. The action of the tyrosinase is destroyed by boiling, does not take place in the cold, is delayed by time, requires the temperature of about 37° C., and also the presence of an activating substance such as ferrous sulphate to start it. The colored substances produced are in accordance with the color of the animals used. Black substances are produced when animals with black pigment in their skins are used, and yellow substance when the skin contains the orange pigment. The colored substances are soluble in alkalis, but insoluble in acids.

Some Physiological Effects of High Altitudes and Low Barometric Pressures.—An expedition was conducted to the summit of Mt. Rosa in the Alps, by A. Mosso, with the object of studying some of the effects of high climates upon the physiology of respiration. The results of these investigations are reported in the *Arch. Ital. de Biol.*, September 7, 1904,

by A. MOSSO, G. MARRO, G. GALEOTTI and A. AGGAZZOTTI. In dogs, as in men, the rarefied air of the Alps does not produce an increase in the frequency and depth of respiration but rather a diminution. There is a diminished alkalinity of the blood and an increase in the number of red corpuscles and the amount of hemoglobin. An increase of temperature causes in dogs a marked polypnea, the respirations reaching 200 per minute. At great altitudes (4,560 m.) the centers that preside over deglutition are functionally modified, manifesting an earlier fatigue and producing more rapid and more active movements in the esophageal musculature. In monkeys as in men the result of the lowering of barometric pressure is to produce sleep and loss of consciousness without any previous excitatory effect, which result shows that the barometric depression does not act like the diminution of oxygen in the blood, nor like the narcotics which always excite the nervous system before depressing it. The effects are due to the diminution in the amount of carbonic acid in the blood. Dogs and monkeys rapidly adapt themselves to barometric depression. The rarefied air causes a slight increase in the amount of carbonic acid excreted, although the amount of oxygen absorbed remains constant. At low barometric pressures the organism has a diminished sensibility to the effects of carbon dioxide, that is, the exciting action of this gas becomes less intense. At the same time the force of the respiratory movements is diminished, showing a mild degree of paralysis of the nerve centers of respiration.

Further interesting observations are reported in *Arch. Ital. de Biol.*, October 31, 1904, by these same investigators. At the summit of Mt. Rosa inhalations of oxygen diminish the depth of respiration and decrease the frequency of the pulse, while they had no effect at the sea-level. Carbonic acid, also, when breathed pure in a rarefied atmosphere and in small doses, also causes a slowing of the pulse. In the presence of a lowered barometric pressure, the percentage of CO_2 diminishes in the pulmonary alveoli. The diminution of the tension of the oxygen in the atmosphere does not suffice to explain the sleep and the other phenomena produced by strong barometric depressions. It is found that alcohol produces physiological effects at high altitudes which are different from those produced at the sea-level. The administration of 40 c.c. of alcohol at Turin caused a slight rise of the rectal temperature, an increase in the force of the cardiac impulse, and a relaxation of the arterial walls, with the production of a true dicrotism; there was also a considerable increase in the frequency of respiration which at the same time became less profound; there was an increased amount of air breathed in a unit of time. At high altitudes alcohol does not cause an increase in the amount of air breathed in a unit of time. There is no change in the pulse, in the blood-vessels, or in the mechanism of respiration. The subjective sensations are reduced to nil, while at the sea-level the same amount of alcohol produces a state of mental excitation like that of intoxication. Under normal conditions a person can hold his breath for a longer time at high altitudes than at the sea-level. While the administration of alcohol at the sea-level diminishes this period of voluntary arrest of respiration, it has no effect upon the latter at high altitudes. The authors conclude that it would appear that at high altitudes the nerve cells of the sensorium as well as of the circulatory and respiratory centers, become less sensitive to alcohol, with the result that their function is not altered, although the blood may at the time contain a comparatively large quantity of alcohol.

The Substitution of Hydrogen for Nitrogen in the Atmosphere.—The question whether life would be possible if the nitrogen in the air were replaced by hydrogen, was put to an experimental test by A. MARACCI (*Arch. Ital. de Biol.*, October 31, 1904). In experimenting upon various animal species, the author found that in such an atmosphere the consumption of oxygen and the elimination of carbonic acid are greatly increased. Moreover the animals suffer a rapid loss of heat, with the result that the bodily temperature falls several degrees below the normal. The hand, when plunged into such an atmosphere, experiences a marked sensation of cold. These changes are attributed to the fact that hydrogen is a good conductor of heat, a property which goes hand in hand with its metallic qualities. The author believes that death in this artificial atmosphere is produced not solely by the subtraction of heat. He believes that hydrogen and oxygen may combine in the organism and that this combination may not be indifferent to the tissues. The greater rapidity in the oxidations that ensues upon respiring a mixture of oxygen and hydrogen, does not suffice to make up for the loss of heat produced by the latter. The author believes that these circumstances furnish the first instance of death resulting from rapid loss of heat produced by a metal, for the hydrogen surrounding an animal may be compared to a closely-fitting metallic armor.

Metchnikoff's Ideas on Old Age and Disease.—An important exposition of this subject is made by L. LEMATTE (*Arch. de Thérap.*, December 15, 1904). Old age is a sort of disease allied to the changes that accompany various chemical intoxications (*e.g.*, alcohol and lead). The same connective-tissue scleroses that occur in old people are also found in the various chemical intoxications (*e.g.*, alcohol and lead). The bacilli of tuberculosis and leprosy may produce a brittleness of the bones which is similar to that which is the result of senility. Old age is not the result of excessive use, but is an expression of a slow auto-infection. In the intestine is to be found the culture medium for those germs whose toxins are the source of senile atrophy. It is well known that birds have a longevity which is greater than that of the majority of mammalia. This is attributed to the fact that birds have no large intestine, in which hordes of bacteria may flourish. Even in old age birds preserve their youthful appearance and agility. The intestinal parasites secrete toxins which in some cases cause a destruction of hemoglobin and of red blood cells, sometimes poison the nervous centers, and sometimes cause an ulceration of the intestinal mucosa. It has been found that the lactic acid bacillus is a redoubtable foe of the putrefactive microbes. Moreover, a lactic acid ferment which is found in Bulgaria seems to be more active than those of other countries. Metchnikoff discovered this ferment in a preparation of milk consumed in large quantities by the Bulgarians, who are reputed for their longevity. It is suggested that this ferment be used in medicine. It precipitates casein, which it also partially digests, which fact explains the ease with which "Bulgarian milk" is digested. The lactic acid ferment found in this preparation of milk continues to live in the intestine, where it destroys unfriendly bacteria. This milk, containing the pure bacillus, has the consistency of white cheese. It has an agreeable, acidulous taste and contains neither alcohol nor carbonic acid. It is well tolerated by dyspeptics. It is indicated in fermentative dyspepsia. Inasmuch as Pawlow has shown that the organic acids are the best excitants of the intestinal digestive juices one may regard this form of milk as an excellent intestinal tonic. It may replace ordinary milk in the fetid diarrheas of typhoid fever and enteritis. The peculiar ferment the Bulgarian lactic acid bacillus, splits up sugar into products which are harmless to the cells. It has been tried in the treatment of diabetes with the result that the amount of glucose in the urine was diminished by two-thirds. Possibly this ferment may replace the diastases of yeast-cells and of raisins used in the treatment of microbic dermatoses. Bulgarian milk may be a useful adjuvant in the forced alimentation of cases of cancer and tuberculosis, used either alone, or mixed with yolk of egg, beef powder, etc.

Functions of the Thyroid and Parathyroid.—It would seem as if preconceived notions as to the importance of the thyroid glands in the animal economy are receiving their deathblow. S. VINCENT and W. A. JOLLY (*Jour. of Physiol.*, December 30, 1904) believes that it cannot be truly said that either the thyroid or parathyroid is essential to life, for it is frequently possible to remove either or both without causing death. The functions of these glands differ widely in animals. Rats and guinea-pigs do not seem to suffer at all from their deprivation, monkeys manifest only transitory nervous symptoms, while cats and dogs frequently suffer and die. In foxes symptoms come on with remarkable rapidity and death occurs early. These differences are to be attributed to physiological and not to anatomical peculiarities. In no animals have the authors been able to produce symptoms resembling those of myxedema. In young animals, although extirpation of these glands causes a temporary cessation of growth, this is not necessarily accompanied by symptoms of a cretinoid nature. Myxedema and cretinism must then be due to causes more complex than simple thyroid insufficiency. When the thyroid is removed the parathyroid appears capable of functionally replacing it to a certain extent and its histological structure changes accordingly.

PRESCRIPTION HINTS.

Nephrolithiasis.—The following rules are given in *Bull. General de Thérap.*, 30 Janv., 1905, for stone in the kidney.

If the colics are of recent date, give during one week

R Sidonal 0.20

half an hour before the two principal meals, twice a day.

The following week, replace the sidonal by

R Urotropin 0.50

twice a day, afternoon and evening. Rest for one week, then repeat as above.

Herpes Tonsurans.—LASSAR (*Med. Klinik*, No. 3, 1905) recommends the following pastes for herpes tonsurans:

R Acid. Salicylic 2.0
Sulphur sublimat. 20.0
Zinc oxid...................... } aa. 14.0
Amyl............................ }
Vaselin flav. 50.0

R Hydragyr. sulph. ruhr. 1.0
Sulph. sublimat. 24.0
Vasel. flav. ....ad. 100.0
Ol. bergamott. ....gtt. 30.0

R Beta-naphthol: 10.0
Sulph. sublimat. 40.0
Vaselin flav.................... } aa. 25.0
Sapon. virid.................... }

THE MEDICAL NEWS.

A WEEKLY JOURNAL
OF MEDICAL SCIENCE.

COMMUNICATIONS in the form of Scientific Articles, Clinical Memoranda, Correspondence or News Items of interest to the profession are invited from all parts of the world. Reprints to the number of 250 of original articles contributed exclusively to the MEDICAL NEWS will be furnished without charge if the request therefor accompanies the manuscript. When necessary to elucidate the text, illustrations will be engraved from drawings or photographs furnished by the author. Manuscript should be typewritten.

SMITH ELY JELLIFFE, A.M., M.D., Ph.D., Editor,
No. 111 FIFTH AVENUE, NEW YORK.

Subscription Price, Including postage in U. S. and Canada.

PER ANNUM IN ADVANCE $4.00
SINGLE COPIES 10
WITH THE AMERICAN JOURNAL OF THE
MEDICAL SCIENCES, PER ANNUM   .   .   8.00

Subscriptions may begin at any date. The safest mode of remittance is by bank check or postal money order, drawn to the order of the undersigned. When neither is accessible, remittances may be made at the risk of the publishers, by forwarding in *registered* letters.

LEA BROTHERS & CO.,
No. 111 FIFTH AVENUE (corner of 18th St.), NEW YORK.

SATURDAY, MARCH 4, 1905.

THE BENEFICENT ROLE OF THE LACTIC-ACID BACILLUS.

THAT branch of bacteriology which deals with the mutual antagonistic relations of pathogenic germs is still in its infancy. The facts already discovered suggest important developments in the future. To what extent clinicians will be able to utilize these antagonisms in the treatment of disease it is difficult to foretell.

A good beginning, however, has been made. It is hardly necessary to recall Coley's work with the toxins of the *Bacillus erysipelatos* and *Bacillus prodigiosus* in the treatment of inoperable sarcoma. Prof. Elie Metchnikoff has contributed to this subject a number of important data which have not yet received practical application. Thus, he has shown that the *Bacillus mesentericus*, the *Bacillus subtilis,* and the bacillus of symptomatic anthrax weaken the toxins of the tetanus bacillus. The bacillus of Eberth destroys the toxins of diphtheria. W. D. Frost has recently shown that mixed cultures of bacteria obtained from the soil and water have a marked antagonism for the typhoid bacillus.

A number of facts which are the offspring not of laboratory investigation but of clinical experience, indicate that the lactic-acid bacillus, which for a long time has been considered a disreputable one, is really one of man's greatest benefactors. As an enemy of the hordes of putrefactive bacteria that thrive in the intestinal canal, this bacillus serves to prevent intestinal autointoxication. It is again to Metchnikoff that one owes important observations in this domain. A firm defender of the theory of intestinal autoinfection, this investigator, whose speculations may be characterized as almost romantic, believes that the atrophic changes incident to old age are to be attributed to toxins absorbed from the food-canal. Metchnikoff observed that natives of Bulgaria, who are reputed for their longevity, consume large quantities of a form of sour milk. He also found that this contains a lactic-acid ferment which is more vigorous in combating the putrefactive bacteria than the ferments contained in the lactic-acid bacilli native to other countries. This ferment may be used in its pure state without the bacilli.

L. Lematte perceives in the lactic-acid ferment a wide sphere of usefulness in medicine. He has found that "Bulgarian milk," which has the consistency of cream-cheese, and has an agreeable acid taste, is well tolerated by dyspeptics. It is indicated in the fetid diarrheas of typhoid fever and enteritis, and has given good results in the treatment of diabetes. Success in the last case would seem to be due to the fact that the lactic-acid ferment splits up sugar in the organism, with the result that the amount of glucose, as Lematte has found, may be diminished in the urine by two-thirds.

It is not only in "Bulgarian milk" that the lactic-acid bacillus has found favor in the eyes of clinicians. Buttermilk, which also contains this bacillus in large numbers, has been used for a long time as an agreeable and easily digested food in various morbid conditions complicated with digestive disorders. As an example, nephritis may be mentioned. But it is only within recent years that buttermilk has found definite applications in therapeutics. By some European physicians buttermilk is considered to be an ideal substitute for woman's milk in infant feeding. Moreover, it has been thought that buttermilk has a marked curative as well as nutritive value in the summer disorders of infants. The experiences of Dr. Flouquet and E. Decherf, in the north of France, merit attention. During a severe epidemic of gastro-enteritis the buttermilk treatment was employed, with good results, while in parallel cases, treated by other means, no improvement was observed. In acute and chronic cases of gastro-enteritis, in cholera infantum, in rickets, in intestinal fermentations, these observers used buttermilk to good advantage. It is administered boiled, one tablespoonful of farina having been added to a quart of buttermilk, the mixture then being boiled for a few minutes, at the end of which time 2½ ounces of sugar are added. It is fed in the same quantities and at the same intervals as ordinary milk-preparations. The beneficial effects of the buttermilk are attributed to the large number of lactic-acid bacilli present, to the small content of fat, and to the fine division of the casein produced by churning.

ALBUMINOUS SYNTHESIS IN THE ANIMAL BODY.

IN a previous editorial we have pointed out that peptic as well as tryptic digestion, when sufficiently long continued, will, in vitro at least, lead to the cleavage of the albuminous molecule to products which no longer give the biuret reaction and hence do not bear an albuminous character.

This, however, does not prove at once that in the gastro-intestinal tract also proteolysis is carried to this extent, and it is quite conceivable that absorption occurs already when the albumose stage has been reached. As a matter of fact there is evidence to show that this is possible. When Neumeister then demonstrated that "peptones" will disappear from solution in the presence of particles of intestinal mucous membrane the inference suggested itself that a reconstruction of the albuminous molecule takes place in the epithelial cells lining the intestinal tract. This view appeared the more justifiable since all attempts to find either albumoses or peptones in the portal circulation had failed.

Cohnheim's discovery of erepsin, however, has thrown a new light upon these older experiments, and now where we know that the ferment in question, although it may occur free in the intestinal juice, is essentially a tissue ferment and will cause the hydrolytic decomposition of albumoses to a point where the biuret reaction can no longer be obtained, it appears rather doubtful that a restitution ad integrum occurs to any marked extent within the cells. On the contrary, it would seem more plausible to assume that albuminous synthesis occurs in the various tissues of the body at large from the fundamental radicles, or at least from products which are simpler in composition than the albumoses.

To test this hypothesis numerous experiments have been undertaken, and while an ultimate conclusion has not yet been reached regarding the nature of the processes involved, there is evidence to show that the animal body is capable of effecting the synthesis of the albuminous molecule from such relatively simple products as result on prolonged tryptic digestion. Some of these experiments have furnished results of great interest. O. Loewi thus found that a dog while being fed on the end-products of pancreatic autolysis, in addition to fat and carbohydrates, stored 0.72 grms. of nitrogen on an average per day during a period of eleven days. This goes to show that the sum of the end-products of pancreatic autolysis, which no longer gives the biuret reaction, *can* take the place of the food albumins. Corresponding results with meat alone show very clearly, however, that quantitatively the end-products do not cover the requirements of the nitrogenous metabolism as readily as the original albumins. Loewi noted a marked tendency, moreover, to diarrhea and vomiting in his animals. Following Loewi's experiments, Henderson and Deane published an account of an analogous investigation, in which the cleavage of meat was effected by sulphuric acid. Here also it was possible, after a while, to maintain the nitrogenous equilibrium of the animal. The writers do not draw the inference, however, that albuminous synthesis occurred; they merely suppose that the material in question acted as a proteid sparer. As in Loewi's case there was a marked tendency to diarrhea and vomiting.

Lesser then took up a similar line of investigations with the end-products of tryptic action on fibrin, but did not succeed in maintaining his animals in nitrogenous equilibrium. With the products of peptic action upon Witte peptone the results were likewise uncertain. He concludes that if it is possible at all to keep animals in nitrogenous equilibrium by feeding with such products it is necessary to give much larger amounts of nitrogen in this form than would correspond to the intact albumins.

The next series of experiments in this direction is reported by Abderhalden and Rona. They worked with mice and gauged the effect of their feeding experiments by the body-weight of the animals. The results are very interesting. They found that animals fed with the products of acid hydrolysis (of casein) lived but little longer than starving control animals, while others which were kept on the products of pancreatic digestion lived as long as the controls which had been fed on native casein. Very curiously intermediate results between the two were obtained with the products of primary peptic-hydrochloric acid and subsequent pancreatic cleavage.

The latest experiments of this character finally came from the physiological laboratory of the veterinary institute of Copenhagen and are reported by Henriques and Hansen. The experiments were conducted on white rats and are quite laborious. These writers also have found that the products of acid cleavage (in the case of casein) are not capable of protecting the tissue nitrogen, even when administered in large amounts. But they find that the end-products of the action of trypsin and erepsin, on the other hand, will not only maintain nitrogenous equilibrium, but can even bring this to a higher level. In one experiment in which the weight of the animal, on the fourth day, had been 68 grms., this increased to 98 grms. by the twenty-fourth day.

This brief survey will show what has already been accomplished in connection with the problem under consideration and in what direction future investigations will have to be carried. It is significant that pancreatic digestion and cleavage by means of erepsin apparently lead to products which the organism can utilize in albuminous synthesis, while acid cleavage manifestly is too extensive. It will be very interesting to observe in future studies to what extent polypeptids are of moment in order that a reconstruction of the albuminous molecule may occur.

MUCH ADO ABOUT NOTHING.

THE American favorite funny story is about the Englishman who cannot see a joke. The tomato story with "They eat what they can and tin the rest" has circled the globe, and "What *was* the matter with the custard pie" is equally famous. But now it is the Englishman's turn to laugh. We fancy that for some years to come no American on English soil can hear the word "chloroform" without feeling silly.

Americans may not know that with all their ability to *see* a joke, they are world famous for not being able to *take* a joke; and a more jovial joker, a more epigrammatic and witty member of society than Dr. Osler never made after-dinner speeches.

The furor that has been raised over his retiring speech at Johns Hopkins reminds one of the "Hobson's kiss" episode, and the "Dewey's house" business. It is on a par with the marvelous facility of the press to kindle a mighty flame from a very little matter, and it illustrates most delightfully our national tendency to take ourselves very seriously. We can ha ha at our neighbor's expense, but not at ourselves.

Now, when Dr. Osler in his dry and genial manner wished modestly to indicate to his fellow-workers that he felt he had lived his best days with them, he facetiously quoted from Anthony Trollope's novel, the Fixed Idea, the scheme on which the plot hinges, of a college into which at sixty, men should retire for a year of contemplation before a peaceful departure by chloroform. He adds, pointing at *himself,* the barb which all the solemn readers of the daily news claim was hurled at their self-respecting selves, these words "That incalculable benefits might follow such a scheme is apparent to any one who, like myself, is nearing the limit and who, like myself, had made a careful study of the calamities which may befall men during the seventh and eighth decade."

He then adds, after recounting some of the well-known follies of the aged: "The teacher's life should have three periods. Study until twenty-five, investigation until forty, profession until sixty, at which time *he should be retired on a double allowance."* The press missed this point.

To round up his playful allusion he says, with affected hesitation, "Whether Anthony Trollope's suggestion of a college and chloroform should be carried out I have become a little dubious, as my own time is getting too short."

Dr. Osler is taking with him to Oxford a curious epistolary collection, for he has been bombarded with letters, telegrams and articles from the senile and the presenile all over the country, stating in good set terms why they should not be chloroformed.

If Dr. Osler was to stay with us much longer we fear that he would have to take to heart the advice of John G. Saxe, who says:

> "Learn to wear a sober phiz,
> 　Be stupid, if you can;
> It's such a very serious thing
> 　To be a funny man."

Honorary **Degrees at Manchester.**—On the occasion of the opening of the new public health laboratory of the Victoria University, Manchester, honorary doctorates of science were conferred upon Professor Calmette, Lille University; Professor Perroncito, Turin University; Professor Salomonsen, Copenhagen University; and Captain R. F. Scott, of London.

ECHOES AND NEWS.

NEW YORK.

Society of Medical Jurisprudence.—Professor Wilhelm Waldeyer was made an honorary member of this Society at its last regular meeting, held February 20, 1905.

Clinic on Cancer.—At the completion of Dr. L. Duncan Bulkley's special course of lectures on Diseases of the Skin, held at the New York Skin and Cancer Hospital, Nineteenth Street and Second Avenue, New York, Dr. William Seaman Bainbridge will give a clinical lecture on cancer, March 29, at 4.15 o'clock. A number of interesting cases will be shown.

For the Treatment of Consumption.—Announcement was made last week that the Health Department's new building in Brooklyn, made necessary by the unsanitary condition of the present quarters in Clinton Street, is to have attached to it a tuberculosis sanitarium of the most modern description. The new building is to be erected in Flatbush Avenue, near Fulton Street, and is to cost $200,000. The scheme of a tuberculosis institution has been under advisement for a long time. It is proposed to build a one-story structure, tiled throughout, without a particle of wood or other material to harbor germs. The tuberculosis ward will be attached to the main building, which will be used for the business offices of the department and fitted for scientific experiments. It is expected that the new structure will be completed within eighteen months.

New Eye and Ear Hospital.—A meeting of the board of directors of the Manhattan Eye, Ear and Throat Hospital, Madison Avenue and Forty-first Street, was held last week to consider the plans submitted by the building committee for the contemplated hospital on Sixty-first Street, running through to Sixty-second Street, between Second and Third avenues. It was found that a suitable hospital would cost nearly $200,000 more than had been appropriated for the building. A letter was read from Frank Tilford, who was recently elected a member of the board of directors, suggesting that the hospital be built upon the original plans, even if a debt must be incurred. He believed there were many who would give large amounts if the need for it were properly presented to them. He backed up this proposition by a gift of $25,000 for the construction of an ear clinic. The board immediately passed a resolution to incur the debt and begin at once with the construction.

A Dettweiler Foundation.—To honor the memory and the works of the late Geheimrath Dr. Peter Dettweiler, the founder of the Falkenstein Sanatorium and the first people's sanatorium at Ruppertshain, it has been decided, by his friends, admirers, patients and pupils, to establish an institution bearing his name which shall be a home for physicians who have served in sanatoria for consumptives and who have become invalidated by disease, accident or old age. For the collection of funds and the final arrangements a committee has been formed under the patronage of H.R.H. the Princess Friedrich Carl of Hesse. This committee is composed of many of the foremost men and women of the German empire. Of the medical men who have signed the appeal for funds we read such names as Besold, the successor to Dettweiler, Professors Kurschmann, of Leipzig, Flügge, of Breslau, B. Fränkel, von Leyden and Pannwitz, of Berlin, General Dr. von Leuthald, physician to the Emperor, Schmidt, of Frankfort, etc. Contributions are to be addressed to Grunelius & Co., Bankers, 16 Gr. Gallus Strasse, Frankfort-on-the-Main, Germany.

Lodging Houses and Tuberculosis.—Mr. Paul Kennaday, secretary of the Committee on the Prevention of Tuberculosis, has made a personal inspection of 101 lodging houses in New York, and publishes the results in this week's *Charities*. No direct evidence of tuberculosis are found, but bad sanitation is the rule. Mr. Kennaday was assured by several lodging-house keepers that all blankets were washed "at least twice a year"! New York's lodging houses—the majority located along the bowery—shelter nearly 20,000 people every night. The Health Department has apparently gone upon the theory that it is impossible to make them keep clean. The old argument against tenement-house reform was that the tenement dweller got as good as he deserved—that he would rapidly defile the most immaculate buildings. But that notion, as we see now, was fallacious. And our floating population is at least entitled to fresh air, an occasional bathtub, and frequent changes of bed linen. If our officials give more careful attention to their duties, and if the few new laws advocated by Mr. Kennaday are enacted, the changes brought about in the tenements may be in some degree duplicated on the Bowery.

Pneumonia in 1904.—State Commissioner of Health, in his annual report, states that, estimated by the death rate from all causes, the sanitary condition of the State for 1904 was unsatisfactory. There were 141,564 deaths reported, which is largely in excess of previous records. The annual average mortality for the past twenty years, including 1904, is 116,600. Of epidemic diseases, cerebrospinal meningitis and measles alone have shown any material increase. This was due to an outbreak of the former disease in the City of New York, beginning in March and continuing several months. Measles has increased in the southern and eastern parts of the State, New York City having had nearly twice as many deaths from this cause as 1903. The chief cause for increase in the mortality of 1904 has been pneumonia. This alone caused 13,500 deaths, against 10,250 in the preceding year. These figures were nearly reached in the years of largest prevalence of the grip, 1891-3, which in the first five months of the year amounted to one-eighth of the total. There were over 14,000 deaths from consumption, the mortality from which is also excessive in grip epidemics, and last year's exceeds any previous year's record.

Subway Signs Not Dangerous.—The subway signs are deadly to bacteria, declares Dr. William H. Park, head of the Health Department division of bacteriology. Dr. Park has embodied his views in an affidavit which the Interborough Company's lawyers will file to-day in rebuttal to the sworn statement of Dr. George A. Soper that subway dust is dangerous to health. This affidavit is one of the last papers to be filed in the plea of the Interborough Company that the City of New York be forbidden to tear out the mural decorations put in by Ward, Gow & Co. Dr. Park, after setting forth his qualifications and stating that he has read Dr. Soper's statement, declares that there is not a sufficient quantity of dust in the subway to be dangerous of itself, and that there are fewer bacteria in the subway dust than in the common or garden variety to be found in the streets above. As to the dust which gathers on the advertising signs, the doctor declares that it dries so quickly there that nearly all bacteria are destroyed. Dr. Park adds: "If the metal frames for the advertising signs in the subway should be moistened they would operate as a positive germicide and destroy practically all the non-spore-bearing bacteria brought in contact with them." In conclusion Dr. Park says: "My conclusion from the experiments above mentioned, and from my knowledge of the conditions in the subway and my knowledge of the subject of bacteriology, is that as a practical matter the presence of the signs attached to the walls in the subway as a menace to the health of the public is so infinitesimal that they may be disregarded entirely for all practical purposes."

A Home for Convalescents.—The fact that three more tents for convalescents are to be erected this week in the Bellevue Hospital yard emphasizes the city's need of a home for convalescents, the building of which is being advocated by the Commissioner of Charities, Mr. Tully, and Acting-Superintendent Rickard of Bellevue Hospital. It is their belief that no relief from the present overcrowding can be brought about until such a home is constructed. "The tents," said Acting-Superintendent Rickard, "are only a makeshift at best. What the city most urgently needs in its hospital work is a capacious home for convalescents. There they could remain until they have received the full benefits of the hospital treatment. As it now is, benefits from treatment are in great measure nullified. It will continue to be so until a home where 5,000 or 6,000 patients may be nursed through the dangerous period of convalescence is provided." Mr. Tully said: "Much of the present trouble could be obviated if we could have a home for the exclusive treatment of tuberculous patients and a home for convalescents. I have asked the Board of Estimate for an appropriation of $500,000 to build the former on our farm of 140 acres on Staten Island, and for another to erect a convalescents' home on our twelve-acre plot on the Coney Island Parkway. If we had these, the relief, both at Bellevue and its allied hospitals, and on Blackwell's Island, would prevent the present crowded conditions at all these places."

Work of the Babies' Hospital.—The sixteenth annual report of the Babies' Hospital, at Fifty-fifth Street and Lexington avenue, has just been issued. There has been a notable decrease in the death rate this year, owing, it is said, to the improved hygienic conditions under which patients are now treated. This in spite of the fact that more than one-third of the total deaths occurred within forty-eight hours after admission, and the majority of these within the first twenty-four hours. The total number of patients admitted during the past twelve months was 929, against 600 for the preceding year. The death rate was 27.7 against 30 per cent. the previous year. The work of the out-patient department shows an increase in the number of patients treated; 5,761 cases were handled last year, and 5,864 during the last twelve months. The report of the treasurer shows receipts of $36,639.99 and expenditures of $30,234.17. The general cost of operating the hospital has been $30,227.17, exceeding that of last year by $118.58. This small excess is remarkable in view of the fact that all the departments have been open the entire year for the first time in the history of the institution. The summer hospital at Oceanic, N. J., was well filled during the three months of its occupancy, the committee securing funds to the amount of $2,000—nearly enough to defray the expenses of the entire season. The income of the Babies' Hospital is in a large measure dependent upon the receipts from its contributors. Checks should be sent to Mrs. John B. Calvert, No. 15 East Fifty-seventh Street.

West Side Doctors Fleeced.—Many physicians on the upper west side complained to the police last week of a handsomely dressed young woman who had succeeded in swindling the doctors out of various sums of money by laying down worthless checks. In each instance the swindler obtained money from members of the doctor's household in the absence of the physician. Just how much money the swindler obtained in the Central Park district could not be learned, but the police came to the conclusion that the woman must have obtained at least a thousand dollars in one day. The woman is described as about thirty years old, of medium build, comely, and of good education. In the majority of cases she described herself as a trained nurse, and said that she was employed by the physician whose house she visited. Her plan was to call in the absence of the physician, and declare that she was there to pay a bill owed by one of the doctor's patients. She offered to pay the bill by check drawn on the Riverside Bank, at Fifty-seventh street and Eighth avenue. At some of the offices she visited she declared that the patient whose bill she was paying owed $5. Then she presented a check for $25, and walked out with $20 of the doctor's funds, handed to her by either the physician's wife or the housekeeper. At a few of the places she said that the sum due the doctor was $20 and presented a check for $50. At the home of one doctor she said she had come to pay the bill of a patient who owed $60, and presented a check for $100, getting $40 change from the housekeeper. On one block alone in West Fifty-eighth Street she succeeded in swindling five physicians out of amounts varying from $5 to $20.

Columbia's Medical Needs.—Dr. Nicholas Murray Butler, president of Columbia University, in acknowledging the recent gift of Mr. and Mrs. William D. Sloane for the endowment of the Sloane Maternity Hospital, points out that "the existence, within the university, of this excellently appointed and well-managed hospital gives a unique distinction to our instruction in obstetrics, and indicates clearly how great would be the advantage to the medical school if the university were in possession of a general hospital of its own." Both the need and the advantage of a university hospital were still more emphatically presented by Dr. John H. Musser in his presidential address at the fifty-fifth annual session of the American Medical Association. He insists that "the final years should be clinical years, and the last should be in a hospital. . . . What has been said regarding the preliminary college training applies equally forcefully to the hospital training. He (the student) is thrice armed who enters the arena thus equipped." Dr. Musser's argument is that public safety demands that each medical school shall have its teaching hospital, and that "every hospital should be a school" in the interests of the patients as well as medical education and broad considerations of humanity. The importance of hospital instruction has always been recognized in the College of Physicians and Surgeons, and in the early days the New York Hospital met the requirements both of the public and of the medical students, who then gathered in New York for instruction. Now too many hospitals in the city are inadequate to the needs of a university course in medicine. Modern medicine demands, both for the instructor and the student, a study of disease from its inception to its close, and this in the full light of all obtainable knowledge.

To this end it is believed there should be established a thoroughly equipped hospital, controlled by the university. European schools of medicine are for the most part founded in connection with the great Government hospitals, and it is for that reason alone that every year such large numbers of students, graduated from the foremost medical schools in the United States, have gone abroad. The opportunities for bedside instruction possessed by the teachers in the medical school at Columbia are considerable, but are inadequate for placing medical education on a university basis.

New York's Dispensary System.—From advance sheets from Annual Report of the Committee on Dispensaries of the State Board of Charities we obtain the following: On October 1, 1903, there were 123 licensed dispensaries in the State. Four dispensaries have ceased work since that date, and no new licenses have been issued during the year. Since October 1, 1904, licenses have been issued to the Italian Benevolent Society to conduct a dispensary at 169 West Houston street, Borough of Manhattan, New York City (license granted October 12, 1904), and to the Bedford Guild, 962 Ber-

Rules.	Yes.	No.	In Part.	Not Applicable.	
I. Public Notice Posted...........	117	2			
II. 1 Registrar	118	—	1		
2 Deputy (not required)........	44	75			
3 Makes and Preserves records..	114	3	2		
4 Receives Applicants	117	1	1		
5 Sees that Rules are Enforced..	18	2	99		
III. 1 Examines all Applicants........	116	3			
superficially 34					
fairly well 31					
thoroughly 54					
are any refused admission	87	32			
a. Emergency cases admitted .,.,...........	119				
b. Poor applicants admitted	119				
c. Doubtful cases admitted upon signing representation card .,....	90	28	1		
d. Subsequent investigation made	41	76	2		
e. Results of investigation filed	32	85	2		
f. Non-signers refused admission	100	18	1		
2 Representation cards in proper form	113	6			
3 a. Pass cards issued......	119				
b. Penalty printed thereon.	110	4	5		
IV. 1 Matron	117	2			
2 Cleanliness and Order Preserved	115	4			
3 Present at gynæcological examinations, etc.	89	3		27*	
V. 1 Contagious diseases excluded..	119				
2 Registrar prevents exposure...	119				
3 Registrar reports to health authorities	118	1			
VI. 1 Clinical or other instruction given	28	91			Instruction permitted by Rules.
2 Treatment conditional thereon.	—	28	91		
3 Consent of patient obtained....	27	1	91		
3 Consent of patient obtained....	27	1	91		
VII. 1 Apothecary (not required).....	107	12			
2 Licensed or medical graduate..	104	3		12†	
3 Appointed under Civil Service Rules	8	—		111‡	
VIII. 1 Board of Health ordinances observed	119				
2 Minute made before September 30	45	74			
IX. 1 Seats for all applicants provided	107	12			
2 Sexes separated in					
a. waiting rooms...........	85	32	2		
b. treatment rooms.........	102	17	2		
3 Suitable equipment and supplies	109	8	2		

* Such examination not held in these dispensaries.
† No prescriptions compounded in these dispensaries.
‡ Applies only to 8 dispensaries connected with municipal hospital in New York City.

gen street, Borough of Brooklyn, New York City (license granted December 21, 1904). Of the 123 dispensaries which were open during a whole or part of the year ending September 30, 1904, 20 were in receipt of public money directly ($11,032.40 all told), 61 were connected with other charities in receipt of public appropriations, and 42 were supported wholly by private contributions. The total property real and personal of the 81 dispensaries in receipt of public funds and reporting annually to this Board was $1,175,436 October

1, 1904; their total indebtedness on the same date $68.996; their total receipts for the year ending September 30, 1904, $125,113, and their total expenditures, $105,642. The work of these dispensaries is of more than casual interest and importance in view of the fact that such work is extensively carried on in this State than in any other part of the country, that here it is more highly organized and developed, and that here, as in no other State, dispensaries are licensed and regulated by the State Board of Charities. The system has now been in operation for a little more than five years, and certain features and results of its workings are set forth herewith. During the year the Inspector of Dispensaries has made a special investigation as to the extent of compliance with the rules of the Board, adopted pursuant to chapter 368 of the laws of 1899, affecting the management of all licensed dispensaries. Four out of the 123 licensed dispensaries in operation at the beginning of the year have been closed, and the accompanying table shows the extent of compliance with the various provisions of the rules on the part of the 119 dispensaries remaining.

It will be seen from the above that with 24 of the 31 requirements of the dispensary rules compliance is practically complete, that in four of these provisions compliance is fairly good, and that in these matters those requiring an investigation to be made as to the ability of doubtful applicants to pay for their treatment, the filing of results of these investigations, and of making a minute showing observance of the ordinances and orders of the Board of Health, compliance is somewhat lax.

Some of the showings of this table are very satisfactory. One hundred and fourteen out of 119 dispensaries examined are keeping reasonably complete records of their work. In 54 cases the examination by the Registrar of applicants for treatment is reported as being done thoroughly, and in 31 additional cases as being done fairly well. In only 34 cases is the work reported as being done superficially. As this is perhaps the crucial point in the proper administration of dispensaries, viewed from the social standpoint, this showing is encouraging though by no means all that could be desired. In 87 dispensaries obviously well-to-do applicants are refused admission by the Registrar after questioning, but without further formality, while in 100 dispensaries, where the Registrar is still in doubt as to the applicant's ability to pay, persons unwilling to sign representation cards are refused treatment. In 90 out of 119 dispensaries doubtful cases are admitted only upon signing representation cards. This would seem to indicate that the doors of the dispensaries in the State are reasonably well guarded in the large majority of cases, that they are partially protected in most of the remaining instances, and that they are not wholly unguarded except in a very small number of cases. In all but two of the dispensaries a matron is employed, cleanliness and order are maintained in all but four, and in only three cases the matron is not present at gynæcological examinations where such are held. In only three dispensaries is the apothecary unlicensed or not a medical graduate, and in every dispensary compliance with the local ordinances of the Board of Health is reported as complete. All but 10 of the dispensaries are reported as having suitable equipment and supplies, and in practically all of them seats are provided for every applicant, and in the great majority of them the sexes are separated both in the waiting and in the treatment rooms. It is interesting to note that the facilities of but 28 dispensaries are used for the purpose of giving medical instruction, and in none of these is the treatment given the patient conditional upon his willingness to submit to an examination before a class. Another item of interest is the fact that but 12 dispensaries are without an apothecary as a regular officer or employe of the dispensary, and that in only three cases such apothecary is not a licensed pharmacist or a medical graduate.

PHILADELPHIA.

Bequest.—The will of Ellen K. Mitchell bequeaths $5,000 to maintain a free bed in the Pennsylvania Hospital.

Donation Day at St. Joseph's Hospital.—The Sisters of Charity who made an appeal for liberal assistance devoted February 22 to receiving donations.

To Open a Private Hospital in the Philippines.—Miss Hicks, formerly chief nurse of the Bryn Mawr Hospital, from which institution she has recently resigned, will in the latter part of March leave for the Philippines, where she will take charge of the first private hospital in those islands.

Anthrax Victim.—A young Jersey farmer, unaware of the dangerous task he was asked to do, removed the hide of a cow which had died of anthrax. The young man soon became very ill; he was taken to the Jefferson Hospital where spreads and cultures were made which upon examination revealed the bacillus of anthrax. The patient was then sent to the Municipal Hospital, where he was isolated with an attendant.

New Hospitals.—The Mount Sinai Hospital, at Fifth and Wilder Streets, will soon be ready to receive patients. This institution will be supported by Russian Jews, who will make monthly contributions of from 10 to 50 cents. The membership at the present is 2,000, but it is soon expected to be 8,000—the number required to maintain the institution according to the above contributions. The building is four stories high. The first floor will be used for the dispensary, accident and drug-room. The second contains four wards, with forty beds; the third floor contains fourteen rooms, five of which are set aside for operating. Upon the fourth floor are the kitchen, dining-room and nurses' rooms. The Union Mission Hospital has also been opened. This institution contains fifty beds, with provisions for twenty-five more. Dr. Charles B. Warder is medical director and Dr. H. C. Weaver is chief surgeon. The medical staff will consist of eleven visiting physicians and a resident.

Bills Introduced into the Legislature.—The first of these provides that after January 1, 1906, the Governor shall appoint one-half of the number of members on the Board of Directors or Trustees of all institutions and hospitals receiving State aid for maintenance or other purposes. The bill does not, however, include the hospitals or asylums for the care and treatment of the indigent insane, which has been erected by any city or county, or any institution or hospital in which all or a portion of the members of the Board of Directors or Trustees are now appointed by the Governor. The other bill requires that in order to practice medicine in Pennsylvania the applicant for licence must have pursued a four-years' course, instead of three as now required by law; but if he has graduated from a reputable literary college, he may be admitted to the second year in the medical college, if he has pursued a four-years' course at that school, two of which having been devoted to science and biology.

Society of Medical Jurisprudence of Philadelphia.—This meeting was held February 26, 1905, with Dr.

Coplin in the chair. Owing to the illness of Dr. Leffman his paper, entitled " A Criticism of the Reid and Crusade Methods of the Enforcement of the Law," was read by Dr. Cattell. Dr. Leffman pointed out that the newspapers try more cases of violation of the law than are actually tried in court. He also noted that in many instances the defence is brought up for prosecution for selling adulterated food or drinks which have never been tested, or which, at any rate, come to trial without a chemical report. The taking up of numerous samples of articles of food spasmodically and subjecting them to tests, he said, is not the intention of the food laws. Dr. Leffman maintained that preliminary examinations of foods and beverages should be made, the dealers be notified of what is required, and then that requirement constantly and steadily forced upon them. The methods of the Law and Order Society is a violation of the law of the government, for it merely scatters vice and crime. Dr. Hirsch moved that the society join the other societies of the city in establishing a pamphlet to be issued every Saturday announcing the official programme of all the meetings the following week. The matter was placed in the hands of a committee to act upon the question.

Section on Ophthalmology of the College of Physicians.—This meeting was held February 21, 1905, at which Dr. H. F. Hansel read a paper entitled: " Some Further Experiences in the Treatment of Ocular Inflammations by Diaphoresis." From his recent experiences he is inclined to avoid the internal administration of pilocarpine to induce sweating and to produce the diaphoresis by means of hot baths. If perspiration is delayed after the bath is begun he gives hot drinks, or, if that fails, he administers a dose of strychnine; and then, if these fail, he gives the pilocarpine as a last resort. He reported three cases in whom good results were obtained by this method of treatment. Very good effects are produced, he said, if the inflammatory conditions are not due to syphilis. The absorption of the exudate, he finds, is hastened by the administration of mercury and potassium iodide.

Dr. C. F. Clark, of Columbus, O., by invitation read a paper on " Astigmatism following the Operation for the Extraction of Cataract." He spoke of the prolapse of the iris and the occasional incarceration of this structure which prevented the healing and favored the production of astigmatism as complication of operation for cataract. When he employed the conjunctival flap and the Snellen wet dressing he had but one case of prolapse of the iris of 30 cases operated. In these cases but 2.92 diopters of astigmatism occurred when the examination was made from nine days to six weeks after the operation. Dr. W. Zentmayer read a paper on " A Case of Paralysis of the Upward Movement of Both Eyes." He gave the history of the case in detail but did not quote literature. Dr. Spiller who saw the case with Zentmayer expressed the opinion that the lesion was in the nucleus of the motor oculi nerves. Dr. de Schweinitz read a paper on " Traumatic Aniridia." The patient of whom he speaks was struck in the eye while wearing spectacles; the glass broke but no foreign body could be located by means of the X-ray. The patient would have attacks of pain in the eye affected, which radiated toward the mental foramen. He was placed upon the salicylates, upon which treatment he improved. The iris could not be found. Dr. de Schweinitz also reported four cases of sarcoma of the choroid and one case of glioma of the retina. Dr. E. A. Schumway exhibited a new ophthalmic outfit for bedside examination.

Course of Instruction in Public Health.—The authorities of the University of Pennsylvania realize the efforts which are being made in communities throughout the country to obtain officials who have had some special training in matters pertaining to public health. Each year the demands for men of this type (either as chiefs of departments or in some subordinate position) is increased, and at the present time there is a lack of men qualified to fill such positions. To meet the needs of such instruction, the University will introduce into its curriculum, beginning October 1, 1905, a course in public health, which will include instruction under the following headings:

Sanitary Engineering.—Including the subject of water supplies, sewerage systems, street cleaning, disposal of waste, etc.

Sanitary Legislation.—A study of the movement for sanitary reform, and of the laws enacted relating to public health, and the methods of enforcement employed in Great Britain and the United States.

Inspection of Meat, Milk and Other Animal Products. —The methods of preparation and preservation of the same, the conduct of dairies, creameries, etc., and demonstrations of the diseases of animals transmissible to man.

The Sanitary Engineering of Buildings.—Including demonstrations of systems of heating, ventilation, plumbing and drainage, the study of plans, etc.

Social and Vital Statistics in the United States.—An examination of statistical methods and their results, with special reference to vital statistics and to city populations.

Practical Methods, Used in Sanitary Work.—Including water, air and milk analyses, studies in ventilation and heating, investigation of the soil, methods of disinfection, sterilization, etc. (This is purely laboratory instruction.)

General Hygiene.—As applied to the community, including lectures upon the causation of disease—exciting and predisposing, methods of prevention—including isolation, quarantine, natural and acquired immunity, protective inoculation, vaccination, and the antitoxic state, methods of house disinfection and the means employed, suggestions for the organization of sanitary work, the influence of water supplies and sewage disposal on the public health, etc.

Personal Hygiene.—Including the physiology of exercise, the adaptation of exercise to the various physical requirements, the use of exercise for the prevention and correction of deformities, the methods of examination and record keeping, the routine physical examination of growing children and the relation of air, food, bathing, etc., to health and development; the hygiene of the school room.

Philadelphia Pathological Society.—At the meeting of this society, which was held February 23, 1905, Dr. R. C. Rosenberger read a paper entitled " Homogenized Cultures of Tubercle Bacilli." He first described his technic. The bacteria, which were originally made from homogenized bouillon cultures, were inoculated from glycerin potato and glycerin agar upon a five per cent. glycerin bouillon. The growth was transferred from the agar or potato by a platinum loop to the side of the tube or flask and then the bouillon, by tipping the tube or flask, was brought in contact with the bacteria—in that way they were washed off and disseminated. When the tubercle bacilli from these cultures were examined they were found pleomorphous, exhibiting

short, nearly coccoid, and long forms, which were filamentous. There were also beaded, club-shaped and branched organisms. Although a few were isolated, the tendency was toward grouping of from six to fifteen elements. In no cultures, even from the third or fourth day to the fourth or sixth week, did he observe motility; Brownian movement was common. The resistance to 25 per cent. sulphuric acid was still maintained. He has not fully worked out the pathogenicity of these organisms, but in one of the two guinea-pigs inoculated with five c.c. of the bouillon cultures caseous nodules developed in the peritoneum; the nodules varied from 5 mm. to 2 cm. in diameter and spreads made from them contained acidfast bacili. Dr. Rosenberger also made homogenized cultures of the Bacillus tuberculosis piscum, Bacillus tuberculosis avian, and of various forms of pseudotubercle bacilli. Dr. D. H. Bergey read a paper in " The influence of Pasteurization on the Chemical and Physical Qualities of Milk." He presented the results of studies on samples of market milk Pasteurized in the laboratory. The bacteria found in milk are the lactic acid and the subtilis group. The bacillus may be present in sufficient quantities to affect the milk. Pasteurization, he said, destroys the Bacillus acidi lactici but not the Bacillus subtilis. From his bacteriological investigations he found that raw milk in the icechest contained 1,260 bacteria; in seventy-two hours it contained 17,000,000, but at room temperature 5,000,000. At the time Pasteurization was completed the milk contained 12 bacteria; at the end of seventytwo hours in the ice-chest it contained 148,000,000. in the room at the end of seventy-two hours 5,000,000. Pasteurizing, he said, removes the most reliable indicator of the changes that occur which make the milk unfit for use. The odor does not indicate the exact condition of the milk. At the time coagulation began he found that the raw milk contained from 50 to 10,000,000 bacteria, while Pasteurized milk contained from 5 to 10,000,000. He maintains that no single test conveys the accurate condition of the Pasteurized milk and that the number of bacteria present is the most reliable. Dr. Bergey stated that the Pasteurized milk should receive greater care at home than the raw article. While the Bacillus subtilis has not been proven injurious, the indications are that under certain circumstances it may be inimical to young children. The next paper was read by Dr. M. E. Pennington on " The Comparison of Pasteurized and Raw Milk." She began her paper by asking the following questions: Are we justified in accepting commercial Pasteurized milk on the findings of laboratory Pasteurized milk? Is Pasteurized milk sold in Philadelphia better or worse than before it is Pasteurized? In the best Pasteurizing plant she obtained the following results from her bacteriological investigations:

	Number of bacteria in fresh milk.	Twenty-four hours later.
Raw milk in reservoir	7,140,000	12,600,000
In milk after leaving cooling coil	3,000	6,000
In milk in pipe to bottle tank	3,333	6,000
In milk when bottled	744,000	785,000

The following are the results from the worst plant:

Raw milk in reservoir	1,504,000	25,000,000
In milk after leaving cooling coil	18,000	360,000
When bottled	2,880,000	45,000,000

From the raw milk of the five dairies supplying these Pasteurizing plants she obtained the following average results: The raw milk contained 5,276 bacteria, and twenty-four hours later it contained 114,542. Dr. Pennington found that Pasteurized milk soured in twenty hours, while raw milk soured in thirty-two hours. Her results seem to indicate that Pasteurizing by the city plants destroys the *Bacillus acidi lactici* present in the milk when delivered, and substitutes the *Bacillus subtilis* from unclean bottles, corks and city dust. Dr. J. Evans read the next paper on "Does Milk Possess Germicidal Properties." He found that in the milk obtained from the tapped cow udder, remained sterile for a week. He inoculated specimens of sterile, raw and Pasteurized milk with streptococci, staphylococci, *Bacillus subtilis*, and *Bacillus coli communis*. The streptococcus inoculation worked out as though the milk possessed germicidal properties. He concludes that raw milk to a certain degree inhibits bacterial growth for from four to eight hours. Dr. Abbott, in opening the discussion on these papers, said that Pasteurizing milk gives the dealers an opportunity to place unclean milk upon the market. Dr. Edsall, in the discussion, said Pasteurizing produced the following changes in the milk: (1) In the taste; (2) in the casein; (3) in the fat; (4) in the lecithin; (5) in the ferments lipase is destroyed; (6) immune bodies, may be destroyed. He states that if the bacteria have produced toxins in the milk heat will not destroy them. Sterilizing the milk damages the nutritional value, while Pasteurizing, he said, does not. He is inclined to believe that it is better to feed children Pasteurized milk than to give them milk containing bacteria.

CHICAGO.

Gift to Presbyterian Hospital.—By the will of Harriet A. Jones, the Presbyterian Hospital of this city receives as a bequest $15,000. Mrs. Jones desired that $10,000 of the bequest to this institution be devoted to the assistance of convalescent patients.

Laboratory for Coroner.—One of the new features in connection with the Coroner's office is the establishment of a laboratory, which will enable the Coroner's physicians to make their analyses, and to constantly be in touch with the Coroner. The Coroner also advocates a law compelling undertakers to refrain from embalming bodies until after death certificates have been issued.

Appointment of Physicians at Dunning.—President Brundage, at a recent meeting of the County Board, submitted appointments to the consulting staff of the county institutions at Dunning. The appointments are as follows: Drs. Frank Billings, Wm. A. Evans, Edward J. Farnum, Alice Hamilton, Arnold C. Klebs, B. McPherson Linnell, John B. Murphy, Hugh T. Patrick, J. Rawson Pennington and Chas. S. Williamson.

Crusade Against Spitters.—During the last few days vigorous efforts have been made to enforce the anti-spitting ordinance. Hundreds of men were arrested and hauled into court for spitting on sidewalks and other places, and fined. It is thought that this will deter others from spitting in public conveyances, public halls, and all similar places, as offenders are liable to arrest and fine under an ordinance of the City of Chicago, which will be enforced from now on by the Department of Police.

Grace Hospital Opened.—This new hospital was recently opened with a reception for the physicians of the West Side and their wives. The new hospital is the result of the united effort of West Side physicians, who felt the lack of a hospital in the district where it stands. Dr. A. M. Harvey is president of the institution. The staff consists of Drs. C. C. O'Byrne, J. S. Nagel, F. A. Phillips, M. D. Bates, J. J. Anderson, A.

E. Bertling, A. A. Whamond, W. F. Duckett, C. W. Harrison, and Howard Crutcher.

GENERAL.

Honorary Degrees at Edinburgh.—The senate of the University of Edinburgh has voted to confer its honorary doctorate of laws on Dr. Alexander Graham Bell, of Washington, D. C., and on Dr. W. W. Keen, professor of surgery at Jefferson Medical College, Philadelphia.

Dr. Willy Merck.—The University of Halle, Germany, has conferred upon Dr. Willy Merck, member of the old house of E. Merck, Darmstadt, established in 1668, a very high distinction, namely, the honorary degree of Doctor of Medicine "in recognition of numerous meritorious contributions looking to the advancement of the therapeutic side of medicine."

Dr. Weir Mitchell.—Dr. S. Weir Mitchell, the eminent physiologist, physician and author, celebrated his seventy-fifth birthday on February 15. Dr. Weir Mitchell presented the candidates for honorary degrees at the celebration of the University of Pennsylvania on February 22. Degrees were conferred on President Roosevelt and on the Emperor of Germany.

Breakers-Up of the Dead.—From *World's Work*, the following account of a peculiar vocation in Lhasa is taken. It is a town of low, uninteresting houses, herded together in an aimless confusion, but beyond question the most ragged and disreputable quarter of all is that occupied by the famous tribe of Ragyabas, or beggar scavengers. These men are also the breakers up of the dead. It is difficult to imagine a more repulsive occupation, a more brutalized type of humanity, and, above all, a more abominable and foul sort of hovel than that which is characteristic of these men. Filthy in appearance, half-naked, half-clothed in obscene rags, these nasty folk live in houses which a respectable pig would refuse to occupy. A characteristic hut is about four feet in height, compounded of filth and the horns of cattle. These men exact high fees for disposing ceremonially of dead bodies. The limbs and trunk of the deceased person are hacked apart and exposed on low, flat stones, until they are consumed by the dogs, pigs, and vultures, with which Lhasa swarms.

Consumption Among Shoe Workers.—An astonishing statement comes from Lynn, as to the number of deaths there from consumption among shoe operatives, there having been 160 within the past three years. Considerably more than half the total number of deaths were from that disease, there having been 297 in all. Hygienic and sanitary conditions must be very much in need of betterment when such a proportion as that is recorded of deaths due to one disease. The savage winds of the East coasts are not soothing or healing to delicate lungs, as many St. Louis people are aware who have lived there, but the deadly effect would hardly be credited except for reliable statistics. There are a number of Lynners in the St. Louis shops. Most of them look solid and hearty, physically. The dry, crisp Western air appears to agree with them. It would appear advisable when such a preponderance of deaths resulted in any community from a single disease, to take prompt steps to improve conditions. There is certainly an appreciable economic loss in a death every week (in the average) from a disease that modern science declares is, to a large extent, preventable.

The Japanese Bath.—The betterment workers of the Colorado Fuel & Iron Co. have encountered some very interesting phases of human nature in their work. An amusing instance of race customs and prejudices is recorded in the March *World's Work* by Mr. Lawrence

Lewis, as follows: Differences in customs, too, require careful study. For example, a gang of fifty Japanese miners, after working two days in one of the large mines, sent a polite message to the superintendent, that it would be impossible for them to continue to work unless provision were made for them to take baths every day when they came from the mine. This made the company's surgeon—who had striven, sometimes vainly, with Mexicans, Slavs and Italians to induce them not to slaughter goats in their sitting-rooms, and at least to throw offal outside the houses where the company's scavenger could get at it on his daily rounds—almost delirious with joy. The superintendent had a large tank constructed of boiler-plate. Every day this was filled with fresh water, which was heated by a fire built beneath and by hot stones thrown into the water. At the change of shifts, all the Japanese, who made no further complaints, went into this tank and thoroughly bathed before going to their houses. The Italians and other "Christian" workmen, who luxuriate in the accumulated sweat and coal dust of years, and whose children are regularly "sewn up" for the winter, spoke with contempt of the "little heathen monkeys" who "must be very dirty since they love to bathe so much."

Annual Meeting of the Instructive District Nursing Association.—A meeting was held at Boston recently by the Instructive District Nursing Association. Mrs. Elizabeth P. Cordner presided, and addresses were made by the Rev. Paul Revere Frothingham, President Robert A. Boit, of the Boston Dispensary, Dr. Arnold F. Furrer, house physician of the Lying-in Hospital; Miss Stark, superintendent of the district nurses, and Helen E. Cary, nurse, the latter outlining her day's work among the sick. In her report the secretary, Mrs. E. A. Codman, said the association was founded nineteen years ago by Miss Abbie C. Howe and Miss Phœbe G. Adams in Boston, and has become a large and necessary body, employing a large number of nurses. The association needs $16,000 for its work in Greater Boston. The cooperation of all the hospitals in Boston has been of great service in developing it. For visits this year the association has received $126.75, which is a great increase over previous years. People able to pay 50 cents a visit or $10 a week generally are referred to the Nurses' Club, which supplies nurses at those rates. The staff last year consisted of a superintendent and assistant, 13 nurses and office agent, and the number of cases attended last year was 8,122, and the number of visits made 75,420. Through the kindness of Dr. G. S. C. Badger, a course of lectures for nurses was carried on. This year Dr. Samuel Robinson has arranged the course. The lectures have been given by Dr. Harris P. Mosher, Dr. C. Morton Smith, Dr. Arthur W. Fairbanks, Dr. Joshua C. Hubbard, Dr. Daniel H. Craig and Dr. Samuel Robinson. During the year a legacy of $100 from the will of Mme. Gaillard, a gift to the permanent fund of $200 from H. E. C., $100 from the Roxbury Charitable Society, and $500 from a member of the Church of the Advent were received. Miss Carey gave $700 for the support of a nurse, in memory of her mother, Mrs. Richard Carey, and in January $1,000 was received from the Society for the Relief of Sick poor in Roxbury, and with the consent of Miss Carey and the Roxbury society two more nurses were named, thus giving the association seven named nurses, leaving three more to be supported.

OBITUARY.

Dr. E. C. W. O'BRIEN, one of the best known physicians in the upper part of the State, died in Buffalo last week. He was curator of the University of Buf-

falo and was an alienist of high reputation. President Cleveland sent his name to the Senate to be Health Officer of the Port of New York, but the nomination failed of confirmation. Dr. O'Brien was about sixty-five years old.

Dr. WILLIAM EDWARD GRIFFITHS, a well-known Brooklyn physician, died last Monday at his home, 320 Schermerhorn street, Brooklyn, N. Y., in his sixty-third year. His great-grandfather, John Griffiths, came from France as a lieutenant under Lafayette in 1777, and served all through the Revolutionary War. Before his graduation from the College of Physicians and Surgeons of New York in 1868, Dr. Griffiths served for two years as surgeon's steward on the United States frigate Colorado in the Civil War. He was visiting surgeon and consulting physician of St. Mary's Hospital and a member of the Kings County Medical Society. He served for fourteen years in the Brooklyn Health Department as a sanitary inspector and chief inspector of contagious diseases.

Dr. JOHN HERBERT CLAIBORNE, one of the best known physicians in Virginia, died at his home in Petersburg, Va., last week, after a brief illness. In June, 1864, when General Lee's army occupied Petersburg, Dr. Claiborne was senior surgeon of the post and chief surgeon of all the military hospitals in Petersburg. He was ex-president of the Medical Society of Virginia, a member of the Southern Surgical and Gynecological Association, of the American Medical Association, a member of the American Health Association and the Boston Gynecological Association, and a Fellow-elect of Victoria Institute of Great Britain. He leaves a widow and several children, among whom is Dr. John Herbert Claiborne, Jr., of New York.

CORRESPONDENCE.

OUR LONDON LETTER.

(From our Special Correspondent.)

LONDON, February 18.

DEATH OF A FASHIONABLE DOCTOR—CHARLATANISM AND SUCCESS—SCHOOL HYGIENE—THE PREVENTION OF SEA-SICKNESS—THE MEDICAL SERVICE OF THE NAVY.

DR. ROBSON ROOSE, who has just passed away at the age of fifty-six years, spent the last few years of his life in a state of what astronomers call occultation. Although he never held a place even among the *minora sidera* of scientific medicine, he shone for a long time in the public eye by a kind of literary flashlight advertisement, and in this way came to be taken by London society for a professional star of the first magnitude. In his early days he walked the trivial round of drudgery in the lower walks of practice, till fortune smiled upon him in the shape of an elderly lady who bequeathed him a comfortable property. His aspiring soul being set free for a loftier flight, he established himself as a quasi-consulting physician at Brighton, a health resort ou the South Coast much frequented by the fashionable world. There, to speak, like Hamlet, " tropically," Roose soon waxed fat, and he soon sought a larger sphere for his undoubted business ability in London. For many years the aristocracy and plutocracy of this country sought counsel of him as if he had been an oracle of God. Nor was it only the "better vulgar," as old Bishop Warburton styled them, that he dragged captive at his chariot wheels. Among his most confiding patients were leading statesmen like Joseph Chamberlain, Randolph Churchill and the Duke of Devonshire; shrewd men of the world like Henry Labouchere, the genial editor of *Truth;* Edmund Yates, founder and for many ears editor of the *World;* Burnand, the editor of *Punch;* Escott, formerly editor of the *Fortnightly Review,* and many other men of light and leading in the political and literary worlds, not to mention bishops, judges and magnates of all kinds. The journalists "boomed" him to such an extent that his name became to judicious readers as great a bore as that of Aristides the Just did to the illiterate voter of Athens. He was privileged to physic the family of our present Gracious Sovereign. And yet the man was looked upon by those who trusted him so much as little better than a fool outside the narrow circle of medical practice. They were never tired of telling stories of his ignorance and ineptitude; they regarded him as intellectually a cipher and treated him at his own table as, from a conversational point of view, a negligible quantity. As a personality he was *nil.* Yet the men who laughed most at him believed in him with unshaken faith as a "good doctor." What then, it may be asked, was the secret of his success? The answer is that, unlike John Arbuthnot, who "knew his art but not his trade," Roose always understood the patient, however little he might understand his disease. He never lost an opportunity of throwing out a line and in this way he landed many a big fish. At a country house he would talk to the people whom he met about their looks and suggest that they should allow him to overhaul them in a friendly way while they were dressing for dinner. To those who rejected these overtures he would discourse warningly about "latent germs of disease." He came to be known as the "touting doctor," but how well Roose understood the average man is shown by the fact that many of those who complained of his touting afterward became his patients. He was a great giver of dinners, always with an eye to business; and he did things in this way that a man of less cheerful impudence would never have dared to attempt. Having got hold of some first rate decoy ducks like the late Duke of Beaufort and Ismail Pacha, he would ask prominent personages with whom he had scarcely any acquaintance to meet them. And as snobbishness springs eternal in the British breast, they accepted his invitations. Political leaders came to look upon his house as a neutral territory where they could meet "without prejudice," as the lawyers say. Another means of keeping his name before the public was the writing of books and articles in the monthly magazines. Roose could hardly put two sentences together, but a man with money can always go into the market and hire a scribe. With the help of an "affable familiar ghost," he gave the world his views on gout, on nerve prostration and kindred matters. There was nothing in his books, but they served their purpose. For a long time Roose was the spoilt child of fortune; then came a cloud of financial trouble which overshadowed the later part of his career. If there was a good deal of the charlatan in him there was much also that was good, or he never could have held so many men of intellect and character in bondage.

After all Roose was no worse than most physicians who achieve what in the eyes of the world is the highest success. Not long ago Sir William Broadbent, in an article published in our leading monthly magazine on the late Dr. T. Maclagan, who introduced the salicin treatment for rheumatism, said that "he lacked one element which goes far to constitute the successful family doctor—a touch of charlatanism." But it is not by any means the family doctor alone whose success is promoted by a touch of charlatanism. Andrew Clark had a touch of it; Charcot and Henry Thompson had more than a touch, while in Gull, Quain and Morell Mac-

kenzie it was an active ingredient. Clark had a certain set of general observations, a regular formula, and a fixed dietary which he invariably used with his patients, contriving to give each of them the impression that the directions for treatment were especially adapted to his case. His power lay largely in suggestion. "You may depend upon it," he would say, "Nature is inexorable. You cannot evade her. Sooner or later she will repay." These platitudes delivered in the tone of Sir Oracle made the dyspeptic, the neurasthenic and the brain-weary feel that they were getting treasures of practical wisdom in exchange for their guineas. Of Gull's power of saying nothing in language that seemed to mean something the stories are innumerable. Sir Samuel Wilks, for many years his colleague at Guy's Hospital, relates how he once gained the confidence of a hypochondriac with whom every other physician had failed. The patient, like all of his class, wished the doctors to believe in his different ailments, but at the same time would have been much alarmed if he had been told that there was anything the matter with him. Gull at once said to him, "You are a healthy man out of health," an explanation which so satisfied the patient that he asked Wilks why other doctors could not have told him that before. Again, a lady much out of health and having palpitation of the heart, believed she had disease of that organ, and accordingly consulted various physicians, at the same time telling them of the unheard of trials and worries she had undergone. They were all agreed that she had nothing the matter with the organ on which her whole thoughts were concentrated. She was dissatisfied, and determined to go to Gull. On her return home she said he at once perceived her ailment, for he said to her: "Madam, you have a tired heart." Perhaps Gull's greatest triumph in this kind of diplomacy was in the case of one of the biggest of Jewish financiers. The patient had Bright's disease, but the physician in attendance did not think it politic to communicate this fact to his wife lest his hated rival Gull should be called in. After pressing in vain for some definite information she insisted on calling in Gull, who, when interrogated, said: "Madam, your husband has a cachexia." "There," said the lady, turning to the discomfited physicians, "I knew Sir William Gull would know what is the matter with my husband." Sir Francis Laking, who has displaced Broadbent in the confidence of the Royal family, though only a practitioner of the most ordinary type as far as scientific knowledge goes, is a consummate diplomat. Broadbent held it to be inconsistent with his duty as a physician to prophesy smooth things; such a man was out of place at Court where unpleasant truths must be conveyed, like M. de Pourceccugnac's clyster, in the blandest and most benign manner.

A conference on School Hygiene organized by the Royal Sanitary Institute with the object of arousing public interest in the matter and so preparing the way for the International Congress which is to be held in London in 1907, was opened on February 7 under the presidency of Sir Arthur Rucker, Principal of the University of London. Among the subjects discussed was physical and mental development during school life. As the outcome of the debate it was resolved that the Council of the Sanitary Institute should be asked to bring the following propositions to the notice of education authorities: (*a*) That for younger scholars, at all events, there should be no home lessons after school hours. (*b*) That the periods for school lessons should be short (twenty to fifty minutes), and that there should be increasing intervals of not less than five minutes between successive lessons, for recreation, taken if possible in the open air. (c) That suitable breathing exercises should be practised at least once during each school session, in the open air or in well-ventilated rooms. (d) That organized drill should be regularly practised by the pupils in every school. (e) That the acquisition of swimming should be encouraged in every school, and should be taught to the pupils wherever practicable. (f) That an efficient system of fire-drill should be compulsory in every school (and in each "house" of boarding schools conducted on the house system), and should be practised at least three times in the course of each school term. (g) That in the opinion of this meeting of the Conference on School Hygiene ample hours of sleep, according to age, are essential to the wellbeing of growing boys.'

The physical inspection of school children was also debated and resolutions were passed that inspectors of schools should be qualified in hygiene and familiar with the development of child life. The attention of the Board of Education was called to the results of an inquiry made both in urban and in rural schools among inspectors and teachers which showed the great importance of appointing properly qualified women as inspectors for infants' and girls' schools of all grades, for pupil teachers' centers and for training colleges. The meeting further expressed the opinion that having regard to the greater susceptibility to infectious diseases among school children, no child should be allowed to begin formal instruction in classes under the age of six years. It further asked that there should be regular and systematic medical inspection of children in schools of all grades.

Another subject discussed was the sanitary inspection of schools, but after much discussion the only conclusion arrived at was that the question should be referred to the Council of the Sanitary Institute for consideration. Mr. Walter Whitehouse, a London dentist, claims to have solved the problem of seasickness. His contrivance is described as a self-levelling bunk. It is suspended in a steel framework from the roof of one of the deck cabins, and the motion of the boat is counteracted by four cords from each corner, which pass through electric brakes. These automatically maintain the cot in a horizontal position. The berth is fitted with a water mattress, and has an electric fan which can be set in motion by touching a button, and drives a delicious draught across the face of the occupant. The berth is said to be motionless, however heavily the sea may be rolling. Two boats, the "Lord Warden" and the "Calais," which carry passengers across the channel, have been fitted with the swinging cots, on the perfecting of which the inventor says he has spent three years. Mr. Whitehouse, who says he is a bad sailor, assures us that ensconced in his swinging cot he thinks no more of crossing the Channel than of drawing a tooth. But things which succeed with the inventor have an unfortunate tendency to fail when tried by other people. The principle of the swinging berth is of course not new. One remembers the *Calais-Douvres*, which was a vessel with a hull within a hull, the inner being swung and balanced so as not to move the outer. That vessel ran for many years between Calais and Dover, but it did not appreciably diminish the amount of seasickness among its passengers. The *Castalia*, another ship which made the same passage a few times some twenty-five or thirty years ago, was another illustration of the difference between theory and fact. The idea was to minimize the pitching and rolling by means of a saloon suspended like a hammock. The public found the *Castalia* a failure, and even its inventors were fain

to admit that if the rolling was lessened the pitching was not diminished. A German inventor not long ago read a paper before the Society of Naval Architects in which he proposed to fit an enormous fly-wheel weighing several tons to passenger steamers; according to the inventor, the "gyroscopic" effect of this apparatus would keep the vessel steady even in rough weather. This dainty device was never, I believe, tried at sea.

Our administrators are never tired of tinkering at the medical services of the Army and Navy. The Navy at present rejoices in a chief, Sir John Arbuthnot Fisher, who is anxious that every one under him should have the strenuous life. There is of course an excellent thing, but the chief himself is perhaps a little too strenuous. Seeking everywhere for outlets for his reforming energy, he naturally comes across the medical service of the Navy. It is only about a year since important reforms were made in that service which have gone far to make its officers contented with their lot—no mean achievement with a body of men who are somewhat difficult to please. It is rumored, however, that Fisher intends to make some further changes of a drastic character. He is credited with the intention of reforming the service altogether—by the summary process of abolishing it. His scheme is said to be to engage civilian practitioners for the length of the ship's commission—usually three years—leaving them at the end of it free to engage again if they think fit. The pay is to be at a uniform rate of five dollars a day, and there will be no pension—only a gratuity of $2,500 after a period of service exceeding five years. Lord Wolseley cherished the idea of providing medical attendance for the army by the same simple plan, but had to abandon it as unworkable. The report seems too absurd for belief. But unfortunately the fact that a project is absurd and impracticable affords no security that administrative reformers will not attempt to put it into execution.

SOCIETY PROCEEDINGS.

CHICAGO SURGICAL SOCIETY.

Stated Meeting, held November 22, 1904.

The President, Arthur B. Hosmer, M.D., in the Chair.

Congenital Deformities of the Knee.—Dr. John Ridlon read a paper on this subject, and said that congenital deformities of the knee are often called congenital dislocations, but in so far as he knows true congenital dislocation does not occur at this joint. The congenital defects and deformities at the knee were mentioned. The cause of them is not known. Many interesting theories have been advanced, but none have been substantiated in any more than a few instances, in fact usually in only one instance. His own opinion is that these conditions are only some of the many instances of defective development of the embryo. The only basis of this opinion is the fact that these knee defects are, as a rule, associated with other congenital defects, such as clubfoot, clubhand, congenital dislocation at the hip, defective shoulders, elbows and wrists. He has had one case of congenital in-knee. The in-knee deformity was associated with an equal amount of flexion deformity, and with congenital talipes equinovalgus. The child is now three years of age, but the patella cannot yet be felt. The knee deformity was corrected about a year ago by forcible hand straightening and prolonged retention in a plaster splint. Congenital out-knee he has not seen. Theoretically, one should treat it on the same principles as in-knee. Both conditions should be corrected by osteoclasis or by osteotomy. In congenital flexed knee the knee cannot be fully extended to the straight line to within fifteen or twenty degrees. Sometimes it cannot be flexed more than for a few degrees. The patella may be present or may be absent. He has had one case of flexed knee in conjunction with in-knee, and two patients, four knees, with flexion deformity without lateral deformity. One of these cases also had congenital talipes equinovarus, dislocation anteriorly of both hips and flexion deformity at the elbows similar to that at the knees. The other child had all these defects and in addition adduction deformity at both shoulders and clubhands. The treatment of flexion deformity at the knee consists in forcible manual straightening, with prolonged retention in plaster splints, followed by massage and passive flexion exercises. The congenitally hyper-extended knee is commonly called genu recurvatum. The knee is in no sense curved or recurved. The deformity is an angular one, with the opening of the angle in front, the shin approaching more or less nearly to the anterior surface of the thigh, it being possible in untreated cases to flex the leg on the thigh not beyond, and sometimes not to, a straight line. During the past twelve years he has seen seven such knees in four patients. In all the patella was absent at birth, and only appeared when, after treatment by passive motion, it was possible to fully straighten, or somewhat flex, the legs on the thighs. One child had both knees hyperextended; one, a sister of first, had both knees hyperextended and one hip dislocated; another had both knees hyperextended and double talipes equinovarus; and the other child had one knee hyperextended, the talipes equinovarus and dislocation of the hip on the same side. The treatment is daily massage and strong passive flexion of the legs on the thighs. In one of these patients, an infant in arms, the mother while making strong passive flexion fractured the femur near its lower end. He was not able to satisfy himself whether the fracture was at the epiphyseal line or just above it. Of outward rotation of the tibia on the femur, he has had one patient, two knees. There was also flexion deformity and permanent outward displacement of the patellæ. This patient was nineteen years old when he came to Chicago from Nebraska to consult Professor Lorenz. Patient gave the following history: He was born with his legs and feet turned backward. When three months old some operation was made to correct the deformity. This left him with legs flexed on the thighs about forty-five degrees. Through subsequent stretching, when he was five years old, and again when he was twelve, the angle was reduced to about fifty degrees. He was unable to voluntarily straighten the legs beyond forty-five degrees, and wore braces to get around. Professor Lorenz, when he examined him, told him that there was no similar case on record. He expressed the opinion that an operation would be of benefit, and referred him to Dr. Ridlon for treatment. Examination at this time showed a flexion deformity of about forty-five degrees. Beyond this point the legs could be flexed normally. There was practically no lateral deformity. The tibæ were rotated outward on the femora about forty-five degrees. The patellæ lay directly to the

outer side of the outer condyles, and we're of nearly normal size. In discussing the case with Professor Lorenz, he (Lorenz) advised using the utmost manual force to loosen up these knee-joints, not only to correct, but if possible overcome, the flexion deformity, and if possible rotate the tibiæ to their normal relations. The operation, with these hopes in view, was made by Dr. Ridlon on December 1, 1902. He was able to fully extend, even overextend, the legs on the thighs, but was not able to rotate the tibiæ into any appreciable extent. The knees were put in plaster splints somewhat hyperextended. He did not see the patient until some four or five days later. At that time both feet were greatly swollen and there was complete loss of sensation and movement in them. The plaster splints were opened up and the knees allowed to flex sufficiently to relieve the tension. The swelling rapidly disappeared from the left leg, and sensation and motion returned after some months. On the right leg there was an enormous blood blister some three inches wide, and extending from the middle of the leg to the heel, and along the entire outer side of the foot. At the knee there was a pressure sore, some two inches in diameter, and at the back of the ankle another some four inches long. In addition to this, the whole foot and two-thirds of the leg showed beginning gangrenous discoloration. Hot boric acid applications gradually cleared up this condition; but sensation and motion did not fully return for more than a year. After the dangerous symptoms had subsided, plaster splints were again applied with the knees slightly flexed; and these were worn with one change until July 13, 1903, about seven and a half months. Since then he has been treated by massage and active and passive movements, and he is now able to walk with a cane. (Patient was exhibited, and walked without a cane.) The immediate results from this operation show very clearly the risks from overstretching blood vessels and nerves; and the final result shows that it is possible to gain a functionally good limb in these cases of permanently displaced patellæ without a radical cutting operation.

Bilateral Torticollis Incidental to Friedreich's Disease.—Dr. Frederick Cleveland Test showed a man, forty-two years of age, who, in 1890, following an attack of grippe, was seized with practically complete loss of voice. Following a second attack of grippe, in 1894, a few weeks after the onset he was awakened during the night by finding that his head had begun a series of spasmodic movements from one side to the other. These movements have kept on, varying, sometimes worse, sometimes better, from that time to this. At present the spasmodic contractions are materially less than they were a year and a half ago, the length of time the patient has been under Dr. Test's observation. The condition, he said, is that of Friedreich's disease, in which the choreic movements of the head, and sometimes of the arms, are usually present in the severer cases of long standing. Ataxia of the legs and of the hands is marked, so that the patient is scarcely able to walk or write; but this was not noticed by him until he came to Chicago from his home in Nebraska; that is, the movements of the head were so markedly severe that they occupied practically all of his attention, so that he cannot tell just when it was he began to walk imperfectly. He walks now somewhat better than he did, but not very much better, and while he has of late years acquired the habit, or devised a method, of holding his head with his right hand to limit the movements of it, still the contractions are so great that when he is not wearing a brace, he needs to hold his head with one hand in order to be able to walk and keep his balance, and see where he is going. He presented the patient because the spasmodic contraction is double in character. Spasmodic torticollis ordinarily is unilateral, while in this case it is bilateral. It is apparently a contraction due to alternate contraction of the sternomastoid muscles, although he was inclined to think that some other muscles were involved ot a varying extent. But the sternomastoid is the muscle that is most affected. Dr. Test said he had some thoughts later on of doing resection of the spinal accessory nerve, but it was at present under advisement.

For the last sixteen months patient has had, with a few interruptions, daily treatments of electricity of the high frequency type, and during the first four months improved greatly, so much so that he was able to write a considerable number of words before his hand began to lose power to guide the pen properly. His ability to walk increased, so that he walked the distance from his house to Dr. Test's office, a mile and one-quarter, in twenty-seven minutes, whereas four months previously it took him forty-five minutes. The head movements decreased in number. Since a third (light) attack of grippe which he suffered last October, thirteen months ago, the ataxia has remained at a standstill; that is, there has been no apparent improvement in the ataxia of the legs or of the hands or arms. The torticollis, however, has improved, slowly, since that time. As treatment, patient has had extract of spinal cord, zinc phosphide, hyoscynamine, lecithin, and two or three other agents that have been recommended by consultants. As usual in these nervous cases the contractions are worse when he is thinking about them; but when he is reading a paper, for instance, with his attention concentrated on something, there is almost a cessation of the contractions; and at night, when he is asleep, the contractions are at a standstill. The muscles involved seem to be those in front of the neck. As is usually the case with Friedreich's disease, this patient has right upper dorsal scoliosis.

Dr. Wallace Blanchard said if his memory served him right, in Friedreich's disease there is very seldom much ataxia; although Dr. Test's case might be an exception to that rule.

Hereditary Ataxia.—Dr. Test said the technical term for Friedreich's disease is " Hereditary Ataxia," which, he thought, would settle the matter as to whether ataxia is ordinarily present or not. There was no family history of ataxia obtainable, but there was one marked neurotic condition present, and that is, the father, mother, and two or three brothers, and sisters of the patient are Christian Scientists! In that respect there is undoubtedly a family neurosis! But there is no spinal neurosis in any member of the family of which he could obtain a history. He believes that in Friedreich's disease, which is the first cousin to locomotor ataxia, the ataxia is a marked symptom. In Friedreich's disease ordinarily the attack comes on in childhood, from ten to fifteen or twenty years of age. In the present case the patient was twenty-eight years old before he lost his voice, and thirty-two years before the choreiform movements or torticollis began.

Dr. Blanchard has seen several cases of Friedreich's disease occur from fright, falls or sudden shock, in adults without any ataxia. At that time he paid very little attention to this subject. But it seemed to him as if ataxia was excluded from Friedreich's disease, the spasmodic condition being brought on, as it usually is, if he understood it correctly, by sudden fright or injury.

Dr. Ryerson said the man had an intention-spasm which simulated somewhat paralysis agitans.

Dr. Test said the patient had been seen by Dr. Daniel R. Brower, who agreed with the diagnosis of Friedreich's disease. In the literature of the subject ataxia is mentioned as one of the earliest and most prominent symptoms, beginning in the feet, and finally involving the legs and body.

Dr. Arthur B. Hosmer concurred in what Dr. Test had said, namely, that Friedreich's disease and Friedreich's ataxia are synonymous terms among neurologists, and during the first four years understood that it was invariably hereditary; although traumatism might be an exciting cause of tuberculosis, he did not think this ataxia was due to fright or traumatism. Ataxia usually of all four extremities is an invariable accompaniment of the disease. It seems strange that the disease should have developed at so late a period as it had in this case. He supposed it had its incipiency at about the age of puberty.

Dr. Ryerson called attention to the patient's gait, saying it was more of a spastic gait than an ataxic one.

Dr. Hosmer said locomotor ataxia was usually regarded as a disease of syphilitic origin, involving the cord, while Friedreich's ataxia involved the cerebellum as well, consequently the gait was more or less spastic from the irregular contractions of different muscles here and there. As to the utility of resecting the spinal accessory, it would stop the spasm in the sternomastoid only temporarily. If, in this case, all of the outer muscles were involved, he doubted very much whether there would be permanent improvement from resection of the spinal accessory.

Two Cases of Hereditary Contracture of the Feet, with Operation.—Dr. John Lincoln Porter stated that although the influence of heredity in the etiology of Dupuytren's contraction of the palmar fascia has been recognized as a factor in many instances, the occurrence of an analogous condition in the feet, with distinct hereditary history, seems to have been observed so seldom as to make these cases of interest. He has found nothing on the subject in the literature. In 1885, Shaffer described under the title " Non-Deforming Clubfoot " a very similar condition, but his cases differed from those of the essayist in several particulars, and so far as the title " non-deforming " is concerned, it would certainly be a misnomer for his cases, as the deformity was marked in both. Shaffer does not mention the factor of heredity in the etiology of any of his cases. Whitman describes the condition more nearly under the title of " Contracted Foot," but neither does he seem to have noticed any hereditary influence in his cases. The condition is also described very closely by other writers under the names talipes arcuatus and talipes plantaris, but perhaps because the patients were younger, the deformity in all cases reported seemed to have been less than in his. To be sure, the disability if more prominent than, and out of proportion to, the deformity, but he believes every case that is allowed to go on to middle life without treatment will result in as much distortion as the ordinary paralytic clubfoot. The condition in an advanced case is as follows: The anteroposterior arch of the foot is increased, producing a hollow foot, and the convexity of the dorsum is correspondingly increased; the foot turns inward, usually in a position of slight varus, although in some cases the foot is everted as in flatfoot. The .toes are flexed, like a hammer-toe, and when the patient stands the ends of the toes come firmly down on the ground. The weight is borne on the heels and heads of the metatarsal bones and the patient walks, stiffly with an inelastic, jarring gait, as in flatfoot. Dorsi-flexion of the ankle is lost and usually the motion in pronation and supination is very slight. The patient complains of pain in the arch of the foot, often extending up into the calf, and also of pain in the transverse arch, which is usually obliterated. The pain grows worse, involving the whole foot and leg upon long standing, or walking, and some of the cases are virtually crippled from the pain and disability and unable to walk but a short distance without rest. Pathology can hardly be discussed, as so little is known.

Case I.—In May, 1903, Mrs. E. F., came under observation with the following history: Aged thirty years; housewife; had for many years had weak feet and painful cramping pains in the feet upon walking. This had grown gradually worse until her first child was born, when it grew worse rapidly. She has had two children in the past four years, and during that time her feet had become so bad that she could scarcely get about to do her housework. She had to sit down and rest and change her shoes several times a day, and did not pretend to walk outside of the house. She could not walk at all without shoes. Her mother is living and well, except for a facial paralysis which she has had since childhood. Father dead; cause of death not ascertained. He had Dupuytren's contraction of palmar fascia and some trouble with his feet which practically crippled him, and for which he had some of his toes amputated. The patient believes her father's trouble was identical with hers. She has a sister, older, who has the same trouble, and a brother, younger, who has trouble with his feet, but not as bad. A still older half-sister by another father has no trouble whatever. Marked increase in arch of both feet; heads of metatarsals very prominent on plantar surface, and covered with calluses. Toes dorsiflexed at first phalanx, and plantar flexed at the ends, and joints covered with calluses. Feet cannot be dorsiflexed beyond a right angle, and only to that degree by great force. Cannot take two steps without shoes, and inner sole of shoes has two rows of deep indentations where heads of metatarsals and ends of toes have made pressure. The plantar fascia feels hard, especially the inner half. The tendo-Achilles prominent; feet slightly inverted in walking, and the ankles tend to turn out.

Operation, May, 1903. Tenotomy of flexor longus pollicis and flexor communis digitorum at the inner malleolus by open incision and of the short flexors at the roots of the toes. Section of the plantar fascia subcutaneously and of all tense tissues that could be felt through the skin. Then the foot was forcibly flattened out and softened as much as possible by manipulation, and the toes extended. Then the

tendo Achillis was divided subcutaneously and the feet dorsi-flexed and put up in plaster. The patient was advised to begin standing on her feet as soon· as possible, which she did in about ten days, and in spite of dissection of the tendo Achillis she was able to walk in the plaster casts in about two weeks. The casts were removed in four weeks, and the patient went home, 'wearing shoes with the toes strapped down to an insole. She has been very greatly improved and able to walk good distances,. and do her work as housewife on a farm. She was instructed to keep all the tendons of the feet stretched by exercises and massage for fear of a relapse. Lately, she has written him complaining of some pain in the feet, particularly in the dorsum of one foot. In June last (1904) her older sister came to him for relief from the same condition. Her disability was even greater than her sister's, and this was made still worse by mutilation, she having had the second and third toes of one foot and the middle of the foot amputated some three years ago. This operation was done under the delusion that the trouble lay in the cramping of the toes, and the patient says that since the toes were amputated the feet had grown rapidly worse. When she appeared for operation she hobbled around and could scarcely stand without shoes on.

Case II.—A similar operation to the one described above was done, except all the flexor tendons were divided at the roots of the toes instead of going after the long flexors behind the malleoli. Even after section of all the tendons and fascia, great force was required to soften up the feet and extend the toes, and one toe was so resistant it had to be attacked three times, and finally the scar tissue about it resulting from the amputations had to be divided freely as well as the skin on the plantar surface. Recovery took longer than in the first case, but the patient is now going about her occupation, very much improved, and very comfortable.

Case III.—The brother, younger than either of the cases reported above, has typical weak feet, though the arches are not flattened. Dr. Ridlon fitted a footplate for one foot two years ago, and he was very comfortable until the past summer, when he began to complain of recurring weakness and beginning trouble in the other foot, when he advised him to have plates made for both feet. After ten days' rest in plaster-of-Paris for the worse foot, a pair of plates with flanges to prevent pronation were fitted, and patient was now on his feet all day, with perfect comfort.

Dr. Porter's cases were discussed by Drs. John Ridlon and A. B. Hosmer.

Dr. Arthur B. Hosmer showed a combination of shoe and brace for supporting weak foot.

PHILADELPHIA COUNTY MEDICAL SOCIETY.

Stated Meeting, held November 9, 1904.

The President, Dr. Roland G. Curtin, in the Chair.

Fibroma of the Uterus, Complicated by Disorders of the Heart and Kidneys. Uremia Without Nephritis from Tumor Pressure.—Dr. George Erety Shoemaker said that later observations of this class of growths had shown that the harmless tumor is comparatively rare, if the past, present, and future of the individual are considered. Some complications are caused by the tumor, others are aggravated by its· presence. Salpingitis, peritonitis, intestinal obstruction, dystocia, diseases of the bladder, secondary anemia, depression of the nervous system from starvation due to hemorrhage, ascending kidney disease, dilatation of the heart from back pressure, and degeneration of the heart muscle may be mentioned. Questions of management in the relatively simple groups which differed from those where serious diseases of other organs exist. The nicest consideration, Dr. Shoemaker said, must be given to individual conditions. Cases having visceral lesions may be operated with advantage, if the presence of the tumor seriously exhausts the vitality or complicates the situation, provided that a reasonable margin of safety can be shown. Careful preparation of the individual is then essential, possibly lasting weeks. Surprisingly good results follow. Cases were given which recovered from hysterectomy, one showing mitral disease, another arteriosclerosis and valvular disease of the heart, another profound uremia without nephritis due to ball valve pressure of an enormous movable tumor intermittently obstructing ureters. Still another case showed serious heart weakness, etc.

Dr. Judson Daland thought that the recurrence of hemorrhage over a period of two years in one case showed the probable effect in heart action. The thing most apparent by the report is that even in those cases in which the conditions made operation necessary there was no serious heart complication, showing that in a number of cardiac diseases, more or less serious, where abdominal section may be demanded, the operative procedure coupled with anesthesia may be performed without serious hemorrhage. He thought that on the whole the danger to such cases was less than has usually been supposed from previous studies of cardiac cases in relation to operation.

The Schott Method of Treating Diseases of the Heart and Blood Vessels.—Dr. James M. Anders pointed out that confusion reigns in the minds of many physicians as to what constitutes suitable cases for the Schott method of treating chronic cardiovascular affections. On the other hand, the Schott method, he believed, had not been as universally appreciated as it deserves. He emphasizes the fact that while a salubrious environment shares in the production of the beneficial effects from this mode of treatment, the principal factors are the methodical use of the saline baths and the "resistance exercises." The baths exert a beneficial influence in various directions in cardiac insufficiency, and prominent among the salient results are a more vigorous systole, with diminution in the size of the dilated heart and a reduction of the pulse-rate.

Especially noteworthy are the effects in impaired nutrition of the myocardium in consequence of a freer, coronary circulation. He had seen all the usual evidences of an impaired circulation presented by the different organs, as the lungs, liver, stomach and kidneys, as well as the anasarca, promptly disappear under the influence of balneologic theraphy. Among the most notable effects of the baths was the distinct clinical evidence of an arteriodilation, as shown by the increase in the volume of the radial pulse. He laid stress upon the "resistence exercises," which form an essential element of the treatment. These require a specially trained operator. Dr. Anders reported cases which were observed by himself while they were under treatment at Nauheim through the courtesy of Prof. T. Schott. He recorded two cases of acute dilatation of the heart following chronic valvulitis, excited by overexercise, in which complete restoration of compensation was effected as the result of the Schott method of treatment. He also reported complete relief in two

cases of chronic cardiac disease with the usual form of secondary dilatation. The method was found especially valuable in arteriosclerosis with embarrassed heart action, and the special effect of the Schott method was most gratifying in cases of angina pectoris. Finally, in that large group of cases in which circulatory disturbances arise from a neurasthenic condition, happy results may be expected from a judicious employment of this now recognized mode of treatment. The metabolic processes also have been favorably influenced to a remarkable extent. Dr. Anders tabulated the contra-indications to the Schott method as follows: (1) Cases presenting fever; (2) advanced arteriosclerosis; (3) far advanced myocarditis; (4) the closing stage of chronic valvulitis, with extreme dilatation of the chambers; (5) aneurisms of the aorta or its larger trunks, except in the insipient stage; (6) in any case in which the blood pressure is lowered by the balneologic treatment; (7) cases in which a tenometric figure as low as 65 or 60 mm. of mercury is found (Schott); (8) cases in which chronic bronchitis and asthma are well marked (Baldwin).

Dr. James Tyson, in the discussion, said he had limited himself to the home use of the Nauheim baths, because in this connection there was the greatest opportunity for its employment, the expense of a trip abroad and treatment at Nauheim being impossible to the majority of persons. He does· not think a bath establishment is necessary and he has used the treatment in private houses in the use of the ordinary bath room appliances.

A person is required to conduct the bathing as well as the exercises, although both may be done by the same individual. The baths, he believed, could be made very much simpler than the paper by Beasley Thorne would lead one to believe. Chloride of sodium and the chloride of calcium were stated to be the two most important constituents. Five pounds of chloride of sodium and five ounces of chloride of calcium are put into the ordinary bath of about forty to fifty gallons of water. The course consists usually of twenty-one baths, three of which are given in succession and then a day skipped.

The proportions of sodium and calcium are increased until in the last five or six baths the water contains about ten pounds of the former and ten ounces of the latter. The carbonic acid element of the bath is secured at home by adding hydrochloric acid and bicarbonate of sodium. The cases that receive the most benefit Dr. Tyson said were those of cardiac weakness with dilatation, chronic dilatation brought about gradually as the loss of compensation is brought about in valvular cases, and also cases in which there has been over muscular exertion. Acute dilatation, he remarked, is best treated by rest in bed and the use of nitroglycerin, etc. In such a case partially recovered improvement may be completed admirably by the administration of the Nauheim bath at that stage. The baths should not be given in cases of edema and general dropsy. Dr. Tyson thought the patient a pretty good guide regarding the continuance of the bath; if he did not feel well after three or four baths, it was a mistake to continue them. Better was it to put the patient to rest. The first bath he makes five minutes in length, the second, six or seven minutes, which time is increased to ten or fifteen minutes. Coincidentally with the increased duration of the bath the temperature is lowered. Eighty-two or eighty-five, he said, was the lowest temperature at which the baths are given at Nauheim.

Dr. S. S. Cohen referred to his demonstration before

the Society of the Schott treatment some eight years ago, by the efficient aid of Dr. Charlotte West, and stated that Dr. West was available for the carrying out of the Schott resistance movements, as well as four other persons whom he had trained. He thought there was no difficulty in having the baths given at home, if the patient and physician were willing to take a little trouble in getting them started, after which intelligent patients can be entirely trusted to carry out the details. In preparing he bath the plan which Dr. Cohen has adopted and which has the advantages of preventing the cooling of the water, and injury to the tub, is to fill the tub half full of hot water, put in the brine and the bicarbonate of soda; let them remain for about twenty minutes so that they are thoroughly disseminated throughout the whole mass of water; then add sufficient water which can be cold or lukewarm, according to the temperature to which the original quantity of water has cooled; then put in the acid sulphate cakes upon the tin foil and there will be a thorough and complete effervescence.

A valuable element in the treatment at Nauheim Dr. Cohen believed was the personality of Dr. Schott. His scientific spirit, his authoritative manner, thorough mastery of routine and of detail, the absolute obedience which he gets from all the attendants he believed count for a good deal. In the home treatment Dr. Cohen's plan is to give the baths in a course of six or eight weeks, interrupting them for eight or ten or twelve weeks and then again repeating them for two or three weeks; then again interrupting them, and again repeating. The best time to give them he considered to be at night so that the patient might have several hours continuous rest afterward. He gives the baths every other day or every third day, giving exercise on the alternate days, if exercise is to be given. Sometimes the baths can be followed by massage, the character of which will vary with the character of the lesion and reaction of the patient. He confirmed Dr. Anders' statement of the value of the method in exophthalmic goiter; but, also stated that there was great danger in its employment in this condition. He would not trust patient or attendant to give the treatment in exophthalmic goiter. In a few cases he believed it would do good if carefully applied and applied by the physician himself.

In cases of arterio-sclerosis, not too far advanced, he has seen very good results; also in angina pectoris, in mitral stenosis and in mitral regurgitation. He differed from Dr. Daland concerning the resemblance between the effect of active exercise on the part of the patient and the gentle resistance movement of the Schott system. In the Schott system there is no muscular exercise on the part of the patient at all. The moment exercise is made the patient defeats the object of the treatment. The method was, he said, "gentle resistance." The benefit obtained was in the starting up of the peripheral muscular pump upon the vessels so that the action of the natural rhythmical contraction of the muscles upon the vessels continued to assist the work of the heart. The carbon dioxide gave to the "skin-heart" a much more active stimulation than could be secured from massage or electricity, though the principle was just the same. the diversion of the blood to the surface and the stimulation of the vasomotor reaction.

Dr. William S. Wadsworth referred to the physiological principles underlying all treatment. In regard to the effect of the various ingredients of the bath on the stimulation of the skin and the effect on the sensory nerves, there was, he said, a very great additional effect,

not mentioned, the effect on the skin itself. For example, putting a piece of skin, alive or dead, into water there was obtained a certain amount of maceration and an entire change in the feeling of the skin. If the finger is put into the water for half an hour the sensations are entirely different from those encountered from the air. All, he said, knew the difference between the sea bath and the ordinary bath. Another factor in the bath, he pointed out, was the suspension of the body in a material which is of a certain specific gravity. Putting the body on a water bed, he considered was also a very important factor. The changes of the specific gravity, he thought, would bear the closest clinical study and would give interesting results. In the resistance movements Dr. Wadsworth stated there was a series of valuable factors developed of a purely mechanical sort. On the chemical side there was another group; a chemical change taking place in the muscle itself. Certain substances were taken up causing change of tone of the whole system. Fatigue stuffs were thrown out which have a distinct effect on every organ that comes in contact with the blood.

Dr. Anders, in closing the discussion, said he was not convinced that the home treatment could be carried forward with much success. To have a suitable establishment in this country would require a specialist in heart diseases to make the treatment a special study and this one should watch the patient daily, noting the effect of every bath and every application of the resistance movements.

Influence of Hunger and Hemorrhage on the Composition of the Blood Plasma.—Dr. Thomas S. Githens stated that by the addition of sodium sulphate to blood plasma it was possible to separate the proteid into four bodies: Fibronogen, euglobulin, pseudoglobulin and serum albumin. He had performed two series of experiments to determine which of these bodies was nearest to the form in which proteid is ordinarily assimilated.

The series showed as a result of repeated bleedings a rapid and steady decrease in the percentage of fibrinogen and a corresponding increase in the serum albumin. Starvation, on the contrary, showed a marked increase in the percentage of total globulin and a corresponding fall in the serum albumin; but after feeding the percentage of albumin rose promptly to normal. Both effects are best explained by the assumption that albumin stands nearest to the form in which proteid is absorbed and therefore is replaced quickly in the food; while fibrinogen being more specialized is more difficult to replace.

On the Use of Methylene Blue in Malarial Fever.—Dr. H. C. Wood, Jr., reported six cases of malaria which were cured by the use of methylene blue. He has collected also from the literature 425 cases with 362 cures. Ivanoff has shown that methylene blue has a destructive action upon the adult malarial parasite, although it has but little influence upon the younger forms. Methylene blue may be given in malaria in doses of 3 grs. every three hours for several days. The treatment should be kept up with small doses for a period of two to three weeks. The unpleasant symptoms which have in many cases been associated with this drug the author thought were perhaps due to the use of the dyestuff instead of the medicinal methylene blue. The latter is the chloride of tetramethylthionin. Methylene blue it was stated rivals in its antiperiodic effect quinine, and has the advantage over the older drug of not causing the unpleasant by-symptoms commonly seen with quinine.

NEW YORK PATHOLOGICAL SOCIETY.

Regular Meeting, held October 12, 1904.

The President, Otto H. Schultze, M.D., in the Chair.

Trypanosoma Hominis and Trypanosoma Brucei. —Dr. F. C. Wood demonstrated stained slides of these. He gave a short discussion of the conditions under which these parasites occur, causing the diseases known as "sleeping sickness" and nagana.

Kala-azar.—Dr. James Ewing presented specimens of a case of this affection recently described by MARCHAND and LEDINGHAM (*Zeitsch. f. Hygiene,* Bd. xlvii). The sections were prepared from material which Prof. Marchand had very kindly presented to him in Leipzig. The sections showed large numbers of the protozoon described by Donovan, Leishmann and others, and which had first been found in the aspirated blood of the spleen. While very scanty in the circulating blood, they were enormously abundant in the viscera. The parasites occupied much enlarged recently described endothelial cells which contained from ten to one hundred in section. The structure of the parasite was very distinct even in the sections stained by hematoxylin and eosin or by Nocht's method. It consisted of a macronucleus and a very densely staining micronucleus inclosed in a protoplasmic envelope from 1 to 2 micra in diameter. It was mentioned that considerable evidence supports the belief that this body represents one phase of the life history of a trypanosome.

Widal Test in Practice.—Dr. John H. Borden presented a paper on this subject, which will be published later in the MEDICAL NEWS.

Dr. W. H. Park, in the discussion, said that it seemed to him that the method described by Dr. Borden was very much easier for the physician than the old method, but he asked whether there was any difference in results with this method of using cultures killed by carbolic acid, and the usual use, in proper proportions, of live cultures.

Dr. Borden said that he had tried a few live cultures macroscopically and they reacted very well. With the method he described the physician did not have to make plants from day to day and keep live bacilli about the house. They reacted, moreover, perfectly well. Widal himself had spoken of using the dead bacilli for his agglutination test.

Dr. F. C. Wood said that he was not willing to give up what had been to him a very important phenomenon—the motility of the bacilli. The bacilli in cases of miliary tuberculosis tested in dilutions of 1-40 and 1-60 showed persistent motility, and it was this motility which differentiated such reactions from true typhoid in which motility ceased early. He asked Dr. Borden if they had had that experience at the Presbyterian Hospital.

Dr. Borden replied that they had.

Dr. Wood asked if they had tried the suspension in cases of miliary tuberculosis.

Dr. Borden said he had tried three cases of miliary tuberculosis by the gross method and did not get the reaction in any of the tubes, 1-40, after standing several hours.

Dr. Philip Hanson Hiss said that he thought Dr. Wood's objection to dead bacilli generally held with the microscopic test. Any action we might get with tuberculosis when using the gross test was not noticeable to the eye, for although we might get very small clumps, he doubted if we would get precipitates.

Dr. E. Libman said that at the Mount Sinai Hospital they had tried the Rüdiger method with formalinized cultures. It was found not to be specific. They had had several cases, not typhoid (in two cases of which there was no fever) and the test gave a complete reaction at 1-20 and 1-50. They had given up the Rüdiger method. Whether this happened when the serum was used alone, he did not know. With the Rüdiger method the blood was diluted. They had obtained microscopic reactions with both live and dead bacilli, and they had found it better to stick to the live bacilli as the results were better. They had had positive reactions with live bacilli when the reactions were absent with dead bacilli. On the other hand, one or two cases were found to give positive reactions with dead bacilli when not positive with live. He said that microscopically, when we do get a good reaction with dead bacilli, it is as a rule better and more decided than we get in the same case with the live bacilli.

Dr. Borden said that the apparent success which he at first had with the bacilli killed with formalin was very deceiving. For a long time the reaction was thought to be specific; it did not always occur in three hours, but in the course of five or six hours a flocculent precipitate would be seen coming down. Rather arbitrarily a standard of three hours was set. This was thought to be all right, but the solutions as made up may have been a little too acid and the reaction comenced to occur before the three-hour limit. Finally, after trying a great many emulsions, the method was decided to be worthless. Whether other observers use a different method in making the suspension, Dr. Borden did not know, but apparently they used about the same. He had gained the impression in reading the articles that they had not done sufficient control work to make their results convincing. He himself had done more controls than cases.

Nerve-Cells in Rabies.—Dr. D. W. Poor reported the results of some studies on the nerve-cells in a number of cases of rabies. He found very constantly in the nerve-cells bodies which have been described by Negri as characteristic of rabies. In some of the brains the bodies were very numerous, both in the cerebrum and cerebellum; in other cases they were few in number, being seen only in the Purkinje cells of the cerebellum. When very numerous they occasionally appeared outside of the cells. The bodies found were round, oval and oblong masses, the largest being 10 to 11 micra, while the smallest appeared as minute granules scarcely visible with an oil immersion lens. The bodies varied a great deal in structure. Some contained from one to a dozen or more small granules each surrounded by a circular clear space; sometimes these filled the corpuscle completely. In other instances but little structure was found except that the periphery stained more heavily at the center, giving the appearance of ring bodies. Dr. Poor was very conservative in his discussion of the nature of these corpuscles. Negri has asserted that they are protozoa. It was suggested by Dr. Williams of the Health Department, that these bodies might be degenerated red cells. It was also possible that the corpuscles might be degenerated forms of some structure, possibly the intranuclear network of the nerve-cell. The hemosiderin reaction for iron was not given. The Negri bodies were not found in the submaxillary glands so far examined, though these glands are infectious.

Dr. Poor thought that as far as he had gone he might say that the bodies were of use in the diagnosis of rabies from a clinical point of view. For diagnostic purposes tissue should be taken from the region of Ammon's horn, the cerebellum and, if possible, from the lumbar cord.

Dr. Anna Williams, in the discussion, said that on first studying the specimens the possibility of the cell inclusions being derived from the red blood-cells seemed great, but the further the study was carried, the less the possibility seemed. The majority of the forms she had seen showed such a constant, definite and characteristic structure, that it seemed almost impossible to consider them derivatives of red blood-cells. Furthermore, a few smears which she had made and stained by the Nocht-Romanowsky method, as recommended by Dr. Ewing, stained the bodies more or less characteristically and showed no evidence of their having been derived red blood-cells or of their being cell degenerations of any kind. Dr. Williams said therefore, that as far as morphological study of stained specimens alone, could help, the evidence was in favor of the inclusions being individual organisms or protozoa.

Dr. James Ewing said that he had the pleasure of looking over some of Dr. Poor's specimens and that he had drawn impressions regarding the nature of the Negri bodies in the reverse order of those expressed by Dr. Williams. In the first cases examined, the very definite structure of the bodies in the ganglion cells, and the fact that they were totally unlike anything he had ever before seen in a considerable experience with ganglion cells examined under a high power of the microscope led him to think that they must be foreign bodies and probably protozoa. After seeing the specimen from the guinea-pig, in which the disease was of slow development, he had found, on the contrary, much evidence that the red cell theory suggested by Dr. Williams, was well founded, and would be a safe one to follow as a working hypothesis. It was well known that the cyanotic blue color of the cortex in rabies was pathognomonic and was referable to extreme distention of the blood capillaries of the gray matter. In the case of this guinea-pig, not only were the capillaries distended, but there was considerable diffuse infiltration of the gray matter with whole and fragmented but otherwise unaltered red cells. Many of these cells lay in the lymph spaces about the ganglion cells, and in the bodies of some ganglion cells there were found unaltered red cells. In this guinea-pig, but not in the other cases he had examined, there appeared to be numerous transition forms between red cells and the parasites.

The argument from such transition forms, however, Dr. Ewing did not regard as free from danger of error, and he had never seen any such degeneration forms of red cells in any other condition. Experience had shown that, whatever their nature, these bodies were diagnostic of rabies. The protozoon theory, Dr. Ewing thought, ought not to be hastily welcomed until less sensational hypothesis had been fully set aside by systematic control work. He had suggested that the staining of cells isolated by teasing and dried on a slide might give some information about the bodies more reliable than that obtained by the study of sections of tissue fixed in complex mixtures of metallic salts and acids. The fact that the bodies were not found in the

parotid and submaxillary glands, and that the virus of rabies passed the Berkefeld filter, seemed incompatible with the view that the Negri bodis were protozoan, and held a definite causal relation to rabies.

Pathological Chemistry of Tumors.—Dr. S. P. Beebe presented the results of some studies on the pathological chemistry of tumors. A striking fact about tumor tissue as compared with normal tissue was that there seemed to be large quantities of material stored up, the results of autolytic processes. In a case of carcinoma of the broad ligament Dr. Beebe had been able to extract from the new growth a considerable quantity of glycocoll. Other aminoacids, leucin, tyrosin, and tryptophan, were found in abundance in tumors which were undergoing degeneration, and also in one sarcoma which was rapidly growing and so far as could be seen not undergoing degeneration. Another substance which Dr. Beebe had obtained was a peculiar type of carbohydrate, in some ways resembling starch, in some ways, glycogen. It gave a color reaction with iodine like starch and was soluble in water. Some of the tumors analyzed contained strikingly large amounts of calcium salts. Others contained large amounts of potassium salts. The speaker did not wish it to be understood that the results given were in any way presented as leading to a new theory as to the cause of cancer.

Dr. F. C. Wood said that Dr. Beebe's findings of glycocoll in the products of autolysis of the tumor cells was especially interesting to him as he had been recently attempting to isolate glycocoll from the urine of a patient with acute yellow atrophy. Leucin and tyrosin had long been known as products of liver autolysis in acute yellow atrophy. Recently Fischer had devised a new method for isolating the amino-acids and by this means glycocoll had been found in the urine in experimental phosphorus poisoning in dogs, but as yet he knew of no records of the finding of glycocoll in acute yellow atrophy. It would be natural to expect, however, that this member of the amino-acid group would be present in the urine.

Regular Meeting, held November 9, 1904

Bile Duct Adenomata of the Liver.—Dr. Eli Moschcowitz presented a case of bile duct adenoma of the liver. The liver was removed from a patient who died at the Roosevelt Hospital on April 27, 1904. No history of the case was obtainable, but the clinical diagnosis was cerebrospinal meningitis. The autopsy was performed by Dr. Ditman. In addition to the characteristic lesions of cerebrospinal meningitis, moderate atheroma of the valves of the heart and a healing tuberculosis of the right apex were present. The liver was larger than normal and yellowish-brown in color. It was uniformly studded with small nodules, gelatinous in appearance and varying in size from the head of a pin to that of a split pea. They were very soft, sharply defined, with no definite encapsulation, and fine prolongations could be seen passing into the liver substance. The organ otherwise showed slight fatty degeneration. Microscopical examination showed an adenomatous structure, the alveoli being round, oval, or tortuous in character. They were lined with low cuboidal epithelium with a large round nucleus, in various stages of degeneration, particularly on those alveoli situated in the central part of the nodule. The lumina of the alveoli were filled with a finely granular or hyaline mass, staining evenly with eosin; but in a few instances were filled with masses of desquamatmg epithelium. The alveoli were enmeshed by dense masses of connective tissue which was fibrillar and non-cellular in the central part but very cellular toward the periphery. The cellular structures of the latter consisted of round cells and many newly formed bile ducts as are ordinarily seen in cirrhosis. These bile ducts in many places could be traced from the various stages of simple canals with no lumen to the cystic changes already described. There was no capsule, the nodules lying directly against the liver substance. There were but few blood vessels. A marked characteristic of these nodules was their intimate relation to Glisson's capsule. The normal bile ducts of the liver showed no changes. In occasional sections the lumen of the portal vein was found to contain large cells resembling in many respects liver cells. There was very little diffuse cirrhosis and the liver cells showed no changes except a moderate fatty degeneration. The picture as a whole was that of an adenomatous hyperplasia of the biliary ducts. The cases in the literature of this character were very few and resembled the one reported in almost every particular, except in the size of the new formations. The livers as usually described were riddled with cystic formations varying in size from a cherry to a child's head. So far as Dr. Moschcowitz could ascertain his case was unique in the number and the uniformly small size of the tumors. The interesting point in connection with the case was their pathogenesis—as to whether the tumors were inflammatory in character or were new growth. Dr. Moschcowitz had at first inclined to regard them as new growths, but after fuller observation had come to the belief that they were an evidence of inflammatory hyperplasia. While it could not be definitely proven that they were not new growths in the strict sense of the term, nevertheless there were many features present that strongly suggested an inflammatory origin. While there was no very extensive cirrhosis present, there was a distinct proliferation of new connective tissue in Glisson's capsule with the formation of new bile ducts such as we often see in cirrhosis. Furthermore, one could easily trace the different stages, from that of the newly formed bile ducts to that of the mature and well formed alveolus. A further evidence of a progressive inflammation lay in the slow transition from the cellular fibrous tissue in the periphery to the advanced and fibrillar connective tissue in the center. The whole picture represented a centripetal process rather than a centrifugal process such as we would expect in a new growth formation. In certain areas, old and degenerated liver cells could be found in the central part of the nodules. This might also be construed as an evidence of old inflammatory changes similar to those found in cirrhosis. There was no evidence of encapsulation as we might expect in non-malignant new growths and as is invariably found in all other adenomata of the liver. An additional evidence that the lesion was an inflammatory one lay in analogy; there was a great similarity in the microscopical picture to that of other inflammatory tumors of the liver, namely, coccidiosis. The majority of observers have regarded these nodules as new growths, but as only the advanced stages have been described this may account for their being so regarded. In an early specimen the inflammatory changes would perhaps be far more apparent than in the advanced stages in which this condition is usually seen. The cause of the dilatation of the newly formed bile ducts was hard to trace. Unfortunately, the history was not obtainable in this case, wherein there might have been found some evidence of an old inflam-

matory process. A distinct history of jaundice had been observed in a few of the cases described. Dr. Moschcowitz thought there was a possibility of there having been a cholangitis or some other form of obstruction of the biliary passages.

Photomicrographic Apparatus Using Ultraviolet Light.—Prof. S. Czapski demonstrated the new apparatus for the use of ultraviolet light for photomicroscopic purposes as manufactured by Carl Zeiss, of Jena. Prof. Czapski first discussed the methods which have been used up to the present time to increase the efficiency of the microscopic objective. He showed that the resolution was dependent upon the aperture and upon the wave length of the light used in the objective. The ordinary objective uses a light of a wave length of about five hundred and fifty millionths of a millimeter. Attempts which had been made to increase the resolving power of the objective by the use of glass of a higher refractive index combined with an immersion fluid of high-refracting power had resulted in the production of an objective of an aperture of 1.60, using monobrom-naphthalin as the immersion fluid. The difficulty of obtaining mounting fluids of this high-refracting index has greatly limited the use of such objectives so that at the present time this means of increasing the aperture of the objective may be considered as having reached its limit. The other method of improving the resolving power of the objective is to use light of a shorter wave length. It has been found possible by the use of quartz lenses, quartz condensors, and quartz slides and cover glasses to obtain an objective the aperture of which by ordinary light, is 2.5, through the use of monochromatic light of the ultraviolet region, whose wave length is two hundred seventy-five millionths of a millimeter. The resolving power of these objectives which possess a numerical aperture of 1.25 is practically twice that of the ordinary apochromatic immersion lens.

The ultraviolet rays are obtained by an electric spark passing between cadmium electrodes. The spark spectrum of cadmium gives a series of strong lines of a wave length of two hundred seventy-five millionths of a millimeter. The light derived from the spark passes through two quartz prisms in order to select this particular group of rays, and is then brought to a focus by a condenser, also of quartz. The light then passes through the object to be photographed, is collected by the objective of the microscope and the image thrown on a photographic plate by means of a quartz eyepiece.

Inasmuch as rays of this short wave length are not visible to the eye, no light in the ordinary sense passes through the microscope. The rays can be rendered visible by the use of a fluorescent screen inserted in the eyepiece. When the image so formed is observed a picture can be seen, the details of which are very imperfect. An approximate focus is then obtained, the camera is swung into place, and the photograph taken. If the focus be correct no further procedures are necessary. If, however, the picture does not appear sharp the focus is slightly changed and a second exposure made. If this is not so good as the first the focus is changed lightly in the other direction, etc.

The mounting fluids which can be used are those which are transparent to ultraviolet light, for example, water, glycerin and a saturated solution of chloral hydrate in glycerin. Prof. Czapski demonstrated a number of photographs taken by means of this apparatus, which showed very remarkable results. Especially striking were photographs of yeast-cells, which showed structures. not visible under ordinary conditions; a photograph of a transsection of a frog's eye, showing that the lens, while transparent to ordinary light, is opaque to ultraviolet light; and also some characteristic photographs of *Pleurosigma angulatum* at a magnification of twenty-five hundred diameters, which showed structures entirely different from those obtained with ordinary objectives.

Vaccine Bodies.—Dr. James Ewing spoke of a new method which he had devised for the differential staining of vaccine bodies in isolated cells, which he designated the "Klatsch" method. The 'slide used was washed in soap and water and then heated in a Bunsen flame, after which it was found that cells adhered to it very easily. Such a slide was lightly applied to a cornea representing any stage of the vaccine lesion and quickly withdrawn without any pressure or lateral motion. The slide when examined was found to have carried the impression of the lesion in the form of isolated cells which have been loosened by the edema of the inflammatory process. Repeated impressions will completely evacuate the ulcer. The cells dry instantly in the air and may be fixed and stained by the same procedures as are used in the study of blood. The best stains are obtained by fixation in 95 per cent. alcohol for ten minutes and staining by Nocht's method for ten minutes. By this means the structures and relations of the epithelial cells are much more easily made out than in sections of hardened tissues. The method had been applied to vaccine lesions in rabbits and rats. Rats are more susceptible to vaccine than rabbits and the vaccine bodies in these animals are usually larger than in rabbits. The first trace of the vaccine body, in "Klatsch" preparations, appears as a thickening and dark-red staining of several adjoining meshes of the cyto-reticulum. This area is usually found near the nucleus, but in superficial cells and in some deeper ones it may lie at some distance from the nucleus. By a gradual extension of this reticular structure almost the whole of the cytoplasm may be transferred into the vaccine body, while the nucleus, without showing signs of compression lies to one side of the cell. During these stages the reticulum of the vaccine body appears to be directly continuous with the cyto-reticulum. In rabbits this cyto-reticulum is finer than in rats and a similar difference appears in the reticulum of vaccine bodies in these two animals. The majority of vaccine bodies in isolated cells show definite connections with the nucleus. In many cases it is difficult to determine where the vaccine body begins and the nucleus ends. The staining reactions of the body also indicate that it contains chromatin. The meshes contain a homogeneous basophile material. After full development of the recticular structures two series of changes appear in the vaccine body: (1) The reticulum breaks into granules chiefly affecting the periphery; (2) basic straining material appears in the center of the vaccine body and the gradual increase of this material at the expense of the red reticulum transforms the body into a homogeneous mass which has the basic staining reactions and the appearance of mucus. The englobement and destruction of one epithelial cell by another is readily followed as is phagocytosis of leucocytes. Besides vaccine bodies other forms of perinuclear cytoplasmic degeneration may be found. In the cornea there are often large numbers of granular or ring-shaped structures from one to two micra in diameter, the nature of which it is difficult to determine. The larger ones look like early ring-shaped malarial parasites and possess chromatin granules, or they may be elongated into rods like bacteria. The smaller members of the series cannot be distinguished from cell

granules which cover the superficial cells. While the structure of vaccine bodies in "Klatsch" preparations offers strong evidence against the protozoon theory of vaccinia, there remain several hypotheses on which it may still be claimed that this body harbors the organized virus of vaccinia. It may be supposed that while the visible vaccine body is a cytoplasmic structure, yet it contains a submicroscopic organism. Or it may be supposed that the vaccine body represents a mixture of the protoplasm of the host cell and the parasitic organism, forming a mycoplasm, such as is believed to exist in wheat-rust by Ericksson and Tischler, in a disease of grape-vines, known as La Brunissure, by Debray, and in crown-gall, by Toumey. But the mycoplasmic theory has not been demonstrated even for plants and the late stages of vaccine bodies show less and not more structure than the early stages. Or, it is possible that some other method of fixation and staining than the one employed in this study may yet succeed in demonstrating some definite protozoon structure or character in the vaccine body. Since more or less specific forms of cell degeneration occur in various infectious processes, it does not seem likely that the vaccine body can be reproduced by another agent than vaccine, and accumulating evidence goes to show that this body is specific for vaccinia and the diseases closely related to it.

Cerebral Lesions.—Dr. Charles Norris presented a series of specimens showing the effect of cerebral lesions. The first specimen was a brain from a woman who died at Bellevue Hospital. Four days before admission to the hospital she had had an attack of partial unconsciousness. The muscles had become rigid and she had fallen to the floor. When picked up she was found to be paralyzed on the right side of the face and in the right arm. She also had motor aphasia. The leg was uninvolved. In the course of several days she was able to walk around and slowly recovered motion in her right arm but never in her face. She never recovered the ability to talk, though she regained almost complete use of her arm. Three weeks after the first attack she had another attack from which she did not recover. The right side of the face was partly paralyzed. She passed without warning into a semi-stuporous condition. The heart action was very slow and slightly irregular. She died about six weeks after the first attack. At autopsy the heart showed chronic mitral endocarditis with stenosis and recent vegetation. There was general congestion of all the viscera. On opening the skull there was complete cystic softening of the precentral convolution, which had practically disappeared except in the upper part, where the leg center is situated. The postcentral and the whole of the third frontal convolutions were likewise softened. The areas of softening involved the first temporal and extended into the supramarginal, but the angular gyrus. Here the softening was less marked. After the second attack in the hospital the patient had been unable at any time to read. She apparently did not understand what was said to her. She had sensory aphasia. It was hard to understand why she had recovered motion in her arm so quickly after the first attack when there was total softening of the arm center in the central convolution.

The second specimen was a carcinoma of the brain following carcinoma of the breast. Very little history had been obtained in this case. The patient had been operated upon elsewhere for the tumor of the breast and successfully, but she had re-entered the hospital for a recurrence. She was thought to be insane and was transferred to the psychopathic ward at Bellevue. She was in a very confused state of mind and had a

.paralysis of the right side. At autopsy the growth was found to involve the motor centers of the arm and leg.

The third specimen was from a case of cerebral embolism. The patient was a man who had been six weeks in the hospital. He was apparently in a very stupid condition during most of the time and after four weeks suddenly became comatose. He had hemiplegia. At autopsy the brain showed an area of cystic softening involving the Island of Reil, the claustrum, the external capsule, and the lenticular nucleus. The origin of the embolism was undoubtedly in the aorta, this being the seat of marked thrombo-arteritis. The valves of the heart were fairly normal.

A Case of Dermatobia Noxalis, with Demonstration of Larva.—Dr. Harlow Brooks presented specimens from a case of *Dermatobia noxalis*, the cases of human infection being so rare as to warrant his calling attention to this instance. He was indebted to Dr. Gillette for the specimens. The patient had been for some time in Panama, where his general health had been good until about six weeks ago, when he first noticed three small lumps, one in the groin, one on the flexor surface of the forearm and the third over the left shoulder. The patient declined surgical attendance on account of insufficient hospital facilities and returned to this country for treatment. Examination showed at the apex of each tumor a small perforation through which a small, moving, black body could be made out. The pain caused by the swellings was considerable and there was a slight rise in temperature. The tumors were opened under cocaine and the worms squeezed out. The largest larva was two cm. long and nine mm. in breadth. There was a considerable collection of pus in one of the tumors, but all of the wounds healed rapidly. Examination of the blood showed a quite marked increase in the eosinophiles. Dr. Brooks said that the larvæ had been frequently seen in the skin of various animals. He had seen it in the skin of the semidomesticated buffalo and in the skin of wild prairie dogs and wild deer. There were some sixty-four different varieties of the bot-fly and consequently sixty-four varieties of the larvæ, and he could not say to just what variety this specimen belonged. Thirteen varieties had been found to infect the skin and many of these had been seen in man. Dr. Brooks showed also a parasite from the skin of the buffalo which differed from the human parasite in the arrangement of the spines. He said that he had been told by travelers in South America that the infection there in man was fairly common.

Dr. James Ewing, in the discussion, said that he was very glad to see the specimen presented by Dr. Brooks and especially to learn the name of the parasite, as it cleared up the identity of a similar parasite which had been sent to the Cornell Laboratory by Dr. Alexander Lambert. This specimen was identical in appearance with the one shown by Dr. Brooks and was removed from a patient who gave much the same history and had recently come from Panama.

SOCIETY OF THE ALUMNI OF CITY HOSPITAL.

117th Stated Meeting, held December 14, 1904.

Tuberculoma.—Dr. Joseph F. Terriberry presented a patient who gave the following history: Russian Hebrew, about thirty-five years of age, who for the past twenty years had been a sewing-machine operator. Very recently the left testicle was removed because of tuberculous degeneration. He was in bed thirty-three days after this operation. Prior to the operation both legs had apparently been normal;

he had, at least, noted no difficulty in walking, nor had he experienced any subjective symptoms whatsoever. When he became convalescent, he noticed that the left leg was tremulous and somewhat stiff. His objective symptoms showed a diminished pain perception in the left foot and an entire absence of heat and cold perception over the same area. Tactile sensation was at this time normal. All the symptoms, both subjective and objective, not alone gradually increased in severity, but ascended the extremity at a very rapid rate. Dr. Terriberry demonstrated that pain sensation was abnormal up to a line just below the umbilicus, and showed the overlapping of perception from above down and from below up. He considered it probable that in view of the symptoms, and of the history, the patient was suffering from a tuberculoma situated in the left side of the cord at about the level of the lumbar segment. This hypothesis is further supported by a marked reaction of the patient to tuberculin injection.

Dr. Morris Manges thought that a possibility of the existence of a syringomyelia in the lower regions of the cord combined with insular sclerosis should be gravely considered, but he agreed with Dr. Terriberry that in all probability the case was a suitable one or would soon become a suitable one for operative intervention.

Pott's Disease.—Dr. J. P. Fiske presented a patient who exhibited an irregular and interesting form of Pott's disease. He had had none of the typical signs of this lesion, but a cyst had appeared in the neighborhood of the eighth costovertebral articulation. This had been opened by a hospital surgeon and appeared as a discharging sinus. When the patient came under Dr. Fiske's care, considering that it probably was a case of necrosis of the rib, he opened the sinus tract up but found the rib normal, the tract disappearing between the vertebræ. The part was disinfected and closed. A noteworthy fact was that it healed by primary intention. The doctor had ordered rubber heels and had put the patient in a very light and beautifully constructed celluloid jacket.

New Instrument.—Dr. George B. McAuliffe presented a new form of adenoid forceps, which were especially designed to protect the uvule and soft palate from injury during operation.

Papillomatous Ovary.—Dr. Brooks H. Wells recited the history of a woman, aged fifty-one years, from whom he had removed a papillomatous ovary. The specimen was thought to be malignant at first, but slides exhibited by Dr. Brooks for the Society showed a fully developed non-malignant tumor.

Gouty Diathesis.—Dr. Charles C. Ransom read a paper in which he related the history of the studies of the so-called "gouty diathesis" and showed in this sketch the gradual evolution of the present conception of the importance of uric acid as a causative factor for gout. He concluded, both as a result of his studies with Herter and from clinical observations in a great many hundred cases, that no time should be lost in discrediting the erroneous and generally accepted view that uric acid has a relation to gout. (This paper will appear in full in a subsequent issue of the MEDICAL NEWS.)

Dr. Morris Manges, in opening the discussion, dwelt on the enormous complexity of the topic and of the confusion of the widely differing views. He alluded to the interesting fact that hogs often develop a form of gout. He said that the existence of the quadri-urate has never been positively proven;

that the modern view that uric acid is a product of nucleinic·acid is probably correct; that no short statement sums the subject up so well as that expressed by Herter who states that in accepting uric acid as the cause of gout we "attribute to ash the quality of flame." He spoke of the clinical importance of nervous symptoms in gouty patients and quoted Sydenham as saying that "a fool never had the gout." In conclusion, he said that there were evidently no true diathetic and diatetic causes for gout.

Aural Affections in Children; Necessity of their Early Recognition by the Family Practitioner.—Dr. Jarecky, after speaking of the frequency of ear diseases in children, said that they should be divided into two types, inflammatory and non-inflammatory. It is an interesting clinical fact that very severe ear disturbances occur in children without any extensive signs of pain, consequently very frequent examinations should always be made when a child is suffering from any of the acute infectious diseases. He concluded that early paracentesis should be performed and that because of the probability of early pus formation in children it should be done earlier and even more thoroughly than in adults. (This paper will appear in full in a subsequent issue of the MEDICAL NEWS.)

Dr. G. B. McAuliffe discussed the relation of the development of the temporal bone in the infant to the causation of mastoid diseases, and concluded that the middle ear was so built that the drum was not in the direction of the least resistance, but that this weaker area was rather toward the mastoid. The infantile drum is highly resistant and the imperfectly closed sutures allow of meningeal infection in the infant much more readily than in the adult. Sixteen per cent. of Chicago children have aural disturbance. He agreed with the writer of the paper that paracentesis should be done early. Inasmuch as there is only $1/100$ of an inch from the stapes to the wall the slightest adhesion only is necessary to interfere with the motion of this bone.

Dr. Jarecky, in closing, said that subsidence of symptoms, particularly in children, must not be expected at once after paracentesis.

HARVARD MEDICAL SOCIETY OF NEW YORK CITY.

Regular Monthly Meeting, held November 26, 1904.

The President, Augustus H. Knight, M.D., in the Chair.

The scientific business of the evening consisted of the reading of a paper by Prof. Theobald Smith, of Harvard University, upon the place of research in the University Medical School.

Research and Medicine.—Dr. Smith said that the laboratory as a part of the teaching of medicine has come to stay. Experiments upon animals make observations more definite and remove many of the uncertain elements in the problem of the causation and the treatment of disease. Modern medicine has gained much by the vivifying touch of modern biology. Research was formerly sporadic, but now there is a definite tendency to organize training of research workers. This tendency is well recognized, and represents undoubtedly one of the best features of modern university life. It takes the question of progress in medicine out of the realm of chance or hazard, and makes the possibilities for discovery much greater than they were before. Laboratories

have done very much for medicine, if it is only considered what comparatively short time the regularly equipped laboratory has been in existence.

Laboratory Development.—The first regularly organized laboratories for the study of disease were those founded and maintained by the United States Government. This is a fact not generally recognized, but of which there can be no possible doubt, and it represents one of the very commendable phases of governmental development in this country. After those in this country came the laboratories of the present institute for infectious diseases in Berlin, the Pasteur Institute in Paris, and then those of other countries. Most of the foreign laboratories were founded with definite ideas of practical work to be accomplished by them. Not long after their foundation, however, their scope was widened so as to have them include the study and investigation of fundamental problems in medicine, and, of course, also in the related biological sciences. It was soon realized that research workers must be spared the details of the medical art. Indeed, the class of mind best fitted for research is quite different from that which is likely to be successful in practice. Nearly the same kind of mind is required for successful investigations in medicine as for new inventions in the arts and in mechanics. The American success in these departments is an earnest of how much may be accomplished in the neighboring field of original research in medicine.

Necessities for Research.—The first and most important need for the research worker is that he shall have a living wage and tools and a workshop. It must not be expected that his discoveries shall have an immediate practical value. As a matter of fact, many great discoveries have been made long before their practical applications were found, and very few important discoveries have come at a·time when science and art were ripe for their use. If the practical application of discoveries be too much insisted on, then ill-advised hurry in investigation inevitably results, with disappointment at the consequence, and even the discoverer himself becomes discouraged after a time. Examples of the harm that has been worked through the development of medicine in this way are not wanting, even with regard to the greatest of medical investigators. The research worker must have a calm attitude, and must learn to look at things dispassionately, estimating them only according to their significance in his chain of reasoning. It seems undesirable that the research worker should be expected to combine anything of the health officer or the physician with his work. These men, in close contact with suffering and death, see the most complex problems of human mortality in all their poignancy, and so are drawn by sympathy away from the simpler observation that might prove the beginning of great discoveries. There is a growing reformation in this country, but much yet remains to be done. There is an immense amount of information that medical students are expected to acquire, and it is sometimes thought that just in proportion to their knowledge of the previously known are they likely to make new discoveries. It must not be forgotten, however, that knowledge stifles the originality of the ordinary mind, and that the accumulation of facts is only desirable because, later, when the real discoverer comes, he is able to recognize the thread of thought running through all the facts that looked quite distant from each other before.

Teaching and Research.—It has sometimes been thought that there is a definite relation between teaching and research, and that it is only the teacher who realizes best the limits of knowledge, while it is only the man who is devoted to original research himself who is able to indicate the present position and the possibility of medical information on points where knowledge is advancing. It is one thing, however, to discover and quite another thing to apply facts and observations. It is the main task of the medical school to train physicians in the practical application of principles of medicine. There is just as much objection to the original investigator having to devote most of his time to such training as to his being a physician directly. Laboratories are meant to give such training, but the director of a laboratory need not necessarily occupy himself much with research unless he has the enthusiasm for it, and time is allowed him for the purpose.

Place of Laboratory.—The laboratory is meant to illuminate facts. Its place in education is for the training of the senses, and in the use of instruments of precision. At the present time there is a distinct reaction against book-learning and the lecture system, which, like all movements in human affairs—especially education—is likely to go too far. As the result of this a superabundance of laboratory work may lead to great waste of time in the learning of mere technic. It must not be forgotten that a servant in the laboratory may sometimes see things that a physician misses, or that a butcher may recognize anatomical peculiarities without any knowledge of anatomy, yet neither of these men is a trained physician. The training of the senses is not the only thing necessary, for the scientific observer must know what he is looking for, and must be able to see the relationship of things observed.

Universities and Research.—The university must encourage researches, hence it must have teachers who are investigators. It must provide stables for animals, so that medicine may be studied by comparative methods as well as in hospitals and clinical laboratories. It is only if the university is engaged in research that teachers are able to judge of the true significance of medical progress. As the result of the disturbance of knowledge, much froth of apparent medical advance may be thrown up, and only the trained investigator can appreciate the insignificance of this. Medical teaching must not as a rule include ideas that are too new, or it will also include many that will eventually prove to be false. An income is needed for research work, however, and without this it becomes impossible. It is better to have no pretense of original investigation than to have poor research workers. How much may be accomplished by research can be realized by the fact that in recent years pathology has become a part of surgery to the great benefit of this practical department of medicine.

Endowments have Created a Trust.—The giving by wealthy men of endowments to university medical schools has created a trust for the benefit of the present and future generations. Hence the necessity that all the information obtained by men working under such a trust should become common property. This is, however, of the very essence of professional work. The physician has learned to give in charity his time and his talent. The university owes it to the public to bring about a development of preventive medicine and of sanitary science. At the same time, if the public is taught to appreciate these advantages, it must be made to recognize the value of the services given by health officers who must, only too often under the present conditions, accept scanty pay. It is among the intelligent classes in the community that renewed interest in sanitary science must be awakened, and this task is worthy of the best men and the best schools of medicine.

Prophylaxis.—The future of medicine will consist much more in prophylaxis of disease than in the treatment and cure of serious affections. Physicians will be sought out before serious disease has begun to make its ravages, and their main duty will be prevention rather than cure. Under these coming conditions undoubtedly the physician will be better paid for his labor than at the present time, when, of course, it is distinctly understood that except for the few very successful professional men, the burden of duty is far ahead of the rewards that come to the medical man. In this last phase of their work, that is, in creating popular sentiment and in educating the general public, a principal duty of the university that has not yet been sufficiently recognized, is involved.

BOOK REVIEW.

PHYSIOLOGICAL ECONOMY IN NUTRITION. An Experimental Study. By RUSSELL H. CHITTENDEN, Ph.D., LL.D., Sc.D., Director of the Sheffield Scientific School, Yale University. Frederick A. Stokes Company, New York.

WHAT to Eat—not as the title of an attractive monthly periodical with photographic reproductions of tempting dishes—but as a problem for the masses and the nation—this is the question taken up by Dr. Chittenden and answered in a manner satisfactory to the test tube, balance and calorimeter, if not to the hungry stomach.

That we all eat too much is well recognized—too much for our own good and more than is necessary to keep well and strong. Yet the question of how much is necessary has been answered by many in numerous ways and according to varying standards. Cults even are founded and maintained on the warmth of dietary discussion, and restaurants and sanitaria prosper as exponents of the only " right living."

The truer answers that science has to offer have proven cold comfort for the aching void of the hungry boy and his descendant, the average man.

In the present series of studies, however, we find enough information to give comfort to the father of large families. He cannot be accused of being a brute and starving his family, even if the children go hungry, for science has decreed that at least one-half of the amount of proteid food ordinarily consumed is more than sufficient for the bodies' needs. The simple life at the family board is after all the road to wellbeing, and economy in diet is certain to bring economy in time—from the better health of the family and an increase in the earning capacity of the workers.

We most seriously commend this work to all physicians. It is timely, full of good experimentation, and the conclusions, if put into practice, would mean a great improvement in the health and wealth of the American people.

BOOKS RECEIVED.

REPORT OF THE SURGEON-GENERAL OF THE UNITED STATES NAVY. 1904.

NORMAL HISTOLOGY AND MICROSCOPICAL ANATOMY. By Dr. J. S. Ferguson. 8vo, 738 pages. Illustrated. D. Appleton & Co., New York.

THE MEDICAL NEWS.

A WEEKLY JOURNAL OF MEDICAL SCIENCE.

VOL. 86.   NEW YORK, SATURDAY, MARCH 11, 1905.   NO. 10.

ORIGINAL ARTICLES.

URIC ACID—ITS INFLUENCE IN GOUT.[1]

BY CHARLES C. RANSOM, M.D.,

OF NEW YORK;

VISITING PHYSICIAN, CITY HOSPITAL.

A FEW days ago a gentleman came into my of-. fice complaining of indefinite pains and general discomfort. He brought with him a specimen of urine. He said that he had been told that he was full of uric acid, that his ills were due to it, and that he wanted me to examine the specimen and also to make an examination of his blood to see how much uric acid he had in it.

Day before yesterday, I received through the mail a magazine called the *Uric Acid Monthly*, the object of which was to set forth the value of various proprietary remedies for the cure of the " uric acid diathesis."

This morning a representative of one of the wholesale drug houses left on my desk a box of sample tablets, which he said were the latest and best uric acid solvent on the market, and which he claimed were a panacea for all ills.

It is this sort of thing that has led me to speak to you to-night upon a subject which is so old, and which has had so much said and written about it. My object is to go over in a brief manner the result of the work that has been done during the past decade upon the subject of uric acid to see what, if any, foundation in fact exists for the belief that uric acid is a cause of gout.

In 1776 Schiele first separated uric acid from the urine; and in 1797 Wollaston found biurate of soda in the deposits about gouty joints. In 1848, Garrod published a paper, in the *London Medico-Chirurgical Transactions*, in which he exploited uric acid as the cause of gout, a theory which was suggested to him by a work of Forbes, some years earlier, who had expounded the " lactic acid theory " of gout. As the causes of gout had long been the object of study, the advent of a new theory which was as reasonable as that of Garrod was accepted almost universally, and the work of physiologists upon the subject of uric acid was stimulated to great activity.

In 1886, Alexander Haig, of London. suffered from headache. He noticed that during these headaches his urine was loaded with excessive urates; he also remembered in this connection that invariably the headaches and the unusual condition of the urine followed the ingestion of large amounts of proteid food. Believing thoroughly in the theory of Garrod, this to Haig's mind was additional evidence of the truthfulness of the theory. Being a clever man and a voluminous writer. Haig did much toward establish-

1 Read before the Alumni of the City Hospital.

ing the present prevalent idea that uric acid is the universal cause of gout.

What is uric acid and what is its influence? Uric acid is a normal constituent of the urine. Great variability in the amount excreted exists among individuals, and also in the same individual under different conditions of diet, exercise and disease. The layman and, I regret to say, many physicians believe that uric acid circulates in the blood, as such. As a matter of fact it is always present in the form of urates, and is almost always excreted as a quadri-urate or amorphous urate. A very pretty theory, but one which is entirely hypothetical as to the form in which uric acid appears in the urine, is that of Roberts, given in the Croonian lectures.

The amount of urates or uric acid found in the urine is no index of the general amount of uric acid held in the blood; neither is the presence of uric acid crystals in any way indicative of an excess of uric acid. It simply means a peculiar condition of the urine which permits it to precipitate. The bi-urate occurs as such, only in gouty tophi or in deposits about the joints.

Since Garrod's time, and before, the origin of uric acid has been a matter of great speculation. Garrod, Latham and others believed that uric acid was derived from proteid matter, and was formed in the kidneys by the union of urea and some other substance, probably glycocin, and that it was thrown directly into the urine.

Another idea was that uric acid is the product of the imperfect oxidation of the acid into urea; that from some disturbance in the general metabolism the nitrogenous elements were held up at the uric acid stage instead of going on by further oxidation into urea.

The generally accepted idea to-day is that developed by Horbaczewski and his pupils. It is called the Nuclein theory. Horbaczewski believes that there is no relationship between urea and uric acid, the former being the terminal product of proteid metabolism, the latter being derived exclusively from the nuclein of the cell. The nucleo-proteid of the cell is broken up, the proteid part undergoing the usual proteolytic changes is converted into urea. The nuclein molecule is oxidized into nucleic acid. The nucleic acid, being further oxidized, forms on the one hand phosphoric acid and on the other the so-called " mother substance." The mother substance is oxidized into uric acid on the one hand and the purin xanthine or aloxur bases on the other.

In confirmation of this work of Horbaczewski are the observations of Williamson. He found that with the destruction of the white blood cells there was a fall in the leucocyte count with a corresponding increase in the output of uric acid and phosphoric acid. The destruction of the white blood cells was confirmed by morphological examination of the blood preceding and during the fall. He further noted that sudden and marked variations in the white blood cell curve corresponded with similar variations in the uric acid and phosphoric acid curve.

Futcher made some observations which showed that in the urine of chronic gout the variation in the uric acid output in the interval and during an attack was accompanied by a similar variation in the phosphoric acid output. Our own observations in such cases of chronic gout correspond with those of Futcher. Another observation which we have made would seem also to be confirmatory evidence of the nuclein origin of uric acid. A number of patients suffering from chronic gout and nephritis were fed upon shad roe, a food rich in nuclein. Corresponding with the ingestion of this food there was an enormously increased output of uric acid which subsided on a return to the ordinary diet. Horbaczewski explains the excessive uric acid output with proteid feeding by the digestive leucocytosis, proving that the excess in uric acid is formed from the increased destruction of the leucocytes and not from the intake of proteid food. This is the generally accepted belief to-day.

Uric acid is present in the urine from two sources: the exogenous uric acid, or that derived with the body from foodstuffs, and the endogenous uric acid, that has its origin in the body cell.

It may exist in the blood from three causes: (1) Through increased production either of the exogenous or the endogenous form; (2) from deficient elimination; (3) from deficient oxidation. The increased production may be due either to disturbance of the general balance of metabolism or from foodstuffs rich in nuclein.

Deficient elimination is due to a loss of the excretory power of the kidney from disease of the organ.

Deficient oxidation may be due to disturbance in the functional activity of the liver, kidneys or other glandular organs, or from lack of muscular activity.

Crofton has demonstrated the power of the kidneys, liver and muscles to oxidize uric acid.

It is in relation to gout that most of the studies of uric acid have been made, and for convenience we will consider it only in connection with that disease.

The first question that naturally arises in considering the influence of uric acid as a cause of disease is, is it ever retained in the blood in excess? Abeles and a few others claim to have found uric acid in small quantities in the normal blood. These observations have not been confirmed by any of the more recent writers, and it is denied by Horbaczewski and many others. More recent methods fail to reveal it.

Magnus-Levy, Hiss, Von Jaksch found it in the blood of leucemia, chronic lead poisoning,

chronic nephritis, chronic arthritis. It is deposited in the kidney and urinary passages as calculi under certain conditions, and in the joint structures and in the skin or gouty tophi in the form of bi-urate. To the first query the answer is yes.

The second question that naturally follows is: Is uric acid toxic when retained in the blood?

Freudweiler and Hiss injected urates about the joints and set up local necrosis. They claimed that the resultant process was too widespread to be accounted for by the mechanical action alone, and believed that it was partly toxic. This was followed by inflammation and subsequent development of fibrous tissue, a similar process to that which we have in the development of a gouty joint. These observations, however, have never been confirmed, and there are many reasons to doubt their accuracy.

As an evidence of the toxicity of uric acid and its relation as a causative factor in gout, Garrod claimed that gouty attacks were accompanied by a retention of uric acid. Our own observations made with modern methods have been exactly the reverse. We find, that is to say, that the low output of uric acid in the interval of chronic gout was invariably followed by an increased output of uric acid coincident with the accession of fever and pain of an acute exacerbation. Futcher has also made similar observations. Magnus-Levy and Hiss showed a light excretion preceding an attack, and a marked increase during the attack. Garrod claimed that there was an excess of uric acid in the blood during an attack, but modern methods have proven this view to be erroneous. He also said that the deposits of uric acid following an attack were due to increased alkalinity of the blood, which permitted of its precipitating out. The observations of Klemperer and Magnus-Levy have shown that there is no increased alkalinity of the blood.

If it were true that uric acid were toxic we would expect to find constantly in conditions where uric acid is known to be held in the body in excessive amounts symptoms which could be attributed to uric acid alone, but this is not the case. In leucemia, pneumonia, chronic nephritis and others in which it has been shown that there is an excess of uric acid, no specific symptoms referable to uric acid are ever seen. Again, in those cases to which I have already referred, in which nuclein holding food was fed in excess and in which the uric acid output was largely increased, there was never at any time during these experiments a disturbance of the system. In a number of cases in which we fed uric acid in large amounts there was never a disturbance of health, although a large part of the uric acid was recovered from the urine. Some of these cases were sufferers from chronic gout and others from chronic nephritis, and we should naturally expect if the uric acid were toxic, especially in the latter cases, to find an aggravation of the kidney disease. But such was not the case.

In carrying on some observations upon rabbits we infused directly into a vein large amounts of uric acid, a large percentage of which was recovered from the urine, but there was no evidence of a disturbance of the health of the animal. We may assume then, I think, that there is no evidence which has been confirmed to show that uric acid is in any way toxic.

In connection with its supposed influence in causing gout various observations have been made. One of the most fanciful perhaps was the mechanical theory of Roberts. Roberts believes that in gout there is a supersaturation of the blood, with the quadri-urates; that the deposits in the joint structure is due to the conversion of the quadri-urates into bi-urate by the excessive amount of sodium salt held in the lymph and synovial fluids. He further believes that the various nerve and other manifestations of gout are due to a crystallizing out of the blood stream into these various tissues of fine needles of uric acid, through which mechanical action alone produce various manifestations. In opposition to such a theory are the following facts: Under no circumstances have crystals of uric acid ever been found post mortem in the tissues. If it were true that the blood were supersaturated there is no reason why in cases of nephritis, for instance, where there is a marked retention of the chlorides and other sodium salts with the supersaturation of the blood with uric acid, there should not be a precipitation in the tissues under such circumstances, as the conditions are ideal for such precipitation. We know that such things never occur.

Again Klemperer has positively shown that the blood is never saturated with the urates, for the serum taken directly from the blood by means of blister is always capable of taking up large quantities of uric acid.

From the foregoing, we are forced to conclude that there is no evidence at all that uric acid causes gout or in fact any other disease; that those who have held so long to this theory have, as Herter has most aptly put it, " attributed to the ash the quality of the flame."

As I have before said, if the uric acid theory were true various conditions showing uric acid in excess would show arthritic changes.

If Koch's theories of specificity are necessary to determine the cause of any infectious disease, should we not by analogy demand that uric acid should comply with some such plan before we accept it as the cause of gout? One might ask what is the cause of gout? If we do not believe in uric acid, can we wantonly destroy this idol without adequately supplying its place? I must confess that we cannot with positiveness say what causes gout, but the most reasonable theory in the light of modern investigation is one of acid intoxication.

My time is too limited to go over this matter in any detail, but there are one or two thoughts I should like to suggest to you in this connection,

which would bear out this theory. Gastro-intestinal disturbance, as you all know, is most common in gouty conditions, and while it is not invariable it is a fact that nearly always an acute exacerbation of gout is preceded by a disturbance of the stomach, and a so-called torpid liver. Then again, the uric acid output during an acute attack is very similar to that during an attack of infectious disease. With the acute exacerbation there is always an increased amount of urea secreted, and this, too, on a milk diet, showing conclusively a considerable waste of tissue. Following an acute attack there is always a diminished amount excreted, following the regeneration of the tissue. This idea is quite consistent with the condition of affairs about the joint, and taken in connection with our accepted nuclein theory as to the origin of uric acid will explain the phenomena which take place in the infection of the joint. Through this trauma a slight inflammatory reaction is set up in the joint structure. The toxic material at once begins its action upon this susceptible tissue. The leucocytes, in the effort to destroy the toxins in this process, come to the joint structures in great number; unable to cope successfully with the toxin, they are destroyed. The nuclein of the cell is oxidized into uric acid, and the result is the gouty joint.

Some observations of Rindfleisch, who has found giant-cells about the joint structures in gout which are capable of taking up uric acid, would seem to have some bearing upon this connection, and the work of Ebenstein which shows a previous necrosis of the tissues before the deposit takes place would coincide with this view.

66 West Forty-ninth Street.

OBJECTIVE AND SUBJECTIVE SYMPTOMS OF SURGICAL DISEASES OF THE KIDNEY.[1]

BY C. L. GIBSON, M.D.,

ATTENDING SURGEON, ST. LUKE'S HOSPITAL.

THERE is to-day a much better understanding of the value of the symptoms—subjective and objective—of kidney lesions, owing to the frequent opportunities to study them in *vivo* during the course of the numerous and satisfactory operations of the kidney, which have become now of daily occurrence.

Notwithstanding the value of increasingly exact laboratory aids and technical adjuvants to be described by others to-night, the main reliance in diagnosis must still rest on these objective and subjective symptoms, although their importance is often seemingly lessened by contrast with the information sometimes obtained with these other means.

The symptoms exhibited by the patient should be most carefully weighed and amplified by further investigation, not only of the main clues so elicited, but also of the routine possibilities of

1 Read at the Annual Stated Meeting of the New York Academy of Medicine, G. U. Section, December 15, 1905. Symposium on Surgical Diseases of the Kidney.

any variety of renal lesion, also of the diseases of other organs as well, particularly of contiguous viscera.

The value of any symptom is relative to its accompanying factors. Familiarity with the particular form of disease and inherent good judgment will best equip the practitioner to decide what weight shall be given to the single equation.

A single symptom may become the central figure from which or toward which we must always work, e.g., the violent typical pain of so-called renal colic. Generally speaking, we shall be on safer ground if we begin by collecting all our evidence dispassionately until we have a complete picture, or a collection of facts which may be further analyzed.

The chief symptoms of surgical diseases of the kidney are: (1) Pain—direct or indirect, or pain and tenderness; (2) variations from the normal on voiding urine and the appearance of the urine; (3) the presence of a tumor; (4) constitutional disturbances, such as fever and abnormal cardiovascular action, and the constitutional condition peculiar to disease of the kidney, uremia. The chief physical signs are the direct, showing anomalies of position, size and shape of the kidney. In addition, we may recognize abnormal mobility or fixation, tenderness to pressure and to some extent the consistency of the kidney.

The indirect signs are those learned by a routine general physical examination, looking particularly for evidences of uremia, dry skin, foul breath, contracted pupil, cerebral disturbances and high tension pulse, and finally the signs of disease or anomaly in the remainder of the genito-urinary system.

The diagnostic significance of pain.—Direct pain is of the greatest value in calling attention to the kidney as the site of a lesion. It is also strongly presumptive of the existence of an acute inflammation. It may be constant and progressive as in malignant disease, it may be characteristically intermittent or variable as in disturbances due to a movable kidney. It is consistently absent in simple hydronephrosis and latent chronic inflammations.

Indirect pain, particularly along the course of the ureter, is of the greatest diagnostic value, and may alone be sufficient to establish the diagnosis of the passage of a stone. Intermittent pain and oliguria followed by polyuria, with a tumefaction of rapidly varying size is characteristic of the occasional kinking of the ureter of a freely movable kidney. Pain may be surprisingly absent. The pelvis and the kidney proper may be full of calculi, yet if acute suppuration is wanting and obstruction of the ureter does not occur, no pain will be felt.

Pain then is a useful positive symptom, but almost any pronounced lesion of the kidney may run a wholly painless course.

The appearance of the urine and disturbances of urination.—Polyuria, except the sudden form indicative of the relief of ureteral obstruction, has some significance in pointing to such conditions as tuberculosis and polycystic kidney in which an interstitial nephritis is regularly present. Diminution is important in indicating a destructive process.

Total anuria without mechanical causes usually means that the kidney's work is done without reference to the particular cause.

Sudden total anuria means either immediate simultaneous obstruction to both ureters or more usually the blocking of the ureter leading to the only sound kidney. Total temporary anuria often means mechanical blocking on one side and reflex suspension of secretion in the other kidney.

Therefore variations in the amount of urine secreted are important chiefly as an index of severity rather than of cause.

Pus in the urine.—The recognition that pus in macroscopic amounts comes from the kidney is proof that a lesion of the kidney exists and of a nature that will ordinarily be best dealt with by direct treatment. To prove that pus comes from the kidney, the absence of suppurative lesions of the rest of the genito-urinary apparatus must be shown.

If a cystitis exists, and can be demonstrated pretty conclusively to be antecedent, the lesion of the kidney is most probably a pyelonephritis and usually bilateral.

Pus from the kidney means for the most part one of two things, a pyelitis primary or secondary to nephrolithiasis or tuberculosis, the differentiation between certain stages of these two conditions also giving rise to the most confusion attending the differential diagnosis of kidney lesions.

Little pus is usually discharged from the kidney proper in ordinary surgical kidney.

Pus appearing in large quantities at variable intervals is more significant of pyonephrosis. Pyuria may point to a destructive malignant process—carcinoma, more rarely in sarcoma.

Blood in the urine has a significance similar to pus, and its origin in the kidney must also be similarly traced.

Renal hematuria as seen in practice is most frequently due to tuberculosis or calculus. In many instances of either condition, the symptom is entirely absent. It is quite regularly present in carcinoma, rarely in sarcoma, it is a symptom in about 25 per cent. of polycystic kidney. It may be due to syphilis, hemophilia, or excretion of irritants.

There is no certain way to distinguish the hematuria occurring in tuberculosis and calculus, the other factors must decide.

Small repeated hemorrhages occurring without previous pain or bodily exertion in a young person of delicate as opposed to the gouty type are more presumably due to tuberculosis, as also the severer exsanguinating hemorrhages.

Presence of a tumor.—The patient is rarely aware of the presence of a tumor unless of large size, such as rapidly growing sarcoma, or a large polycystic kidney. Unusual mobility of the normal or abnormal kidney is generaly readily felt.

Constitutional disturbances.—Acute inflammatory lesions of the kidney regularly have symptoms of acute sepsis. Fever is marked, in the acute suppuration it is more continuous though it may have abrupt exacerbations. Chills are frequent but not characteristic. Irregular chills and fever of the pyemic type are more typical of the chronic pyelonephritis especially if there is an acute lighting up of the process.

Sudden lowering of the temperature to subnormal and remaining there, usually betokens uremia of a fatal type.

A regular evening rise of temperature, even if slight, is very suspicious of a tuberculous kidney.

Physical signs.—Given a very pronounced lesion, involving marked changes in size and shape of the kidney in a very thin person, the diagnosis can be made usually largely from the physical signs. Exactly the same condition may be overlooked or unrecognizable in a corpulent person with a resisting abdominal wall. Again a kidney may be palpated with ease and show nothing abnormal although extensively diseased.

With the exception of congenital anomalies, increased size is for the most part due to distention of the pelvis. Tumors and polycystic kidney are the notable exception, the kidney retaining its general shape, while distention of the pelvis gives a more globular surface. The larger kidneys will generally be sarcomata in children or hydronephrosis, simple or infected. Calculus of the kidney, unless complicated with suppuration or obstruction, generally causes no appreciable enlargement. Tuberculosis with inconsiderable infection of the pelvis produces little or even no enlargement. Tenderness of the kidney to the touch generally means suppuration of the acute type. Fixation of an enlarged kidney generally implies active suppuration, tuberculosis or malignant disease. An easily perceptible fluctuation generally means a simple hydronephrosis,—purulent collections seldom are so manifest. Irregularity of surface is fairly frequent in tuberculosis, it may be marked in malignant disease and polycystic kidney.

The following are in brief the chief diagnostic factors of the important surgical diseases of the kidney in their order of importance:

Anomalies.	*Physical Examination.*
Abnormal mobility	History. Recognition of displacement by examination. Associated neurasthenia and gastro-enteroptosis. Direct and indirect pain.
Tumors	*Age.*—Sarcoma in infancy, carcinoma in later life. Cachexia. Tumor. Pain. Hematuria.

Congenital polycystic kidney.	Large kidney shaped tumor; irregular surface,—sooner or later bilateral. Chronic diffuse nephritis. Pain and discomfort from dragging and pressure. Occasional hematuria.
Hydronephrosis, *Unilateral*	Antecedent history of blocking of one ureter, usually by a calculus. Large painless, rounded fluctuating tumor in the loin. Absence of constitutional and uremic symptoms. Compensatory hypertrophy of other kidney.
Hydronephrosis, *Double*	History usually of chronic obstruction to the escape of urine from the bladder, or of malignant growth pressing on both ureters. Recognition of the source of obstruction.
Pyonephrosis	Antecedent history of infection and obstruction. Large globular and fixed tumor in the flank. If process is *active*, febrile and other constitutional symptoms.
Pyelonephritis or surgical kidney	Usually history of long obstruction, *plus* infection,—mostly elderly men with obstructing prostate and men in middle life with stricture. Recognition of the obstruction and cystitis. A low grade chronic sepsis,—occasional acute exacerbations with chills and febrile disturbances. Chronic diffuse nephritis. Seldom any enlargement or tenderness of the kidney. Usually bilateral.
Tuberculosis	History of constitutional tuberculosis. Other tuberculous foci especially of the genito-urinary tract. Persistent evening rise of deep temperature. Very insidious and latent course of symptoms. Polyuria from chronic diffuse nephritis. Frequency of urination even in earlier stages before marked changes in bladder. Irregular hematuria without apparent cause. Pus thoroughly mixed with the urine which has an *acid* reaction.
Renal calculus	The passage per urethram of sand gravel, or small calculi. Typical renal colic. Attacks of hematuria,—especially if accompanying renal colic.

Renal calculus
$$\left\{\begin{array}{l}\text{Symptoms of suppuration in the kidney,—local pain and pyuria.}\\\text{Recognition of an enlarged kidney due to pyelitis or hydronephrosis.}\\\text{Excess of crystalline sediments.}\\\text{Temporary oliguria followed by polyuria.}\\\text{Gouty or rheumatic diathesis and chiefly in middle-aged individuals.}\end{array}\right.$$

LABORATORY FINDINGS IN SURGICAL DISEASES OF THE KIDNEY.[1]

BY FREDERIC E. SONDERN, M.D.,
OF NEW YORK.

IT is an undisputed fact that recent years have witnessed many advances in practical urine analysis; many long cherished ideas have been completely overthrown, importance has been found to attach to observations formerly noted but not considered significant, and many additional diagnostic and prognostic signs have been described.

As in everything else, *method* should exist in a urine analysis, and as our knowledge of the subject increases, this methodical routine procedure becomes correspondingly more complex and time consuming. The clinician with proper laboratory training in exact chemical technic is best fitted for the work, and the results of his efforts are not only scientific from the laboratory point of view but practical from the clinical standpoint as well. Practice in this ideal way is impossible in most instances for two reasons: (1) The clinician has not the time at his disposal, and (2) the laboratory expert who must be ready to do the simplest or most intricate task at a moment's notice, requires such an array of delicate apparatus in perfect adjustment, and carefully standardized reagents, which he cannot afford to maintain unless this character of work occupies his entire time. When the relationship between the clinician and the laboratory expert is like the ideal association of the physician and surgeon, then diagnosis, and in many instances prognosis, are as scientific as they can be made to-day.

Before considering the typical and atypical pictures presented by the urine in the different surgical diseases of the kidney, I beg your attention for a few minutes to some of the more important generalities. It is both undesirable and impossible to mention here all the phases of this work, and as it is, I am afraid of being accused of the commonplace.

Concerning the quantity of urine, 24-hour specimens teach many significant points not learned in any other way. In considering the significance of a polyuria, that due to neurosis, diuretics, ordered intake of much fluid, a previously removed kidney or an occlusion of one

1 Read at the Annual Meeting of the New York Academy of Medicine, G. U. Section, December 15, 1904. Symposium on Surgical Diseases of the Kidney.

ureter should not be forgotten. In oliguria or anuria, that due to unilateral painful lesions in or about the kidney, reflex and without obstruction, must be kept in mind.

Concerning the chemical analysis of urine, it is here that routine work is so essential. Owing to the omission of a test for glucose because the specific gravity created no suspicion in this direction, a post-operative diabetic coma has often come as a surprise. The usual tests for glucose are made much more sensitive by keeping the tubes on a water bath in preference to simply boiling.

Pentosuria is by no means the uncommon condition formerly believed, and its occurrence in presumably healthy persons is not at all rare. Many a case of pentosuria is called glycosuria because a differential test is not made.

In testing for albumin, the methods selected should be such that nucleoalbumin, albumose and Bence-Jones albumin are not overlooked or confused. It is needless for me to add that albuminuria does not necessarily indicate a nephritis or that a nephritis must present even traces of albumin at all times. Concentrated urines show faint traces of albumin much more clearly if they are diluted with water before testing.

Concerning the daily excretion of urea, the belief has long been abandoned that an output of 6 or 8 grams means an impending uremia, or one of 40 grams necessarily healthy kidneys. On the other hand, Cabot's statement that a knowledge of the daily excretion of urea is not of the slightest use, is the other extreme. The usual text-book statement that the daily excretion of urea is normally from 25 to 40 grams is an heirloom. From 16 to 28 grams are much better figures, in this city at least, and Koranyi has stated that in his opinion 16 grams is the normal minimum for a well-built male.

The relative and absolute excretion of chlorides has had renewed attention of late; in this connection the method by incineration must be advocated and the direct method condemned.

Concerning the microscopical examination of urine, the great value of the centrifuge, aside from its time-saving advantage, is established. The absurd statements that renal elements are destroyed by its proper use, or structures formed that simulate casts, have been disproven. The microspectroscope will demonstrate the proper bands from one red blood cell.

Concerning the presence of casts it is needless to add that a granular cast does not necessarily indicate a chronic nephritis, or that a nephritis demands the constant presence of casts. Structures derived from the prostate simulate casts and particularly so-called cylindroids, but with care the differentiation is not difficult.

An erroneous laboratory diagnosis of an inflammatory or malignant lesion based solely on the structure of one or a number of epithelial cells, has annoyed almost every clinician. While it is far from me to deny the value of the information gained by a close observation of the epithelial cells in the urine, modern writings justly show less attention to this particular feature. Text-books are very vague on the subject and usually present plates copied and recopied from the older authors. Tumor particles are sometimes found in the urine and justify a conclusion, but a diagnosis of carcinoma or sarcoma of the kidney based on the presence of a "cancer cell" or a "sarcoma cell" is simply absurd, although it is done daily.

Concerning methods for determining the functional ability of the kidneys, much of what has been advocated has proven decidedly useful, though like most other things not infallible. Molecular concentration determined by cryoscopy of the blood is perhaps the best procedure; it is an important factor in the prognosis when a diseased kidney must be removed, it lends much weight in deciding if a kidney is to be removed or not, and it is of value in determining the functional ability in bilateral kidney disease. Cryoscopy of the urine applied to any given specimen or to a 24-hour specimen teaches little or nothing. G. Fuchs[1] and others claim better results by multiplying the freezing point by a factor learned from the gravity and the daily quantity of urine. On the other hand, cryoscopy applied to specimens of urine collected from each kidney separately, is perhaps as good a guide to the relative functional ability as we have. Previous intake of large amounts of fluid is not advisable if this test is to be used.

The electric conductivity of the urine teaches nothing in addition to cryoscopy, and the results are for practical purposes identical. The phloridzin, methylene blue, indigo carmine and similar tests have never gained the popularity in this city that they have enjoyed abroad. Their value seems to decrease from year to year and their use does not seem without risk.

Determining the functional ability by means of the toxic quality of the urine has been advocated by Bouchard. He figures a urotoxic coefficient, but I have no experience as to the value of the method.

To return to the subject at hand. The following brief conclusions are based chiefly on personal laboratory experience, the exact data of which I cannot present in the limited time at my disposal. In acute catarrh of the renal pelvis, the urinary picture is somewhat different if the lesion is due to a local cause or to an ascending infection. In the event of a local cause, calculus or pronounced crystalline deposit, the daily amount of urine is decreased, there is corresponding concentration, normal output of solids, blood cells according to local irritation, few leucocytes, some mucus, characteristic groups of epithelial cells, and an amount of albumin and casts according to the degree of hyperemia of the parenchyma which invariably accompanies the condition. In the event of an ascending infection,

1. Zeitsch. f. angew. Chem., 1902.

pyogenic, gonorrheal or colon bacillus, the urine, showing the evidences of the bladder lesion, suddenly becomes scanty, with some increase in the albumin and the presence of few casts, and, if one is fortunate enough to recognize them, epithelial cells referable to the pelvis, but with a normal daily output of solids. In either class this condition does not last long; the evidences of the acute catarrh disappear or the picture soon becomes that of a pyelitis.

In pyelitis with hyperemia of the parenchyma, the daily amount of urine is increased, the gravity lowered and the daily excretion of solids is normal. The microscopic picture shows pus in addition to the elements found with catarrh of the pelvis. In pyelonephritis the urine presents the same features as in pyelitis with the addition of the elements referable to the parenchyma, i.e., albumin and casts. In the event of a compensating excretory action of the other kidney which usually exists, the daily excretion of solids remains normal or nearly so. Purulent exudates from the kidney do not form a coagulum nearly as frequently as those from the bladder, and are always much poorer in epithelial cells.

Renal hematuria, unless the bleeding is very profuse, also lacks the tendency to coagulation, and much of the hemoglobin is dissolved in the urine, while in vesical hemorrhage most of the coloring matter is in the sediment of corpuscles which are usually in clots.

In hydronephrosis and pyonephrosis with occlusion of the ureter, the urine passed may be perfectly normal but usually shows a little polyuria and evidences of slight hyperemia of the parenchyma doubtless due to the additional excretory labor of the acting kidney. An emptying hydronephrosis, especially if there is an accompanying hematuria, by no means rare, presents a very confusing urinary picture often of little value in diagnosis.

The microscopic picture of the urine obtained when a pyonephrosis is discharging into the bladder may also be quite meager, but a corroborative diagnosis can frequently be made by the necrotic character of the pus.

Aspirated fluid from a hydronephrosis or pyonephrosis is very easily identified and needs no further comment.

In cysts of the kidney, in the syphilitic hyperplasia simulating malignant tumors as well as in the cystic degeneration of the kidney, urine analysis presents little or nothing of value in the specific diagnosis.

In renal actinomycosis the urinary picture is that of a pyelitis with hyperemia of the parenchyma or of a pyelonephritis, with more or less frequent hematuria of renal origin. The fungus is usually rather difficult to identify positively.

In floating kidney the urine discloses no characteristic features, but in these cases transient neurotic polyuria is very frequently observed.

In malignant tumors of the kidney, intermittent hematuria often of very short duration is the most frequent abnormal feature in the urine. This hematuria is usually quite profuse and in consequence frequently presents clots and even casts of the ureter or pelvis. In typical cases the urine is otherwise normal or perhaps more frequently shows the evidences of a slight hyperemia of the renal parenchyma. The presence of microscopic blood between the attacks of pronounced hematuria is a very suggestive feature. Even if the hemorrhage is quite slow the blood looks red and is very seldom smoky as in acute nephritis. The coexistence of a pyelitis or pyelonephritis is really foreign to the condition under consideration, and when present is brought about by an ascending infection perhaps due to lack of resistance on the part of the mucous membrane, or it is the result of a local suppurating lesion in the tumor. A few cases present a marked albuminuria without corroborative evidence of a corresponding lesion of the remaining healthy parenchyma. As a matter of fact, the urine analysis in malignant renal tumors teaches less of diagnostic value than is usually held. When sufficiently preserved shreds of tumor are passed the conclusions are obvious, but this occurrence is by no means as frequent as generally believed, in which particular considerable experience makes me agree with Israel. I have already expressed my opinion as to the value of a diagnosis based on single "cancer cells" or "sarcoma cells" which seems to be Israel's conclusion as well.

In renal tuberculosis the picture at first is that of a pyelitis with a hyperemia of the parenchyma, an almost invariable presence of at least a few blood cells and a distinct polyuria ; and later there are the evidences of a pyelonephritis.

Finding the tubercle bacilli in the sediment has been much improved by the introduction of the centrifuge, and success is largely due to the patient and painstaking search made for them. The cases of renal tuberculosis in which bacilli are not found when a number of specimens have been examined are not as numerous as many will have you believe, and the fault usually lies in the examination of but one specimen. There are cases, however, in which bacilli cannot be found on repeated search, and in these animal inoculation is often, though by no means invariably successful. Tuberculous urine as a rule does not show a macroscopic bacteriuria, and usually has an acid reaction. When, however, a mixed infection occurs and the specimen is foul, an attempt should be made to get it into a sweeter condition before animal inoculation is attempted. In the event of animal inoculation, one should not be satisfied with the macroscopic result, but the presence of tubercles microscopically must be demonstrated. I recall one case where the animals died at the proper time and presented the gross appearance of a tuberculosis, but the microscopical examination revealed no tuberculous lesion.

A word concerning the differentiation between tubercle bacilli and smegma bacilli. In the usual specimens there is no difficulty in the use of the standard methods, but where there is a marked alkaline fermentation, tubercle bacilli do not withstand the action of alcohol as well. An opinion based on the presence of single bacillus must remain guarded, but where the organisms occur in groups, fortunately the case in the majority of instances, these present evidences clearly characteristic of either tubercle or smegma, which specific grouping has been emphasized in the older writings, but is often overlooked in articles on the subject to-day. The diagnosis of tuberculous renal disease can usually be made from the urine, and success is due rather to patient investigation than to particular skill. Statements to the contrary usually originate from the fact that the search for bacilli has been confined to one or two specimens.

In cases of renal calculus the urinary picture is most varied. On the one hand, perfectly normal urine may be voided or there may be the evidences of a slight hyperemia of the parenchyma, and on the other the most severe pyelonephritis and cystitis with a marked alkaline fermentation may be seen, in which it is often difficult to find any structural elements in the vast amount of very offensive coagulated pus.

At the time of a renal colic, the picture ordinarily is that of an acute catarrh of the pelvis, with more or less hyperemia of the parenchyma, the amount of blood being in direct proportion to the mechanical injury. After the attack of pain these evidences disappear more or less quickly, or a pyelitis is developed, to remain or gradually clear up, as the case may be. In the chemical analysis of specimens from cases of renal stone, I was impressed years ago by an almost constant high relative, as well as absolute nitrogenous output, and have gradually come to look upon these features as an important point in differential diagnosis with almost constant success. It stands to reason that a patient whose mode of life has been suitably corrected does not present these characteristics or only to a moderate degree. The presence of pronounced crystalline deposits, while forming a link in the chain of evidence, justifies absolute conclusions in only a small number of cases. Triple phosphate deposits are the result of an alkaline fermentation due to any cause and merit no consideration in this connection.

Intermittent hydronephrosis often empties with a colic, tenesmus and frequent micturition, and at this time is apt to show some blood. The differential point between it and a stone colic is, that in the former the amount of urine is usually large and the gravity low, whereas in the latter the opposite is an almost invariable rule.

In nephralgia and allied conditions, the etiology of which seems but little understood, the urinary findings may so closely resemble those of other diseases, that a differential diagnosis is usually difficult and at times impossible. The absolutely pessimistic view held by many is often due to the negative outcome of one or two specimens, while the clinical examination is repeated over and over, with no better result. Careful and often repeated analysis, while possibly leading to no positive result, tends to exclude other conditions, and is oftentimes of greater practical utility than the clinical work. During a nephralgia the urine may be perfectly normal, but this is also true in renal colic due to stone, though much less frequently. A neurotic polyuria may occur at the time of a neuralgic pain, whereas no simulating condition is observed in stone colic. On the other hand, cases of neuralgia with hematuria and scanty urine are not unknown, but in my observations they never show the almost immediate evidences of inflammatory lesions noted in the same conditions due to calculus. The pronounced hematuria at times seen with contracting kidney and quite different from the bleeding of an acute nephritis, or an acute exacerbation more properly, must be kept in mind when seeking a cause for a renal hematuria.

In subcutaneous renal injuries the first urine shows a pure hematuria and the subsequent picture depends largely on the nature and result of the injury and on the presence or absence of a bacterial infection.

Time does not permit me to continue this review, but before closing my remarks I beg your attention to a few additional points. In contemplated kidney surgery in diabetes the surgeon should be influenced more by the evidences of intoxication than by the percentage of glucose.

Postanesthetic nephritis is to-day a much less frequent condition than it was fifteen years ago, an improvement which can doubtless be ascribed to the more careful use of anesthetics, quicker operating, the free administration of water by mouth or rectum after operation and proper early attention to the bowels.

A routine blood examination teaches much in forming an opinion as to the necessity and urgency of operation in septic kidney lesions. Here, as in other septic processes, many observers have attempted to fix the degree of leucocytosis at which an inflammatory lesion without exudate may be suspected, and that at which a suspicion of the presence of a purulent exudate is justified. Leucocytosis is, however, largely dependent on body resistance toward infection; thus good resistance will occasion pronounced leucocytosis in slight infections, and poor resistance little or no leucocytosis in grave infections. As there is no method of determining this body resistance with sufficient accuracy, the inferences drawn from a leucocytosis of given degree must remain questionable, except perhaps in unusually excessive counts.

For some years I have been impressed by the fact that the differential count of leucocytes offers a far better guide to the status of the inflammatory process, one which is not influenced to a perceptible degree by body resistance, and furthermore, that the leucocytosis with a given differential count may be an indicator of this body resistance, but unfortunately I cannot here enter into the details of this subject.

I will close with a new motto on an old subject: "The man who makes every diagnosis in the laboratory is as short-sighted and liable to grave error as the man who ignores microscope and test tube."

THE X-RAY IN KIDNEY DISEASE.[1]

BY LEWIS GREGORY COLE, M.D.,

OF NEW YORK;

SKIAGRAPHER TO ROOSEVELT HOSPITAL.

LAST spring it was my privilege to read a paper on X-ray before the G. U. section, and I greatly appreciate having an opportunity to supplement it at this time.

Until recently X-ray was used only as a possible aid in diagnosing renal and ureteral calculi. If it confirmed the diagnosis, well and good; if not, the operation was performed just the same.

Within the last year or so there have been improvements in the apparatus and technic which enable us to make skiagraphs of moderate-sized subjects, by which the diagnosis may be made regardless of signs or symptoms. By diagnosis, I mean the negative as well as positive diagnoses of calculi.

In order to do this, however, we must have what I demonstrated here last spring, viz., the ray of selective absorption. At that time I thought it was an easy thing to get but it is not. Since then, I have spent many hours of hard work getting, losing and getting it again, each time, however, learning facts about it which shortly I am going to publish. This ray is absolutely essential for the negative diagnosis of renal and ureteral calculi.

It is perfectly possible to show some renal calculi in skiagraphs made without this ray, but such plates are worthless in making negative diagnoses.

Last spring I spoke also of the necessity of short exposures on account of the motion of the kidney during respiration and because of the danger of burning the patient. There is still another danger, not to the patient but to the plate, viz., fogging the plate by the rays that go *around* the patient instead of *through* him. At the time I mentioned the remarkably short exposures of seven and fourteen seconds for a patient weighing 100 lbs. Since then, for all patients weighing 150 lbs. or less, my rule has been from five to fifteen or perhaps twenty seconds in making an exposure.

With the improvements in the apparatus and technic and with the ray of selective absorption,

[1] Read at the Annual Meeting of the New York Academy of Medicine, G. U. Section, December 15, 1904. Symposium on Surgical Diseases of the Kidney.

we are able to show finer gradation of shadows and greater contrast between the different soft tissues. As these shadows increase the difficulty of reading or interpreting the plate increase. For instance, in an X-ray plate there is not only bone, muscle and calculi to be seen; but perhaps also feces, undigested food in the intestine, calcareous nodules or arteries, or tuberculous deposits in the kidney. Carcinoma of the lower end of the esophagus shows distinctly and I have every reason to believe it would show in an affected kidney.

You will readily see that any or all of these shadows might be misinterpreted as renal or ureteral calculi. In order to make a diagnosis of calculi you must be able to make out the size and shape of the calculi.

Near the lower end of the ureter there are shadows cast which very closely resemble those of ureteral calculi both in size and location. These at first were all supposed to be ureteral calculi; but occasionally we found them on both sides and sometimes on the opposite side from the symptoms and in most cases multiple.

The first case we were sure of was operated on by Dr. Brewer at Roosevelt Hospital. The plate showed several shadows on the left side. The ureter was opened and only one of these shadows proved to be a calculus. What the others were, we do not know—probably vein-stones, or sesamoid bones in the great sacrosciatic ligament, or in some muscles.

Dr. Brown will tell you how we may solve the problem of which are ureteral calculi and which are not.

The range of positions of the renal calculi is the thing that I want to emphasize most in reading skiagraphs.

In all cases I have the tube 18 inches from the plate, vertically over the umbilicus, and I will show that the variety of positions of the stones is astonishing. Some are within one-half inch of the tip of the third lumbar vertebra, others are above and external to the tip of the last rib and in other inconceivable regions.

In order to make a negative diagnosis, the spine and transverse process of the lumbar vertebra must show distinctly clear-cut edges all the way to the tip. The last rib and psoas muscle must also show. The kidney and wall of the intestine may show but are not really necessary for even a negative diagnosis.

In 179 cases I have failed once to show a renal calculus when it was present; this failure was due to the plate not extending high enough to cover the kidney region, and twice I have made a diagnosis of a possible renal calculus where it did not exist. One of these was in a case of a man weighing 217 pounds and the mass was found to be feces; the other, a woman weighing over 200 pounds, and the shadow was covered by gallstones and carcinomata of the head of the pancreas. In neither of these cases was I able to detect the size or shape of the supposed calculus.

THE CYSTOSCOPE AND URETER CATHETER IN THE DIAGNOSIS OF SURGICAL DISEASE OF THE KIDNEY AND URETER.[1]

BY F. TILDEN BROWN, M.D.,

OF NEW YORK.

EVEN a ten minutes' talk on this topic need not omit a salutation to Nitze and his coworker Leiter, but for whose incentive and genius we know not how far behind the present status the diagnosis of renal disease would be to-day. Certainly no single agent has done so much to expand the field of our specialty and given to it dignified recognition, as has the cystoscope and ureter catheter.

As an outline for discussion we may consider in the first place, what importance attaches to cystoscopic pictures of the ureter mouth in the diagnosis of affections of the upper tract? Secondly, what can be employed in like cases from the cystoscope when employed in its secondary capacity, as a medium for ureter catheterization?

The cystoscope may show a ureter mouth which, either in an active or quiescent stage, looks like any one of the various kinds experience has led us to regard as normal, such as a faintly pinkish slit in a low papilla of yellowish white mucosa; in another instance a conical dimple capping a more pronounced papilla, or but one noticeable lip at the anterior base of which lies the nearly concealed but normal ureter mouth. Although such oscula are not calculated to arouse suspicion of any trouble beyond, nor excite doubt by anything seen to issue from them, still there may be disease of an associated kidney.

On the one hand the ureter mouth may impress us at once as abnormal, in that a tumor-like body occupies its site, or, on the other hand, a decided excavation. In either case the meatus may be invisible or conspicuously gaping. When tumor-like, the color varies from a reddish opacity to a glistening white; the latter being caused by the electric light transillumination of every edematous tissue, the same combination causing a brilliant central pink effect if one can look into the ureter at its moment of gaping emission.

Perhaps in the mouth of a bulging ureter we may see imbedded a brownish body recognized at once as one pole of a calculus, quite naturally by reason of this experience when we next encounter a similar sort of protruding edematous ureter, but see no stone, we will infer its presence at some little distance beyond.

When a lesser grade of ureteric protrusion occurs, with more or less marginal inflammation of the meatus, we may picture its cause as some antecedent infection of the kidney.

If at some part of the inflammatory zone a ulcer exists we are prone to believe in a particular kind of renal infection—the tuberculous, as the cause—and still stronger this belief, if in place of any protrusion there is a marked retraction and an irregular ulcer near where the ureter

[1] Read at the Annual Meeting of the New York Academy of Medicine, G. U. Section, December 15, 1904. Symposium on Surgical Diseases of the Kidney.

mouth should be seen, such an ulcer has some surrounding hyperemia and a base so uneven as to make it difficult to know which of its various recesses will give a lead for the catheter into the ureter.

When undulating mounds of opaque reddish mucosa cover the trigonum and obliterate all trace of the ureteric papilla, and, in the midst of this nodular field, every trace of a meatus is lost, we may infer that the ureters have been for a long time discharging from faulty kidneys some sort of irritating débris or gravel upon the surfaces so disfigured.

When translucent ovoid bodies beset the mucosa about the bladder meatus or that of a ureter, we may think of some extravesical neoplasm.

When the ureter mouths are atypical in location or number we may infer some congenital abnormality higher up.

Only two of these foregoing pictures are of particular moment—the tuberculous ulcer and the imbedded calculus.

As to what may be seen issuing from the ureter. Here a fluid turbid with pus or blood admixture, mucopurulent or mortar-like material;

Fig. 1

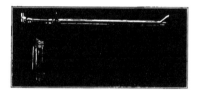

The author's double catheterizing cystoscope, with bottles for collecting separate urines.

all mean a pathologic state above and in conjunction with other exterior data might be enough to indicate surgical intervention, but not to give us the etiology, consequently steps should be taken to collect this abnormal efflux for examination and the same opportunity seized to gather by catheter the excretion of the other supposedly healthy kidney. Cases of traumatic hematuria in general call only for cystoscopy. As an instance, a hospital male was observed for three days in the alcoholic ward as a case of ruptured bladder—cystoscopy showed the bladder to be intact and that blood was coming from the left ureter. Diagnosis was changed to ruptured kidney which was confirmed at autopsy.

If we were compelled, or as not a few appear to be, content, to stop investigation of the renal and ureteric conditions after a wizard-like interpretation of various pictures of the ureter mouths, diagnosis of affections of the upper urinary tract would be nothing like so complete as they easily can be made, when, with a short flexible catheter lying a couple of inches within each ureter, we obtain the individual renal products for micro-

scopical, chemical and cultural examination and perhaps supplement this test by a long ureter catheter for determination of any anatomical abnormality of the ureter and renal pelvis.

To Brenner is due the credit for first adapting the cystoscope to affect ureter catheterization. We assume whatever is due for the first bilateral cystoscope making synchronous collection of the urines feasible. The evident advantages of this need not here be rehearsed; it being understood that in renal affections, particularly of a surgical nature, it is just as necessary to know the competency of a remaining kidney as it is to know the full pathological condition of the one to be removed.

As a means of diagnosis the ureter catheter is valuable (1) by reason of what comes through it; (2) by reason of its contemporaneous service as a sound, and (3) by its use as an X-ray landmark, with which to compare other questionable X-ray shadows, or questionable and palpable tumors.

Of all our bilateral catheterization tests, those which demonstrated a unilateral renal tuberculosis were probably as a class more gratifying than any, on account of the accurate and early diagnosis, together with the practical results attending nephrectomy which substantiated the pre-operative estimate as to adequacy of the other kidney. In three of the renal tuberculous cases no abnormality was noticeable in the condition of the corresponding ureter mouth, while on the other hand the catheter secured urine containing tubercle bacilli, and the removed kidney showed the lesions.

Among the least satisfactory results from catheterization were those in cases of renal hematuria, although the doubtful source of bleeding was determined in all, the etiological factor in more than 50 per cent. was not made out, despite that in a number of the cases a reinforcement of the usual urinary tests was sought by inoculation, cultural, and X-ray tests. Such negative results naturally supported the inference of neoplasm, and this tentative diagnosis was verified in 80 per cent. by operation or necropsy.

In two male patients with symptomless, marked unilateral hematuria of moderate duration the urines were sterile. Bleeding ceased after catheterization, which, while but a probable coincidence, was still an interesting fact. Neither of these cases were among those of suspected neoplasm.

In a sixty-seven-year-old male patient of symptomless unremitting right hematuria, of long duration, the only additional right urine abnormality was a colon bacillus culture. This patient was given several pelvic lavages of adrenalin with not even a temporary effect. Although he declined operation, he bequeathed us his kidneys just before death some two weeks ago, fourteen months after onset of hematuria. He died of acute anemia and exhaustion. The only post-mortem lesion found being a hypernephroma of the upper pole of the right kidney (Fig. 1).

An ambulatory forty-year-old male patient with excessive and continuous hematuria had a large left-side abdominal tumor—considered spleen, kidney or retroperitoneal lymphoma by different observers. A surprise attended the catheter test in that his left urine was normal while the right was densely bloody. Later developments showed that the patient had right renal neoplasm and great splenic enlargement.

We may review a few cases belonging to the class where the catheter served also as a sound in measuring the distance of an obstruction:

1. Thirty-year-old female; had right lumbar tumor; pain and some fever; voluntary urine normal. Diagnosis, pyonephrosis. Ureter catheterization gave normal left urine, but the right catheter remained dry and its progress was

Fig. 2.

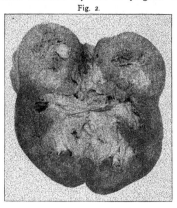

Hypernephroma right kidney unilateral hematuria, fourteen months.

checked at 4½ inches by impacted calculus; hemorrhagic complications following nephrotomy necessitated nephrectomy. Two years later this X-ray plate showed the stone still in its original location just below the iliosacral brim.

2. Twenty-two-year-old female; intermittent right lumbar tumor; pain and fever; voluntary urine variable in quality. Diagnosis, intermittent pyonephrosis. The right ureter catheter remained dry until it was finally twisted through a stricture three inches below the pelvis, when turbid urine came continuously in rapid drops. Nephrectomy. Cure. Dr. Eliot's case.

3. Thirty-four-year-old female; left lumbar pain; sharp chill followed by fever at first every ten days, later, every month. The first such septic manifestation followed some three weeks after protracted labor and instrumental delivery. Catheter in left ureter gave no flow and its insertion was checked at six inches from

the bladder. Diagnosis, traumatic stricture and complete occlusion of ureter. Septic attacks became less frequent. Now, a year after inception, three months have elapsed without one. Probable atrophy of the kidneys.

Three cases where the styletted ureter catheter was used in conjunction with X-ray pictures to elucidate diagnosis:

1. Twenty-seven-year-old female; some bladder and other urinary symptoms together with a tumor in region of appendix; thought by her physician to be displaced and diseased kidney. In evidence to the contrary was this X-ray photograph by Dr. Johnson, which shows our styletted ureter catheter extending well beyond the tumor to the normal position of the kidney. Subsequent operation proved this organ to be insequent operation proved organ to be intact.

2. Thirty-four-year-old female; where there was disagreement in regard to the organ involved by a large left abdominal tumor dipping into the pelvis. That it was not the left kidney all were satisfied when synchronous ureter catheterization gave identical and normal urines and when an X-ray of the styletted left catheter showed the kidney pelvis to be on a line with upper margin of tumor and in a normal position.

3. Forty-nine-year-old female; obscure symptoms referable to pelvic organs and left urinary tract. Ureteral catheterization suggested partial stricture of lower left ureter. Then two X-ray pictures, taken independently, showed in each a shadow easily referable to the lower part of the right ureter but a little nearer the ischial spine than a normal ureter might be expected. To determine whether this opaque object was in the ureter or not, the styletted ureter catheter was then X-rayed in position by Dr. Cole, and the resulting two shadows are seen to be more than half an inch apart. Another similar X-ray plate, but taken with oblique rays, showed the object to be behind as well as to the outer side of the ureter.

EXPLORATORY OPERATIONS RELATING TO THE KIDNEY.[1]

BY HOWARD LILIENTHAL, M.D.,
OF NEW YORK;
ATTENDING SURGEON TO MT. SINAI HOSPITAL.

WHEN inspection, palpation, auscultation and percussion, the cystoscope, the separator, and the ureter-catheter, the X-ray and the cryoscope and the microscope have done their work, then comes the turn of the scalpel. Sometimes the operation is for the purpose of doing what the other methods of research have found necessary, and sometimes it is avowedly for the purpose of pure diagnosis, the treatment to be determined upon later.

In my experience nearly every operation on the kidney, like every abdominal section, is more or less exploratory in character, but the surgeon in addition to making and clinching the diagnosis

[1] Read at the Annual Meeting of the New York Academy of Medicine, G. U. Section, December 15, 1904. Symposium on Surgical Diseases of the Kidney.

must be prepared to deal, more or less radically, with conditions as they present themselves with the patient on the table. Let us take, for example, such a disease as hypernephroma. Here hematuria may be the only really striking symptom. Palpable tumor may be absent and all that the cystoscope and allied instruments can tell us may be directed toward determining which kidney is affected and whether there is a second kidney to do the work in case the diseased one should have to be removed. The actual diagnosis can be revealed only at operation when, as a rule, nephrectomy is indicated and should be at once performed.

As to this matter of the presence or absence of the "other" kidney, it is well to remember that about one person in 2,500 is what may be termed "mononephric" that is, has but a solitary kidney, which naturally forbids nephrectomy, so when the cystoscope fails to disclose two ureters it is safer to make a quick exploratory incision in the suspected loin to assure ourselves of the presence of the necessary "other" kidney than to remove even a hopelessly diseased solitary one —an accident which it was the writer's fortune to witness in a case operated upon by a colleague. When once encountered, such a disaster makes a profound impression and the possibility of the danger is not likely to be again overlooked.

Another condition in which the presence of a second kidney healthier than the suspected one cannot be demonstrated by the cystoscope, is that of nephrocystosis. Here a rapid exposure of the apparently normal side may reveal a condition so much like the one for which operation was undertaken, that it would be better to abandon further surgical steps. Certain renal cysts are very apt to be symmetrical, in which case nephrectomy would probably do no good.

Obese individuals, in whom tumor has been palpated on the right side because of the greater mobility of the right kidney, may have a tumor of equal size on the left and yet its situation beneath the ribs and behind a thick abdominal wall may prevent its discovery without incision.

In most infections of the kidney, in palpable tumors and in calculus, the various clinical nonoperative methods will yield, in the great majority of cases, a general diagnosis. The actual extent of the disease, however, it may be impossible to foretell without operation, and therefore I repeat, that in a wide sense, every operation upon the kidney is exploratory in character. Surgical exploration must often be very thorough so that small but important points may not be overlooked. Indeed, when a case is not perfectly clear on exposure of the organ, the kidney must be drawn out of the wound, its vessels compressed by an assistant and systematic search made for abscesses, cysts, small calculi or tumors the existence of which is suspected. It may even be necessary to incise the kidney from the ischemic line in its convex border into the pelvis in order to make a diagnosis by exclusion.

Hemorrhage from the kidney is often a most obscure symptom, which nothing short of operation will clear up and which even a most careful operation may fail to explain.

A few years ago a woman, of thirty-five years of age, was admitted to my service at Mount Sinai Hospital with severe hematuria. The hemorrhage was intermittent, ceasing entirely for days at a time. During periods of quiescence the cystoscope was valueless except to demonstrate that the blood did not come from the bladder, and during the active hemorrhage bleeding was so profuse that no cytoscope could show whence it came. The clear urine showed an apparently mild nephritis. The patient became anemic to the verge of exsanguination, when during a sharp hemorrhage suprapubic cystotomy was done and the blood in great spurts was seen to come from the right ureter. Right nephrotomy was at once performed and nothing found. An olive-tipped, soft woven urethral bougie was passed through the urethra and guided into the right ureter with the help of the finger in the suprapubic wound. The instrument was large enough to fill the ureter completely and check the hemorrhage. The kidney was then carefully packed, the wound left open and the patient put to bed.

She died of acute anemia. A careful autopsy by Dr. Libman, of the Pathological Department, failed to show one single break in continuity from the pelvis of the kidney to the bladder. The mucosa of the pelvis and entire ureter was most carefully inspected and no abrasion or ulceration found. The microscopical examination of the kidney showed what the urine had already indicated,—that there was nephritis. This then was a fatal case of pure hemorrhagic nephritis which could not have been absolutely diagnosed by anything short of a microscopic examination of a piece of the kidney *plus* the exclusion of all other causes for the hemorrhage by means of a complete examination of the entire urinary tract. Even exploratory nephrotomy was useless except to aid in exclusion. I have seen other cases of hemorrhagic nephritis in which nephrotomy permanently checked the bleeding.

To sum up we may state that

A. Exploratory operation is probably the surest method of diagnosis in suspected surgical disease of the kidney.

B. The indications for its performance are: (1) In hemorrhage from one or both kidneys when other measures have failed to check the bleeding and the danger signals appear. (2) In palpable tumor with symptoms pointing to renal disease. Sometimes even to establish whether the tumor is kidney, gall-bladder or some other organ. (3) Without palpable tumor when there is reason to suspect surgical renal disease and when medical, hygienic and local treatment fail to give relief.

C. Exploratory incision may be necessary to demonstrate the condition of solitary kidney.

MEDICAL PROGRESS.

SURGERY.

Etiology and Pathology of Coxa Vera.—The number of cases of this disease, in which an anatomical or microscopical examination has been made, is relatively small. and for this reason considerable interest to the report of a case in which it was necessary to do a resection of the head of the femur. A. SCHLESINGER (*Archiv f. klin. Chir.*, Vol. 75, No. 3) studied the specimen very carefully, and found that this was an instance of a purely traumatic separation of the ephiphysis. Reference to the history showed that the patient, a girl of fifteen years, had never had any pains previously, but that the symptoms came on immediately after the injury, a fall on the side, and continued up to the time of operation. There were no other evidences of disease. The relation of traumatic separation of the epiphysis to coxa vera has never been definitely cleared up, and an effort is made by the writer to gain some conclusions from the few cases reported in which anatomical and histological studies were made. Of these there are twelve. It seems that in no case of coxa vera at puberty were any evidences found, either macroscopical or microscopical, of rachitis or osteomalacia. Furthermore, the softening of the spongy tissue in the head of the bone is due to an insufficient nutrition of the displaced segment. In healthy individuals the locus minoris resistentiæ is the epiphyseal line, whereas in rachitic children it is the entire neck of the femur, because an epiphyseal separation occurring in a rachitic child has never been recorded. The author believes that in ordinary cases it is the continued trauma which gradually bring about a displacement of the head of the bone at the epiphyseal junction, and that this is the cause for the advancing deformity, as the nutrition of the head of the bone suffers.

Prostatectomy Under Local Anesthesia.—The problem of prostatic hypertrophy, even with the many resources recently introduced and developed, still offers in certain cases many difficulties in its solution. Prostatectomy, when carefully performed, is generally recognized as the ideal procedure, but the dangers of the operation are chiefly from the anesthetic and hemorrhage. Spinal cocainization has been largely given up on account of its uncertainties, and now M. B. TINKER (*Jour. Am. Med. Ass'n,* February 11, 1905), with a proposition to employ local anesthesia. He advocates a solution of beta eucaine, 1 to 500, with an addition of adrenalin chloride to make it 1 to 120,000, or even weaker, where large quantities are found necessary. The use of the adrenalin not only limits the amount of bleeding, it also prevents the absorption of the anesthetic drug, and reduces pain and congestion after operation, and finally acts as a stimulant. It is necessary to have an accurate knowledge of the anatomy of the region in order to employ this method effectively, and the first step is the infiltration of the main trunks from which the various nerve branches take their origin. Taking the tuberosity of the ischium as a landmark, the needle of the syringe is inserted in the skin about one inch in front and internal to the tuberosity. After the superficial tissues are infiltrated, a stronger solution of cucaine (0.5 per cent.) is injected at a depth of from one to two inches in the region of the ischiorectal fossa. Finally, a weak solution is injected along the line of the proposed skin incision. The operation itself is practically that described by Young in the *Journal* of the American Medical Association of October 26, 1904. A case is reported in which the method was used with very satisfactory results, in a very much emaciated and weakened patient, and a second case is merely noted, in which equally good results were obtained.

Syphilis of the Liver in the Diagnosis of Abdominal Tumors.—The fact is becoming gradually established that syphilis of the internal organs may play an important rôle in the diagnosis, even when the clinical picture points to functional disturbances of inflammatory processes accompanied by fever. For a long time specific disease of the internal organs was always associated with the other classical symptoms of the disease, but it has more recently been admitted that such lesions of various organs may appear without any other symptoms which might be designated as luetic. For it must not be forgotten that the original infection may have escaped notice, and likewise the primary and secondary stages of the disease may have been marked by very slight disturbances. An interesting contribution to this subject has lately been published by Prof. KÖNIG (*Berl. klin. Woch.,* February 6, 1905), who reports three cases who suffered from attacks of pain in the hepatic region, but who presented no evidences of functional liver disturbances, no loss of appetite or weight. In each instance a diagnosis of hepatic tumor was made, and in one case a movable mass was made out, which was believed to be connected with either the liver or the kidney. An exploratory laparotomy showed that the tumor was a lobe of the liver, which, together with the rest of the organ, was covered with grayish nodules. As the liver and stomach were adherent, it was assumed that a carcinoma of the stomach furnished the primary focus for the supposed multiple metastatic deposits in the liver. After the patient recovered from the operation, a treatment with mercury and the iodides was instituted, and all the symptoms, including the tumor, disappeared. No history of syphilis could be elicited. Similar conditions were found in the other two cases, in which operation had also been done for the relief of symptoms. Impressed by the importance of this subject, König made some further studies, and now believes that the luetic growths of the liver may be divided into two classes—the first consisting of flat, hard, irregular swellings on the surface of the organ and within the percussion boundaries; and the second, of masses apparently separated from the liver, which are often movable, nodular, round or kidney-shaped, attached to the viscus by a pedicle and representing a large portion of the same. The question of operation in these cases is a very important one. Where the least doubt exists, a mercurial treatment may be tried, although it must not be forgotten that in isolated cases no results are obtained. Moreover, in one of the author's cases, no effect was secured with mercurials before operation, but a very pronounced one followed the employment of the same means after laparotomy. There may be circumstances which urge operation and the dictum, "do not operate because the condition is due to lues," should not be overdone. In the one case which the author reports it was certainly justifiable to remove the pedunculated growth, and he concludes with the statement that where an exploratory celiotomy reveals the presence of syphilitic disease, any removal of affected tissues must be entirely governed by the findings in each individual case.

Strangulated Hernia in the Very Old.—D. C. PEYTON (*Am. Med.*, February 18, 1905) believes the process of inflammation of the imprisoned loop offers a satisfactory explanation of the cause of strangulation. The obstructive venous congestion is the first step in the inflammatory process, and this inflammatory process, begun in obstruction, by pressure engorgement is the result of the increased activity and virulence of *Bacillus coli communis,* and several varieties of the staphylococcus and streptococcus, which, if not arrested, results in gangrene and death. The treatment is operative only, and the earlier the operation the more satisfactory will be the results. He believes taxis is not only a mistake but a menace to the life of the patient and should never be resorted to. Extreme age should be considered a bar to operation, the patient's general condition should be considered only. In the very old, the minimum degree of general anesthesia is desired, so that the injection locally of Schleich's solution along the line of incision has proved of great advantage by reason of its local effect. When the heart is weakened, the use of oxygen alternating with ether is an excellent precaution. Old people do not stand confinement to bed, so it is of greatest importance to get your old patient out of bed and into an invalid chair in not longer than four or five days. Turn them to the sound side in twenty-four hours after operation. Frequently success may be determined by this fact. Less that a year ago Peyton operated on a woman of eighty-four less than eight hours after strangulation of a femoral hernia. The sac was opened and extensive adhesions broken up, the omentum well pulled down, ligated and cut off, the intestine returned to the cavity, and the ring closed with the pursestring suture. The patient made an uninterrupted recovery, was out of bed and in an invalid chair in four days, and in seventeen days walked.

Simultaneous Stenosis of the Pylorus and Intestine.—This combination of lesions has been observed by E. PAYR (*Archiv f. klin. Chir.*, Vol. 75, No. 2) in eight cases and from a careful study of the subject, he lays stress on the following points. He finds that this double form of stenosis occurs most frequently with round ulcer of the stomach which is complicated with perigastric changes, and the lumen of the gut is narrowed by the resulting adhesions. Fibrous strictures of a syphilitic character may also occur in the stomach and intestine of the same individual, and where this is the cause, treatment is very satisfactory. Therapeutic measures are of little value, however, where malignant neoplasms cause the gastric stenosis and where the intestinal stenosis is due to metastases. Aside from these there are also a large number of other etiological factors in the production of this condition. There are definite forms of perigastritis, which may bring about stenosis of the gut either close to or at some distance from the stomach. A very typical form of constriction of the large intestine is caused by the retraction of the transverse colon toward the region of the ulcer, while those which involve the small gut are more irregular in character. There are well-marked distinctions, both clinical and anatomical, between a cicatricial constriction of the pylorus and these adhesion and compression deformities, in the latter case, the higher grades of ectasia are often absent. A stenosis of the pylorus may mask to a great extent that of the intestine, and after its removal, occlusion of the intestine may suddenly come on. In the extreme degrees of intestinal stenosis, a pyloric constriction may be masked by the threatening intestinal symptoms, and where a chronic stenosis of the gut exists, the gastric symptoms may be readily overlooked and do not become prominent until the intestinal occlusion has been relieved. Cicatricial stenosis of the pylorus do not constitute any hindrance to the retrograde flow of the intestinal contents into the stomach, the rigidity of the tube preventing a complete closure of the lumen. With the aid of various diagnostic measures, which he describes, it is often possible to make a differential diagnosis, the most effective being the test for gastric ectasia by Boas' method and the presence of hyperperistalsis in the gut, in a different direction and at a different time than in the stomach. If operation is undertaken, the twofold nature of the trouble may often be recognized under certain circumstances by the hypertrophy of that section of gut lying between the pylorus and the site of the intestinal constriction. If an operation is decided on, it is necessary that both obstructions be removed at once. Where perigastric adhesions exist, no matter what their etiology, it is imperative that the remainder of the intestinal canal be carefully examined, as constriction in the small or large intestine may readily be overlooked and in this way invalidate the results of a gastro-enterostomy.

Traumatic Rupture of the Intestine Without Injury to the Abdominal Wall.—C. P. FLINT (*Med. Rec.*, February 18, 1905) is an advocate of prompt exploratory incision in doubtful cases of abdominal trauma. His conclusions are summarized as follows: (1) Any injury to the abdomen may be associated with drainage to the intestine or other viscera; (2) an exploratory operation is justifiable in cases with distinct rigidity; (3) an operation is absolutely indicated when there are, besides rigidity, pain, tenderness, vomiting, shock, dulness, or other symptoms indicative of some intra-abdominal disturbance. (4) Cases not operated upon are lost. (5) The importance of early operation cannot be emphasized too strongly. (6) At present the death rate is about 75 to 80 per cent. (7) When early operation is the rule the death rate will be much lower.

Diabetes in Surgery.—Ephemeral traumatic glycosuria and the induction of narcosis in diabetics are two subjects discussed by W. KAUSCH (*Archiv f. klin. Chir.*, Vol. 74, No. 4) as of particular moment at the present time. He has observed an increasing number of cases where glycosuria followed injuries, nine of which were fractures and two contusions. In every case the urine shows the presence, soon after the injury, of not more than one per cent. of sugar, the entire quantity of which during twenty-four hours may run up to 15 grams. The other manifestations of diabetes were usually absent, due most likely to the small amount of sugar present, and the condition lasted from one to eight days. Kausch found that these cases were not of the so-called latent variety, during the course of which the trauma has brought about an exacerbation of the diabetes. He was also able to show that these patients manifested a well-marked tolerance to carbohydrates, and failed to exhibit any alimentary glycosuria within a few days after the injury. The writer's observations show that there are individuals who are perfectly normal under ordinary circumstances as regards their metabolism of sugar, but who present a distinct glycosuria under the influence of a trauma. The condition depends on two

possible explanations,—there is neither a reflex action
of purely mechanical concussion on the nervous
system, or the effect of the trauma is a psychical
one. The author is inclined to accept the latter theory, and believes that as the result of this same disturbance a true diabetes may even be developed.
In discussing the question of narcosis in diabetic
cases, Kausch submits the following statements.
In the first place, general anesthesia should be restricted as much as possible and local anesthesia employed, unless specially contra-indicated. Narcosis
for purely diagnostic purposes should be avoided, and
successive anesthesias without sufficiently long intermissions cannot be permitted. Ether is preferable to chloroform. The quantity used and the length
of the anesthesia should be contracted as much as
possible. Inhalation anesthesia in diabetics had best
be done early in the morning, so that the time of abstinence from food shall not be prolonged any longer
than is absolutely necessary. Particular attention
must be given to the nourishment both before and
after the operation. Every case, even where the
local anesthetic is employed, must be given a preliminary treatment with the bicarbonate of soda
method, until the urine has an alkaline reaction.
By this means the acid intoxication of true diabetic
coma may be neutralized to a certain extent. When
possible the anesthetic should be given when the
patient is free from sugar excretion, but not until
this has been established for some time. If coma
threatens, or is present, the soda administration must
be pushed, per os, anum, subcutaneously and intravenously.

**The Effect of the Removal of the Thyroid on the
Genital System.**—The relation between the thyroid
gland and the genitals has been studied by
Lanz (*Archiv f. klin. Chir.*, Vol. 74, No. 4) in a series
of animal experiments. He found that in dogs, rabbits, hens, and goats, procreation was usually impossible after thyroidectomy. Two human subjects were
also under observation. A man, ten years after total
thyroidectomy, presented the picture of cretinism.
At the age of twenty-eight years he had never had
the slightest sexual desire, no erections and no pollutions. Three months after the administration of
thyroid extract was begun he began slowly to manifest sexual desires, which he was able to satisfy by
coitus. Later he married, but the union remained
childless. Within a few weeks after the administration of the thyroid was stopped his other symptoms
returned, and the sexual desire declined. In the
other case, that of a woman, amenorrhea was present, but after the use of the thyroid extract for several months, the menses gradually appeared. The
girl remained unmarried.

MEDICINE.

Aloin Test in Typhoid.—The feces of 18 cases of
typhoid were examined systematically with the aloin
test for traces of blood by C. Petracchi (*Zeitsch f.
klin Med.*, Vol. 56, Nos. 1 and 2). The more severe
cases were postitive more often than the milder ones
and the greatest frequency occurred during the second and third week. It is possible to predict a large
hemorrhage by this method, since the first trace of
blood may often be detected one to five days before. Frequently the pulse increases 12 to 22 beats
per minute with the first appearance of blood and
a hemorrhage is then almost certain. In such cases
the baths should be used more carefully or stopped
altogether until the dangerous period has passed.

Cryptogenetic Fever.—Fevers of obscure origin
are divided by C. Bozzolo (*Wien. klin. Therap. Woch.*,
January 1 to 8, 1905) into the following classes: (1)
Fevers where the origin can only be detected at
autopsy. The most common example of this class
is endocarditis ulcerosa. (2) Fevers whose cause
is detected during life, though late. This interesting
group includes the recurrent rises of temperature so
common with leucemic and pseudoleucemic glandular enlargements. The focus may be extremely
small as in prostatic abscesses after gonorrhea or
intra-urethral manipulation. Obscure abscesses may
also form about the anus, and the antrum of Highmore should not be overlooked as possible source.
The possibility of a chronic septic endocarditis or
of a pyelitis in young subjects should not be forgotten. (3) There is a special form of glandular
fever, suggesting a tuberculous fever and accompanied only by glandular swelling. Occasionally,
hypertrophic tonsils will give rise to fever which
disappears when the tonsils are removed. (4) Another type of fever may be termed "precarcino-
matous." The tumor (generally carcinoma, more
rarely sarcoma) may not yet be evident, especially
when it develops in the deeper part of the abdomen.
The curve is often intermittent, suggesting malaria.
Carcinomata of the stomach, liver, ovaries, uterus
and mediastinum most frequently run with fever.
In one case observed by the author, a specific germ
could be isolated, both from the tumor and the circulating blood. (5) Very frequently, tertiary syphilitic manifestations will be responsible for an obscure fever. The type is generally quotidion, intermittent and irregular, without very high rises, and
long periods of apyrexia may be interposed. Antisyphilitic treatment is very prompt in its action. (6)
Nervous and hysterical fevers are characterized by
great irregularity both as far as height and duration
are concerned. The highest temperatures on record
are recorded in hysteria, but the fever is rarely distributed uniformly over the body. (7) The last
group, cryptogenetic fever proper, includes all forms
of bacteremia or septicemia with late localization,
which are generally cleared up by a bacteriological
examination of the blood. The course is usually
acute but may also be so chronic as to suggest a
malignant tumor somewhere in the body. This class
may be again subdivided, according to the germ
found in the circulating blood, as follows: (*a*) in pure
Streptococcus mycosis, there is an irregular, intermittent course, with moderate fluctuations, but exceptions are common. A regular, continuous fever
is, however, rare; (*b*) staphylococci generally give
rise to a continuous or slightly remittant fever; (*c*)
pneumococci behave like staphylococci; (*d*) *Bacterium coli* and the gonococcus generally cause an exquisitely intermittent fever, with rapid rise and falls;
(*e*) mixed infections also give rise to an intermittent
curve. These rules only apply in a general way, since
the amount of bacteria and their localization also play
a prominent rôle. In simple bacteremia without localization, the type is continuous or remittant, while
in puerperal sepsis with numerous metastatic abscesses or in ulcerating endocarditis, the type is more
intermittent. Occasionally a sepsis may follow an
infectious disease and need not necessarily be caused
by the same germ as the infectious disease. The author has observed streptococci, staphylococci and
diplococci in the blood after typhoid, and in one rare
case diplococci and staphylococci were isolated during different periods. The therapy of sepsis is as yet

in its infancy, and it is to be hoped that ere long serum-therapy will advance so that a remedy will be at hand for every given case. Little can be expected from quinine or the endivenous application of sublimates, but collorgol is sometimes followed by good results.

Endemic Occurrence of Myelogenous Leucemia.— Since three cases of myelogenous leucemia from the same town were treated in the clinic at the same time, LANSPERGER (*Münch. med. Woch.*, January 3, 1905) took a trip to the surrounding country, and was surprised to encounter eight more cases. It is very difficult to explain these endemic cases, but some common infection seems to be probable. The following important facts could be obtained: The entire valley was visited by a severe typhoid epidemic a few years ago. It is therefore possible that toxic or mechanical insults to the spleen predispose to a disease in which the spleen plays so prominent a part. The hygienic conditions were very poor and the supply of water not of the best, since the inhabitants relied chiefly upon wells.

A Review of Recent Literature on the Relation of Human and Bovine Tuberculosis.—D. BOVAIRD (*Med. Rec.*, February 25, 1905) discusses the experimental work done, and the results obtained, by American and European investigators in their attempts to settle the question raised by Koch in 1901, when he affirmed the independence of human and bovine tuberculosis. After considering the evidence pro and con, the author sums up his views by saying that it appears that human tuberculosis can be transmitted to cattle but with difficulty, and it seems highly improbable that such transmission plays any great part in the production of the disease among cattle. Bovine tuberculosis can be transmitted to man, but the evidence that such transmission occurs under ordinary circumstances is extremely scanty, and it is highly improbable that such transmission plays an important part in the spread of the disease in man. An important feature in the research work done, has been that relative to the infection of children through the intestine, and of this the author says that despite the discordant results noted, it seems that it can safely be said that the greatest weight of evidence is against frequent infection of children through the intestine, that is through food, and that one cannot, therefore, consider that tuberculous milk is frequently the means of conveying the infection.

Classification of Gastric Ulcers.—A. L. BENEDICT (*Am. Med.*, February 18, 1905) urges the same general use of the term ulcer in the case of the stomach, as of other parts of the body, first because there is no unanimously accepted definition of gastric ulcer and, second, if there were, it would be impossible to make all cases correspond to it. Without hemorrhage or opportunity for inspection, the diagnosis of ulcer can only be tentative, but a diligent search should be made for small hemorrhages. If hemorrhage is clinically demonstrated to be from the stomach, it almost always means an ulcer in the proper general sense of a solution of superficial continuity. He classifies ulcers of the stomach, including certain conditions associated with hemorrhage, as follows: (1) Peptic ulcer, the most frequent, occurs in patients who do not have apoplexy, thrombosis, embolism and organic vascular lesions elsewhere and in whom a primary organic basis for the necrosis is untenable. He asserts that the digestion of the necrotic area is not simply an erosion by excess

of HCl and he is also skeptical as to the uniform association of hperchlorhydria and peptic ulcer. (2) Superficial erosions due to chemic and thermic caustics. (3) Ulcers due to vascular lesions, occurring in syphilitics and in elderly persons. He reports such a case in detail and alludes to others. (4) "Catarrhal" ulcers, analogous to eczematous ulcers of the skin, not strictly separable from the foregoing, but without definite, conspicuous, local vascular lesions. (5) Varicose ulcerations, due to venous obstruction and, practically, almost always to hepatic sclerosis. (6) Toxemic diapedesis, as in scurvy, purpuras, etc. (7) Vicarious menstruation. (6 and 7 are not true ulcers.) (8) Gangrenous ulcer. Such cases usually illustrate 3 and 4 and, still more frequently, cancerous ulceration and do not really constitute a distinct, pathologic type. (9) phlegmonous ulcers. Unless due to pyemia or subphrenic or other abscess contiguous to the stomach, such ulcers are usually due to iodin poisoning. (10) Specific ulcers include exanthematous, pneumococcic, tuberculous, syphilitic actinomycotic and similar conditions due to special germs and, by an extension of terms, those due to the breaking down of neoplasms, especially cancer. (11) Traumatic ulcers, due to foreign bodies, hard particles in food, crushing injuries, gross parasites, etc.

Copper Foil in Destroying Typhoid and Colon Bacilli in Water.—HENRY KRAEMER (*Am. Med.*, February 18, 1905) carried out a series of experiments for testing the efficiency of the copper method for the purification of drinking water. The experiments were made mostly with copper foil rather than copper sulphate. It was found that in every instance colon and typhoid bacilli were completely destroyed in less than four hours by placing strips of copper foil in water containing pure cultures of these organisms. In the duplicate experiments, namely, in those in which no copper foil was used, it was found that the organisms persisted and continued to multiply even for sixty days. Kraemer considers it extremely fortunate that in the copper treatment of water a method has been devised which is so effective in destroying intestinal micro-organisms and which can be applied so easily on a large scale and so safely by the average householder. The method suggested for domestic purposes consists simply in placing a piece of copper foil 3½ inches square in a quart of water, allowing this to stand from six to eight hours, or over night, at the ordinary temperature, and then removing the foil or drawing off the water.

Intestinal Putrefaction in Catarrhal Jaundice.— The amount of ethereal sulphates present in the urine has been considered a means for estimating the intensity of intestinal putrefaction in any given case. It is claimed, however, that not all the aromatic bodies which are produced in the intestine take this form—only a part appearing as ethereal sulphates, the other as glycuronic acids, etc. The proposition was therefore made to make quantitive estimates of one product, such as indican. F. BLUMENTHAL (*Berl. klin. Woch.*, January 30, 1905) reports a case of catarrhal jaundice in which this test would have shown the intestinal putrefaction to have been abnormally diminished in degree, because on certain days the indican excretion in the urine was practically nothing, and not until couvalescence was established and a sufficient quantity of bile was present in the gut were any considerable amounts of indican present. The quantity of phenol excreted, however, was sometimes more than double the normal amount. The writer believes that the volatile fatty acids in the urine afford a better means of making an estimate as to the degree of intestinal acid fermentation, but that an absolute index cannot be obtained from a mere estimation of the indican, phenol and ethereal sulphates as to the degree of intestinal putrefaction in the gut. In addition to these, it is also necessary to determine the amount of volatile acids, in order to find out whether acid fermentation may not be taking the place of the production of aromatic bodies.

PHYSIOLOGY.

The Selective Action of Cocaine on Nerve Fibers. —Two hypotheses may be advanced to explain the action of cocaine, according to N. E. DIXON (*Jour. of Physiol.*, December 30, 1904). He first considers cocaine a general protoplasmic poison; the sensory nerves are affected because they are more exposed, the motor ends are not affected because cocaine does not reach them. The second hypothesis holds that cocaine specifically affects the sensory nerve endings, just as curare affects only the motor end-plates. The experiments of the author show that cocaine applied distally to nerve-fibers picks out and paralyzes some fibers before others, the sensory before the motor, the vagus fibers conducting upward before those conducting downward, the vasoconstrictors before the vasodilators, the bronchoconstrictors before the bronchodilators. It is suggested that the local application of cocaine to the vagus may be the means of combating death during early chloroform narcosis. Drugs which affect the central nervous system almost invariably attack the sensory cells and fibers before the motor. There is no reason to suppose that cocaine has a specific action in the sensory nerve-endings.

Relation between the Thymus and Sexual Organs. —For some time an intimate relationship between the thymus and the sexual organs has been recognized. According to D. N. PATON (*Jour. of Physiol.*, December 30, 1905), who submitted this observation to an experimental test, Paton and Goodall noted that in guinea-pigs the thymus increases in size during the first two months and begins to atrophy only when the animal reaches sexual maturity. J. Henderson found that castration in cattle delays the onset of atrophy of the thymus. From these observations the conclusion was drawn that the life history of the thymus is closely related to that of the testes; the onset of atrophy of the thymus is dependent on or is determined by the maturation of the sexual organs. The question which the author asks himself, and to the solution of which he devoted a series of researches, was, Does the thymus in turn exert any influence upon the sexual organs? The results of his experiments show that in male guinea-pigs weighing less than 300 gms. (*i.e.* before the time the thymus begins to atrophy), the removal of the organ is followed by a more rapid growth of the testes. Hence there is a reciprocal relationship between thymus and testis, each checks the growth of the other. In females, on the other hand, removal of the thymus does not markedly accelerate the onset of sexual maturity.

The Effect of Alcohol upon the Viscosity of the Blood.—That the viscosity of the body-fluids is one of the important determining factors in the metabolic exchanges in the body, may be gleaned from the recent experiments of Traube, Overton and others. The question as to whether alcohol would effect this viscosity is not, would therefore be of considerable importance from many points of view. R. B. OPITZ (*Jour. of Physiol.*, December 30, 1904) found that while 0.770 Na Cl solution causes a very distinct decrease in the viscosity of the blood, as determined by means of capillary tubes, a similar amount of alcohol causes an increase in viscosity. This occurs whether the alcohol is injected directly into the circulation or into the digestive tract. The effect is quick and marked when the alcohol is injected into the stomach or duodenum. The maximum increase occurs five to ten minutes after the injection, and the effect lasts at least one and a half hours.

The Gaseous Metabolism of the Kidney.—The production of diuresis is accompanied by a marked increase in the absorption of oxygen by the kidney, but not in proportion to the degree of diuresis produced, according to J. BANCROFT and T. G. BRODIE (*Jour. of Physiol.*, December 30, 1904). There is no definite relationship between the amount of oxygen taken in and the amount of CO_2 given out at any moment. Moreover, the latter is in excess of the former. This is especially the case at the beginning of the experiment before diuresis has been set up. The onset of diuresis is not necessarily accompanied by an increase in the rate of blood-flow through the kidney. If an increase of the latter is ever present it is never in proportion to the acceleration in the flow of urine.

The Universal Presence of Erepsin in Animal Tissues.—A peptone-splitting ferment, erepsin, was discovered by Cohnheim in the intestinal mucosa, and has been supposed by this investigator to be in distinct relationship to the digestion of the partially hydralyzed proteids. H. M. VERNON (*Jour. of Physiol.*, December 30, 1904) finds that this ferment is present in all the tissues of a large number of animals examined, from the fresh-water mussel to the cat; the higher up in the scale of animal life the species is, the richer are the tissues in the content of erepsin. The same tissue in various animals shows the same relative amount of erepsin. The ereptive value of a tissue is subject to change. The various tissue-erepsins are probably to some extent specific. The universality of erepsin indicates that the theory that erepsin is concerned in the digestion of the partially hydrolyzed proteids in the intestine is probably incorrect.

The Pancreatic Lymph-Flow.—The interest which has been aroused within recent years in the physiology and pathology of the pancreas, particularly with reference to derangements of glycolytic metabolism, gives a certain degree of importance to every study, however limited, into the metabolic phenomena that accompany pancreatic activity. An investigation into the nature of the lymph-flow from the pancreas was made by F. A. BAINBRIDGE (*Jour. of Physiol.*, December 30, 1904). The recent discovery of an activating substance extracted from the mucous membrane of the small intestine, and called "secretin," which when injected into the circulation causes an increased flow of pancreatic juice, enabled the author to study the effect of secretin upon the flow of lymph from the pancreas. The injection of secretin caused an increase in the flow, even after ligation of the portal lymphatics. There is evidently a close relationship between the secretion of pancreatic juice and the increased flow of lymph. This is derived entirely from the pancreas, and is probably formed as the result of metabolic changes occurring in the pancreas during the secretion of juice.

The Mechanism of the Storage of Poisons in the Liver.—The anatomical position of the liver and its great size suggest for this organ an important filtering function, depriving the blood coming from the intestines of poisons that may have been absorbed. A careful study of the manner in which the liver takes up and fixes these poisons was made by ZOLTAN DE VÁMOSSY (*Arch. Internat. de Pharmaco, et de Therap.*, Vol. XIII, Nos. 3 and 4). Copper, injected into the portal vein, is fixed by the nucleo-albumins and albuminoids of the hepatic cells. Mercury is stored up in the globulins of these cells, the nucleo-albumins and the nucleins. The nucleo-albumins principally and also the nucleins have the power of fixing arsenic. In fatty degeneration of the liver, the capacity of storing up the metals is diminished. This is also the case during starvation. The liver stores up half of the alkaloids that traverse it. The tetanizing dose of strychnine that must pass through the liver is just twice that of the drug when introduced under the skin. Toward atropine the liver behaves in the same way as toward strychnine. The amount of glycogen in the liver has no effect upon its storage capacity with respect to poisons. The nucleins hold the alkaloids not merely mechanically, but fix them in chemical combination.

PATHOLOGY AND BACTERIOLOGY.

Changes in the Trachea in Advanced Age.—If the trachea be filled with plaster-of-Paris before it is opened at autopsies, it will be found that a saber-shaped organ is very common in old age. The shape is similar to that found with compression by a goiter, but involves almost the entire tube, down to the bifurcation. Frequently there is also a moderate degree of torsion. Ossification of the treachea is also common and can be easily demonstrated by examination with the Roentgen rays. Chronic catarrh of the tracheal mucous membrane and emphysema of the lungs are frequently combined with stenosed trachea and are probably a direct result of the constriction. Dilatation of the trachea may also occur, but is less common, according to M. SIMMONDS (*Virchow's Archiv*, Vol. 179, No. 1). It is due to insufficient resistance on part of the tracheal cartilages, aided by frequent coughing.

Experimental Migration of Lymphocytes.—It is known for some time that mononuclear leucocytes are able to migrate, though to a less degree than polynuclear cells. F. PRÖSCHER (*Virchow's Archiv*, Vol. 179, No. 1), now reports a method whereby one may obtain an exudate which contains lymphocytes almost exclusively. A suspension of intracellular tuberculotoxin in normal salt solution is prepared in the usual way and then injected into the peritoneum of guinea-pigs. Several hours later, some peritoneal fluid is removed by means of a glass pipette, and examined under the microscope. A large number of perfect lymphocytes will be encountered and in addition, the formation of lymphocytes from endothelial cells may be observed. A similar process goes on in every tubercle, the toxin stimulates the fixed tissue-cells to form the so-called epitheliod cells; the succeeding layer of small round cells results from the epithelioid cells, while the peripheral layer of round cells is directly due to chemotactic action.

Tuberculous Processess and Lymphocytes.—From clinical and experimental observations, C. J. FAUCONETT (*Deutsch. Arch. f. klin. Med.*, Vol. 82, Nos. 1 and 2)

concludes that the lymphocytes are not specifically affected by tuberclin or by the presence of tuberculous processes in the body. The tuberculous toxins, like other bacterial toxins, may exert chemotactic action solely upon the polynuclear, neutrophile cells. It is true that a preponderance of lymphocytes occurs in most tuberculous exudates, and as cerebrospinal and pleural fluids, yet they merely show the local influences of the tuberculous process. If the blood be examined in such cases, polymorphous cells will generally predominate.

Origin of Blood-platelets.—The so-called spindle cell found in frog's blood do not correspond to the platelets of man, but are more closely related to leucocytes. According to E. HELBER (*Deutsch. Arch. f. klin. Med.*, Vol. 82, Nos. 1 and 2) frogs and even birds do not possess platelets; the blood of the mammals, on the other hand, contains platelets but no spindle cells. In the rabbit embryo, at first only mother cells containing hemoglobin are found. After the thirteenth day, the nuclei are extended, generally without affecting the protoplasm, yet sometimes the nucleus dissolves in the protoplasm, destroying the cells. Leucocytes are not present at this stage, but blood-platelets are abundant. These latter make their appearance as soon as the nucleus is cast off, and, like this, are made up of a chromatic and an achromatic substance. After the twentieth day platelets are no longer formed in the blood itself but chiefly in the liver and red bone-marrow. The author distinguishes between plasma platelets, originating from the cell-protoplasm, and nuclear platelets. The number of platelets present will give a good idea of the function of the bone marrow, thus, in anemia with many platelets, the regenerative powers are good, and vice versa.

Abnormal Pathological Processes in Carcinoma.—It has been shown that the X-rays have the property of modifying the fermentative processes in carcinoma cells and also that in the autolysis of hepatic cancer a characteristic substance is formed, free reducing pentose, which does not occuur in the autodigestion of the normal tissue. The same author, C. NEUBERG (*Berl. klin. Woch.*, January 30, 1905), has now made some further studies, using in addition to the metastatic deposits in the liver also material from the primary focus in the stomach. It was found that autolysis showed no free pentose when the primary growth was subjected to the process, but that the hepatic growths yielded abnormally large amounts. It must, therefore, be assumed that, in the migration of the original cancer cells from the stomach to the liver, some change in the original ferments were produced or else new ones were acquired. Tests were also made of the action of the hepatic tissue on the lung tissue of the same individual. the autopsy showing that the latter was absolutely free from cancerous deposits. The digestion experiments showed that an exact reverse of the normal conditions was present. The carcinomatous extract produced an abnormal decomposition of the pulmonary albuminoid bodies, but is not able to break up the albumoses, as occurs normally, and these probably reach the circulation. The author intends to bring forward further proof of these claims, but thinks that this transposition of important cell functions, acquiring new fermentative processes on the one hand or loosing specific enzyme properties on the other, has an important bearing on the production of cachexia.

Diagnostic Importance of Bactericidal Action of Blood in Typhoid.—If the bactericidal action of the blood is to be determined instead of the agglutination test, to insure a diagnosis of typhoid, the procedure would be as follows: The serum to be examined is diluted 1:50. A number of small test-tubes are filled, each with one c.c. of physiological salt solution except the first one, which · contains only one c.c. of the diluted serum; a number of dilutions are thus prepared, which are then mixed with half a c.c. of broth culture of typhoid bacilli and half a c.c. of diluted (1:10) normal serum obtained from the ear-vein of a rabbit, which acts as complement. The test-tubes are placed in the incubator for half an hour with several controls, and then mixed with agar and poured into Petri dishes. After twenty-four hours the degree of bactericidal action can be easily determined by noticing in which plate a development of typhoid germs still goes on. The same method must be repeated with the two forms of paratyphoid germs. The bactericidal test is not always positive even in cases of typhoid where the germ has been isolated from the blood; positive results are, however, more frequent than with the agglutination test. The earliest period during which the germs were killed by typhoid serum was the eighth day. One great drawback of the method, according to KLAUBENHEIMER (*Zeitsch. f. klin. Med.;* Vol. 56, Nos. 1 and 2), is the amount of time and apparatus necessary; thus, for a single case, no less than 35 agar-plates are required.

The Physiological Differentiation of Pneumococcus and Streptococcus.—It is impossible, by current cultural methods and by morphological examination, to clearly differentiate between pneumococci and streptococci, according to P. H. HISS, JR. (*Jour. of Exper. Med.,* February 4, 1905). Well-marked capsules may occur on organisms which have with reason been classified as streptococci. The author's experiments show well-marked differences between the metabolic activities of pneumococci and streptococci, which may prove useful in the differentiation of these organisms. These differences become apparent when the pneumococci and streptococci are cultivated in an alkaline serum medium, or in a serum medium to which the carbohydrate inulin has been added. Pneumococci slowly produce acid in the alkaline serum. They ferment the inulin and thus rapidly give rise to acid. Streptococci do not form appreciable acid in either of these media, nor do they ferment the inulin. The penumococci coagulate the serum of these media while the streptococci do not. Starch and glycogen media are coagulated by pneumococci and by some at least of the streptococci. Lactose, saccharose, and maltose are fermented by pneumococci with the production of acid. Certain members of the *Streptococcus pyogenes* also ferment these disaccharids. In serum media, especially starch-bouillon serum, sterilized at 68° C., pneumococci usually develop well-marked capsules. In some of the serum media streptococcus cultures may at times have demonstrated capsules. All the streptococci classified as streptococci have been found to possess capsules. The same stains are applicable to the demonstration of pneumococcus capsules.

Cause of Carcinoma.—An interesting review is given by E. COHN (*Zeitsch. f. klin. Med.,* Vol. 56, Nos. 1 and 2) of the various forms of protozoa that have been held responsible for malignant growths at one time or another. The lowest organism described in this connection is an ameba, the *Leydenia gemmipara,* but it has been shown since then

that an ordinary body cell may closely simulate all the details in the structure of an ameba. An ameboid stage is also found in the life-cycle of another subdivision of the rhizopoda, the *mycetozoa,* and one particular form, the *Plasmodiophora braissica,* has frequently been mentioned in connection with cancer. The next class, the *Magistophora,* are only known as parasites of the blood (especially in cattle), but attention has been frequently directed to the sporozoa in that they are preeminently parasites of the epithelial cell. Their life-cycle is very complicated and they have been frequently encountered in various tissues of the higher animals. It is true that certain cells in carcinomatous tissues closely resemble certain phases in the development of these parasites, but absolute proof is lacking, since we do not possess any methods for cultivating them outside of the body. More recently still, various forms of pathogenic yeasts have been described in carcinomatous tissues, but these are most likely artefacts or secondary infections, since most attemps at inoculation have been unsuccessful. There are a few diseases undoubtedly caused by yeasts (*Blastomycosis cutis,* the lymphangitis epizootica of horses, etc.), but these bear no resemblance whatever to carcinoma. All in all, the parasitic theory of malignant growths rests on insufficient evidence, especially since it has been shown that Plimmer's bodies, and other structures supposed to be characteristic of lower forms of life, are nothing but vacuales in the protoplasm formed during a peculiar process of degeneration.

NEUROLOGY AND PSYCHIATRY.

The Epileptic Criminal: With Report of Two Cases. –T. H. EVANS (*Med. Rec.,* February 25, 1905) gives the histories on an epileptic who, in a period of depression, committed a murder, and a woman belonging to the borderland epileptic type who, in an access of jealousy, attempted to kill her lover. Taking these instances as a text the author concludes that (1) The essence of crime, is in the intention, and the ability not so to intend. (2) No punishment is adequate to any crime; restraint not only after a crime has been committed, but effort to hinder any such deed, is preferable always. (3) The victims of epileptics ought to have legal ground for suit against the community as well as those in charge of the epileptic. (4) Reservations ought to be established in which degenerates and the morally irresponsible could be colonized and treated, allowing all possible freedom of initiative for useful and safe pursuits therein. (5) Marriage of neurotics should be regulated. We can afford to lose the few sane descendants if we could also cut out their degenerate progeny. Democratic principles encourage, in this as in other matters, the average, and discourage the exceptional or abnormal—great or small. (6) All epileptics are to be viewed with suspicion. Many cases of psychic erraticism, cranks, and mistaken reformers, are to be taken as examples of epileptic psychic equivalents. The major forms of epilepsy may not prove so dangerous to the community as these veiled manifestations.

Prognostic Value of the Formula of Leucocytes Found in the Cerebrospinal Fluid.—The histological examination of the cerebrospinal fluid is an easy method, according to GOGGIA (*Gazz. deg. Osped.,* January 29, 1905), and if the formula of the cells found in condition of disease is correct, it gives an extremely valuable method of diagnosis. In cases of acute meningitis due to the pneumococcus, meningococcus, and streptococcus, polynuclear leucocytes are in evidence and in the majority, especially in the fatal cases, while in the curable cases the polynuclear leucocytes are gradually replaced by the mononuclear elements. This fact is emphasized by the recent French writers. The author urges that this must not be confused with the lymphocytosis of the cases of tuberculous meningitis. In two adult patients suffering from acute meningitis one recovered and one died. They were both treated by Quincke's puncture of the cerebrospinal canal for therapeutic purposes. The daily microscopical examination of the fluid demonstrated the following facts: (1) The constant predominance of small mononuclear cells in the patient who died, in whom the diagnosis was confined by autopsy. (2) The constant presence of polynuclear elements even in the early days of convalescence of the patient who survived. The writer believes that the various observations on this subject make the formula of the French school very exact. But one must remember that the prevalence of lymphouytes in the cerebrospinal fluid is not a positive evidence of tuberculous meningitis, for polynuclear leucocytes may also be seen in abundance, and indicates that the proportion of leucocytes does not alone contribute a sure guide for prognosis and diagnosis.

Peripheral Facial Paralysis.—Seven cases of this affection were described and illustrated by PALESE (*Gazz. deg. Osped.*, November 15, 1904), demonstrating a certain family heredity, which makes it possible to speak of a true family type of the disease not dependent on cold for a cause. Charcot described three such cases. Concerning prognosis the presence or absence of pain does not modify the course. One case of facial paralysis, without being preceded or followed by pain, lasted eleven months without being cured.

Researches in Dementia Præcox.—A. D. ORMEA and F. MAGGIOTTO (*Gazz. deg. Osped.*, January 22, 1905) report the following observations on the urine óf cases of dementia præcox. They believe a definite relation may be established between the limination of methylene blue and the clinical symptoms of depression and excitement. They arrive at the following conclusions: (1) In dementia præcox there is a special and characteristic alteration of the process of excretion, which shows (a) by means of the elimination of methylene blue through the kidneys, which begins and reaches its maximum intensity with great delay and is prolonged far beyond the time customary in normal individuals; (b) by the character and composition of the urine, in which the total quantity is diminished and the specific gravity is reduced; with a great reduction of urea, uric acid, phosphates, sulphates, nitrogen, and total acidity, with a slight increase of chlorides. (2) The elimination of methylene blue in other psychoret, manic-depressive insanity, hysteria, phrenasthenia, melancholia, of involution and dementia paralytica, is always more rapid than in normal individuals. (3) These types of mental disease do not show the same variation in the urine corresponding to the symptoms of depression and excitement. (4) These observations suggest that dementia præcox is an idiopathic form of disease, quite distinct from other kinds of psychoses, and based on the alteration of the excreted materials,. probably produced by the blood vessels in the sexual organs—resulting eventually in a systemic and partial degeneration of the brain. (5) The elimination of methylene blue in this characteristic way shown in dementia præcox can be used to diagnose this disease.

PEDIATRICS.

A Case of Noma Cured by Means of Red Rays.—Another triumph of phototherapy is recorded in the successful treatment of that dread malady, cancrum iris, by W. O. MOTSHAN (*Arch. f. Kinderheilk.*, Vol. 40 Nos. 4 to 6). The patient was a nine-year-old boy, who after having passed successively through scarlatina, varicella and measles, developed noma of one cheek, which went on to perforation. Immediately upon the admission of the case to the hospital, the local use of red rays by means of a 16-candle-power incandescent lamp with a red globe, was resorted to. The wound alone was exposed to the rays. The results of this treatment were soon apparent. On the third day pain disappeared. Seven days later the anterior half of the wound was filled with granulations. The necrotic areas gradually diminished. Two months later the patient was presented before the Pediatic Society of St. Petersburg, entirely cured.

Treatment of Gastro-enteritis with Buttermilk.—During a severe epidemic of gastro-enteritis and of cholera-infantum in the north of France, buttermilk was largely employed as a medicament. The conclusions which have been drawn by Dr. Floquet from the results of his experiences are reported by E. DECHERF (*Arch. de Méd. des Enfants* (January, 1905) as follows: Buttermilk is generally well taken by infauts, who prefer it to sweetened boiled water. Its use was followed by good results, while in parallel cases, treated by other means, no improvement was observed. while acting in these cases as a specific, buttermilk is also a food and causes an increase in weight. It is indicated in both chronic and acute cases. It produces excellent results in rickets; it combats the intestinal fermentations which give rise to chronic auto-infection. Some practitioners have administered the buttermilk raw, but the majority who have used it prefer to give it boiled. The following is the method of preparing the buttermilk: One tablespoonful of farina to a liter of buttermilk, which is then slowly boiled in an enamelled or porcelain vessel, at the same time that it is constantly stirred. The mixture is kept boiling for several minutes, at the end of which 75 grams of sugar are added. It is then ready to be fed to the infant, either in the bottle or with the spoon or cup. In cases of either acute or chronic gastro-enteritis, it is given in the same doses as milk, every three hours. In the beginning it is best to give it in fractional doses of a tablespoonful every fifteen minutes. Although during the first few days the child may vomit after taking the buttermilk, the stomach soon gets used to this acid food. In children over a year old, sometimes large doses are necessary. The good effects of buttermilk are to be attributed to the large amount of lactic acid present, which counteracts intestinal fermentation. The small amount of fat contained, and the fine division of the casein, thanks to churning, render the preparation very digestible.

Incontinence of Feces in Children.—Three instances of this rather rare condition, of which only about a dozen cases are on record, are reported by M. OSTHEIMER (*Univ. Penn. Med. Bull.*, February, 1905) as occurring in boys ranging from four and a half to ten years. In one case the incontinence had followed diphtheria and scarlet fever and persisted for two years. In six months upon nutritious food, tonics, and fresh air, he made a complete recovery. The other two boys were otherwise well, with the exception of a general nervousness in one of them. The latter after a time also developed paroxysms of pain with micturition, and often passed bloody urine. After removal of a vesical calculus, he became perfectly well. The author found the best results attended the administration of strychnine and atropine, up to one-tenth of a grain of each daily. Relapses are common and must always be treated in the same manner. Tonics and good food, together with plenty of fresh air, are very important.

Standardized Gruels.—H. D. CHAPIN (*Med. Rec.,* February 18, 1905) says that with the increased knowledge that has resulted from a careful study of the use of gruels in infant feeding it has become recognized that they have other values than as attenuants of the curd of the cow's milk. They may often be employed to economize the enery of the body that is being used in the effort to prepare food for assimilation, and by taking advantage of this fact it is frequently possible to keep the body well nourished on a quantity of food much smaller than is theoretically indicated. It is highly desirable, therefore, that there should be some uniform standards for use in preparing gruels, and that their food values and possibilities should become better known. With this object in view the author had made gruels containing varying amounts of pearl barley, prepared barley flour, wheat flour, and rolled or flaked oats, which were then assayed to determine their composition in order to show the relative properties of tissue-building and heat and energy producing elements. The tables obtained are reproduced, as well as others showing simple methods of preparing gruels of any desired strength.

Fresh Cold Air Treatment of Pneumonia in Infants.—W. P. NORTHRUP (*Med. Rec.,* February 18, 1905) reports two cases of pneumonia in infants in which the windows of the sickroom were kept open day and night; both children recovered. He believes it will become more and more the rule to treat pneumonia in this way. Cool, pure air, he says, reddens the blood, stimulates the heart, improves digestion, quiets restlessness, and aids in overcoming toxemia. He concludes with the following prescription for killing a baby with pneumonia: Crib in far corner of room with canopy over it. Steam kettle; gas stove (leaky tubing); room at 80° F. Many gas jets burning. Friends in the room, also the pug dog. Chest tightly enveloped in waistcoat poultice. If child's temperature is 105° F. make a poultice thick, hot, and tight. Blanket the windows, shut the doors. If these do not do it, give coal-tar antipyretics and wait.

PRESCRIPTION HINTS.

Early Treatment of Consumption.—The therapeutic arsenal for the treatment of pulmonary tuberculosis is well stocked, and even overstocked, remarks Prof. Renon. Neither the tuberculin of Koch nor the new tuberculin T.R. have given decisive results. The same may be said of the series of serums recommended by men of good faith and of undeniable scientific standing.

One of the best remedies to be utilized in phthisis is arsenic. It may be given in very small doses:

R Arsenate of soda...................... 1 gr.
Water ....10 oz.

A tablespoonful twice a day at meals, and continued twenty days a month for three or four months. There are other preparations of arsenic, such as cacodylate of soda and arrhenal. The former is employed by the mouth, the rectum or subcutaneously. M. Renon prefers the latter mode. He injects one grain dissolved in twenty drops of sterilized water every two days, or eight injections in sixteen days. He then suspends them for eight days and recommences the series. Arrhenal may be employed in the place of cacodylate of soda, but M. Renon thinks it inferior. The *raison d'etre* of the arsenical treatment is to keep the patient in good condition and increase his weight if possible, but it should be used with prudence, especial care being taken to avoid even the semblance of any gastro-intestinal disturbance, as such would act prejudicially in the matter of feeding the patient.

Creosote was considered a kind of specific for phthisis for many years, but it frequently aggravates the condition of the patient by fatiguing the stomach, and, on the other hand, it has frequently provoked hemoptysis. In certain torpid forms of phthisis, however, creosote might be given by the rectum in twenty to thirty drop doses. Synthetic preparations, such as guaiacol or thiocol, they replace creosote. Thiocol given in 10-grain wafers three times a day has much benefited some patients.

Besides creosote, and acting in a different manner, is urea, utilized first by Harper in England, which has a favorable action in all forms of tuberculosis. It can be employed in subcutaneous injections and by the mouth. Prof. Renon gives it in wafers containing 12 grains each, two to four daily. Tannin is also an excellent preparation, but, unfortunately, this is ill tolerated by the stomach. It is best given in the form of wafers:

R Tannin .... 5 grs.
Phosphate of line.....................10 grs.
For one wafer; five daily.

Tannigen is a good substitute in the dose of 4 grains three times a day. The glycerophosphates have a good action on the general nutrition. Two or three 5-grain doses daily before meals. Lately M. Renon has been employing with much benefit a new phosphated substance called phyline, described by Posternak, which is a phospho-organic principle of vegetable grains. It is well tolerated, improves the appetite, and favors sleep. He gives 10 grains of it before the two principal repasts.

One of the complications of pulmonary consumption is fever. For this rest in bed will frequently be sufficient. Otherwise antithermics must be given. Of these there are a host, but those which have given the best results are aspirin and cryogenin, discovered by Lumière, of Lyons. Either of these agents may be given in four-grain doses twice a day, at three o'clock in the afternoon and at six o'clock.

Two other symptoms frequently require attention—hemoptysis and diarrhea. The former will be treated by the classical remedies, needless to mention. The diarrhea is best treated with:

R Cotoin ....2 grs.
For one wafer; two daily, or,

R Methylene blue ....2 grs.
Lactose ....4 grs.
For one wafer; two daily.

For the cough M. Renon recommends a half grain of opium two or three times a day.

THE MEDICAL NEWS.

A WEEKLY JOURNAL
OF MEDICAL SCIENCE.

COMMUNICATIONS in the form of Scientific Articles, Clinical Memoranda, Correspondence or News Items of interest to the profession are invited from all parts of the world. Reprints to the number of 250 of original articles contributed exclusively to the MEDICAL NEWS will be furnished without charge if the request therefor accompanies the manuscript. When necessary to elucidate the text, illustrations will be engraved from drawings or photographs furnished by the author. Manuscript should be typewritten.

SMITH ELY JELLIFFE, A.M., M.D., Ph.D., Editor,
No. 111 FIFTH AVENUE, NEW YORK.

Subscription Price, Including postage In U. S. and Canada.

PER ANNUM IN ADVANCE	. . . .	$4.00
SINGLE COPIES	. . . . .	.10
WITH THE AMERICAN JOURNAL OF THE MEDICAL SCIENCES, PER ANNUM	. .	8.00

Subscriptions may begin at any date. The safest mode of remittance is by bank check or postal money order, drawn to the order of the undersigned. When neither is accessible, remittances may be made at the risk of the publishers, by forwarding in registered letters.

LEA BROTHERS & CO.,
No. 111 FIFTH AVENUE (corner of 18th St.), NEW YORK.

SATURDAY, MARCH 11, 1905.

THE RATIONAL BASIS OF NARCOSIS.

THE greatest triumph in the physician's art is his almost absolute control over pain. Yet numerous and varied as are the means at his disposal for putting to sleep the sensory cells of the brain, his practice in this respect has not yet passed beyond the stage of empiricism. To say that these drugs inhibit vital activity is merely to re-state the problem in different language.

If one review the vast list of narcotics from ether and morphine to chloretone and veronal, the thought is aroused that possibly all of these drugs have some physical or chemical character-istic in common. The discovery of this common principle would not only simplify but would also impart scientific distinction to the treatment of pain. A glance at the recent literature concerned with the experimental pharmacology of narcosis reveals that Science has begun to grapple ably with a problem worthy of its steel.

A year ago, we referred editorially to the novel theory propounded by Wedensky, who regards narcosis as a stage of vital activity. There are four stages of the latter, namely, rest, activity, inhibition or narcosis, and death. The same phys-ical or chemical stimulus may, according to the strength or duration of its action, give rise to any one of these stages, or may even produce them all successively. As an example, ether first stim-ulates the ganglion cells of the brain, then causes inhibition or narcosis, and if the action is too intense or too prolonged, causes death. The same sequence of events is true of nearly all other nar-cotics and of most poisons. This theory suggests that possibly the real explanation of narcotic action will be found in the physiology of the nerve-cells.

Most of the investigations on narcosis have been concerned mainly with the chemical aspects of this problem. S. Baglioni studied a group of compounds related to phenol, including benzyl-alcohol, benzaldehyde, acetophone, and benzoic acid. These are all built up from a benzol-nucleus to which a methyl side-chain is attached. The latter is easily oxidized to CO_3H. The more oxy-gen present in the side-chain, the less is the nar-cotic effect. Thus, benzyl-alcohol is a powerful depressant, while still less so is benzaldehyde, and least of all is benzoic acid. Baglioni concluded that the narcotic power of these substances de-pends upon their ability to draw oxygen out of the protoplasm of the nerve-centers,—in other words, upon their power of reduction. There are other facts which tend to support the view that if the tissues are deprived of oxygen, narcosis re-sults. Asphyxia results in unconsciousness. C. A. Herter found that ether, chloroform, and chloral diminish the reducing capacity of the tis-sues. They thus impair the ability of the tissues to reduce the oxyhemoglobin of the red blood cells, with the result that oxygen-starvation oc-curs. The narcotic effect of cold may be ex-plained in the basis of the further discovery made by Herter, namely, that cold diminishes the re-ducing power of the tissues.

A. Jolies has found that the reduction of oxy-hemoglobin is brought about by means of a spe-cial ferment, katalase, and that the amount of this ferment in the blood is diminished in coma-tose conditions. He suggests that the symptoms here are in great part due to insufficient supply of oxygen in the nervous centers. Moore and Roaf have found that chloroform and other an-esthetics form compounds with hemoglobin and serum-proteid; they hence limit the physio-logical activity of the hemoglobin. All the above results lead to one conclusion, namely, narcosis and oxygen-starvation are identical.

Of closely related interest are the researches recorded by P. Bergell and R. Pschorr. These investigators sought to determine to what extent the action of morphine may be explained by means of the substance from which it is derived, phenanthrene, and its derivatives. Phenanthrene is a cyclic hydrocarbon having the symbol $C_{14}H_{10}$, and is in itself quite inert. But oxy-phenanthrene or phenanthrol produces tetanic seizures. The derivatives of phenanthrene equinone show a decided power of forming methemoglobin; likewise epiosin, a methyl derivative of phenanthrene, also produces methemoglobinemia. The above observers believe that there is evidently some connection between the narcotic manifestations of morphine and the methemogbinemia produced by some of its derivatives.

Within recent years attempts have been made to explain narcosis upon the basis of physical rather than chemical action. A. R. Cushny, one of the ablest defenders of the physical theory, refers to the experiments of Kionka, who found that although CH_4 has no narcotic action, CH_3Cl has some effect, the Cl being evidently responsible for this activity. Yet while $CHCl_3$ is four times more powerful than CH_3Cl, CCl_4 instead of being still more powerful, is only half as depressing as $CHCl_3$. Kionka concluded that the depressing qualities of this series are not determined by their molecular structure, but by some physical characteristic which is present in most of this group.

It is hardly necessary to recall the theory proposed three years ago by A. P. Matthews, that chloroform and ether owe their narcotic power to the fact that they dissolve the fatty constituents of the nerve-cells. Closely related to this is the theory advanced by Overton, that the ease with which narcotics pass into the cells is dependent upon the degree of their solubility in the lipoids (fat, cholesterin, lecithin), contained in the cell-wall. Overton and Meyer found that the good narcotics, anesthetics and antipyretics have a high osmotic power. J. Traube finds that there is a close relationship between surface-tension and narcotic power. He found by experiment that if two liquids are separated by a membrane, such that the surface-tension of one is less than that of the other, the former will osmose into the latter. He attributes the ease with which narcotics penetrate the walls of the ganglion-cells of the brain, to the fact that the narcotics have a remarkably low surface-tension. He also distinguishes between two classes of narcotics,—the toxic and the non-toxic. The latter dissolve in the lipoids without uniting with or decomposing the proteids or other substances of the cell. The other class includes the toxic narcotics,—nicotin, allyl-alcohol, pyridin, anilin, phenol, acetaldoxim, and methyl-acetate, whose toxicity is attributed to the fact that they enter into chemical combination with some of the cellular constituents. All other narcotics partake to a slight extent of this toxicity.

HOSPITAL EXAMINATIONS AND MEDICAL TEACHING.

FOURTH-YEAR medical students are now approaching a turning-point in their lives. During the coming month competitive examinations will be held by the hospitals of New York to determine who shall be granted the inestimable privilege of serving as internes in these institutions. Men who entered medical school calmly, almost thoughtlessly, tremble as the time approaches for leaving it; for no one knows better than they how inadequate is the instruction which has been imparted to them, if it be regarded as a final preparation for professional practice. This instruction is not a completed edifice; it is a mere assemblage of building materials—valuable if ultimately cemented together by clinical experience, but little more than useless rubbish if not supplemented by the binding power of knowledge gained at the bedside.

With the annual hospital examinations, class distinctions appear where none should exist; to a favored few is granted as a precious privilege that which all should receive as a right. Next fall we shall read in the college catalogue the proud statement that " 50 per cent. of the members of the class of 1905 received hospital appointments "—a good recommendation for a " quiz " class, perhaps, but a sorry confession for a supposedly great and representative seat of professional learning. Where, may be asked, will the remaining 50 per cent. acquire that clinical knowledge which is indispensable to one who is to undertake to practice independently the art of medicine? Some will ruthlessly trample over the bodies of poor and helpless victims, and thus at last will escape from the mazes of their enlightened ignorance and attain real proficiency. Others, beginning with deeply rooted misconceptions, are doomed to perpetual blunders which will cost the public dear. A third group, affrighted at the dangers that beset them, will quickly abandon medicine for some less difficult field.

It is not to be wondered at that the " regular " school of medicine does not monopolize public confidence. With all its vaunted superiority of scientific attainment a great many of its followers are wretchedly trained. Medical schools vie with each other in building and equipping laboratories where a few research scholars may carry on investigations in bacteriology, chemistry or pathology; but the hospital is the laboratory which is needed most, and the " college hospital " is not a feature of the equipment of the medical schools of New York.

Shall appeals again be made to the charitable hospitals of the city to open their doors to undergraduate medical students? Again and again such appeals have been rejected, though its advocates were leaders and teachers of wide renown and influence; and to-day there is no new force within the hospitals themselves to set aside the objections which repeatedly have been brought forward. Yet medical schools must do their duty. Somehow, somewhere, they *must* find the means to build their own hospitals; and when built, these hospitals must be so conducted as to win the unqualified favor of the benevolent public. Let us have but one notable demonstration of the worth of such an institution, and the permanent and general success of the movement will be assured. If but a small fraction of the annual income of existing institutions is once diverted to the training of a college hospital, other hospitals will soon fall into line, and New York will be fairly launched on the path to preeminence in medical science and teaching. It is our prayer that the beginning may soon be made.

THE DYSENTERY BACILLUS.

THERE is perhaps no micro-organism, not even excepting the meningococcus, which became notorious in 1902 and 1903 through the polemics of Albrecht and Ghon, which has given rise to so much dispute within recent times as has the so-called dysentery bacillus.

The title to this discovery, its biological and cultural peculiarities, its agglutinative reactions, its pathogenicity, its unity, have successively been the subject of such violent dispute that it has seemed to many workers as if light could never come out of such confusion worse confounded. The identification of the dysentery bacillus in the summer diarrheas of children and in other native enteric diseases, while it emphasizes the extreme importance of the organism as a factor in the

every-day experience of the working physician, only served to complicate the difficulties of the initial problem.

It was suspected even by the earlier investigators, notably Kruse, that the organisms isolated under these various conditions, namely from the patients suffering with epidemic dysentery in the Philippines by Flexner, and from similar cases in Japan by Shiga, were of a different type from those found, for example, in the epidemics of dysentery in the insane asylums of Germany. With the method employed by them, however, it was quite impossible to formulate these differences in definite terms of biological and cultural expression. Only by means of the more exact criteria offered by the fermentation tests and the agglutination methods, has it become practicable to differentiate these various organisms with any degree of facility and certainty.

Perhaps the most impartial review of the entire literature, and the most thoroughgoing comparative investigation extant of the various types of so-called dysentery bacillus is to be found in a recent article by Prof. Hiss, in the *Journal of Medical Research*. In his fermentation studies, he made use of dextrose, maltose, saccharose, dextrin, and mannite, dissolved in various media, such as serum water, pepton water, pepton asparagin, and so forth. In all of these tests, the degree of acid production, if any, and the rapidity of its production, was the point to be determined. As a result of these experiments, it was found that all the organisms might be divided into two groups, namely those which do not ferment mannite with acid production, and those which produce acid from mannite. The first group contains the *Bacillus dysenteriæ* of Kruse and Shiga; the second group, all the other forms.

Further tests of all these organisms were made by means of careful comparison of the quantitative agglutination reactions in immune sera, and of the absorption of agglutinins.

These tests developed the fact that the agglutinins produced in the serum of animals inoculated with representations of the various groups are probably distinct and specific, thus supporting the classification indicated by the differences in fermentative activity.

The important question to determine is the actual relationship of these organisms to the diseases in which they are found to occur. That there is not necessarily an etiological relationship goes without saying. The changes in the chemical reaction and constitution of the intestinal juices which accompany all forms of enteritis might conceivably be the factor at work in the alteration of the bacterial flora. The potency of this factor is best illustrated by the marked changes which accompany the substitution of cow's milk for mother's milk in nurslings; the Gram-positive bacilli which had almost usurped the microscopic field under the previous conditions are practically substituted by Gram negative forms. As is conservatively stated by Hiss: "What the etiological significance of these various organisms is has not as yet been satisfactorily determined. So far as their occurrence in abundance in the digestive tract, coincident with the development of certain inflammatory conditions and the increase of apparently specific agglutinins in the blood of the patient, goes, they all at present, it seems, have an equal claim to be looked upon as possible inciters of dysenteric and diarrheic diseases. Whether one or all, or indeed any of them, will continue to hold this claim only further observation and experimentation can determine."

ECHOES AND NEWS.

NEW YORK.

Medical Ethics.—Two lectures on the above subject will be delivered by Dr. A. Brayton Ball at the College of Physicians and Surgeons, March 22 and 29, at 5 P.M. This follows out an old system that was discontinued for a couple of years and is to be taken up again, as decided upon at a recent meeting of the Faculty. Dr. Ball's lectures have always been of great interest to the students.

The Charaka Club and Dr. Osler.—Last Saturday, at the invitation of Dr. C. L. Dana, the president, the Charaka Club, of New York, known largely for its interest in medical, historical and literary pursuits, gave a farewell dinner to Dr. William Osler, one of its own members. The dinner at the University Club was a great success. Next week the MEDICAL NEWS will present a summary of the evening's proceedings.

New York Academy of Medicine. Section of Laryngology.—A meeting of this Section will be held March 17 at 8.15 P.M., in honor of the one hundredth birthday of Signor Manuel Garcia. The following is the interesting program: (1) Manuel Garcia: Teacher, Discoverer and Man, by James E. Newcomb, M.D.; (2) Address, by Walter Damrosch, Esq.; (3) "The Future of the Laryngoscope and the Study of Laryngology," by John N. Mackenzie, M.D., of Baltimore.

To Study Meningitis.—The Board of Health has empowered Commissioner Darlington to ask the Board of Estimate and Apportionment for a small sum to pay a commission to investigate the matter and try to find some remedy to retard, or, if possible, to stamp out the disease. The Commissioner said that the

disease could be conveyed by contact, as it is a germ disease, but though many patients had been sent to hospitals he had never heard of a case being contracted in a hospital. In January, 1904, there were twenty-five deaths, while in the same month this year there were 107. In February, 1904, there were twenty-six deaths, while in February, 1905, there were 149. There have been printed 2,700,000 pasters, which will be placed in all school text-books warning scholars against spitting on sidewalks and floors of public places.

PHILADELPHIA.

Charitable Bequests.—Two institutions, the Women's Home Mission Society of the M. E. Church and the Maternity Hospital, will each receive $200 according to the will of Margaret Frank, late of 4324 Westminster Avenue, Philadelphia.

Spinal Cord Sutured.—This operation was performed at the Medico-Chirurgical Hospital March 4, 1905; the following day the patient was doing well, and it is thought that he, Edward Farrel, will recover, although there seems to be some doubt whether the paralysis in the leg will disappear.

Meeting of Philadelphia Obstetrical Society.—At the meeting of this society, held March 2, Dr. W. R. Nicholson read a paper on "The Indications for Slow Methods of Inducing Labor." Dr. George M. Boyd spoke of "Accouchement Forcé." Dr. Richard Morris read a paper on "The Slow Methods of Inducing Labor," and Dr. Barton Cooke Hirst on "The Methods of Inducing Labor."

Election of Officers.—The Auxiliary II of Free Hospital for Poor Consumptives, which was organized December 8, 1904, with a membership of thirty-one, and which now has a membership of seventy-nine, elected Miss Anna Morris, chairman; Mrs. Talcott Williams and Mrs. M. P. Ravenel, vice-chairman; Mrs. C. J. Hatfield, secretary; Mrs. D. L. Edsall, treasurer. Before the election they listened to a lecture on the future plans of the organization by Dr. Talcott Williams.

Hospital Reports.—The following statements have been issued by some of the hospitals of Philadelphia:

Name of Hospital.	Patients Admitted in Feb.	Patients Discharged in Feb.	Patients remaining Mar. 1.	Patients Treated in Dispensary
Presbyterian	185	173	215	1,709
Germantown	109	114	85	1,132
Women's Homeopathic	91	65	52	971
Howard	39			572

The Charity Hospital treated 273 medical cases, 258 surgical, 26 eye cases, 59 ear, nose and throat, and 165 cases of diseases of women and children.

New Measure to Prevent the Spread of Infectious Diseases.—For the bill recently introduced by Senator Gransback he has now substituted a new one which not only gives to the authorities the power to make rules for the care and control of persons suffering with acute infectious diseases, but also gives them power to govern the sanitary control of the premises where such diseases exist. The bill also empowers the authorities to make rules governing the burial of bodies having died of acute infectious diseases, and it fixes fines and penalties for violating any rule made. It stipulates that the rules shall cover the following: (1) Reports from physicians; (2) Quarantining and disinfecting; (3) Treatment of infected bedding, clothing, etc.; (4) Care and burial f the dead in cases of contagious diseases; (5) Disinfection of conveyances; (6) Governing the admision and attendance of persons at public or private chools, asylums, hospitals, and compulsory vaccinaion and revaccination.

Philadelphia Neurological Society.—This society iet February 28. Dr. J. D. McCarthy presented "A ase of Tuberculosis with Graves' Syndrome." In iscussing the case he said about five per cent. of ie advanced cases of tuberculosis present von raefe's symptom. Dr. Pemberton presented for r. Spiller "A Case of Lumbo-thoracic Syringoiyelia." The condition began with weakness of the gs, difficulty in walking and alteration in her menstrual functions. On the right side the tendon reexes are lost, ankle clonus is marked and the Babinki reflex is present; heat and pain sense is lost. Dr. piller then exhibited "A Case of Progressive Musular Dystrophy with Atrophy of the Bone;" "A ase of Tabetic Facial Palsy;" "A Case of Chronic Iercurial Poisoning." Of the first case Dr. Spiller aid the condition began about the second year of fe, it came on gradually and the patient has never ad any pain. There is a marked diminution in the ize of the muscles of the left side and the size of the ones of the same side are much decreased. The econd presented a marked Argyll-Robertson pupil nd a weakening of the left side of the face and the aralysis on the right side. The patient who was resented as the third case works in a hat factory ·here mercury is used, and the dust with which the tmosphere of the room is laden is constantly being ihaled. The man presents a tremor which by use f the part becomes exaggerated. In discussing this ise Dr. Dercum called attention to the difference in ie symptom complex produced in mercurial poisonng when it is inhaled and when it is introduced into he system either by the mouth or hypodermically.)r. Weisenberg showed two patients. "A Case of Iemorrhage in the Pons;" "A Case of Hemorrhage n the Floor of the Aqueduct of Sylvius." Of the rst case he informed the society that both external ecti muscles of the eye are paralyzed but the eyerounds are normal; the knee-jerks are exaggerated ut there is a chilly feeling constantly running up nd down the left leg and a feeling of pricking of ins and needles in the left arm. He found aneshesia of the tissues supplied by the upper branch f the fifth and hypolgia of the tissues of the middle ne. In the second case ptosis came on very suddenly; he finds that all the muscles of the eye except he external recti are paralyzed. Dr. Geo. E. Price eported "A Case of Malaria Infection Presenting ymptoms of Multiple Neuritis." The patient of /hom he spoke had malaria eighteen months before e saw her. When she came under his care there /as numbness of the right leg, the reflexes were /eak, and in walking she dragged her feet. Microcopical examination of the blood revealed the stevo-autumnal parasite. Dr. Alfred Gordon read paper on "Clinical and Pathological Report of a ;ase of Lead Poisoning with Remarks on the ·Pathgenesis of the Disease." The case presented all he clinical symptom of the disease. He found the ells of the anterior cornua involved and degeneraion in the anterior columns, posterior roots and osterior columns. These changes were most 1arked in the lumbar region, but the columns of the ervical cord were involved. He infers from his tudies.that.the changes in the reflexes does not deend upon the alterations in the posterior roots

alone. He also states that lead has no selective affinity for a special structure and that all elements of the nervous system are simultaneously affected by the lead. He does not believe that the changes in the blood vessels alone can account for the lesions produced.

College of Physicians of Philadelphia.—This society met March 1. Dr. Robert H. Willson reported a number of cases of uremia in which the symptoms had been materially ameliorated by the withdrawal of cerebrospinal fluid. In some cases the procedure failed, in others the relief was prompt and most gratifying. In the discussion Dr. William E. Hughes, in whose wards at the Philadelphia Hospital the work was done, referred to two cases in private practice, in neither of which had any noteworthy benefit resulted. In one case there was reason to believe that the puncture wounded a vessel and led to a hemorrhage around the cord. Dr. James Tyson expressed a willingness to try the method but thought it did not seem to promise more than venesection with hypodermoclysis or saline transfusion. Dr. W. M. L. Koplin referred to the recent work of Krönig and others on the value of lumbar puncture in the treatment of eclampsia, in which condition it had been taught to be of benefit to cases of markedly elevated cerebrospinal tension. He expressed the one in which the symptoms depended upon heightened tension while in the other group there was present in the cerebrospinal fluid an excess of one or more of its normal constituents, or the presence in noxious quantities of one or more abnormal bodies upon the action of which the symptomatology of the condition in question depended. He referred to a number of French observers who have shown that in certain cases of Bright's disease the cerebrospinal fluid contains an excess of urea and while it is not probable that this substance alone was responsible for the symptoms it might be an index to the presence of other poisons for which there are no accurate tests. Dr. T. L. Coley gave an interesting review of "The Famous Controversy Concerning the Internal Use of Cantharides—an Historic Sketch." Dr. Alfred C. Wood reported "Removal of Gall-stone by Operation which Obstructed the Intestine." He relieved the obstruction by opening the intestines and excising the stone, at the same operation he removed a concretion from the gallbladder. So far as he is able to find, his was the first case in which simultaneous removal of the obstructing calculus within the intestine and also a second calculus in the biliary passages, had been practised. Dr. John B. Roberts read a paper on "The Gardener's Spade Deformity and the Silver Fork Deformity in the Fractures of the Carpal End of the Radius." He called particular attention to fractures in this locality in which the lower end of the fragment is displaced toward the palmar aspect of the arm, giving rise to a special contour which he designates "The Gardener's Spade Deformity."

Philadelphia Academy of Surgery.—The meeting of this society was held March 6. Dr. John Gibbon read a paper on "The Matas Operation for the Cure of Aneurism," showing a case. He informed the society that this operation was done within the sac and did not interfere with the anastomosis. In this case he found that the aneurism extended under the gastrocnemius muscle and that of the opening· of the artery into the sac and the outlet were very close together. He opened the sac, after applying a tourniquet, closed both openings of the artery with chromicized catgut, then pulled in the sac by double row of sutures. His case became infected and he noted that many of the cases reported were similarly affected. Dr. William J. Taylor read a paper on "Varicose Veins Simulating Femoral Hernia. Operation: Death from Heart Clot, Believed to be due to Chronic Gastric Ulcer." The mass in the femoral region presented an impulse upon coughing and disappeared when the patient was placed in the recumbent position. At the operation when he exposed the mass he found he was dealing with a dilated vein, which he ligated above and below the dilatation and then sutured the sac. Sometime later the patient began to complain of distressing symptoms in the gastric region which were attributed to gastric ulcer. About a month after the operation the patient died suddenly, and at post mortem there was a clot in the heart, a hemorrhagic pericarditis and old healed gastric ulcers. Dr. Mitchell exhibited a stomach upon which he operated for perforating gastric ulcer, but the patient died from a second perforation. Dr. R. P. Reynolds then read a paper on "Cysts of the Pancreas, with Report of a Case." The diagnosis of these cysts, he said, is not easy. There is usually a history of a slowly growing tumor in the abdomen which is hard, but may fluctuate, and by dilatation of the stomach with gas or air it is found to be retroperitoneal. The presence of sugar in the urine is of little value in diagnosing these cases. If the fluid from the cyst can be obtained and the presence of pancreatic ferment demonstrated the diagnosis at once becomes clear. The cyst in his case filled the greater portion of the peritoneal cavity. He was unable to remove the entire sac. He maintains that the fluid of these cysts will not infect the peritoneum. Dr. Geo. Erety Shoemaker read a paper on "Spindle-Cell Sarcoma of the Ovary, not Yielding to Coley's Fluid nor to X-ray." He first gave a short sketch of one of his cases that was cured by the combined treatment of Coley's fluid and the X-ray. Of the case referred to in the paper he said there was present an inguinal hernia and that the tumor in the abdomen was thought to be a fibroid of the uterus, so both conditions were to be treated at the same operation, but after the operation on the hernia had been completed and the abdomen opened he found the tumor mass involved the uterus, bladder, part of the rectum and the right ovary were not identified. The condition was considered inoperable and the treatment with Coley's and X-rays was instituted but without beneficial results. Dr. W. W. Keen then exhibited an apparatus to maintain the position of the patient during an operation.

CHICAGO.

Visiting Nurses' Report.—At the regular monthly meeting of the Board of Directors of the Visiting Nurses' Association, Miss Harriet Fulmer, Superintendent, reported 963 patients cared for and 4,159 visits made by the nurses. The Association gives special attention to the care of tuberculosis cases in the homes of the poor and to all chronic cases not eligible to hospitals.

Annual Meeting of Stockholders of Chicago Eye, Ear, Nose and Throat College.—At this meeting of the stockholders, the following were re-elected Directors: Drs. Wm. A. Fisher, Adolphus G. Whippern, Thomas Faith, H. W. Woodruff, and John R. Hoffman. Dr. Wm. A. Fisher was re-elected by the

Directors as President and Treasurer, while Dr. Adolphus G. Whippern was elected Vice-President, and Dr. John R. Hoffman Secretary.

Columbus Hospital.—A new North Side hospital bearing this name was opened February 26. Addresses were delivered by Dr. John B. Murphy and Judge Theodore Brentano. The institution was dedicated with appropriate ceremony by Archbishop Quigley. The staff of the hospital includes Drs. Gustav Fütterer, Julius H. Hölscher, H. H. Brown, Thomas S. Crowe, Willis G. Storer, A. Biankini, Wm. P. Verity, Randolph Brunson, A. C. Garvy, Harold N. Moyer, David Lieberthal, Frank Byrnes, and John B. Murphy.

Nurses Receive Diplomas.—Twenty nurses received their diplomas at the annual commencement of the Chicago Hospital Training School for Nurses, February 28. Dr. Alexander Hugh Ferguson presented the diplomas. In addition to the regular number, two honorary diplomas were awarded to Miss Martha L. Giltner, Superintendent of Nurses at the school, and to Mrs. Margaret Guerley, of Waukegan. The Rev. John Archibald Morrison and Dr. Alfred C. Crofton spoke. At a banquet at the hospital in the evening, Dr. Alfred S. Henning acted as toastmaster. Responses to toasts were made by Drs. Wm. N. Hardin, Alex. Hugh Ferguson, Alfred C. Crofton, H. W. Gentles, Philip Kreissl, A. McDermid, John T. Binckley and Miss K. Donahue. The graduates were the guests of honor.

Campaign Against Tuberculosis.—Members of the State Legislature are receiving a flood of literature devoted to arguments in support of the passage of Mr. Glackin's bill appropriating $200,000 for the erection of a sanitarium for consumptives. A circular letter was received by members of the two houses from the Illinois State Association for the Prevention of Tuberculosis, with headquarters at Chicago. A large delegation from Chicago and other parts of the State will go to Springfield to urge the passage of the bill. It is argued that statistics show that in 75 per cent. of patients treated in similar institutions the disease is arrested. The enactment of this bill into law will provide the State with an institution, which, in importance, not only to thousands of sufferers, but to people at large, overshadows any other institution. A list of prominent citizens of the State who have endorsed the bill is appended to the circular.

Early Diagnosis of Tuberculosis.—The State Board of Health has just issued for distribution to the physicians of the State, a circular on "The Early Diagnosis of Tuberculosis," which will bring to the physician in concise and systematic form all of the information on the diagnosis of the disease to be obtained from a most exhaustive review of American or foreign medical literature. The great interest in consumption, manifested during the past few years, has resulted in extensive scientific investigation, and the importance of early diagnosis, both in saving the life of the patient and in protecting those with whom he comes in contact, has directed much of this investigation to the earliest reliable signs of the existence of the disease. Unfortunately, much of the most valuable material has not yet found its way into the standard text-books and lies hidden away in the pages of the hundreds of medical journals and monographs, unavailable to the busy practitioner. It was especially with a view of placing this later information in the hands of the physician that this circular was prepared. In taking up the newer methods of diagnosis, however, the utmost care has been taken to eliminate all that is still questionable or speculative, and those signs and symptoms whose value are under discussion were omitted altogether. One subject on which there has been some difference of opinion on the part of medical men, however, is discussed in the circular with considerable emphasis, and that is in regard to advising the patient as to the character of the disease. It is the belief of the State Board of Health that, after the diagnosis is established, the patient should be fully advised of the nature of the disease, what he can reasonably expect in the way of cure, what he must do to bring about the best results, and, far from least important, what he must do to protect those who are about him. According to the circular, "A frank statement of fact is not unkindness, nor will the knowledge act prejudicially to the physical welfare. Withholding this information removes from the patient and the public their greatest safeguard." Attention of the medical men of the State is directed to the laboratory of the State Board of Health at Springfield, and it is announced that examination of sputum of patients supposed to be tuberculous, will be made without cost at any time. The establishment of container stations, for the distribution of mailing cases for specimens, one in each county of the State, is also announced and special attention is drawn to the fact that, wherever consumption is found by physicians to exist in unusual numbers, inspectors will be sent to assist in the investigation of the cause and in taking necessary steps to check its spread. The circular also contains a reproduction from a photograph of the laboratory of the board.

GENERAL.

Association of American Medical Colleges.—By vote of a two-thirds majority of all the colleges voting, it is decided that the next meeting of the association is to be held in Chicago Monday, April 10, 1905. Detailed information as to place of meeting and program will be issued later.

Gift to Westminster Hospital.—The sum of £1,000 has been presented by Mr. Edward Heron-Allen to the Westminster Hospital, London, to endow a bed in one of Dr. Murrell's Wards "in recognition of his valuable contributions to pharmacology and his researches on the action of remedial agents in the treatment of disease."

American Laryngological, Rhinological and Otological Society.—The eleventh annual meeting of this society will be held under the Presidency of Dr. Frederic C. Cobb, at Boston, Mass., on Monday, Tuesday and Wednesday, June 5, 6 and 7, 1905. The profession are cordially invited to attend the meeting and take an active interest in the papers and discussions.

The Prevention of Malaria.—At the request of the Society for the Study of Malaria, the Italian Minister of Public Instruction has sanctioned the distribution among the teachers of evening and holiday schools for illiterate adults of pamphlets containing simple explanations of the mode of origin and spread of the disease, and instructions for the use of the quinine supplied by the State for prophylactic purposes. The object is to secure the co-operation of the teachers in the work of prevention.

Atlantic City Medical Library.—A medical library has been established by the Atlantic City Academy of Medicine and this society has entered into an arrangement with the Atlantic City Free Public Library by

which a room has been set apart for its books and periodicals. These will, however, only be given out to members of the Academy and their friends, as it is deemed unwise to allow the public free access to medical books. Physicians visiting Atlantic City will be extended every courtesy the library can offer. Contributions on medical subjects will be gladly received and may be directed to Dr. Wm. Edgar Darnall, President of the Academy, or Dr. Philip Marvel, Chairman of the Committee.

The Supply of Midwives.—The English Association for Promoting the Training and Supply of Midwives held its annual meeting on February 14, when the report of the Council for the year 1904 was presented and adopted. It recorded the acceptance of the position of patroness by Her Majesty the Queen, a fact which was deemed to emphasize the national character of the Association's undertaking, and stated that among the accessions to the Council were the medical officers of health for several counties. Propaganda work throughout the country had been actively carried on, and twenty-three pupil midwives had been trained, the fees of eight being paid for by the Association. In return for free or assisted training the pupils bound themselves to do district midwifery for not less than two years, the Council retaining their certificates meanwhile. Steps were being taken which it was hoped would result in the Educational Authority for London adding lectures for midwives to its technical courses. It was stated that to carry on and extend the work further financial aid from the public would be necessary. The Secretary of the Association is Miss Gill, Dacre House, New Tothill Street, Westminster.

An Ancient Strike.—Last Sunday, states the *British Medical Journal*, the *Observer*, which is printing paragraphs extracted from its issue for the corresponding week a hundred years ago, published the following taken from its issue of Sunday, February 17, 1805: "A dispute has arisen between the physicians and surgeons of Worcester, in consequence of which the former have written to the apothecaries that they shall decline acting as consulting surgeons, and that they *will not* meet the surgeons on medical cases. 'Who shall decide, when doctors disagree?'" We should like to know a little more about this dispute, how it arose, and how it ended. Apparently the question must have been raised by the surgeons, for the notification given by the physicians, although it was evidently intended as a snub to the surgeons, was in effect a self-denying ordinance. It looks as though the surgeons had objected to the physicians being consulted in surgical cases, and that the physicians, feeling themselves compelled to agree to this, tried to cover their retreat by professing their intention not to meet the surgeons in consultations on medical cases. It was obviously an unwise notification, and we suspect that the plan was soon found to be unworkable.

Congress for Internal Medicine.—The twenty-second Congress for Internal Medicine will be held in Wiesbaden, April 12-15, under the Presidency of Dr. Wilhelm Erb, of Heidelberg. Heredity will be the subject under discussion for the first session. H. E. Ziegler, of Jena, will treat of the present-day position of Heredity in Biology; Dr. D. Martins, of Rostock, will discuss the Relationship of Heredity and Predisposition in Pathology, particularly with regard to Tuberculosis; Drs. A. Hoffmann and Paul Krause will discuss the Treatment of Leucemia by the X-Ray; Dr. Schütz, of Wiesbaden, will discuss the question of the Mucous Secretion of the Intestines; Dr. H. Matthes, of Jena, will talk on Autolysis; Dr. Cleum, of Darmstadt, will speak on Plaster Bandages for the Stomach; Drs. S. Kaminer and E. Meyer, of Berlin, will discuss Diagnostic Injections of Tuberculin; Dr. A. Bickel, of Berlin, will speak on the Researches of Normal Salt Solution on the Gastric Secretions; Dr. A. Laqueur, of Berlin, will dilate on the Uses of the Bath in Heart Diseases; Dr. Aufrecht, of Madgeburg, speaks on the Successful Use of Tuberculin in Almost Hopeless Consumptives; Dr. Rumpf, of Bonn, will talk on Nephritis; Dr. L. Gürisch, of Parchwitz, will demonstrate Rheumatism in the Joints; Dr. O. Hetzel will speak on the Early Symptoms of Tabes Dorsalis; Dr. Bernhard Fischer, of Bonn, will speak on the Results of Adrenalin Injections; Dr. Lüthje, of Tübingen, will talk on Experimental Diabetes; Drs. Homberger, Kohnstamm, Goldmann, Pick and Turban will also read papers. There will be an exhibition of instruments, apparatus and preparations relative to Internal Medicine. Parties who desire to read papers or information regarding this meeting should address their inquiries to Dr. Emil Pfeiffer, 13 Parkstrasse, Wiesbaden, Germany.

Panama's Yellow Fever.—Dr. Charles A. L. Reed, a member of the joint commission appointed by the United States and the Republic of Panama to adjust property values in dispute between the two countries, and who has just returned from the Isthmus, says that the sanitary conditions in Panama are being improved as rapidly as could be expected. The delay hitherto, the doctor believes, has been due to the non-arrival of construction material, ordered in the United States. Dr. Reed said that the health authorities apparently had the situation well in hand when he sailed from Colon a week ago. "There have been just thirty-six cases of yellow fever in Panama, with twelve deaths, since July 12 last, when the first case was reported," said Dr. Reed. "Colon is not infected, or at least was not when I left there. Sensational reports of the widespread prevalence of the disease are due chiefly to the fact that every case of fever that is sent to Ancon, where all fever cases are sent, is at once supposed to be yellow fever. As a matter of fact, all such cases, unless so fully developed that diagnosis is unmistakable, are held until all doubt is cleared up. In this way seventy or eighty suspected cases have been proven not to be yellow fever, but no account is taken of this fact, and all are charged up to yellow fever. I lived two weeks at Ancon Hospital, visited the yellow fever ward, attended autopsies on those who had died of yellow fever, and was in close touch with the yellow fever board. This body consists of Colonel Gorgas, Major De Garde, Captain Lyster, and Dr. Carter, the strongest aggregation of yellow fever experts in the world. They meet daily in consultation over suspected cases, and their verdict, which is arrived at only after every scientific resource is exhausted, is authoritative. Everything that intelligence and energy can do with the limited facilities available is being done to stamp out the disease. The waterworks and sewerage system that ought to have been in place last December are not yet installed, simply because of dilatoriness in getting pipe to the Isthmus. The first cargo was being discharged when I left. This delay makes it impossible to suppress water-barrels and other disease-breeding centers.

The city is, however, being very thoroughly fumigated, the streets are being kept clean, and garbage is being disposed of by our sanitary officers."

A Martyr of Science.—Tito Carbone, Professor of Pathology in the University of Pisa, died late last year of Maltese fever, acquired while studying the parasite of that disease. The *Archivio per le Scienze Mediche* has recently contained a biographical sketch by his friend, Prof. Foá. Born in 1863, the son of a poet of some fame, Carbone took an early interest in biological studies, and like F. Poupart, the outlines of whose life were given last month, devoted himself to the study of small animals. But while Poupart's researches extended over several classes of invertebrates, Carbone did not venture to aspire to the title even of an entomologist, but was proud of achieving a high reputation as "lepidopterist." On taking his medical degree he distinguished himself by energy and self-devotion during the cholera epidemic, 1886-87, and then became assistant to Prof. Lombroso as gaol surgeon. The enthusiasm with which he adopted the teaching of that great founder of criminal anthropology, and insisted on treating his charges as moral as well as physical "patients," brought him into opposition to legal prison officials and resulted in his resignation. After a visit to America he devoted himself specially to pathology, of which he became a professor at Cagliari, Modena, and finally at Pisa. Prof. Foá gives brief abstracts of his principal works in this capacity, e.g., on the pigments of melanosarcoma and Addison's disease, on the pathology of gout, on the coagulation of the blood, etc. In the summer of last year he succeeded in isolating the *Micrococcus melitensis* from the body of a soldier who had died with obscure febrile symptoms, and his last work forms the most valuable contribution yet made to our knowledge of its pathological action. Both in animals and man the two dominant characters are the marked congestion of the abdominal viscera and the rapid destruction of the red and white blood corpuscles. This is accompanied by great dilatation of the blood vessels and the conversion of their endothelial cells into phagocytes, which rapidly absorb and remove the products of the decomposed cells. Hence, probably, the relative benignity of Maltese fever in patients all of whose organs are healthy. Unfortunately, in spite of spending his vacations butterfly hunting in the Alps and Apennines, Carbone was unable to escape a natural tendency to corpulence and emphysema accompanied by cardiac weakness. Consequently, when he appeared to be already convalescent from the disease he had so thoroughly investigated, he died suddenly from heart failure at the age of forty-one, leaving us to mourn the loss of a brilliant leader on the battlefield between disease and science.

Medical Defense in Great Britain.—A great deal has been heard lately about Medical Defense and its adoption by the British Medical Association. A somewhat elaborate scheme, writes the *Medical Magazine*, February, 1905, was submitted last year but has ended in collapse. At the present time there is a lull in the usually disturbed atmosphere of Medical Defense, and so it may be appropriate to consider a few of the salient features of this question, past and present. It was not till many years after artisans and laborers had learned to acquire, by combination, that power which individually they altogether lacked, that the medical profession began to recognize the weakness resulting from want of union. Twenty or thirty years ago the overcrowded state of the profession, the senseless lowering of fees, the steady encroachments of the friendly societies and medical clubs, combined with the glaring injustice so often meted out to their medical servants, and the frequent blackmailing of unprotected medical practitioners, led some of the more vigorous spirits in the medical profession to plan means by which they might join together for mutual protection. It was thought also that if some body were formed capable of enforcing the law a stop might be put to the practice of innumerable quacks who competed with medical practitioners, robbing and lowering the medical profession, and working much injury to the health of the public. One of the earliest of the Associations formed for purposes of Medical Defense entered into a costly conflict with quackery, and succeeded in doing little more than proving the utter inadequacy of the existing medical laws to check the practice of unqualified or even of fraudulent practitioners. Want of success in its legal enterprises, and consequent want of funds, brought the career of this pioneer society to an early end. Subsequently the society from which the present Medical Defense Union developed was inaugurated, and its career was at first none too brilliant. The way had, however, been explored, and in stronger hands the Medical Defense Union soon entered upon a line of action which showed that medical men had sufficient business capacity to guard their own interests. The growth of the Union under the presidency of Mr. Lawson Tait was rapid. In fact it grew so fast that it became unsuited to the autocratic government which Mr. Lawson Tait had established. Hitherto the headquarters of Medical Defense had been at Birmingham. London, which seldom takes the initiative in anything, when the movement began to become an unequivocal success, commenced to assert its overpowering influence. A split resulted, and many of the leading members of the medical profession in London, who had looked askance at the Birmingham organization, now readily joined in the new movement. Its leaders did not hesitate to take advantage of experience already gained, and new ideas and new vitality were infused into this long-needed brotherhood of medical practitioners, ready and able to defend any of their number who might be unjustly attacked, and to protect the material interests of the medical profession generally. In many respects it was greatly to be regretted that there should have been more than one society formed for the defense of medical men, but, on the other hand, the good effects of a healthy rivalry have been more apparent than the weakness resulting from a division of forces. Be this as it may, there can be no question but that the formation of the latter society—the London and Counties Medical Protection Society—gave much fresh impetus to the effort of the medical profession to assert its proper power and influence or, at least, to maintain its dignity and to check the degradation which was fast overtaking it. Naturally, the British Medical Association, which had now established its pre-eminence among existing medical societies, did not remain unaffected by the prevailing sentiment. In 1886 an effort was made to induce the Association to undertake Medical Defense. The dominant section, if not the majority, of members was, however, averse from the Association becoming anything more than a scientific society, and the difficulty of taking up Medical Defense, under the

existing Memorandum of Association, was gladly brought forward as a fatal obstacle to the proposed development. In 1897 a special meeting of the Association, by a very narrow majority, decided in favor of the general principle that the Association should actively maintain the honor and interests of the medical profession. The Council of the Association gave no effect to this resolution, and it was subsequently reversed by another general meeting of the Association. During the last three years, under the new constitution of the Association, the movement in favor of the taking up of Medical Defense by the British Medical Association has been vigorously renewed, but in the meantime the existing societies, formed for that specific object, have increased greatly in numbers and in influence. Without the consent of the existing societies to merge themselves in the British Medical Association it is doubtful whether the Association can do more than create a third combination with the same objects. What could have been done years ago without any difficulty has now become a complicated and difficult enterprise. A majority of the Association is no doubt now in favor of the general principle that the Association should defend its members, but there is the greatest diversity of opinion as to essential details. The present machinery of the Association, in the striving after perfection, has been rendered slower than ever, and while it grinds away one obstacle, ten others are developing. If the Association could see its way to offer fair terms to existing societies for taking over their members and for granting them proportionate representation and privileges, and, having made such offer, proceeded at once to establish a department for Medical Defense it could probably still obtain control of this important movement. But it was very nearly, if not quite, lost its opportunity, and in a year or two it will no longer be able to assume the lead to which its great numbers and influence might even yet seem to entitle it. The British Medical Association has failed to take the tide at its highest point, and its opportunity is fast ebbing away.

There is no insuperable obstacle to prevent the British Medical Association from forthwith successfully forming a Medical Defense Department, with a special subscription, admitting to this department all registered and qualified doctors and dentists whether voting members of the Association or not. If it does so, it may even yet possibly absorb the existing societies and consolidate Medical Defense. If it spends years over forming such a department, and does it feebly, and in a narrow, exclusive spirit, it will merely weaken societies which are now doing good work, and it will confer no benefit on the medical profession.

As regards the attitude of the existing societies toward the British Medical Association, it must be remembered that they have never yet obtained any definite expression of opinion from their members. The Council of a society cannot be said to represent the society itself. The matter must go to a general meeting and be voted upon. No poll of their members on this question has been taken either by the London and Counties Medical Protection Society or by the Medical Defense Union, and as so few members can be got to attend and vote at general meetings such a poll would be the only real test of the views of the society. No doubt the societies are a good deal influenced by the decisions of their Councils. In the case of the Medical Deiense Union, its Council has definitely resolved to reject all advances from the British Medical Association. The Council of the London and Counties Society, on the other hand, has decided that any communication or scheme or proposals from the British Medical Association shall, at any rate, have full and courteous consideration.

OBITUARY.

Dr. IVAN AMILON, of Chicago, died last Wednesday in that city. Dr. Amilon was in practice in Philadelphia previous to his going to Chicago, as an examiner for the Equitable Life Assurance Company.

Dr. WILLIAM G. ROBINSON, of 142 East Fortieth Street, New York City, died at East Freetown, Mass., on March 2. Dr. Robinson was about fifty-four years of age, and had been ill for some time.

Dr. WARREN ELI REYNOLDS, for many years a physician in Harlem, died last week in a sanitarium, where he was taken two weeks ago from his home. He was a native of New York, fifty-six years old and unmarried.

Dr. CORDELIA POST HICKOX, the first woman to practise medicine in Iowa or west of the Mississippi River, died at her home in Cedar Rapids, Iowa, on Monday last. A graduate of the Cleveland Homeopathic Medical College, she went to Iowa in 1862. She was born in New York in 1827.

Dr. ADOLPH ZIPERLIN, an honorary member of the Faculty of the University of Tübingen, Germany, from which university he was graduated more than fifty years ago, died at his home, in Cincinnati, Friday last, aged nearly ninety years. He was a surgeon in the Union Army during the Civil War.

Dr. JOHN J. PRENDERGAST died last week at his home in Brooklyn. He was born in Boston in 1847, graduated from Seton College in 1864, and from the New York College of Physicians and Surgeons in 1868. He also took a course in the Columbia College Law School. Dr. Prendergast was for several years connected with St. Francis Hospital in Jersey City, and, with Dr. Thomas R. Poorley, he founded in 1888 the Manhattan Eye and Ear Hospital.

Dr. WALTER S. CHRISTOPHER, a well-known pediatrician, of Chicago, died of heart failure March 2 at his residence. He had been ill since last August, but in January it was hoped he would recover. He was forty-six years old, and was born in Newport, Ky., in 1859. He was educated in the public schools of Newport and Cincinnati, and was graduated as a doctor of medicine from the Medical College of Ohio in 1883. During the last year of his course in the college he was an interne at the Cincinnati Hospital. In 1884 he became demonstrator of chemistry, and continued in this relation until 1890. In 1890 he was called to the Chair of the Theory and Practice of Medicine in the University of Michigan. After a year's service he came, in 1891, to Chicago, and was appointed Professor of Diseases of Children at the Chicago Policlinic. A similar appointment to the College of Physicians and Surgeons was made in 1892. For two years, 1898-1900, Dr. Christopher was a member of the Chicago Board of Education. He was instrumental in establishing the system of medical inspection for the schools, and the child study department. He was a member of several local medical societies, the American Medical Association. and of the American Pediatric Society.

CORRESPONDENCE.

OUR LONDON LETTER.

(From Our Special Correspondent.)

. LONDON, February 25.

QUEEN ALEXANDRA AT THE COLLEGE OF SURGEONS—THE RELATION OF LONDON HOSPITALS TO MEDICAL SCHOOLS—THE TREATMENT OF INCIPIENT INSANITY—PROFESSIONAL SECRECY.

THE newspapers announced that the Queen paid a visit to the Royal College of Surgeons on February 15 and "expressed herself delighted with all she had seen, and hoped the good work which the college is accomplishing would long continue." This reminds one of Marshal MacMahon's famous remark to the colored student at the Military College of St. Cyr. The Marshal, who was then President of the French Republic, was as little of an orator as another famous soldier and president, General Grant. He had to deliver the prizes to the cadets and was supposed to say a graceful word of encouragement to each. But the poor man could only give all who came before him the stereotyped advice "Go on." When, in due course, the colored youth was presented to him, the President delivered himself of the sapient remark, "Ah, vous êtes le nègre: eh bien, continuez!" It is probable that after such encouragement from royalty the College of Surgeons will continue. My respects for the Veracities, however, compels me to state that Her Majesty did not appear to some of those who were present when she inspected the scientific treasures of the College to take a particularly intelligent interest in what she saw. She is very deaf, and Sir Frederick Treves, who played the part of showman, had to shout his explanations into the royal ear. She was shown specimens of diseased appendix, but seemed to be more interested in freaks and deformities. Her thick, drawling speech makes it not altogether easy to catch what she says, but as her comments were for the most part limited to such exclamations as "How hawrible!" this did not matter much. Her most original exclamation was in reference to a specimen of congenital syphilis in a child, which she said looked "like a mongkey." One thing which was noted in the Queen may interest your lady readers. On close inspection she looks just as youthful as she is represented in her photographs; there is no trace—at any rate, none visible to the masculine eye—of make-up by enameling or the grosser arts of the toilette. Her skin is wonderfully fresh and healthy-looking; but whether this is altogether natural or a masterpiece of "face massage" this deponent will not take it upon himself to say.

For years past Mr. Stephen Coleridge, the leader of the antivivisection agitation in England, has striven to divert the subscriptions of the charitable from hospitals with medical schools attached on the ground that these contributions were applied toward the maintenance of the school, and thus to the support of vivisection, as well as toward the relief of the sick poor. In this endeavor he has not been very successful, because, although it was thought by many that he had a good case, it was felt that he only made it a pretext for attacking a method of research which he dislikes. Some time ago a committee was appointed by the Prince of Wales, as President of King Edward's Hospital fund, to inquire into the financial relations between the hospitals and the medical schools. The committee consisted of Sir Edward Fry, Ex-Lord Justice of the Court of Appeal, the Bishop of Stepney, and Lord Welby, for many years Permanent Secretary of the Treasury and sometime Chairman of the London County Council. Their report was issued a few days ago, and their findings are generally in favor of Mr. Coleridge's contention. Of the twelve hospitals in London which have medical schools in connection with them only two (University College and King's) are completely absolved; while in the case of two others (Guy's and the Royal Free, which is the hospital where the students of the London College for Women gain clinical experience) the charge is declared to be not proven. In the case of the eight other hospitals—Charing Cross, London, Middlesex, St. Bartholomew's, St. George's, St. Mary's, St. Thomas's and Westminster—the Committee find that contributions, either direct or indirect or both, have been made to the schools out of the funds of the hospitals. On the question whether the hospitals derive any counterbalancing benefit from the schools in return for these contributions, the Committee find that, in some cases, the fact that a large body of students and of medical men are being, or have been, educated in a hospital diffuses a wide interest in that institution and thus tends to aid the finances of the hospital. Moreover, "the presence of a body of eager young men watching the proceedings of their teacher has the tendency to keep the medical man on the alert, and to counteract the effects of the daily routine of duties;" and "the opportunity for teaching a large number of pupils attracts to hospitals with schools the gratuitous services of the most eminent men in the profession." The Committee further express the opinion that the publicity which attends the work of a hospital where there is a body of young men in attendance tends to maintain at a high level the whole work of the institution. The Committee think, however, that no saving of expense can be attributed to the presence of medical students who act as clerks and dressers. With regard to the welfare of the patients, the opinion is expressed that "probably, in cases of great obscurity and difficulty, the presence of a large number of students may at times be useful." On the other hand the Committee think that the quiet of an hospital without students must often be a comfort to patients. As regards the advancements of medical science and the consequent benefit to the public, the existence of a medical school is in their opinion of the highest value. "London," they say, "probably offers the greatest facilities of any city in the world for clinical teaching and for surgical and medical research, and we regard it as of the highest importance that the greatest use should be made of these facilities." The general conclusion at which they have arrived is that "the schools confer certain considerable benefits on the hospitals, and the hospitals confer on the students a very great benefit, because without admission to such institutions the students could obtain little or no clinical teaching. These mutual benefits may, the Committee think, be fairly set off the one against the other. If that be done it follows that in the case of the schools which last year received benefits in money or money's worth from the hospitals over and above the benefits last alluded to, there is no return made by the schools to the hospitals which can be treated as recouping this expenditure of the hospitals, and that the schools still remain debtors to the hospitals in respect of these pecuniary contributions." For the future the Committee proposes that the distinction between the hospital and the school should in every case be drawn with such clearness that it may be understood by the general public, so that no question may arise as to the destination and application of moneys contributed whether by the King's Fund or from any other source. The Com-

mittee do not limit their pronouncement to the terms of the reference, but go on to say that they have formed the opinion "that a broad line of distinction ought to be drawn between the studies of the first three years of a medical student's curriculum and the studies of the last two years, or, in other words, between the preliminary and intermediate studies on the one hand and the final studies on the other; and that while the latter studies can only be pursued with advantage within the walls of a hospital, and nowhere in the world with more advantage than in London, the earlier studies have no real relation with a hospital, and are therefore more properly to be pursued in an institution of a university character; and, further, that the attempt of many hospitals to associate with themselves schools teaching the preliminary and intermediate subjects is a great, if not the chief, source of the exhausted condition of the funds of many of the schools and the consequent demand of the schools on the funds of the hospital." The report· has naturally been hailed with jubilation by Mr. Coleridge and his followers. But his victory is a hollow one, for after all the findings of the Committee are in accord with what has been for many years the feeling of those most actively interested in the improvement of medical education and the advancement of science. The multiplicity of schools imperfectly equipped and inadequately staffed in point of quality as well as quantity has been recognized as a source of weakness and hindrance of development. The doom of the hospital schools pronounced by the Committee will be accepted with satisfaction by all but those having a vested interest in these institutions. Most of them are on the verge of bankruptcy; some indeed, it is whispered, are suspended over the abyss by so slender a rope that the clinical teachers, so far from receiving any emolument, have to pay for the privilege of imparting instruction. In regard to schools of constitution so dilapidated as to need all this artificial support, reformers may well say, "Cut them down: why cumber they the ground?" They are worse than superfluous, for they give the enemy cause to blaspheme. The difficulty has hitherto been largely want of money; but the Committee express the hope that the University of London may now get sufficient funds to enable it to provide scientific teaching in anatomy, physiology and other preliminary subjects of a kind and on a scale worthy of a great university.

At the annual meeting of the Neurological Society, held on February 16, Sir John Batty Tuke, expert in mental diseases and Member of Parliament, pleaded strongly for the treatment of insanity in its early beginnings. Our whole conception of the nature and causes of acute insanity has, he said, been revolutionized by the advance in knowledge of the action of toxins on the structure and functions of the nerve cell, and especially the cortical cell. There is now, he holds, the strongest evidence of toxemia in certain forms of acute insanity and of the rapid implication of structure as a result of these poisonous agents. Physicians are being forced to the conclusion that the mental symptoms in the acute psychoses are manifestations of a toxic physical condition just as the delirium of fever is a symptom of certain phases of intoxication of the nervous system. The existing Lunacy Laws are based on the older notions of the nature of insanity as being something different from corporeal disease. Their general tenor is toward the protection of the mentally afflicted rather than toward the cure of sick persons. On this ground Sir John Tuke said he had urged on the Government the appointment of a Royal Commission to consider whether a change in the law is or is not necessary in the public interest. In England at present incipient cases among the poorer classes of the community cannot be treated till they are so far advanced as to be certifiable, that is to say, till the morbid action has gone so far as to make recovery tedious and difficult and often impossible. To the accumulation of unrecovered insane persons Sir John Tuke thinks the alleged increase of lunacy to be mainly due. He appealed to the experience of those whom he addressed to confirm his statement that if treatment were applied in the initial stage recovery would be far more frequent and relapse far more rare. He urged the establishment of hospitals in which cases of incipient insanity could be kept under observation and treated like other cases of disease. He pointed to the example of Glasgow, where some years ago special wards were set aside in one of the city hospitals for the treatment of lunatics. Of 1,345 persons admitted between 1899 and June, 1904, 1,052 were discharged "recovered" or "relieved," 86 died and 183 were sent to asylums. Encouraged by these results the civic authorities built a pavilion in connection with one of the general hospitals for the reception of insane persons. From June to December, 1904, 260 were admitted to this institution, of whom 155 were discharged "recovered" or "relieved," 62 were at once sent to asylums and 13 died. It has been said that the majority of these cases were "drunks." Sir John Tuke, as the result of personal inquiry, says that of the total number of cases admitted since 1890 only 28 per cent. are alcoholics. He pointed out that the treatment of lunatics in special hospitals or in special wards of general hospitals is carried out extensively in Germany and to a less extent in Austria, Italy, Switzerland and the United States. He added that a bill amending the existing Acts and providing for the early treatment of incipient cases will be submitted to Parliament in the present session.

At a meeting of the Medico-Legal Society on February 14, Dr. A. G. Bateman, Secretary of the Medical Defence Union, read a paper on Privileged Communications and Professional Secrecy. He pointed out that in this country the medical witness when giving evidence in a court of law can claim no privilege in regard to matters relating to his professional attendance or secrets pertinent to the issue before the Court that may have been confided by him by patients. In the famous case of the Duchess of Kingston it was laid down by the great judge, Lord Mansfield, that "a surgeon has no privilege when it is a material question on a civil or criminal cause to know whether parties were married or whether a child was born, although his introduction to the parties was in the course of his profession and in that way came to his knowledge." "If a surgeon," the judge went on to say, "was voluntarily to reveal these secrets he would be guilty of a breach of honor and of great indiscretion, but to give that information in a Court of Justice which by the law of the land he was bound to do, will never be imputed to him as any indiscretion whatever." Many other English judges have given similar rulings. Judges differ, however, as to the consequences to a medical witness who should refuse matters confided to him in his professional capacity when ordered by the Court to do so. He may be sent to prison by one judge while by another he may be upheld. Most authorities hold that a doctor is bound to give information if it should come to his knowledge in the course of his practice that a crime has been committed. But Mr. Justice Hawkins, in the case Kitson vs. Playfair, said it would be "a monstrous cruelty" if a doctor called to attend a woman who had attempted to pro-

cure abortion were to inform the police of the fact. In English courts actions for breach of secrecy are unknown, but in the Scottish Court of Sessions it has been judicially decided "that secrecy is an essential condition of the contract between a medical man and his employers, and breach of secrecy affords a relevant ground for an action for damages." The Society was invited to consider the following questions: (1) Can the medical profession obtain the same or a similar measure of privilege which attaches to a lawyer, and would it for the public benefit if this were conceded? (2) Given the commission of a crime such as abortion, is it right for a medical man to give information to legal authorities? (3) Is there any danger, should a medical man not disclose the fact of a crime having been committed, of his being guilty of concealment of a felony? (4) Is the mere concealment of the knowledge of a felony sufficient to make a person particeps criminis? Dr. Bateman's paper gave rise to an animated discussion which, however, threw no particular light on the problem of professional secrecy and left his conundrums unanswered.

"DE MORTUIS NIL NISI BONUM."

To the Editor of the Medical News:

DEAR SIR: In letter appearing in your issue of this date, and from your London correspondent, very grave injustice is done to my dead friend, Doctor Roose.

Doctor Robson Roose is of an excellent family, one branch of which is titled, he was of liberal education, widely traveled, of polished manners, splendidly certificated as a medical student, and he was the protégé of Sir William Jenner, physician to Queen Victoria, as well as the friend and physician of Sir Michael Hicks-Beach, and other British ministers.

I walked with him, in Paris, the wards of the Beaujon Hospital, in 1869, just before he entered upon his practice at home, and I have known him intimately ever since. He succeeded in families of every grade, up ao and including royalty, *because he deserved to succeed,* because he was a true Christian gentleman, "with malice toward none," an indefatigable student, and an intuitive physician.

This presents him in a very different light from the sneering commentary of your correspondent, to whom other successful British medical men, otherwise venerated, also seem to give special offence.

If it were ever permissible to dip one's pen in gall, and write venomously of one's colleagues, methinks it would hardly be so in the presence of the maxim, "*De mortuis nil nisi bonum.*"

Yours very truly,
FREDERICK WOOSTER OWEN, M.D.
Morristown, N. J., March 4, 1905.

SOCIETY PROCEEDINGS.

NEW YORK ACADEMY OF MEDICINE.

Regular Meeting, held December 15, 1904.

The President, Andrew H. Smith, M.D., in the Chair.

SYMPOSIUM ON THE SURGICAL DISEASES OF THE KIDNEY.

The Diagnosis of the Surgical Lesions of the Kidney and Ureter.—Dr. L. Bolton Bangs, in opening the discussion, said that the profession was more inclined to form its opinions and base its practice upon its personal experience rather than upon hearing and reading the experiences of others, but there was no question regarding the value of such a symposium as had been presented this evening and, although it was ifficult to select from such a feast, he wished to make few remarks upon one or two points that had occurred ɔ him during the reading of the papers. He was impressed with the fact that the more experience one ad with renal surgery the greater the value of making precise diagnosis preliminary to operation. He had een struck, in reading the books of the great operars such as Israel, with how emphatically it was stated ιat prior to operation a careful and, if possible, define diagnosis should be made. Notwithstanding the nportance of this, he confessed that he had met with ases where it was impossible to make a preliminary, efinite diagnosis the group of symptoms not being clear nough. In such he had found it necessary to make an xploratory operation in order to make a diagnosis ossible. After listening to Dr. Sondern's paper one ust not infer that it was an easy matter to determine e functional capacity of the kidney. This is highly nportant and should be determined if possible. Dr. angs said he had been much interested in reading a ery clever book by Caspar and Richter, who recomended in all cases the catheterization of one ureter r both in order that an examination of the urine from ach kidney might be made. Moreover one should be ery careful to know whether or not a second kidney present. In the hands of the most careful men uring the earlier days, before the introduction of the ιore precise means of diagnosis which were now at and, one kidney had been operated and, at autopsy, was found that one kidney was congenitally absent. s to the question of skiagraphs, Dr. Bangs said that ɛ had had a rather mixed experience and he was very ateful to Dr. Cole for the enlightenment he had given. r. Bangs said he had come to the conclusion that he ad not the requisite training of the eye to define the hadows cast and he believed that this should be left ɔ the expert.

Dr. F. Tilden Brown, in the discussion, said that although the evening's topic did not include the ϳherapeutic uses of cystoscope, he would like permission ɔ announce an innovation in this field which he beeves to be of promise, namely the ureter catheter and ome other material as agents in the dislodgment of ιreteral calculi. In a patient of Dr. Alvarez, the stones ϳeing clearly shown in an X-ray picture made y Mr. Caldwell, and where the speaker had inerted a fine ureteral catheter beyond the lowest stone nd given a warm boric acid injection, the patient two ays later presented Dr. Alvarez, when about to operte, with a box containing the stones. Dr. John L. \ndrews, knowing the facts in this just previous case, ϳished the efficacy of catheterization and injection ried on a patient of his before submitting him to oper-.tion which the man—a long-time sufferer—was preared to undergo, the same gratifying result was here lso attained. Encouraged by such an experience the peaker is prepared to state that some stones, lodged ven for years, may be freed and passed from the ιreter after a dilatation of the distal portion of the anal by catheters of increasing sizes and some aqueous ιedium, oil or glycerin, injected. Whether a catheter an be passed beyond the stone or not the injection of ome warm sterile solution to distent the upper ureter nd renal pelvis will tend to increase the vis-a-tergo nd enhance the chances of successful expulsation on he withdrawal of the catheter. It is probable that he majority of lodged ureteral calculi do not completey obstruct the canal. Consequently the catheter, if ntroduced only as far as the stone and if of as large size as the ureter will admit, so as to have no leakage bout it, can be turned to additional advantage by in-

jecting through it or when its lumen is temporarily closed with a rubber cap or plug, by thus damming back the urine for its distending as well as increased expulsive effect on withdrawal of the catheter. With a view to accomplishing a more rapid dilatation of the ureter Dr. Brown is now experimenting with dried laminaria in tubular and solid forms. This water plant, formerly much used for dilatation of the uterine cervix, under the name of tents, was at times not free from serious consequences, but the absence of asepsis in those days was clearly the main cause. If this substance can be sterilized without detriment to its drying and later hygroscopic qualities, the first requisite will have been obtained, for it will be quite feasible to pass one of these small cylinders with the ureter cystoscope, the bladder being best distended with air so as to avoid any fluid contact with the laminaria tent until this is in the ureter, where in a very short time, influenced by the urine or the injected fluid, it can dilate the caliber of this tube to three or four times the original size. By being made tubular, with a spiral wire center, urine can flow through the ten under control of the operator, and the whole be withdrawn at any desired moment. Any one who has cut for or seen the operation for calculus in the lower segment of the ureter is well aware of its magnitude; and to all, except those most dexterous surgeons who revel in difficult feats, a procedure which offers promise of relief without the knife will probably be viewed favorably. In the newer adaptations for ureteral catheterization and the rapidly growing number of expert cystoscopists we see sufficient reason to anticipate affirmative reports following such undertakings in the near future.

The particular cystoscope, according to the testimony of a number of disinterested users, which has rendered ureter catheterization so comparatively simple is shown on page 443, in one of its several forms. This instrument is made by the New York firm of Wappler Brothers. Its original features and mode of use were described in the medical and surgical reports of the Presbyterian Hospital for 1902.

Dr. Francis C. Wood said that he heartily agreed with Dr. Sondern regarding the slight value of the leucocyte count in many cases of severe sepsis, and the great value of the relative count of the different forms of leucocytes. He would like to add that the determination of the presence or the absence of an iodophilic reaction in the leucocytes was also of great importance in a decision as regards operative procedures. A number of cases which he had been enabled to observe in the wards of St. Luke's Hospital had shown that even if the total leucocyte count were low, when the polynuclear leucocytes were relatively high and an iodophilic reaction was present, pus had been invariably found on operation. With regard to cryoscopy, he could not take so favorable a view of the results as that expressed by Dr. Sondern. If one relies upon the brilliant papers of Kümmell, the diagnosis of a renal insufficiency would appear to be a simple matter, and the determination of the possibility of an operation equally easy from the freezing point of the blood. The speaker's own experience of the method, extending over a period of about five years, had led him to think very highly of it; but he recognized that there were a considerable number of exceptional cases. In all such work the general look of the patient, the findings on physical examination, and the skill of the surgeon were the most important points. If, for example, the blood froze at -.60° to -.63° C., it has been stated by many of the German surgeons that it was unwise to operate, for the reason that such patients frequently suffered from anuria after any operative procedure or even after the administration of an anesthetic. A case of this type with double pyonephrosis and a low freezing point had recently been operated upon with the most brilliant results, the freezing point of the blood returning to normal as soon as the kidneys were drained. Another point in the general use of cryoscopy is that the technic is exceedingly difficult and the results, unless determined with the greatest care, were of no value. The examination of the urine obtained from each kidney by catheterization of the ureters was a valuable aid in diagnosis. The freezing point, however, gives nothing especial in determining the efficiency of the secreting power of the kidney which is to be left in. That kidney, though passing a urine of fair quality, may still be insufficient when the other organ is removed, or on the other hand, may prove to be capable of sustaining life even though the quality of urine passed may have been very poor before operation.

Dr. B. Farquhar Curtis said that the general surgeon often received great assistance from the progress made in the art of special diagnosis. But too frequently when a case was brought before him he had found that these complicated methods of diagnosis failed. In many instances the ureters could not be catheterized. His personal experience was limited to the Kelly method, and when he found that he could not enter the ureter, he had called in an expert in male cystoscopy and ureteral catheterization, and yet he had failed to gain an entrance. The difficulties of catheterization seemed to him still to be great, but when it could be done and a good specimen of urine obtained it was a very valuable adjunct in diagnosis. He would urge the necessitiy of simplifying the methods or increasing the skill of the expert, so that the patient would not suffer so much in the manipulations.

Regarding the examination of the urine he had found too that the laboratory findings did not answer his questions: sometimes the tubercle bacilli could not be found in the urine and yet a tuberculous kidney existed; sometimes the urine was decomposed, or filled with pus and other deposits, which would obscure the microscopical examination. But it must also be acknowledged that the simple and ordinary clinical symptoms were often misleading; oftentimes pain existed without apparent cause. In some of these cases the kidney had been opened under the supposition that a calculus was present, causing the pain, and the patient had been relieved, although no cause for the pain could be found, the result justifying the operation.

Dr. Eugene Fuller said that there was one special point in Dr. Sondern's paper that interested him, and that was the question of urea, albumin and casts. There was a time, not very long ago, where a diminution in the amount of urea, or the finding of casts, were sufficient indications to prevent one from operating upon the lower urinary tract. Where urgent symptoms were present he did not think it necessary to postpone operations simply because urea was diminished or because of the presence of casts or albumin. If the kidney was working against an obstruction it was far better to operate promptly than to wait for the kidney to be still further damaged. Even though a patient had had uremic attacks and was suffering from uremia when coming under observation, the trouble being caused by an obstruction, he said it was wonderful in how many cases the kidney lesion would repair itself when the obstruction was relieved. With regard to the presence of tubercle bacilli in the urine, he in-referred from what Dr. Sondern said that many people got tired of searching for them before they found them.

He said he was much interested in the beautiful skiagraphs presented by Dr. Cole. The introduction of the catheter into the ureter and then taking the skiagraphic picture, as suggested and practised by Dr. Brown, was a very valuable aid. Dr. Fuller was not inclined to be so pessimistic as Dr. Curtis regarding ureteral catheterization; he did not think it was a very painful procedure in the hands of an expert. He believed the passing of the cystoscope through the deep urethra was the painful part of the procedure, while the actual catheterization of the ureter was not so. It was wonderful the amount of tolerance the ureter had, and how little reaction followed catheterization of it.

Dr. John F. Erdmann said he would limit himself in the discussion to considering the question of intercurrent or concurrent diseases, and presented four specimens of stones with the photograph of one as it looked when properly mounted. Of these four stones, three were removed by operative procedure, the fourth being passed voluntarily. The large stone (the one accompanied with the photograph), when he was called, was supposed to be a case of intestinal obstruction with all of the profound symptoms which accompany such a condition; pulse 140, temperature 103° F., abdomen distended, no movement of the bowels for three days, the latter easily explained by the fact that she had morphine, with a large tumor in her left side which occupied the entire left loin and extended down into the iliac fossa. In taking a careful history, evidences of having passed a small calculus and urine with pus for some time before were obtained. A specimen passed that day contained considerable pus, sediment, and also one small calculous body. The tumor on palpation appeared to be retroperitoneal, fluctuant in its main portion and boggy in the lower portion. A diagnosis of perinephritic abscess was made and emergency operation done, an immense quantity of urine and pus were liberated as soon as the fat capsule of the kidney was entered, and perforation of the pelvis of the kidney was observed through which the pus and urine were escaping; this was drained. Six days later it was necessary to remove the kidney owing to the continued sepsis; twenty small stones were found in the kidney. A period of three or four months later, the same symptoms attacked the patient on the right side. An X-ray showed a very large calculus (the one shown tonight) and nephrotomy was done through the pelvis of the kidney, and this large stone removed. Patient made recovery. The second case was from a male, four years old, who gave all the symptoms for a number of years of appendicitis and a history of an attack early in life. No blood was found in the urine at this time. He had been in consultation with numbers of the best general practitioners and surgeons in the city and surrounding neighborhood. He was seen by Dr. Nathan Potter, who, after a series of urine analyses obtained evidences of blood. Dr. Potter felt that he had no appendicitis, but that his trouble was stone. I personally felt that he had appendicitis with the bare possibility of stone. An explorative operation on the appendix was advocated at the same time exploring the ureter. This was done and a badly diseased adherent appendix was found, and a large number of adhesions removed from the cecum, but nothing was found in the ureter. A pronounced feature in favor of the diagnosis of appendicitis after operation was the fact that the patient was able to eat foods, that he had not been able to for a period of years. At the end of about three or four months, pain again appeared which was absolutely in the region of McBurney's point. This pain was so intense as to require chloroform to produce relief.

Urine examined at this time showed free blood. An X-ray taken before the first operation proved negative, an X-ray taken at this time showed evidence of stone in the pelvis of the kidney. A nephrotomy was done removing the stone through an incision in the pelvis of the kidney, with recovery. The third specimen stone, passed voluntarily, was obtained from a medical student six years ago in whom there was no question at the time of the diagnosis. This patient, though, also had digestive symptoms, and within a short time after passing his stone he was seized with an attack of gangrenous perforating appendicitis, for which he was operated on with recovery. The fourth specimen was removed three weeks ago from a male twenty-two years old, who gave absolutely sharp evidences of both diseases, appendicitis and kidney stone. There was no question in regard to the double diagnosis, although it required four X-rays before the stone was shown. It was then found to be in the pelvic portion of the ureter near the spine of the ischium. The patient was operated upon through a transverse skin incision just below the line of the usual appendix site. The muscle fibers were separated in their axis until reaching the transversalis fascia. This was divided in the axis of the rectus. The appendix which was adherent and involved was removed, the ureter explored, a stone located one and a half inches from its bladder entrance, the ureter opened extraperitoneally, two sutures taken in the ureter opening (peritoneal cavity having been closed previous), a small rubber tissue drainage down to the site of the operation in the ureter and the rest of the abdominal wound closed. The patient was discharged on the 14th day. All the cases had marked digestive disturbances. Two had pronounced hematuria, and one had pyuria, and one had ureter catheterization.

Dr. Frederic E. Sondern, in reply to Dr. Wood's statement regarding cryoscopy, said that Koranyi and his followers believed that when the freezing point was low it did not mean that no operation should be performed, but that no renal parenchyma, however diseased, should be removed. Probably, in cases of this kind, operation should be incision and drainage, but *not* removal of renal parenchyma, which would further jeopardize the patient's life.

Dr. Lewis Gregory Cole, in reply ti Dr. Bang's remarks, said that out of 179 cases examined by him during the last eighteen months only three occurred in which he could not make either a negative or positive diagnosis, or where the diagnosis had been incorrect. In one of these the patient, a man weighing 217 pounds; another was a woman who weighed over 200 pounds. In the third the plate was not high enough to show the presence of a stone in the kidney. In one of these cases only a partial diagnosis had been made, the mistake being made because he had been unable to see the edge of the stone; he could see a definite shadow, but the edges were not clear cut.

Dr. F. Tilden Brown said he wished to have it placed on record that he believed the improvements made in the cystoscope would enable men to relieve those distressing cases in the future where there was an impacted stone in the ureter. The surgical procedures attending the romoval of calculi in the lower segment of the ureter was accompanied by many difficulties, and if something could be substituted for such an extensive operation it certainly would be of great value. He felt much encouraged in this because of the results he had already had in catheterizing the uterus. He said there was but little reason to doubt that these calculi which became lodged in the ureter for some time could be dislodged if the catheter, in many cases, could be passed in and irrigation practised. His scheme would be to have ureteral catheters of increasing sizes, and, where calculi were seated in the ureters low down, to introduce spongiopile or laminaria tents and dilate this portion so as to enable the stones to escape. With the improvements in sterilization today this seaweed could be so prepared that they could be left in the lower part of the ureter to distend the canal to the size required without danger of ill effects. Dr. Brown wished to express his approval of the work Dr. Fuller was doing.

Election of Officers..-President, Dr. Charles Loomis Dana; Vice-President, Dr. T. Mitchell Prudden; Trustee, Dr. Abraham Jacobi; Treasurer of Board of Trustees, Dr. Reginald H. Sayre; Committee on Admissions, Dr. William C. Lusk; Committee on Library, Dr. L. Emmett Holt; Delegates to State Medical Society, Drs. David Bovaird, James Ewing, Charles L. Gibson, Homer W. Gibney and Edward L. Keyes, Jr.

NEW YORK ACADEMY OF MEDICINE.
ORTHOPEDIC SECTION.

Regular Meeting, held December 16, 1904.

The President, Homer Gibney, M.D., in the Chair.

Tumor from the Shaft of the Left Femur.— This specimen was presented by Dr. Homer Gibney, who said it was from a patient operated on recently by Professor Bull. The history of the case is, briefly: Male, thirty-three years of age; specific history at the age of twenty years; treatment continued three years. At the age of twenty-nine years he began to have twinges of pain in the left knee, very slight, thought to be rheumatic. A small nodule appeared on the inner aspect of the knee, which gave him no discomfort, and little attention was paid to it. During the following three years he was conscious of the increasing size of the knee, but this was so gradual and painless that he did nothing for it. Two years ago, however, he found he could flex it with difficulty, and soon thereafter was unable to do even this. Meantime, his leg was becoming noticeably larger, and infrequent paroxysms of pain during the night were relieved by standing or the upright position. For the past six weeks the pains have been more frequent and more lasting, discomfort greater, locomotion interfered with.

Examination.—He presents a large irregular mass on the left leg, extending from below the knee three inches upward and including the knee to about the upper third of the femur, terminating abruptly, and a distinct nodule on either side of the knee, one over the inner tubercle of the tibia and another on the outer lower third of the femur. The comparative measurements are: Right knee above the patella, 16 inches; over the patella, 15¾ inches; below the patella, 14½ inches; left, 21½, 23, 16 inches, about 5 degrees of motion. The mass was hard and no fluctuation could be detected. A diagnosis of osteosarcoma was made. Advised exploratory incision—amputation. X-ray showed a rather uniform mass completely encircling the knee-joint, and extending to about the line of the upper third of the femur. The line was a trifle lighter than the shaft presented. Subsequently he went to the hospital and amputation was done. Good hard bone was met and he stood the operation well.

The tumor was sent to Dr. Norris who makes this report: "The specimen is a tumor of the left femur. The shaft of the femur is completely surrounded by a cylindrical or fusiform shaped growth of firm, bony tissue. The specimen measures 51 cm. in its greatest circumference, just above the condyles, and extends from the condyles, upward along the shaft of the femur, for a distance of 19 cm. It measures 43 cm. in its middle part; in its widest portion, 16 cm. in breadth. The new growth consists of very firm, bony tissue, which measures 19 cm. in length, and extends from the shaft anteriorly, 4½ cm. in its greatest width. Posterior to the shaft there is likewise an extensive formation of new bone, which extends into and involves the muscles and tissues behind the bend of the knee-joint.

" The cortical portion of the shaft has become rarified, but, nevertheless, remains distinct throughout the course of the tumor. The cartilages of the knee-joint are not eroded. The marrow of the shaft has apparently not been involved. The patella is not involved, but the articular surfaces for the patella are the seat of a growth which, in appearance, is chondromatous. The peri-articular tissues are very much thickened, firm in consistency, and have all the appearances of a fibrosarcoma. In several places there are, most notably on the anterior portion of the tumor, nodules 1 cm. in size, which, in appearance and consistency, appear to be chondromatous. In places, the new growth is sclerotic, whereas in many places it is much softer in consistency. The tumor is periosteal osteoscaroma of the femur."

Tuberculosis of Knee Joint Following Gonorrheal Arthritis.—Dr. George R. Elliott reported this case. He said the patient had had the knee resected, and was wearing a plaster splint, so he could not show very much to the section. The case was of interest to him on account of the difficulty in making a diagnosis, and others had experienced a similar difficulty. Man, aged forty-five years, gave a history of having had gonorrheal arthritis eighteen years ago. The knee-joint was opened at one of the hospitals and drained, and he recovered. Has been going on without much disability and no pain ever since, until about a year ago, when he began to feel a certain amount of disability and pain, accompanied by considerable irregular swelling. The symptoms continued to increase in severity. Dr. Elliott saw the patient in June. At that time he had irregular swelling of the left knee, with fluctuating mass on the external and posterior surface. He had about one inch atrophy of the thigh, and very little pain upon moving the joint. There was no reflex spasm present, but there was tenderness of the head of the tibia. The speaker had some of the fluid removed and sent for pathological examination, and this was reported negative. A fixation splint had also been applied, but the symptoms increased so that it became impossible for the man to stand and walk, and at that time a diagnosis of osteomyelitis albuminosa following gonorrheal arthritis was made. This was based on the character of the fluid examined, tenderness of the head of the tibia, contour of the joint, absence of reflex spasm and general history of the case. The well-marked symptoms of tuberculosis were absent. The patient was admitted into the service of Dr. A. A. Berg, Mt. Sinai Hospital, and an X-ray showed tremendous exudate about the joint and great irregularity of the head of the tibia and condyles of the femur. From the examination of fluid and X-ray it was supposed to be an osteomyelitis of the type mentioned. Dr. Berg resected the joint and found a tuberculous mass with very extensive exudate. Union had taken place. Interest lies in the fact that the disease followed gonorrheal arthritis of years ago; a clinical picture of periostitis or osteomyelitis albuminosa with, however, well-marked tuberculous findings.

Pott's Disease with Some Unusual Features.—Dr. P. W. Nathan described this case. He presented the third and fourth lumbar vertebræ, removed from the body of M. P., female, aged twenty-four years. The vertebræ were firmly united by bony anchylosis. Not alone the bodies but also the articular processes are united by dense bony tissue. The height of the left half of the third lumbar vertebra is diminished by half, and it contains a tuberculous focus on its anterior surface. Where the two surfaces of the vertebræ come together, on the right side, there is a tuberculous focus about the size of a lima bean, which contains a large sequestrum. The posterior surface of the body of the third lumbar vertebra contains two foci about the size of a pea. All these foci communicate with the interior of the bone. On longitudinal section of the bodies of the vertebræ the intervertebral disk has been completely destroyed, and that the two bodies are united by very dense bone. The spongy tissue of the body of the third lumbar vertebra has been almost entirely replaced by dense bone, and more than half the body of the fourth lumbar vertebra is similarly affected. Clinically, this case was interesting because all symptoms of Pott's disease were absent before the appearance of a psoas abscess. In fact, back symptoms were not manifest until some time after the abscess was incised. The disease lasted about three years from the time of the abscess, but there never was any kyphosis. The absence of the kyphosis is accounted for by the fact that the disease was confined entirely to the lateral portions of the third lumbar vertebra. It is remarkable that the foci in the posterior part of the body of the third lumbar vertebra did not cause symptoms of paraplegia. These are, however, not apparent during life. The compensating proliferation in ostitis so common in other inflammatory conditions of bone is quite unusual in tuberculous disease. At any rate it almost never occurs to the extent found in the specimen presented this evening. Undoubtedly the disease had existed long before the advent of the psoas abscess in our case, but the new bone formation compensated for the very gradual destruction of the vertebræ, and for this reason the external signs were never pronounced. The bony anchylosis, which is somewhat rare in Pott's disease, was another hindrance to the usual forward tilting of the spine.

Dr. H. W. Frauenthal read the paper of the evening, entitled "Gonorrheal Arthritis." Will be published in a subsequent issue of the Medical News.

Dr. Wm. P. Northrup, in the discussion, said that he was much interested in the kind of joint. In all infectious diseases there is found the same kind of joint occasionally as that seen in scarlet fever. He was interested in the paper on this subject, because it had been his personal experience that the practitioners think of this cause of isolated joint affections last of all. A year ago he went on duty at the Presbyterian Hospital, and being a little more than generally interested in joints of this kind, he unearthed three gonorrheal joints that had been treated for rheumatism six weeks and eight weeks. They were taking ordinary rheumatic treatment, and passed as rebellious rheumatic joints. These joints were treated by immobilization and gradually recovered. At one time there was coincident occurrence of several gonorrheal joints at the Presbyterian Hospital. One of the first cases to attract attention was that of an old Irish woman who had an acute arthritis of the elbow. The speaker looked at it—at that time he did not know much about elbows of that style. Exquisitely sensitive—one could not touch the bed without her making some Hibernian remarks—swear profusely. She was very rebellious, and would not submit to treatment of any kind. She wanted to go home—said she would not stay. The speaker had never seen anything more exquisitely sensitive. No fever—a fusiform swelling from wrist to shoulder. Beneath the elbow it was boggy, brawny, red. If touched it became white, and the blush returned slowly. Patient was not ill otherwise. One surgeon looked at it; he wished to open it for pus, but her Hibernian blasphemy broke loose; he left the ward and she went home. Dr. Northrup said he was very much interested in this elbow. Soon another case came in, quite like it, and it was pronounced gonorrheal joint. The speaker looked up the Hibernian woman of blasphemy and irritability. Told her he would like to help her—would put on a plaster splint—it could do no harm. She said she would have nothing of it; that she had seen a homeopathic physician who had lanced it. It would get well. Dr. Northrup saw nothing but a spot, a place where the doctor had pricked it and got a drop of fluid. The woman was no better. Finally she allowed the application of a plaster splint. That made two cases which began to get better immediately upon the application of the splint. Several similar cases followed, and among them a man came into a private ward with a similar affection of the knee. His urethral history was satisfactory; he had an old discharge which stopped before the swelling began. He wished to know how long he would be sick, whether he would get well and have a good knee. He must have an answer. He was told that he would be sick about six weeks; would have a perfectly good joint. He recovered in six weeks with a perfectly good joint. Another knee case came in just at this time; he was told the same story, and was also good enough to get well with a perfectly good knee-joint. He could take it in his hands and put it up to his chin. Then came a short series of cases similar to those described by Dr. Frauenthal in his paper—exquisite sensitiveness, fusiform swelling, apparently edematous, about the joint, with serous exudate in the joint. No destruction of tissue, no adhesions, perfectly good joints resulting. One was somewhat stiff, with little or no fever. They all ran this course, improving very much by immobilization in a plaster splint. Unless put up in plaster, these inflamed joints had not done well. That led the speaker to think every kind of rheumatic joint should be put in a bandage or something to immobilize it. Orthopedists may think it a primitive conclusion on the part of a medical man, but at present every kind of sore joint that comes under Dr. Northrup's care is put into plaster. Cases of rheumatism coming in fresh and sore are put up in guaiacol and glycerin, and improve, but the minute they are absolutely immobilized they do better. In the Willard Parker in scarlet fever cases it was interesting to note that most postscarlet fever joints were of the same nature, and recovered under the same immobilization, without destruction of tissue. In all discussions speaker's seem to be talking about different lesions; one speaks of a lesion with destruction of all tissues about the joint, recovering with permanent anchylosis, another of pus in the joints, etc. It did not seem to the speaker that this particular joint, pariarticular cellulitis, had been very well described. In looking at the books he could not find one, at that time, which gave him a good picture of the eight or nine joints he had been seeing in those three months' service. Dr. Northrup thought the acute gonorrheal mono- or poly-arthritic joints deserved a favorable prognosis if properly treated.

Dr. L. E. Holt mentioned an epidemic of gonococcus infections at the Babies' Hospital in which 120 cases had occurred in a period extending over more than a year. In 17 children the joints were involved. All the cases were observed in infants and very young children. The joint inflammations as a rule were multiple, and involved most frequently wrists, ankles, knees and small joints of the fingers and toes. The process in the joints was a superficial one, and complete recovery of function occurred in a number of instances.

Dr. Gibney said the subject was very interesting, and he felt much indebted to Dr. Frauenthal for his paper and for calling attention to the acuteness of the pain. He also was indebted to Dr. Northrup for his remarks as to immobilization in joint disease. Orthopedists have so often been accused of too much immobilization and told that they have anchylophobia, that he was glad to have a man like Dr. Northrup say he immobilized every joint, even rheumatism; it was encouraging, and made one feel that he had not been working in vain.

As to the question of diagnosis, since the last case he had presented at the Section, which Dr. Frauenthal had suggested might be the effects of gonorrhea, he had been much interested. To-day he had a case of gonorrheal peri-arthritis of the spine, and eight years ago of the feet. He had not been quite so successful in his treatment of the joints in gonorrheal infection as Dr. Northrup, although he had used plaster-of-Paris, nor had he gone into it so thoroughly as Dr. Frauenthal in his cases. He could recall some of the most distressing cases in his practice—multiple arthritis with anchylosis, which never recovered. He did not know whether they were still going about. Sometimes one does make prompt recovery. If he could give his promise that they should recover in six weeks' time he would feel very happy.

Dr. B. Lapowski said he was very much interested in the remarks of Dr. Holt, and he regretted that they had not been made before the Academy instead of before the more limited Section. Dr. Lapowski suggested that Dr. Holt ascertain how the spreading of the disease in hospitals took place. Flies might have something to do with the spreading of the diseases, as Dr. Welander, in a similar epidemic, demonstrated that flies are carriers of gonococci. The next point is that it is not safe to rely upon microscopical examination alone, even if made by the best man. Gonococci, when injected into the muscle, produces an inflammation, edema, redness, but not pus, as shown by Wertheim, and the cases mentioned by Dr. Northrup can be brought into this category. It would be interesting to know whether the cervix uteri and other parts as urethra, rectum, were involved in the process. In women the vagina is not the usual localization of the gonococcus. It is doubtful whether even in children the vagina alone is affected.

Dr. Nathan said that he wished to fully substantiate what Dr. Lapowski had said. He had seen a great many of those gonorrheal joints, and would say that when they were purely gonorrheal they never suppurated, there was no destruction of tissue. Only where there was mixed infection and pus was there destruction of tissue. In regard to treatment of purely gonorrheal joints, without mixed infection, they would recover with rigid immobilization in a great many instances.

As to operating joints, no matter how careful the teachnic, all know that in some instances one gets infected joints after opening, and, as a consequence, stiff joints. With a mixed infection, where one is positive there is pus, the joints should be opened and drained. He had seen a number of cases of purely gonorrheal arthritis treated by general surgeons, in which the joints were opened and drained, resulting in complete anchylosis of the joints. To have opened these gonorrheal joints when there was no pus present was a grave error and a wrong to the patie t.

Dr. Sayre said he had been very much interested in the discussion. He thought there was no question that the different joints described *were* different, and that one has a simple gonorrhea or a mixed infection with different results. In some of these joints there had been complete cure, although his cases had not been of the six weeks' kind more particularly spoken of by Dr. Northrup.

He had also seen the kind where there was great destruction of tissue of the joints. Dr. Sayre had seen several cases in the spine where there was anchylosis of almost the entire spine, and as he read accounts of those cases reported as spondylose rizomelique, the majority of them seemed to be gonorrheal arthritis affecting the spine. He had seen several such cases which were apparently classical spondylose rizomelique. The advantage of immobilization of any inflamed joint has not been appreciated by the profession at large as by orthopedists.

The speaker said he was very glad to hear Dr. Northrup say it is a good thing to keep inflamed joints still, as ophthalmologists consider it a good thing to keep inflamed eyes still, as orthopedists think it a good thing to keep any inflamed part of the body still. The reason a great many of these joints are a burden, a terrible cross, and last so long, with great destruction of tissue, is because they are allowed to wobble around; every treatment except rest being tried while the joint is progressively going from bad to worse. Some of these cases are extremely slow in recovering, in the experience of the speaker, certainly if not treated properly in the beginning. If they come to our notice after the patients have had them for a long time, the condition is invariably intractable. Many broken down feet, painful feet, tender feet of one kind or another, with not much apparently to account for the condition, have their origin in gonorrheal arthritis of the tarsal joints, and they are extremely intractable in the experience of the speaker.

Dr. Fiske said that in making a diagnosis of some of these cases one ought to bring to his aid every scientific means; still, a diagnosis of gonorrhea is often made without the microscopical slide in the same way that one is able to make a diagnosis of gonorrheal joint without making an aspiration of such joint. In every case the speaker made the statement to the patient that he might be well in three months—he thought that a reasonable statement to make. Most of these gonorrheal joints represent a self-limited disease; if the urethritis, the original focus be attended to, the joint will recover without treatment. Immobilization is a grand thing for these joints, or for any sensitive joint. Hot air—baking—is of great value. Some of the gonorrheal joints Dr. Fiske had seen had been cured in a remarkably short time, within two or three weeks, by baking. The joints are exposed to a temperature of 250° to 300° F. Dr. Fiske thought these joints should undergo this treatment. He still thought that if the original focus be attended to, the gonorrheal joint would go on to recovery; then it would be a self-limited disease.

Dr. Frauenthal said that the condition of the joint differs with differing contents, as explained by König's classification, and that is what makes the difference of opinion of various physicians as to the nature and prognosis of gonorrheal arthritis. Those containing plain serous effusions will as a rule recover in three, four or five weeks.

NEW YORK OBSTETRICAL SOCIETY.

Stated Meeting, held December 13, 1904.

The President, J. Riddle Goffe, M.D., in the Chair.

Double Fibromata of the Ovaries.—Dr. Bache McE. Emmet presented two solid tumors of the ovaries —one the size of a full-term fetal head, the other of a lemon, he had removed from a single woman, forty-four years of age, whose menses had ceased seven years previously. The appreciation of the presence of a tumor for two years, occasional pains, lately becoming almost continuous, and moderate emaciation were the chief symptoms for which she sought relief. The operation showed the larger tumor to be firmly adherent to the omentum, and to be twice twisted upon its pedicle. The smaller tumor was not adherent. The tumors are so markedly calcified that they had to be cut with a saw. A specimen removed for histological examination has been treated for two weeks with sulphuric acid to render it fit for microscopic section.

Dr. Clement Cleveland, in the discussion, asked if a microscopical examination had been made of these tumors, as several cases he thought to be fibroids proved by microscopical examination to be sarcomata. Most of his cases were accompanied by ascites, and he would also like to ask Dr. Emmet if ascites were present in his case. He had recently removed a small pedunculated fibroid of the uterus, the surface of which was calcareous, but its center was soft and necrotic. The menorrhagia, from which the patient suffered, was found to be due to a partially submucous tumor, so that he thought it is possibly wiser to advise laparotomy in a larger number of such cases than is the present custom.

Dr. J. Riddle Goffe asked if these are the ovaries themselves, or if they were simply attached to the ovaries as their seat of origin.

Dr. George E. Brewer (guest) asked if calcified fibromata of the ovary are common, as he had removed a tumor much like the one presented by Dr. Emmet from a woman seventy-three years of age, who had an acute intestinal obstruction from an incarceration of the tumor in the pelvis. A carcinoma of the sigmoid was afterward found, which was removed by tying a ligature about the base of the sigmoid and severing. A colostomy was performed. Subsequent examination showed the ovarian tumor to be a sarcoma, which evidently occurred independently of the carcinoma of the sigmoid.

Dr. Edward Reynolds (guest) made a plea for a more exact pathological examination of apparently simple fibroids than has usually been made. He stated that for three years he had had every fibroid submitted to gross serial sections, and if any were at all suspicious they had been subjected to microscopical examination. He had discovered in this way that many cases of apparently benign tumors showed centers of sarcomatous degeneration, although experience had shown that one should not be too prompt in giving too much clinical significance to such pathological phenomena.

Dr. Emmet, in closing the discussion, said that calcified fibromata of the ovary are not common. There was no ascites in his case, although he thought the presence of the twists in the pedicle might itself cause fluid to be present. No ovarian structures were present other than the tumors. The presence of the calcification, he thought, pointed to a slow growth, and precluded the possibility of its being sarcoma. He referred to a fibro-sarcoma of the ovary that he had previously reported to this society, in which, from the solidity of the tumor, it was first thought no sarcomatous tissue existed.

He also recalled a case which he first thought to be a uterine fibroma, but from its extensive connections and the presence of a rectal stricture, he finally concluded was malignant and did not attempt its removal. Subsequent observation showed this diagnosis to be correct.

Ventral Fixation and Labor; Laparotomy at Term to Free Adhesions.—Dr. R. L. Dickinson gave the history of a patient, thirty-four years of age, upon whom he had done a ventral suspension according to the method of Kelly, seventeen months previous to the beginning of her present pregnancy. A hematoma had formed in the abdominal wound but no suppuration occurred. During pregnancy the fundus remained close to the thin abdominal wall with only a little mobility. A dragging pain was noted toward the end of pregnancy when the uterus was found to be symmetrically enlarged and extremely tense with the abdominal scar depressed. The fetal head in the L.O.P. position was far above the inlet and below it, and behind the pubes was a soft mass that might be either fluid or the thick and vascular uterine wall. At 8½ months the smallest Voorhees bag was passed into the cervix, and the largest into the vagina, and left for eight hours. Moderate pains began and during the uterine relaxation between the pains a rigid band could be felt extending just above the abdominal scar. Only moderate uterine activity was induced, and the internal os was out of digital reach at about the level of the promontory. An examination under chloroform upon the fourth day confirmed the diagnosis of the false band, which was cut through an incision made above, and to the left of the old one. No real ligament was present, but an adhesion, one inch long by one half wide, dragged obliquely downward on the uterine peritoneal covering and upward upon the parietal layer. The omentum was lightly attached to it above. The uterine stump was covered with a Lembert suture. The abdominal wall was sutured in layers with catgut, reinforced by four figure-of-eight silkworm-gut sutures. Pains began spontaneously in five hours, and an easy labor occurred ten hours later. Of the three methods he has tried for these extreme cases of fixation—manual dilatation with forcible extraction, Cæsarean section, and freeing the adhesions, the last he considers infinitely preferable.

Dr. E. B. Cragin, in the discussion, said, we all admit that dystocia following ventrofixation occurs, but the treatment must depend upon the condition that is found in each case. In two cases that he had seen the entire anterior uterine wall was adherent to the abdominal wall and Cæsarean section had to be performed, but with such a condition as was present in Dr. Dickinson's case, he would do as he did. In both of his cases, too, suppuration had occurred in the wounds at the time the ventrofixations were done and was the cause of the extensive adhesions.

Dr. Henry N. Vineberg recalled a case he had previously reported to this society of adhesions between the uterus and abdominal wall following an operation for ectopic pregnancy. When first seen by him on the third day of labor, no advance had been made and the cervix was above the promontory and beyond digital touch. A thin membrane covering a defect in the abdominal wall where a drain had been passed was ruptured while preparing the abdomen for operation, and a small portion of omentum presented. The adhesions were broken up through this opening, after which an assistant pushed up the fundus and brought down the cervix, and delivery was accomplished naturally.

Dr. Clement Cleveland thought that the opportunity should not be lost by those who are opposed to either the operation of ventral fixation or suspension of pointing out that such a case as Dr. Dickinson has here reported offers a very potent argument against either of these operations.

Dr. Bache McE. Emmet would not absolutely do away with this operation, but in case future pregnancies were expected would never antevert the uterus and attach it to the anterior wall, and also would make a slight suspension but not abrading the peritoneal surfaces.

Dr. R. L. Dickinson, in conclusion, said these accidents are relatively rare, and the arguments are not sufficiently strong to make us abandon the operations. He referred to cases he has reported of patients going through the pregnancy smoothly.

Antepartum Measurement of the Fetal Head.—Dr. W. S. Stone made a preliminary report upon a method of measuring the fetal head with the ordinary pelvimeter. The two poles of the head—the occipital and the frontal—are first palpated in the ordinary way for determining the position. An assistant standing at the foot of the table, places the ends of the pelvimeter between the ends of the ring and middle fingers of the palpating hands, and presses them in as the one who is palpating directs, and reads off the measurement upon the scale. He has now collected 42 cases in which this method has been tried, and the measurements compared with the occipitofrontal measurements after delivery: 27 proved to be exactly right; 13 showed an error of .25 cm.; 2 showed an error of .50 cm. Further measurements are to be made, and a more detailed report of the cases will be published at another time.

Nephrectomy for Early Tuberculosis of Left Kidney and Stricture of the Intravesical Portion of the Corresponding Ureter.—Dr. H. N. Vineberg showed a kidney he had removed from a woman, thirty years of age, who began to complain last summer of lassitude and general malaise, with an evening temperature of about 100° F. Examination was negative except for a moderate prolapse of the right kidney and the presence of a trace of albumin in the urine. Treatment for a marked constipation seemed to promptly improve her condition, and an extended sojourn in the mountains caused an entire disappearance of the symptoms and a marked gain in weight. Two weeks after returning to the city the old symptoms reappeared, and the urine began to be turbid and contained pus. There was slight vesical tenesmus and the urine contained tubercle bacilli. The right kidney now seemed to be slightly enlarged and moderately tender on deep pressure. The lower pole of the left kidney could be barely felt on deep inspiration, but no tenderness could be elicited on the deepest pressure. Although a diagnosis of tuberculosis, probably of the right kidney was made, cystoscopic examination showed the right ureteral orifice to be normal and 15 c.c of urine collected from the right kidney was practically normal. The left ureteral orifice presented a nipple-like projection with a slit in the center. The trigonal area was considerably injected, and a few small tubercles were seen irregularly scattered in the interureteral space. The catheter passed into the left ureter was arrested about an inch from the bladder entrance. At a second examination the catheter was directed through the stricture, and the urine collected from the left kidney contained a large amount of pus and tubercle bacilli. The freezing-point was .89° C. The ureter was removed as far as the pelvic brim with the kidney, which shows an abscess the size of an English walnut, situated between the cortical and medullary portion, and at the junction of the.

lower with the middle third. The abscess involved
chiefly the posterior wall which was considerably
thinned.

**Nephro-ureterectomy for Tuberculous Disease with
a Description of the New Technic for the Operation in Women.**—Under this title, Dr. Edward Reynolds, of Boston, read the paper of the evening. He
earnestly deprecated the indiscriminate application of
nephrectomy to all cases of venal tuberculosis, and
would only select cases for operation after careful
study and usually after long preparatory and constitutional treatment. He divided the cases into two
classes: (1) Those in which the course is rapid and
the constitutional failure marked. As such cases usually have tuberculous foci outside of the urinary apparatus, he would treat them constitutionally and would
only operate for the relief of otherwise irremediable
suffering. While the chances of cure in this class by
constitutional treatment are few, he noted such improvement in two cases that operations were refused. (2)
Those in which the progress of the disease is slow,
the constitutional condition is fairly good, and in which
the tuberculosis is not only limited to the urinary tract
but also can be demonstrated by cystoscopic examination to be limited to one kidney, its ureter and perhaps
the bladder. In this class of cases he considers that
a combination of constitutional and operative treatment a radical cure may be expected. The selection
of the cases for operation should depend upon repeated
examinations, and, if the bladder is diseased, by a preliminary local treatment before catheterization of the
uterus is attempted. Of a large number of cases of
renal tuberculosis he has operated upon eight. Two
belong to the first class, and were distinctly improved
for some time. Six belonged to the second class; nephrectomy upon two; one had a nephrectomy with subsequent ureterectomy; three had nephro-ureterectomy.
One suffered from prolongation of symptoms due to a
vesical cause, but at the end of four years was in an
improved condition of health. Of the five others, four
were in perfect health at periods ranging from eighteen
months to seven years. One had a subsequent tuberculous abscess but is again convalescing. All of the
eight made surprising gains in weight, color and
strength during the first six months following the operations. After performing nine nephrectomies for
tuberculous and other suppurative diseases, and seven
complete nephro-ureterectomies, Dr. Reynolds is convinced that whenever a renal tuberculosis is held to
indicate nephrectomy, the ureter should also be completely extirpated, because after the incomplete operations the symptoms persist longer, and in two of nine
cases he had been obliged to subsequently perform
ureterectomy. He thinks the superiority of the complete operation has been shown especially in tuberculous
disease, in which the ureter is so often the seat of extensive disease.

Technic.—The chief features of Dr. Reynolds' technic
are the doing away with the traditional nephrectomy
pillow, and so placing the patient that through a moderate incision, about 3½ to 4½ inches long, extending
from one-half inch anterior to the lower costal cartilages downward and outward to a point about an
inch inside of the anterior superior spine, the entire
operation can be performed under the eye by the aid
of retractors, and the dilatation of the wound from the
negative abdominal pressure. The patient is placed
upon her side on a hard table with the legs extended
nearly in line with the body, and is rolled as far backward as is possible without losing the negative abdominal pressure, which is shown by the appearance of a

transverse concavity in the outline of the abdominal
wall. A thin patient is best placed almost exactly on
the side, while a stout one should be rolled farther
backward, and may even need to have the hips raised
by a cushion. The table may be advantageously tilted
at its foot. After division of the muscles and fascia,
a retractor in the upper angle of the wound enables the
operator to recognize the perinephritic fascia and free
the kidney, which, after removal of the contractor, is
delivered, if the vessels are of the normal length. If
not, it may be pressed posteriorly and elevated by the
fingers of an assistant so that the vessels may be recognized. The kidney is then fastened to the edge of
the incision in order to prevent any injurious dragging
upon the ureter during the remainder of the operation.
The ureter is freed by separating the peritoneum from
the lateral abdominal wall until the pelvis is reached,
when a Sims' speculum with a long and flat blade is
introduced into the lower angle of the wound, and the
ureter is freed under the eye to its insertion into the
bladder. The stump is disinfected with 95 per cent.
carbolic, and the entire wound is usually sutured without drainage. If the ureter is so diseased that it is
broken during the operation, the wound is drained
through the vagina.

Dr. F. Tilden Brown, in the discussion, stated that
he had tried all of the various postures for nephrectomy, including the one described by the reader of
the paper, except he had cushioned the sound ilio-
costal space, so as to render the kidney more acceptable,
while Dr. Reynolds had omitted it in order to render
the pelvic part of the ureter more accessible. Except
in one instance, he had never done the complete nephro-
ureterectomy, chiefly because in some of his early operations, in which extensively diseased ureters were left,
the cases progressed so well as to suggest that such
organs on becoming functionless were rendered more
or less inert as foci of tuberculosis dissemination. A
realization in later cases that surgical precepts should
be better observed by a total removal of the ureter was
offset by the possibility of extensive traumatism and
protracted operation. Two cases, in which the ureter
was severed seven and nine inches from the kidney, the
dip at the sacral brim limiting easy accessibility, five
years later presented no evidence of urinary tuberculosis, unless a suggestion of Addison's disease in one
might be called such. In another instance, after nephrectomy the vesical symptoms persisted and a ureterectomy with partial cystectomy was contemplated,
but a compromise suprapubic cystotomy to permit of
curettage of the bladder and ureter by means of specially constructed curettes passed through the urethra,
was followed by marked improvement so that now,
two years afterward, no vesical symptoms exist. While
his views differed from the essayist as to what constitutes a feasible limitation, he was wholly in accord
with him regarding the advantages attending the removal of as much of a tuberculous ureter as is feasible. He could not agree, however, to the necessity of
making this complete operation in all cases of renal
tuberculosis. Such objection may be recognized in
Dr. Vineberg's specimen of beginning disease and early
diagnosis in which a part of one pyramid has a small
necrotic lesion, although the small lesion noted at the
vesical extremity of the ureter may or may not demand
some later attention. His only nephro-ureterectomy
was performed upon a man with bilateral renal tuberculosis after a lumbar transplantation of the right ureter
had been made to relieve extreme suffering two months
previously. Although the transplantation had relieved
the vesical and ureteral pain, his condition was so

threatening that the kidney and ureter were removed. A surprisingly good convalescence occurred and he remained in fairly good health for two years while living on a farm, but after returning to work on a canal boat the other kidney became worse and he died after two months' stay in the hospital.

Dr. George E. Brewer believes these are cases in which the operation described by Dr. Reynolds is the rational one to perform, but does not agree with him entirely in his statement regarding operative interference in limited cases. He considers an ideal case for primary nephrectomy is such a one as has been presented here by Dr. Vineberg, in which an early diagnosis of an abscess can be made, before extensive infiltration has occurred through the pelvis or ureter. Tuberculosis of the intermediary portion of the ureter is seldom found, but the intravesical portion frequently becomes first involved so that in no operation can this portion be removed. In Dr. Reynolds' operation there is left a tuberculous stump. He also considers tuberculosis a disease that may be overcome by sufficient resistance of the individual after the primary focus has been removed as in tuberculosis of the kidney, testicle or joint. He referred to a plea of Dr. Willy Meyer before the New York Surgical Society for early diagnosis so that such principles may be carried out. A quick operation with less damage to the tissues, he considers, best carries out this principle, and in those cases which have an extensively diseased ureter, the complete operation should not be done with the idea of completely removing the disease. He stated his surprise that the reader of the paper could so readily reach the lower part of the ureter through his incision, because in his experience even in an incision extending along Poupart's ligament he had found it very difficult to follow the ureter, and in one case he found that a probe from the pelvic brim passed five inches before entering the bladder. Tuberculosis is nearly always a blood infection and tuberculous deposits reach the kidney through the blood in the majority of cases from the bronchial lymph nodes so that the kidney does not represent the primary lesion. He thinks in all of these cases cryoscopy is one of the most reliable means for making a precise diagnosis.

Dr. H. N. Vineberg, in closing, stated that his patient had been away to the country but had returned with evidently more disease of the kidney than before. He does not believe in treating the bladder before nephrectomy, and recalled a case in which he had done a nephrectomy after treatment of the bladder had been carried out at different hospitals for some time. Rapid disappearance of the symptoms and a marked gain in weight followed the operation. He agreed with Dr. Brewer of the uselessness of removing the ureter in cases similar to that which he presented to-night, because of the inability of removing the intravesical portion. He had reported six years ago a case of nephrectomy for early renal tuberculosis, in which a stricture of the ureter gave the first indications of the presence of the disease. Complete recovery followed. He believed, however, that an attempt should be made to remove a ureter that is extensively thickened. He referred to Kümmel's series of seven cases in women, in which an early diagnosis was made without bladder or renal symptoms, except general malaise, pains and the passage of turbid urine, in which tubercle bacilli were found to be present. Each case presenting foci in other parts of the body must be judged by itself. Tuberculosis of the kidney is more frequent in women than in men and is limited to one kidney more frequently than is generally supposed. Bladder infections are secondary.

LAENNEC SOCIETY OF THE JOHNS HOPKINS HOSPITAL.

Stated Meeting held 'December 15, 1904.

SYMPOSIUM ON TUBERCULOSIS OF THE URINARY APPARATUS.

Pathology of Kidney Tuberculosis.—This phase was discussed by Dr. William Welch. There were, he said, two forms of kidney tuberculosis, the scattered miliary and the chronic localized types. The former was usually associated with general miliary tuberculosis, but it was noticeable that the kidney, though sometimes crowded with tubercles, usually contained fewer than other organs (particularly the liver and spleen), a fact found not only at the autopsy table but in experimental work as well. Perhaps the kidney is particularly resistant to this infection. Certainly miliary tuberculosis here is of no clinical importance for it produces no recognizable symptoms. The disease is probably perivascular though its embolic origin has been suggested.

Chronic Localized Renal Tuberculosis.—This was said to be the more interesting form clinically, much light having been shed on it by surgical advance. It may begin in the pyramids, sometimes at the papilla itself. An extensive caseous mass is then formed, there is marked tendency to cavity formation and nephrophthisis results. Sometimes only one pyramid is affected; but often more than one, and then the picture is that of a pyelonephrosis. The pyramids are destroyed but the columns of Bertin persist. The process extends as do similar cavities in the lungs. A caseous mass is formed. This is surrounded by a layer of granulation tissue, and outside of this is a fibrous layer containing many tubercles. Another type of the condition is, however (though less commonly), seen. Here several large caseous areas form and the whole organ becomes fibrous; but no real cavities appear. The disease may, though not commonly, begin at the cortex.

The Source of Renal Tuberculosis.—Dr. Welch said there was no doubt but that both ascending and hematogenous forms occur. Cohnheim was the first to show that not all renal tuberculosis was of the ascending type and to suggest the Ausscheidungstuberkulose. If, as stated by some, injection was always hematogenous, it was difficult to see why the disease was more frequent in males than in females—as autopsy statistics undoubtedly showed. The speaker's opinion was that infection took place by both routes—in females most frequently through the circulating blood.

Clinical Features of Renal Tuberculosis.—Dr. Futcher spoke of the varieties and symptoms of the disease, having drawn his facts largely from a complete monograph on the subject shortly to be published in the *Johns Hopkins Hospital Reports* by Dr. George Walker, who was unavoidably absent. Of 753 patients dead of tuberculosis in the Charité Hospital in Berlin, 25 per cent. showed renal infection. In 19 cases the bladder was involved and the prostate and testis in 13. Of 1,369 cases autopsied at the Johns Hopkins Hospital 784 showed tuberculosis. In 25 the kidneys were involved. Of 36 miliary cases all showed renal involvement. Primary tuberculosis of the kidney was not demonstrated in any case. Liver and spleen were involved about as frequently as the kidney. In the medical department of the hospital there had been 16,000 admissions. Of these 1,085 were tuberculous, the infection being renal in 17. Most of the cases occurred in the third decade. Tumor was palpated in 7 cases; pyuria present in 13; hemorrhage in 8; acid urine in 15; and tubercle bacilli found in the urine in 9. The condition was secondary to tuberculosis of the lower genito-urinary tract in 9 cases.

Symptoms of Renal Tuberculosis.—The condition has often been latent and presents no additional symptoms when a part of acute miliary tuberculosis. Tilden Brown has reported cases without symptoms, but with bacilli in the urine. Polyuria has often been the earliest symptom. Its cause is not known. Frequent urination has usually been present early. With it there have been burning in urethra and bladder during or at the end of micturition. This is present without vesicle tuberculosis and may be due to the action of acid urine on a slightly inflamed trigone. Hematuria is always an early and may be the first symptom. The amount of blood is usually not large but the hemorrhage continues throughout the twenty-four hours—differing in this respect from calculous hematuria. Pyuria always appears sooner or later—the pus being abundant or only microscopical. Pain is common over the kidney. It is usually dull and radiates to groin, abdomen or scrotum. It may be paroxysmal (due probably to lodgment of a clot or a caseous mass in the ureter) and at this time the urine may be quite clear. Tumor is palpable in many of the cases, is usually tender and may either preserve the kidney outlines or be quite irregular. Walsham and others have found tubercle bacilli where no kidney infection was present, and this possibility must be borne in mind. The urine for microscopical examination should be collected by catheterization with careful technic as the tubercle and smegma bacilli are practically indistinguishable by ordinary stains. A portion of the second urine should be centrifuged and the smear stained by Grethe's method (carbol fuchsin, decolorization with 20 per cent. HNO_3, followed by absolute alcohol, counterstain with alcoholic solution of 'methylene blue) or by the method of Bunge and Trautenroth (absolute alcohol, chromic acid, carbol fuchsin, sulphuric acid, counterstain). Fever is 'a constant symptom. It is continuous, but irregular, and may rise quite high if the ureter be blocked. Sweats are frequent. Cystoscopic examination with ureter catheterization may be necessary to localize the disease. Injections of methylene blue and of phloridzin, together with cryoscopy, have been used to determine the condition of the unaffected side.

Operative Treatment of Renal Tuberculosis.—Dr. Kelly discussed the results of a series of 41 cases treated surgically by himself, Dr. Cullen and Dr. Hunner. In this series no case of ascending infection was noted, and it is probable that infection usually passes in the direction of secretion, going from kidney to bladder in the female and from epididymis to bladder in the male. Vesical tuberculosis without renal involvement occurred in only three cases of this series—being secondary to rectal involvement in one, and to hebal involvement in a second—the transmission being direct in these cases. In the third case no renal involvement could be proven though the patient always reacted violently to tuberculin. The route by which the bladder and then the oposite kidney are infected is not known. Probably it is the blood current, though disease of the urethral orifice may allow ascending infection from the bladder. Albert in 1890 pronounced nephrectomy for renal tuberculosis a flagrant error. but the disease is now undoubtedly curable. If allowed to go untreated there may be healing, or the enclosure of the kidney in a sclerotic sac or obliteration of the ureter. These processes will protect the general economy from involvement. Advance of the disease in the

kidney, transmission down the ureter, secondary infections and tuberculous involvement of other organs are, however, the dangerous and frequent results of neglect. Surgical treatment may be conservatively done and cure has occasionally followed currettage. If the disease is sharply defined a wide excision might be possible; but as a matter of experience it is usually too extensive for this procedure. Nephrotomy is never a curative operation, but is admirably suited for patients too ill to undergo nephrectomy. The examination of urine for tubercle bacilli is a difficult matter. Catheterization does not necessarily avoid the entrance of smegma bacilli and guinea-pig injection may be necessary. A persistent acid pyuria without other organisms is always ·suggestive. Animal inoculation may be positive in cases with no kidney lesions, but the absence of urinary symptoms will make the diagnosis. The kidneys should always be palpated, but the possibility of a hypertrophied sound kidney should always be kept in mind if a tumor is felt. Palpation of the ureter per vaginam is most important. Cystoscopic examination of bladder and urethral orifices will often make the diagnosis. Tuberculous reaction is valuable when pain is localized in the affected kidney. Nephrectomy should be done through the kidney triangle, and when the capsule is thickened and adherent Olliei's intracapsular operation should be done. The next step in advance in this subject is earlier diagnosis. Localization of tuberculosis in the kidney is the most favorable one in the body; and vesical tuberculosis does not contra-indicate surgical treatment. Nitrous oxide is the anesthetic par excellence for these cases. Dr. Noble, of Philadelphia, said that his experience had convinced him that kidney tuberculosis was never the result of an ascending infection—first, because the disease was always more advanced in the kidney than in the bladder, and secondly because the bladder always healed after nephrectomy. Dr. Osler referred to the importance of early diagnosis and said that hematuria and pyuria should always suggest the possibility of tuberculosis. He congratulated Dr. Kelly on his brilliant results and spoke of three cases in the series known to him personally who are now in excellent health several years subsequent to operation.

JOHNS HOPKINS MEDICAL SOCIETY.

Regular Meeting, held December 19, 1904.

A Case of Aortic Embolism.—Dr. Osler showed the specimens from a patient who had died with this condition. Aortic embolism was, he said, an extremely rare occurrence, being only less rare than embolus of the heart. The patient was a girl of twelve years, with ulcerative endocarditis. She had been ill for six weeks with a high, irregular fever, but with no embolic features, and the diagnosis had been made on the heart signs. One week before death paralysis of the legs with sensory disturbances appeared. The limbs became cold but did not change in color nor did gangrene supervene. At the autopsy emboli were found in the aorta and in the spleen and kidneys.

A Case of Meningism.—This case was reported by Dr. Cole. A child. with a history of one week's illness (abdominal pain, fever and chill of onset) had become acutely delirious after admission to the hospital. The knee-jerks were increased and Kernig's sign present. Widal reaction was positive and *Bacillus typhosus* was cultivated from the blood. At autopsy lymphatism was extreme—thymus, general glands and Peyer's patches being much enlarged. Meningeal symptoms without lesions and in the absence of organisms in the cerebrospinal fluid have been called "meningism." Dr. Osler referred to the possibility of occurrence of all the symptoms of cerebrospinal meningitis with simple acute congestion of the cerebrospinal centers.

Puerperal Gas Bacillus Infections.—Dr. H. M. Little reported 10 cases of infection with this organism occurring in obstetrical practice. The case of physometra reported by Dobbins in 1897 was the first of this kind to be accurately worked up. Several organisms had been reported as the cause of this condition, among them the vibrine septique of Pasteur, the *Bacillus phlegmoni emphysematosus* of Fankel and Ernst, the *Bacillus emphysematosus vaginæ*, etc. Uterine infections with the *Bacillus aerogenes capsulatus* might, according to Dr. Welch, occur as emphysema of the fetus, as puerperal emphysema, as endometritis or as gas sepsis—the last being probably often preceded by endometritis. The *Bacillus aerogenes capsulatus* does not normally occur in the vagina, and hence auto-infection is not possible. Of the ten cases reported by Dr. Little, in one the organism was isolated from a breast abscess following a saline infusion, and in the other nine from the uterus. Infection of the organs through a typhoid ulcer seemed probable in one case. The organism occurred alone in only two cases and its association with others made it apparently a more serious infection.

Arteriovenous Aneurism.—Dr. Osler reported a case who had developed this condition immediately after a pistol-shot wound of the thigh. The tumor, which reached from the ankle to thigh, was accompanied by a vibratory thrill and a continuous humming-top murmur accentuated at systole. Dr. MacCallum briefly reviewed the subject of arteriovenous aneurism. The classification of Orth was said to be the best, the condition being divided into (1) arteriovenous aneurisms (aneurisms which have later broken into a vein); (2) varix aneurismatica (varicose vein connecting with an artery), and (3) aneurisma varicosa (hematoma followed by later connection with the vessels). The cause is usually an injury, and particularly a stab or revolver wound. Complete rupture of the artery with simultaneous wound of the vein may take place and the condition prove fatal before a sac can form. Or bruising of the walls of artery and vein with later union may occur and few symptoms follow. Or there might be a small wound of each vessel with extravasation. Distention of veins and arteries, and chronic passive congestion result. Operative treatment has not proven satisfactory. Dr. Osler referred to a patient who had developed an axillary arteriovenous neurism, and is now, years later, living an active life. He had seen another case of arteriovenous aneurism involving the subclavian vessels. Dr. Bloodgood said that the treatment for these cases was suture, not ligation.

Ovariotomy at the Extremes of Life.—This subject was reviewed by Mr. Wiel. Dr. Kelly had, he said, removed the ovary in 115 patients over seventy years of age, and felt that the age of the patient was no contra-indication to the procedure. As to the character of ovarian tumors, dermoids were more frequent in children and rarer in the old, while the reverse was true of multilocular cysts. There were only three cases of carcinoma in the literature under ten years of age. The patient reported had come to the dispensary complaining of a vaginal discharge. The girl was five years old. The family

and previous history were negative, except for a fall at one year. On examination there was an offensive discharge, the genitals were red and excoriated, the breasts somewhat large and a tumor was felt which under ether proved to be a movable, circumscribed tumor of the left ovary. At operation the other ovary was found normal and there were no glands. The tumor, which was removed, proved to be a cystic adenocarcinoma. Dr. Kelly said that too little emphasis had been laid on gynecology in children. They were, he said, particularly easy to examine and the vagina could be more satisfactorily explored by examination through a vesical speculum than with the finger.

Regular Meeting, held January 16, 1905.

A Case of Arteriovenous Aneurism.—Dr. Osler showed a patient exhibiting this condition. The patient, a male, now thirty-one years of age, had, in his eleventh year, received a knife-wound just above the right knee. This was soon followed by swelling of the calf of the leg, and a little later pulsation was noticed along the femoral artery with the development of a swelling in that region. The patient's health had remained good and he was exceptionally vigorous except for some disability in the right lower limb and for attacks of hemorrhage from varicose veins in the lower leg. Along the outer thigh, ran huge, tortuous varicose veins, and the whole right leg was enlarged. Thrombi were palpable in the the veins, some of them organized and a few probably calcified. There was a pulsating swelling in Scarpa's space and along the femoral artery. Over this a thrill was felt—most intensely about the middle of the thigh. In the abdomen was another pulsating tumor, eight inches across and occupying most of the hypogastrium and right ilias fossa. The pulsation here too was expansible in character, and over it a thrill could be feebly felt. The abdominal tumor was thought by Dr. Osler to be a large venous sinus associated with the enormous venous dilatation above a traumatic arteriovenous aneurism. Its origin was, however, not perfectly clear and, so far as he knew, there were no other cases like this one in literature.

The Immunization of Mice to Cancer.—Dr. G. H. A. Clowes made a preliminary report of recent work on this subject done by him at the New York Cancer Laboratory in conjunction with Dr. Gaylord. The work started from the study of two mice infected with cancer brought to this country from Professor Jensen, of Copenhagen. These animals—which were suffering from subcutaneous carcinoma simplex—died before reaching Buffalo, but inoculations from their tumors, though unsuccessful in the first and second experimental series, finally "took" in a large percentage of the descendants of these inoculated animals (hereditary predisposition?) and the investigators then had cancer experimentally produced on which to work. In the inoculations the tumor material was macerated in twice its weight of sodium chloride and injected subcutaneously. A tumor appeared locally (on the average in about 40 per cent. of selected cases), the animal became cachectic, the blood count fell and the growth became, in a few months, nearly as large as the experimental animal. During the course of the work the cancer material became attenuated and a certain number of animals with small tumors recovered spontaneously. It was from these recovered mice that immunizing serum was obtained for subsequent experimentation. A series of mice were inoculated with the cancer; half of this number then received a dose (2 c.c.)

of immunizing serum and the other half were kept as controls. This experiment was tried on animals with small, with medium and with large tumors. In almost every case the difference between the history of the immunized mice and the "controls" was quite marked. In the former small tumors disappeared in about five days, larger tumors diminished to half their original size; in the latter, the disease took its usual progress. All the control animals are now dead; all the immunized animals (with the exception of one dead from infection) are still alive. Later corroboratory experiments, while not quite so satisfactory as the earlier ones, gave in a general way always the same results. Tumors larger than a small cherry were never cured, but treatment reduced their size and rendered them more easily operable. Mice cured by serum immunization had sera capable of further curing, or at least counteracting, the disease. The sera of animals whose tumors had been improved by X-ray treatment were studied but they proved not to be protective. The protecting body of this immunizing serum was not a cytolysin, possessed no particular hemolytic activity and precipitice tests all gave negative results. Its protecting activity was not great and a large dose was necessary. The hope for the application of these results to human cancer lay, of course, in obtaining a case of spontaneously cured (or possibly even improving) cancer and then testing the serum of this patient for protective or curative powers.

Pathological Changes.—Dr. Welch discussed the microscopical features of the specimens showed by Dr. Clowes. The tumor produced in the mice was, he said, of the solid or simplex type, without acini and made up of polymorphous cells. The stroma was well developed and the connective tissue quite cellular. In the immunized animals the microscopical picture showed a striking change. In the larger tumors retrogressive metamorphosis was shown by necrosis of many cells at the center and by diminution in size of both protoplasm and nuclei of cells still preserved at the edge. In the smaller tumors it was almost impossible to tell that a carcinoma had ever been present, the picture being almost that of an inflammatory granulosa with multinuclear giant cells, necrotic center and vascular connective tissue shell. The observation of Drs. Clowes and Gaylord was, he said, a new and most important one. It offered at least a ray of hope for the treatment of human carcinoma; and while there was, as Dr. Clowes had said, a mathematical possibility that the results had been accidental, he felt this chance to be almost infinitesimal and the experiments practically conclusive within their own limits.

Apparatus for the Treatment of Fracture of the Femur.—This was described by Dr. Theodore Dunham, who devised it ten years ago and has been using it successfully ever since. It consisted of a plaster spica of the hip, connected with a plaster bandage of the lower leg by two long metal plates incorporated in the two plaster dressings and fastened together by seizing. In applying the apparatus the plaster bandages were first put in and the metal plates incorporated. Extension was then made in the required direction and the two metal plates lashed together. Coaptation splints might be added for older children, but were not indicated for young infants, in whom the thigh might be put up at right angles. giving the natural positon for nursing. The apparatus gave a constant extension, was simple and easily applied. did not necessitate keeping the patient in bed. did not interfere with the routine of life. allowed the thigh to be frequently examined without removing the dressing, and had given excellent results. It was necessary to reapply the seizing

at intervals in order to take up slack and keep extension perfect. Size and muscularity made the treatment unsatisfactory in adults.

Treatment of Esophageal Stricture.—Dr. Dunham also demonstrated a method of treatment of "impassable" stricture. A silk thread was passed into an ordinary drinking tube and its loose end allowed to float in a glass of water. The water was then sucked from the glass by the patient through the tube and the silk thread was then washed down the esophagus. Its lower end could then be caught through a gastrostomy wound and the stricture sewed by the method of Abbé. If regurgitation occurred or the patient resisted with his tongue the thread could be passed through a rubber tube inserted into the nostril, and could then be washed down by pouring water into an attached funnel. The lower end of the thread could then be caught through a gastrostomy and the upper end fished out from the pharynx. An instrument for cutting strictures was also shown consisting of a guide bougie on which was locked an olivary-tipped dilator. Through the olive ran a cord the two ends of which were brought out through the patient's mouth. The filiform guided the dilator, the stricture being thus put on the stretch by the olive and sawed by the string. This allowed further dilatation and was followed by further sawing. A wire and spindle dilator was also shown provided with rubber protecting tubes for portions of the esophagus both above and below the stricture; and demonstrations of the use of the thread method were given on an apparatus constructed to represent esophageal stricture. Dr. Finney said that the great difficulty in these cases was in once getting something through, and that Dr. Dunham had made an important contribution to the solution of this problem. He himself had modified Abbé's method by simply tying knots in the cord, and after passing these through fastening larger and larger bits of gauze for the purpose of dilation.

Peripancreatic Abscess.—The case reported by Dr. Thayer was of a woman, aged fifty-one years, who had been taken in June with epigastric pain and jaundice. From this she recovered, but shortly afterward had an attack of very severe abdominal pain accompanied by jaundice, fever, nausea and vomiting. Fever was intermittent in character and there were night sweats. She complained of a "sore pain" in the left abdomen where there was a slight prominence, especialy above the iliac crest. A deep mass could be felt which did not reach to the perinephric region. Two weeks later, however, it had reached the hip and the kidney. Operation was performed by Dr. Finney, a peripancreatic abscess with fat necrosis being found and drained. Four similar cases had been seen at the Johns Hopkins Hospital characterized by abdominal pain (the onset being, in some cases, exceedingly severe), usually jaundice, fever, sweats, sometimes chills and, on palpation, a deep mass. This might be felt in the pancreas region, but in some cases extended much beyond it, even going well over to the right side. The clinical symptoms were fairly characteristic and the diagnoses could usually be made without urine and stool examinations, which, to be of value, would be quite complex chemical procedures. Possibly the test for a fat-splitting ferment in the urine might be used.

Surgical Treatment.—In peripancreatic abscess Dr. Finney said, the surgeon could either do nothing or accomplish much by doing little. Opening and drainage were the essential features. If the case was seen early it was better to do this in two stages, the tumor being isolated by gauze in the first and opened in the second after peritoneal adhesions had formed.

MEDICAL AND CHIRURGICAL FACULTY OF MARYLAND.

Stated Meeting, held December 16, 1904.

Anchylostoma Duodenalis.—Dr. Smith showed a patient infected with this parasite. There was a history in youth of having suffered with ground itch, but otherwise the previous record was clear. Accidental discovery of an eosinophilia in a differential count made on his own blood (the patient was a medical student) led to an examination of the stools and anchylostoma eggs were found. Dr. Smith reviewed the morphological and cultural features of this parasite referring to the skin lesions (ground itch) caused by the entrance of the larvæ.

Primary Pernicious Anemia.—Dr. McCrae opened the symposium on this disease with a discussion of the clinical features. The symptoms were, he said, few and not characteristic. Weakness, dyspnea and pallor were the first to be mentioned. Then should come loss in weight—a feature seen in 50 per cent. of the cases in spite of the opposite statement of the text-books. Gastro-intestinal symptoms (dyspepsia, vomiting and diarrhea) were frequently seen. Hemorrhages also occurred. The nervous manifestations (numbness and tingling in the extremities, weakness of legs, ' tabetic'ᵡ gait) were not unusual and might be most confusing. Nothing in the symptom-complex was pathognomonic. As for the signs of the disease the color should be mentioned first. This might be a diffuse lemon yellow, a true jaundice, a local pigmentation or a pigmentation due to arsenic. In the mouth an infectious pyrrhea was sometimes seen—a feature greatly emphasized by William Hunter and his followers. Circulatory signs were not uncommon. The pulse was often rapid, moderate dilation occurred and hemic murmurs were common. In the stomach hydrochloric acid was often absent but lactic rarely present. The liver and spleen might be enlarged, ascites was sometimes seen and edema of the ankles occurred. Here again no feature was pathognomonic.

Diagnosis of Pernicious Anemia.—This of course could only be positively made from the blood examination and the most significant feature there was the color index. Confusion could arise from a group of diseases which ought to be distinguished from pernicious anemia and from another group impossible to differentiate. Under the first heading were included jaundice, cardiac disease, certain gastrointestinal conditions, kidney disease and some nervous affections. The blood count would, of course, make the differentiation. Cancer of the stomach, certain other anemias, spastic paraplegia (in early cases) and tabes dorsalis (in late) might be impossible to tell from pernicious anemia. In cancer of the stomach the red count was rarely below 2,000,000, and in pernicious anemia rarely above it. A high hemoglobin was also found in the former condition.

The Blood Picture of Pernicious Anemia.—This, said Dr. Emerson, was really the whole disease. The features were a low count, a high color index, increase in the size of the reds, presence of nucleated reds in large number, evidence of blood destruction (poikilocytosis, blood pigments in the urine, jaundice, iron in blood and internal organs). The diagnosis might often be suspected from the fresh smear,—the size and dark color of the red cells, the variation in their size and shape and the lack of leucocytosis being noticeable. The average red count at the Johns Hopkins Hospital had been

1,500,000. The color index was over one in eighty per cent of the cases. It must be remembered that hemoglobin estimations are only approximate and not so accurate as blood counts and too much stress must not be laid on the color index. The large red cells of pernicious anemia are not "dropsical" like the chlorotic cells. The cause of the dark color of the red cells is not clear. It is probably due to degeneration. The symptoms of the disease do not bear any relation to the blood count. At the Johns Hopkins the lowest count was 454,000. The leucocytes as a rule average under normal and there is a relative, but not an absolute, lymphocytosis—due really to changes in the granular cells. Megaloblasts (red cells with nuclei at least as large as normal erythrocytes) are found in fifty per cent. of the cases at a low estimate. Blood crises,—when a large number of nucleated reds suddenly appear in the blood,—were once thought to signify regeneration and to be always followed by a rise in the count; but the attempt at regeneration is often abortive. High color index, poikilocytosis and megaloblasts are occasionally seen in other conditions but are fairly characteristic of this disease.

Pathology of Pernicious Anemia.—Dr. C. H. Bunting reviewed this phase of the subject. The disease was said to be a general one (except for an apparent immunity in Prague and Munich), to affect all races, to occur most often in middle life and among robust people. Addison regarded the disease as a general anemia without discoverable cause; Biermer defined it as a progressive anemia due to diseases associated with hemorrhage, to long diarrhea, to unhygienic conditions and occasionally to unknown cause. It is not yet certain whether pernicious anemia is a pathological entity or a symptom-complex associated with many conditions. Iron deposit in the viscera, yellow fat, unusually red muscles, and charged bone marrow are among the pathological features. Atrophy of the stomach, cord degenerations and infections of the gastro-intestinal tract are also seen. The cause of the disease has been the subject of much dispute. Cohnheim thought there was a reversion of the bone-marrow to the embryonic type. Possibly the process consists in absorption of toxins from the intestine, hemolysis and resulting poor function by the bone-marrow. In certain rabbit experiments, made by Dr. Bunting, hemolysis was produced by the injection of ricin which seemed to bear out this explanation.

Treatment of Pernicious Anemia.—Dr. Brown said that this varied somewhat with the physician's theory of the cause of the disease—mouth antisepsis being emphasized by some, administration of bone-marrow by others. Transfusions of defibrinated blood should probably be reserved for extreme cases. Arsenic, given as Fowler's solution, as cacodylate of sodium or as atoxyl, was the drug par excellence. Improvement with it might be striking. The combination of other drugs usually availed little. Absolute rest, fresh air, a moderate climate (possibly a slight altitude) and great care as to the diet were essential features in the treatment.

Stated Meeting, held January 3, 1905.

Pathology of Nephritis.—Dr. MacCallum, in opening a symposium on this subject, referred to the unsatisfactory nature of all classifications. The most classical and fundamental paper since the one of Bright had been Weigert's. The disease is a diffuse and not a local one and degeneration rather than inflammation is the essential point. It is due to toxins (probably not usually bacterial), to poisons (alcohols, etc), to intestinal absorption, to constitutional diseases (gout, lues, etc.) and follows the acute exanthemata and pregnancy. Variations in the intensity of the toxins explains variations in symptoms, course and pathology. All the tissues of the kidney are affected simultaneously in the disease, the degenerative change being the first. Then follows a reaction, inflammatory in character. Attempts at regeneration occur and there is healing with a scarformation and shrinkage. The interstitial is therefore a secondary form, and the various clinical varieties should be thought of as transitions in a large series.

Acute Nephritis.—Here the kidney is swollen, the capsule fairly normal, the glomeruli prominent and cortical striations opaque. There is epithelial degeneration, exudate in the tubules, and inflammatory reaction in the glomeruli.

Chronic Nephritis.—No really definite types can here be separated, the various forms grading into one another. Epithelial degeneration is extensive, there is marked infiltration with wandering cells and there is local scarring. The capsule adheres, and under it are wedge-shaped areas of atrophy separating areas of hypertrophy and active function. This is the typical picture; other forms differ only in the relative amount of degeneration and scarring.

The Symptoms.—In the acute form, said Dr. Futcher, the onset was abrupt, and there were fever, headache, pain in back, nausea and vomiting, and prompt edema. The chronic might often follow, being characterized by pallor, a pasty putty face, chronic persitent anasarca, high blood-pressure and the well-known vascular and urinary changes. Many of the interstitial cases were unsuspected and came to the physician first with severe symptoms. Headache, vertigo, pallor, nausea, vomiting and high blood-pressure taken with the urinary changes made the diagnosis. The symptoms might be grouped as the cardiovascular, the uremic, the respiratory, the sensory and the urinary. A continued unexplained diarrhea should always make one suspicious of nephritis.

Urinary Changes.—These were described by Dr. Whitney. Nephritis, and not mere albuminuria, being taken as the subject. In the interstitial form the quantity, nearly normal at first, becomes larger and subsequently smaller. In the parenchymatous variety the amount is reduced. Albumin is in a rough way inversely proportional in amount to the amount of urine. A decrease of albumin with an increase of urine is approximately a good prognostic sign. but only approximately. It is probable that there is no marked retention of urea over a long period of time and urea determinations have a very limited value. So, too, of the various methods of functional diagnosis.

The Eye Changes.—The most important early changes were said to be subconjunctival hemorrhages and arteriosclerosis of the retina (the so-called Marcus Gunn vessels).

BOOKS RECEIVED.

VITAL STATISTICS OF THE CITY OF CHICAGO,· 1899 to 1903, inclusive. Chicago, 1904.

ESSENTIALS OF ANATOMY. By Dr. C. B. Nancrede. 12mo, 419 pages. Illustrated. W. B. Saunders & Co., New York, Philadelphia and London.

BOOK REVIEWS.

BACTERIOLOGY AND THE PUBLIC HEALTH. By GEORGE NEWMAN, M.D., F.R.S.E., D.P.H., Metropolitan Officer of Health of the Metropolitan Borough of Finsbury. Third Edition. P. Blakiston's Son & Company, Philadelphia.

THIS is essentially a popular treatise. Not of that type commonly so designated by many writers in this part of the world—and which may be translated into the general word "rubbish," but a popular work of a high order, written by a man of the highest repute and with a large experience as a health officer.

Looking through the pages of this work the reviewer is tempted to ask—How long, O Lord, how long—shall the sanitation of our large municipalities be delivered up into the hands of the spoilsman and fowler. When, throughout the land are we to have men of this type of qualification at the head of our sanitary affairs—not sporadically as we do have, and a few in a decade, but everywhere and at all times.

The problem of public health is one of the most important in the domain of the physician. It should not be soiled by the dirty hands of the political contractor. We commend to our health officers and students of public sanitation this excellent volume.

The mechanical get-up of this work is everything to be desired.

TEN LECTURES ON BIOCHEMISTRY OF MUSCLE AND NERVE. By W. D. HALLIBURTON, M.D., F.R.S., Professor of Physiology, Kings College, London. P. Blakiston's Son & Co., Philadelphia.

DR. C. A. HERTER, of New York, in accepting the chair of Pharmacology at Columbia University, founded at the University and Bellevue Medical College a Herter Lectureship on questions concerned with clinical physiology or chemical pathology. Dr. Halliburton was the first to give these lectures, and the present volume represents the substance of the lectures in an elaborate manner.

The series are of intense theoretical as well as of practical interest. They review practically all that is known of the intricate changes that go on in these structures under the many diverse conditions of both normal and abnormal functioning. We cannot hope to pass in review the results here set forth. We can only commend them as readable and profitable to student and practitioner alike.

A TEXT-BOOK OF HISTOLOGY. By FREDERICK R. BAILEY, A.M., M.D., Adjunct Professor of Normal Histology, College of Physicians and Surgeons, Medical Department Columbia University, New York. William Wood & Company, New York.

THIS is essentially a student's book—and a very excellent one. From first to last it is evident that the author has in mind the needs of the student in the classroom, and has given him a descriptive manual of high excellence.

In general the treatment of the subject is straightforward and direct. Controversial matters are omitted, and abundant illustration makes the text very simple and effective.

We feel that the chapters on the blood might have been more fully treated and better illustrated, but this is the only subject that does not seem to have received a full share of attention. The mechanical work on the book is excellent.

THE MEDICAL NEWS.

A WEEKLY JOURNAL OF MEDICAL SCIENCE.

VOL. 86.   NEW YORK, SATURDAY, MARCH 18, 1905.   NO. 11.

ORIGINAL ARTICLES.

HE FRESH AIR TREATMENT OF SURGICAL TU-
BERCULOSIS.[1][2]

BY LINSLY R. WILLIAMS, M.D.,

OF NEW YORK;

TTENDING PHYSICIAN TO SETON HOSPITAL FOR CONSUMPTIVES AND
HOUSE OF REST FOR CONSUMPTIVES, ETC.

It is with considerable trepidation that I speak) you to-night on the subject of tuberculosis. 'or speaking upon any phase of this broad sub- ect I apologize most humbly. I have nothing ew to offer, nor have I any elaborate or scien- fic report, but I will confine myself only to the reatment and to the Fresh Air Treatment of urgical Tuberculosis in Children, with especial ttention to the work that is being carried on y the New York Association for Improving 1e Condition of the Poor at its temporary hos- ital at Coney Island.

You are all familiar with the treatment of pul- 1onary tuberculosis according to the methods utlined by Brehmer, Dettweiler and Trudeau, nd the strict hygienic rules laid down by them. ut I think that some of you are less familiar ith the application of these same principles in 1e treatment of surgical tuberculosis.

Through the efforts of Bergeron[1] in France, 1e first hospital at Berck sur Mer was begun 1 1861, and the original hospital of 100 beds as been enlarged to accommodate 600, and since 1en other hospitals have been built there and sewhere in France.

Cazin,[2] in 1885, published the results of thir- en years' experience at Berck, and the results 'ere very satisfactory.' Since this beginning 1ere have been built in Germany, Austria, Bel- ium, Holland and in Italy sanatoria for the reatment of surgical tuberculosis in children, 1e majority of them being on the seashore. .ugland has only Margate, built in 1796, for pul- 1onary as well as other forms of tuberculosis.

The French writers speak enthusiastically of 1e results, claiming (d'Espine[3]) 93 per cent. 1ccessful cases at Asile Dollfus and 87 per cent. 1ccessfully treated cases at St. Pol. In 1900, Espine,[4] of Geneva, said "Everyone is agreed 1at salt air and sea-baths constitute the best reatment for scrofula."

In 1902, Tubby[5], in London, compared the tses treated in the London hospitals and those eated at Sevenoaks, at a hospital where hy- .enic measures could be satisfactorily carried 1t. He concluded that it was not justifiable treat these cases in the city. It has gradually

---

[1] Read before the Academy of Medicine, January 19, 1905.
[2] With especial reference to the work being carried on by 1e New York Association for Improving the Condition of the 'or, at its Seaside Hospital, Coney Island, N. Y.

become recognized that country air is needed, and by some that the sea air is better. The importance of fresh air, rest, good food and sunshine is mentioned in the most modern books on sur- gery, and orthopedics and particularly empha- sized by Gibney and Whitman[6] in this city in the treatment of surgical tuberculosis. In a paper read before the section on surgery of the Academy of Medicine, in the winter of 1903, Knopf[7] insisted on this treatment of surgical tuberculosis, especially in postoperative cases, and strongly urged the establishment of sanatoria for this purpose at the seashore. In this coun- try there has been little sanatoria treatment for surgical tuberculosis. The fresh-air treatment of septic cases was commenced about thirty years ago at the Boston City Hospital, and, so far as I know, was the first treatment of the kind for any septic cases. Lately Burrell[8], of that city, has successfully treated numbers of cases of surgical tuberculosis by treating them on the same general plan as consumptives. Some of our hospitals in this city where surgical tuber- culosis is treated, have country homes where post- operative cases are sent to convalesce, they also make use of the various summer homes and float- ing hospitals near the city, but the accommo- dations for them are far too small.

During 1903 some of the members of the Board of Managers of the Association for Improving the Condition of the Poor felt that the time had come for the establishment of a maritime sanatorium for surgical tuberculosis. In the summer of 1903, Mr. J. S. Ward, Jr., of the Association, visited all the important sanatoria in France, and returned, making an enthusiastic and satisfactory report of the results obtained in France.

During the winter of 1904 the Association appropriated sufficient funds to build a tent camp at Coney Island upon rented land in close prox- imity to their Fresh-Air Home, "Sea Breeze." The tents were opened on June 6, 1904, with some 20 patients. There were, of course, con- siderable difficulties, as with every new institu- tion. Hospital management and tent life were not very familiar, but, notwithstanding many trials, the scheme was satisfactorily pushed through. The tents suffered from lightning and wind, and on an afternoon in August they were all unroofed, and two of them demolished dur- ing a violent thunderstorm. The Association had appointed a medical advisory board, consist- ing of Dr. W. B. James, chairman; Dr. John W. Brannan, of New York City; Dr. L. F. Flick, of Philadelphia; Dr. E. L. Trudeau, of Saranac Lake; Dr. Hermann M. Biggs, Dr. Virgil P. Gibney, Dr. Newton M. Shaffer, and Dr. E. G.

Janeway, of New York City, who gave wise counsel and personal effort to make the venture a success. Much credit is due especially to Dr. Brannan, who gave much time and almost daily valuable advice in all matters. With the advent of the fall, the association felt that the experiment had been so far successful, yet realized that in order to prove it beyond criticism the work should be continued during the winter. The Association did not desire to run a hospital further than to prove this point, and the question was first raised, " Is there any conceivable way of continuing the work for the winter?" But as October drew near the question became, " Have we the moral right, after the short period of upbuilding, to condemn those children to the undermining conditions of their homes, or even to the best indoor hospital life that can be provided within the city limits?" Letters were written on behalf of the association by Dr. Brannan[9] to the various members of the Medical Advisory Board asking if, in their opinion, there would be any danger to future occupants if these cases of surgical tuberculosis occupied one of the Association buildings at Sea Breeze (the Fresh-Air Home). The answers were unanimously negative, Dr. Biggs[10] saying: " Of course any statements as to there being danger to the other children next summer from their presence in the building during the winter is perfect nonsense. I should have no hesitation whatsoever in saying this with the utmost emphasis." The Board of Managers of the Association then decided to use the so-called service building at Sea Breeze for winter quarters. This building needed but a few alterations, including the installation of a heating plant, and it was ready for use, and the treatment there is being carried on in the same manner as at the Tent Camp.

The treatment of surgical tuberculosis is hygienic, medical and surgical, and I can best describe it by telling of the treatment being carried out at Coney Island. The children are treated much like pulmonary cases as regards fresh air, good food and an abundance of it, and rest. During the summer the tents were always open, and various adjuncts to ventilation were carried out according to suggestions made by Drs. James and Biggs. The children were also given daily sea-baths until October, when the air and water grew too cold. The windows in the wards are kept always open except for a half hour before and during the time the children dress and undress.

The children spend the entire daytime out of doors, except for meals. Since the opening of the school term, the Board of Education has given us the services of a teacher, who holds school for the older children. The most any child has is two hours, five days a week, and only one hour continuously, in a bright, airy room. Those children that are able, have calisthenic exercises out of doors. The morning lunch, consisting of crackers and milk, is taken out of doors.

If for any reason a child is unable to run about, he is kept in his crib, but out on a bright, sunny piazza, and not exposed to the wind. During the cold weather the children are warmly clad. At night they wear outing flannel nightgowns, knitted wool slippers, hoods and flannel jackets. These measures keep them perfectly warm. During the day they do not complain of cold, the circulation being good in almost all of these surgical cases, and the association is able to supply them with suitable clothing, which is so often lacking in our charitable institutions for pulmonary tuberculosis.

Considerable stress is placed upon the care of the mouth and teeth. The children brush their own teeth under supervision, twice daily, using a good tooth powder. The services of a dentist are also called in when necessary. The children take good care of their noses, and are taught to use gauze handkerchiefs, which are all burned after use. Strict regard is also paid to cleanliness and to the care of the skin.

The food is of the very best, and a good, substantial, varied diet is given, such as is suitable for children. Soups, milk, eggs, plain meats and vegetables forming the main articles of diet. The daily routine is as follows: 6 o'clock, windows closed by night nurse; 6.30 to 7, dress; 7. breakfast; 7.30 to 9, outdoors; 9 to 10, school for older children (5 to 12) ; 10 to 10.30, lunch; 10.30 to 10.45, singing; 10.45 to 11.15, school; 11.15 to 11.30, exercise out of doors; 11.30 to 11.45, school; 12 M., dinner; 12.30 till dark, out of doors. at present till about 4 P.M; 2 to 2.45, teacher gives a few backward pupils fifteen minutes each; 5 P.M.. supper; 6, smaller children to bed; 7.30, larger children to bed.

Dietary.—Breakfast, 7 A.M., farina or one of the following: Flaked rice, wheat biscuit, hominy, malta vita; cocoa, milk, bread and butter ; minced beef or soft boiled egg.

Lunch, 10 A.M., crackers, soda or Graham, and milk.

Dinner, 12 M.. soup: beef or other broths; meat; roast beef. lamb, chicken, stewed beef, stewed lamb, or fresh fish: vegetables: potatoes, and two others: beans, peas, lettuce, tomatoes, macaroni. or rice. Dessert: Ice cream twice a week or milk puddings: bread and butter and milk.

Lunch, 3 P.M., crackers and milk.

Supper, 5 P.M., gravy. bread or milk toast; stewed fruit, pears, blackberries, raspberries, plums, or peaches: bread and butter.

The children in good health, especially those who do not have joint disease of the lower extremity, have considerable freedom as to play outdoors, and it agrees with them. Those wearing braces and some of the cases of Pott's disease take enforced rest, sometimes dressed, and sometimes in their cribs on the piazza.

Not believing in any specific medicine. no special plan of medical treatment has been adopted. The use of tonics, such as arsenic and iron, has en given a trial, in certain cases with apparent nefit, and some cases which have not gained tisfactorily in weight have been given coder oil and Russell's emulsion.

The surgical treatment is conservative and der the advice of the Advisory Medical Board. ie necessity for absolute asepsis is well realized, d in the dressing of even a small sinus the most pains are taken and thorough cleanliness iisted upon.

The treatment of tuberculous wounds has been ven too little attention, but the recent knowlge that they heal comparatively quickly, proied they do not become infected with pyogenic ganisms, should enable us to give these wounds tter care.

The bacteriological findings in opened and opened tuberculous abscesses has been ably monstrated by Petroff[11] and others, and there now no excuse for lack of asepsis in the case tuberculous wounds. The point has been too ten overlooked.

The orthopedic treatment I need not go into rther than to say that it is carefully carried out Dr. Charlton Wallace, under the supervision the Advisory Board.

The question you now ask is, ' What are the sults after carrying on this work for seven onths? I do not intend at this time to give u a detailed report of cases cured and imoved, nor do I intend to give you the gains in :ight. I only will tell you that the results are markable, the cases have, almost without exption, improved, though we have cared for ery variety of case, the far-advanced as well the incipient, the latter cases doing better than e advanced. One infant aged two years came us in June with, apparently, tuberculous perinitis, his parents refusing operation. He was scharged much improved the last of September. e was examined January 14, and was found be apparently in perfect health, the signs of iid in the abdomen having disappeared. Anher boy with hip disease and abscess has what ? have diagnosed as anyloid disease of liver and dneys. He has improved somewhat and we do t as yet despair of his recovery.

Now you may ask, what is the cost of this exriment? Naturally large. The total cost while the tent camp was $12,056.84, accommodating . children.

The daily per capita cost from June 6 to ptember 30, inclusive, including cost of conuction, equipment and repairs, was $2.44, exisive of equipment, construction and repairs, .13. Total number of children, 63; 4,926 ys.

The daily per capita cost for November at 5ea Breeze " was $1.45. There is no cost of nstruction or rent in this building, 35 children r a total of 915 days. The daily average per pita cost for December was $1.32 for 31 chilen for a total of 953 days. A large item expenditure during these two months was for

coal, which could be diminished, if coal could have been bought earlier and in bulk.

Does it Pay?—I think so, decidedly, even at a far greater financial outlay. If you could have seen the children in June and see them now, you would believe that almost any expense to demonstrate the improvement in those poor children was decidedly worth while.

For those of you who are interested in surgical tuberculosis I wish you would see the results for yourselves, for seeing is believing. Visit the wards of any hospital in the city and see the poor children suffering from various forms of external tuberculosis, then take the trouble to visit the children at Coney Island. You will be amply repaid for your trouble. I know of no other way for you to realize how good the results are. Ten of the children, discharged in October, reported for examination January 14. They had all maintained their good health and all but one kept or gained in weight.

I think that the Association has proven definitely that there is but one treatment of surgical tuberculosis, namely, constant fresh air, not neglecting orthopedic and conservative surgical treatment, and that the sea air is the best, we believe, though we cannot prove.

The time has come that some definite action should be taken for the establishment of a permanent seaside sanatorium for the treatment of the 3,000 to 5,000 poor children of this city afflicted with surgical tuberculosis. New York is foremost in the prevention and treatmest of pulmonary tuberculosis, and foremost because of a most efficient Board of Health. The Board of Health still hopes for a municipal sanatorium for consumptives, but is unable to obtain a suitable site owing to the Goodsell-Bedell bill. Sites, however, for a suitable sanatorium for surgical tuberculosis are available within the city limits. I hope that the day is not far off when we can have such a sanatorium for the city, preferably under municipal control.

I thank you for the honor you have done me in listening to my paper.

REFERENCES.

1 Bergeron. d'Espine's article. No. 4.
2 Cazin. d'Espine's article. No. 4.
3 d'Espine. d'Espine's article. No. 4.
4 d'Espine. Congres Internat. Med., Paris, 1900. Vol. V., p. 264 et seq.
5 Tubby. Rep. Soc. Study Dis. Children, London, 1902. Vol. 111, p. 263.
6 Whitman. Text-Book on Orthopedic Surgery, p. 256.
7 Knopf. Articles published in N. Y. Med. Jour., 1903, p. 108.
8 Burrell. Boston Med. Surg. Jour., Vol. 148, p. 692. Vol. 149, p. 1.
9 Brannan. Sixty-first Report New York Association for Improving the Condition of the Poor, p. 24.
10. Biggs. Sixty-first Report New York Association for Improving the Condition of the Poor, p. 27.
11 Petroff. Translation, Ann. de l'Institute Pasteur, 1904, XVIII, p. 502.
12 Gibney. Jour. Am. Med. Ass'n., 1904, p. 1276.

A Physician as a Deputy.—At the recent supplementary elections in Italy, Dr. Giovanni Battista Quierolo. professor of Clinical Medicine in the University of Pisa, obtained a seat in the Chamber of Deputies. Professor Quierolo is one of the leading physicians in Italy.

AURAL AFFECTIONS IN CHILDREN; NECESSITY FOR THEIR EARLY RECOGNITION BY THE FAMILY PRACTITIONER.[1]

BY HERMAN JARECKY, M.D.,

OF NEW YORK;

VISITING OTOLOGIST, HARLEM HOSPITAL; EYE, EAR AND THROAT SURGEON, SYDENHAM HOSPITAL; ASSISTANT SURGEON, MANHATTAN EYE AND EAR HOSPITAL, ETC.

CHILDREN and infants being susceptible to the exanthemata, intestinal disorders and various inflammatory disturbances, are naturally subject to the ear conditions which complicate and follow in the wake of these affections. The family practitioner is usually the first to be consulted, and a prompt recognition of an aural disturbance, admits of immediate treatment with relief to the patient, and a consequent freedom of subsequent embarrassment to the doctor.

In considering the subject generally, we might divide the whole into two types, the inflammatory and the non-inflammatory.

The inflammatory type consists of the ear conditions in those who complain, or where there is evidence of pain or of a persistent unaccountable fever. In this category belong all cases of exanthemata, intestinal and respiratory disturbances, in fact all febrile affections.

In the second class belong all those that are caused by pathological conditions in the nose, throat, and mouth. Thus are included nasal obstructions, as exostoses, foreign bodies, deviated septi and polypi; throat conditions as enlarged tonsils, adenoids, edema, abscesses and ulcerations and oral affections as dentition and decayed teeth. Here also belong neuralgias due perhaps to exposure, malaria, rheumatism, etc.

The family doctor being called to see a child or infant with any acute inflammatory trouble should not consider his examination complete without including the ears. This is usually, except in very young infants, easily accomplished. Any furuncle in the external canal is readily seen. To examine the middle ear a large sized speculum is generally the best, except, perhaps, when viewing the extreme upper part of the drum membrane, then a small one is very often preferable. The warmed instrument is inserted with a gentle rotatory movement, the auricle in older children is drawn backward, whereas in infants, it is drawn downward and one must look upward. This straightens the canal, which must be cleared of any discharge, epithelial flakes, cerumen, or vernix to obtain a distinct view. Sometimes the drum membrane may appear white from exfoliated epithelium or discharge. This can be easily discovered by wiping with a cotton-tipped applicator when the reddened membrane will appear.

There may exist two types of inflammation, either catarrhal or purulent. In the catarrhal variety the symptoms are milder usually. The membrane may be reddened with slight or marked degree of swelling, caused by the in-

flammatory exudate. Sometimes it is of a peculiar yellowish color through which the level of the exudation may be seen. The symptoms in the purulent variety are generally more marked. The upper part of the membrane becomes hyperemic, the congestion extending down along the malleus handle gradually the whole membrane becoming involved, edematous, swollen and all the landmarks obliterated. The pus occasionally burrows between the mucous membrane and the bone.

In the mild catarrhal variety the process may end and the inflammatory products may become absorbed. Not so, however, in the purulent variety. Here, unless paracentesis is performed, either the membrane ruptures spontaneously with a large enough opening to admit of drainage or else an extension of the process takes place.

From the anatomical structure of the child the pathological process may involve the meninges through the partially ossified sutures or from the prolongation of the dura mater which lines the upper part of the cavity. Thus the brain may be infected with abscess formation. Internally through the fenestra rotunda and ovale the labyrinth may become affected, causing partial or complete mutism. Below, through a thin plate of bone which is occasionally absent, the jugular bulb may become infected and pyemia ensue. Backward, the mastoid process and the lateral sinus may become the seat of purulent infection.

A discharging ear must be attended to, and always regarded as a menace to life and health. Mastoid involvement may be suspected if the discharge is excessive and does not improve under treatment, if a swelling appears back of the auricle, causing its projection, one beneath it along the sternocleidomastoid, a continued temperature, constant pain or continued tenderness over the bone. An irregular fever with systemic disturbance occasionally will denote an infection of the jugular bulb, or of the lateral sinus.

In all cases of earaches the membrane must be examined and if normal the nose and throat and nasopharynx should receive attention. Decayed teeth or dentition is a very common cause. Adenoids and enlarged tonsils frequently cause recurrent earaches.

Backward children should be examined to see if there is a loss of hearing power and the cause removed if possible. Foreign bodies are quite frequently found. If the case belongs to the class of nasal and throat troubles a retracted drum membrane will exist and the parents should be warned that if not attended to the condition will grow worse and may become permanent.

It is impossible in a short paper to consider the symptoms in the various kinds of cases, except in a general way. With middle ear involvement the patient may or may not complain of pain, be restless, put its fingers to its ears, bury its head in the pillow, or show an increase in temperature.

---

[1] Read at the Meeting of the Society of the Alumni of the City (Charity) Hospital, December, 1904.

Prompt paracentesis has cured what appear to be attacks of meningitis, pleurisy, pneumonia, typhoid, colitis, malaria and various other diseases. In the exanthemata, especially scarlet, where aural mischief is rapid and severe, repeated examinations should be made. Any unexpected or continued rise of temperature during a febrile disease, or any unusual restlessness should attract attention to the ears.

In looking over my records at the Sydenham Hospital Dispensary I find about 33 per cent. of the ear patients were children under fourteen years of age, half of whom were suffering from suppurative ear troubles. Of the adults 25 per cent. were suffering from ear trouble contracted during childhood from suppuration or the so-called chronic catarrhal condition, due to the neglect of the nose and throat in their early years.

Any swelling of the drum membrane, especially in its posterior part, calls for a paracentesis. It should not be allowed to rupture spontaneously as the opening may not be sufficient for drainage, and may have to be enlarged and also because a clean cut wound heals easily and prevents loss of hearing power.

In concluding, I wish to draw attention to the following:

1. That an early recognition of an ear affection may prevent pus formation which in children proceeds rapidly.

2. If pus has formed, the attention to it may prevent its toxic absorption.

3. Early paracentesis may prevent extension from the tympanum to the mastoid cells, brain, internal ear, and sinuses as well as the partial loss of audition.

4. Partially-deaf children should have the nose and throat examined and pathological conditions removed.

5. All cases of earache and discharging ears should be properly attended to.

6. In all inflammatory diseases children's ears should be repeatedly examined during the course of the disease.

115 West One Hundred and Twenty-first Street.

THE WIDAL TEST FOR PRACTISING PHYSICIANS.[1]

BY JOHN H. BORDEN, A.M., M.D.,

OF NEW YORK;

CLARK SCHOLAR AND ASSISTANT IN BACTERIOLOGY, COLLEGE OF PHYSICIANS AND SURGEONS, N. Y.; ASSISTANT ON PNEUMONIA COMMISSION.

SINCE the demonstration of the value of Widal's test as an aid in the diagnosis of typhoid fever, various modes of applying it have been in vogue. Dried blood has been used largely for clinical work. For scientific study, the separated serum which permits more accurate dilution, has been employed. Hanging drop preparations observed with a high power of the microscope have been as a rule a part of the clinical technic. Until recently no method which could be applied readily

1 Read before the meeting of the New York Pathological Society, October 12, 1904.

and safely by each physician to his own cases had been suggested, but within the past few years several attempts have been made to introduce a macroscopic Widal test. In each instance the advantages claimed have been: (1) Ease and simplicity of technic; (2) independence of the microscope; (3) the use of a permanent suspension of dead bacilli.

In April, 1902, Pröscher[1] described a new Widal technic. He used an emulsion or suspension of twenty-four-hours bouillon-grown bacilli killed with formalin. This he mixed with the diluted serum in little transparent dishes, set them in the incubator at 37° C., and at the end of an hour or two observed the result with a low

Fig. 1.

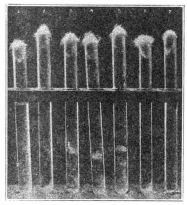

Different Stages of the Reaction.—Dilutions— Tube 1, $^1/_{200}$; 2, $^1/_{100}$; 3, $^1/_{70}$; 4, $^1/_{60}$; 5, $^1/_{40}$. These five tubes have stood at room temperature for five hours. Tube 6 represents a completed reaction. Tube 7, a control made with normal serum in a dilution of $^1/_{40}$. The control has stood twenty-four hours. Note the haziness as contrasted with the completed reaction. Photographed by Dr. A. J. Brown.

power of the microscope. The method is hardly adapted to use outside of a laboratory.

In 1903, Ficker,[2] of Darmstadt, published a notice of a typhus diagnosticum devised by him and possessing all the advantages of general availability suggested above. He failed to state how he prepared the suspension which was the essential feature of his method, but intimated that it involved a lengthy and complicated process and that it would not be wise for others to try to make a similar solution. Ficker gave no reports of cases in which his diagnosticum had been tried but said it had been used with success.

In August, 1904, Walter[3] reported a series of 22 cases tested with Ficker's diagnosticum. Of these, 15 caused agglutination in high dilution.

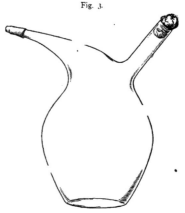

Of the 15, 12 were undoubted typhoids, 2 were probably typhoid, and 1, which reacted only in a dilution of 1:50, gave no other sign of typhoid fever. The remaining 7 non-typhoid cases did not react. All of the cases were tried at the same time by the usual microscopic method and grossly with a solution which Walter made with agar-grown cultures suspended in a mixture of salt solution, glycerin and carbolic acid. The results of the three methods coincided.

Ruediger,[4] in a recent number of the *Journal of Infectious Diseases,* reports a long series of gross reactions done with formalinized emulsions

Fig. 2.

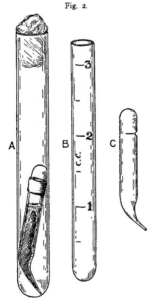

A—Small test tube containing the collecting bulb filled with blood. A convenient method of transporting. *B*—Graduated test tube for rapid dilution. *C*—Collecting bulb showing vent and file mark for breaking end.

and states that certain typhoid sera diluted 1/20,000 caused visible agglutination in 5 to 8 hours. This is perhaps possible, but after our experience with formalinized cultures it seems likely that owing to insufficient control work he was deceived by albumin precipitations.

Buxton[5] also has met with success while using cultures of bacilli killed with formalin.

Rolly[6] has worked to advantage with a solution in which the organisms are killed with formol or toluol. The preparation of Rolly's emulsion necessitates several weeks' time and much care.

Graman[7] and Kasarinow[8] have reported favorably on Ficker's diagnosticum.

Early last spring, in the Presbyterian Hospital laboratory, we began working with suspensions of typhoid bacilli which had been killed with formalin. With one particular stock of solution we met with marked success, testing a large series of cases of typhoid fever and thoroughly controlling the work with many different non-typhoid sera. All the typhoid cases agglutinated our formalinized emulsion and only two of over 100 different control sera caused apparent clumping within the three-hour time limit. One of these cases had certainly had typhoid fever, the other possibly. An approximate dilution of 1/100 was used in each case and if there was no clumping visible to the naked eye at the end of three hours the result was considered negative. The average day of reaction was the seventh to

Fig. 3.

Dropping bottle for sterile salt solution.

eighth day of the patient's sickness in bed. Many of the control tubes showed clumping on standing six to twelve hours.

We never made another formalin solution which abundant control work did not prove unreliable. We attributed this to the instability of the formalin and to the fact, pointed out by Gatrona[9], that this reagent in the presence of a very slight trace of acid constitutes one of our most delicate tests for albumin.

After several further unsuccessful attempts to compound a satisfactory suspension, we made one in the following manner:

A well-tried strain of typhoid bacilli is grown for twenty-four hours on slant agar in large tubes.

The bacilli are washed from the medium with a mixture of sterile salt solution, 450 parts, glycerin, 50 parts, 95 per cent. carbolic acid, 2.50

arts. Fifty c.c. of the solution are sufficient to ash one large agar tube.

This solution is at first cloudy, but after standig for one week becomes translucent and the acilli on being transplanted fail to grow. It is nen ready for use, and is permanent if kept in erile bottles in a moderately cool and dark place. he small percentage of carbolic acid, equal to /200, renders contamination difficult, and the lycerin by increasing the specific gravity serves) keep the bacilli in suspension. The stock bote should be shaken occasionally.

With such a suspension and five others preared in the same way, 30 cases of typhoid fever id 27 controls were tested. Of the 30 cases, 29 zglutinated in an accurate dilution of 1/100. he one case which failed to clump died in the :cond week after his blood had been twice tested. one of the controls reacted with the serum dited only 1/40. The controls included 3 cases of ephritis, 2 of malaria, 1 of appendicitis, 2 of iberculosis, 1 of abscess of the liver, 1 of chole-thiasis—both with jaundice—and several surgi-il cases. The reaction if positive occurred ithin twenty hours. Six controls stood for eight ays without apparent change of any sort, and iany others from forty-eight to seventy-two

may be carried any distance. The point is sealed by the drying of the blood in it.

2. From a modified Shuster dropping-bottle with a very small lumen in the spout, a small graduated test tube is filled to the 1 c.c. mark with sterile salt solution. The large end is broken from the bulb at the file mark and with a capillary tube drawn to a long point and gradu-ated in one-hundredths of a c.c., enough serum is diawn up to make with the salt solution the dilu-tion required. The pipette with the contained serum is then inserted into the test tube and thor-oughly washed out with the salt solution.

3. From another dropper enough of the ty-phoid suspension is added to bring the fluid in the test tube to the 2 c.c. mark. The mouth of the tube is then stopped with a plug of non-absorb-ent cotton, inverted once or twice and set aside in a dark place.

Within one-half hour to twenty hours, if the reaction is positive, depending upon the dilution of the serum used and its agglutinating power, a marked granularity of the fluid in the tube will be noted. Following this there will be seen dis-tinct clumps beginning to sink toward the bottom, and at the conclusion of the reaction, the fluid above will be limpid and free from clumps and

Fig. 4.

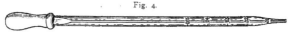

Graduated pipette.

ours. The average day when the reaction was btained first was the patient's seventh day in bed. our reacted on the second day in bed, 1 on the iird, and 1 on the fourth. Twenty-five cases ere positive on the first examination,—the irliest possible on admission. The different so-itions were uniform in their susceptibility to zglutination except that one made with bacilli rown for eight days was much slower in react-g than the others. Coincident examinations sing Ficker's diagnosticum and the microscopic ethod gave similar résults. Ficker's suspen-on was slower and less delicate, doubtless be-iuse his diagnosticum is less dense. At the ex-ration of three months' use the solution reacted i well as on the first day. Our technic has been ie following: All tubes and pipettes are cleaned :fore using with water, alcohol and ether.

1. The blood is collected in bulbs with a small :nt-hole at one end and drawn to a capillary be at the other. (Fig. 1 C.) It is only :cessary to prick the ear rather briskly with a agedorn needle and keep the tip of the bulb to e exuding drop. Milking (not squeezing) the be of the ear will facilitate the flow of blood. /hen the bulb is two-thirds full, it is held for one inute in a slanting manner and laid aside for one two hours. At the end of this time about 0.2 c. of serum will have separated. By covering e vent-hole with a broad elastic band the bulb

the point of the test tube will contain a small, white, flocculent, mass of agglutinated bacilli.

In conclusion:

1. The method is to be adapted to use by the practising physician because its technic is simple and free from danger, and because the reading of the reaction is absolute. It is either positive or negative. For the diagnosis laboratory it seems specially fitted because requiring so little time for its application.

2. It is possible that a similar suspension of appropriate bacteria may be used in the diagnosis of diseases other than typhoid fever.

3. The methods of collection and dilution here suggested are thought to be simpler and more rapid than those heretofore employed.

Finally, I wish to thank Dr. T. Hastings for valuable suggesions, and Miss Selma Granat, of the Prebyterian Hospital laboratory, for material aid in preparing the suspensions.

BIBLIOGRAPHY.

1. Prüscher. Zur Ausstellung der Widalischen Reaction, Zen. tralblatt f. Bakt., No. 31, 1902.
2. Ficker. Ueber ein Typhus-Diagnosticum. Berl. klin. Woch., No. 45, 1903.
3. Walter. Zur Diagnose. Deut. med. Woch., August, 1904.
4. Ruediger. Journal of Infectious Diseases, Vol. I, No. 2, 1904, p. 236.
5. Buxton On Agglutination, Journal of Medical Research, July, 1904.
6. Rolly. Zur Diagnose des Typhus abdominalis, Münch. med. Woch., 1903, No. 45.
7. Gramann. Zur Serodiagnose des Typhus abdomin. Mittels des Fickerschen Diagnosticum, Deut. med. Woch., No. 22, 1904.
8. Kasarinow, Russk. Wratsch, 1903, No. 52.
9. Gatrona, Gatrona Test for Albumin, La Riforma Med., 1903.

THE TECHNIC OF PERINEAL PROSTATECTOMY.[1]

BY GEORGE RYERSON FOWLER, M.D.,

OF BROOKLYN, N. Y.

HOWEVER well founded the claim that the suprapubic or intravesical route is the one of choice in prostatectomy, it must be acknowledged by the most ardent advocates of this method that there are cases to which the perineal route is best suited. In fact, no hard and fast rule can be laid down in this respect, but it is the belief of the writer that the great majority of cases of hypertrophy of the prostate can be most easily reached and safely dealt with by the natural route of the perineum. Without entering into an elaborate argument upon this phase of the subject at this time, it will suffice to call attention to the following:

1. Intravesical enucleation will almost necessarily demand total enucleation. A conservative operation designed to spare the ejaculatory ducts in younger subjects is scarcely possible by the suprapubic route. This is the more important since there is a growing belief among progressive surgeons that the best results will be ultimately obtained by instituting operative interference earlier in the case than in the past, in which case a preservation of the sexual function will present a far more important phase of the subject than at the present time, when either the patient's age is such as to relegate this consideration to a position of secondary importance, or his sufferings so great as to impel him to sacrifice this, as well as everything else, in the effort to obtain relief. In the perineal operation, on the other hand, either an enucleation, or a resection of the lateral lobes with preservation of the parts adjacent to the urethra together with the ejaculatory ducts is possible.

2. The perineal is the natural route, both anatomically and physiologically. The prostate is not an intravesical organ in any sense, and both freedom from urinary extravasation and infection, as well as drainage, are best accomplished by this route. In the case of the suprapubic intravesical operation the ease with which the capsule is entered depends upon a problematical thinning of this structure at the points of union of the lateral lobes above and below the urethra. On the other hand, the capsule can be entered anywhere by the perineal route, and the " shelling out " process carried on from the direction which proves the easiest of accomplishment.

3. It is possible to perform a relatively complete prostatectomy by the perineal route without entering the urethra. A simple tampon of gauze in the wound will enable the patient to sit upright in from twenty-four to forty-eight hours following the operation, a most important point in the after treatment, particularly in the more elderly patients. Even in cases in which the urethra is opened this course may be followed in selected cases. At the most the presence of a drainage

tube for forty-eight hours will suffice. Further, with traction properly applied, it will not be necessary to make pressure from the rectum in perineal prostatectomy, as is frequently the case when the suprapubic method is employed. The gain from the aseptic point of view in the case of the latter is worthy of note.

4. The fears of infection of the deeper pelvic planes is an ever present one when the suprapubic method is employed. While it is true that a skillful operator may in time acquire the dexterity of a Freyer, and enucleate the prostate in a comparatively large number of cases without tearing through the prostatic capsule proper other than at the points mentioned (vide infra), yet it is more than likely that many lives will be sacrificed before this manipulative skill can be acquired by any considerable number of operators. On the other hand, while it is extremely desirable that the enucleation should be carried out without lesion of the capsule other than the opening made for the introduction of the finger, if this does occur no harm will result other than moderate bleeding from the prostatic plexuses lying between the fibrous sheath derived from the pelvic fascia and the true capsule of the organ.

The steps of the operation include the following: The patient is placed in the exaggerated lithotomy position, or a combination of the usual lithotomy position and the elevated pelvis position of Trendelenburg. Either a general anesthetic or spinal analgesia may be employed. M. B. Tinker employs local eucaine or cocaine anesthesia by infiltration and intraneural injections at the ischial tuberosity, anesthetizing the internal pudic and long pudendal nerves. The bladder is irrigated beforehand, and, if resection or partial prostatectomy is to be attempted, the largest possible soft-rubber catheter introduced and left in situ. If enucleation is intended a lithotomy staff is introduced. The incision is carried from the root of the scrotum to the external sphincter of the anus. If the prostate is deeply placed the additional branching incisions passing in the direction of the tuber ischii, constituting the ⅄ (inverted Y) incision of Young, are made. If enucleation is to be performed the urethra is to be opened upon the staff. If resection is to be performed the opening of the urethra is to be omitted and accidental injury of this structure avoided. In enucleation the prostatic capsule is incised transversely at the point where this lies adjacent to the membranous urethra, and the finger entered at this point for shelling out both lobes. In resection the perineal fascia is split and the posterior part of the gland exposed by blunt dissection. The wound edges are well retracted and the capsule incised at a distance of six millimeters from the median line upon either side, in order to preserve the ejaculatory ducts, and at the same time guard against injury of the urethra.

In enucleation, once the capsule is entered the

1 Read before the Medical Society of the State of New York, February 1, 1905.

ass is slowly worked loose by the finger tip. The latter readily recognizes the feel of the capule, and the process of intracapsular enucleation is somewhat comparable to turning an orange ut of its enveloping rind. In resection the sepration of the capsule is stopped at the proper istance from the urethra and a long clamping orceps applied to the mass parallel with the later; the loosened portion is then resected (Rydyier). This is repeated on the other side. The leeding from the divided prostatic mass is slight. In the operation as thus outlined it will be noced that no reference is made to methods of aking traction upon the organ to aid the enuleation or resection. I do not believe that any ppliance employed to make traction from within he bladder is necessary, and that certain of these ay be responsible for the paralysis of the vesical phincter so frequently observed. It is my own ractice to grasp the corresponding lobe through he opening in the capsule as soon as sufficient as been exposed for the purpose by means of a ouble tenaculum forceps. Once this has been one the control of the situation is absolutely in he hands of the operator.

The after-treatment of perineal prostatectomy is simple. Tamponade of the wound without refrence to any injury of the urethra, avoiding the se of a perineal drainage tube entirely; the reservation of cleanliness by frequent changes of he soiled dressings and irrigation of the wound urfaces; and, most important of all, getting the atient out of bed and sitting up at the earliest ossible moment, embrace, in the main, the inications. If a drainage tube is employed it hould be removed not later than forty-eight ours.

UPERFICIAL INGUINAL HERNIA, WITH REPORT OF A CASE.[1]

BY ALBERT E. SELLENINGS, M.D..

OF NEW YORK;

SSISTANT ATTENDING SURGEON TO GOUVERNEUR HOSPITAL; ASSISTANT DEMONSTRATOR OF ANATOMY, IN UNIVERSITY AND BELLEVUE HOSPITAL MEDICAL COLLEGE.

So MUCH has been written concerning hernia at it would seem the subject had been exausted, and had become devoid of any attracons. But the more unusual forms always exite interest and certainly merit a description, specially if, as in this instance one more case of uperficial inguinal hernia is added to the comaratively small number reported. Undoubtedly ore cases have been observed than one would e led to believe from the number one finds reorded in literature. For this reason it would be naccurate to base a percentage of occurrence n the cases we find described and reported.

In a paper published in the *Annals of Surgery* June, 1903), Coley records 937 cases of inguinal ernia, and of this number five cases are menoned of the superficial inguinal variety. No ndividual operator with the exception of Mac-

ready, reports as many as does Coley, who, as stated, reports five. Erdmann, in his article on Strangulated Hernia,[1] reports three cases. If we take Coley's statistics we arrive at a frequency of occurrence as represented by one to about 187. This proportion based on the experience of a single operator will not, however, stand the test of accuracy, and will not represent the true relative frequency, as can be readily understood.

Superficial inguinal hernia was first described by Küster in 1887, and in his first communication he describes three cases. The reported cases as far as I am able to find them are to be credited as follows: Küster 3, Hulke 1, Moynihan 1, Macready 6, Wahl 1, Goebell 1, Moschcowitz 1, Fano 1, Curling 1, Erdmann 3, Coley 5, and Warren 1. The case of Warren is included in a recent article on " Undescended Testicle," by Odiorne and Simmons.[2] Moschcowitz, in an article published in the *Medical Record* of January 10, 1903, adds to his series another case. He credits it to Salzman, who found the condition on autopsy. Thus we find including the Salzman case a total of 26 cases, not including the case herein reported. To Moschcowitz is credited the collection of 17 cases, to which number are to be added those of Coley, Erdmann, Warren and the one of the author. The total number of cases then is 27.

This hernia may be considered as a congenital variety, not in the sense, necessarily that it exists from birth, but that the conditions leading to its production are most favorable. In other words, the cavity of the tunica vaginalis remains patent and communicates with the general peritoneal cavity. With this non-closure of the vaginal process and the testicle lying in an abnormal position it is readily understood how a hernia may protrude into the open and receptive pouch.

Macready, in his Treatise on Ruptures, classifies superficial inguinal hernia among the interstitial herniæ. and gives the following variations as regards these: (1) The viscera may be placed between the parietal peritoneum and the fascia lining the abdominal muscles; (2) between the internal and external oblique muscles; (3) on the surface of the external oblique, between it and the skin. The relations in superficial inguinal hernia are as given in the third variety. The essential features of this type then, are a condition in which the hernia and testicle lie directly upon the aponeurosis of the external oblique and having a covering of only skin and superficial fascia. The infundibuliform fascia and the cremaster muscle are but little developed, which facts, perhaps. are in keeping with the etiology of the condition. A reference will be made to this point later on.

Eccles is authority for the statement that interstitial herniæ may be associated with imperfect

---

1 Read before The Society of Alumni of Bellevue Hospital, ew York, February 1, 1905.

1 Medical Record, March 12, 1904.
2 Annals of Surgery, December, 1904.

or abnormal descent of the testicle. On the other hand they may be found in males whose testicles have descended into the scrotum. Further, interstitial herniæ occur in females in a greater proportion than in males. The proportion, according to Langton's statistics is as two to one. In 129 cases of interstitial hernia, observed during a period of twenty-four years, Macready found that some abnormality of the testes existed in $73^4/_{10}$ per cent., and in $67^1/_{10}$ per cent. the testis was completely retained or had only partially descended. What proportion of superficial inguinal hernia is associated with imperfect descent of the testis I am unable to state accurately, but I think it may be safely said that nearly all cases have some degree of cryptorchism.

There are at least five varieties of inguinal hernia associated with imperfect descent of the testicle—bubonocele, scrotal, interstitial, cruroscrotal, and superficial perineal (Eccles). Of all the conditions found associated with imperfect descent of the testicle, hernia is the most frequent complication. Perhaps 50 per cent. of the cases are thus complicated. Of the varieties as given above, bubonocele is the most frequent form of hernia that is encountered, and it is the form which would naturally be expected, for it is but an earlier stage of several other varieties.

In trying to discover a possible explanation of this condition, a great number of theories has been expressed by various authorities, and this very fact of divers opinion, shows that as yet, none has been satisfactory or really meets the conditions. Sufficient it is, to state in the scope of this paper, that more than likely an abnormal development of the scrotal portion of the gubernaculum has something to do with its production and must be considered a factor in the genesis. By reason of this deficiency or insufficiency of the gubernaculum the protruding mass escaping through the external ring and finding its way into the scrotum blocked, goes in the plane of least resistance, or in other words, dissects between the skin and the aponeurosis of the external oblique. In addition we must take into consideration that in many instances of interstitial hernia there is to be found an abnormal development or certain retrograde changes in the structures forming the abdominal parietes. The fact that interstitial hernia occurs so frequently in females who have borne a number of children and in whom the musculature has become deficient and flabby, attaches special importance to this point. In males, then, given a tardy development in the muscular structures of the abdomen and a non-descent of the testis complicating, superficial inguinal hernia has at least a partial solution.

As to the proper procedure with imperfectly descended testicle complicating hernia, again there is a diversity of opinion. The remarks on this point are confined to adult cases. It is generally held that an abnormally placed testicle

has no function, at least as far as the production of spermatozoa is concerned. Some there are who believe in the internal secretion of even an atrophied testicle and for that reason never remove it. Reports of single cases in which the testicles has been transplanted to a scrotal bed are to be found, and the results are seemingly satisfactory. On the other hand, more cases abound in which the testicle much atrophied has retracted after a time, to a position high in the scrotum, just outside of the external ring and even into the canal itself. In a review of these unfavorable cases, pain is a most predominant symptom. Some authorities are firm in the belief that if for any reason orchidopexy cannot be performed, as for example, by reason of a short cord, then the proper procedure is to replace the testicle into the abdominal cavity. This has the objection that the testicle may again find its way into the canal, with a recurrence of original conditions. Again, there are cases in which testicles placed in the scrotum by operative measures, have gone on to full development. Others again consider orchidectomy the proper procedure. In view of these conflicting observations, it is clear that no one plan can be formulated to apply to the treatment of all cases. In every case, peculiar and distinctive conditions obtain and operative measures must be employed as best suit the occasion. In cases of radical procedure on one side, there is the satisfaction of knowing that a single properly descended testicle of normal development will carry on the bodily functions. Given a much atrophied testicle, with a shortened cord, firmly adherent to the sac, there is to my mind, but one treatment—orchidectomy. Further, it is to be remembered, that an undescended testicle after the age of puberty, atrophies more and more, is a constant source of pain and is liable to undergo inflammation and malignant change.

To Dr. Ladinski I am indebted for the privilege of reporting this case. During his service at Gouverneur Hospital the patient was admitted and referred to me for operation:

Case.—S. M., twenty-seven years of age, was admitted to Gouverneur Hospital on the evening of September 20, 1904. He is married and the father of several children. Right scrotum has always been empty. Three months ago patient began to be troubled with a " rupture " on right side. This " rupture " has been getting larger, but never had caused any great amount of trouble. It was always reducible. The undescended testicle at times caused inconvenience. At 4 P.M. on the date of admission, after some heavy lifting, the tumor suddenly became larger and he was unable to return it as before. The tumor increased in size, became more and more painful, and he began to vomit. At this time he was brought to the hospital. The case was reported to me as a strangulated femoral hernia. The description of the House Surgeon was that a tumor about the size of a large fist occupies the region of the right external ring, somewhat above the usual location of an inguinal hernia and extends downward on the thigh to a point corresponding to the saphenous opening. The tumor is dense and the overlying tissues are very thin and somewhat movable. He gives the signs of strangulation. His temperature is 97° F. and pulse eighty. An examination some thirty minutes later revealed a tumor as reported, and the man presenting signs of strangulation. The tumor extends in part below Poupart's ligament, but upward pressure shows the femoral canal free, and the protrusion really comes from above the ligament. The right scrotal sac is empty. An incision four inches in length above and parallel to Poupart's ligament was made. Skin and superficial fascia having been passed through, the tumor presented itself as lying above the external ring and resting directly upon the aponeurosis of the external oblique. Inspection revealed that it was composed of intestine and a small almond-sized structure which upon later examination proved to be the testicle. The diverging pillars of the external oblique tightly encompassed the whole protrusion. The external oblique aponeurosis was the slit and the inguinal canal seemed entirely obliterated, that is, the internal and external rings were almost in a straight anteroposterior axis. The sac being opened the hernia revealed itself to be of the congenital variety. The point of stricture was found to be at about the site of what should be the internal ring and was due to a narrowing of the lumen of the peritoneal sac. The stricture was divided and the gut which showed signs of gangrene was treated with hot saline applications, and after about ten minutes, was deemed viable and was returned. Great difficulty was experienced in the attempt to separate the sac from the attenuated cord and atrophied testicle, and they were therefore sacrificed. The sac was ligated and returned to the abdomen. The steps of a Bassini operation were followed with the exception that there was no cord to deal with. The patient reacted well from the operation and made an uneventful recovery, being discharged on the twenty-first day.

The special point of interest attaching to this case, aside from its being of the rare superficial inguinal type, is the fact that on first examination it had all the aspects of a femoral hernia. The first diagnosis as reported to me, it may be inferred, was made without the careful examination which should always be made of a large hernia in the inguinocrural region. The ability to displace the mass above or below Poupart's ligament will establish the diagnosis as either inguinal or femoral hernia as the case may be. Macready moreover, has this to say regarding interstitial hernia: "The ventral swelling of interstitial hernia is not always confined to the area of the abdomen. When it becomes prominent it may fall over the thigh and simulate femoral hernia."

As to the diagnosis of the conditon of superficial inguinal hernia, it is believed that it can be but speculative and not positive. This is to be said, however, that perhaps additional stress can be put on the possibility of the existence of such a hernia when there is a mal-position of the testicle complicating.

102 East Thirty-first Street.

REFERENCES.

Coley. Annals of Surgery, June, 1903.
Moschcowitz. New York Medical Record, January 10, 1903.
Eccles. London Lancet, March, 1902.
Erdmann. New York Medical Record, March 12, 1904.
Macready. "Treatise on Ruptures."
Kuester. Archiv für klinische Chirugie, Band XXXIV, page 202.
Odiorne-Simmons. Annals of Surgery, December, 1904.
Langton. London Lancet, December, 1900.

THE IMPORTANCE OF THE PHYSICAL EXAMINATION OF THE BACK IN GENERAL DIAGNOSIS.

BY JOHN P. ARNOLD, M.D.,
OF PHILADELPHIA.

IN the physical examination of patients one very important part of the body is almost entirely neglected, and in general diagnosis this neglected part of the body is one of the most important to be examined, namely: the back.

In every case of disease, whether acute or chronic, marked indications will be found by a careful examination of the spine in the region supplied by the posterior primary divisions of the spinal nerves corresponding to those segments of the spinal cord from which the affected parts derive their innervation. No part of the body can be functionally or structurally diseased without there being a disturbance either primarily or secondarily in those segments of the cord from which the part receives its nerve supply, and these diseased conditions invariably express themselves by indications which can be readily detected along the spinal column by a careful examination.

The question will be immediately asked by the readers of this paper as to what physical signs may be elicited which indicate these conditions? In the first place I may state that there are so few people in perfect health that it is seldom that one sees a perfectly symmetrical back. There are few people who are not compelled at some time during their lives to seek the advice of a physician, and in all of those cases in which the individual struggles through life with some crippled organ there will be found expressions of distinct impairment of the nervous mechanism of the parts involved which are invariably indicated by a careful examination of the back. In all of the cases of chronic disease which have come under my observation there have been disturbances of the nervous mechanism of the disordered part, usually dependent upon a deficient tonus of its blood vessels which is the result of a deficient blood supply to the segments of the spinal cord from which the vasomotor nerves arise.

If the back of a perfectly healthy individual is examined it will be found that, with the body placed in an upright, sitting posture, with the hands placed symmetrically upon the knees, the spinous processes will present a vertical line without deviation. There will be no indications of prominent or depressed spinous processes aside from those normally found in the two anterior and two posterior curves in the spinal column. There will be no tendency to an abnormal separation of spinous processes due to relaxed ligaments or disturbances of the erector spinæ group of muscles, and the normal back will be found to be symmetrical if we make due allowance for the rather greater development of the musculature on the right side of the body, especially of the arm and shoulder.

If the patient is then placed in a recumbent position on the right side, with the head slightly elevated, there will be found in the normal individual a smooth, well developed group of muscles along the left side of the spinous processes all along the vertebral column, and there should be an absolute absence of tenderness or contracted bundles of muscle fibres which roll under the palpating finger, and vary in size from that of the diameter of a knitting needle to the thickness of the thumb. The same should be found along the right side of the vertebral column when the patient is placed upon the left side. The palpating hand should be placed upon the side of the spinous processes toward the physician when he stands facing the patient. The object of placing the patient in the lateral recumbent position, with the head slightly elevated, is to relax the muscles of the part examined.

After the thorough examination of both sides of the back the patient should be placed in a dorsal position, with the head upon a level with the trunk, and an examination made of the muscles of the neck, which, as those of the spine, should be in a normal individual perfectly elastic, smooth to the touch and painless upon moderate pressure.

These remarks apply, of course, to a perfectly normal, healthy person. As has been said before, these conditions are rare, and those who come to seek the physician's aid come because they have some complaint. It will, therefore, be found in these cases that the examination of the back and neck will reveal conditions very different from those found in the normal, healthy person.

A very common class of cases which come under the doctor's observation are constipation and disturbances of the digestive apparatus. Many of these cases, of course, are due to excessive or injudicious eating, lack of exercise, bad habits, etc., but in all cases of disturbances of functions of the stomach indications will be found by an examination of the back between the fourth and tenth dorsal segments of the spinal cord; and in cases of chronic constipation, accompanied as they are most frequently by disturbances of the functions of the stomach, additional indications will be found in the lower dorsal, lumbar and sometimes in the sacral regions of the cord. This class of cases is simply quoted as an example of

what may be found in an examination of the back, and is applicable to all of the diseases, acute or chronic, which come under the observation of the physician, varying only in the localization along the vertebral column which corresponds to the disturbed part. These indications are marked by slight lateral deviations of the spinous processes, atrophied erector spinæ muscles, irregularly contracted bundles of muscle fibre, which are nearly always tender to the touch when rolled under the palpating finger, and relaxed interspinous ligaments indicated by prominence or depression of one or more spinous processes. As these indications are always found in the region of the posterior primary divisions of the spinal nerves which arise from the segment of the cord which supply the organ or part affected, it seems logical to assume that they are indications of disturbances of the functional activity of those segments, and this assumption is borne out by our more recent knowledge of the functions of the spinal cord.

It is very difficult in a brief paper to elucidate this subject clearly and I would advise that each reader thereof in caring for his patients carefully examine the spine, when he will be able to satisfy himself that these statements are borne out by experience, and that a careful examination of the back will very often enable the physician to determine the existing conditions in the patient's body with little reference to what the patient may have to say in the way of a description of symptoms, etc.

With an intelligent class of patients the physician will have no difficulty in persuading them to allow him to make the proper physical examination, and they will often be grateful for the care that he has taken in investigating their cases.

In the examination of male patients it is seldom necessary to have the patient do more than remove the coat, vest and collar, as the condition can readily be palpated through the other clothing.

In female patients, of course, no satisfactory examination can be made without the removal of the corset, and in dealing with these patients it has been the author's habit to have the patient, after the removal of the corset, put on a light dressing saque or kimona, when the examination can be satisfactorily made. Of course, where possible, direct inspection of the bared back should be made.

I believe that if the readers of this paper will make an earnest endeavor to investigate this matter for themselves they will find much of interest and profit, and will be in a position more rationally to treat their patients.

As it is somewhat difficult to find in the ordinary text-books the data essential to the location in the spinal cord of the nervous mechanisms of different parts of the body, I have appended hereto a brief description of the nervous mechanisms of the different parts of the body and the segments of the cord from which they arise.

It must be borne in mind that the segments of the cord physiologically considered are thirty-one in number and correspond to the thirty-one pairs of spinal nerves and not to the vertebræ. Further, the indications to be found on examination correspond to the exit of the spinal nerve and not to the location of the segment of the cord in the spinal canal. For example, the sacral segments of the cord are located about the second or third lumbar vertebræ, but the indications are found over the sacrum at the exit of the nerve or in the muscles supplied by it.

All of the functions of the body are regulated by a mechanism consisting of an orderly arrangement of neural cells with their prolongations—the neuraxones, and dendrons with their branches the dendrites—so that messages are sent into the nervous system by the dendrons and dendrites, and messages are sent out from the central nervous system by the neuraxones: messages which regulate the functional activity of the various parts of the body and which change in response to alterations in external conditions surrounding the organism.

In the interpretation of this article it should be borne in mind in contradistinction to the ordinary anatomical consideration, that dendrites and dendrons are used exclusively in reference to those processes which carry messages to the neural cell body, while the term neuraxone is used exclusively to those processes which carry messages away from the cell body.

One of the most important parts of the nervous system, and the one upon which the functional activity of all of the cells of the body depends, is the circulatory system, which includes the circulation of the blood and lymph. The mechanism which controls the contraction and dilatation of the blood and lymph vessels is called the vasomotor mechanism. It consists of dendrons arising in all parts of the body which go to neural cells in the central nervous system, and neuraxones from cell bodies in the central nervous system which go to muscle cells of the vascular apparatus by which the supply of nourishment and oxygen to every part is controlled and the waste products removed. As typical of the general arrangement of this nervous mechanism that which supplies the blood vessels may be referred to. In this we have to consider two sets of ingoing paths and two sets of outgoing paths. In the medulla oblongata, in the floor of the fourth ventricle, there is a collection of neural cell bodies arranged in two groups. One group, which has the control of vaso constriction, and the other which controls arterial dilatation. The first is called the vasoconstrictor nucleus and the second the vasodilator nucleus. These two nuclei taken together are called the vasomotor nucleus.

The neuraxones of these nuclei pass downward through the spinal cord probably chiefly through the anterolateral descending tracts and come into contact with neural cells in the anterior horns of the spinal cord. One neuraxone, by means of

collaterals, may come into contact with neural cells in a number of segments of the cord. The vasomotor cells in the cord send their neuraxones through the anterior roots of the spinal nerves. They leave the spinal nerve a short distance beyond the junction of the anterior and posterior roots and pass through the rami communicantes to one of the ganglia of the sympathetic system of nerves, and have been named by Langley the "preganglionic paths." In the ganglion the preganglionic paths end in contact with one or more neural cells whose neuraxones, as "postganglionic paths," are distributed to the muscle cells of the blood vessels.

The neuraxones from the constrictor nucleus to the muscle cells of the blood vessels are in a constant state of functional activity keeping up a partial constriction of the muscle cells of the blood vessel walls and thus preserve arterial tone, which is necessary for the proper distribution of the blood.

Postganglionic paths of both constrictor and dilator neural cells are, as a rule, found together except in the case of certain of those supplying the blood vessels of the head and those supplying the blood vessels of the abdominal and pelvic viscera and the external organs of generation. The postganglionic paths of neural cells supplying the blood vessels of the skin, the muscles of the leg, trunk and arms follow the paths of distribution of the spinal nerves, reaching the spinal nerves through the rami communicantes between the sympathetic and spinal nerves. Those which supply the blood vessels of the muscles follow the distribution of the musculomotor nerves, and those supplying the blood vessels of the skin through the paths of distribution of the sensory nerves.

Practically all of the vasoconstrictor neural cells, so far as we know, are found between the second dorsal and the second or third lumbar segments of the cord. Those for the brain, face, scalp, eye, ear, mucus membrane of the nose, mouth, pharynx, tonsils, larynx and salivary glands are found in the second, third and fourth dorsal segments of the cord. All vasoconstrictor neural cells for the esophagus and stomach are found in the fourth to the ninth dorsal segments. Those for the small intestines from the sixth dorsal to the second lumbar. Those for the liver from the sixth dorsal to the first lumbar, but chiefly in the tenth, eleventh and twelfth dorsal The vasoconstrictor neural cells for the pancreas, spleen and suprarenals in the eighth to the twelfth dorsal, although some are found in segments above the eighth though less numerous in these regions. The vasoconstrictor cells for the large intestines are found from the eleventh dorsal to the second lumbar. Those for the bladder, the external organs of generation, the uterus, Fallopian tubes, ovaries, testicles and prostate gland are located chiefly from the eleventh dorsal to the second lumbar segments, but it is probable that occasionally they may be found in the third and fourth lumbar segments. Those for the external organs of generation and the skin of the anogenital region in the second and third lumbar segments.

The vasodilator neural cells, with the exception of those supplying the blood vessels of the skin and muscles of the trunk, are found chiefly in the nuclei of the cranial nerves and in the sacral segments of the cord, those for the skin and muscles of the trunk being found throughout those segments of the cord which supply these regions. The vasodilator neural cells for the blood vessels of the eye are found chiefly in the nucleus of the third cranial nerve, probably also to some extent in the nuclei of the third and sixth. Those for the face and scalp are in the nuclei of the seventh and ninth cranial nerves; those for the mucous membrane of the nose, the hard palate, the soft palate, the mucous membrane of the upper lip and upper gums in the nucleus of the seventh. Those for the floor of the mouth, the lower lip, the mucous membrane of the cheeks, the lower gums and the tongue in the nucleus of the ninth cranial nerve. Those for the parotid glands in the nucleus of the ninth, and for the submaxillary and sublingual glands in the nucleus of the seventh. Both vasoconstrictor and dilator cells for the bronchial arteries (supplying nourishment to bronchi and lungs) are probably located in the third to seventh dorsal segments of the cord. The vasodilator neural cells for the stomach and small intestines, the liver, pancreas, suprarenals, spleen and probably the first half of the large intestine are found in the nucleus of the tenth. The vasodilator neural cells for the Fallopian tubes, uterus, ovaries, testicles are found chiefly in the third, fourth and fifth sacral segments of the cord. For the bladder, external organs of generation and the skin of the anogenital region in the third and fourth sacral segments.

The neural cells, both constrictor and dilator, for the blood vessels of the spinal cord and its membranes are probably found throughout the entire length of the cord, and they send their preganglionic paths to the coresponding vertebral ganglion, from whence postganglionic paths pass to the corresponding spinal nerve to be distributed to the blood vessels of the cord and its membranes.

In addition to the importance of a knowledge of the location in the cord of vasomotor neurons it is important to know the location of the visceromotor neurons which control the involuntary muscles aside from those of the vascular walls.

The visceromotor cells for the iris and ciliary muscles are located as follows: Those which bring about a constriction of the pupil, in the nucleus of the third cranial nerve. The dilator cells for the pupil are found chiefly between the sixth cervical and first or second dorsal. The visceromotor mechanism for the bronchi and bronchioles are found of the constrictor type only so far as we know in the nucleus of the tenth cranial nerve, and it is probable that there may be

an opposing group of cells in the spinal cord between the third and seventh dorsal segments for the reason that the proper manual treatment in this region of the spinal cord is of great value in relaxing the bronchial spasm in asthmatic conditions. The heart also has a double visceromotor mechanism which consists of an accelerating set of neurons found chiefly from the sixth cervical to the first or second dorsal segments of the spinal cord. The inhibitory neural cells for the heart are located in the nuclei of the tenth and eleventh cranial nerves and send their paths to the heart through the tenth nerve.

The entire alimentary canal is also provided with a double mechanism consisting of those neurons which accelerate peristaltic movement and those which inhibit peristaltic movement. The accelerating cells for the esophagus, stomach, small intestines and probably the ascending portion of the large intestines are found chiefly in the nucleus of the tenth cranial nerve, possibly also to some extent in the eleventh. Their paths are also distributed through the tenth. The inhibitory neural cells for the parts just named are found chiefly in the spinal cord in segments which correspond to the vasoconstrictor neural cells which supply them. (It is also probable that some inhibitory paths exist in the tenth cranial nerve, and some accelerators in the cord.)

The neural cells which bring about inhibition of the muscular coat of the fallopian tubes and uterus, with contraction of the cervix, the vagina and perineum, are located chiefly in the second, third and fourth lumbar segments, while those that bring about a constriction of the Fallopian tubes, the muscular coat of the uterus, accompanied by dilatation of the cervix, vagina and perineum, are found in the second, third and fourth sacral segments, the paths to the perineum and the vagina passing by way of the internal pudic nerve. Neural cells which bring about inhibition of the muscular coat of the bladder, accompanied by contraction of the sphincter of the bladder, are found in the second, third and fourth lumbar segments; while those that bring about contraction of the muscular coat of the bladder accompanied by a relaxation of the sphincter, are found in the second, third and fourth sacral segments.

The mechanism of the rectum and its internal sphincter are of similar character to those of the bladder, and occupy practically corresponding segments of the cord, while the neural cells for the external sphincter are probably in the last sacral and to some extent in the coccygeal segments.

This in a general way will cover the location in the spinal cord of the mechanisms that control practically all of the important functions, but of necessity has had to be brief, and for more detailed information the reader must be referred to the more recent large text books on physiology, especially Langley's article on the sympathetic and Sherrington's article on the spinal cord, to be found in the second volume of Schafer's physiology. Much information may also be found in Tigerstedt and the American text-book. In addition to these text-books reference may be made to the various papers of Langley and Langley and Anderson, Bayliss and Starling, Sherrington and various others, which appeared within the last few years in journals of physiology.

NOTE.—Vasodilator cells located in the nucleus of the seventh cranial nerve send preganglionic paths to Meckel's and the submaxillary ganglia. Those in ninth send preganglionic paths to the otic ganglion. The postganglionic paths of both the seventh and ninth are in the main found in the fifth cranial nerve.

LOCAL ANESTHESIA BY CATAPHORESIS AND BY MECHANICAL PRESSURE.[1]

BY WILLIAM JAMES MORTON, M.D.,
OF NEW YORK.

THE three great discoveries of modern times in medicine—vaccination, anesthesia and antisepsis—are those around which respectively cluster great advances. Vaccination presses on into the great doctrine of "immunity." Anesthesia which, like Minerva of old, sprung forth full grown and fully equipped, with ether anesthesia in 1846, was in 1847 supplemented by the substitution agent, chloroform, and has since excited many efforts toward a practical local anesthesia. Antisepsis suggested asepsis and modern methods of resisting microbes.

In this discussion there has been assigned to me but a brief leaflet out of the great volume of anesthesia, namely, local anesthesia by cataphoresis and by mechanical pressure.

I will consider the two subjects in their historical order.

Cataphoresis.—Cataphoresic medication implies that medicaments may, by electric pressure or voltage, be caused to penetrate the sound skin or mucous membrane and thus exert their characteristic effects. If these medicaments have anesthetic or analgesic properties, we have then established a local anesthesia or analgesia.

But the penetration of the skin may begin at either pole and we therefore must speak of an anaphoresis. For this reason I have suggested calling the entire process, electric medicamental diffusion.

Privati, of Venice, in 1747 was the first to claim the transportation of medicine by electricity into the system. He employed static electricity. His views were, however, apparently fantastical. Following the advent of galvanic electricity, Reuss in 1807, observed that ordinary osmosis of fluids of differing densities, separated by a membrane, was accelerated by the battery current. Porret, in 1815, demonstrated that the direction of the flow was almost always from the positive to the negative terminal of the battery

circuit; he was the father of electric osmosis. Fabré-Palaprat, in 1833, was apparently the first to introduce medicines into the animal body by the galvanic current. He employed a compress, saturated with the medicine and covered with a platinum disc on each arm. Klenke and Hassenstein, in 1847, and Hassenstein in 1853, successfully repeated the experiment with iodide of potassium and with solutions of mercurial salts. G. Wiedermann in 1853, formulated the laws governing the diffusion or transportation of liquids by the current.

In 1859, Dr. (later Sir) Benjamin Ward Richardson, endeavored to introduce into practice a method of local anesthesia by the use of electricity and narcotics, terming the procedure "voltaic narcotism."

The medicines employed were aconite and chloroform, as follows:

R Tinc. Aconiti .... ʒiii
　Ext. Aconiti.......................... Əi
　Chloroformi .... ʒii
Mix.

Using this mixture at the positive pole and applying it to the leg of a dog, complete anesthesia was produced in eleven minutes, and later the leg was amputated without pain. So much opposition led by A. Waller, was developed toward Richardson's claims, that he abandoned his position, compensating, however, for his abandonment by introducing a method of local anesthesia by the ether spray as at present in use.

The above mentioned efforts, extending over a period of about one hundred years, produced no effect in practice, partly because of fundamental defects in technic, and partly because of universal scepticism as to the validity of the facts. The modern revival of electric pressure anesthesia followed the advent of the use of cocaine as an analgesic. Wagner in 1886, suggested electro-cocaine local anesthesia. Erb, in 1884, introduced medicines through the intact living skin by the aid of the continuous current, and demonstrated their presence in the saliva and the urine of the subject. Lewandowski did the same. Boccalari and Manzieri introduced strychnine, atropine, quinine, and iodide of potassium, through the unbroken skin. In 1886, Adamkiewicz introduced chloroform into tissues and thereby produced local anesthesia. J. Leonard Corning, of New York City, in 1886, punctured the skin with the Baunscheidt needle apparatus, and then used the electric current to introduce cocaine. Frederick Peterson, in 1888 and 1889, undertook a series of exhaustive experiments, which settled definitely many disputed points, and used cocaine and other alkaloidal compounds for the relief of neuralgic pain. His experiments, however, did not extend to the point of the production of local anesthesia for the performance of surgical operations.

In 1889, Mr. Newman Lawrence and Dr. A. Harris, both of London, described the cataphoric

1 Read before the Annual Meeting of the American Therapeutic Society, June 2, 1904.

method of medication. Cagney, of London, followed their plans. In 1890, Mr. Thomas A. Edison wrote a paper upon the employment of cataphoresis for the relief of gout, using chloride of lithium salts. In later years, excellent papers upon the subject were published by Danion, Labatut, Destot, Tommassi, Bergonié, Grosheintz, Imbert de la Touche, Gärtner and Ehrmann, Leduc, William J. Herdman, and many others.

In 1885, Mr. Vergnes, an electroplater, discovered that medicines could be extracted from the human body by the galvanic current as well as introduced into it, and was thus the originator of the process of " cataphoric demedication," as I have termed it. A system saturated with mercury, can thus be freed from the mercury. This plan was further advocated and published by Poey, of Paris. McGraw, of California, in 1896, applied electro-cocaine anesthesia for the purpose of benumbing the pain of a sensitive tooth, inserting the electrode upon a pledget of cotton saturated with cocaine within the cavity of the tooth.

Westlake, Gillet, and the writer, took an active part in the further introduction of cataphoresis into dentistry. The writer's contribution to electro-cocaine anesthesia was to add guaiacol or some similar agency, like carbolic acid, to cocaine. This addition decreases the time of administration upon a surface of the skin, from fifteen minutes with an aqueous solution as formerly employed, to two minutes with a guaiacol or carbolic acid solution, and decreases the amount of current required from fifteen milliampères for a one inch surface of electrode, to two milliampères. The advantages of this combination are, that the toxicity of the cocaine is reduced, that its effect is enhanced, and that the application sterilizes.

The writer also invented a new form of cataphoric electrode, consisting of a metal, like block tin, perforated all over its surface with drill holes, in order to form honeycomb-like recesses for the fluid, thus providing a continual feed to the intervening piece of blotting paper between the skin and the metal. The drill holes, one-thirty-second of an inch in diameter, should not entirely perforate the metal. A further advance by the writer was to use cataphoric anesthesia for minor surgical operations, in a first case, December, 1891, Dr. Howard Lilienthal operating, employing proper electrodes and an aqueous solution of cocaine.

The modern process of cataphoric local anesthesia is an absolutely simple and practicable one, and has been entirely wrested from the realm of uncertain and doubtful procedures.

Physical Basis.—Many early experiments from 1750 onward, have demonstrated beyond a question, that material particles are conveyed by the electric current, whether static or galvanic, from the positive to the negative pole. If we place glycerine or syrup or any other viscid material upon the positive discharging rod of an influence machine, we may observe that the fluid is carried directly across the intervening gap to the negative pole. This is an actual transportation of matter from the positive to the negative pole. If, as the writer has done by actual experiment, very finely ground particles of graphite, are held in suspension in " water glass " (silicate of sodium solution) and applied to the arm at the positive pole of the galvanic current, the graphite particles are driven into the sweat glands, and remain visibly imbedded for a week or two. There can, therefore, be no doubt of the actual transportation of both fluids and solids from the positive to the negative pole.

On the other hand it is equally positive that in the act of electrolysis, the respective ions are transported with their respective speeds from the positive to the negative, and from the negative to the positive poles. Following the doctrine of Arrhenius, we would say that in dilute solutions only the free ions were thus transported, and this is undoubtedly the fact. From this point of view, certain medicines must be used at the positive pole, and certain others must be used at the negative pole. Most modern authors explain the phenomena of cataphoresis, therefore, on the ionic doctrine. It seems to me that both explanations as above given, must be taken into account and I have suggested that while the free ions obey the electrolytic law, that the neutral molecules obey another electric law of transportation from the positive to the negative pole. For example from the electrolytic point of view, if iodide of potassium is placed upon the positive pole, the iodine, being electronegative, will remain there, while the potassium being electropositive, will move toward the negative pole, but from the transportation point of view, the free neutral molecules of iodide of potassium, will move from the positive to the negative pole. From an electrolytic point of view, therefore K. I. should be placed upon the negative pole to secure the introduction of iodine but not of iodide of potassium.

The currents from influence machines, as well as " battery currents," may be successfully employed.

Drugs Available.—The most favorable drug for electric local anesthesia, is, of course, cocaine; eucaine follows next. Other possible drugs are acoin, holocaine, orthoform, orthoform-new, nirvanine, anesin, tropacocaine, hemicranin, and chloreton.

Method and Technic.—These may be best illustrated by the relation of a single case, namely, the removal of a large pigmented nevus, suspected to have a sarcomatous tendency. The nevus was nearly three inches long by one-half inch wide, situated upon the thorax. An ordinary galvanic battery of, twenty-four cells was employed. The electrode was of block tin, three and one-half inches in length by two inches wide, and one-quarter of an inch in thickness, and perforated thoroughly but only half way through the metal with drill holes. This metal plate is set in an ebonite frame projecting beyond the metal the width of a piece of blotting paper. A piece of blotting paper cut to fit the metal and its surrounding ebonite ring served to hold the anesthetizing solution. This solution was prepared freshly, according to the following prescription:

R Guaiacol 5i
Cocaine hydrochlorate anhydrous........gr. vi
Mix.

Of this solution sufficient was put upon the blotting paper to wet it thoroughly, while some was also placed beneath the blotting paper in the honeycomb cells. The skin of the proposed operation was washed with soap and water. The electrode was then applied, six milliampères of current were allowed to flow for six minutes. The surgeon then made two deep linear incisions, each about three inches long and half an inch deep, in such a manner as to include the nevus. The nevus and the including parts of sound skin were then dissected up from the subcutaneous tissues, the dissection extending at least an inch deep. Five small arteries were subjected to torsion and ten deep stitches closed the wound. No pain whatever was produced either in procuring the anesthesia, making the incisions and dissections, twisting the arteries, or inserting the stitches. The patient, himself a physician, watched the operation and said that he had experienced no pain. There were no subsequent toxic effects of the cocaine. The wound healed by first intention.

It is well immediately upon removing the electrode, and before making any incision, to wash off the part thoroughly with alcohol, in order to obviate any possible absorption of the guaiacol, and cocaine solution into the incision. Also catgut ligature should not be used, since it may be acted upon by some remaining guaiacol.

Uses.—The uses of a complete and perfect local anesthesia, like the one above described, are obvious, and it is remarkable that this method has not come into more general practice, though, of course, the fact that a battery of from twenty to thirty cells, is required, has been unfavorable. In hospital practice, or in the practice of electro-herapeutists, this objection would not hold good. In my own practice, I use electro-cocaine-guaiacol local anesthesia, in a great variety of minor surgical operations, as, for instance, the removal or treatment of a nevus, a facial blemish, the incision of a carbuncle or furuncle, or felon, for all cases where electric needles are to be applied with pain, etc. The principal value of the method, herefore, is in minor surgery, but I have no doubt that incisions for laparotomy and larger operations might in the same manner be painlessly made.

Of late years I combine adrenaline chloride with cocaine and find that the effect is superior to that of cocaine alone—using both, of course,

with guaiacol or carbolic acid. This mixture may be diluted with oils.

Pressure Anesthesia.—The term "pressure anesthesia" was invented by the writer in 1897 to define a new method of local anesthesia, presented by him at that time. This method was based on the idea that medicamental solutions, especially anesthetizing solutions, might be forced into the tissues by the pressure of vapors or gases, or by mechanical pressure. The following language, used at that time in an address published in the *Dental Journal* entitled "Items of Interest," Vol. 19, pp. 717-18, describes the main idea involved. "It occurred to me that I might dissolve hydrochlorate of cocaine in ether and produce anesthesia, but I tried it and found that the cocaine salt would not dissolve in ether. I finally dissolved my cocaine in guaiacol. I made a strong solution and added half and half of sulphuric ether, and there was no precipitation of the cocaine. I had a very small test tube on the table and I put some of the guaiacol sulphuric ether and cocaine solution into that tube, pressed the mouth of the tube on my arm and asked my assistant to time me; I held it there for five minutes, and taking a needle I found my skin was numb. I had made an experiment that established a new order of things, which I have christened "pressure anesthesia."

This plan was immediately put into practice by many of the dental profession, in the following manner: A pledget of absorbent cotton saturated with the anesthetizing solution was introduced within the cavity of the tooth, when it was desired to benumb the pain or extract the nerve, and this pledget was then immediately sealed in closely with a soft rubber stopping. In a very few minutes the sensitive contents of the interior of the tooth were anesthetized and the operator could then proceed to excavate without pain, or even to extract the nerve painlessly. It would appear that the evaporation of the sulphuric ether into the closed cavity forced the anesthetizing solution into the sensitive tissue of the tooth cavity. It also was plain that the mechanical pressure of forcing in the rubber stopping had much to do with disseminating the contained anesthetizing fluid.

The method above outlined has now become wellnigh universal in dental practice, so much so that a recent editorial in *Items of Interest* of the date of November, 1903, refers to it as "An Era in Dentistry" as follows: "The perfection of any new and valuable discovery constitutes an era in the history of the art or science to which it applies. That such an event has occurred in dentistry does not appear to be sufficiently appreciated." The editor then discussed the treatment in vogue in dentistry for more than a century of "killing the nerve" in teeth by means of arsenic, and points out the disadvantages of the removal of the pulp of the tooth, both with and without arsenic. Referring to the fact that cataphoresis had lost its popularity and that arsenic had again become dominant, he states that finally this method of pressure anesthesia had solved the problem. There still remains, however, as an occasional difficulty in the removal of the nerve, the fact that sometimes hemorrhages occur, and to control these, Dr. Clyde Davis had recommended the use of adrenalin in connection with the cocaine pressure anesthesia. The editorial concludes by saying: "The dental profession has now at hand a ready means of removing pulps painlessly and without the use of arsenic."

In the actual practice of pressure anesthesia in minor surgery I have frequently made use of a cupping glass, a watch glass, or a test tube, as described in the experiment above quoted, that is to say, utilizing the pressure qualities of ether or alcohol vapors. The process is exactly opposite to that of cupping, for the pump may be used to fill the cupping or other glass, as well as to abstract air from it.

This method, of course, has nothing to do with the infiltration method of Schleich, where the solution is injected into the tissue. The pressure factor of the operation, which I had christened pressure anesthesia, refers to the method of introducing the agency into the tissue, rather than to its action after it has been introduced.

While, therefore, pressure anesthesia, as first proposed by the writer, has at the present moment its principle utility in dental practice, it is by no means impossible to say that further experimentation in the direction of demonstrating its practicability, may not find it a valuable adjunct in surgical local anesthesia.

MEDICAL PROGRESS.

MEDICINE.

New Physical Signs in Diseases of Chest.—A number of new physical signs described by A. GROBER (*Deutsch. Arch. f. klin. Med.*, Vol. 82, Nos. 3 and 4) are considered by him as far more valuable in the diagnosis of intrathoracic disease than diascopy. It is but little known that difference in the size of the pupils is a common symptom of apex tuberculosis. The pupil of the affected side is generally wider since the sympathetic nerve is irritated by the inflamed pleura. Another valuable sign is the behavior of the veins of the chest if an expiratory effort is made with closed glottis as in Valsalva's method. Normally the vessels on both side swell equally, but with tumors, aneurisms, etc., the veins which are affected by the compression, will be more prominent. Normally, the pupils will contract somewhat during expiration and dilate slightly with inspiration; with Valsalva's method, there will be a gradual, slight dilatation during the deep inspiration preceding the expiratory effort and a gradual, slight contraction during the latter. The following variations occur: (1) Only one pupil will show the normal contraction; the other will dilate. On the side of the latter, pathological lesions of definite localization will be found in the thorax. (2) If both pupils dilate instead of contracting during forced expiration, the disease is bilateral. (3)

If there is a difference in the size of the pupils during normal respiration and the dilated pupil widens still more during Valsalva's experiment, while the contracted one will become normal, intrathoracic disease on the side of the wide pupil is probable. (4) If the pupils differ in size with quiet respiration but dilate with Valsalva's method, bilateral intrathoracic affection is probable. If the smaller pupil becomes equal in size or larger than the second one, the disease probably also affects both sides, if local disease or organic disease of the nervous system can be excluded. Absence of all these phenomena does not argue against intrathoracic disease. The percussion note obtained over the manubrium sterni is also of the greatest value. In real or inflammatory tumors of the mediastinum there will often be dulness with closed mouth and dull tympany with open mouth, or dull tympany with closed mouth and Wintrich's change of percussion with open mouth. If the posterior mediastinum is chiefly affected, the note will be purely tympanitic with closed mouth; with distinct Wintrich's change on opening the mouth.

Spastic Diplegia During Pertussis.—J. H. W. RHEIN (*Journal A. M. A.*, March 4), reports the case of a child, thirty months old, who had spastic diplegia in the legs with nystagmus. Later a similar condition of the arms gradually developed, with difficulty in swallowing, etc. The child became greatly emaciated, and finally died after numerous general convulsive attacks, worse on the right side. The autopsy revealed numerous small hemorrhages in the right and left frontal cortex, slight thickening of pia in the paracentral region, with a few small cortical hemorrhages. There were areas of distended perivascular spaces containing many round mononuclear cells, which were also distributed everywhere throughout the cortex; their protoplasm was granular. In the occipital region there was thickening of the pia and intense red blood cell infiltration. Microscopically, marked degeneration was observed in one cerebral peduncle. The general appearance was that of a hemorrhagic meningoencephalitis. Rhein believes that the widespread lesion of the cortex was due to a toxin acting on the vessels and setting up an inflammatory process. This caused local destruction of fibers, especially in the paracentral region, followed by degeneration in the pyramidal tracts. The minute cortical hemorrhages he attributes to the convulsive attacks preceding death.

Fear in Cardiac Disease.—W. R. DUNTON, JR. (*Journal A. M. A.*, February 18), incited by a statement that all cases of alienation showing apprehension revealed cardiac disease, examined the twenty-five most recent admissions in the Sheppard and Enoch Pratt Hospital and some twenty cases in the Johns Hopkins Hospital. He concludes that the cardiac lesion is not the primary factor in causing the associated state of apprehension. What we may call, for want of a better term, the idiosyncrasy of the patient, is largely responsible for apprehension associated with cardiac lesions. In neurasthenic types a lack of vagus control is an important etiologic factor. Our knowledge of the subject is still not yet exact, and he asks the cooperation of clinicians in the investigation.

Mortality of Pneumonia in High Altitudes.—Major CHARLES F. KIEFFER (*Am. Med.*, March 5, 1905) refers to the very common belief that pneumonia is more fatal in high altitudes than at the sea level

Several recent papers are reviewed. The paper is a study of the cases occurring at Fort D. A. Russell, Wyoming, at an elevation of 6,195 feet above sea level, during the period between 1868 and 1905. During this time among 26,569 admissions for all causes, there were 127 cases of pneumonia with 20 deaths; a mortality of 15.74 per cent. The fatal cases are classified according to the anatomic location of the disease. The writer calls attention to the prognostic import of syphilis on pneumonia. The figures are compared with those of the entire army. In the period between 1868 and 1893 the total admissions in the army for pneumonia were 7,078 with 1,105 deaths; a mortality of 15.61 per cent. During the same year at Fort Russell, there were 123 cases with eighteen deaths; a mortality of 14.63 per cent., the advantage in favor of high altitude being one per cent. Charts are included showing the incidence of the disease by months and a chart showing the mortality and ratio of incidence in the army for thirty-six years. The paper concludes that the figures, as far as they go, seem to show that altitude has very little influence on the mortality of pneumonia.

Carbonic Acid and Tuberculosis.—A treatment of tuberculosis by means of drugs which increase the amount of carbonic acid in the blood, is recommended by E. FUNKE (*Wiener klin. therap. Woch.*, January 29, 1905). The tubercle bacilli cause a secondary destruction of the tissue-proteids. Hydrogen is set free and acting as a reducing agent, attracts oxygen, which brings about vigorous oxidation of the tissue proteids. It is desirable to prevent this action of oxygen, by having the blood which bathes the tuberculous areas contain a large amount of carbonic acid. This is accomplished by the administration of sodium bicarbonate, and formic acid (CH_2O_2). The use of the phosphates of calcium will accelerate the process of calcification of old tuberulous areas.

Poisoning by Potassium Bichromate.—FRANCIS E. FRONCZAK (*Am. Med.*, March 5, 1905) describes fully a case of attempted murder by poisoning with potassium bichromate, which is rarely used for such purpose, only a few cases being reported in the literature. The patient, a woman of fifty-eight years, was given the poison in port wine, and in a mixture of alcohol with raspberry syrup. Later, her husband prepared her a strong solution of the chemical in water, calling it "tea." The woman took altogether about 6.5 gm. (100 grs.) At first she vomited heavily, had convulsions, pains in the stomach, dizziness, headache, cold sweats, and diarrhea. Her face became later ghastly pale, eyes dilated, respirations very slow and labored, about 8 to 10 per minute, pulse 56, weak and compressible. Urine contained considerable blood. The woman recovered after a week, but complained of occasional pains in the stomach and of backache; for some time albumin was found in the urine. The author reviews the subject of potassium bichromate and recommends treatment, which consists in giving alkalies and milk to counteract the irritating poison, and anodyne for the pain. Some very simple methods of finding all soluble chromates are fully described.

SURGERY.

Exploratory Abdominal Section.—JOHN YOUNG BROWN (*Journal A. M. A.*, March 4), insists on the importance of exploratory section in all cases of penetrating wounds of the abdomen, when multiple perforations exist, or when the blood supply is cut off resection of the bowel is imperative. For this purpose, in case of gunshot wounds, he considers the Murphy button the ideal method. In severe abdominal contusions, he agrees with Bottomley, that operation is generally advisable, especially when there is pain, tenderness and muscular rigidity. In cases of strangulated hernia, when there is any question as to the integrity of the bowel, he believes that resection should be performed. The distended loop should be drained above the constriction. As soon as the gut has been delivered through the supplementary incision he clamps it off and ties a glass tube, to which is attached a rubber hose, into its proximal end, and then proceeds with the resection. This is time saving and drainage is effected without soiling the field.

Acute Intussusception in an Infant; Resection of Gangrenous Intussusceptum; Murphy Button Anastomosis; Recovery.—E. W. PETERSON (*Med. Rec.*, March 4, 1905) reports what he believes to be the first successful operation on an infant, for the relief of intussusception, in which resection of the gut was performed. The patient was an infant of four months and twenty days, with typical symptoms pointing to an intussusception of about thirty hours' duration. Four inches of the ileum, the cecum, and an inch of the ascending colon were resected and an end-to-end anastomosis made by means of the Murphy button. Convalescence was stormy, but the patient was discharged cured on the fifteenth day. The button was expelled on the fourth day. The author considers that it is of importance to avoid the systematic use of opium in the postoperative treatment of these cases, owing to the risk of the drug's aggravating the enteritis and toxemia usually present.

Prosthetic Treatment of Fracture of the Mandible.—F. A. FAUGHT (*Med. Rec.*, March 4, 1905) says that fracture of the mandible is usually compound, and that probably in one-fourth of the cases the injury is multiple, but that the prognosis is generally favorable except in extreme old age. Complications must be guarded against by frequent cleansing of the wound and mouth, and removal of all fragments of bone which show the slightest tendency to produce suppuration. The problem of securing adequate fixation of the fragments without interfering with mastication. and the proper care of the mouth, is often difficult, and some of the plans employed are open to serious objections. Among these is the use of the upper teeth as a splint and guide for maintaining the fragments in place, because it is uncertain in result and entails much discomfort. The continued use of a fixation bandage passing around the front of the chin is also unsatisfactory, and may lead to positive and permanent harm. The introduction of wire sutures through holes drilled in the bone is to be resorted to only after all other methods have failed. The author describes the steps necessary to produce a metallic cap splint, which is accurately modeled on the restored cast of the injured jaw and is cemented to the teeth. This offers the advantage of introducing the least amount of foreign substance into the mouth, is contained entirely within the mouth, and affords a rigid support for the fractured bone, while permitting of free movement of the mandible with easy access to the oral cavity from the first.

Iodoform Bone Plugging.—This subject has aroused a good deal of attention in this country, and judging from the reports presented from the surgical section of the Academy, it is well merited. MOSETIG MOORHOF and SEYMOUR JONES (*Lancet,* January 21, 1905) in an extensive monograph on the subject, report as follows: The mixture consists of 60 parts of the finest pulverized iodoform and 40 parts each of spermaceti and oil of sesame, a compound which at the ordinary temperature of a room forms a stiff yellow mass; at 15° C. it becomes fluid, and on allowing it to stand, the oily constituents rise and the iodoform sinks. It must therefore be well shaken before using. Moorhof began his researches on bone cavities five years ago. He then used an iodoform paste of the consistency of putty. He soon discovered, however, that hermetic sealing of the cavity, the desired result was to be obtained only by pouring in a thoroughly fluid mass. This mass must adhere to every portion of the wall filling every fissure and interstice. To accomplish this, the cavity must obviously be entirely dry and should be treated precisely as though it were occurring and being treated in a tooth. This implies that the part must be made not only as aseptic as possible, but practically dry. Silbermack has contrived a very simple apparatus by means of which sterile, cold, dry air can be blown in. The air is carried through a formalin solution and then through calcium chloride. When the walls are free from moisture, they appear dull. If electrical power is available, drills run by motor are preferable to any operated by hand power, although this is not a necessary part of the technic. The plugging material should be poured in slowly and for well plugged cavities, no special drainage is required, for they neither bleed nor discharge. A small amount of lymph may be secreted by the soft parts, but if no sinuses are present, it is sufficient to depend on rather wide stitching of the wounds for drainage. The secretions are invariably of a lymphoid character, being obtained almost entirely from the divided lymphatics. It is interesting to note that here as elsewhere in the case of paraffin and other materials introduced into the tissues, the filling has but a relatively short life in the cavity. It stimulates granulation tissue very actively and may be pressed out by the growth of this from below. Even more fortuitous is the absorption of the mass by phagocytic action, occurring after primary union of the soft parts. This process may be demonstrated in two ways. It may be seen under the X-ray, for iodoform throws an excellent shadow, or it may be determined by the amount of iodine reaction in the urine. This iodine is absorbed very slowly and there can therefore be no danger of intoxication or iodoform poisoning even in the case of very large cavities. The production and gradual growth of bone tissue are effected by a primary formation of new connective tissue. Later the lime salts are deposited. The bone thus formed has been derived from the granulation tissue and the process is not unlike that seen in callous formation. In connection with this, Silbermack has made extensive investigations with animals since the beginning of 1903, the results of which he will soon publish. The time which is required to complete the organization of the bone is very variable. It may take more than a year, or it may be accomplished in less than one-quarter that time. Moorhof, in 220 cases, has never seen any ill effects arising from the technic. The exploitation of the method has not been remedied to ordinary osteomyelitic cavities, it having been used freely and successfully in the treatment of tuberculous joints. It is obviously necessary that the freest possible incision should be made to gain access to the joint, and that it should be most thoroughly cleaned before any effort is made to use the wax. Suc-

cessful operations have been performed upon the wrist-joint, the elbow, the shoulder, the ankle and the knee, and the hip-joint. Moorhof proceeds according to the following rule, which is applied in all cases to children. He removes the cartilage piecemeal with a heavy knife and then proceeds to cut out the affected bone. There is no advantage of sawing off thick slices, for this interferes immediately with the gait of the patient. A thorough scooping process and a getting of the part absolutely dry usually being much preferable. Further use of the material is found in face lesions, such as dental cysts and empyemata of the antrum of Highmore. Moorhof has also reported a case in which he plugged the mediastinum in a fourteen-year-old girl. There was present in the middle of the sternum an ulcer. The apices were not involved. On opening the chest, it was found that a cavity existed which required 200 grams to fill it. The results were extraordinary. The evening temperature ceased and the patient was outdoors on the seventh day. Dyspnea, however, occurred and could be relieved only by hypnotics. It was found furthermore that the air made its entrance and exit through the lower wound.

Report of Eighty-four **Operations on the Kidney and Ureter.**—G. E. BREWER's (*Med. Rec.,* February 18, 1905) list comprises twenty-seven nephrotomies, the same number of nephrectomies, nine nephrorrhaphies, ten decapsulations, five operations on the pelvic portion of the ureter, and six emergency operations on traumatic cases. These classes are discussed in detail, and the diagnosis of renal calculus is treated at considerable length. From a review of the conditions present in his cases the author feels justified in stating that there is no single symptom nor sign, nor any group of symptoms or signs that is absolutely pathognomonic of renal or ureteral calculus, unless the calculus lies in the lower ureter and can be touched by a metal bougie or catheter. The most important factors to be considered are pain, tenderness, hematuria, the results of radiography, cystoscopy, and ureteral catheterization. While vomiting, vesical irritability, pyuria, fever, and the presence or absence of a renal tumor are important and will often help us to confirm or lead us to exclude other pathological conditions, too much reliance must not be placed upon them in the diagnosis of calculus. While pain and tenderness were present in practically 100 per cent. of the author's cases of stone, there were also present in a large perecntage of the cases in which no stone was found, and calculus may, and often does exist without pain. Hematuria was known to be present in 52 per cent. of the author's stone cases, but it was also present in 45 per cent. of the cases without stone. Spontaneous hemorrhage occurring during rest and sleep generally means new growth. Hemorrhage following active exercise or jolting and accompanied by characteristic colic, in the absence of other demonstrable pathological conditions is strongly suggestive of calculus. Excluding imperfect plates and those in which the edges of the shadow were not distinctly defined, the X-ray gave accurate indications in 95 per cent. of the cases, and must therefore be regarded as the most reliable means of examination which we possess. Cystoscopy helped to a correct diagnosis in 60⅔ per cent. of the cases examined, while it was misleading in 33⅓ per cent. Ureteral catheterization proved valuable in confirming the diagnosis, in definitely determining the side of the lesion, and in estimating the competence of the opposite kidney.

Purgation Before and After Operation.—I. S. STONE (*Am. Med.,* February 25, 1905) discusses this subject at length, he asserts excessive purgation should be restricted because it is enervating to the general system. It produces great irritation to the mucous lining of the bowel. It may add to the danger of ileus and paresis. Purgatives have very little effect in limiting the amount of extraperitoneal exudate and fluids. Instead of calomel and saline purgation, bland evacuants such as castor oil should be used before abdominal section. The use of suitable bland nonfermentative foods is desirable until just before operation in weak patients. After operation limit peristalsis; give only small quantities of food and drink by mouth. Rarely give opium. Enemas should be administered to relieve distention and cause peristalsis in downward direction, after normal peristalsis laxatives should be given as required.

OBSTETRICS AND GYNECOLOGY.

The Use of the Modified Champetier De Ribes Balloon.—Many measures have been advocated for inducing and shortening the duration of labor; none have given better results than the use of a conical cervical dilater, a Champetier De Ribes balloon, which best simulates nature's bag. J. W. Voor-hees (*Am. Jour. Obstet.*, January, 1905), who has suggested modifications of the balloons to increase their strength, advocates their use in dry labors in that the bags quickly start strong pains, rapidly dilate the cervix and plug the os, thus preventing the loss of more liquor amnii. In breech presentations it is not necessary to bring down a foot so soon and thereby prolonged pressure on the child is avoided. A bag should be introduced if pains do not start within twenty-four hours after the rupture of the membranes. In protracted labors the balloon strengthens the pains and shortens the first stage, thus saving the woman's strength and rendering the cervix in better condition for any operative procedures that may be necessary. In certain emergencies only should manual dilatation be resorted to. For the induction of labor the balloon is the most reliable of all methods. When the cervix is long and but little dilated and an anesthetic contraindicated, a bougie should be used in preference. In albuminuria and eclampsia the uterus is inert and a bougie often useless. If a bag is used even though there are no pains, dilatation can be brought about by traction on the tube. The plan advocated in treating eclampsia is to insert a bag at once, stimulate all the excretory organs, reduce arterial tension, temporizing only until the cervix is soft enough to stand an accouchement forcé without tearing and with little shock to the patient. In placenta praevia the balloon is also very reliable; it stops the hemorrhage, starts pains, softens and dilates the cervix and prepares the way for an easier and less dangerous delivery, for, when the largest balloon comes through, forceps can be readily applied or a version performed without difficulty. The gauze lampan is an efficient adjunct during the time required for getting ready for the introduction of the bag. In considering objections to the use of the balloons the fact that the membranes are occasionally ruptured is of no consequence. The placenta may be separated in placenta praevia but the bag arrests the hemorrhage. The presenting part may be displaced if the introduction is faulty and the bag too rapidly filled. Where the bag is expelled a long cord or one loosely coiled about the neck may prolapse, a complication that should be watched for. The balloons can be boiled and should give rise to no infection. No special introducing forceps or syringe are necessary. An anesthetic is employed only

when it is necessary to dilate the cervix to insert the bag or when the cervix is very high, the patient very nervous, or the vulvular orifice narrow and sensative.

Perforation of the Uterus During Curettage.—Curettage is considered by the average practitioner a simple and easy operation, belonging to minor surgery—every beginner performs it. Perforation of the uterus during this operation has occurred at the hands of experts but is usually the result of carelessness and inexperience. W. Hessert (*Am. Jour. Obstet.*, January, 1905) says that conditions which result in atrophy or softening of the uterus predispose to perforation. Among such conditions may be mentioned lactation, senile and postoperative atrophy. Hyaline and fatty degeneration and necrosis of muscle fiber may result from infection. In poorly nourished women after numerous pregnancies a softening of the uterus may occur, due to a separation of the muscle fibers by an edematous infiltration without degeneration or inflammation. Carcinoma, myoma, pelvic tuberculosis and pelvic abscess may also be associated with uterine atrophy and softening. General diseases, as leucemia, diabetes, nephritis, Addison's disease, tuberculosis, pernicious anemia, as well as acute infectious diseases, may be followed by uterine atrophy. When the uterus is soft and offers no resistance the expert operater may perforate, but will recognize the condition and act accordingly; a novice is likely to fail to recognize the perforation and inflict fatal visceral injuries. Perforation may be accomplished with a probe, sounds, curette, douch point, dilators, sponge tent or other instruments. The result of perforation depends on whether or not fluids have been injected (liquor ferri, lysal, sublimate, iodine, etc.) or infection carried into the peritoneal cavity, or visceral injury has occurred. In general the following principles should be observed to guard against perforation: (1) Accuracy of pelvic diagnosis as to size, position, mobility and consistency of uterus: presence of tumors and condition of adnexa. (2) The direction of the cervical canal and uterine cavity should be accurately determined by means of a graduated sound before introducing dilators. Dilitation should be done slowly, turning the instrument around in all points of the circle. (3) A sharp curette is best in the hands of the experienced. (4) Except in the presence of septic endometritis the use of the irrigator is considered superfluous. The treatment of such an accident should be expectant if it occurs after antiseptic precautions and has been done with a blunt instrument. Irrigation should be omitted and the uterus packed. If there is evidence that the intestine has been pulled down or otherwise injured by curette, placenta or volsellum forceps, the abdomen should be opened and the entire intestine examined. If there is an infection endometritis present an hysterectomy had best be done.

Subcutaneous Emphysema during Labor.—Cases of emphysema under the skin of the chest and the throat from rupture of some of the pulmonary alveoli from straining in labor have been reported, but an emphysema from any other source in this condition is thus far unknown. What is apparently the first instance of this kind is reported by H. T. Herman (*Zeitschrift f. Geb. u. Gyn.*, Vol. 53, No. 3) where the air gained access to the tissues under the skin not through the lungs, but through the nose or one of its accessory cavities. The patient, a primipara suddenly developed, in the later stages of her labor, a swelling of both eyelids, which gradually extended over the forehead, the face and the neck, and then invaded the abdomen down to the navel, the back and one arm. The characteristic evidences of subcutaneous emphysema were present, but the normal conditions returned on the seventeenth day of the puerperium. The author believes that there was some ulcerative process in the wall of the nose or the accessory sinuses which allowed the air to enter, as the patient admitted having had more or less trouble with her nose since her early life.

THERAPEUTICS.

The Toxic Effects of Formaldehyde and Formalin. —The widespread use of drugs in internal medication which generate formalin in the tissues, imparts great value to the researches of H. M. FISCHER (*Jour. Exper. Med.*, February 4, 1905). The results of his investigations show that the inhalation of formaldehyde gas in even small quantities is followed by bronchitis and pneumonia. Formalin belongs to that rare group of poisons which are capable of producing death suddenly when swallowed. The introduction of formalin into the stomach is followed by the production of a gastritis which varies greatly in character. The duodenum and jejunum may also be involved in the inflammation. Intraperitoneal injections of formalin causes peritonitis of a fibrino-hemorrhagic character. The injection of formalin into the lungs is followed by pneumonia and bronchitis. The inflammation which follows subcutaneous injections of formalin is characterized by intense exudation. In whatever way introduced into the body, formalin is absorbed and is then capable of producing lesions in the parenchymatous organs. The injection of formalin or the inhalation of the vapors of formaldehyde produces cloudy swelling of the parenchyma of the kidney.

Treatment of Sciatica.—There is hardly any method of treatment, from simple rest in bed to articulation at the hip, which has not been tried to alleviate the pains of sciatica. According to J. LANGE (*Münch med. Woch.*, December 27, 1904) the best results are obtained from injecting 70 to 100 c.c. of Schleick's solution into the sciatic nerve, directly where it issues from the sacrosciatic foramen. The injection is made after the skin has been infiltrated, and most patients will experience a sensation resembling an electrical shock as soon as the needle has entered the nerve. Occasionally it is necessary to give a second injection, but the relief in most cases is remarkable, even where morphine and other analgesics have been used for a long time. After effects are rare, but sometimes the patients complain of slight pain over the site of injection.

Treatment of Acute Suppuration by Bier's Compression.—Over one hundred cases of acute suppuration have been treated by A. BIER (*Münch med. Woch.*, January 31, 1905), by the method of venous hyperemia, so successful in chronic conditions. The technic is as follows: The limb above the suppuration is surrounded by several turns of a rubber bandage, so as to compress the venous but not the arterial circulation. The affected part should give the appearance of a fiery red edema, but should never look blue. The parts peripheral to the affected area are not bandaged, but participate in the swelling. In acute suppuration, the bandage should be worn ten hours daily; in very severe cases at least twenty to twenty-two hours. Thus for a suppura-

tive tenosynovitis, the Esmarch is applied at ten o'clock in the morning and worn continuously until eight or nine o'clock in the evening. It is then removed and reapplied somewhat higher or lower At eight in the following morning, the bandage is again removed and the limb elevated until ten o'clock. In some cases, frequent intermissions of one and a half to two hours are necessary. The presence of a lymphangitis in the affected limb is not a contra-indication. As a rule, pain disappears very soon after compression, pus will be absorbed or changed into serum, or else it will be converted into a cold abscess. In suppuration of the larger joints, the pus was never evacuated, nor were fistulous tracts, already present, enlarged, since passive motion, combined with compression, is the best method of removing pus.

The Night-Sweats of Tuberculosis and Their Cure, Especially by Veronal.—It was most plausible to take Cornet's view as to the cause of night-sweats, that they were to be looked upon as a symptom of the action of tuberculous toxins. Hr. v Schrötter properly distinguished between sweats in the initial stage and in severe cases. In cases with fever, there was mostly a connection between fall of temperature and the outbreak of perspiration. In contrast to pneumonic cases, in which the outbreak of sweat brings relief, in feverish phthisical patients it caused extreme discomfort and weakened them to complete exhaustion.

Most medical men were in favor of endeavoring to overcome night-sweats. Salter, however, was an exception; he was of opinion that they should not be suppressed, as they excreted tuberculous toxins

The patient should get accustomed to sleep in a cool room, lightly covered, and with open windows regular and not too warm baths, or lukewarm o cold rubbings night or morning, or both. Salicy powder, tannoform dustings, and painting with 50 per cent. formalin solution. Brehma recommended a quarter of a liter of milk, with seve spoonfuls of cognac.

Of internal medicine the antipyretics did not d much. Atropine was in the front rank; it ofte did good, but it sometimes failed altogether. Afte atropine came agaricine in the form of a pill. I also relieves cough, but patients got accustomed t it. Camphoric acid also did good and guai camphol, also camphorate of pyramidon. Of oth remedies he only mentions veronal, which in r duced doses is a very active remedy for nigh sweats. It was given before bedtime, either dry in tea. in doses of 0.3 grm. The first doses act scarcely at all, with the second the night-sweat w generally less; after the third it usually ceased alt gether. Sometimes one had to wait longer for tl effect. In a few cases the dose had to be raised t 0.6 grm.

Treatment of Enteritis.—In enteritis, especiall the tuberculous form, M. PERROTE (*These de Pari* 1904, No. 228) praises highly the action of meth lene blue. It is not only a parasiticide; it also prov analgesic in the various nerve troubles and acts . cholagogue. The following formula is recom mended:

R Methylene blue ....0.05 gme.
     Sugar of milk ....0.20 gme.
Three or four times daily one powder.

After three days of the above treatment tl diarrhea will generally cease. The drug should l pure and free from chloride of zinc.

THE MEDICAL NEWS.

A WEEKLY JOURNAL
OF MEDICAL SCIENCE.

COMMUNICATIONS in the form of Scientific Articles, Clinical Memoranda, Correspondence or News Items of interest to the profession are invited from all parts of the world. Reprints to the number of 250 of original articles contributed exclusively to the MEDICAL NEWS will be furnished without charge if the request therefor accompanies the manuscript. When necessary to elucidate the text, illustrations will be engraved from drawings or photographs furnished by the author. Manuscript should be typewritten.

SMITH ELY JELLIFFE, A.M., M.D., Ph.D., Editor,
No. 111 FIFTH AVENUE, NEW YORK.

Subscription Price, Including postage In U. S. and Canada.

PER ANNUM IN ADVANCE	. . . .	$4.00
SINGLE COPIES	. . . . . .	.10
WITH THE AMERICAN JOURNAL OF THE MEDICAL SCIENCES, PER ANNUM	. .	8.00

Subscriptions may begin at any date. The safest mode of remittance is by bank check or postal money order, drawn to the order of the undersigned. When neither is accessible, remittances may be made at the risk of the publishers, by forwarding in *registered* letters.

LEA BROTHERS & CO.,
No. 111 FIFTH AVENUE (corner of 18th St.), NEW YORK.

SATURDAY, MARCH 18, 1905.

PHYSICAL EXERCISE WITHOUT APPARATUS.

THIRTY-FIVE years' experience as an instructor of students in Harvard's Hemenway Gymnasium and "as adviser of business and professional men, and twenty-three years as director of a normal school for the preparation of teachers of physical culture" combine to make the advice of Dr. Dudley A. Sargent, of Cambridge, worth having, and of promulgating, even among the medical profession—nominally experts in such affairs. This is theoretically. Practically, the actual book ("Health, Strength and Power" by name) bears out the *a priori* probabilities of its author's fitness to advise. Three elements especially of the substance of this popular manual are noteworthy from the medical view-point and commend it as worthy even of editorial discussion. First, its author is a soundly scientific and fadless physiologist and hygienist; second, it makes possible adequate exercise without apparatus, that is, at any time and any place; third, it emphasizes what is physiologically certainly the essence of neuromuscular exercise: "the chief essential of physical training is *voluntary* movement."

The first two of these, although of much importance and rare among the numerous recent "systems" of bodily exercise, need no special notice, but to even some physicians it may not be at once obvious that voluntary movements (that is movements made with an effort of adjustment), are of more value than routine exercise which soon becomes habitual and more or less reflex. The physiological conditions seem to be somewhat as follows:

The benefits of physical exercise arise from its stimulation of the lymph-flow (which stands for a heightening of body-metabolism generally), of the respiration, of the circulation, of the muscles (constituting more than half the mass of the body, and last, but certainly not least, of the nervous system. The muscles and nerves constitute together the neuromuscular mechanism, the two parts always working together, never either alone; indeed, they are properly one, *the master mechanism of the organism.* But just as a child learning to read develops its reading-faculty much more rapidly by reading always unfamiliar matter, and that not only because new words are thus more quickly acquired but also because of the additional effort thus necessarily expended, so in exercising this neuromuscular mechanism additional benefit accrues to both the nerves and the muscles by using a large variety of easy exercises requiring a degree of conscious effort if they are to be perfectly performed. In this way the part of the neuromuscular organ constituted by the central nervous system gets exercised beneficially and in a way quite otherwise than that of mental exertion. Exercise of this sort in fact approaches the benefits of outdoor games of exercise and skill such as tennis and golf, without being limited by the time and place and outfit these latter demand.

From a recital of a few of the fifty-six exercises which Dr. Sargent describes, may be most readily seen their interesting variety. There are imitations of wood-chopping, swimming, striking the anvil, rope-pulling, fencing, throwing the discus, windmill, mowing, pitching hay, grand salaam, fire engine, sawing wood, rowing, rocking the boat, bowling and locomotive; these will suffice and serve as types of the remainder also. It is obvious that movements like these, fifty-six of them, run well through the range of possible extensive bodily motions, and that if performed repeatedly, from five to a hundred times in various cases, furnish a very wide range of muscular exercises coordinated into the desired postures by effort of the central nervous system. It is told in separate chapters which of these are best adapted to children and which to youth, girls, and women. while special stress is laid on the adaptation of exercises for persons advancing beyond middle-life, and for those passing into old age. But for Dr. Sargent, as for the rest of the world, these set exercises are considered only necessary substitutes and complements of the more useful outdoor pursuits they represent. Who, indeed, would advise a weak pretense of pitching hay in one's bathroom save in winter when the hay fields of one's country home are deep beneath the snow; and who would saw wood beside his bed if there were cord-sticks piled high in the yard outside? On the other hand, windmill, fire engine and locomotive would certainly impress the neighbors less humorously if done indoors (unless, indeed, the exerciser be a small boy), whereas rocking the boat in the bathroom is obviously less foolish than rocking the boat out of doors.

More than a hundred photographic illustrations made from these exercises, as performed by a skilled model, show excellently the various attitudes and expressions involved, illuminating the descriptive text in a very satisfactory and pleasing manner.

One cannot help believing that all persons of sedentary habits, could they be induced to systematically practise such comprehensive movements as these, would promptly feel the benefit in every organ of their bodies. But as every physician knows only too well, the majority of those persons who need most such activity are so deep in the slough of habitual inactivity that not even the thought of a needlessly early death itself is strong enough to drag them into the habit of exercise which would save them. Habit is life's great law, and laziness is many a man's life-habit still, despite the awakening to physical culture, which is passing over the earth, despite, too, his doctor's warning of hardening arteries and of weakening digestive muscles. Yet here, if anywhere, during the larger part of the year when outdoor activity is impracticable, lies the "way out," namely in such a wide range of interesting, easily learned, general bodily exercises so various as to require voluntary effort to acquire them and as not to become monotonous and altogether mechanical. It seems to us indeed that the medical profession must welcome Dr. Sargent's little book as a substantial, because practicable, contribution to the aids to longer and more vigorous and happy living. It inculcates and well illustrates that harmonious adjustment of part to part and of part to whole wherein bodily health chiefly consists. And in a vast majority of cases it is

only necessary to keep the bodies vigorously well and the minds will find no excuse to quarrel with the evils of a world even as wearisome as this,— for thus, fortunately, are we created.

PAVLOW AND DIGESTIVE PHYSIOLOGY.

THE recent announcement of the award of one of the Nobel prizes to Professor Pavlow, Professor of Experimental Medicine at the Imperial Institute of St. Petersburg, brings once more into prominence the work of a man who has done more perhaps than any other in our generation to throw light on the complex processes of digestion. His experiments and observations included every portion of the digestive tract from the salivary glands to the intestines, and on every one of them he has succeeded in shedding new light.

While it is not generally realized the progress thus made is much more significant for clinical medicine than advances, so-called, in physiology usually have been. His observations have shown especially the importance of the individual element, of what the difference in the preparation of food and in the form in which it is consumed means to the digestive tract, and how wonderfully varied can be the reaction of various digestive glands not alone to food itself, but to the varying conditions of food administration.

An excellent example of the character of his work is to be seen in his investigations with regard to the salivary glands. Notwithstanding the fact that the mouth is said to water when particularly pleasing food is presented to an animal, practically no saliva at all appears in the mouth of the dog during the eating of raw meat, though the dog relishes this class of food very much. If the raw meat, however, be given powdered, then saliva is secreted in large quantities. The same thing is true for all forms of dry food, so that the secretion from the parotid gland at least is dependent not upon the kind of food, but on the form in which it is consumed. If small stones are given to the dog, there is no secretion of saliva, even though he may play with them in his mouth and apparently thus be sure to excite salivary secretion. On the other hand, if sand be given, there will be a large amount of watery saliva secreted, evidently in order to help the animal in getting rid of the offensive material. Almost the same observations can be substantiated with regard to the submaxillary gland, and it is evident that a large amount of watery saliva means not so much a help to digestion, as an effort of nature to get rid of materials in the mouth that are not easy to swallow.

With regard to the glands of the stomach, very interestingly varied secretive reactions to various kinds of food are found. If to dogs meat be given, then a gastric juice containing the highest degree of acidity is secreted. For a milk diet a distinctly lessened degree of acidity of the gastric juice is always to be observed, while for food composed mainly of cereal products, the lowest amount of acid is secreted. In a word, the character of the gastric secretion is specific for each kind of food. The character of the secretion is different also as regards the length of time and the rate at which it appears. When the main element of the feeding is bread, the secretion continues for nearly ten hours. With milk it lasts for only six hours, and the meat gastric secretion is for an intermediate time. With meat, the maximum of secretion is reached toward the end of the second hour. With bread the maximum occurs during the first hour, while with milk it is during the third hour. It is thus seen that the stomach reacts in its own way with a sort of instinct, and that hard and fast lines as to the character of the stomach secretion cannot be drawn without great risk of error, unless the specific reaction in the individual has been observed.

It has been the custom of physiologists generally to insist that the mechanical irritation caused by food is sufficient to arouse gastric secretion. Such experiments conducted under Professor Pavlow's direction seem to prove entirely futile. Irritation, for instance, with a feather, or with a quantity of sand, though the mucous membrane of the stomach might be expected to be particularly susceptible to such forms of irritation, do not give rise to a single drop of secretion. The reason for the mistakes in the older cases was that the psychic element which entered into all digestive processes had not been eliminated with sufficient care. If a dog is placed in the neighborhood of food, then a certain amount of secretion in preparation for that particular kind of food is sure to take place. This element of the digestive function Professor Pavlow has put on a clearer plane than ever before, though showing that it is not so important as some of the exaggerated notions have suggested.

The digestive mucous membrance has, in Professor Pavlow's experience, a distinctively selective action and sort of capacity for recognizing the qualities of substances presented to it. Any one stomachic selective action may be the result of innate natural qualities or may be acquired. Digestion thus becomes eminently individual in character, and the existence so commonly noted of likes and dislikes, whose influence for facile digestion or the opposite, becomes easier to understand. It is not so much that the gastric juice may be lacking in some important element, but that the specific reaction of the digestive glands which furnishes just the proper gastric juice for a special kind and form of food is lacking, that constitutes the problem of digestive disturbances. This takes away much of the value of the investigation of stomach chemism, always an unsatisfactory subject, but it sends us back to the clinical study of the patient once more, and this is ever a fruitful field for important and enduring progress.

A LARGE ORDER.

THERE was a time in the history of medicine when the physician was chemist, botanist, pharmacist and healer. But that was many, many years ago. Since that time social relations have become very complex, but none more so than the relations of pharmacy to medicine.

We venture to assert that there are few, if any, physicians or pharmacists, or bodies of the same, who are conversant with the many complicating phases of these relations.

From time to time certain features that concern the medical profession very closely have received no small amount of criticism on the part of reformers, and sporadic attempts have been made to adjust certain questions which have been deemed prejudicial to the best interests of medicine.

One of these problems has concerned the ethical stand that the profession, as a whole, should adopt toward the exploitation of proprietary remedies. At first sight it seems an easy problem to solve, but in reality it has shown itself to be one of extreme difficulty to grasp in its entirety. A beginning, however, has to be made, and the most radical step that has thus far been contemplated has been recently outlined by the *Journal of the American Medical Association* (March 4, 1905).

Writing on " The Secret Nostrum *vs.* The

Ethical Proprietary Preparation," it plunges at once into one side of the subject with a courage that deserves praise and an insight that commands the highest respect for its intelligent grasp of an intricate social question.

A sharp distinction is drawn between the "patent medicine," which is exploited to the public, and the "proprietary" manufactured for the physician's use—not a distinction, however, from one point of view, since both are "patented," or "copyrighted," as to name or as to contents. With the so-called "patent medicines" we have nothing to do. A careless government permits their exploitation and we may have our opinions as to their effect on the people, but with that side of the question the *Journal* does not at this time concern itself. It would examine the other group, the group which it proposes to consider was originally intended as examples of elegant preparations of standard formulæ and were expected to reflect the advances of the pharmaceutic art, but in many instances they have, in late years, fallen from grace, and are neither a credit to their makers nor is their use a credit to the intelligence of the prescriber.

But degrees of degeneration are inevitable, since biological laws hold sway even in commercial evolution, and how may the sheep and the goats be separated is the problem at hand.

For more than a year the officers of the Association have considered the plan which they offer —namely, a "Council on Pharmacy and Chemistry" composed of fifteen members, all reputable men, who will examine the "composition and status of the various medicinal preparations that are offered to physicians and which are not included in the United States Pharmacopœia or in other standard text-books or formularies." Such examination is to be thorough and exhaustive, else it is of little value. This Council is to prepare a book on "New and Non-Official Remedies," to be published by the *Journal,* which shall "supply necessary and desirable information concerning those which it considers unobjectionable." Such information is made in accordance with ten rules which we publish in our news column in this issue, page 511. The Council will not pass judgment on the therapeutic value, but on the ethical status only of these preparations. Pharmacologic and therapeutic data are, however, to be included.

Such in brief is the scheme of the *Journal* of the Association to bring some light out of the present darkness.

That we as practising physicians need light there is not the slightest doubt, and we welcome most heartily the effort on the part of the *Journal* to pull our chestnuts out of the ethical fire. We are at one with it in its efforts to in any manner improve certain unfortunate tendencies in modern pharmaceutical practices, and while we feel that the plan outlined has many admirable features, we regret that the Association has been hastened in its formulation by the cackle of some young and eager reformers, and has presented to us a scheme which we believe to be very incomplete and one that will lend itself to much injustice, to distrust and to misconception.

It will be impossible to prejudge such a comprehensive plan in its entirety, but certain points that appear on the surface offer themselves for discussion, since "criticism and suggestion will be welcome."

If the book "does not pass judgment on therapeutic value," and yet is to be "an accessible authoritative work of reference," why include therapeutic data, particularly if the first edition is to be hurried and to contain only a small portion of the field? Does the Council recognize how big the field is likely to be, and is the Association to furnish the funds to pay for a small army of analysts? One "competent chemist" is ludicrously inadequate. Organic analyses are not things of a day or a week.

May we suggest that we are under the impression that certain of the members of the Council are known to be the "Consulting Chemists" for some manufacturing houses, a fact not reprehensible in itself, yet certainly not a desirable factor.

While the Council enumerated is to pass judgment on the status of the preparations more particularly from the standpoint of the contents, we would like to see some practising physicians on the list of the Council.

Laboratory pharmacologists and chemists are too far away from the problems of the practice of medicine to enjoy the confidence of the practitioners of the country. It is true that a subsidiary staff of medical consultants "is to be formed," but nothing should be done until the staff is formed," and if therapeutic data are to be included, certain of their number should be on the Council to keep it along practical lines—not figure-heads, and above all, not men well known to be so busy that they hardly have time to eat between consultations, and who go through their wards in a whirlwind.

Other problems arise by the score; they must be thrashed out one by one, and we defer them until a later time. We are in most hearty accord with the hopes of the *Journal* in its proposed plan. We trust, however, that it will make haste slowly, else by foolish counsel a worthy conception may end in abortion.

ECHOES AND NEWS.

NEW YORK.

Meningitis Increasing.—According to the report of the Board of Health for last week, the total of all diseases except meningitis decreased, as compared with the previous week. Epidemic cerebrospinal meningitis showed an increase. There were 57 deaths from this cause last week, against 49 for the previous week, in the Borough of Manhattan alone. In the whole city the number of deaths from the cause last week was 78.

Resign from Lying-In Hospital.—A governor, a director, three deputy directors, five attending physicians, and two pathologists have resigned from the management of the Lying-in Hospital, at Seventeenth Street and Second Avenue, as a result of dissatisfaction with the methods of Dr. J. W. Markoe, the governor, who is most closely allied with J. Pierpont Morgan, who built and partly endowed the hospital. Dr. Markoe has always been a figure of importance in the institution, and since the absence in Europe of the superintendent, Dr. W. H. Spiller, has been more powerful than ever. Several of the younger doctors connected with the hospital, are said to have complained that his treatment of them was not such as was called for by professional etiquette. As a protest against these conditions, the following resignations have been sent to the board of governors: Richard T. H. Halsey, governor; Dr. H. McN. Painter, director, Dr. R. C. James, Dr. A. E. Brown, and Dr. W. S. Stone, deputy directors: Dr Robert Watts, Jr., Dr. Fellowes Davis, Jr., Dr. Percy H. Williams, Dr. James I. Russell, and Dr. A. S. Morrow, attending physicians, and Drs. Walstein and Farley, pathologists.

Medical Inspectors Organize.—At a meeting of the Medical Inspectors of Schools of the Health Department of the City of New York, held on Friday, March 3, 1905, at the Academy of Medicine, a society was organized for the promotion of good fellowship, and the study of problems of hygiene and public health, under the name of the Society of Medical Inspectors of the City of New York. Medical inspectors of any of the divisions of the department, and in any of the boroughs, are eligible to membership. The first meeting was held under the auspices of a Committee on Organization, headed by Dr. Edward M. Thompson, as Chairman, who presided at the meeting. A constitution was adopted and the following officers were elected: President, Dr. Augustine C. McGuire; Vice-President, Dr. Otto Jahn; Secretary, Dr. Edward M. Thompson; Treasurer, Dr. Leopold Marcus. Executive Committee: Dr. Joseph Baum (Chairman), Dr. Helen Knight, Dr. Samuel A. Buchenholtz, Dr. Thomas A. Neafsey and Dr. DeSantos Saxe. The society will hold monthly meetings and will invite the higher officers of the Department, as well as other sanitarians of repute, to address it on various special topics.

Scientific papers will also be read by members, and good fellowship will be promoted by means of annual dinners, etc.

Pure Food in New York.—Under the above caption the New York *Times* prints this editorial: "Men become doubtful of the system of government of which they naturally desire to be proud when the only way in which a bill establishing standards of purity in food can be passed is to make it a party measure and pass it—not because it is right and will make for good, but because it can be turned to party advantage. Recent investigations by the Department of Agriculture show very clearly that the country is flooded with food preparations unfitted for use and involving more or less danger to life and health. The bills drafted to safeguard the public interest in this respect, through the regulation of inter-State commerce, were defeated in the United States Senate by a lobby so powerful that it made of no effort the clearest proof that such laws were imperatively demanded to check the inter-State traffic in adulterated and poisoned food preparations. These same investigations further showed that the laws of New York are deficient in this respect and do not adequately protect the consumer against expedients in dilution and adulteration from which he suffers more than pecuniary injury. The Health Committee of the New York State Senate seems to recognize its duty in this matter, and will report a bill which it hopes to pass by making it a party measure. It will endeavor to make the present regulations more effective by fixing specific standards to which merchandise of this character must conform. Such a law should be passed, even if incomplete and in certain details unintelligent, but there should be a higher reason for passing it than that a partisan advantage may be gained therefrom. However, this may be an instance in which the result is of more consequence than the method by which it is reached. New York State should lead in legislation of this character. As it is, it is far behind many States of less commercial consequence."

Some Aspects of Commercialism.—The *Evening Post* in commenting on professional commercialism and the evil of the spread of the money-making spirit, writes:

"The evil also spreads from commercial life, where making money is the avowed ideal, to the professions, in which there is presumably a somewhat less selfish aim. A lawyer who would plan and help to execute a fraud on the Government is obviously unfit for the bench; and yet a special meeting of the State Bar Association was necessary in order to muster a majority against whitewashing Justice Warren B. Hooker. The medical profession boasts a very strict code of ethics. Curiously enough, according to *American Medicine*, the physicians of Providence are receiving the following letter from a company which manufactures drugs:

Dear Doctor:—"There are a few physicians in Providence that have not taken advantage of our recent, liberal, profit-sharing offer, and we regret to say that you are one of them. This ought not to be so. The plan should appeal to you, as nothing is asked of you but what is strictly ethical, namely, prescribe our preparation whenever indicated only when you believe it to be equal or better than any other similar preparation. See that your patient gets the genuine article, keep a memorandum on the blank sent you, and when full, sign and send to us, receiving in return our check for $10.' A very simple matter, and as one physician wrote us, after having received several such checks, 'your plan is a good one and ought to be productive of good returns both to the company and to the physicians.' We agree with him. Do you?

Hoping to hear from you, we remain,

Fraternally yours,

"——— ——— ———,"

Evidently enough doctors are working for this 'strictly ethical' graft to make it worth while for the company. If this circular means anything, it means that in the presence of some physicians the old jest about an alliance with the druggist and the undertaker is twitting on facts."

PHILADELPHIA.

Election of Resident Physicians.—The following members of the senior class of the University have been elected as resident physicians, each to serve two years in the University of Pennsylvania Hospital: Eldridge L. Eliason, S. W. Moorhead, G. M. Pearsol, Frederick Prime, Jr., and H. G. Schleiter.

Sale of Patent Medicines to be Curtailed.—Senator Charles L. Brown will introduce a bill into the legislature which provides to regulate the sale of patent and proprietary medicines containing alcohol. According to the bill no person, firm or corporation shall sell any of these medicines except upon a written prescription from a regularly registered physician.

Court's View of Insanity.—In giving instructions to the jury, how to discriminate between a crime committed by an insane person and one who pretends insanity, Judge Schwartz, of Norristown, said: "A man may act queer and talk foolish, yet if he knows the difference between right and wrong, if he can restrain himself from committing wrong acts, when he wants to, the law will not excuse him if he commits a crime."

Governor Vetoes Food Bill.—The bill which prohibited the sale of fruit syrups prepared fruits and fruit products containing more than one-fourth of one per cent. of sodium benzoate or the same amount of color obtained from harmless vegetable substances, was vetoed by the Governor upon the ground that this bill contained nothing which is not in the Act of 1895 bearing upon this subject. The Governor holds this bill unconstitutional because it repeals an act but does not refer to the act which is to be repealed.

The Pennsylvania State Veterinary Association.—At the annual meeting of this organization, Dr. Leonard Pearson, of the University of Pennsylvania, read a paper entitled "Vaccination of Cattle against Tuberculosis." In this paper he gave an account of the experiments of injecting into 100 heads of cattle virulent bacilli of bovine tuberculosis. Recently four of the injected animals and two not injected were killed. The six head having been stabled for two years with highly tuberculous cows. At the post mortem he found that the injected cows were free from the disease, while those not injected were tuberculous.

Panama and Yellow Fever.—In a lecture before the College Club, Miss Dora Keen, after giving a description of Panama and Colon and pointing out the enormous undertaking of the canal to be constructed, called her hearers' attention to the sanitary problem before this country. She informed the audience that yellow fever was the most difficult

question to be solved. Owing to the inadequate supply, much of the water must be brought from the interior of the country in tanks which are, in many instances, allowed to stand uncovered in the open air, consequently favorable sites for the develpment of mosquitoes are established. Then too, she points out, that in order to limit the travels of the ants, the legs of chairs and tables are placed in cans or cups of water; these serve also for breeding places.

Philadelphia Pathological Society.—This society meeting was held March 9, 1905. The scientific discussion was opened by Dr. Allen J. Smith who, with R. S. Beeder, presenting specimens of the *Solenophorus megacephalus.*" Dr. Smith, in the course of his talk, stated that this was a parasite of the snake. The head of the parasite has two cups which are tubular, and each opens into an alimentary canal. This parasite, he said, was described in 1825, and since that time at least 25 other authors have written of it. He stated that the worm is slender, measures sometimes seven inches in length. The links are broader than they are long, except toward the end of the parasite they are nearly round. He has never seen the eggs. All the links which he obtained were sterile. The suckers, he merely suggests may have a cell lining, which secrete a toxic substance that is responsible for the anemias which occur in the parasitic diseases. Dr. H. R. Alburger presented (1) Secondary Sarcoma of the Liver. Of this growth, he said, the primary tumor was in the eye where it has been seen ten years before death. (2) Hypertrophy of one Kidney and Atrophy of the Opposite Organ." From his talk it was elicited that the latter is to be regarded as a hypoplasia instead of an atrophy. (3) Amyloid Disease of the Liver Due to Potts' Disease. Dr. H. Fox then read a paper on "The Nature of Paratyphoid Fever and Its Allied Infections." During the course of his paper he referred to an instance where the paratyphoid "B" was isolated for gallstones. The frequency of the two types of the disease are five cases of the paratyphoid 'B'" to 1 of the "A." Hemorrhage is more frequent in the type due to the "A" bacillus; "B" often produces suppuration while "A" may suppurate. The "B" bacillus, he said, stands nearer the bacteria of meat poisoning. Shotmüller and one other author, he stated, have found interagglutination of the paratyphoid "B" and "A" and the *Bacillus typhosus*, which incident he has found in his experiments and observations. The bacillus paratyphoid "A" resembles the *Bacillus typhosus,* while the paratyphoid "B" produces a condition very much like septicemia. Dr. Riesman exhibited four specimens of "Ulcerative Endocarditis." The first case presented symptoms like typhoid fever, at one time the patient developed severe pains in the abdomen, and the diagnosis of perforation was considered. His second case was purely cardiac in type, while the third presented symptoms of pyemia.

Philadelphia Medical Examiners' Association.—The meeting of this organization was held March 7, 1905. Dr. E. H. Hammill, medical director of the Prudential Insurance Co., addressed the society upon what he entitled "Cullings from the Desk." He spoke of the following: (1) The Responsibility the Medical Examiner Bears to the Company. He dwelled upon that point but a short time. (2) Perfunctory Service was the next point. He would discard the printed blank because it tends to make the examiner mechanical, so that he neglects orig-

inality. (3) Latitude of Inquiry. He claims that
Medical examiners are too narrow; they neglect to
ask questions which should have been asked but
were omitted because they were not specified in the
blank. Here again, he asserts that the blank is a
disadvantage. He maintains that 20 per cent. of the
cases reported at the home office need further correspondence because the reports sent lack points
that need emphasizing. (4) The Moral Hazard of
the Applicant. The information necessary to clear
up this matter can be obtained from the environ-
ments, business, home, and manner of dress of the
applicant. This point many examiners fail to consider. (5) Haste of Conducting Examinations. He
spoke of the bad risks that are assumed by the
company as a result of it. (6) Incomplete Medical
Reports. Further communication consumes time
and may produce prejudice. (7) Insufficient Inform-
tion in the Report. This, he said, places the director
at the home office to take too much for granted. (8)
Occupation of the Hazard. Very often the name of
the occupation is too technical, so that the director
has not the slightest idea of character of the applicant's work. (9) Height and Weight. Upon
this point examiners left too much unsaid. They
do not designate how much below or how much
above the standard table. (10) Examiner's Lack of
Knowledge of the Home Office, Usage and the Instruction Book. (11) He laid a great deal of stress
upon legible writing. (12) He urges that concise
statements be given. (13) Relation of the Agent to
the Examiner. This should be cordial and can be
accomplished and maintained by diplomacy on the
part of the examiner. (14) Thoughtful Advice.
This will assist the director very often in deciding
what to do with an applicant. (15) Prompt replies
are of great benefit to both the examiner and the
home office. (16) He advised the examiners to visit
the home office whenever possible. (17) He cautioned the examiners about giving the agent knowledge of the examination, and reticence of the cases
to be examined. (18) He thought that the home
office should be advised at what time the patient
was examined and at what time the report was
mailed. (19) He dwelled long upon the identity of the
applicant, this can be done by means of a card, occupation, manners, letters or initial on the clothes.
A lengthy discussion followed.

Philadelphia County Medical Society.—The meeting of the organization was held March 8, 1905.
The scientific part of the meeting was opened by
Dr. Charles W. Burr, who "Exhibited a Patient
with an Old Fracture of the Cervical Spine." He
informed the society that the patient fell from a
wagon in 1898, from which fall he was made unconscious for some time, and when he regained
consciousness he was found paralyzed in the arms,
but had slight motion in the legs. Priapism did
not occur. When Dr. Burr saw him some time
later he could walk but could scarcely use his arms.
There was some disturbance of the bladder muscles,
which improved later. After a long stay in the hospital he gained considerable strength in his arms,
and when he left could use them fairly well. After
leaving he had several attacks of severe pain in
the arms and shoulders and back but these soon
passed away. At the present time the patient has a
traumatic pachymeningitis of the cord. The X-ray
pictures taken showed a fracture of the fifth cervical spine and lamina, a forward displacement of
the fourth and backward displacement of the fifth

cervical vertebra. Dr. J. Madison Taylor then read
a paper on "How Can the General Practitioner
Profit by Preventive Medicine." In considering this
question he maintained that preventive medicine
could not be succesfuly accomplished until the physicians and the people cooperated, not until the
doctors are so skilful that they can predict that
certain conditions in the individual will lead to disease, and not until they are able to recognize pro-
dones of disease. He suggests that physicians be
allowed access to homes to examine members of the
family that are apparently in health with the view
of determining derangements which may lead to
disease. Especially should this be done with children. Doctors should be allowed to go to the nursery. The physicians acting as inspectors of the
public schools, he thinks, should have greater authority. He condemned very strongly the use of
what are known as tonics. and he also condemned
narcotics and the use of proprietary preparations.
Dr. W. Wayne Babcock read a paper on "The
Osmic Acid Treatment in Tic Douloureux." He
stated that although many failures, cases have been
injected with this substance with complete anesthesia and relief of the pain for periods of time varying
in length, some being four years. There is no danger of absorption of the osmic acid. The nerve is
exposed and the aqueous solution is injected directly into the nerve trunk at different points and it
is advisable, he said, to inject some at the foramen where the nerve escapes from the skull. The
operation can de done through the mouth
so that no scarring results. The last paper
was read by D. G. B. Harlan on "Problems
of the Treatment of Tuberculosis of the Larynx. He maintained that the tuberculous condition
in the larynx is most frequent on the cords and the
arytenoid folds. He announced that this condition
affected the larynx as (1) a superficial ulcer; (2)
infiltration of the mucosa: (3) tuberculoma; (4)
deep ulceration. When in tuberculosis the larynx
is affected by no other disease the prognosis is good.
He reported an obstinate case of tuberculosis of the
larynx, which was treated with the X-ray; the results were very good. Upon the ulcers he applies
lactic acid.

CHICAGO.

Dr. Lydston Honored.—Dr. G. Frank Lydston
was recently elected a Fellow of the London Society of Authors.

Hospital Fire.—On March 2, a fire broke out in
the Chicago Union Hospital. during which the
nurses and attendants carried fourteen patients safely from the burning building, and then assisted in
preventing the spread of the flames until the fire
companies arrived. The extent of damage to the
building was about $25,000.

Medical Bills Introduced into the Senate and House
of Illinois.—A bill (No. 171) providing for the appointment on the State Board of Health of two regular. one homeopathic, one eclectic, one physiomedical and one osteopathic member, has been
favorably reported on by the Committee on Judiciary Department and Practice. Senate Bill No.
171, revising the present medical practice act, and
providing for the regulation of regular, homeopathic. eclectic. physiomedical and osteopathic practice, is being considered by the Committee on License and Miscellany. Senate Bill No. 225, for an
act to establish a State Board of Examiners of

Registered Nurses, and Senate Bill 226, for an act to regulate the practice of dental surgery, have been approved by the committees to which they were referred. Dr. M. G. Reynolds, of Aledo, Ill., a member of the State Legislature, has introduced a bill making it the duty of the State Board of Health to see that diphtheria antitoxin be kept in each county seat in the State for sale to physicians, and that supplies be furnished to the poor free of charge on the order of the overseer of the poor. The State Board of Health has endorsed this bill.

GENERAL.

University of Michigan.—Founders' Day, the anniversary of the founding of the medical department at the University of Michigan, was celebrated February 22 by the Medical Society. The meeting was held in Sarah Caswell Angell Hall. A portrait of the late Dr. A. B. Palmer was presented to the University.

Medical Study Tour in Germany.—The medical study tour in Germany this year will start from Munich on September 13. The tour will comprise visits to the following watering places and health resorts: Ischl, Reichenhall, Berchtesgaden, Gastein, Gossenass, Levico, Roncegno, Riva, Gardone, Solo, Arco and Meran, where the tourists will arrive in time for the meeting of the German Association of Scientists and Physicians which is to be held there this year.

Society of Medical Phonographers.—The January number of the Phonographic Record of Clinical Teaching and Medical Science, which is now issued quarterly instead of monthly as formerly, contains a paper by Mr. G. W. Cathcart, dealing with the subject of recent methods of diagnosing the relative conditions of the two kidneys in surgery, which is well worth study, and one by Sir William Gowers on syphilitic disease of the brain. The number also contains the annual report of the Honorary Secretary, Dr. Fletcher Beach, of the Society of Medical Phonographers, which shows that, although the society is doing good work, it is in want of new members, who may be either qualified medical men or students.

Russian Universities.—The festal celebration arranged in honor of the one hundred and fiftieth anniversary of the foundation of the University of Moscow, which fell on January 25, was postponed, writes the British Medical Journal, on account of the disturbed state of the political atmosphere. At the beginning of the present year the total number of students was 5,489; of these 1,349 belonged to the Faculty of Medicine. The teaching staff comprised 72 ordinary and 17 extraordinary professors; of the former category 25, and of the latter 9, belonged to the medical faculty. The University of Charkoff completed its first century of existence on January 27, but, as at Moscow, the anniversary was allowed to pass without formal celebration. The number of students is 1,486.

Need Not Wed Infected Person.—"If tuberculosis is an infectious disease which passes from parent to offspring, then it is against public policy for such marriages to be permitted, and no person should be mulcted in damages who breaks a promise he has made to marry such an affected person." That was the opinion rendered by Superior Judge Albertson yesterday in passing upon a motion to strike out an interrogation propounded to Rosena Grover by Mayor Zook, of Ballard, in a suit in which the young woman seeks to recover from him $5,000 damages for breach of promise. In the answer filed by the Mayor he admitted that he had promised to marry the woman, and would have done so had he not discovered, after the promise was made, that she was affected with tuberculosis.

Medical Sociology.—A society for the study of questions of social medicine and hygiene and medical statistics was formally constituted in Berlin on February 16 at a meeting attended by a large number of medical practitioners, political economists and sociologists. Prof. Mayer, of the Imperial Statistical Bureau, Dr. Dietrich, of the Russian Cultus-Ministry, and Prof. Lassar were elected presidents. Dr. Rudolph Lennhoff, editor of the *Medizinische Reform*, and Dr. A. Grotjahn, medical editor of the *Jahresberichte für soziale Hygiene und Demographie*, was appointed secretaries, and Dr. George Heimann, of the Statistical Office of the city of Berlin, treasurer. The membership of the new society already amounts to 89, and includes medical practitioners, official statisticians, and persons interested in social politics.

Cremation in France.—The report recently presented by MM. Georges Salomon and Bourneville to the Société pour la Propagation de l'Incineration states that the number of bodies cremated in France increases year by year. The total number of cremations carried out in Paris from August 5, 1889, when the method first came into use in France, to December 31, 1903, is given as 67,286. While the total for 1890 was 3,388 that for 1903 was 6,654. It must be pointed out, however, that these figures, taken at their face value, give a very misleading impression as to the progress of cremation in France. In one-half of the total number of cases, the remains cremated were limbs and other fragments of humanity from the hospitals, and of the other half a large proportion consisted of stillborn children and fetuses. Of cremations in the proper sense the total number was 3,151; the number of dead persons whose bodies were disposed of in this manner, which was 46 in 1889, rose in 1903 to 306.

Clinical Meeting at the Massachusetts General Hospital.—A clinical meeting was held March 10, at the Massachusetts General Hospital. Dr. J. G. Mumford presided. Dr. Arthur Cabot showed a case of sarcoma of the prostate and described the very few other cases which he had been able to find in the hospital records. The symptoms, operation, pathology and results were carefully gone over.

Dr. James M. Jackson spoke on Neutral Bromide of Quinine in the Treatment of Exophthalmic Goiter. He showed five cases, the severest ones, which he had had under this treatment. All except one who had not followed treatment faithfully were markedly improved. He gave the results in detail in the 50 cases he had seen, and in the 25 which he had been able to follow through in detail. He did not claim any specific action for bromide of quinine, but thought that it did work better than any remedy which he had yet found.

Dr. R. H. Fitz spoke on Pericardial Paracentesis. He had looked up the cases in the hospital, and those in which the condition was found not diagnosed at autopsy. He described in detail a case in which although the signs were unmistakably those of a large pericardial effusion, yet after repeated tapping nothing was found. After death a needle was put in the xyphoid angle and a pint of pus obtained. On autopsy that remarkable and rare condition was found, an interpleural lipoma of large size, which had prevented all former attempts at tappings from succeeding. He described one other case of this condition. Dr. E. A. Codman gave a preliminary report in a paper on Periarthritis of the Shoulder Joint, showing several patients.

Dr. Oscar Richardson spoke on the bacteriological basis of the surgical technic in wounds infected with tetanus. He described some experiments which he had done along this line.

Dr. C. L. Scudder spoke on Stenosis of the Pylorus in infancy.

French Doctors before Molière.—In an article on French doctors before Molière, which appears in the *Practitioner* for February, it is stated that the practice of wholesale bleeding was introduced in the fifteenth century by Leonardo Botalli, who was physician to Charles IX. and Henry III. If a man was ill he was bled to let out the evil humors; if he was well, to prevent their formation. It was an accepted dogma of the medicine of the day that the human body contained twenty-four pounds of blood, of which twenty pound could be withdrawn without causing death. Botalli being asked whether the removal of so much blood did not weaken people, replied that the more stagnant water was withdrawn from a well the more fresh pure water came up: the more a nurse suckled a child the more milk she had. Even so, he held, was it in regard to the blood. Strong young men were bled every month, old people from four to six times a year. Ambroise Paré bled a man of twenty-eight years 27 times in four days, and records the fact "to encourage the young surgeon not to be timid in drawing blood in cases of acute inflammation." Louis XIII. was bled 47 times in one year by his physician Bouvard, and in the reign of Louis XIV. that "sanguinary pedant" Gui Patin, boasts in his correspondence of his exploits with the lancet. He calls bleeding "one of the principal mysteries of our art." He showed the strength of his faith in the mystery by ordering his wife to be bled 12 times in the course of a pneumonia and his son 20 times during a continued fever. He bled an infant three days old and a child of seven years 13 times in a fortnight. Patin had himself bled seven times for a common cold, and he relates like things of other physicians. He records with indignation that a physician—Guy de Labrosse—died without having been bled. Venesection had been suggested, but the dying man preferred to die unbled. For this Patin treats him as a blasphemer—and worse. "The Devil," he says, "will bleed him in the other world as he deserves to be—the scoundrel, the atheist!"

Council on Pharmacy and Chemistry.—The following ten rules are adopted to guide the Council on Pharmacy and Chemistry of the American Medical Association: (The term "article" shall mean any drug, chemical or preparation used in the treatment of disease.)

Rule 1.—No article will be admitted unless its active medicinal ingredients and the amounts of such ingredients in a given quantity of the article, be furnished for publication. (Sufficient information should be supplied to permit the Council to verify the statements made regarding the article, and to determine its status from time to time.)

Rule 2.—No chemical compound will be admitted unless information be furnished regarding tests for identity, purity and strength, and, if a synthetic compound, the rational formula.

Rule 3.—No article that is advertised to the public will be admitted; but this rule will not apply to disinfectants, cosmetics, foods and mineral waters, except when advertised in an objectionable manner.

Rule 4.—No article will be admitted whose label, package or circular accompanying the package contains the names of diseases, in the treatment of which the article is indicated. The therapeutic indications, properties and doses may be stated. (This rule does not apply to vaccines and antitoxins nor to advertising in medical journals, nor to literature distributed solely to physicians.)

Rule 5.—No article will be admitted or retained about which the manufacturer, or his agents, make false or misleading statements regarding the country of origin, raw material from which made, method of collection or preparation.

Rule 6.—No article will be admitted or retained about whose therapeutic value the manufacturer, or his agents, make unwarranted, exaggerated, or misleading statements.

Rule 7.—Labels on articles containing "heroic" or "poisonous" substances should show the amounts of each of such ingredients in a given quantity of the product.

Rule 8.—Every article should have a name or title indicative of its chemical composition or pharmaceutic character, in addition to its trade name, when such trade name is not sufficiently descriptive.

Rule 9.—If the name of an article is registered, or the label copyrighted, the date of registration should be furnished the Council.

Rule 10.—If the article is patented—either process or product—the number and date of such patent or patents should be furnished. If patented in other countries, the name of each country in which patent is held should be supplied, together with the name under which the article is there registered.

Boston Medical Library.—The meetings of this society, in conjunction with the Suffolk District Branch of the Massachusetts Medical Society, was held at the Library, March 1, on the general subject, "The Surgery of Renal and Ureteral Calculi." Dr. B. F. Harrington was in the chair. Dr. J. H. Cunningham, Jr., spoke on the actual results of cases at the Boston City Hospital. Dr. Hugh Cabot reported the results obtained at the Massachusetts General Hospital. Dr. H. F. Hewes spoke on the diagnosis of renal calculi from examination of the urine, and Dr. Benjamin Tenney discussed other means of diagnosis. Dr. Paul Thorndike approached the subject from the point of view of the operation for renal and ureteral stone.

On March 8, the last meeting of the Boston Medical Library, in conjunction with the Massachusetts Medical Society was held. Dr. Geo. W. Gay presided. Dr. John H. McCollom gave a long and interesting report of nine years' experience in the treatment of diphtheria with antitoxin at the South Department of the Boston City Hospital. He first went over the history of the disease, the discovery of antitoxin, the violent opposition to it at first and its gradually increasing use. By means of carefully prepared charts, he demonstrated the wonderful results in lowering the former frightful mortality in this disease. He spoke at length on the relative merits of intubation and of tracheotomy in cases of laryngeal diphtheria, showing results by means of charts. Both operations were discussed and described. Antitoxin, dosage effects, and the resulting skin lesions were carefully described. The effects on house officers and nurses of their stay in the infectious wards was spoken of.

Prof. William T. Sedgwick, of the Massachusetts Institute of Technology, next spoke on the Present State of Opinion Concerning Sewer Gas and its Effects. He spoke of sanitation and its history, the rivalry between the two schools, headed respectively by Koch and by Pettenkoffer, of Munich, and the effects of the teaching of these schools on the subject of sewers and sewer gas. He described the advancement of house sanitation up to a certain stage; then the sudden sickness of a very prominent family in a dwelling where the plumbing was defective, the results of this on the public mind, and the marked reaction that followed ending in the putting up of sewer gas as a cause of almost any disease. At present in the minds of quite the majority of people a normal state had been reached, and the public realized as well as the profession that, first, there is no such thing as sewer gas, a distinct entity, and, second, that air from a sewer is not necessarily and usually is not found to be more impure or as impure as air found in most dwellings to-day.

In the discussion that followed these two papers, Dr. Thomas M. Rotch told about the results of the use of antitoxin in the children's and the infants' hospitals, and described how the present state of affairs had been reached, whereby it was considered best to give antitoxin every twenty-one days to every patient entering the hospital.

Dr. David Cheever, in a most interesting five-minute talk described the changes that had taken place during his own professional career in the treatment of diphtheria. Dr. F. H. Williams spoke on the subject of tracheotomy versus intubation, advising the former in cases in the country far from skilled medical help, and when careful nursing and watching could not be obtained.

Dr. Charles Harrington spoke on the subject of the cause of the dread of sewer gas. He thought that the Pettenkoffer school was not at all to blame for this state of affairs, but that it was due to an unfortunate coincidence.

The Isthmian Canal Commission's Mismanagement in Sanitation.—Dr. Charles A. L. Reed, on his return from Panama, March 1, filed his report with the Secretary of War, and the report is printed in full in *Journal A. M. A.*, March 11. Dr. Reed states that he has given every facility to study the condition of organization and the details of administration as they relate to the public health interest. He says that he was impressed with the efficiency and zeal of the sanitary staff and with the fact that much has been accomplished in the way of sanitation, but states that much remains to be done which can not be done unless better facilities are afforded. He states that the governments of Panama and of the United States both recognize the importance of efficient sanitation. At the meeting of the commission held at Ancon, August 28, 1904, Mr. Grunsky, as the committee on a proposed health department, presented a report, which began by stating that "After repeated conferences with" Colonel Gorgas and with practically the entire sanitary staff, "it has been agreed," but which should have stated that "in certain important particulars Mr. Grunsky has agreed with himself," for much of the report was formulated over the respectful protest of the medical men who were invited to the conference. By this report, the commission, more especially Mr. Grun-

sky, provided for the creation of a board of health, with power to formulate regulations, which would become effective only after approval by the Commission, or, in cases of emergency, only on approval of the governor of the canal zone. Thus the chief sanitary officer had his discretion limited to the enforcement of regulations which had first been adopted by the Commission or by a board of health, in which latter event it had to be sent generally to Washington to be endorsed by the Commission, or, in cases of emergency, might be approved or rejected by the governor of the zone. It thus came about, says Dr. Reed, that the chief sanitary officer whom, and whose department, the medical profession had asked to be made largely autonomous, and which the President himself had obviously intended to be so, became, by action of the Commission, more especially of Mr. Grunsky, subordinated to the governor of the zone; to the chief disbursing officer; to the chief of the bureau of material and supplies; to Mr. Grunsky; to the Commission; to the Secretary of War; to the President; subordinated, in fact, in the seventh degree from the original source of authority, and this, says Dr. Reed, is the state of affairs on the Isthmus to-day. Dr. Reed states that if the superintendent of the Ancon Hospital makes a requisition for supplies, he must take it for approval to the chief sanitary officer; then to the governor of the zone; then to the chief disbursing officer; whence it goes to the Commission at Washington; then to Mr. Grunsky as committeeman; then back to the Commission; then, if allowed, bids are advertised for; awards are made; the requisition is filed under the supervision of a purchasing agent notoriously ignorant of the character and quality of medical and surgical supplies; the material is shipped to the Isthmus; consigned to the chief of the bureau of material and supplies; who notifies the disbursing officer; who notifies Colonel Gorgas; who in turn notifies the superintendent; who applies to the quartermaster—"the boss of a corral—for transportation, and so much of the stuff as in the judgment of the first, the governor, next the chief disbursing officer, next the Commission, next and more particularly Mr. Grunsky, ought to be allowed to the superintendent of the hospital, finally arrives or does not arrive at its destination, and this, Dr. Reed says, is no fanciful picture; and what is true at Ancon Hospital is true at Colon, at Culebra, at Miraflores, and at all other points that require supplies of this description. In case of emergency, certain purchases are permitted to be made at Panama, but, of course, at greatly increased prices. Dr. Reed cites examples of the littleness of the Commission, showing how the Commission consumed its time with the minutiæ of administration that ought to have been intrusted to the men employed for that purpose. Dr. Reed states that the Commission visits on the sanitary department unnecessary and unreasonable restraints and confronts it with petty antagonisms, and he quotes instances showing how requests for necessaries have been treated. For instance, doors and windows for the hospital at Culebra were asked for in January, but are not in place. Materials for disinfection work were asked for last September; the Commission, more especially Mr. Grunsky, cut the estimate down to one-fourth, and sent the material in small lots from time to time. The Commission established interneships in the hospitals in the zone, incumbents to be paid $50 a month, the same salary that is paid to nurses, and in this way the sanitary

minute. In addition to these symptoms, there was tremor, general nervousness, sweating and insomnia; also occasional headaches. Dr. Booth said the interesting feature of the case was the early age at which the disease had manifested itself. It was usually observed between the fifteenth and the twenty-fifth or thirtieth year. There were four other children in this patient's family, who were all enjoying good health.

Adenoma of the Pineal Gland, Occluding the Aqueduct of Sylvius, with Escape of Cerebrospinal Fluid Through the Nose and Perforation of the Frontal Horn of the Right Lateral Ventricle.—This case was reported by Dr. Adolf Meyer. The patient was a male. In 1894, when diving, he struck the top of his head. Following this, he complained of headache. He became blind in 1898, with chiasma symptoms. In 1899 he had transitory attacks of numbness on the left side of the face, leaving out part of the area of the middle branch. From that time there was difficulty in moving the lower jaw toward the left. There was no atrophy of the masseter. In August, 1900, cerebrospinal fluid began to drip from the right nostril, with considerable relief of the general symptoms. On the few occasions when the flow stopped, the patient would become sleepy and stuporous for two or three days. During May and October, 1902, the patient, who was then twenty-two years old, had several general convulsions. It was during that year that he was presented by Dr. Meyer at one of the meetings of the New York Neurological Society. In January, 1904, death occurred in a status epilepticus. The only permanent symptoms had been weakness of the left side of the jaw, a small area of loss of pain sensation of the lower corner of the mouth, and subjective numbness in the left side of the tongue. The gait remained normal; the knee jerks were both increased; there was no clonus. At autopsy a tumor was found in the form of an adenoma of the pineal gland. It had pressed itself through the roof of the midbrain behind the posterior commissure, protruding into the third and fourth ventricle and displacing the posterior corpora quadrigemina; the adenoma had practically no sand and but slight pigmentation. The right lateral ventricle had a funnel-shaped depression in the anterior end, with a perforation through the cortex. In the case reported by Wollenberg (*Arch. f. Psychiatrie und Nervenkrankheiten*, 31, p. 206) there was a tumor of the occipital lobes, but there was no occlusion of the ventricle to help account for the perforation. In connection with the case reported by Dr. Meyer, photographs made by Dr. C. I. Lambert were presented, and Dr. C. B. Dunlap demonstrated some microscopic sections.

Dr. Meyer, in reply to a question, said the only motor symptoms the patient presented were those of the masticatory segment, which showed in the deviation of the jaw to the right whenever the mouth was opened. In other words, there was a weakness of the left pterygoid muscles. It was impossible to demonstrate any atrophy of the masseters. There was no motor symptoms referable to the upper extremities.

Case of Old Fracture Dislocation of the Spine.— This case was presented by Dr. J. Ramsay Hunt. The patient was a man forty-five years old, a laborer. Twenty years ago he had a venereal sore followed by a suppurating bubo. He received internal medication for one month. No secondary symptoms were noted. He has had numerous attacks of gonorrhea, followed by the development of strictures. At present a stricture of small caliber existed in the membranous portion of the urethra. In 1895 he met with a severe accident, falling three stories through an airshaft. He was unconscious for a few minutes, and was taken to Bellevue Hospital in

an ambulance. Following the accident, he complained of severe pains in the back, and both legs were paralyzed, although not completely, as he could move them slightly in the bed. It was necessary to catheterize him a few times after the injury, but this difficulty soon passed away. After the accident an angular deformity of the spine was noted, which still exists. It was located about the level of the twelfth dorsal vertebra, and it was safe to assume that the spine had suffered a fracture-dislocation at that point, and that the spinal cord had been injured at the same time. After remaining in bed for two months, the legs began to improve. This improvement continued, and six or seven months later he was able to resume his occupation as a truckdriver, a laborious one, which necessitated the lifting of heavy weights. One year after the injury he was able to do a full day's work, and was suffering no pain or inconvenience. He admitted however that his legs were not quite as limber nor as strong as they were before the accident. He could not run as fast as formerly, owing to a slight stiffness in the knees. There was no sensory nor vesical symptoms during this period. For four years or more the patient remained in this condition. He drove a truck, and led the vigorous outdoor life of a laboring man. About three years ago there developed, very gradually, symptoms of trouble in the lower extremities. He began to complain of sensations of numbness and cold in the feet and legs, accompanied by stiffness and weakness. Upon stooping, he felt a numbness in the lower portion of the back, extending down the posterior thighs and legs. During the past two years these symptoms had progressed slowly and steadily, without any sudden exacerbation, and without acute pain. The left leg was weaker than the right, and it was important that this was true of the initial paralysis and the long period of disability during convalescence. At present the patient's condition is as follows: He had a well-marked kyphosis, the tip of which corresponded to the twelfth dorsal vertebra. Corresponding to this, there was a posterior bilateral band of hyperesthesia at the same level. The spinal column was fairly mobile, and was not tender to direct pressure or on jarring. There has been no change in the degree of the kyphosis since the accident. There was spastic paraplegia of the lower extremities, with the spasticity and clonus more marked on the left side. Babinski's phenomenon was present on both sides. The skin reflexes were present, and there were distinct objective sensory disturbances in the lower extremities, including touch, pain and temperature, more pronounced on the right side. The man was able to stand fairly well with his eyes closed. He had considerable difficulty in urination, with occasional incontinence. He also complained of sharp, painful sensations and prickling down the posterior aspect of the thighs and legs, and on stooping he felt numb from the hips down. His sexual power was apparently unaffected. Coarse myokymic twitchings were present in the back below the level of the lesion; also in the buttocks, thighs and legs, especially their posterior aspect, after exertion and exposure to the cold. Occasionally during the past year he had sharp, shooting pains in the course of the sciatic nerves, causing reflex movements in the legs; these were more pronounced on the left side.

Case of Fracture Dislocation of the Spine, Causing a Unilateral or Partial Lesion of the Cord.—This case also was presented by Dr. J. Ramsay Hunt. The patient was an elevator operator, twenty-two years old, who about two months ago fell six stories with his elevator. He was unconscious fifteen minutes after the fall. He was removed to the Gouverneur Hospital, where it was found that he had suffered a fracture dislocation of the spine, the deformity corresponding to the eleventh and twelfth dorsal and the first and second lumbar vertebræ. In addition there was a fracture of the internal and external malleoli of the left ankle-joint. The case was seen by Dr. Hunt six weeks later, through the courtesy of Dr. John Rogers. At that time there was an oval area of anesthesia to touch, pain and temperature over the anterior and lateral surfaces of the right thigh. The right knee-jerk was absent; the right Achilles-jerk was present and not exaggerated. The left leg was weak and spastic, with clonus. The Babinski reflex was not elicitable on either side. A girdle sensation was felt in the lower abdominal region, especially on the right side. There was difficulty on urination. Dr. Hunt said the case was a good example of a unilateral or partial lesion of the cord, resulting from a fracture-dislocation of the vertebræ.

The interesting features of the first case were the recovery from the initial paralysis, the long interval of comparative normal function, during which period a laborious occupation was practiced, and then the gradual reappearance of cord symptoms referable to the same level of the cord. The progression of the disease had been most insidious, but always steadily advancing, and of such a nature as to suggest a very gradual compression of the spinal cord. It seemed reasonable to infer in such a case that the cord was undergoing gradual compression in the spinal canal, already narrowed by the fracture dislocation, and produced by an osseous outgrowth (chronic proliferating osteitis) plus pachymeningeal thickening and adhesions. Spinal syphilis or chronic inflammatory changes within the cord could be excluded, Dr. Hunt believed that surgical measures should betaken to relieve the marked symptoms of compression.

Dr. Joseph Fraenkel, in the discussion, said it was rather difficult to decide the exact nature of the lesion in Case I, shown by Dr. Hunt. Pressure on the cord due to an osseous lesion he thought would give rise to more severe symptoms than were present in the case, and he suggested the possibility of a post traumatic hematomyelia.

Dr. Hunt, in closing, said that in studying the case, the possibilty of a posttraumatic syringomyelia had been considered, as well as syphilis, or a chronic inflammatory condition of the cord, originating at the site of the old injury. The theory that symptoms followed a hematomyelia he thought could be discarded from the fact that such a lesion was generally found in the gray matter of the cord, and that it would have given rise to dissociate sensory symptoms. In the first case shown it is true there were coarse myokymic twitchings but no atrophies and no dissociate sensory symptoms. The symptoms were those of a gradual compression of the cord. In cases where the compression was of insidious onset, sharp pains were often absent. In the case shown there were pains of sufficient severity to suggest involvement of the posterior roots. The differential diagnosis was important in cases of this character, Dr. Hunt said, because of the treatment. The symptoms were growing progressively worse, and if they were the result of compression, osseous or otherwise, the advisability of an exploratory operation was worthy of consideration. This would he decided the speaker said, on further observation and after an X-ray picture had been taken of the area involved.

Diffuse Cauliflower-like Puckering of the Cortex in Arteriosclerotic Epilepsy.—Dr. Adolf Meyer demonstrated a brain that he had obtained through the courtesy of Dr. M. C. Ashley, of the Middletown State Hospital. The specimen showed a form of vascular affection, principally of the cortical terminals, in a patient fifty-five years old. This patient gave a history of having had syphilis at the age of twenty years. There was mental deterioration, with epilepsy, for twelve years, and slowly progressive left hemiplegia during the last year of life. The small vessels of the pia in the affected regions were generally and diffusely occluded.

The lesions affected principally the occipital lobes; the The lesions affected principally the occipital lobes; the temporal and parietofrontal regions were also affected, leaving, however, intact the convolutions bordering on the Sylvian fossa. The case belonged to a group of which Dr. Meyer had described two instances in the Pathological Report of the Illinois Eastern Hospital for the Insane at Kankakee, in 1896. The condition was frequently called diffuse sclerosis, but presented a distinct variety of a progressive disorder of middle life or senescence, akin to the cases reported by Pozzi, Hess, Prout, Blackburn and probably also by Greiff. The term cirrhosis was used instead of sclerosis because the latter referred more to the broader lesions taking in the white substance, whereas cirrhosis, as applied to the kidney and liver, directed the attention more to the parenchymatous portions, and in this case to the cortex itself.

Dr. T. P. Prout said in one case he had observed where the early history was obtained, it was found that it belonged to the realm of the infantile cerebral palsies, upon which epilepsy was subsequently ingrafted. This was the light, the speaker said, in which he had during recent years come to regard these cases. The epilepsy was ingrafted upon an early cerebral palsy, in the same way as we saw it ingrafted upon other brain lesions.

Dr. Fraenkel said he had seen quite a number of cases in which epileptiform seizures developed late in life, accompanied by some mental deterioration. The diagnosis was of importance, because in a younger person such a condition would be regarded as a general paresis. It was interesting to study the onset of these seizures, which could usually be differentiated from those of ordinary epilepsy by the slight focal symptoms.

Dr. Meyer, in closing, said he did not think it was justifiable to assume an infantile lesion in these cases, because it was possible to demonstrate all degrees of more recent and older foci, with numerous granule cells. In reply to the suggestion made by one of the speakers to call these cases pseudoparalysis, Dr. Meyer said this would be apt to involve them in the general confusion of that term, which for a while stood for the cases of general paralysis on a demonstrable syphilitic basis, but which we had since learned to recognize as the backbone of that disease from the etiological standpoint.

The following officers were elected for the ensuing year: President, Dr. Joseph Fraenkel; First Vice-President, Dr. J. Arthur Booth; Second Vice-President, Dr. Smith Ely Jelliffe; Recording Secretary, Dr. J. Ramsey Hunt; Treasurer, Dr. G. M. Hammond; Corresponding Secretary, Dr. F. K. Hallock.

A New York Physician Knighted.—The King of Italy, at the recommendation of the Italian Minister of Foreign Affairs, has made Dr. Antonio Fanoni, of New York, a knight (chevalier) of the Order of the Crown.

MEDICAL ASSOCIATION OF THE GREATER CITY OF NEW YORK.

Stated Meeting, held December 12, 1904.

The President, T. E. Satterthwaite, M.D., in the Chair.

Mucous Colic.—Dr. R. C. Kemp read a paper on this subject. As to the pathology of this affection, variously known as mucous colitis, pseudomembranous enteritis, membranous colitis, tubular diarrhea, etc., he said that except in rare instances mucous colic is engrafted on a catarrhal colitis, it is the consensus of opinion that no inflammation exists. Microscopically the membrane discharged consists of a structureless matrix with columnar epithelium, and its chief constituent is mucus. Dr. Kemp's investigations have led him to believe that the principal factor in the etiology of mucous colic is ptosis of the colon with associated gastroptosis. In ten cases examined by him, enteroptosis was found invariably associated with gastroptosis. Enteroptosis and associated gastroptosis, with gastro-intestinal disturbances and auto-infection, he places as the factors of mucous colic, and the neurasthenia so commonly met with in these cases as the result of the auto-infection. He considers, therefore, that mucous colic is one of the manifestations of Glenard's disease. In the treatment, consequently, proper abdominal support he regards as a most important feature. Other means, however, should not be neglected, and he gave in detail the methods he employed both during the attacks of colic and in the intervals.

Dr. William H. Thompson, in the discussion, said he knew of scarcely any trouble which was so vexatious both to the patient and the physician. This is particularly the case because the condition is specifically characterized by low spirits, and if it lasts for any length of time in a woman it is accompanied by an appalling variety of distressing symptoms. The most important point is the etiology, and what has most impressed him is the one story of chronic constipation, lasting perhaps ten, fifteen or twenty years. It is not difficult to understand that the continued or repeated presence of what may be termed a foreign body (the hardened feces) in the intestines must have a most pernicious effect upon the innervation of the whole alimentary tract. This, then, is the primary and most common cause, resulting in the production of auto-infection and toxemia. Here we have the reason why the disease has so often been pronounced a neurosis. Instead of being a primary neurosis, however, it is the local condition which causes the neurotic trouble so frequently present. Other factors, in exceptional instances, are such exercises as excessive horseback and bicycle riding. In the treatment great assistance may often be obtained from the replacement of the displaced stomach and bowel, just as relief from distressing symptoms may be secured by the replacement of a displaced uterus or kidney. As to drugs, probably the best results may be obtained from the use of castor oil as an alterant, in doses not exceeding one-half drachm. To this may often be added with advantage asafetida, or sodium benzoate.

Mucous Colic and Gastroptosia.—Dr. A. Rose remarked that one author had said of gastroptosia: "The descriptions in the books of the symptoms of gastropsia are hopelessly obscure and chaotic; characteristic and diagnostic points are few and misleading." To this may be said: The symptoms in gastropsia are indeed manifold and numerous, but if we keep in view that there is only one factor, and that this factor is relaxation, we have a characteristic and diagnostic point which

is not misleading, but indicates at once a rational method of treatment which in most, if not all, cases will cause the symptoms to disappear or to become ameliorated. This applies to some extent to mucous colic, which is not a disease *sui generis*, but is, at least as far as Dr. Kemp's and my own observations go to show, one of the manifestations of gastropsia. By this term should be understood abdominal ptosis, atony, or relaxation. For scientific as well as for practical purposes it is best to employ Greek terms in our onomatology in their original meaning. The question whether gastroptosia is the cause of mucous colic in all cases will have to be decided by further observation. While some writers have paid attention to the coexistence of gastropsia. Gastropsia is very frequent and mucous colic is rare, but this does not exclude the fact that mucous colic may be one of the many kinds of manifestations of gastroptosia. The relation of certain ailments to gastropsia has been recognized only since abdominal strapping has been practised. Dr. Rogers and Dr. Rose found that cases of dysmenorrhea in which uterine flexions or ovarian troubles existed along with gastroptosia were promptly relieved by this strapping. Relief of gastroptosia was relief of dysmenorrhea. German colleagues, who during the last two years have made extensive use of the strapping, state that this method did better service in many instances of uterine flexions than all the pessaries. Gastroptosia in women does not always cause dysmenorrhea, nor in men and women always mucous colic; but mucous colic, as well as dysmenorrhea, may be caused by gastroptosia. Gastroptosia is very often the cause of disorders of circulation, as well as of nervous disturbances, and these disorders may in some instances cause mucous colic and in others dysmenorrhea. The relief of gastroptosia, therefore, is relief of mucous colic and relief of dysmenorrhea in the cases in which such relations exist. In Germany it was Dr. Walther Clemm who introduced what Dr. Kemp has named the Rose belt. What is thought of it may be learned from a paper by Dr. Weissmann, of Lindenfels, in which he says: "There exists a large number of chronic cases going from Pontius to Pilatus, and not a small percentage of their ailments is connected with gastropsia. Physicians should, in cases of gastric disorder, neurosis, neuralgias, look for gastric atony, because they may, in many instances, relieve their patients from persistent and painful sufferings by means of the simple Rose belt."

Appendicitis and Intestinal Obstruction.—Dr. Robert Abbé opened a discussion on this subject with remarks on Obstruction Following Operations for Appendicitis, which were illustrated by diagram. The subject, he said, was one of growing importance. In his private practice during the last few years there had been ten cases of which he had exact notes, and it was upon this personal experience that he would base his remarks. It was an accident which no doubt occurred more frequently than was generally realized, as the symptoms resulting from it had formerly been attributed to other causes. Out of the ten cases, he had been able to save seven, and all would certainly have proved fatal had not timely operative interference been made. The obstruction is a mechanical one, and usually occurs in the form of a simple adhesive band. Formerly it no doubt resulted more frequently from the appendectory itself than is now the case. This was due to the elaborate "toilet of the peritoneum" which was then considered necessary. Fixation of the intestine was liable to result from the presure of the iodoform gauze employed. At the present time, however, a simple washing out with saline solution is believed to afford the best results. Drainage is abandoned to a large extent, and hence one cause of the accident has now been eliminated. In the cases under consideration no such gauze application was employed. The date at which the obstruction commenced was as follows: On the second day, one case; fourth day, two cases; fifth day, one; sixth day, one; twelfth day, one; in one wéek, one; in five weeks, one; in two months, one; in seven months, one. In one case that had come to his knowledge, the obstruction did not occur until after five years.

Symptoms.—The patient is supposed to have made a good recovery from the operation, when suddenly a new train of symptoms make their appearance. They do not have, however, the intensity of those caused by a strangulated hernia. First there is colicky pain, usually referred to the navel, which may come on gradually and have sharp exacerbations. The countenance becomes ashen, the eyes hollow, and the tongue furred. Usually there is albuminuria, and then anemia. All these symptoms are due to the circulatory condition, a capillary anemia, probably associated with cardiac weakness. The colicky pain, if long continued, is apt to be associated with vomiting. Such is the case if there is a kink in the intestine. With simple adhesions, the vomiting occurs later. Experience has shown that black vomit is not necessarily a fatal sign. From the local condition we might expect asymmetry of the abdomen, but this is not usually the case. As a rule it is dome-shaped. In such cases the search for indican in the urine is a waste of time. With pain, swelling of the abdomen, hiccough and regurgitation, there can be little question of the existence of intestinal obstruction. Loss of desire for food is one of the earliest signs. If the abdominal wound is unhealed, the secretion of the wound becomes altered, This is not because there is a septic wound, but is due simply to the loss of secretion resulting from the general circulatory condition.

Prompt Operative Interference Demanded.—in from two or three days to an unlimited period after the operation, as has been seen, the obstruction may come on. The average time is five days to three weeks. As time goes on, the chances of intestinal obstruction become less. It is interesting to know whether acute obstruction can be overcome without operation. In exceptional instances it may. One such, the case of a girl of fourteen years, in whom the obstruction developed on the fourteenth day after the operation for appendicitis, was mentioned. This is not the rule, however, and the earlier the operation, the greater the chances of success. Up to the second day almost every case can be saved, and the great point therefore is to operate early. In nine out of Dr. Abbé's ten cases the obstruction was located near the caput coli (within two feet of the ileocecal valve). An adhesive band was found there, and when such a band is divided, the contents of the intestine are at once allowed to pass down, and the patient is usually safe. In one case, however, a second operation was required, as it was found after the first that there was another adherent stricture of the intestine lower down. Before operating it is always well to empty the stomach with a tube. It is important to remember that, notwithstanding the existence of a stricture near the ileocecal valve, a patient may sometimes pas feces and gas; these coming simply from the colon. After an obstruction has lasted more than two days a case may not do well, even if operated upon. The gut may by that time have become so thickened and altered in character that it cannot be restored to its normal condition. In operating for appendicitis the chances of a subsequent intestinal ob-

struction will be diminished if as large an amount of saline solution as possible is left in the abdominal cavity.

Intestinal Obstruction Following Attacks of Unoperated Appendicitis.—This was the title of a paper by Dr. C. A. McWilliams. He has been able to collect 33 cases reported in medical literature.

Dr. Algernon T. Bristow said that personally he had met with only one or two cases of intestinal obstruction following the operation for appendicitis, and this had also been the experience of his colleague, Dr. George R. Fowler, who had operated more than two thousand times. The symptoms of obstruction, as described by Dr. Abbé, were practically those met with in septic peritonitis. The important point to note was that these symptoms occurred in a patient previously doing well, while in the case of peritonitis they occurred in one doing badly. In some cases of angulation of the intestine, Dr. Bristow had had good results from the formation of an artificial anus. This was done under local anesthesia with cocaine, as he did not deem it safe to use a general anesthetic.

Dr. Carl Beck said that not so very long ago intestinal obstruction was regarded as an unknown quantity, and that even twenty-five years ago any attempt to remove such obstruction by operation would have been condemned by the profession. He spoke of the diagnosis of interstitial adhesions from distended gallbladder and other conditions, and said the X-ray had proved useful in his hands. In certain chronic cases of adhesion characterized by extensive cobweb-like formations, of which he had seen three or four instances, the prognosis was very bad.

Dr. Forbes Hawkes said that in the differential diagnosis between sepsis and adhesive bands the condition of the right rectus muscle was of importance. When bands are present there is a much greater amount of rigidity. As to the danger of causing adhesions by the leaving of gauze in the abdominal cavity for drainage, he thought this could be practically obviated by placing rubber tissue around the gauze. Before operating for appendicitis it was always good practice to thoroughly clean out the lower bowel, for if that were done, even a small movement after the operation indicated that peristalsis was renewed and that the proper function was established.

Dr. Robert T. Morris said that Dr. Abbé was to be congratulated on his results, which were certainly much more favorable than the average. He felt, as Dr. Bristow felt, that cases of strangulation occurred frequently, and he believed that such could be relieved by means other than operative. His plan of treatment consisted of (1) massage, (2) posture (elevation of the hips), and (3) the use of ergot. In many cases of postoperative ileus these three agencies would save the patient's life. Frequently he had seen within thirty minutes pronounced evidences of the relief afforded by them. In his hands this mode of treatment had proved practically more successful than operation, and he had seen cases relieved by it which would ordinarily have been operated upon.

Annual Meeting, held January 9, 1905.

The President, T. E. Satterthwaite, M.D., in the Chair.

Report of the Statistical Secretary.—This showed a membership of 657.

Professional Responsibility in the Diagnosis and Care of the Insane.—Dr. A. C. Brush read a paper on this subject. The responsibility for the early recognition of insanity, he said, clearly rests with the general practitioner. Insanity has never been successfully defined, and wisely the law of this State makes no attempt to define it. It has, however, established a well-defined line between responsibility and irresponsibility from insanity and other causes. It is the duty of the family physician to detect abnormal mental processes in the young, and advise proper mental and physical means for their correction. The classification of insanity is purely clinical, except in the case of general paresis. The Kräpelin classification, imperfect though it be, is an improvement over the older ones. Dr. Brush adopted this in describing the diagnosis of the various abnormal mental conditions which form the basis of the insane condition.

What the State of New York is Doing for the Insane and for the Advancement of the Science of Medicine.—This was the title of a paper by Dr. Frederick Peterson. Having referred to the duties of the State Commission in Lunacy and of the medical officers of the hospitals, he said that there are no better public hospitals for the insane than those of New York, and no others where at the present time more purely scientific and medical work is being done. During the past three years, under the direction of Dr. Meyer, director of the Pathological Institute on Ward's Island, much attention has been paid to the matter of stimulating new medical interest among the 130 physicians constituting the staffs of the 14 State Hospitals. Courses of lectures and demonstrations have been attended not only by the assistant physicians, but also by the superintendents of these institutions. In addition, Dr. Meyer and his assitants have spent some time at each hospital, working over clinical and pathological material with the staff. The accumulation of the elaborate histories now made must become of incalculable value to investigators in psychiatry; but quite as important is the fact that the very work of the preparation is an education to the young men performing the service—stimulating their understanding, improving their powers of observation, and sharpening their scientific judgment. The practice of having staff meetings once or twice a week, for the discussion of conditions of patients and for the presentation of new and interesting data in the domain of medicine, has become general. Nothing has been spared in the way of well-equipped working medical libraries or of making each institution equal in facilities and modern appliances to any general hospital. Where these hospitals are located sufficiently near to large towns or cities, consulting boards of medical men, active in various specialties, have been secured in order to bring the members of the staffs into relation with all lines of medical progress. The result of all this has been to make each hospital a nucleus for a large amount of genuine clinico-pathological work. Each has on its staff both a salaried ophthalmologist and dentist, and over a thousand nurses have now been graduated from the hospital training schools. It is designed to have as soon as practicable a psychopathic reception hospital in connection with each of the State hospitals situated in or near a city or large town. The concluding part of the paper was devoted to an enumeration of some of the improvements which have been made in the treatment and care of the insane, particularly as regards the amelioration of their condition.

Dr. C. F. MacDonald, in the discussion, said that a wide difference was recognized by all between the medical and legal definition of insanity. In the code of criminal procedure the law does not concern itself, except as regards the commission of some crime, and confines itself explicitly to the question of responsibility. The tendency is always to cling to precedents. Medical men are fully aware that not infrequently the very insane know perfectly well the abstract difference between right and wrong, and especially is this the case with paranoiacs. But medical science says that it is not a question of the recognition of right and wrong, but of the ability of the individual to resist the impulse to do wrong. The medical and legal definitions of insanity, therefore, are widely different. Dr. MacDonald said he differed somewhat from Dr. Brush as to the definition of insanity. Many of the definitions which have been brought forward have been mere attempts at condensed psychological descriptions, and are impracticable. For the purpose of teaching psychiatry to students and medical practitioners he would say that insanity is a disease or disturbance of the brain in which there is a prolonged departure from the individual's usual methods of thinking, feeling and acting. This disease may be functional, as well as organic. The important point to be recognized is that an insane person, however robust he may appear, is always suffering from a disease of the brain. Insanity is therefore characterized by mental derangement. Our lawmakers have entrusted to the medical profession the power of depriving individuals of liberty by declaring them insane. Hence it is very important that the practitioner should be familiar with the prodromata of insanity, for it is in the early stages that the most can be done in the way of treatment. By the inauguration of early and appropriate treatment confirmed insanity can often be prevented. The stage of *alteration* always precedes the stage of *alienation*. It is therefore most essential, in determining insanity in its early stages, to compare the patient with himself, and thus see if there is a prolonged departure from his usual methods of mental operation. It is a common notion that there is a general standard, any deviation from which constitutes insanity. This is not the case, however. Every individual must be judged from his own personal standard. In obscure and doubtful cases, therefore, it is very important to determine what the normal standard of the individual is as regards heredity, environment, habits, etc. Hence, in the matter of early diagnosis, the great importance of this method of comparing the patient with himself, in order to determine whether there is any prolonged departure from his usual manner of conducting himself. As regards classification, he said he had not been able to accept that of Kräpelin. He thought it open to more objections than some of the older ones. He had been accustomed to regard those as the best which were founded on the mental symptoms and had substantially as their basis the old classification of Pinel. As far as he was aware, that of Kräpelin had not as yet been generally accepted by alienists.

Dr. Adolf Meyer said that as a rule hospital physicians were very anxious to make advances in the scientific character of their work, and he believed that on the whole the medical profession underrated the value of what was being accomplished in the State hospitals. It was to be said, however, that during the period of strenuous economy in the State administration the hospital staffs had been so reduced in numbers that the physicians in these institutions labored under a great strain. There were not enough of them to properly carry on the work required of them. The effort was being made to train the hospital physicians both in autopsy and clinical work. If adequate records are kept, the autopsy findings can be carefully compared with the conditions that existed during life. In this respect he said he had met with a great deal of encouraging enthusiasm in all the State hospitals. The matter of classification he thought was now constantly being regarded as of less and less importance. For commitment a diagnosis is not necessary. It is the mental and physical symptoms that are required—the facts of the case. Among the facts most important to ascertain is the question of deterioration. Hence, one of the principal points to investigate is whether the condition present is likely to require the permanent care of the State or whether the case is a recoverable one. Classification is, therefore, not essential. What we want is facts, facts which will enable us to prognosticate as to the future and to determine the kind of care required.

Dr. E. D. Fisher said it was fortunate that Dr. Peterson was able to speak from a double standpoint, that of the interne and that of the administrator of hospitals. He was, therefore, peculiarly well adapted to present this subject. From his personal knowledge he could verify all that Dr. Peterson had said of the immense improvement which had taken place in the practical care of the insane, the hospital equipment, and the class of physicians during the last few years. The Pathological Institute has accomplished a most admirable work. In former years the asylum physician was not on a par, as regards scientific attainments, with the outside alienist. There had also been a great improvement in the dietary of the patients during the incumbency of Doctors MacDonald and Peterson in the Lunacy Commission. This was a very important point because there was always exhaustion in insanity, and hence he thought extravagance in the matter of food would be decidedly preferable to parsimony. He felt very much inclined to agree with Dr. Meyer that the hospital staffs were not sufficiently large, and that the physicians were consequently overworked. As to local boards of managers for the State hospitals, he had been very much opposed to their abolition, and he was glad to hear that the present Governor proposed to restore such boards. He hoped that the measure would go through. Boards composed of intelligent persons of high standing in the community, he thought, were especially desirable for the hospitals outside of New York City. In these State hospitals the care was excellent, and he would much prefer to have a patient treated in one of them rather than in a private sanitarium at a charge of $15 to $20 a week, or even more. In regard to the classification of Kräpelin, he would be disposed to agree with Dr. Macdonald that it would not be advisable to accept it absolutely.

Dr. W. M. Leszynsky said it was pleasant to compare the present with the past, when superintendents were appointed on account of their political pull. In former years there was a constant cry of improper management in the city hospitals for the insane. Even before the establishment of the State hospitals, however, there had been a great improvement, and this had steadily continued down to the present time. He thought that if Dr. Peterson's paper could be widely promulgated it would have an excellent effect in removing the prejudice which now exists in the minds of many in regard to the State hospitals.

Dr. E. C. Dent said he was a thorough believer in the Kräpelin classification. He thought that in the future it would be productive of admirable results, and even at the present we are able by means of it to make better classification. He realized very keenly that there were some drawbacks to Kräpelin's theory, but he felt assured that in time these would be overcome. At the present time it was quite impossible to make a perfect classification. It would take a long time to arrive at definite conclusions. He believed he voiced the sentiments of all the other superintendents in stating that very considerable progress had been made at the State hospitals under Dr. Meyer's guidance. Furthermore, the Commission in Lunacy invited all the medical profession to visit the various hospitals and give the physicians in them the benefit of their advice. He quite agreed with Dr. Meyer that the staffs were too small. In some of our best hospitals there were not half enough physicians to properly do the work called for. The examination of patients often necessarily consumed much time, and there was a great deal of clerical work required in carrying out the present methods. In conclusion, Dr. Dent gave a brief summary of the history of the care of the insane in New York City. This, he said, showed what progress had been made, and it was a slow and gradual evolution. One of the essentials of proper treatment was good nursing, and a great advance had been made in the establishment of training schools for nurses.

Dr. R. T. Morris thought that in the line of progress came the idea of having a competent surgeon on the staff in the hospitals. In every large assembly of the insane there is a certain percentage of cases (not large, it may be) which can be cured by surgery. That is, before neurotic habits have been established—after this has occurred it is too late to act. He did not claim that psychoses were caused by surgical lesions, but he believed that certain psychoses were *precipitated* by such lesions. He would not operate except in cases where an operation was demanded on the ground of common humanity. In illustration he mentioned some cases in his own practice. One was that of a patient suffering from melancholia who had auto-intoxication dependent on a floating kidney. As soon as fixation of the kidney was done the melancholia was promptly cured. There were a number of major psychoses and a great many minor psychoses in which he believed an operation would be of service. In reply to Dr. W. V. Hayes, who inquired whether neurasthenia with depression might not result from surgical operations, Dr. Morris said it was a fact that insanity is sometimes precipitated by an operation, and particularly hysterical insanity.

Dr. Brush said that the law does not attempt to define because the medical profession does not, but it has to define responsibility and non-responsibility. He had adopted the Kräpelin classification because it was the latest and seemed to him the best. In some cases it had given him great assistance.

Dr. Peterson said that, as to the matter of diet, a few years ago Dr. Flint was authorized to devise a schedule, and this was used for some time. Subsequently a ration recommended by Professor Atwater was adopted. This proved too great a reduction, however, and still later a combination of. the two was tried. This had proved adequate, and was still in use. In reply to Dr. Morris he would say that a whole volume might be written of the surgery during the past year in these institutions. In the Manhattan State Hospital, West, no less than 150 capital operations had been performed. Doctors Bryant, Bickham, and other well-known surgeons were in attendance, and operations were done because operations were indicated. As to the inquiry of Dr. Hayes, he said that insanity was especially apt to follow ovariotomy, and particularly double ovariotomy. In undertaking such operations, therefore, he thought the question of insanity should always be taken into consideration.

CHICAGO MEDICAL SOCIETY.

Regular Meeting, held December 14, 1904.

Pneumonia, Typical and Atypical.—Dr. C. S. Williamson read a paper on this subject. After discussing briefly the onset in the typical cases of pneumonia, the author discusses in detail the aberrant forms where the onset does not directly point to the lung.

1. *Abdominal Cases.*—It is a comparatively old observation, but one which has been but little heeded, that pneumonia frequently begins with sharp abdominal pains. This fact was first impressed upon the author by seeing a distinguished surgeon operate a case for supposed salpingitis, because of intense pain in the lower abdomen, the case dying within twelve hours and the autopsy revealing no abdominal or pelvic disease, but a double croupous pneumonia. The commonest group of these abdominal cases are those where the pain and tenderness are localized at McBurney's point for the first two or three days (appendicular form). He agrees with Massalongo as to the frequency of this form in childhood. In other cases the pain is localized to the gall-bladder region, and may mimic biliary or even renal colic or gastric ulcer for the first twenty-four or thirty-six hours. It is not justifiable to recognize, as some foreign authors would do, separate groups of cases in accordance with the localization of the pain at the onset. What is needed is not so much hyper-refinement of classification, but careful exploration of the chest by physician and surgeon before every abdominal operation. The explanation of these reflected abdominal pains is that the six lower intercostal nerves in their passage downward to the abdominal wall, give off filaments to the diaphragmatic, and possibly also the parietal, pleura. Irritation of these filaments may, by a well-known law, be referred to the end distribution of other branches of the same nerve.

2. *Senile Pneumonia.*—The author calls particular attention to the fact that the onset in old people is apt to be entirely latent. In some cases there is a chill, but very slight elevation of temperature. A chill occurring in old people without apparent cause should be always regarded as suspicious of pneumonia. In the terminal pneumonias the onset, frequently the entire course, is latent. In alcoholics the same statements apply.

3. *The Onset in Pneumonia Due to the Friedländer Bacillus.*—A small portion of cases of croupous pneumonia are due to the pneumobacillus of Friedländer. The clinical symptoms do not ordinarily differ from those of cases caused by the pneumococcus except in one important point, namely, in regard to the character of the sputum. In the Friedlander pneumonia the sputum is so characteristic that from it alone a fair diagnosis of the form of pneumonia may often be made. It is intensely mucoid, ropy, and stringy, and when lifted upon a knife-blade or similar instrument, it can be drawn out in long threads.

This is a point which has hitherto escaped general observation. Attention is called to the fact that the Friedländer pneumonia may be readily recognized post mortem by observing the character of the cut surface. This, instead of being dry, as in the pneumococcus form, is bathed with a ropy, tenacious, rusty-looking mucus which is highly characteristic of cases produced caused by the pneumo bacillus.

4. *General Pneumococcus Infection.*—Very much rarer than the above cases, but much more important, are the cases where the onset is with a pneumococcus septicemia. The author quotes a case seen by him in consultation where the onset was with a bloody discharge from the nasopharynx and middle ear (through an old perforation in the drum), and where the lung findings were entirely negative. Examination showed a nearly pure culture of pneumococci in the bloody serum from the nasopharynx and the ear; the cultures from the blood revealed the pneumococcus in pure culture. Twenty-four hours later a pneumonia developed. In this case the march of events was undoubtedly that the infection occurred from the nasopharynx and ear, from which sources bacteria were taken into the blood to produce, several days later, a croupous pneumonia. Cases of this kind have a very great theoretical as well as practical interest, since they demonstrate, for some cases at least, the hematogenous origin of pneumonia.

Physical Basis for Diagnosis in Pneumonia.—Dr. Robert H. Babcock presented a contribution on this subject, saying that the pulmonary findings on which the diagnosis of acute croupous pneumonia may be based are determined by the pathological conditions within the lung, and as this latter varies much in extent and in character during the different stages of the process, the physical signs display corresponding differences in definiteness and character. There are three propositions, therefore, which he regards as fundamental to a correct understanding of the data furnished by examination of the chest in this affection: (1) The exudate is not necessarily lobar in extent, but may be lobular or patchy, and hence the objection to the term lobar pneumonia. This is especially true of this disease in children and old or debilitated subjects. It is ignorance of this fact that is responsible for the failure on the part of some practitioners to always recognize the disease in the class of cases referred to. (2) The inflammatory exudate does not always form rapidly and uniformly throughout the affected lobe, and hence three or four days may elapse before the exudate beginning deeply spreads to the surface so as to become clearly recognizable at the bedside. This fact accounts, he thinks, for many a disastrous delay in diagnosis, and hence has an important bearing on the treatment. (3) There may sometimes be a striking contrast between the severity of constitutional symptoms and the results of physical examination of the lungs. For this reason a practitioner should make repeated examinations of the chest early in the course of the affection. Later on frequent and careful examinations are also necessary because of the liability to extensions and the importance of their recognition. In fact, he believed the state of the lungs should be ascertained at each professional visit, since only by so doing can the physician have an accurate knowledge of what is going on.

Dr. Babcock then discussed the stage of engorgement, the stage of hepatization, mensuration, palpation, percussion, auscultation, and the microscopic inspection or examination of properly stained sputum. Recently he was asked to see in consultation a man of

sixty years who was suffering from cardiac insufficiency. He had been having a cough of chronic bronchitis, and two weeks ago was edematous. Treatment
had improved his condition, but for the last three
days he had been slightly delirious. He found a heart
lesion, to be sure, but the pulse was only 96, and signs
of stasis were not present. The thing that struck him
at once was the character of the respirations, which
were shallow and forty to the minute. Mouth temperature was normal, but in the rectum the thermometer registered 103° F. The lungs were then carefully
examined, with the result that on the left posterior
axillary line, not far from the scapula, was discovered
a small patch of dulness, with increased resistance,
slightly exaggerated tactile fremitus and bronchial
breathing. On these findings a diagnosis of pneumonia was made. Without the loss of normal pulse
respiration ratio, he should not have suspected acute
pneumonia, but with this and the rectal temperature
he was led to go over the lungs with more than ordinary care, and with the result just stated.

Cardiac and Renal Aspects of Pneumonia.—Dr.
Arthur R. Elliott read this paper, saying that on the
heart and kidneys rested the safety of the pneumonia
invalid. Owing to special conditions imposed by the
disease, circulatory considerations take precedence of
all others in importance. General agreement exists
that cardiac insufficiency is the usual cause of death.
The author distinguished between symptomatic involvement of the heart and inflammatory lesions of the
cardiac structure occurring as complications, and confined himself to a discussion of the former. Three
forms of cardiac failure are observed in pneumonia, *i.e.*,
collapse with a high temperature, collapse occurring at
the time of crisis, or soon after, and collapse following
exertion during convalescence. Various explanations
have been advanced to account for the cardiac collapse
in pneumonia. The author proceeded to discuss the various theories, taking up serially the ideas of von
Jürgenson, regarding the importance of pyrexia in
bringing about circulatory crisis, the importance of the
direct action of pneumococcus toxins in the production
of cardiac asthenia, the effect upon the heart of the obstruction of the pulmonic circulation in causing right
heart paralysis, and the vascular theories of Romberg
and Passler and Rolly. Blood pressure observations in
pneumonia were analyzed, and the author concludes
that heart failure is probably due to several causes, the
principal of which are vasomotor paresis, paralyzing distention of the right heart, and the direct action of toxins
on the myocardium. The clinical signs of cardiac collapse were next reviewed, and attention was drawn to
the importance of studying the pulse and pulse respiration ratio in pneumonia. A pulse in the adult of over
120, and in children of over 130, especially after the first
day, is of bad omen, although no arbitrary rule of
prognosis can be followed in interpreting the pulse.
Delirium and coma in association with high pulse rate
is grave. A dicrotic, irregular pulse occurring at the
height of the disease is a bad omen; occurring after the
crisis it is of less note. Attention was directed to the
great clinical value of the pulmonic second sound as
furnishing a reliable indication of the state of the right
heart. The author briefly discussed the renal aspects
of pneumonia, regarding which but little information is
current. Pneumonia complicating Bright's disease is
frequent, but acute nephritis as a complication of pneumonia seldom occurs. One is not warranted by experience in ascribing to the pneumococcus any more important influence in the production of nephritis than is
possessed by other infective organisms. Cloudy swell-

ing and other slight degenerative changes have been
noted in the kidneys in a majority of cases of pneumonia examined, and more or less albuminuria is observed during the course of the disease when systematically tested for. Statistics show the association of a
high death rate, and albuminuria is probably because of
resulting renal inadequacy. From this standpoint albuminuria may be regarded as an unfavorable development. Pus, blood and casts in the urine point to mycotic endocarditis or a local pneumococcus infection of
the kidney. Other urinary considerations are of less
importance.

Regular Meeting, held January 25, 1905.

The President, John B. Murphy, M.D., in the Chair.

**The Therapeutic Use of the X-rays: Three Years
After.—Dr.** William Allen Pusey read a paper on
this subject. Reference was made to his contributions on this subject in 1900, 1901, and 1902. He reviewed the subject and his cases treated at that time
by means of the X-rays, and undertook to estimate
from the results the therapeutic limitations and possibilities of this agent. Its use for the permanent
removal of hair had not equaled his early expectations, as in his experience the results were only satisfactory in 50 per cent. of the cases, and even to obtain these requires long treatment. In sycosis and
tinea sycosis the results of the X-ray were exceedingly satisfactory. Acne offers a good illustration of
the value of the X-ray. He has treated a large number of cases of acne and his results have been very
satisfactory in most cases. Occasionally there may
be recurrences of the lesions, but even when relapses occur the cases are amenable to treatment.
X-ray treatment in cases of acne, however, must be
carried out with great care. He has not seen unpleasant after-effects from the rays in this condition.
His results in rosacea had been quite as satisfactory
as in acne. However, some of these cases show a
slight tendency to relapse, but the ultimate outcome
is satisfactory. He reported one ugly, stubborn case
that had practically remained well for three years
without treatment. The X-ray in chronic inflammatory dermatoses has been valuable, particularly in
eczemas of the hands. Satisfactory results have also
been obtained in chronic indurated eczema of other
parts. It relieves itching, but occasionally fails to
do so. In subacute or chronic inflammatory disease
of the skin, such as psoriasis and lichen planus, the
effect of the X-ray is markedly beneficial. However, it does not offer striking advantages over
other methods of treating these conditions. In
pruritus ani and vulvæ he has not seen the benefit
from the use of the X-ray mentioned by other observers, and he is not sure that any case has been
permanently cured. In pigmented and vascular nevi
his experience with the X-ray in a few cases has
been favorable. As to keloid and scars, there has
been no return of the keloid in one case treated for two
years after treatment. He has treated successfully
eight or ten typical keloids, most of them being on
the chests of women. His experience in treating
lupus vulgaris with the X-ray corroborates that of
other observers, namely, that it is of great value.
He mentioned one case that failed to heal satisfactorily with the X-ray, and this was a lupus of the
face which occurred after an extensive plastic operation. The results from Finsen's method are good,
but the author says he can duplicate any of the results obtained by the Finsen method with the X-ray.
He believes that the X-ray has decided advantages

over Finsen's light method. He has had considerable experience in the treatment of tuberculous glands of the neck. In the treatment of cervical adenitis without involvement of the skin, he has succeeded in many cases in reducing the size of the glands and by long-continued treatment has caused them to diminish almost to the point of disappearance. In other instances he has not observed much improvement. In cases of cervical adenitis in which there was involvement of the skin, the results were more positive. The X-ray in tuberculosis of the joints seems to have no appreciable effect in his experience, although in some positive benefit was noted. In blastomycosis his experience with the X-ray, extending over half a dozen cases, has been uniformly favorable. He has treated successfully by this method two large suppurating papillomatous tumors, one over the knee, one on the thigh. The patients were women, and had resisted other methods of treatment for two years. In a case of actinomycosis of the jaw, the patient having been referred to him by Dr. Ochsner, X-ray exposures combined with twenty grains of iodide of potassium, t.i.d., were followed by complete and permanent resolution in a few weeks. His results in treating superficial epitheliomas and cutaneous carcinoma have been satisfactory, with some failures. In 19 cases out of 20 of epithelioma of the lower lip, referred to him by surgeons, there was no palpable involvement of the glands. Nineteen cases gave healthy scars, and all of the 19 patients are well. He discussed at length the use of the X-ray as a therapeutic measure in cancer of the neck, pseudoleucemia and leucemia. He has treated a number of cases of goiter with the X-ray without any benefit. He has not been able to convince himself that the use of the X-ray is of any value in the treatment of goiter.

Treatment of Lymphatic Leucemia with the X-ray. —Dr. Joseph A. Capps and Dr. Joseph F. Smith contributed a joint paper on this subject, which was accompanied by numerous tables and charts. The first case of leucemia treated by the X-ray was Dr. Pusey himself. The patient was treated for one month, but did not show improvement, probably because the treatment was not carried on long enough. The patient refused further treatment. Fresh interest was aroused on the subject in 1903, when Dr. Nicholas Senn reported a case of leucemia symptomatically cured. Dr. Senn had given the essayists permission to follow out the case. When first seen by Dr. Senn, patient presented the typical symptoms of splenomyelogenous leucemia, and had been ill for fourteen months. Treatment was begun daily and every other day by Dr. Senn, through the latter part of January, February, March, April and May, and at the time of Senn's last observation, the white count came down to 10,000, and the spleen was almost of normal size. This does not mean, however, that the disease itself was cured, although the patient felt perfectly well. Patient was subsequently treated by the X-ray, but died later with symptoms of toxemia apparently, and not from an X-ray burn, as one might suppose.

Another case of splenomyelogenous leucemia is still under treatment. The first case of lymphatic leucemia they had seen reported was treated by Dr. Pusey for several months, and improved symptomatically, but patient died in ten months. It was a chronic case.

Another case of lymphatic leucemia was reported by Senn in an article on Hodgkins' disease. The

case was followed for a time, was much better under X-ray treatment, but died in about seventeen months.

A case treated by Churchill, an infant, died in a comparatively short time, although the X-ray treatment had been faithfully carried out in this instance.

The authors reported three cases of lymphatic leucemia treated by the X-rays, two of which were of the acute form. In one case there was no effect on the blood or the glands. Patient died in six days. In a second case there was no effect on the blood or glands, and the patient died in ten days.

Of the subacute cases, there were two. In the first the blood showed improvement under the X-ray treatment; the spleen and glands diminished in size, but patient died in the course of nine months. While the X-ray exerted a beneficial effect, it did not control the disease. The second subacute case died in six weeks after treatment was begun. Better results were obtained in treating the chronic cases by the X-ray, and of these the author reported three instances.

In summing up, the authors stated that splenomyelogenous cases of leucemia should receive X-ray treatment, because they are greatly benefited. They respond more slowly than do cases of chronic lymphatic leucemia. These patients feel that they are cured, but in the light of Senn's case and of other cases reported as symptomatically cured, some of which have since died, physicians must not be too sanguine in regard to pronouncing cures. It is altogether probable that some of these cases are not cured, but that the process is held in abeyance. Oftentimes in leucemia the spleen will diminish in size and the blood count come down under X-ray treatment, and the patient, as far as the leucemia is concerned, is very much better symptomatically, but the disease reasserts itself always, and the case cannot be regarded as cured. The X-ray, in the opinion of the authors, exerts a wonderful modifying effect, and is a very good method of treatment for the alleviation of symptoms in cases of lymphatic leucemia and of splenomyelogenous leucemia, but probably it does not effect an absolute cure.

Dr. Oliver S. Ormsby, in the discussion, referred to cases treated in the laboratory and in the practice of Drs. Hyde and Montgomery. Their observations extended over three and a half years, and covered more than two hundred cases of epithelioma treated by the X-ray. The cases that had been relieved most perfectly were of the superficial rodent ulcer type. The results were uniformly good. In two cases there was a mild recurrence. They had treated nineteen cases of superficial epithelioma of the lip with excellent results. They had used the X-ray in over one hundred cases of psoriasis. It was a convenient and clean method to use, but they did not select the X-ray in all such instances. Psoriasis of the scalp could be removed with the X-ray without removing the hair. Their results in acne and acne rosacea were excellent. Brilliant results had followed treatment by the X-rays in cases of eczema. In seventeen cases of sycosis the results were good, one-half of the cases being entirely well. In two obstinate recurrences took place. In keloid their results in eleven cases had been the same as those mentioned by the essayist, Dr. Pusey. Thirty-five cases of lupus erythematosus were treated, combining radial with phototherapy, with excellent results.

Dr. E. A. Fischkin stated that in cases of sycosis they reacted beautifully to X-ray treatment. The same could be said of cases of keloid. He spoke of the idiosyncrasy of different patients to the X-ray. He mentioned two patients who had psoriasis, a brother and sister being sick at the same time. It was about two years since psoriasis appeared in both instances. They were given the same treatment. The sister was cured after six or eight treatments, and it was now about two years since the last treatment was given, with no recurrence. The brother still had the disease. Although he had had over one hundred treatments, the psoriasis had increased all over the body. There was no evidence of cure of any of the lesions. This case illustrated that there is a decided difference in the reaction of patients to the X-ray.

Dr. R. R. Campbell stated that in two cases of blastomycosis which he had treated by the X-ray without the administration of iodide of potassium his results had been the same as those of Dr. Pusey. The cases of epithelioma of the lip he had selected for X-ray treatment were of the superficial type. In two cases out of twelve in which there was some slight induration he failed to get any beneficial results from the X-ray. When one had a case of epithelioma of the lip in which it became necessary to curette, he thought the domain of the X-ray ceased, and the case properly belonged to surgery. His results in lupus erythematosus had not been satisfactory with the X-ray. In lupus vulgaris, he believed the X-ray was eminently the best means of treating that form of tuberculosis. In acne his experience had been gratifying.

Dr. David Lieberthal corroborated what the other speakers had said in regard to the treatment of acne, lupus vulgaris, acne rosacea, etc., with the X-ray, as well as the results obtained. He emphasized the importance of carefully selecting and classifying cases.

Dr. Pusey, in closing, speaking of idiosyncrasy, stated that, contrary to the statements of some gentlemen, he had noticed a marked difference in the susceptibility of patients to the X-rays. The variation in individuals was so great that much care had to be taken in treating a lesion like an epithelioma.

Administration of **Oxygen Gas.**—Dr. H. J. Burwash read a paper with this title. He referred to a paper by Kellogg, of Battle Creek, Mich., entitled "Oxygen Gas Per Enema," which was published in 1887. In this paper Kellogg discusses at length experiments on guinea-pigs, showing that gas per enemata is readily absorbed, and that dark venous blood was noticed to be immediately changed into bright arterial blood by its application. He therefore recommended this method for the treatment of diseases of the liver and digestive organs. He reports many cases, nearly all being of digestive troubles. Dr. Burwash has made a new application of it by using it in the treatment of the acute respiratory diseases, particularly pneumonia. This method was first used by him in August, 1891, in a severe typhoid fever case, after failing to resuscitate the patient by the usual method by inhalation. The patient was a young girl, sixteen years of age, who, from the persistent high temperature, became profoundly toxic, delirious and cyanotic. The gas by inhalation did not appear to revive her from the stupor, and then it occurred to him to administer the gas per enema. He gave her one gallon; after two minutes' duration the respiration became more exhilarated, and the deep cyanosis turned to a beautiful pink condition. The patient recovered after a very protracted illness. Since that time he has con-

tinued to use oxygen per enema in all his critical cases, especially pneumonia. He mentioned two recent cases of pneumonia. The first was that of Mr. K., aged thirty-five years, brewery worker, who developed a double pneumonia of the apex on the one side and base on the other, in which the temperature varied from 103° to 106° F., rectal; the toxemia increasing, as a result the patient became delirious with extremely rapid respirations and weakened heart. About the sixth day of the disease the oxygen gas was used after the usual cold bath had been administered, which was necessary to reduce the high temperature. The bowels were first thoroughly evacuated by normal salt solution. The gas was administered for from one and a half to two minutes' duration hourly until the condition indicated the relief desired. At each administration about one gallon of the gas was consumed, though the amount used was determined by the patient's condition rather than by measure. Immediately following each administration the usual physical phenomena appeared. In this case the high temperature continued until the eleventh day, when the crisis appeared, and thereafter he continued to uninterrupted recovery. The administration of gas was continued until the heart's action was assured. He reported another similar case of pneumonia treated by oxygen gas, with recovery. Why does oxygen gas administered by the intestinal canal oxygenate the blood, and tissues so much more efficiently than when given by inhalation? It is plainly apparent that the introduction of a large quantity of oxygen gas into the intestinal canal not only neutralizes and deodorizes the noxious gases that are frequently present there, but also by this direct method introduces oxygen through the portal system to the liver, whose cells are not only stimulated to greater activity, but are nourished as well. Besides this, the already overcharged lungs are assisted in their function of aeration of the blood by this condition of reenforcement.

Normal Salt Solution and Other Local Analgesics in the Office Treatment of Anorectal Diseases.—Dr. J. R. Pennington read a paper on this subject, in which he stated that recent discoveries and improved technic in the use of local analgesics obviate the necessity for patients suffering from hemorrhoids, fissure and many other forms of anorectal disease, to forego all business and social obligations, go to a hospital, take chloroform or ether, be operated upon and remain there for two or three weeks before convalescence. Such patients, with few exceptions, are now operated upon by him at his office. They then go home and return the following day or the day thereafter for their dressings, or return to their country homes. Before operating, if there are no contra-indications, about the only question he asks the patient is: Did your bowels move to-day? If so, and an operation is indicated, or necessary, and the patient so desires, he prepares the field and proceeds at once to operate, using either normal salt solution or eucaine-adrenalin solution as the local analgesic. Heinze, of Dresden, found that pure water alone is an intense irritant to the sensory nerves, and that anesthetic solutions diluted with it beyond a certain extent have the same effect, and render the injections painful. He also demonstrates that the addition of salt entirely obviates this source of irritation. Hence, it occurred to the author that a salt or some other isotonic solution would be a better agent than water with which to produce pressure or mechanical analgesia, as it is desirable that the-solution injected shall give as little pain as possible and also that it shall not be harmful to the tissues. Should it be desirable, as it is in some instances, especially when the injections must be made into the deeper tissues and the operation necessarily prolonged, to secure the specific action of some drug as eucaine or cocaine alone, or in combination with the distension of the tissues, he then adds to the salt solution a small quantity of eucaine and adrenalin chloride.

In internal hemorrhoids the salt solution is injected directly into the tumor until it becomes white, when it is grasped with a pair of forceps and the mucosa carefully divided down to the sub-mucosa; this tunic, which contains the principal blood vessels, is then ligated with a very fine ligature, and the major portion of the tumor cut off. As the lymphatics and circulating blood rapidly removes isotonic solutions from living tissues, the anesthesia is of short duration and the operation must be performed very quickly. In polypi the solution is injected into the base of the pedicle, a ligature thrown around it and the tumor cut off. Interno-external piles are treated similarly to the internal variety. In prolapsus ani the injection is made into the mucosa and deeper structures; sections of these tunics are then ligated and cut off. The author prefers a knife to the use of scissors as it causes less pain. The cases in which he has successfully employed one or the other of these solutions to produce local analgesia include radical operations for protruding and nonprotruding internal hemorrhoids; interno-external, thrombotic and cutaneous hemorrhoids; polypi, anal prolapse, fissure, ulcerations, abscesses, sacral dermoids, lipomata, condylomata, and secondary operation for colostomy. It is important that the solution should be warmed to the body temperature. Rapid injections should be avoided, as sudden distension of the tissues may be painful; for the same reason neither solution should be used when too cold or too hot. Strange as it may seem, most cases complain of but little pain on the days after the operation. He has operated on seventy-five cases by this method of anesthesia, and presented a brief report of twelve, six of whom were physicians.

OBSTETRICAL SOCIETY OF PHILADELPHIA.

Stated Meeting, held December 1, 1904.

The President, Richard C. Norris, in the Chair.

Chorio Epithelioma Malignum.—This paper was read by Dr. P. B. Bland. His patient was thirty-one years of age. One maternal aunt died of cancer of the uterus. The patient herself always enjoyed comparatively good health. She was married at eighteen years and had five labors. The first four were normal; the fifth occurred at the eighth month and was hastened or produced by sustaining a severe fall. Her symptoms began about four months after her last labor and six months before admission to the hospital. These consisted in more or less vague and indefinite pains in the lower portion of the abdomen, which were of a dull, aching, boring character. Two months prior to admission she suffered from a rather free, serous and offensive discharge which soon became tinged with blood. The bleeding progressively increased in intensity. Patient on admission was extremely pale and anemic and had lost considerable flesh. Examination revealed the uterus twice its normal size. It was more

or less soft in consistence, the cervix was large and the os admitted the tip of the index finger. There was no palpable pathological alteration in the tissues outside of the uterus. The patient was prepared for operation, but before opening the abdomen the uterus was dilated and a nodular mass discovered in its interior. Some of this was removed and resembled so strikingly malignant disease that hysterectomy was decided upon and performed.

Morbid Anatomy.—The uterus was possibly two or two and one-half times its normal size; the enlargement was uniform. The uterine wall was thickened and showed changes found in subinvolution. Occupying the interior of the uterus on its posterior wall and in the fundal region, a large irregular nodular mass was found. This was of a greenish blood coagula color and of rather tense consistence. The nodules varied in size from a pea to a man's thumb. The mass did not show any line of demarcation between itself and the uterus, but apparently infiltrated the uterine wall to the extent of three-eighths of an inch. The ovarian vein of the right side was distended greatly by an organizing thrombus. A portion of this was protruding from the vessel after removal. Microscopical examination of sections of the nodules revealed the tumor to be a typical chorio-epithelioma. The patient was living and well eight months after the performance of the operation without any subjective manifestations of recurrence of the disease. The writer reviews the early history of chorio-epithelioma and believes from his observations and study of the genealogy, that there should be no controversy as to the nomenclature of these tumors. He believes, with Marchand, that they develop, as was recognized in his case, from the epithelial coverings of the chorionic villi, and, therefore, that chorio-epithelioma malignum is an appropriate term. He thinks, in discussing the pathology, that the line of invasion in chorio-epithelioma is distinctly characteristic of the tumor, differing from carcinoma in that it is soft, mushy and sloughing. In carcinomatous tumors the lines of invasion as is well known is hard, dense, and firm. He also spoke at some length of other neoplasms containing choriomatous cells, and believes with the late observers, that they should be classed with the teratoma and not considered as true chorio-epithelioma; for it would be better, he thinks, to adopt a nomenclature which would distinguish those closely connected with gestation and those arising independently of it. The author also discusses in detail the etiology of these tumors, reviewing all the theories thus far advanced as to their causation. He strongly inclines to Ehrlich's side-chain theory. The high type of malignancy exhibited by these tumors the writer also believes to be due to the time of its occurrence or its association with the preceding pregnancy. He discusses in full the symptoms and diagnosis of the condition, and also the prognosis. The latter, he says, is extremely grave. It is perhaps the most malignant of all tumors, occurring as it does during the full physiological activity of the patient, and with the physiological process of pregnancy, in an organ in which the blood vessels are greatly multiplied and enlarged, and, therefore, in a state highly favorable for the transportation of malignant cells throughout the body. The outlook for the patient suffering with this condition cannot positively be asserted, however, to be either good or bad, in view of the fact that spontaneous healing has occurred in some, and that even in extensive cases of metastases after removal of the primary site of infection, patients have recovered. The treatment for the condition should be the same as for malignant disease elsewhere in the body—complete extirpation of the uterus in the field of healthy tissue at the earliest possible moment should be the only operative resource considered.

Dr. B. C. Hirst, in the discussion, said he had seen two cases of chorio-epithelioma, one of which began immediately after labor and ended fatally in three months. The patient had refused operation at first, later returned to the hospital soliciting it, but it was then too late. The second case was a metastatic tumor in the brain following hydatidiform mole from which the patient died about six months after expulsion of the diseased ovum. There was nothing in the intra-uterine examination to indicate malignancy. The most interesting question in this connection to the practical man is that of diagnosis. He had a case last year of which he had a good drawing. He was called to see a woman who had been bleeding off and on during pregnancy; she was delivered prematurely between the sixth and seventh month. Three or four days after delivery she began to bleed, and the hemorrhage continued so profusely that her physician thought Dr. Hirst would scarcely arrive in time. Dr. Hirst found the woman in a desperate condition. The vagina was packed, and she was sent to the University Hospital. In commenting upon the case the next day, he called the attention of the class to the causes of hemorrhage from the uterus after childbirth, and mentioned among the causes retention of some portion of the ovum, and, as the rarest of all causes malignant growth in the womb. He said, however, that while it was rare, it should be borne in mind, and if no other cause could be found malignancy should be thought of. He then proceeded to examine the interior of the woman's womb, and found to his surprise that he had removed with the placental forceps a curious brain-like material, which microscopically was most suggestive of malignancy. It looked exactly like the material removed from cases of adenocarcinoma of the endometrium. Specimens were submitted to three different pathologists. Two thought it was chorio-epithelioma. The third did not think it was, but as the history was so suggestive, and the appearance of the specimen under the microscope was so suspicious he recommended hysterectomy. On the advice of the three pathologists, and prompted by his own feelings, he removed the uterus. Inside of the womb, near the fundus, but not at the placental site, was to all microscopical appearances a well-developed neoplasm. He had this studied carefully under the microscope, and all the pathologists to whom it was submitted agreed that it was not a chorio-epithelioma, but they were unable to tell what it was. There was an infiltration of necrotic material and granulation cells, which formed a well-marked tumor extending above the endometrium about half an inch, and reaching into the myometrium about one-quarter of an inch. He had, therefore, removed the woman's womb on a diagnosis of chorio-epithelioma, and the operation proved to be unnecessary. Fortunately the patient made a good recovery. He cannot see how this mistake is to be surely avoided in the future. It is easy enough to make a diagnosis in well-marked cases that are already inoperable. What is wanted, however, is to make the diagnosis early. In the present state of knowledge, he does not see how this can be done with certainty. In every case of pathological condition of the endometrium after childbirth one may see the same multiplication of syncytial cells and the same inversion of the myometrium as in chorio-

epithelioma, and no one yet has been able to tell me how to distinguish between the two. By the microscopical appearances of scrapings from a case of retained placental fragments the diagnosis of chorio-epithelioma might be justifiable. The only light there is, that, in addition to the microscopical findings, one must have a large, exuberant neoplasm in the uterus, profuse hemorrhage, evidence of erosion of the uterine wall, and, in addition, possibly metastasis. If, however, one waits for all these symptoms the operative results are not going to be particularly brilliant.

Dr. Bland, in closing, said that the diagnosis of chorio-epithelioma is somewhat difficult, but from the history of the case and the microscopical findings he thinks one should, as a rule, be able to make a reasonably positive diagnosis. One should not, however, depend upon the microscope alone, for the clinical manifestations are extremely valuable, indeed. To his mind a digital examination of the interior of the uterus would be the best means at command to establish the true character of the lesion, though he does not think, just as in other departments of medicine, an absolutely positive diagnosis could even be made by the execution of this procedure. A characteristic of the growth that should help one is that it is almost always in the fundal region and on the posterior wall. Moreover, the peculiar and characteristic conformation of the basal portion of tumor is so entirely different from other neoplasms that it in itself should strongly suggest the presence of this tumor.

Posttyphoid Ovarian Abscess and Suppurative Cholecystitis with a Gall-stone and an Intraperitoneal Abscess.—The subjects were treated by Dr. Barton Cooke Hirst. He said that the first patient was a young woman who was admitted to a Philadelphia hospital with the symptoms of typhoid fever. One month subsequently marked pelvic pain developed; two months from time of admission she was discharged. The pelvic pain continued for three months after leaving the hospital, when she consulted the writer. He found marked abdominal tenderness, fever, a weak, rapid pulse, and to the right of the uterus an inflammatory mass the size of an orange. A diagnosis of posttyphoid ovarian abscess was made, based upon the history and physical signs. Upon operation the ovary was found converted into a single-chambered cyst, which on bacteriological examination contained a pure culture of colon bacilli. The second patient was a young woman who had recovered from an attack of typhoid fever, three months previous to the author seeing her, she had noticed a lump below the ribs on the right side. On pelvic examination a retroverted uterus and prolapsed ovary were found. The following operations were done: Dilation and curettement, ventrosuspension, shortening of the infundibulopelvic ligament. The gall-bladder was incised, a stone and several ounces of pus were removed, an abscess in the peritoneal cavity below the gall-bladder was also evacuated. The patient made an excellent recovery. The pus was submitted to a bacteriological examination, and contained a pure culture of an unidentified bacillus of the colon group.

Dr. Müller, in the discussion, said that the typhoid bacillus is probably always an inhabitant of the gall-bladder during the attack of typhoid fever, producing a slight degree of cholecystitis in many cases, which disappears on subsidence of the attack, and requiring in the great majority of instances no treatment whatever. Sometimes suppurative cholecystitis occurs after typhoid fever, usually in a few weeks or months after the disease has subsided. In the last 55 bacteriological examinations in the German Hospital of bile aspirated during operations, performed by Dr. Deaver, 32 cultures were obtained from the 55; seven of which were typhoid bacillus in pure culture; of the others, in 21 the colon bacillus was obtained; in three the staphylococcus, and in one streptococcus. The typhoid bacillus produces widespread lesions of the gall-bladder walls, cholecystectomy being invariably required in the cases examined. Histologically the gall-bladder shows ulceration of the mucous membrane, serous and cellular infiltration of the walls and a plastic exudate covering the serosa. In one case a fistula existed between the gall-bladder and stomach. He recalled an interesting case on the service of Dr. Frazier, at the Philadelphia Hospital, of a young girl of fifteen years who had had an attack of typhoid fever a year, previously and entirely recovered. She became pregnant, was delivered at term, and two weeks afterward she developed symptoms of severe cholecystitis. Here to all appearances she was perfectly well, yet a 'calculus had developed within the gall-bladder, and did not give rise to trouble until a subsequent infection with the colon bacillus drove it into the cystic duct. In cases in which there is a distinct history of typhoid fever it is readily understood how the infection would be carried to the gall-bladder by the blood, either of the general or portal circulation. In the other cases to which he had referred there was no history of typhoid, yet there was pure culture of the typhoid bacillus found in the gall-bladder, and in these cases a consideration of the source of infection makes it evident that there is some point of focal necrosis within the intestinal canal, not sufficient to give rise to any intestinal lesion, from which the bacillus is carried to the gall-bladder by the portal circulation giving rise to the cholecystitis.

Exhibition of Specimens.—Dr. Barton Cooke Hirst presented these. The first exhibit is an illustration of that rather rare condition, myxomatous degeneration of an adenomyoma of the uterus. This is only the second case he had seen. Myxomatous change ranks among the rarest degenerations of fibroid tumors. Primary carcinoma of the clitoris is likewise rare. Carcinoma of the vulva anywhere is rare, but carcinoma of the clitoris is the rarest of all. He had seen six cases of carcinoma of the vulva and only one of carcinoma of the clitoris. Primary carcinoma of the vagina is also rare. In this case the disease attacked the posterior vaginal wall within the posterior commissure and extended two-thirds of the way up the vaginal canal, leaving the anterior third of the vagina free of the disease. The most interesting question in this connection is whether the uterus must in all cases be removed. He resected three inches of the rectum with the posterior two-thirds of the vagina, but did not remove the uterus. The remnant of the vagina was made into a narrow canal to carry off the menstrual discharge. The patient recovered from the operation, but has been lost sight of since.

Dr. A. J. Downes also exhibited specimens. The first one was a uterus which was removed from a woman sixty years of age. It shows the features which in some cases are considered to be inoperable. The woman came from the South, and in April last she had the first sign of hemorrhage after ten years cessation. She was examined by a doctor in the city. A correct diagnosis was made but advice given against operation. Then she consulted an eminent gynecologist in New Orleans, who made the same diagnosis and advised against operation. Dr. Downes saw the woman a short time ago, and she appeared to him to be in very good condition physically from general inspection. Upon examination he found a small mass protruding

below what should have been the posterior wall of the uterus, extending an inch down on the posterior wall. The anterior lip of the uterus could be made out. By both vaginal and rectal examinations there was a fixed mass at the side of the cervix. Owing to the woman's good general appearance, he thought he would give her a chance by operation, and thereupon did a panhysterectomy. He first sterilized the vagina and did not touch it again. The fundus of the uterus was perfectly normal, the cervix was twice the size of the fundus. He removed the uterus through the abdominal incision without the use of a ligature, and the closing part of the operation consisted in clamping off the vagina and leaving it shut. Six months ago this would have been an easy operation and practically curable, for there was evidently no cancerous tissue left on the removal of this. This was taken out by the electro-thermic clamp, the method of heat and pressure for hemastasis, and practically without loss of blood.

MEDICAL AND CHIRURGICAL FACULTY OF MARYLAND.

Regular Meeting, held January 6, 1905.

Symposium on Immunity.—Dr. Welch opened the meeting with a brief historical résumé of the development of immunity. The question has always been of interest to medical men and immunity to a second attack in the case of certain diseases has long been known. The first example of experimental immunity was variolization which was successful but dangerous. Then followed Jenner's great triumph marking the first era in the history of the subject. Pasteur was able to show the possibility of vaccinating (or "Jennerizing," as Behring has suggested) against several organisms, particularly against anthrax and rabies. The scientific studies of Metchnikoff, leading to the phagocytosis theory of immunity marked the next epoch. Then followed Nuttall's work on the blood sera which resulted in the humeral theory. The discovery, by Roux and Yersin, of a toxin, and of an antitoxin by Behring cleared up the subject of antitoxic immunity, the production of which has only a restricted application (the best examples being diphtheria and tetanus). Following the work of Pfeiffer all the problems of bacteriocidal immunity were opened up and the "antibodies" (precipitins, agglutinins, etc.) began to take attention.

Production of Active Immunity.—This may be effected by the injection of organisms, living or dead (Jennerization) or by the injection of specific toxins. If micro-organisms are injected bacteriolytic immunity results; if toxins, "Giftfestigkeit" or "poison-proofness." In the latter case it must be possible to obtain soluble toxins and as this is only possible in the case of a few organisms (notably diphtheria and tetanus) this sort of immunity cannot always be produced. Immunity may practically be produced (1) by injecting germs alive and fully virulent (only possible when the animal is not very susceptible to the given germs). (2) By injecting attenuated cultures. This involves a risk and is not always applicable to human beings. (3) By injecting dead organisms. (4) By injecting toxins when these are obtainable. After the reaction caused by their injection the blood acquires a new bacteriolytic or antitoxic) property and immunity results,— an immunity which may be transferred with the transfer of the serum producing *passive* immunity. The second method is used in smallpox and rabies though the specific organism is known in neither case. In the case of rabies it seems probable that the organism of the fixed virus is more virulent but less resistant than that of the virus of the streets. Statistics show a high though not perfect immunization possible for rabies. In animals similar immunization is possible against anthrax and (following Koch's investigations) against Rinderpest; and the pecuniary results from these discoveries alone outweigh all the outlay for scientific medicine since the world began. Trudeau, Smith, Behring and Pierson have shown that the bovine tuberculosis is more virulent than the human form and have undertaken to immunize animals by injecting the human disease. It has been hoped that human immunization might be possible if tuberculosis from cold-blooded animals were used. The injection of killed cultures has been attempted in plague, cholera and dysentery, but with only a limited success. Wright, of London, has made extensive experiments in typhoid and the results have been definite but not uniform. The three requirements for this method of immunity are (1) assurance of success; (2) absence of serious dangers; (3) the presence in the community of a danger of general exposure to the disease. In smallpox alone are these requirements met.

Agglutinins.—These result when bacterial or other cells are injected into the animal body and they cause a clumping of these cells. They were first studied by Pfeiffer. Grüber and Grünbaum discovered the reaction in the case of typhoid fever but Widal, who published somewhat earlier, has had his name, quite unjustly, attached to the phenomenon. The reaction is of very great use bacteriologically, in the diagnosis of organisms and clinically in the diagnosis of disease. It is of great value clinically in typhoid fever. In other diseases clinical features make the agglutination reaction superfluous, or the reaction is inconstant or it does not occur.

Passive Immunity.—This was defined by Dr. Marshall as that type of immunity conferred by the injection of an immunized serum. The original immunity must be experimental, for natural immunity cannot be transferred. Antitoxin is a specific reaction product to the organism which unites with the toxin somewhat as acid and base; and the materials which destroy the toxins are not the same as those which destroy the bacteria in bactericidal immunity. Practically, passive immunity is best illustrated by the case of diphtheria, where the mortality has fallen from 50 to 15 per cent. by the use of antitoxin. Doses of 2,000 to 14,000 units should here be used and be given intravenously if the case is not seen early.

Hemolysins and Precipitins.—The former, said Dr. Stokes, are substances capable of separating hemoglobin from the stroma and their action is seen in the anemias of acute infectious diseases. Precipitins are substances formed after the injection of material into animals, capable of clotting the injected material. They are only specific for the injected substance and Nuttall has applied the precipitin reaction to forensic medicine in attempting to distinguish the blood of different species of animals in this way. Dr. Hemmeter referred to the early foreshadowing of Ehrlich's theory in the work of Emil Fischer, who called attention to the necessary configuration of enzymes in ferments and used a phrase to express this fact, which has since been a favorite of Ehrlich's: "Wie ein Schlüssel in das Schloss."

The theory itself is so colossal that it is bound to meet opposition, but it is certainly a most satisfactory, if not an infallible, guide.

BOOK REVIEWS.

STUDIES FROM THE DEPARTMENT OF PATHOLOGY OF THE COLLEGE OF PHYSICIANS AND SURGEONS, Columbia University, New York. Vol. IX, for the Collegiate Year 1903-1904.

THIS characteristic volume again appears, gathering from the various periodicals the most important studies published by the workers in the pathological department of the university during the year, and giving evidence of great and varied industry. It forms a very desirable series of reprints, and the director is to be congratulated upon the appearance and significance of the new volume.

ESSENTIALS OF MEDICAL CHEMISTRY, Organic and Inorganic, containing also Questions of Medical Physics, Chemical Philosophy, Analytical Processes, Toxicology, etc. Prepared especially for Students of Medicine, by LAWRENCE WOLFF, M.D., Formerly Demonstrator of Chemistry, Jefferson Medical College; Physician to the German Hospital, of Philadelphia; Member of the German Chemical Society of Philadelphia College of Pharmacy, etc. Sixth edition, Thoroughly revised by A. FERREE WITMER, Ph.G., formerly Assistant Demonstrator of Physiology, University of Pennsylvania; Neurologist to the Out-Patient Department of the Hospital for Ruptured and Crippled, New York City. W. B. Saunders & Company, Philadelphia, New York and London.

THE fact that this book has reached its sixth edition in so short a time, will prove beyond a doubt its usefulness. Recent discoveries in physics and inorganic chemistry, almost epoch-making in their importance, have made a new edition necessary. The subject of organic chemistry, especially organotherapy and the substituted ammonias, has also been carefully revised and much new matter added.

BEING DONE GOOD. By EDWARD B. LENT. Second Edition. Brooklyn Eagle Press, Brooklyn-New York.

THIS cheerful volume in which Mr. Lent describes in a style worthy of Mark Twain his varied and thrilling experiences with doctors and remedies uncounted, during a protracted siege of rheumatism, deserves a place in the library of every man who ever had ache or pain. Its irrepressible, audacious humor could scarcely be so effective were it not for the accompanying conviction that genuine courage is at the bottom of it. A man might *entertain* with secondhand experiences, but this is a book which will not only amuse those in health, but lend real cheer and stamina to the sick, who find in it undeniable evidence of actual experience. One would like to add another topic to Mr. Lent's list of things by which the sufferer is "done good," and with the conviction that this little volume will be more efficacious than patent medicine or Spanish flies.

BOOKS RECEIVED.

MENTAL DEFECTIVES. By Dr. M. W. Barr. 8vo, 368 pages. Illustrated. P. Blakiston's Son & Co., Philadelphia.

MEDICAL LABORATORY METHODS AND TESTS. By H. French. 12mo, 152 pages. Illustrated. W. T. Keener & Co., Chicago.

THE MEDICAL NEWS.

A WEEKLY JOURNAL OF MEDICAL SCIENCE.

VOL. 86.   NEW YORK, SATURDAY, MARCH 25, 1905.   NO. 12.

ORIGINAL ARTICLES.

ROOF GARDENS ON CITY PRIVATE HOUSES.[1]

BY W. P. NORTHRUP, M.D.,

OF NEW YORK;

PROFESSOR OF PEDIATRICS, THE UNIVERSITY AND BELLEVUE HOSPITAL MEDICAL COLLEGE; ATTENDING PHYSICIAN TO THE PRESBYTERIAN AND FOUNDLING HOSPITALS; CONSULTING PHYSICIAN TO THE HOSPITALS OF THE HEALTH DEPARTMENT.

How may we multiply safe and sunny playgrounds for children dwelling on Manhattan Island? The object of this communication is to suggest how city roofs may be adapted to such needs, to give illustrations of one such approved playground, and to describe the excellent results shown in the health of the children concerned.

Fig. 1.

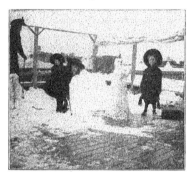

Snow lady.

A friend bought a house on the East Side uptown, abreast of Central Park, determined to try the experiment of keeping a family of children aged three, five and seven, in town. The last three winters they had spent on Long Island. The parents chose the locality near the Park and on high ground, with the thought of approximating the conditions of country air, hoping that an added year on the life of the children might make the experiment successful.

The children had regularly each fall returned to town in robust health. They gradually lost their appetite, became listless, sallow and languid, caught cold, were confined to the house, were classed as grip patients, went from bad to worse, till the parents picked them up and fled to the country house again. This had been repeated in all three times. Once in the country the children spent much of their time in the open air, and became well and hearty.

1 Read before the New York Academy of Medicine (Pediatric Section), March 2, 1905.

"Why were they not sent out into the Park half a block away?" someone will ask. They were sent to the Park daily. Soon they came to loathe the thought of going out. In the country they had been accustomed to feed their chickens and rabbits when out of doors. In short, they loitered many hours in the open air, playing quietly, pleasantly entertained. They took no notice of the time they were out. It was not done by the watch. They *lived* in the open air.

In town they must be dressed fit for the Park, the nurse must dress herself properly, and by the time they are all ready to go out they are too

Fig. 2.

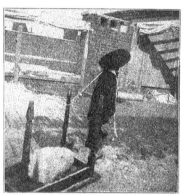

Trolley-car.

warm in their wraps, impatient, pulling in divergent directions. After twenty minutes perhaps they emerge from the house. In the short walk to the Park they must dodge automobiles, boys on roller skates, grocer carts, bicycles, baby carriages and all varieties of out-of-temper, hurrying people. Within the Park they must "keep off the grass," must not "pick flower, fruit or leaf," must not get up on the iron benches with their feet. What they may do is to trail along with the nurse till the time is up and they can go home. Their wildest diversion is to hang to the leash of an eager dog, and see that he does not get away and get shot by the police.

If one direct that children spend as many hours in the Park as possible on all but positively bad days, the resulting report is usually this: "Oh, yes, the children are in the Park all-day." What does "all day" mean, when really figured out in hours? After the children have been in the

Park an hour they begin to be tired and look tired. They get home, having successfully dodged the self-moving bolts hurtling along Fifth Avenue, also other nerve and life destroy-

Fig. 3.

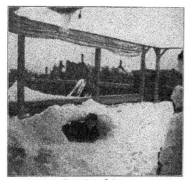

Tunneling—Subway.

ers. After an hour and three-quarters they return to their home cross, tired, the youngest jaded and pale.

The often-heard statement " Out all day in the Park " frequently means, when figured out, an hour and three-quarters in the morning and an hour in the afternoon. This, then, is the life to which many children return after six and eight months in the country, where it is exceptional for them to be indoors at all in sunlight hours.

I was asked to see what could be done for this family who had spent three winters on Long Island. Their new house faced south, on rising ground, was five stories high, and upon the top was a half story for servants. In front of this half story, and facing south, was a tin roof 24x24 feet, without a nuisance. The vent pipes opened above the half story. Here was an area of 576 square feet, 60 to 70 feet in air, flooded with sunshine, above the dustline, free from noise, and confusion. From its surface Central Park, less than half a block away, lay as a private lawn under the eye, the view south was unbroken to Murray Hill, the New Jersey shore and Long Island Sound were distinguishable. In short, there was an unbroken horizon south, west and east, and permanent protection on the north. Upon this area the sun shone all day, the clear upper air fell without its usual admixture of dust : no noise and no confusion could intrude.

Carpenters were put to work to cover the tin roof, laying a floor of narrow strips, boards four inches wide, with an interval of a quarter of an inch between. The floor was laid in sections which could be taken up as desired, to repair the tin roof or recover lost toys. The open flooring allowed the boards to dry quickly.

While this work was just beginning the youngest boy seemed more than ever drooping and run down, and it was said, " He looks very white when he comes in from the Park." "Hurry up the roof." was the reply, " and when a quarter of the flooring is laid, put him on it. The carpenters will entertain him, and the ends of boards and bits of timber will please him. Loitering in the open air is what he wants. *Air with ease* is his prescription."

The floor once laid, the area was surrounded with a wire net, and the enclosure, pen, or " chicken house," as some friend named it, was ready for use. This enclosure was quickly and inexpensively constructed. In anticipation of vigorous winter weather a permanent partition was raised on the northern half of the west side, nearest the half story, the " deck house." Canvas slides were adjusted in such a way that, at will, the " chicken house " could be converted into a pen. Cold winds could thus be shut off (" modified " is a favorite word just now,) while the sun could always shine in.

One more precaution was taken. An awning was spread over the northern third, rolling down from the house cornice upon a frame. This could be put up or let down at will. Again, in case of drizzling weather, an apron was ready to be extended from the point where the awning ended on the north, nearly to the southern limit. The result of this was that the children could play out in all weather. If it rained or snowed heavily, the strong awning protected eight or nine feet of the north end and kept it dry, the permanent board partition protected from the prevailing

Fig. 4.

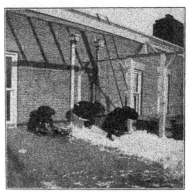

Street cleaning.

west wind. In drizzling light rain the apron protected nearly the whole floor.

The roof playground has stood the test, and proved available for all weathers.

What has been the result? It is now five

months since the beginning of the experiment. Within two weeks the smallest boy was pronounced better than he had been since he was eleven months old. He had always been fatigued in getting the amount of outdoor exercise which he was supposed to need. He dragged about, and was rather a quiet, demure little man. Any other child could take his toys away from him without remonstrance. At present writing it is said he used to be too tired to have a character, now he has rather too much. He is obstinate and self-willed. Last night he was put to bed without saying good-night to his parents, because he flew into such a fury and was so obstreperous.

For five hours every day, the blizzard days included, these now vigorous children have been out on the roof, playing at making snow men and snow ladies, houses, tunnels, etc. They have a toboggan slide, a cave, mounds and tunnels in the snow. It is not easy to get them to keep on their mittens. They are so warm-blooded that they complain that they feel too hot, they can't breathe with their mittens on. Most of the time the mittens hang by their sides.

The net result of the experiment is that the three children have been able to spend the winter in town, the family is undivided. To use the words of their best friend, they have been able to live a civilized life for at least one more winter. Not only have the children kept well, but they have been better than in all their lives before. The air of New York City is really good after one gets above the drifts and swirls of dust of the street level. Probably, too, the food has been more pleasing than the country markets supply. They have consumed vast quantities of food material. The children have not taken any medical treatment. The habitual colds of winter have not been present. It is impossible to find in town or country a more exuberant family of three, so entirely emancipated from the ills of town dwellers, so absolutely unsusceptible to cold, so savagely hungry, such sound sleepers. One can only think and speak of them as young polar bears. In the days of the blizzard the youngest was prevailed on to wear mittens for a time. Their complexions are of such bright hue that when the two elder children are on the street passers stop and turn to look at them. The Park policeman asked how long they had been over, and if they were Irish or English. No one could deceive him, he assured the nurse, no such color ever showed in American faces. The roundsmen, the snow-plough men and the street-cleaners know these little uptown fresh air children, and designate them in their own way as little polar bears and St. Bernards.

An interesting observation has been the fondness the children have shown for their aerie. Until the ice skating in the Park put a new attraction before them, the older two begged to stay and play on the roof. They tired of dragging and "keeping off the grass." On the roof their imagination converted ordinary toys into fire engines, wild animals, etc. Probably the one plaything which has given more prolonged pleasure than any other is an upturned wooden table and a cord which figured as a trolley car. With this the three have played for hours, pushing, pulling, filling their lungs with good dust-free air. With sled and wheelbarrow they are a street-cleaning department. With shovel and spade they mine and tunnel. Indeed, they really work hard. They occasionally vary the angelic mood with terrible displays of temper, they so far forget their long ancestry of good blood as to descend to furious battles among themselves. The small boy who was formerly "too tired to have a character", has steadily advanced to second place, and is now trying for first. He has fought it out with his sister, and now struggles for supremacy with his older brother. They love well, eat like wolves, sleep well and fight gloriously. Indeed, the proud mother must many times feel, before her friends with their well-

Fig. 5.

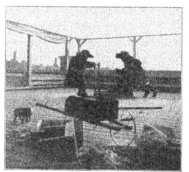

Trouble brewing.

behaved, anemic children, that her young thoroughbreds are in the eyes of her visitors wild things from the polar regions.

These children spend nineteen hours a day in outdoor air, five hours on the roof, fourteen hours in a sleeping room with windows open. The room is cold. Water freezes in it, the screen blows over, snow drifts in but does not melt.

Child No. 3 shows the greatest improvement. It will be remembered that the "roof paddock" was constructed largely for him. He has been on the street but once, and he has now grown so much that he has within a week been mistaken for the older boy.

Many odd nooks and angles are easily adapted to the purpose of a playground in an inexpensive way. There are but two essentials: the sun must come in, and the harsh winds stay out. A pen with canvas sides answers the purpose.

A word of testimony from the graduate nurse in charge of these children. In November last she looked " worn out " with all the significance of the expression as applied to a nurse who has been at her work steadily for ten years. Last week she informed me spontaneously that she had for the first time in her life gained weight in winter. She had gained five pounds in five months, the same that each of the growing children had. Furthermore she was not nervous, was so stupidly sleepy at nine o'clock at night that she went to bed soon after the children did, and in the morning, which surprised her more than all, her appetite for breakfast was such as she had never known since adolescence.

I mention these details because it is true, word for word, with the testimony of four other nurses.

One word of caution on the part of the parents. In inaugurating this new and radical treatment, a wise nurse is a necessity. For the first two weeks children unaccustomed to such a regimen should be carefully watched until they become accustomed to it. After two weeks the children and nurses are not susceptible to cold.

In this connection I may add that parents with " sand " are a necessity. It requires courageous parents to follow implicitly such a course. They may encounter adverse criticism, and be called " mad as March hares," as were these. Those who called them mad, now add the clause, " The children are wonders ! "

The total cost of this roof playground was a little more than $150. The saving in the wages of one attendant and in the difference of cost in clothing necessary to play on a retired roof garden and to go into the Park would fully equal this amount in five months.

57 East Seventy-ninth Street.

FIFTEEN YEARS' EXPERIENCE IN THE TREATMENT OF TYPHOID FEVER AT THE ROOSEVELT HOSPITAL.

BY WILLIAM HANNA THOMSON, M.D., LL.D.,
OF NEW YORK;
PHYSICIAN TO ROOSEVELT HOSPITAL.

THERE is no acute disease which seems to afford better opportunities than typhoid fever for testing the question whether we can beneficially modify its course by measures of treatment. This is because its onset is usually gradual, with a subsequent prolonged course, during which it progresses deliberately through definite successive stages, with dangers or complications so characteristic of each that they may be foreseen or expected, till finally it ends as gradually as it began.

In each of these respects it markedly contrasts with pneumonia, which commonly sets in abruptly, and then often develops severe symptoms so rapidly that its fatal issue may practically be decided in less than a week. If a patient should succumb to a surgical injury in so short a time as some do to a croupous pneumonia, it generally would be inferred that nothing could have saved him. Likewise in pneumonia, it is often doubtful whether it be not beyond our power to

counteract the blow to vitality already inflicted before we can begin to do anything.

Not so typhoid fever. Its dangers ordinarily arise from definitely timed derangements of one function after another, each contributing a greater or less share to the condition, according to the particular case. We, therefore, appear to be furnished with special indications for lessening the effects of these different derangements each in turn, and by so much improving the chances of the patient.

Nevertheless, the question is often raised whether the treatment of typhoid fever is any more successful now than it was thirty-five years ago. In England, judging from their hospital statistics, the mortality from this fever seems to remain about the same that it ever was. In a paper read before the Harveian Society, November, 1899, Dr. Sidney Phillips, physician to the London Fever Hospital, maintains that the chances of recovery of a person contracting typhoid fever to-day are little or no better than they were fifty years ago, notwithstanding the advances in medical knowledge, improved nursing and hygienic conditions. Murchison found that the mortality of patients in the London Fever Hospital during the ten years ending 1862 was 18.5 per cent., and Dr. Phillips says that all the figures available to him in the same Fever Hospital and in other London institutions, as well as the Registrar-General's returns, show that the mortality from 1890 to 1897 still remained over 18 per cent. The inference which Dr. Phillips draws from these figures is that typhoid fever will be found to kill 18.5 per cent. of its victims in London no matter what the treatment may be.

Whatever progress, therefore, has been gained in the last fifty years in medical knowledge, and that has been great, so far as these figures go, the treatment of serious acute diseases has made no advance at all.

As regards pneumonia, we must regretfully admit, I think, that there has been little diminution, if at all, in its mortality in the practice of our generation. It still remains the same dread disease as ever. But I hold that it is far otherwise with typhoid fever, the mortality of which, according to my recorded experience in hospital practice for the past thirty years, should not be much over three per cent. among those patients who give us an opportunity to treat them. I make this statement at the outset, with full recognition of the fact that no such conclusions should have weight, unless they are based upon carefully made and recorded observations extending over prolonged periods. Typhoid fever shares with other acute infections a varying severity according to what is termed the epidemic constitution of the particular season. The experience of one year, therefore, is no criterion of what it will be the following year. Hence, I submit this review of fifteen years' experience in its treatment in my wards at the

Roosevelt Hospital, with results, which I do not think can be only by accident or coincidence, so much better than the above cited statistics of the London hospitals. For the compilation of these statistics I am indebted to my former House Physician, Dr. E. V. Hubbard.

	Total.	Males.	Females.
Total admissions to my wards at the Roosevelt Hospital, during four months, from May to July, and September to November, each year, from May 1, 1889, to November 1, 1904	574	398	176
Total number of deaths........	40	31	19
or, 7.05 per cent. of total number.			
·But the total number of patients who died within a week after admission was.........	23	15	8
or, 57 per cent. of all deaths, and 80 per cent. of these did not survive the fourth day.			

Of the remaining 551 patients who were in the hospital for more than a week, there were 17 deaths, or 3.09 per cent.

It readily can be shown that the percentage of the fatality in the total number of admissions to the hospital in this period, viz., 7.05 per cent., affords no just criterion of the results of treatment, for the following reasons: A large proportion of the patients are not sent to hospitals with this fever until the disease is in advanced stage. Some, in fact, in my service were practically moribund on admission, and only served to swell the mortality figures. When the question, therefore, is about the efficiency or otherwise of any line of treatment, some distinction should be made between patients who gave some opportunity, in respect to time corresponding to the usual length of the disease, for the treatment to be tried, and those who were so far gone on admission that practically there was no chance to test in them that or any other form of treatment.

Thus, of the total deaths, 23 or 57 per cent. died within the first week after admission, and 80 per cent. of these did not survive the fourth day; only two of the 23 reached the seventh day of their stay in the hospital, the beginning of the illness in all of this class ranging from fifteen days to nine weeks before they came in, while no less than seven succumbed to perforation within four days after admission. These facts only confirm me in my belief that the proper management of the patient, as hereinafter detailed, within the first week or ten days of the illness, can materially modify its subsequent course. The above percentage of the total number of deaths, however, should be borne in mind in comparison with the 18.5 per cent. of the London hospitals, as it is to be presumed that the London figures also cover all deaths occurring in those institutions, whether among those admitted early or late in the disease.

One drawback to the completeness of my report, however, should be ·mentioned, namely, that, in common with my colleagues at the Roosevelt Hospital, my terms for service cover only two months at a time, May and June, and then September and October. According to the returns of the Health Board, the first two months correspond to the time of the least prevalence of typhoid fever in New York, while in September and October it is at its highest. In order, therefore, to make the test of treatment by my method as complete as I can, the number of deaths includes any which occurred up to November 14, or two weeks after my service terminates, as I presume that this subsequent period would fairly balance the exclusion of the first week above mentioned.

Statistics of mortality, however, are not the only test of the efficacy of any method of treatment, and particularly·so in typhoid fever. How the patients pass through the attack in respect to the occurrence and to the gravity of its various accompaniments, and in what condition it leaves those who recover from it, are much more satisfactory indications whether the disease is amenable to certain remedial measures or not. Whether any progress, therefore, has been gained in the past thirty-five years in the management of typhoid fever would be best illustrated by a comparison between the incidence and the degree of the leading symptoms of typhoid fever as they are described in such text-books as Watson's and Bristowe's of forty years ago, and those found in the clinical histories now presented.

Therefore, following Bristowe's enumeration of symptoms we will first note the diarrhea. He speaks of it as generally associated with the initial symptoms, though sometimes absent then, to become a striking feature of the disease, and rarely absent from the second week on. He deprecates, on this account, the use of laxatives, unless perhaps a small dose of rhubarb or of castor oil during the first week, and he regards the recommendations of Trousseau and of George Johnson, that the diarrhea should be allowed to run its course, as erroneous and dangerous, preferring to check it by the systematic administration of tannic acid, sulphuric acid, lead and opium, etc.

In my own records, diarrhea occurring at all after the first week after admission is reported in only 39, or 12 per cent., and in the majority of them it was not severe, so that there are very few prescriptions recorded as administered for this symptom. On the contrary, constipation, which had to be relieved by enemata, was of frequent occurrence. The absence of diarrhea in typhoid fever is not confined·to my hospital experience, but has been reported of late years as common in American hospitals generally, and to a less extent in the English reports. I would ascribe this change in a large measure to a change in the feeding of the patient. Thirty years ago the use of beef tea in typhoid fever was almost universal. I believe that hardly any articles are so prone to fermentation in the alimentary canal, and nothing is so apt to induce tympanites, as the continuous administration day and night of meat broths in febrile conditions.

Thirty years ago tympanites was so constant a symptom that it was rated as a diagnostic feature of the disease. As Watson says: "If you make pressure on the abdomen, you will find it hard and unnaturally resisting, as though its walls were much distended, but whether large or not, Dr. Jenner states that its shape is invariably the same and peculiar. The patient is never pot-bellied, but tub-shaped."

As I have always placed a good deal of store upon this symptom, I have had its occurrence noted in every case, so that even its temporary presence might not be overlooked. According to my impression, so infrequently had it been a marked symptom in any but the fatal cases, that I was surprised to find it recorded in 101, or 18 per cent. On reviewing this record, however, it was found that about 40 per cent. of the whole number of instances of tympanites occurred in September and October, 1898, and were noted in 39 soldiers admitted for typhoid fever contracted at various camps in our own country and in Cuba during the Spanish-American War. Of these, six had malaria as well, in four of whom *Plasmodium malariæ* permanently disappeared after the typhoid fever ran its course, while in two others chills and fever, with a reappearance of the plasmodium, took place after they had fairly convalesced from typhoid. It was probably owing to the reduced physical condition of these soldiers from the poor food and other hardships of camp life that they so generally presented this symptom on admission. Deducting, therefore, these soldiers, the occurrence of tympanites in all is recorded at most in only about 62 patients, or about 26 per cent. Its presence is generally noted in the histories of those who were admitted late in the disease, and in the majority of those it disappeared soon afterward under treatment. The prevention of this particular symptom, I believe not to be without bearing upon our question, whether we can favorably modify the cause of the fever, for tympanites is both a sign and a complication. It is a sign of weakened innervation and loss of the normal antiseptic power in the gastro-intestinal secretions, on the one hand, and the direct cause of cardiac and of pulmonary circulatory enfeeblement on the other; while it cannot be without some effect in increasing the tendency to accidents at the seats of the intestinal ulceration. I always regard a persistent tympanites in a typhoid patient with uneasiness, and any method of treatment in which this symptom becomes a rarity I cannot but consider as materially beneficial.

Hemorrhage from the bowels occurred in one per cent. In no instance was it directly fatal, and it was readily controlled by measures to be mentioned. It is always, however, a complication of some moment, as it may oblige us to suspend the Brand bath at a critical period of the hyperpyrexia. One man, while sitting up convalescent on the thirty-second day of his disease, began to bleed from nearly every mucous membrane of his body. He died in two days after excessive hematuria.

Among the 31 deaths of male patients, seven succumbed to intestinal perforation. One case also occurred in a woman during a relapse, after she had been in the hospital five weeks, another in a boy who had been in the hospital ten days. All the others occurred in patients who had been there less than a week after admission. The boy was operated upon and recovered. Five others were operated upon, but died.

To continue our comparison with the descriptions of former text-books: Dr. Bristowe proceeds to describe the classical "typhoid condition," into which he states a large proportion of the cases pass in the second week. "The elevation of temperature continues, the rash still comes out, the diarrhea still persists, the tongue becomes dry and brown and traversed by deep fissures; the lips and teeth covered with sordes; the mind grows dull and apathetic, and delirium, sometimes violent, sometimes busy, sometimes muttering, supervenes; tremors, subsultus and involuntary passage of evacuations takes place," etc.

I have no hesitation in saying that our present forms of treatment have done away with the "typhoid condition" here described so entirely that repeatedly successive house physicians have said to me that they had not seen cases of the kind and would have to go elsewhere to find them. That this picture of a patient's state should become a rarity is certainly an evidence of improved therapeutics, and is shown by the following reports of the incidence of its constituent symptoms. Thus, as to delirium: Out of the whole number admitted it was noted in 60, or 16 per cent. But of these 26, or nearly 50 per cent., were delirious on admission, 12 of whom died within that week, whereas the rest recovered from their delirium in a week or less. The entire absence of delirium at any period of their illness in the remaining 517 patients, or 94 per cent. of the whole number, is at least an indication that they hardly passed into the "typhoid condition" at any time in the course of the disease; while on the other hand, nothing testifies so clearly, in my opinion, to the benefits of treatment as the absence of all signs of mental disturbance in the majority of these ward patients. Some of them were drowsy, but tremors and subsultus were too rarely observed to figure among the clinical symptoms. The state of the tongue was always carefully noted, but fissure is not once recorded. Sordes on the teeth and lips were present in some patients on admission, but in every case soon disappeared, and is never recorded as developing in patients after admision. Of this fact I feel quite sure, for it has seemed to me that a remedy soon to be mentioned is commonly quite efficacious in preventing general dryness of the tongue if administered at the first appearance of this symptom at the tip.

Of other complications in our series, pneumonia occurred in 11, or 1.9 per cent., bronchitis in 65, or 18 per cent., but it was an initial symptom in more than 40 per cent. of the cases and was easily controlled.

Peripheral neuritis occurred in 28, or not quite even per cent., and in each case was limited to the feet. The causation of this symptom in typhoid is apparently purely mechanical, from the foot drop induced by prolonged relaxation of the leg muscles, thus causing the nerves to be put upon a continuous stretch. I, therefore, am always particular to direct that the feet have a foot rest in the third week, with care that the weight of the bedclothes should be taken off them by a cradle. Neglect of these precautions may make the recovery of the power of walking very slow during convalescence. The best local application to relieve the tenderness and pain in the feet is to wrap them up twice a day for half an hour in cloths wet with an infusion of red pepper, one dram to the pint of hot water. The peripheral neuritis in many patients long confined to bed with phthisis has much the same characters.

Phlebitis occurred in 11. In two of them it was very troublesome, and much prolonged the convalescence. Local applications of the strong tincture of iodine, or of silver nitrate, 20 grains to the ounce, should be applied over the affected vein very early.

Relapses occurred in 62, or no less than 18 per cent. of all cases. Though some of them seemed to occur in close sequence to some imprudence in eating during the hungry period of convalescence, yet in many instances no such cause could be assigned. Moreover, the tendency to relapse is much more marked in some years than in others, rising in one year to 30 per cent. of all cases, so that the etiology of these recrudescences is obscure. In London also it is noted that the three per cent. of relapses given by Murchison has now risen to 13 per cent. As a rule, the prognosis is not unfavorable, except in those patients who begin the relapse with vomiting. It seems to me, however, that relapses are more frequent in that class of patients in whom the brunt of the attack appears to fall on the intestine, more so than with those characterized from the beginning with tendency to hyperpyrexia. A patient with the symptoms of pronounced abdominal lesions, such as persistent tympanites and tongue tremor, should not be allowed solid food in any form for ten days after his temperature has fallen to normal.

The treatment of typhoid fever should be both of a general kind, to be prescribed in all its details for every case from the beginning, no matter how mild the type may seem to be (for we are never sure but that a mild case may at any time develop severe symptoms) ; and particular, according to the special tendencies developing in the course of the disease. Those special tendencies should be early recognized and definitely dealt with, for routine treatment is no more justifiable in this than in any other serious complaint.

The general line of treatment, which in the majority of cases is the only treatment needed, I would describe as follows:

First, early attention to the state of the kidneys. During the first week or ten days there is a marked tendency to a diminution in the secretion of urine. This I regard as an initial complication, whose effects may render the subsequent course much more severe, by favoring the increased multiplication of the typhoid bacillus in the blood, owing to the retention of excrementitious matters in it from the early failure of renal elimination. Late researches show that the typhoid bacilli, instead of developing only locally in the intestine, may charge the blood as early as the end of the first week. I would recommend, therefore, a recourse in all cases in the first two weeks of the fever, to the most certain diuretic which we possess, namely, rectal irrigation with hot normal saline, twice a day. Kemp's rectal irrigator is the best instrument for this purpose that I know of, using with it about four gallons each time, at a temperature of 115° to 120° F. The flow should run out as fast as it runs in, and it so constantly increases the urinary secretion that I have no doubt now, from numerous comparative observations between those who had it and those who were without it, that the course of the fever is distinctly changed for the better by this measure.

In some cases acute nephritis develops comparatively early in the disease, and then constitutes a serious complication, with a tendency to death from uremic coma with pulmonary edema. The causation of this complication is a septic invasion of the kidneys by the *Bacillus coli,* and should be promptly dealt with by the administration of ten grains of urotropin, always along with ten grains of sodium benzoate, to prevent irritation of the kidneys by the urotropin. It is striking to note how soon this remedy lessens the percentage of albumin in the urine, and lessens the number of casts along with improvement in the general symptoms of a uremic kind. When improvement occurs, the intervals of the dosing should be lengthened.

One of the best procedures in the first stage of the fever is intestinal disinfection by a calomel purge, given every other night till the middle of the third week. My usual dose is five grains of calomel and thirty-five grains of compound jalap powder. It promptly stops diarrhea, if that be present, and is remarkable for lowering the febrile temperature in the first week, often from one to three degrees compared with its previous range. It acts well also in promoting the secretion of urine. After the middle of the third week it is omitted owing to risk of hemorrhage from cathartics.

How to feed the patient is a prime question. There is nothing so preventible in the majority of these patients as the extreme wasting and general weakness which is so conspicuous in convalescence with many who have been inadequately or imperfectly fed during their long experience of fever. The starvation plan of treatment is preposterous, for we ought always to aim to maintain the nutrition of the muscular tissues, as that includes the nutrition and strength of the heart, on which so much depends, and it is the muscular tissues which suffer most in all pyrexias. It happens, however, that there is a special difficulty in this disease to secure the proper digestion, and hence the assimilation of food. That difficulty is due to the fact that typhoid fever diminishes the peptic power of the stomach more than any other known disease, including gastric cancer itself, as was shown by Fenwick, who on scraping the mucous membrane of patients dying with this fever, found that it had less pepsin than the stomachs of the others dying after the most wasting of diseases, such as phthisis, diabetes, etc. In some of the typhoid cases, not a trace of pepsin could be found.

Bearing this fact in mind, we should regard the stomach of a typhoid patient as having reverted to the weakness of a newly born infant. The only food for such a condition is fluid food, and of that, therefore, milk is the sole article which contains every ingredient to support life. But cow's milk, as such, cannot safely be given to an infant, nor is it any better suited for a typhoid patient. Cow's milk should invariably be diluted, for them, with lime water in the proportion of fully one-half, and in some cases, as shown by the presence of undigested curds in the passages, with even two-thirds of lime water, with the addition of salt, as it is a peculiarity of typhoid, as also of pneumonia, to have the chlorides entirely disappear from the urine. I choose lime water because it is also an antiseptic, and thus counteracts gastric tympanites. The administration of simple pure milk in this fever, I am sure, is responsible for many untoward developments. Besides lime water, I have for many years kept up the stated administration of five grains of scale pepsin, or of ten grains of saccharated pepsin, every three hours for the twenty-four, and I am sure that it shows the good results in practice, which we would expect from it on theoretical grounds, in the maintenance of the nutrition of the patients. I have often heard it remarked by visitors, that the patients in my wards did not in their appearance show much effect from the serious disease which they were passing through.

The systematic employment of intestinal antiseptics is of great importance. Some reasoners claim that it is impossible to disinfect the alimentary canal, because it will still contain millions of bacteria whatever we do. It is difficult to have patience with this talk, because it assumes that disinfection is synonymous with sterilization, whereas we are, while in the best of health, daily kept from being fatally poisoned by our own intestinal contents, through the normal check to the action of putrefactive bacteria by the antiseptic properties of healthy digestive secretions. Those normal secretions are so diminished in typhoid fever that decomposition of the gastro-intestinal contents proceeds apace, with its accompaniments of generation of gas and diarrhea from the acrid character of the intestinal contents. Disinfect, and then both tympanites and diarrhea cease.

Much the most serviceable of all these disinfectants is bismuth, owing to its non-irritating character, and its locally sedative properties, which cannot be said of other agents often employed, such as salol. I use ten to twenty grains of the subcarbonate, given along with the pepsin every three hours, or from 80 to 160 grains a day. Occasionally, if tympanites is persistent, five grains of the sulphocarbolate of soda is added to each dose.

With the first sign of dryness at the tip of the tongue, the oil of turpentine in 15 to 20 minim doses is added, given in mucilage every three hours till the tongue is moist again.

When cardiac weakness develops, alcoholic stimulants are given in the form of whisky. I object to repeated small doses, such as half an ounce, and much prefer an ounce at a time every three hours, given after milk. At first alcohol should be given only after midnight, then, as the fever continues, in the evening, and then in the afternoon. It is better to omit it in the forenoon, for that is the natural period of lessened fever and prostration. The secret of giving alcohol is not to look upon it as possessing any continuous sustaining power, but only that of a temporary stimulant for times of prostration, and hence the dose should be large enough to produce stimulation.

Strychnine is very commonly regarded as a needed cardiac stimulant in this affection. Its routine and persistent administration is mischievous, and it is well to suspend it every few days, and note the effect. Occasionally in pronounced cardiac debility, I prescribe it in combination in a pill of

℞ Strychnine sulph...... ....gr. ss
 Caffeine citrat ....grs. xxxvi
 Sparteine sulph....... ....grs. xv
 Ext. taraxici .... .q.s.
M. Div. in pilul. xx. S. One every three hours.

Much the most certain of all cardiac stimulants, however, is camphor given subcutaneously in 7½ gr. doses dissolved in 20 minims of sterilized almond or olive oil. I have seen it succeed in conditions of collapse in typhoid, as well as in pneumonia, when every other heart stimulant had failed. It may be repeated once an hour in urgent cases, or once in three hours.

Such has been my treatment for all ordinary cases so far as medicines go. But for thirty years I have regarded the Brand bath as the most effective of all agents at our command in typhoid fever. Without it, I should not care to treat a typhoid patient; and as will be noted, I have not feared to keep a patient in a bath at 70° F. for forty-seven minutes, because her temperature would not give in before. After that we had no further trouble, because from a condition which threatened death from hyperpyrexia, she changed to a case of mild typhoid and progressed steadily to recovery. I am sure that when the physician finds the temperature either increase after the cold bath, or begin very soon to do so, instead of losing heart he ought to grow bolder, till the thermometer shows that he is carrying the day with this invaluable remedy.

About the action of the Brand bath, it ought to be emphasized at the outset that is is not simply because it lowers the temperature. We have in the coal tar derivatives as certain antipyretics as it is, with this difference, that with antifebrin, antipyrin, or phenacetin, we can bring down the temperature, but, with them we bring down the patient too. I never prescribe either of them at any stage of this fever. The chief efficacy of the cold bath is that it is a potent eliminator of the typhoid toxin to the kidneys. It has been abundantly demonstrated that the toxicity of the urine, when injected into animals, is more than oubled after a bath than before it, a fact which ; clinically illustrated by the subsidence of the orst nervous symptoms after the patient is re- urned to bed.

This potent remedy should be used with all he discrimination which all remedies call for in roportion to their potency. It should be begun o soon as the temperature reaches 102.₅° F. t is often put off too long, for the earlier its liminating property is resorted to, the better for he subsequent course. The duration of the bath hould be wholly according to the effect. If he temperature drops from one to two degrees hile in the bath, the patient should be taken out hough he has been in it only five minutes. It should never be allowed to drop to 100° F., or t goes on falling after he is put back to bed. Otherwise, if instead of falling, it tends to go up ifter he has been in ten minutes, he must be left n it till it begins to fall, thought it may require over half an hour to do so. Severe shivering is not to be paid any attention to, but a good measure to shorten this after the bath is a dram of Hoffman's anodyne in an ounce of camphor water, and in some who show this symptom with every bath, this stimulant may be given just before, as well as after it. The frequency of the baths should be according to the subsequent rise of the temperature, for the bath should be repeated so soon as the thermometer reaches 103° F. Active friction should be kept up during the

bath, and in some very nervous patients the water may at first be tepid and then cooled afterward by ice. In private practice, where the patients can afford it, I think very well of the Nauheim salts being added, with their free production of carbonic acid, as it has seemed that the effect is more prolonged than after the ordinary bath.

A few patients cannot take cold baths. The only criterion of this fact is that the pulse remains weaker after the effects of the bath have been recovered from, than before it was taken. In them, a warm bath from 95° to 98° F. may be tried instead, and occasionally it acts as favorably in such cases as the cold bath does in others. If, however, the temperature does not fall after a warm bath, but rises instead, the cold bath should be resumed and pushed fearlessly. I have seen many more bad results from timidity in using cold baths than from excess in their employment.

The only condition which should interrupt the administration of the Brand bath is the supervention of intestinal hemorrhage. This complication is unfortunate chiefly ou that account, for I have never seen intestinal hemorrhage directly fatal at Roosevelt. With the first sign of its occurrence, a dose of three pills is at once administered, of the following prescription:

R Argent. nitratis ....grs. v
    Pulv. opii ....grs. v
    Terebinthinæ resin..................... ʒiii
    Liq.. kali............................. ʒi
M. Div. in pilul. lx.

The object of the turpentine is to prevent the silver salt from being absorbed until the pill is well on its way down the intestine. Sometimes these pills are voided unchanged, in which case they are rubbed up with more licorice powder in the making. I have used these pills for years in the treatment of ulcerative colitis, or ulcers in chronic dysentery, intestinal tuberculosis, etc., with such good effects that I have no doubt that besides checking intestinal hemorrhage in typhoid, they may be of service in preventing perforation. After there have been no signs of hemorrhage in typhoid for thirty-six hours, the baths are resumed again.

In the third and fourth weeks, the patients are often restless from a general aching of the body. This is due to the absorption of the subcutaneous cushion of fat leaving the nerves (which never waste) so exposed to pressure against the bones, as at the sacrum, scapulæ, knees, etc., that intolerable neuralgic pains often results. This aching is markedly relieved, and sleep thereby promoted, by spreading sheepskins with the wool on them, or buffalo robes, on the bed, and then over that a sheet for the patient to lie upon. In all conditions of emaciation, such measures to relieve pressure on nerves should be employed. Rubbing the patient all over with warm lime water liniment, to which Ol. cinnamoni, one dram to the pint, has been added, is very soothing after the second week; and if well applied to the back twice a day is a good prophylactic against bed sores.

As typhoid fever progresses in its course, about the middle of the second week the symptoms often indicate in which of three directions the chief danger of the patient lies. The first of these is death due mainly to continued hyperpyrexia. The temperature tends to reach a high grade in the mornings, as well as at night, and is not affected, unless it be to be increased, by the cold bath given for fifteen to twenty minutes. Severe nervous symptoms develop, such as active delirium, and if the fever be not broken, general tremors occur. Death, preceded by coma and general cyanosis, ends the scene. It is in these cases that the patient should be dealt with just as we use the ice bath in sunstroke, or in the hyperpyrexia of acute rheumatic fever. I have kept such typhoid patients in an ice bath for 33, 40, 45 and 48 minutes, with full recovery in each case; and unlike the hyperpyrexia of rheumatism, when the fever is once broken, in my experience, its subsequent rises are as easily controlled as in ordinary cases.

The second tendency which should be noted, has for its symptoms an early development of tympanites, with or without diarrhea, with pronounced tremor of the tongue, as well as dryness. The expression of the face is that of settled anxiety, with the corners of the month persistently turned down. In these patients, as already remarked, the brunt of the attack is upon the intestinal tract, and they are more liable than others to hemorrhage, to extensive slow-healing ulcers, to relapses, or to perforation often while they seem convalescing. These patients should have only about one-half the average amount of milk given to them, and in smaller quantities at a time. Five grains of resorcin given in an ounce of sweetened water t.i.d., with the dose of bismuth doubled, and in some cases with the addition of five grains of the sulphocarbonate of soda with each dose of bismuth, is the modification of the ordinary medicinal prescriptions which I follow for such patients, and as above remarked, they should abstain longer than others from taking solid food on the subsidence of the fever.

The third class are the least promising of any, their symptoms being those of severe toxemia and of general prostration from the beginning. The temperature instead of keeping up at a high range may, on the contrary, show a comparatively low average. But the chief features are those of weakness of all functions; the heart remaining feeble, and the effect of baths, whether cold or warm, is plainly not beneficial. Deaths occurs from pure asthenia. I would give such patients twenty drops, four times in the twenty-four hours of the tincture of the chloride of iron, with three grains of quinine each time, and one-sixth of a grain of the calcium sulphide, while the cardiac stimulant of camphor, hypodermically, is to be used constantly.

On the other hand, some patients, especially after a prolonged course, owing to the experience of a relapse, suddenly develop alarming attacks of severe rigors, during which they appear to be actually dying. The temperature rises to 105° F. or more, but after a few hours it drops to 101° F., or even to normal. These rigors are not at all periodical, for they may return any time. If the urine is examined after the attack has subsided, it will be found loaded with immense numbers of the *Bacillus coli*. This disturbance is doubtless due to this mixed infection, and the prognosis is not necessarily fatal, for four out of five of the last examples in my experience got well. The urotropin with sodium benzoate mentioned in connection with nephritis complicating typhoid, should be immediately resorted to.

Lastly, mixed infection causes some patients to remain with febrile symptoms for many weeks subsequent to the usual duration of typhoid fever, even after a relapse. As Prof. Francis Delafield has shown, these patients should not be considered as suffering from typhoid fever then, nor be so treated. He recommends that they be allowed to sit up and to take more liberal diet, whereupon they soon improve in their general symptoms, and their fever leaves them.

23 East Forty-seventh Street.

CLINICAL STUDIES IN BLOOD-PRESSURE AND SHOCK IN TRAUMATIC SURGERY.[1]

BY JONATHAN M. WAINWRIGHT, M.D.,

OF SCRANTON, PA.;

SURGEON-IN-CHIEF TO THE MOSES TAYLOR HOSPITALS AT SCRANTON, PA., AND BUFFALO, N. Y.

ACCORDING to the bulletin of the Department of Labor, Pittsburg has the highest percentage of deaths from trauma of all the cities in the United States. Scranton is third from the top in this respect. It is probable that the same high percentage of deaths from trauma obtains in all the coal or railway towns in the State. Since in nearly all the deaths from trauma the real cause is shock or its ally, hemorrhage, there are few societies to whom the study of shock, its causes, its prevention and its treatment, are more important to this one.

This study is more important still on account of the fact that the recent observations very strongly assail the value of our previous well-worn methods of treatment. And also because of the recent introduction of instruments of comparative accuracy by which the essential phenomena of shock and the effects of treatment can be more accurately determined. Up to within the last few years it was the unquestioned practice, at least in most hospitals in New York, to treat shock resulting from severe accidents and operations by the most active hypodermic stimulation. Not a few patients during this period were subjected to a hypodermic stimula-

---

[1] Read before the Fifty-fourth Annual Meeting of the Medical Society of Pennsylvania, held at Scranton, September 29, 1904.

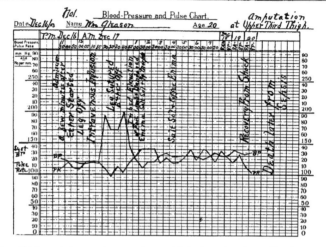

Chart I.—Thigh caught between bumpers of cars. Admitted two hours later. Hopeless crush at middle of thigh. Immediate amputation of upper third. Intravenous infusion of 2,000 c.c. salt solution with one dram adrenalin (1-1,000). This sustained pressure at high point during operation. Fall afterward but not to an alarming degree. Note gradual improvement after being put to bed with abdomen and extremities bandaged, salt solution enema and morphine. No "stimulating" drugs. Temperature after operation 103.4° F. by rectum. Recovery from shock but death later from sepsis.

tion of some sort every hour and, as Crile well says, synergists, antagonists, and drugs which have no effect at all or are even harmful were combined regardless of their physiological action.

A reaction against, or, at least, a rigid questioning of, these methods was started, in this country at least, principally by Crile's prize essay on "Blood-Pressure in Surgery," appearing in 1903. Crile has conclusively shown that the essential factor in shock is a low blood-pressure, and that the heart is little if any at fault. Crile considers the low blood-pressure entirely due to exhaustion of the vasomotor center in the medulla. He shows that nervous impulses such as handling the abdominal viscera or burning the extremities first cause a rise in blood-pressure. If these stimulating impulses increase in severity or continue over a considerable time, the vasomotor center finally becomes exhausted and a fall in blood-pressure follows. In this exhausted condition he considers it as illogical to attempt a further stimulation by drugs as to add to the cutaneous or visceral insults.

To support this theory, Crile cites some two hundred and fifty experiments on dogs which he first reduced to more or less profound shock and then submitted to various forms of treatment. The results of these experiments show that strychnine and digitalin increase the blood-pressure only in mild grades of shock. In deep grades they would seem to be useless. Saline

infusions and adrenalin were of doubtful effect and alcohol and the nitrite group were harmful.

The vasomotor centers then being beyond the aid of the ordinary stimulating drugs, Crile places his sole reliance in combating the low pressure on supporting the peripheral circulation. This he accomplishes to a very remarkable degree by means of a pneumatic suit which can be inflated so as to exert an equable pressure over the whole body or any chosen part. The same result can be brought about though less efficiently by elevating the foot of the bed and bandaging the extremities and the abdomen.

Since adrenalin acts locally as a powerful stimulant to the muscle fibers of the peripheral vessels, it was employed in the treatment of shock with great hopes of its value. Its clinical place, Crile and others consider, is yet to be determined.

While fully acknowledging the great importance of Crile's work, one must remember that the great volume of evidence is drawn from laboratory experiments. Before clinical surgery can accept these teachings and lay aside measures which for years competent clinical observers have considered of value, it will be necessary to submit these ideas to rigid scrutiny at the operating table and bedside.

It is fortunate that the introduction of sphygmomanometers of the Riva Rocci type has given to clinical surgery instruments of sufficient accuracy to observe closely the phenomena of shock

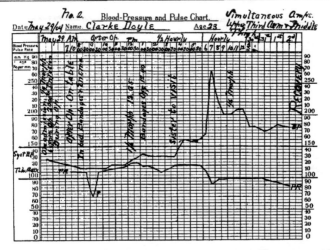

Chart 2.—(Case referred to in text). Run over by train about midnight. Was not seen and lay at side of track for three hours. Admitted five hours after accident. No tourniquets or medical attention before admission. Profuse hemorrhage. Upper arm crushed at middle and thigh just above knee. Immediate simultaneous amputations. Fair pressure on admission. Intravenous infusion of salt solution prevented marked fall during or after operation. Temperature after operation 101.2° F. by rectum. Gradual satisfactory recovery after very severe injury without "stimulating" drugs. Note rise in pressure after each injection of morphine and after sister's visit. Note high pressure as reaction is complete.

and the influence of various therapeutic procedures.

In applying laboratory results to clinical work, it must be remembered that, clinically, hemorrhage is nearly always a factor in causing the depressed state, and also that in contradistinction to comparatively brief laboratory experiments we have in the depression after severe trauma a condition lasting many hours. It is very probable therefore that other vital functions besides the vasomotor centers after a time take part in this depression and require support even if they were not at fault at first.

Moreover, the physiologists are not at unity in exempting the heart from participation in shock. Howell, writing in Vaughn's Festschrift, considers that there are two kinds of shock, a cardiac and a vasomotor form apparently agree with those of Crile but he considers that this form is always accompanied by the cardiac variety. (For probable example of the cardiac shock, see Chart 8.)

However the question of drug treatment may turn out, there are two very important facts in regard to shock which the work of Crile and others has demonstrated. These are: (1) The cause of shock is overwhelmingly irritating nerve impulses of some sort, and (2) the important condition to combat is the low blood-pressure. On these facts the question of treatment is based.

The first attention, therefore, should naturally be given to removing or diminishing the causative nerve impulses. For this reason morphine is now to be considered the most important drug in shock. Crile's work shows that animals receiving morphine before anesthetization are more resistant to artificial shock. Clinical experience also bears this out. In our own accident room the routine injection of strychnine into a patient as soon as admitted has now practically given place to an almost equally routine injection of morphine. Even during recovery morphine seems to be a most important drug. The sensory impulses are still kept blunted and even an increase in pressure may follow morphine as some of the charts show.

To remove the nerve impulses after trauma an immediate repair of the injury, if at all feasible, is very important. For this reason our own view is strongly in favor of primary amputations in limbs hopelessly mangled. Leaving a mangled, oozing limb with crushed and exposed nerves in the hope that delay will give a more favorable opportunity for intervention will, in many cases, by allowing the cause continually to act, only drive the patient into a condition beyond all hope. A well-covered stump with oozing checked, on the other hand, will give a patient in whom the cause of shock is stopped and to whom the administration of therapeutic measures will not be like pouring water through a sieve.

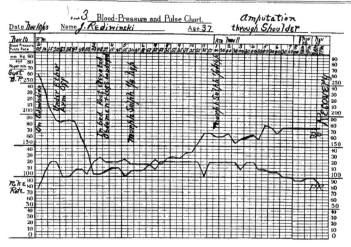

Chart 3.—Arm run over by loaded mine car two hours before admission. Immediate amputation through shoulder. Note high primary pressor period. Slight fall after nerve impulses were blunted by ether. Marked fall after operation. Temperature after operation 103.1° F. by rectum. Note pressor effect of each injection of morphine. A typical case of gradual recovery from severe shock without "stimulating" drugs.

The causative nerve impulses having been as far as possible removed or blunted, the low blood-pressure must next be overcome. It is now a condition in which, as Crile says, the control of the blood-pressure is the control of life itself. The truth of this must, it would seem, be admitted by all who review the literature or who with modern instruments observe for themselves the blood-pressure in shock. Equally convincing is the fact that, to control the blood-pressure the most effective means at hand are the so-called mechanical ones. By this is meant pressure over the dilated peripheral blood-vessels either as noted above by Crile's suit, or lacking this by elevating the foot of the bed and by bandaging the extremities and the abdomen. The bandage to the abdomen by means of a tight Scultetus bandage is especially important as it has been shown that in shock the blood especially collects in the splanchnic area forming the condition which has been called intravenous hemorrhage.

That these mechanical means may be markedly effective even in the most desperate cases, is shown by a case recently in our wards. This was a man twenty-three years old. He had been run over by a train about midnight. The wheels of one or more trucks passed over the left arm midway between the shoulder and elbow and over the left leg just above the knee. The bones in each limb were ground into fragments and the soft parts were terribly crushed. The man was not seen by the crew of the train

which ran over him and in the above condition he lay at the side of the track in the cold of early morning for three hours. At the end of this time he was seen by a passing freight and brought to the hospital, a distance of thirty miles. He arrived at the hospital about five and one-half hours after the accident, having had no medical aid, not even a tourniquet, and having as noted, spent three hours lying beside the track. That the condition of shock under these circumstances was severe will be admitted. An immediate simultaneous amputation was performed. The arm had to be taken off just below the shoulder and the thigh at its middle. A hypodermic of one quarter of a grain of morphine was given before the operation and a 2,000 c.c. intravenous infusion during the operation. The operation did not add to the shock. On being returned to bed the remaining extremities and the abdomen were bandaged and the foot of the bed elevated. The gradual progress to recovery is shown in Chart 2. No hypodermic "stimulation" was used.

While the value of the previous methods of drug stimulation is justly questioned, our own clinical experience in regard to the value of intravenous infusions of salt solution is far too favorable to allow our reliance on it to be at all shaken by any evidence yet adduced. In spite of the theoretical and experimental evidence to the contrary, we have seen so many cases in our wards which were almost pulseless and apparently on the verge of death come up under

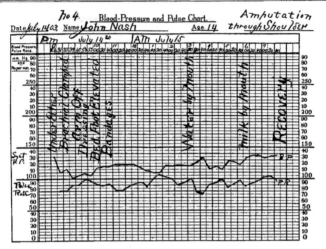

Chart 4.—Arm run over by mine cars two and one-half hours before admission. Immediate amputation through shoulder. Fall of 35 mm. during operation. Temperature after operation, 99° F. by mouth. Note ether being put to bed with elevation of foot and bandage of extremities. Note pressor effect of water and milk by mouth. Gradual progress to recovery without "stimulating" drugs.

an infusion and never again sink to a disquieting condition that we consider its practical value in certain cases demonstrated beyond assault. A nine-tenths per cent. salt solution should be used instead of the old six-tenths per cent. Matthews' formula, here given, is probably better still:

R Sodium chloride .... .09
  Potassium chloride .... .03
  Calcium chloride .... .02
  Water 100.00

From our own observations we are not yet able to say whether or not adrenalin increases the efficiency of a salt solution infusion. We have used it a number of times in the proportion of one dram of the 1/1,000 solution to 2,000 c.c. of the nine-tenths per cent. salt solution.

In regard to the value of digitalin and strychnine in practice, we are still somewhat uncertain. Some of our blood-pressure determinations do seem to show that they have a real value. Cook and Briggs' work also indicates that they have. If we accept Howell's idea concerning the part played by the heart in shock, they would theoretically have a place. Clinically, too, we have no way of telling whether the vasomotor centers are really exhausted beyond improvement or whether their depression is only partial and temporary and whether they would not be better for medicinal treatment. Crile's experiments show that strychnine and digitalin do exert a favorable influence in shock of mild grades, and it is very possible that in severe cases, after the peripheral circulation has been mechanically supported, we

create this mild condition in which these drugs are useful. It is now chiefly this phase of the question, i.e., what, if any, is the value of digitalin and strychnine that now requires the most careful and exhaustive clinical study aided by the sphygmomanometer. (It may be said in regard to these two drugs that they are seldom given in large enough doses when their use is considered necessary. If one expects to get an effect in severe cases, the dose of each should be one-tenth grain, its repetition to be guided by its effect on the pressure. We began using digitalin in this dose about four years ago and often obtained what we thought were excellent clinical results.)

That alcohol is of real value in shock can now be denied from all standpoints. Personally, however, we are far from banishing it from use in surgical conditons. We frequently see people who have recovered from the primary shock and may have a normal pressure, but still on the second, third or fourth day are far from being in a satisfactory condition, the event being still in doubt. The digestive organs, like all vital forces, seem below par, and in this general failure the ordinary foodstuffs are not absorbed and the body lacks fuel. In this condition alcohol offers itself as a very diffusible food of high potential energy, which is easily absorbed and furnishes the body with the fuel it needs to carry on its struggle. The condition is allied to that of asthenic pneumonias and typhoids and the exhaustive bronchopneumonias of children where alcohol is used by clinicians the world over.

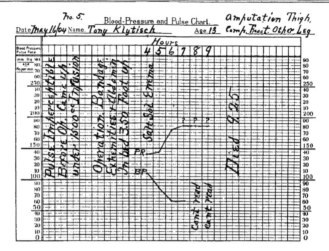

Chart 5.—Boy run over by cars in mine about two and one-half hours before admission. Pulseless and nearly dead on admission. Pulse brought up temporarily by infusion. Rapid sinking of general condition and fall of pressure after operation. Temperature two hours before death 103.4° F. by mouth. A typical death from shock.

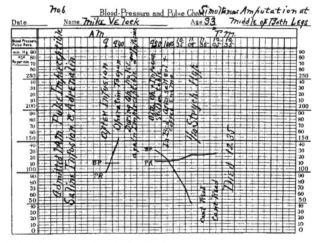

Chart 6.—Both legs run over by train 60 miles from hospital. Admitted eight hours later. No medi-cal attention. No tourniquets. Great hemorrhage. Hopeless case from start. On admission barely conscious, pulse imperceptible. Infusion of 2,000 c.c. salt solution, with one dram adrenalin (⅟₁,₀₀₀) brought pressure up to 115 mm. at which it was sustained for nearly an hour. During operation pulse again imperceptible. A second infusion brought it up to 135 mm., from which it rapidly fell. No response from any measure in dying patient.

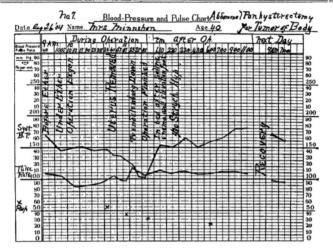

Chart 7.—Abdominal panhysterectomy for fibroids. Removal of both tubes and ovaries. Much debilitated from repeated hemorrhages. Before operation red cells 3,200,000, hemoglobin 40 per cent. High pressure on first reading in etherizing room from excitement. Reading after ether is probably normal. Gradual fall in pressure during long operation with moderate hemorrhage. Marked increase in fall after Trendelenburg position is let down. Condition at end of operation is serious. Marked rise in pressure after patient is put in bed with foot elevated and one pint of saline enema given. Temporary rise of 15 mm. after strychnine hypodermic. Later gradual rise without further attention. High reading on full recovery. Temperature after operation 97.6° F. by mouth.

While most of Crile's brilliant work in regard to shock can be accepted unconditionally, in actual practice a few vitally important points must be submitted to careful clinical observation. The final chapter in regard to treatment is still far from being written, and it must wait till observations on the human being after severe trauma or surgical operation permit a reliable consensus of opinion.

My own views, after carefully observing many cases with the aid of the Riva Rocci apparatus, are still unformed and hazy on many points. Tentatively, I have formed as a temporary working basis the following conclusions:

1. There is one drug, morphine, of which the value is unquestionable.

2. The most effective treatment is the mechanical one. This suffices in many desperate cases. After it has been carefully applied strychnine and digitalin may possibly be of value. These drugs alone without mechanical treatment are probably of no value in severe cases.

3. Nitroglycerin, atropine and alcohol are inert or harmful, though alcohol is valuable in after-conditions.

4. Intravenous infusions are of real and great value. The efficiency of adrenalin in addition is doubtful.

(The ordinary detailed attention to avoidance of exposure, the application of artificial heat, full and even anesthesia, with ether and not chloroform, rapid operative work without unnecessary handling, the copious administration of water by mouth or rectum, etc., have the same great value as always.)

Appended are charts illustrative of various phases of this subject. The legend with each one is probably sufficient explanation. Charts 11 and 12 have nothing especial to do with shock but are included to show the value of the sphygmomanometer in diagnosis.

These determinations were all taken with Cook's modifications of Riva Rocci's apparatus. The armlet is 5 cm. wide. This apparatus usually gives readings about 20 mm. higher than actual but it is sufficiently accurate for comparative work. Our own experience with this instrument with active, hard-working railroad men and miners would show that for them about 150 mm. is an average normal reading.

A large part of the data is due to the enthusiasm of various generations of internes who have frequently continued these readings all night.

It may be added that the use of the instrument has been of the greatest practical value in the care of severe traumatic cases and there is no way in which the operator can so easily keep informed as to the true condition of the patient, both on the table and after, as by the use of this

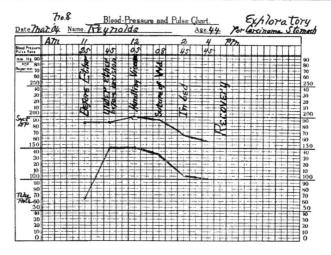

Chart 8.—Operation for carcinoma of stomach. Condition found inoperable and interference stopped. First reading in etherizing room is high from excitement. Note increase in pressure on manipulation of iscera during exploration. Important point in this chart is the marked increase in pulse rate without hange in pressure. This is an example of Howell's cardiac shock. Recovery from operation. Death several weeks later from carcinoma.

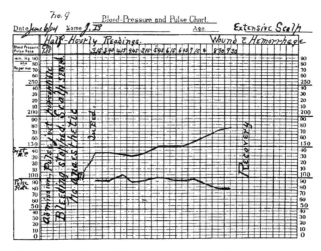

Chart 9.—Case corresponding to Crile's collapse. Extensive scalp wound two hours before admission with profuse hemorrhage. Pulse barely perceptible on admission. Temperature on admission 99° by mouth. Scalp sutured in accident ward without anesthetic. Chart shows gradual recovery after itient is put to bed without any treatment at all.

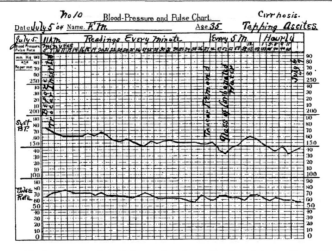

Chart 10.—Blood pressure readings during tapping of an ascites from cirrhosis. Ten quarts removed. High pressure before tapping from intra-abdominal tension. Gradual fall of pressure during tapping with no disturbance of pulse-rate. Note marked rise in pressure after taking a glass of carbonated water. While tapping this man on another occasion a fall of 35 mm. was caused by making him sit up during the tapping.

instrument. It is no longer a laboratory toy but it is now a very important addition to a surgeon's outfit.

The charts here reproduced (Janeway's model) do not of course represent all our recent observations. They are single more or less typical illustrations of phenomena which many observations in our own wards or by others have taught us to accept as true.

The points which we would emphasize from the teachings of these charts are as follows:

1. *The Primary Pressor Period.*—It has been indicated above that the sensory impulses which finally cause shock at first cause a stimulation of the vasomotor centers and a rise in pressure for a certain period before exhaustion supervenes. We not infrequently have cases of severe accidents, which when admitted are in this primary pressor stage. (See Chart 3.) This, we consider, is the ideal stage for operative repair of the injury: *i.e.*, primary amputation, etc. This high primary pressure is generally markedly reduced when the sensory impulses are blunted by full anesthesia. (Also see Chart 3.)

2. *The value of Intravenous Infusions.*—Chart 2 shows that after a preliminary infusion with one-fourth grain of morphine a simultaneous amputation of the upper arm and thigh could be performed with a fall of only 20 mm. in the blood-pressure. Compare this with Chart 3 in which without these preliminaries a fall of over one hundred mm. was caused by the much less severe shoulder amputation and with a fall

of 35 mm. in a similar operation in Chart 4. Chart 1 shows a remarkable pressor effect of an intravenous infusion begun during an amputation at a time of falling pressure. The pressor effect was maintained until after the patient was returned to bed. A fall did occur later but it was only temporary. Chart 6 shows a temporary raising of an imperceptible pulse to a pressure of 135 mm. by an infusion during an operation.

3. *Excessive Reaction.*—In many cases even when simple mechanical or no treatment at all has been employed after reaction the blood-pressure reaches an unusually high point. The explanation for this is not yet evident. It is illustrated in Charts 2, 3, 7 and 9.

4. *Cardiac Shock* (Howell).—While this clinical condition is still questionable, Chart 8 is a good example of its possibility. In this exploration which was attended by no loss of blood, the handling of the abdominal viscera increased the pulse rate from 70 to 150 and if this condition had been observed by the finger on the pulse only it would have caused the gravest apprehension. The sphygmomanometer, however, showed an actual rise in the pressure and no alarm was felt.

5. *Morphine, Water by Mouth, and the Visits of Friends.*—The pressor effect of morphine is definitely shown in Chart 2. In Chart 3 it is absent. The pressor effect of water by mouth is shown in Charts 4 and 10. This is due to reflex action, and not to the mechanical effect of

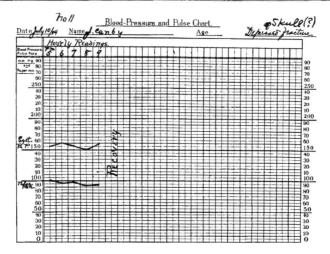

Chart 11.—Showing value of blood pressure determinations in diagnosis. Man fell from top of box car four hours before admission. Four inch scalp wound over frontal area. First attendant had palpated through this and thought there might be a depressed fracture. Wound had been sutured before admission and local examination was unsatisfactory. Cerebral pressure was not considered to be present, and this was corroborated by stationary normal pressure. Uneventful recovery.

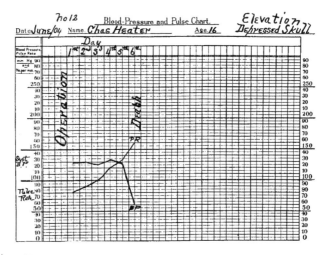

Chart 12.—Value in diagnosis. Fall of roof of mine on head. Open depressed fracture in parietal region with laceration and protrusion of brain tissue. Skull elevated. Daily readings show that there is no cerebral pressure. Marked fall before death. Death from injury to brain substance. Temperature at time of death 108° F. by rectum.

the water absorbed. The effect is greater after carbonated water than plain. The pressor effect of a visit of a friend is seen in Chart 2. This particular case is not very conclusive as the curve is ascending. That this is a true effect has been shown by the Boston Committee, and is probably from mental excitement.

6. *Strychnine and Digitalin.*—The charts, which it has been convenient to reproduce here, throw only a negative light on this question, as they show how much can be done without them in severe cases by mechanical methods. Chart 7 shows a pressor effect of 15 mm. Chart 6 shows an absence of effect in a dying case with a large dose. Our other observations on this point are not yet sufficiently numerous and complete to be instructive.

NOTE ON THE TEMPERATURE CONDITIONS IN SHOCK.

At the suggestion of Dr. B. Farquhar Curtis the cases herewith reported were further reviewed with regard to the temperature changes. Kinnaman (*Annals of Surgery*, December, 1903) has made an elaborate laboratory study of the temperature in dogs which had been reduced to shock and found that the temperature is always reduced, and that the amount to which it is lowered is fairly proportional to the degree of shock as measured by blood-pressure.

Kinnaman's experimental data is so complete that little doubt can remain as to the truth of his deductions in experimental animals. Clinically, however, the behavior of the temperature in shock is very inconstant. Sometimes it is reduced and sometimes it is elevated. For instance, in Case V, which was a death in a typical condition of shock about eight hours after the boy's legs were both run over by a train, the temperature shortly before death was 103.4° F. by mouth. In Case I, on return to bed after amputation of the thigh the temperature was 103.4° F. by rectum. The next evening when the shock had been recovered from the temperature was 99.8° F. In Case II, on return to bed after a simultaneous amputation of the thigh and upper arm the temperature was 101.2° F. by rectum. This was the man who had lain beside the railroad track from midnight till 3 A.M. before being found. He had ample opportunity for the loss of body heat. In the two shoulder-joint amputations, both of which healed per primam, the temperatures immediately after operation were 103.1° F. by rectum and 99° F. by mouth, respectively. Neither of these two cases had infusions, though the first three noted in this connection did.

The only case in this series which showed a reduction of temperature was Case VII, in which, immediately after an abdominal panhysterectomy, the temperature was 97.6° F. by mouth. At noon the next day, when the shock had entirely disappeared, it was 98.6° F.

The high temperature in Case XII was due presumably to the brain lesion, either a septic meningo-encephalitis or a simple laceration of the brain.

The reason for this varying of the temperature conditions in clinical cases, as well as its departure from laboratory results is as yet very obscure.

THE PURPOSE OF EYEGLASSES.
BY ELLICE M. ALGER, M.D.,

OF NEW YORK;

OPHTHALMOLOGIST TO THE NEW YORK DISPENSARY; INSTRUCTOR AT THE NEW YORK POSTGRADUATE MEDICAL SCHOOL.

IT might seem at first sight that the discussion of such a topic was superfluous, yet every oculist must have noticed that the majority of his patients have the most rudimentary ideas on the subject, while it is the most difficult thing imaginable to get even the postgraduate medical student to abandon the popular belief that the only function of glasses is to improve the sight. The family physician is also firmly convinced that when vision is keen glasses are unnecessary, and ascribes manifest discomfort to "granular lids," a term which, like "malaria" and "uric acid," suggests to the victim patience and resignation. The refracting optician is also deeply imbued with the same idea and generally adds to it the still more harmful belief that any glass which will improve the sight should be sold the patient in as expensive a frame as possible.

It goes without saying that improvement of vision is one of the ends of properly fitted glasses; but probably half of the prescriptions given patients who use their eyes steadily are not for the improvement of vision but the relief of strain. The first often requires very little skill, and it is a notorious fact that the laity select their own glasses with the same cheerful confidence with which they buy their patent medicines. The relief of headache and reflex disorders on the other hand is a matter often involving very complicated problems and a much higher grade of skill.

Many persons are born into the world with eyes the capacity of which for receiving visual impressions is perfect, but through optical defects of the eye do not have a clear image formed on the retina. For instance the hyperopic or far-sighted individual has an eyeball that is shorter than normal, in which case the rays of light come to a focus behind his retina instead of upon it and the image instead of being sharp and clear is like that on the ground glass of an ill-focussed camera—dull and indistinct and lacking detail. And just as in the camera the focus is adjusted by changing the position or strength of the lens, so in the human eye the accommodation is brought into play, the lens becomes more convex, the rays focus on the right spot and distinct vision results at once. As long as this compensation takes place without any appreciable effort the patient feels no need of any artificial help. But it must be remembered that every act of accommodation requires an expenditure of muscular energy and that what is mere play to one person may be exhaustive labor to another. A young person may have a short eyeball and with the vigorous accommodation of youth have perfect vision, but as age increases and the elasticity of his lens diminishes his need of a glass becomes more and more imperative. Some eyes are so hyperopic that even in the vigor of youth the accommodation is not sufficient to secure clear vision, and a convex glass is needed from the first. Even with normal eyes, after the age of forty years the accommodation has diminished so much that the patient though still able to see distant objects as well as ever is no longer able to see small objects close at hand and has passed into the state of presbyopia or old sight. These are almost the only patients who require glasses because they cannot see well, and fitting them is often a matter of patience rather than of skill.

A much larger class is composed of people who see perfectly and yet ought to wear glasses to relieve them of troubles which they do not ascribe to their eyes at all. Suppose for instance the case of a young and healthy patient with a moderate hyperopia; with his eyes completely at rest, images of distant objects are focussed behind his retina, but by a moderate and unconscious use of his ciliary muscle his vision may be even a little better than normal and he often takes pride in the keenness of his sight. But when an evening at the theater calls for several hours continuous action of his accommodation his eyes get very tired and he not infrequently pays for his overwork with a raging headache. As he gets along into middle life and his accommodation gets weaker and weaker the keenness of his vision can be depended on for shorter and shorter periods and he finally graduates into the class of those who cannot see even distant objects without glasses. If this tiring of the ciliary muscle is true for distant objects it is even more certain when near vision brings its additional strain, and the man whose shooting is the envy of his friends may not be able to finish the first chapter of a novel without a headache.

· We often see children with well-marked squint which the fond parents ascribe to a fit or a fright or some special accident, since the eyes were perfectly straight at birth. Such children often have perfect vision in each eye but in order to get this perfect vision have to strain the accommodation. They find it easier to make this increased effort by turning the eyes in, since there is a normal relation between accommodation and convergence. Inasmuch as eyes that cross cannot both see the same object they look with one eye and disregard what they see with the other, and if it happens that both eyes are equally good the eye which first catches sight of the object fixes while the other squints. Such children therefore squint sometimes with one eye and again with the other. When they are fitted with suitable glasses they can see without straining the accommodation and therefore they no

longer find it necessary to squint. It is common enough to see children whose eyes are perfectly straight while they wear their glasses and which instantly cross when they are taken off. It is less common in adults. If glasses are not worn they begin gradually to use one eye in preference to the other, the squint becomes a fixed one and the squinting eye from lack of use may loose its keenness to a large degree. At the same time the muscle which turns the eye in becomes hypertrophied from overuse and the squint is present even when the eye is completely at rest. Such cases have got beyond relief from glasses alone, since the eye has become so much poorer than its fellow that it makes no instinctive effort at fusion and even if it did the muscle which should keep it straight has no longer the requisite power.

In the myopic or near sighted person the eye instead of being too short is too long, and the rays of light are focussed in front of the retina, the image being correspondingly indistinct. In this case vision is best when the accommodation is completely relaxed. But even this will not cause the focus to fall on the retina and myopic patients always have defective vision at a distance though they can obviate this difficulty by bringing objects nearer to them. Thus it often happens that the patient needs a glass for use on the street or at the theater while he can read his book or paper without. Glasses are generally given in myopia therefore to aid vision rather than to relieve strain though this is not always the case. Inasmuch as the myope sees things at a distance best with his ciliary muscle relaxed, it is from simple lack of use very much smaller and weaker than that of the far sighted patient. When he picks out his own glass or has it fitted to him by the trial case alone he invariably selects a glass which overcorrects his error since this allows him to exercise his ciliary muscle somewhat and gives him splendid vision for a time. But unfortunately this muscle from lack of use is small, gets easily tired and headache results. As a rule the ciliary muscle eventually becomes stronger from the exercise and the headache disappears. In a respectable minority however the muscle becomes cramped so that the focus is again in front of the retina and the patient again ceases to see clearly till a still greater overcorrection is given. This vicious circle eventually gets the patient into a condition where the eyes are not only very painful but for the time absolutely useless, and it often takes weeks of rest and care to rid the ciliary muscle of this tendency to cramp when put to any use. This same weakness often makes any unusual near work more tiresome to the myope than to his hyperopic brother. Still another factor is present in very high degrees of myopia in which the patient has to hold his book or work within a few inches of the eyes which have to converge abnormally to fix on the same object. This may not only cause great discomfort but eventually lead to changes in the balance of the ocular muscles. In myopia, then, it follows that glasses are to be ordered very carefully and that the glass that gives the patient the best vision is not by any means the best for him to wear.

The subject of astigmatism is much more complicated. In the astigmatic eye the refracting media are so disposed that rays of light are not refracted alike in different meridians and consequently do not come to a focus at the same spot. Just how the eye adjusts itself to conditions of this sort we do not know, but in low degrees of hyperopic astigmatism distant vision may be normal and near vision painless. The correction may be made by changing the shape of the lens through an uneven action of the ciliary muscle, or perhaps by tilting the lens slightly in its fossa, but in either case it involves extra work for the accommodation, and work which is all the more trying, because it is unevenly distributed among the fibres. Just as in simple hyperopia, when the accommodation is strong, the patient may be unconscious of any ill effect, and may have good vision, but he is liable in an increased degree to all the disabilities of hyperopia, the difficulty increasing progressively as the work is continuous and nearer to the eye. In hyperopic astigmatism of low degree, therefore, glasses are prescribed to relieve strain, while in the high degrees, which are beyond the powers of the accommodation, they not only accomplish this, but improve vision.

In myopic astigmatism distant vision is always impaired, since it is not corrected by even the most complete relaxation of the ciliary muscle and by the same token it is painless, though the reverse is often true of near vision. The patient brings the object near enough to get a clear focus in his most myopic meridian, and then focusses the other meridian by unevenly straining the accommodation, just as though he were hyperopic and with the same result. In myopic and mixed astigmatism, then, glasses serve to improve vision at a distance and to relieve the strain of near work.

Without going further into the subject, enough has been said to justify these conclusions.

1. That improvement of sight is only one function of glasses.

2. That relief of eyestrain is fully as important.

3. That eyestrain is often responsible for headache and other reflex nerve phenomena.

4. That one may have perfect vision and still be subject to eyestrain.

5. That small errors of refraction often cause more strain than large ones, since there is a more constant effort to overcome them.

6. That strain can generally be relieved by properly fitted glasses.

7. That glasses which give the best vision may simply increase the strain, and that therefore the patient cannot safely select his own glasses; and that, as he will not buy of an optician glasses which do not improve vision, he very seldom gets the correct glass and therefore fails of relief.

THE TREATMENT OF CHRONIC EMPYEMA OF THE ANTRUM, BOTH SIMPLE AND WHEN COMBINED WITH EMPYEMA OF THE ETHMOID AND SPHENOID.[1]

BY R. BISHOP CANFIELD, M.D.,
OF ANN ARBOR, MICH.
CLINICAL PROFESSOR OF OTOLOGY, RHINOLOGY AND LARYNGOLOGY, UNIVERSITY OF MICHIGAN.

I HAVE chosen to consider the treatment of chronic empyema of the antrum under these two heads because in my experience, in fully 40 per cent. of all cases of antral disease, the disease process is limited to the antrum alone, while in the remaining 60 per cent. a favorite combination is with disease of the ethmoid and sphenoid. In such cases the treatment of the antrum includes the treatment of the other cavities affected.

The patient presenting himself suffering from disease of the nasal accessory sinuses exhibits symptoms not only of a local, but also of a general character. The physician realizes that the sinus disease has been the cause of the general symptoms, and that relief of the local condition will have a beneficial effect on the general health. He should also realize that attention to the general health will assist materially in hastening the improvement of the local disease. A course of tonic treatment and personal hygiene will sometimes yield gratifying results in cases previously obstinate.

In considering the local treatment of antral empyema, one should remember that the disease is essentially one of extension. It is exceedingly doubtful if empyema ever originates in the antrum itself. It is much more logical to believe, and clinical evidence and pathological findings bear out the supposition, that empyema is a result of some disease process previously existing.

There has been, I think, a line too sharply drawn between the so-called conservative and radical treatment of accessory sinus disease. Some operators make the mistake of adhering too closely to conservative methods, while others hasten on too rapidly to radical measures, before they have exhausted other resources at their command. There is, to my mind, a general scheme for the treatment not only of empyema of the antrum, but also of disease of the other accessory sinuses, a combination of radical and conservative measures, careful attention to the details of which offers better results than adherence either to one or to the other.

The first step in the successful treatment of empyema of the antrum is to learn definitely the exciting cause. Examination of considerable numbers of cases teaches the observer that nearly all cases of empyema of the antrum arise from one of two causes; that is, they arise either by extension of disease from the nasal cavity or they come from a carious tooth. Cases of syphilis, tuberculosis and malignant growth are, of course, excepted.

1 Read before the Wayne County Medical Society, Detroit, Mich., January 23, 1905.

To consider first the treatment of the second class.—Naturally the first step to take is to remove completely not only the diseased tooth but also the carious bone in its neighborhood. This is easily done with a pair of dental extracting forceps, and a sharp curette. From this point on the treatment should be the same as if the disease had arisen from intranasal causes.

Many operators treat such a condition by boring through the alveolar process in the cavity previously occupied by a tooth. The opening is made large to admit either a wick of gauze or a drainage tube. Through this opening irrigation of the antrum is carried on. Such a procedure is, to my mind, generally only a waste of time. It is applicable to those cases only in which the antrum alone is diseased, and must be considered insufficient as soon as it is learned that other cavities are affected. Then, too, any communication between the antrum, whose resistance against additional infection is already lowered by disease, and the mouth cavity the secretions of which are laden with pathogenic bacteria of all kinds and degrees of virulence, is certainly to be deprecated. I have under treatment at present a patient with a most foul-smelling empyema whose antrum, previously healthy, was infected through such an opening made by extracting a tooth.

After a certain time the operator is confronted by the fact that he must either insert an obturator to maintain a permanent opening or he must allow the wound to close. If he choose the former, he forces the patient not only to wear a foreign body in his mouth for the rest of his life, but also to extend the daily toilet of his teeth to his accessory sinuses. If he choose the latter he may fairly expect a recurrence. By this method careful control is impossible and success is doubtful. Cases do clear up, but they are ones that would have yielded to other and more scientific methods. Statistics of several large throat clinics show a surprisingly large percentage of failures in cases treated in this way, not only as to complete success, but also in keeping the patient comfortable and free from pain. I have had a number of patients who had been treated both by this and by intranasal methods, each of whom has told me that he preferred infinitely the latter. Not only is the former more painful, but the continual draining of pus into the mouth has a bad effect upon his health, his spirits and his mental attitude toward life.

Another method of treating empyema, and one that appeals to me much more strongly, is the intranasal, to the successful use of which belongs not only treatment of the accessory sinus, but also the treatment of the entire nose and nasopharynx. In this connection I hope I may be pardoned if I quote to some extent from an article which I read some time ago before the American Laryngological, Rhinological and Otological Society. Careful rhinoscopic examination of empyema cases impresses one with the fact that in such cases pathological nasal conditions of importance, such as hypertrophies, polypoid posterior ends, spurs and adenoids are almost always to be found, and it is generally true that permanent results are not secured until they are corrected. It may be interesting in this connection to consider briefly the influence that such pathological conditions have upon empyema, both as etiological factors and as factors to determine the chronicity of the disease.

These hypertrophies, either congenital or arising from external conditions, occupation, mode of life, etc., particularly predispose to influenza, diphtheria, scarlet fever, measles and repeated head colds, which are themselves most important in the causation of empyema. It is continual coughing, sneezing and hacking that loosens the mucous membranes from the nasopharyngeal wall, and predisposes to polypoid degeneration, polyps and to severe infection.

Nasal hypertrophies not only predispose, but also act as direct etiological factors and may be considered to act in one of two ways. A posterior end or a mass of adenoid may become a depot for the formation of pus and so become a continual feeder of infective material, which may easily find its way into any one of the accessory sinuses and so set up an empyema essentially chronic from the start. The condition, then, which is so important in causation is naturally an important factor in determining the chronicity of the disease, for as long as such a source of reinfection exists, treatment of the sinus itself is but of slight value.

Hypertrophies act then as sources of infection and reinfection. They act in another way equally important. That is they prevent free nasal respiration, without securing which one cannot expect to bring his case to a successful termination. This truth, I believe, I am one of the first in this country to advance. The value of free nasal respiration can scarcely be overestimated. Two years ago M. Halle, of Berlin, advanced the theory that the air passing in and out through the nostrils was acted upon as in a chimney, drawing out from the accessory sinuses not only the air, but also any secretion that might be in them. That this theory was founded upon fact I have demonstrated to my own satisfaction upon patients. For I have observed if the natural antral orifice which has previously been occluded be made patent, or if an artificial opening through the middle meatus be made into the antrum, that the antrum will soon be emptied of a certain amount of its fluid pus, and that with the patient in a sitting position. Antra opened radically not infrequently show strings of pus extending out through their ostea into the nose. These and similar observations go to prove that proper nasal respiration is of great assistance in securing free ventilation and drainage of the antrum.

As early as possible, then, in the treatment of antral empyema free nasal respiration should be established and the pathological conditions which could possibly bear upon the case should be corrected. If the symptoms referable to the antrum permit, this can be accomplished at the first few sittings. For the sooner these two ends are accomplished the sooner one can attack intelligently the seat of disease.

In proceeding to treat the antrum itself one finds it accessible through both the middle and inferior meatuses, through either of which he may enter the sinus. As many successful operators prefer one while others equally successful choose the other it has small worth to discuss at length the various opinions upon the subject. One should, I think, be governed by the anatomical conditions and features of the particular case he is treating. Sometimes the middle meatus is small from above downwards or it is situated on a higher plane than usual. These conditions render it less easily accessible, and make the inferior meatus the one of election. Again the inferior meatus is sometimes found to be on an unusually low plane, even considerably below the floor of the nose. Manifestly in such a case the middle meatus should be chosen. If one chooses to enter the antrum through the middle meatus he must first remove the anterior end of the middle turbinate and probably a good share of the uncinate process. This gives free access to the cavity and has the advantage that it lays bare the ethmoid to further operative interference should it become necessary to attack it.

In general, however, the inferior meatus is the easier of access and is the one usually chosen. Free approach to the lateral wall of the nose should be secured by removing the inferior edge of the inferior turbinate. This is especially true when a part of the after treatment is to be carried out by the patient himself. An opening should then be broken into the antrum by means of a drill or a mallet and chisel. This opening can be enlarged by means of a Cordes double chisel until it is exactly the size desired. I have found the most satisfactory size to be about three-quarter inch by one-half inch. This is quite large enough to allow free ingress to the antrum and, in the majority of cases, to remain permanently open. Care should be exercised in making this opening. Most of the instruments, trocars, drills, etc., splinter the bone badly, leaving the edges of the wound rough and irregular and often forcing pieces of bone into the antrum. The electric drill is not open to these objections and grinds the bone into such small bits that they can easily be washed away. For enlarging the opening a Cordes chisel does very well as it brings away the bone fragments in its grasp.

When once the communication has been established satisfactorily a suitable curved tube is inserted into the antrum and the antrum is vigorously inflated from a compressed air tank, if possible. By this first inflation pus is generally found. Air under considerable pressure is then allowed to pass through the antrum for a minute

or so, after which the cavity is thoroughly irrigated and again dried thoroughly with air heated to a temperature as high as can be comfortably borne by the patient. Iodoform powder may then be insufflated. I wish to say a word concerning the instrument through which one irrigates. To be efficient it should possess a curve different from that peculiar to the great majority of instruments used for that purpose. The ordinary Krause trocar and most of its modifications are bent in a curve representing an arc of a circle of about three inches diameter. When such an instrument is inserted into the antrum it passes directly across the cavity. Consequently fluids entering through it are forced across to the lateral wall, fall to the floor and finally without exercising any particular scrubbing action, flow out through the ostium. Fluid entering in this way has but an unsatisfactory cleansing function. A curve much better adapted to the necessities of the case is the one belonging to the instrument suggested by Halle. It is, to be sure, a modification of the Krause trocar but it is a very useful one. When this instrument is inserted into the antrum it lies along the inner wall in such a manner that fluid passing from it is forced round and round the cavity in a rapid current finally passing out of the sinus through the ostium, emptying it not only of its fluid contents but also of the tough strings of pus often fastened to its walls. That that is not merely theory one can demonstrate by using a Krause and then a Halle trocar. When the pus is tenacious and stringy the latter is generally more successful in removing it than is the former more widely accepted instrument. I lay considerable stress upon drying the antrum thoroughly after the irrigation. It is left in better condition and regeneration of the mucous membrane and formation of scar tissue must be encouraged. After the first few treatments the details of the succeeding ones depend largely upon the course of the disease. It is often necessary to make irrigation a part of the treatment for some considerable time. I think it should be discontinued as soon as the character and quantity of the discharge will allow. It is often wise to omit irrigation for a few days and then to return to it in order to keep the antral condition under control, for it must be remembered that although the antrum sound dry a considerable amount of dry pus may be adherent to its walls, which, of course, must be removed. As soon as irrigation is omitted the treatment consists of careful but vigorous inflation, which to be most efficient must be kept up two or three minutes.

Uncombined antral empyemas generally show immediate and marked improvement under such treatment. If such be not the case, one of two conditions may be suspected. Either the antral disease is combined with disease of some other of the accessory sinuses, from which reinfection is taking place, or the condition in the antrum is one that will not yield to this kind of treatment.

The former supposition should be the one acted upon first, and careful examination should be made of those sinuses most commonly affected, the ethmoid and sphenoid. If the ethmoid is found diseased, or perhaps in order to find out if it is diseased, the anterior half of the middle turbinate and the ethmoidal bulla are removed. This gives access to an ethmoid cell, generally the second, through which others may be reached. In this way the various accessible cells can be examined and somewhat satisfactorily cleaned out through the nose. As Killian has said, his speculum for median rhinoscopy is an invaluable instrument for such examination and operative procedure. I am surprised to find this instrument in such limited use. In operating upon the ethmoid one goes no further than he can see clearly. Above the plane of the attachment of the middle turbinate he should proceed with the greatest care and should never venture in this direction more than a quarter of an inch. By such intranasal methods small ethmoids of typical shape can be fairly well cleaned out. There remain, of course, in a great many cases infraorbital and anterior cells not to be reached in this way. To reach the posterior ethmoid cell necessitates the removal of the rest of the middle turbinate, after which it is open to inspection and treatment. The posterior ethmoid cell, it must be remembered, is subject to great variation in size, position and shape, and may be easily mistaken for the sphenoid. While laboring under the delusion that he is treating the sphenoid, the operator may have cause to wonder at the pus which continually reinfects his field of operation from an unknown source. These two cavities, posterior ethmoid cell and sphenoidal sinus, should, in this connection, not be confounded, as in obstinate empyema of the antrum knowledge of the condition of the latter is important, for in thirty per cent. of all cases it is infected.

Any intranasal operation upon the sphenoid presupposes the correction of any septal deviation obstructing a view of its orifice. However early in the course of treatment, its condition should have been learned. If the orifice is visible this is, of course, simple, as a probe or catheter can be inserted without difficulty. When on account of septal deviation or hypertrophied turbinate, this is impossible, the condition of the sinus can be ascertained by passing a slender canula over the hypertrophies or deviation along the cribriform plate until it reaches the nasopharyngeal wall. A little manipulation enables one to enter the sinus although it be invisible.

If the sphenoid be found diseased, the deviation must be corrected and turbinate removed in order to give free approach to the anterior wall which is to be completely removed. Pus and polyps can then be wiped out. Of course only that part of the sinus immediately opposite the anterior wall can be reached. When the cavity is large, extending as it sometimes does into the wings of the sphenoid bone, one must trust to other means.

Here again irrigation is useful. This can be carried on successfully through a cannula or a long Eustachian catheter. A half liter can be used to advantage. After this the cavity is thoroughly dried and a dusting powder insufflated. The sphenoid can in most cases be reached and treated in this way through the nose quite as successfully as by some other route.

If the empyema has not yielded to painstaking treatment of this kind, or even before this, in many cases, one is warranted in undertaking more radical measures. It must now be suspected that the cause of the obstinate character of the disease lies either in the character of the pathological changes in the antrum or in involvement of the infraorbital and anterior ethmoid cells. To reach these more successfully one has to resort to the so-called Luc-Caldwell operation or to some modification of it which gives freer approach to the antrum. In determining the course to be followed it is of the greatest value to know as far as may be the character of the pathological changes with which one has to deal, and in this connection I have found the X-ray of very considerable value. The fluoroscope or better, the plate not infrequently shows exactly the cause of the intractability of the case; for it may reveal the antrum filled with hyperlastic growth or extending into the cavity the hidden root of a tooth, long since covered by mucous membrane and forgotten.

This operation may be performed under general or local anesthesia. A lasting and satisfactory anesthesia may be secured by the use of a one-fourth to one-half per cent. solution of cocaine in a solution of adrenal 1-1000. Two or three drams of this solution injected into the mucous membrane of the alveolar process both inside and out, into the soft tissues of the cheek, and into the lateral wall of the nose causes a sufficient anesthesia for from one to two hours. Being an isotonic solution it is, of course, absorbed slowly. One very satisfactory feature of this method is that it makes the operation almost bloodless. If a general anesthetic is chosen I think ether is to be preferred as one may operate with it under much more shallow anesthesia than would be considered safe with chloroform, which fact allows the patient to retain his throat reflex which is of great value in operations during which a hemorrhage into the throat may be expected. The injection of adrenalin is helpful also when using ether although its action is not so satisfactory as when cocaine is employed. If a general anesthetic is employed it is a good plan to pack a wick of gauze into the angle of the jaw to prevent unnecessary sponging of the throat.

The operation itself includes the total resection of the facial wall of the antrum through an incision in the mucous membrane above the tooth line and extending from the first molar to the first incisor. This enables one thoroughly to remove all new growths and diseased mucous membrane. From the antrum the ethmoid cells not accessible from the nose are reached and curetted. Infra-orbital and anterior cells are obliterated. If the sphenoid has not been treated through the nose it may now be found by passing through the posterior ethmoid cell. Its treatment is as outlined above. The median wall, that is the body lateral wall of the nose, is more or less completely removed and if desired a flap of mucous membrane corresponding in size to the opening in the bone is made, its base being its anterior extremity. This flap is then turned into the antrum and sewed to the median end of the first incision. This procedure leaves an opening large enough to be permanent through which intranasal treatment can be carried out. The question of closing the wound for primary union is an interesting one and must be decided according to the character and extent of the pathological changes found.

When the mucous membrane is entirely destroyed and its place taken by new growth or granulation tissue, or when bone caries exists one must consider the advisability of leaving it open and the antrum free to inspection. In this case the after treatment is much shortened by the application of skin grafts. These may sometimes be applied at the time of operation, especially if the hemorrhage is slight and if the antrum can be thoroughly cleaned out. A simple way of applying the grafts successfully is to slip them from a solution of normal salt on a thin spatula to the walls of the cavity, where they are tamped firmly in place and covered by one layer of iodoform gauze cut in small pieces. This layer of gauze is allowed to remain indefinitely as it protects the grafts while any attempt to remove them brings the graft away also. As soon as there is evidence that the healing process is progressing satisfactorily, the buccal wound may be sutured and any further treatment carried out through the nose.

The after-treatment is essentially the same as described before. Now that regeneration of mucous membrane and formation of scar tissue are going on satisfactorily irrigation may generally be discontinued and the dry treatment resorted to. That is, the antrum may be kept free from secretion by frequent inflations and insufflations of a dusting powder, with an occasional irrigation to serve as control of its condition.

The duration of the after-treatment varies greatly and depends upon several factors. It is influenced greatly by the size and shape of the cavity, for the larger the sinus and the more irregular and atypical its form, the longer the time required to accomplish its epidermatization. Again the condition of the patient and the rapidity with which he responds to treatment are important. If he is in poor physical condition his convalescence will naturally be longer. It is characteristic of some patients that they refuse to heal while others require only the slightest assistance in order to conquer their disease. Sometimes the formation of exuberant granulations, fibrous septa and pockets of pus give rise to a condition quite as difficult to treat as the previous one. Such cases require reoperation and

much careful and prolonged treatment. Again the character of the infection must have a certain influence, although after years of existence the infection is always so mixed that the importance of each different germ is difficult to determine. The character and extent of the pathological change are factors of the greatest importance in this connection, and stand in closer relationship to the time required for the after-treatment than does the duration of the disease, for while it is commonly true that difficulty in hearing is in direct ratio to the duration of the disease, it is by no means always true, but depends rather upon the disease process. Some empyemas of years' standing are cured by a few weeks' treatment, while others of a few months' standing resist all treatment. Again the extent of the after-treatment depends upon the combination with disease of the other accessory sinuses, and is in inverse ratio to the ease with which those cavities are reached. Lastly the duration of the after-treatment depends upon the care with which it is carried out. For this reason it is better that it be in the charge of the physician who can note any change from day to day. At times, however, it is wise to hand it over to the patient himself. He should then be furnished with a suitable curved tube, a rubber syringe, and a Politzer bag; be taught how to insert this to the tube, to syringe and inflate the cavity, and to report at intervals to his physician.

Finally in choosing a method of treating chronic empyema of the antrum one should remember that the disease as a rule causes the patient much pain, discomfort and inconvenience, but in the majority of cases does not imperil his life. The percentage of deaths from untreated empyema of the antrum is comparatively small as metastasis and extension into the brain cavity are rare. Perfect cure in the chronic combined cases is difficult and often impossible to secure even by skilful treatment carefully carried out. Therefore, it is the duty of the physician to select that method of treatment which relieves the patient most easily of his symptoms and to resort to radical methods only after conservative ones have been given a thorough trial.

MEDICAL PROGRESS.

MEDICINE.

The Indiscriminate Use of Cathartics.—The idea is firmly rooted in the lay mind and also in that of many physicians, that any arrested bowel action must be promptly restored by the administration of a cathartic. M. L. HARRIS (*Jour. Am. Med. Ass'n.* February 25, 1905) comments on the dangers attending this procedure, especially in the presence of acute intestinal conditions, and calls attention to the fact that no patient ever dies simply because his bowels do not move. The danger lies in the condition which produces the obstruction, and the idea of giving a cathartic with the thought of forcing a movement of the bowels is irrational and harmful. Where there is a mechanical obstruction, the increased peristalsis above the seat of the obstruction simply makes the condition worse and finally leads to fecal vomiting and an increase in the severity of the local pathological lesion, be it intussusceptin, strangulated hernia, peritonitis, etc. Where there is present some acute abdominal condition which cannot be definitely determined, with nausea, vomiting, prostration, etc., no cathartics should be given, as the stomach and intestines absorb very little at this time. The author recommends washing out the stomach with normal salt solution or soda solution, and then to keep it empty, not even giving water. The lower bowel may be emptied with enematas. For the thirst, Harris advises salt solution subcutaneously, 1,000 to 2,000 c.c. in twenty-four hours. It must be understood that this treatment is preliminary and must be supplemented by the proper operative measures as soon as a mechanical obstruction can be diagnosed or even thought to be probable. This procedure places the entire intestinal tract at rest and places the patient in a better condition for operation.

Congenital Pyloric Stenosis.—The most common pathological condition underlying the pyloric stenosis of infancy, according to J. J. SCHMIDT (*Münch. med. Woch.,* February 14, 1905), in a muscular hypertrophy of the pyloric sphincter combined with spasm owing to irritation from errors of diet or too large meals. The common symptoms are projectile vomiting during or shortly after feeding in otherwise healthy infants, crying spells owing to painful spasms, and rapid loss of weight. The vomitus does not contain any bile, the stool is chiefly made up of mucus and excretion of urine soon becomes deficient. If peristaltic movements of the stomach can be detected and if a tumor is palpable, the diagnosis is easy, but this is the exception. In moderate cases internal treatment is in place (hot applications to the stomach, moderate amounts of milk every three hours, and small doses of opium); in the severe cases, however, only an operation will save the life of the child. The best results are obtained from gastro-enterostomy; the fatal cases reported after this operation are solely due to the wretched condition of the patients owing to too prolonged internal treatment.

Latent and Ambulatory Plague.—In a recent proclamation, the governor of Hongkong has pointed out the great danger from the so-called latent plague, that is, a form of plague where the afflicted are hardly ill yet where the blood, when examined is found to contain very many plague bacilli. The great danger from this form of disease, should it exist, is very evident. Blood cultures from a large number of cases from the Philippines, which were not sick but had come into intimate contact with plague patients, were made by M. HERTZOG (*Virchow's Archiv,* Vol. 179, No. 2) to settle this question, but the results were negative in every instance. The constant repetition of epidemics is therefore not due to unrecognized cases but to the apathy of the Chinese who do not abide by the ordinary rules of hygiene. In conclusion, mention is made of a very mild case which died very suddenly. At autopsy, a metastatic bacillary focus was found in the pulmonary artery and a rather recent tuberculous process in the lungs.

Aspergillosis of the Lung Cured by Operation.—An interesting case of aspergillus infection of the lung is reported by G. SCHWARTZ (*Zeitsch. f. klln. Med.,* Vol. 56, Nos. 1 and 2). The patient complained of fever, loss of strength, purulent expectoration and occasional hemoptysis. The physical examination revealed consolidation in the lower portion of the right lung, and after many futile attempts, pus was found

after aspiration. The patient was at once transferred to the surgical division, where a pneumonotomy was done. A piece of necrotic lung, the size of a small apple and containing many mycelia of *Aspergillus fumigatus,* was removed. The patient made a perfect recovery in a very short time. The portal of entry of the fungus was probably the nose, since the patient remembered having been troubled with crusts there, which on examination showed the same fungus. The latter grew well on artificial media and proved strongly pathogenic when injected into mice.

Valedictory Address at Johns Hopkins University. —the *Journal of the A. M. A.,* prints in full, March 4, the valedictory address of Dr. Osler, of Johns Hopkins University, which has been quoted and misquoted in the daily press. He deals with some of the problems of university life and states that the loss of a professor may be of benefit to a university. He stated that to a man of active mind too long attachment to one college is apt to breed self-satisfaction, to foster a local spirit, and to promote senility. He said that much of the phenomenal success of the Johns Hopkins University has been due to the concentration of a group of intellectual men, without local ties, whose operations were not restricted and who were willing to serve faithfully in whatever field of action they were placed. Dr. Osler advised the interchange of teachers, both national and international, and even advised the changing of college presidents now and then "for the good of the exchequer." He said that intellectual infantilism and progeria were two appalling maladies due to careless habits "of intellectual feeding." As a prophylactic measure he advises visiting other universities and colleges, both at home and abroad. He said that it is a very serious matter to have all the professors in a university growing old at the same time, and said that there should be a fixed period for the teacher, either of time of service or of age. He spoke of the comparative uselessness of men above forty years of age, and said that to modify an old saying, "A man is sane morally at thirty, rich mentally at forty, wise spiritually at fifty—or never." He said that the young man should be encouraged and afforded every possible chance to show what is in him, and that the chief value of the teacher, who is no longer a productive factor, is to determine whether the thoughts which the young men are bringing to the light are false idols or true and noble ideas. He said that it would be of incalculable benefit, in commercial, political and professional life if men would retire from work at the age of sixty. He said that the teacher's life should have three periods, study until twenty-five, investigation until forty, professional until sixty, at which age he would have him retired on a double allowance. He went at some length into the history of the Johns Hopkins Medical School, mentioning the strict entrance requirements and the scientific teaching in laboratory work especially. He dwelt on the necessity for practical training in the hospital wards as well as in the laboratories and class rooms. He said that the faculty of Johns Hopkins University has been blessed with two remarkable presidents, who had been a stimulus in every department, and that the good fellowship and harmony among the faculty has been delightful.

Obstruction of Retinal Arteries. —ALLEN GREENWOOD (*Journal A. M. A.,* March 11) considers at length the three principal causes of obstruction of the retinal arteries, viz., arterial disease, embolism and spasm. He thinks that primary thrombosis is rare, though thrombosis is frequently a complication of the above conditions. The most important arterial disease is arteriosclerosis, and he points out the earliest danger signals of this condition. They are a slight increase of arterial reflex, slight irregularities in the size of the arteries, slight congestion of the disk, and feathery outline. Where the artery crosses above a vein the latter may be compressed. A little feathery exudate is often seen beside the arteries which should not be mistaken for the opaque nerve fibers often observed. With thickening of the central artery venous pulsation may sometimes be observed ophthalmoscopically; one or all of these conditions may be present. In more advanced cases the light reflex is increased, the arteries become beaded, retinal lesions appear and, finally, we have the full picture of albuminuric retinitis. The early stages of arterial degeneration require the careful inspection of the upright image for their detection. Spasm, the author believes, most frequently occurs in the early stages of arteriosclerosis, and should be looked on as a warning of future obliterating endarteritis. The treatment of arteriosclerosis is mainly a well-regulated life and avoidance of nerve strain and excesses and keeping elimination and digestion unimpaired. Greenwood has been in the habit of advising long-continued use of small doses of iodide of potash. The treatment of embolism is rarely prompt enough to save the function of the retina, but Greenwood advises the early use of vasodilator drugs and deep massage to carry the embolus, if possible, into the smaller branches and to reduce the field defect. For spasm the treatment for arteriosclerosis should be carefully followed. Nitrate of amyl might be used to cut short an attack.

Treatment of Epidemic Cerebrospinal Meningitis by Diphtheria Antitoxin.—E. WAITZFELDER (Med. Rec., March 11, 1905) reports the results following the treatment of seventeen cases of epidemic cerebrospinal meningitis by the injection of large doses of diphtheria antitoxin according to the suggestion of A. J. Wolf. Five of the patients recovered completely; three died, of whom two were adults, and nine cases are still under treatment. Of these, five show such marked improvement as to indicate probable recovery, four being convalescent. Of the remaining four cases, all are in a serious condition and prognosis is impossible at the present time. Most of the cases were severe in their onset with well marked evidence of profound constitutional infection, as is to be expected in the early periods of an epidemic. The doses of antitoxin given were 6,000 units to children less than five years of age; 8,000 units to those between five and twelve, and 10,000 units to adults. This amount was injected under the scapulæ on alternate days. In some severe cases it was given daily. Usually the injection was followed by a fall of temperature and pulse, and great improvement in the general symptoms. No bad effects developed as the result of the administration of the antitoxin. Should the results in these cases prove to be consistently repeated in others, the author believes that to Dr. Wolf belongs the credit of having discovered the remedy for one of the most fatal diseases, and of having evolved a plan of treatment not second in its effects to the antitoxin treatment of diphtheria.

Case of Cicatricial Stricture of the Esophagus.— A. B. ATHERTON (Med. Rec., March 11, 1905) describes a case of obstinate cicatricial stricture of the lower end of the esophagus which when first seen admitted only an olivary French bougie two millimeters in diameter. By gradual dilatation it became possible to introduce an instrument of twice this size, but after this no further stretching could be effected. The stomach was therefore opened and the stricture softened by the use of the string and bougie procedure of Abbe,

after which gradual dilatation became possible so that a short red rubber bougie one centimeter in diameter could be permanently worn. The upper end of the bougie lay at the junction of the pharynx and esophagus and was secured by a silk thread fastened to a tooth or to one ear. When last heard from, a year after the operation, the patient was still obliged to continue the daily use of the bougie, otherwise the stricture soon contracted.

Advances in the Physiology and Pathology of the Pancreas and Their Application to the Diagnosis of Pancreatic Diseases.—JOHN C. HEMMETER (Am. Med., March 11, 1905) in a lengthy article, fully considers this subject. Of special interest are his observations concerning the diagnosis of relative pancreatic insufficiency from defective protolysis, amyolysis, and adipolysis. He believes the effort to determine the degree to which protolysis is interfered with is rendered futile by the presence of erepsin, secreted in the intestinal juice, and which can break down proteids very rapidly after they are once attacked by gastric juice. Defective fat digestion as a gauge for pancreatic insufficiency is equally disappointing. However, he believes great aid can be obtained from the method of Adolph Schmidt. This is based upon the physiologic fact that only gastric juice can digest connective tissue (collagen) and only pancreatic juice can digest the nuclear substance of meat fiber. Hence the presence of remnants of undigested connective tissue in the feces indicates insufficiency or absence of gastric secretion and the presence of nuclei in the cells of meat fibers points to insufficient pancreatic secretion. Hemmeter tested the stools of two patients, one suffering from pancreatic cyst, comprising the duct of Wirsung and the other from a stenosis of the duct caused by an old pericholecystitis. In both cases the stools contained muscle fibers, showing well-preserved nuclei.

Medical Treatment of Gastric Ulcer.—FREDERICK P. HENRY (Am. Med., March 11, 1905) says: The tendency of gastric ulcer is toward recovery as proved by the frequent presence of cicatrices in the stomach post-mortem. The object of treatment is, therefore, to assist nature. This is best achieved by rest, general and local. The patient is confined to bed and nourished for a longer or shorter period, according to the idiosyncracies of the case, by rectal enemas. Opium is advised during this period for the purpose of allaying pain, quieting peristalsis and obtunding the sense of hunger. Milk and milk-gruel should be the sole articles of diet for one, two, or more weeks after nourishment per os is resumed. The milk should be mingled with lime water. Sodium bicarbonate is not recommended because of the evolution of gas attending its use. The formation of hard, indigestible curd may be prevented by mingling the milk with flour previously well boiled with milk or water, or, this failing, the milk may be peptonized. Buttermilk is sometimes an excellent succedaneum for milk. As the case progresses favorably, row or soft-boiled eggs, meat broths or beef peptone are added to the dietary, but the diet of health is not resumed until several weeks after the beginning of treatment. Among medicines, bismuth subnitrate, in large doses, suspended in barley water or mucilage, is believed to be of benefit. Silver nitrate is inert, because of its immediate conversion, in the hyperacid stomach, into the insoluble chloride. Mercurials are emphatically condemned. Vomiting is treated by cessation of feeding per os, by morphine hypodermically, and by cocaine hydrochlorate; hematemesis by ergot and adrenalin hypodermically and by the administration of ice, gallic acid and acetate of lead.

Carlsbad water or Carlsbad salt, dissolved in a large amount of water, should be slowly swallowed during the early morning hours. Anemia, or chlorosis, if present, is to be treated with iron albuminate which may be prepared extemporaneously after the formula of Ewald. Leuhe's method of treating gastric ulcer by continuous poulticing is discussed and recommended with some modifications which consist in "nourishing the patient during the first week of treatment either entirely or partially by rectal enemas and in the pro re nata employment of opium and its derivatives." Henry has seen "nothing but advantage in the judicious employment of opiates in gastric ulcers."

THERAPEUTICS.

Serum-therapy of Hay-fever.—The manufacture and use of pollantin, the antitoxic serum recommended against hay-fever, is given by A. LÜBBERT (*Therap. Monatschft.*, December, 1904). A toxalbumin is isolated from the pollen of the grasses liable to set up a catarrh, and this is then injected into horses in gradually increasing doses. After two to three weeks a high degree of immunity is established and the blood is withdrawn and allowed to express its serum. The subcutaneous use of pollantin is not recommended since the immunity is only partial, and of short duration; it is much better to apply the serum directly to the nose, eyes or pharnyx (one to two drops every morning during the season). If a reaction sets in, the dose is to be repeated. Very obstinate cases should carry a small bottle with dropper with them every day and resort to an instillation as soon as the first irritation is noticed. If the attack has already set in, the pollantin should be used every ten minutes and the patient instructed to stay indoors.

Specific Treatment of Recurrent Fever.—Since all treatment of recurrent fever is without avail, G. GABRITSCHEWSKY (*Zeitsch. f. klin. Med.*, Vol. 56, Nos. 1 and 2) has attempted to obtain a specific antiserum, according to the following method: The blood from patients known to contain the specific spirilla is defibrinated and injected in quantities of 5 c.c. into mules and zebus, since these animals are said to be especially susceptible. After three weeks the animals were bled and the blood then used for subcutaneous injections in man. A decided cure was never obtained, but after total amounts of 40 to 60 c.c. the frequency of the recurrent attacks was considerably diminished. Good results were also seen from removing a certain amount of blood from the vein at the elbow, defibrinating it and warming it to destroy the spirilla and then reinjecting into the patient. Better results would no doubt be obtained if all these experiments could be made with pure cultures of the spirilla, but it has not yet been possible to grow them outside of the body.

The Action of the Vagus on the Respiration of the Tissues.—The researches of Stefani have shown that in the higher animals the cardiac inhibitory action of the vagus increases with the rise of temperature, and in this way, by moderating the action of the heart, the vagus protects it from the exhaustion produced by fever. F. SOPRANA (*Arch. Ital. de Biol.*, October 31, 1904) has supplemented the above researches by demonstrating that the vagus furnishes a complex mechanism, defending the tissues from the effects of high temperature. It serves to moderate the intensity of the oxidative processes, which are otherwise augmented by an increase of the bodily temperature.

The Auto-digestion of Pepsin.—It has been found by A. HERLITZKA (*Arch. Ital. de Biol.*, October 31, 1904) that pepsin placed in the thermostat with hydrochloric acid, slowly loses its activity, with the formation of peptones. It is assumed that one part of pepsin acts upon the other, peptonizing it, and that this process is a true auto-digestion of pepsin. These results contribute anew to the conclusion that pepsin is a true proteid.

The Diuretic Action of Theobromin.—This drug is effectual in producing marked diuresis in cases of hydrops in which the cardiac action has previously been insufficient according to V. PLAVEC (*Arch. Internal. de Pharmaco. et de Therap.*, Vol. XVVV, Nos. 3 and 4). It is therefore no genuine diuretic, but is really a cardiac drug, increasing the contractile power of the heart-muscle. In exceptional cases, the vasomotor nerves are affected in such manner as to cause a moderate fall in blood-pressure, which neutralizes the effect of the heart. The rise in diuresis produced by theobromin results in consequence of the increased blood-stream through the kidneys.

Treatment of Laryngeal Tuberculosis with Sunlight.—Sunlight will influence favorably tuberculosis of the lungs, but it will also exert a marked action upon a focus located in the larynx. A novel scheme for introducing the rays of light into the throat, is suggested by L. KENWALD (*Münch. med. Woch.*, January 10, 1905). An ordinary hand-mirror is fixed on a level with the mouth of the patient, who is in a sitting position, with the back toward the sun. The rays of light are reflected into the mouth; the patient then pulls out his tongue with the left hand and introduces a laryngeal mirror so that he can see the reflection of his own glottis in the hand mirror. With a little practice even an unskilful patient will soon acquire this technic. The good results of this treatment are best demonstrated by a patient who never succeeded in illuminating the entire portion. The parts which had been exposed to the rays of light appeared healthy, with remarkable retrogression of the tuberculous foci, while the unilluminated portion still presented the original appearance.

Investigation of Magnesium Dioxide.—J. WINTERBERG (*Med. Blätter*, 1904, Ne. 43) calls attention to Ehrlich's early investigations on the oxygen requirements of the organ in which he shows the essential value of cell respiration, and the use of oxygen internally in enhancing such oxidations. The recent work of Ehrlich on reduction of methylene blue in the organism seems to show that magnesium dioxide taken internally is capable of splitting off a certain amount of oxygen which can be utilized in cell respiration, and following these investigations there has been a marked increase and interest taken in the internal administration of such products. At the present time magnesium dioxide is widely used in the form of biogen, and clinical results substantiate the bearing of the indicated pharmacological researches.

Treatment of Skin-Cancers with Fluorescent Substances.—Six cases of superficial cancer of the skin and mucous membrane have been treated by A. JESIONEK and H. v. TAPPEINER (*Deutsch. Arch. f. klin. Med.*, Vol. 82, Nos. 3 and 4) by impregnating (topical applications and injections) the ulcerating tissues with fluorescent substances, usually eosin, and then exposing the patient to sunlight. The concentration employed was 0.01 to 5 per cent. A decided improvement was observed in all cases; in four, the ulceration cicatrized and the tumor-masses disappeared completely.

Atropine in Gynecology.—D. DRENKHAHN (*Therap. Monatschft.*, February, 1905) speaks very highly of the use of atropine in diseases of women, particularly in septic conditions of the uterus. Puerperal fever is at first a purely local condition for which the chances for a cure are exellent, if the uterus is kept at rest. Contractions of the uterus will force the germs through the lymphatic channels into the blood and thus bring about a general sepsis. Atropine is the best remedy known to stop the contractions and will also diminish absorption from the large surface of the puerperal uterus.

Fibrolysin.—Thiosinamine was first recommended for lupus but its use has been extended to all morbid conditions due to scar tissue (urethral stricture, parametritis, pyloric stenosis, etc.). One great disadvantage of the drug is its insolubility in water. Injections of alcoholic solutions are exceedingly painful and the application of plasters, etc., is less efficient. F. MENDEL (*Therap. Monatschft.,* February 1905) has therefore placed on the market the double salt of thiosinomine and sodium salicylate, to which he has given the name fibrolysin. This is perfectly soluble and may even be injected directly into a vein. It is rapidly split up into its component parts and posseses a remarkable elective action upon scar tissue, no matter where this may be. Even after a single injection, swelling and softening occurs, but to bring about a permanent cure, repeated injections will be necessary. In certain conditions, such as stricture of the urethra and esophagus, fibrolysin will soften the thickened tissues, but mechanical treatment will be necessary to bring about the necessary dilatation.

Fibrosarcoma Treated by Roentgen Rays.—C. E. SKINNER (*Arch. of Electr. and Radiolog.,* October, 1904) gives an account of a patient, afflicted with a large fibrosarcoma, deeply seated in the abdomen, which yielded in a remarkable way to the Roentgen rays. The case had been pronounced inoperable by competent surgeons and erysipelas toxin had been used for ten months with only temporary success. After 46 applications during a period of 125 days the size of the tumor had increased appreciably but considerable improvement was noticed in the general condition. After this, the tumor began to diminish slowly in size and when the total number of applications had reached 136, it had disappeared entirely. The original dimensions of the spindle-cell sarcoma were: horizontal, 10 inches; vertical, 8 inches; anteroposterior, 5 inches.

Treatment of Pertussis.—Excellent results are reported by H. STEPP (*Therap. Monatschft.,* November, 1904) from the use of fluoroform in whooping-cough. As a rule, the disease lasts about thirty-five days, but with this drug the duration was reduced to eighteen. Another advantage is that even very young infants show no bad after-effects. The solution generally employed contains 2 to 2½ per cent. fluoroform dissolved in water. Very young infants receive two teaspoonfuls every hour, while older children may take as much as a tablespoonful. The treatment should be continued for three to four weeks.

The Action of Ergot and Ergotinine Upon the Cardio-Pulmonary Circulation.—The intravenous injection of the fluid extract of ergot produces in the dog a marked elevation of blood-pressure in the pulmonary artery, according to L. PLUMIER (*Jour. de Physiol.,* January 15, 1905). This is caused by an ehergetic constriction of the blood-vessels of the lungs, through a direct action upon their walls. The dog's heart, removed from the body and nourished by means of Locke's solution, is at first weakened by ergot, and then strengthened and its action accelerated. The transient fall in carotid blood-pressure is due to the primary depressing action on the heart. The ergotinine of Tanret has almost no effect upon the heart and pulmonary blood-pressure.

PRESCRIPTION HINTS.

Infantile Bronchopneumonia.—Bronchopneumonia is a much graver affection than pneumonia in children, generally secondary, as a complication of smallpox, grippe, diphtheria, typhoid fever, or measles. When children are affected by any of these maladies, rigorous antisepsis of the natural orifices should be enjoined. In children of a certain age antisepsis of the nasal fossæ will be obtained by inhalations of

℞ Menthol	grs. iii
Boric acid	℥ss

For one powder dissolved in an infusion of the leaves of the eucalyptus tree and inhaled through a funnel. In young children, these inhalations can be replaced by instillations of

℞ Menthol	grs. xx
Oil of sweet almonds	℥ii

The mouth should be frequently rinsed with a solution of boric acid, and the eyes bathed with the same liquid, while oxygen water, reduced to half strength should be instilled into the ears.

When in the absence of such prophylactic measures, or in spite of them, bronchopneumonia does set in, the treatment varies according to the intensity of the disease. If the child is not too depressed a vomitive will clear the large bronchi of mucosity, but if dyspnea with tendency to cyanosis be present, a teaspoonful of the following mixture every hour should be given:

℞ Acetate of ammonia	℥ss
Rum	℥iv
Syrup of ether	℥iv
Water	℥iii

To control the fever cryogenine might be ordered:

℞ Cryogenine	grs. xx
Rum	℥iv
Syrup of tolu	℥iv
Syrup of cinchona	℥iv
Water	℥iv

A dessertspoonful three or four times a day.

Hydrotherapy is one of the best means we have of treating bronchopneumonia. The wet sheet, warm or cold baths, according to the judgment of the attendant.

The warm baths, on the other hand, should be given at 100° F., in which the patient remains from ten to fifteen minutes. Cold should be applied to the head while the child is in the bath to prevent cerebral congestion. In cases of collapse, mustard should be put in the bath.

Revulsives consist in mustard poultices and small blisters left on four hours and renewed.

As to a curative method, none has yet been found. Netter appears to have obtained good results from

℞ Collargol	grs. xxx
Vaseline	℥iii
Lanolin	℥i

Rubbed into the axilla or the groin for about fifteen minutes, then wiped off and the place covered with oiled silk.

If at the end of a month or six weeks the patient has not quite recovered, tonic treatment should be ordered and the air cure.

THE MEDICAL NEWS.

A WEEKLY JOURNAL

OF MEDICAL SCIENCE.

COMMUNICATIONS in the form of Scientific Articles, Clinical Memoranda, Correspondence or News Items of interest to the profession are invited from all parts of the world. Reprints to the number of 250 of original articles contributed exclusively to the MEDICAL NEWS will be furnished without charge if the request therefor accompanies the manuscript. When necessary to elucidate the text, illustrations will be engraved from drawings or photographs furnished by the author. Manuscript should be typewritten.

SMITH ELY JELLIFFE, A.M., M.D., Ph.D., Editor,
No. 111 FIFTH AVENUE, NEW YORK.

Subscription Price, Including postage in U. S. and Canada.

PER ANNUM IN ADVANCE $4.00
SINGLE COPIES 10
WITH THE AMERICAN JOURNAL OF THE
MEDICAL SCIENCES, PER ANNUM . . 8.00

Subscriptions may begin at any date. The safest mode of remittance is by bank check or postal money order, drawn to the order of the undersigned. When neither is accessible, remittances may be made at the risk of the publishers, by forwarding in *registered* letters.

LEA BROTHERS & CO.,
No. 111 FIFTH AVENUE (corner of 18th St.), NEW YORK.

SATURDAY, MARCH 25, 1905.

THE NEW YORK LYING-IN HOSPITAL.

THE open discussion in the recent daily press of the condition of affairs at the New York Lying-in Hospital must necessarily tend to lower a very serious matter to the level of a routine hospital schism. It is a very unusual event, however, when practically the entire medical staff of a long-established hospital, including the pathologists, and even a member of the Board of Governors tender their resignations in a body, leaving a small, peculiarly intrenched minority in nominal control of the situation.

It is not a pleasant task to discuss the very peculiar features of this situation, but it appears to be of such importance to the medical profession of New York City, to the art of obstetrics, to the general community, and especially to the patients who seek this hospital, that it becomes a plain duty to point out some of the abuses which have long been practised at the institution, and to urge their removal.

It is a matter of record that during the last few years no less than sixteen physicians who had been attracted by the apparent possibilities offered by the institution, have resigned, and it is an unsavory fact that these resignations have resulted from dissatisfaction with the arbitrary behavior of the one man whom the generous donor placed in absolute control of the new building. Now comes the resignation of eleven more of the staff, so that twenty-seven men, including most of the prominent younger obstetricians of New York, have registered their refusal to tolerate the conditions prevailing.

From the excellent quality of the original studies in the annual report for 1897, unfortunately almost the only one, and from the initial equipment of the new Lying-in Hospital, pronounced the best of its type in existence, it was confidently predicted that the institution would become the leading scientific obstetrical center of the country. Instead, there has been an absolute lack of scientific work in obstetrics, charges, too well founded, of startling incompetence in the routine clinical work in certain wards and operating rooms, open ruptures between the medical director and any progressive colleague who attempted to introduce modern methods, and finally complete disintegration with the stigma of having been tried and found wanting by a score of the most active obstetricians of the city. Not the least of the unworthy chapters in its history has been the attempt made to employ the great possible value of the institution for instruction of students to further professorial aspirations which must otherwise have seemed chimeras to all but the aspirants.

Not even the nurses have escaped the baneful effects of whimsical and abused authority, for an enforced attendance at the "Lying-in" has long figured as one of the greatest of prescribed trials in various training school circles.

It is well-known that the Board of Governors have not been wholly ignorant of the state of affairs. In fact, it is betraying no secret to admit that their troubles have been severe, especially since in the words of one of these, the hospital became "the laughing stock of the country." For it is impossible to obtain bequests from general sources for an institution which is everywhere known to exist for selfish professional interest, and hence the directors have faced the alternative of closing the hospital or keeping it open upon the old plan. At least one of them has indicated by his resignation that it were better to close it.

It is seldom that the airing of soiled linen is decent or justifiable. We realize the unsavory character of the foregoing references, but we hold it justifiable to protest without let or hind-·

rance where the progress of obstetrics, at present a lame duck in medical science, the obstetrical teaching and professional chairs in metropolitan universities, and the lives of indigent women in labor appear to be menaced for purely personal considerations.

Contrary to the impression given by one of the daily papers, we can assure the governors that neither the Lying-in Hospital nor any other can be rescued from condemnation upon any such plans as theirs, and that after the present upheaval no self-respecting physician can afford to hold a position on its staff. We would further remind the Board of Governors that the Society of the Lying-in Hospital was handed down to them by such men as Alexander Hamilton, DeWitt Clinton, Frederick de Peyster and Nicholas Fish, and that their office, now become public, is a public trust.

"IT MIGHT HAVE BEEN CAESAR—IT IS SMITH."

THE blessings that pertain to a paternal government do not appear to be of the variety that brighten, particularly when they take their flight across the Western Ocean. In the good old days of yore, when knighthood was in flower, or when the patriarchal Arab sheik pleasingly combined the duties of the midwife with the functions of the undertaker and watched over and assumed the personal charge of his followers from the cradle to the grave, affairs were naturally conducted with a high hand. But the world "do move" and customs change with its revolutions and though free trade may or may not be desirable in business undertakings, there is no necessity for "protection" or for the official vaunting of foreign medical quackery.

It now appears that the United States Consul at Nottingham, England, has reported a "new treatment for defective eyes" and that this having been published in the Daily Consular Reports of the Department of Commerce and Labor, the craze which has caused the greatest excitement in England has been transplanted and has taken violent and sudden root in this country. Mr. F. W. Mahin, the consul, writes: "This locality is much interested in a remarkable new method of treating defective eyesight. It is described briefly as "Manipulation of the eye," and was thought out and developed by Dr. Stephen Smith, surgeon to the eye department of Battersea Park Hospital. The precise method of treatment is not disclosed, remaining the inventor's secret. The treatment

is described as gentle and gradual, a few minutes daily, causing no pain and having no injurious effect of any sort. Some patients are cured in a week, and in all cases improvement is rapid. Thirty patients who previously had to wear spectacles have so far been treated by Dr. Smith and with one exception it is stated all have discarded glasses and can now read at either long or short distances as easily as people who have never needed glasses. The cures applied to myopia (short sight), hypermetropia (long sight) and astigmatism (irregularity in the shape of the eye) and are claimed to be permanent, which, of course, remains to be demonstrated. Optimists assert that the general use of this method will practically abolish eyeglasses."

Now, in examining into the merits of any alleged original procedure in the practice of medicine, two things are to be taken into consideration. First; if the application *is* new, and second the standing and professional position of the person presenting it. In regard to the originality of Dr. Smith's "discovery" he may have achieved, though we doubt it, a success that other experimenters in the same direction have failed to attain, but he is not by any means the first worker in that particular field. The *British Medical Journal*, which is generally a most conservative and carefully edited paper, is singularly ill informed when it states, that "massage has not, so far, been credited with the power of altering the shape of a living elastic globe," and if the rest of the conclusions on this theory are based on a similar want of knowledge of the facts, it will hardly be necessary for American ophthalmologists to enter the lists to tilt with windmills. For a great deal has been written on the influence of massage upon the errors of refraction by Darier in 1899, by Gradenigo in 1894, and by Domec, of Dijon. In Darier's *Leçons de Thérapeutic Oculaire*, published in 1892, a full description is given of the effect of pressure massage upon hypermetropia, myopia and other errors of refraction, while Richey, of Washington, D. C., has repeatedly called attention to the beneficial effects of massage in the treatment of glaucoma. This, however, is another matter, and is probably due to the relief of venous stasis by the softening of the rheumatically stiffened sclera, rather than to any expansion with a consequently increased cubic capacity of the eyeball.

For it has been, since the days of the publication of Donder's classical work on "The Accommodation and Refraction of the Eye," a cardinal point in mathematical optics, that the lenticular and refractive system of all eyes is practically one and the same thing, and that the optical deviations from the standard emmetropic eye are due to an increased or lessened length of the antero-posterior diameter of the globe and not, as hitherto believed, to an increased or deficient lenticular activity. Such being the case anatomically we do not see how Dr. Smith could have "thought out" a rule of three (myopia, hyperopia and astigmatism) that is good enough to work both ways. If his "gentle massage" will cause the shortened hypermetropic eye to gradually elongate, until the retina is pushed back to the position where the refracted rays will meet on its accurately adjusted surface, well and good. But how will the *same* manipulation induce the distended tissues of the myopic eye to contract until the distant retina has been drawn up to the focal point? All this seems more blind than the professor's glass-needing patients, but we confess that we do not understand the modus operandi and must, therefore, be content to let it remain the "author's secret" until this modern sheriff of Nottingham, with his eagle eye and massive brain, is either more comparative in his elucidations or less positive in his prophecies.

With regard to Dr. Stephen Smith, himself, he seems to be pursued by the proverbial fate of prophets in their own country, as he has been thoroughly damned by the English medical press without even the customary amelioration of faint praise. Thus the London *Ophthalmoscope* says, editorially, that "Mr. Stephen Smith, who has leaped into such notoriety, should be handled without gloves. This public proclamation of what he claims to be a scientific discovery to a knot of newspaper reporters, is an outrage on the traditions that govern medical life, which undignified procedure has proved a huge advertisement for himself and incidentally to the antivivisection hospital over whose ophthalmic department he presides." Meanwhile he seems to have entered into a sort of free-for-all, catch-as-catch-can public fight with an optician, one Aitchison, while an "ophthalmic surgeon," a Dr. Wm. Ettles of 141 Minories, is apparently to hold the stakes and to act as umpire between surgeon and tradesman.

After all, it is not what Mr. Smith has or has not done that is remarkable, but the effect that its publication has had on the community at large

Even the tulip craze was second to it in the excitement that the belief that eyeglasses were to be done away with has produced and the succeeding depression will be vast in extent and cerulean in hue. In fact, as the "discovery" is old and as Smith's pretentions are undeniably new, while the scheme is adapted from the experiments of others and will prove unquestionably disappointing to the masses, the whole "new method" can be poetically summed up in the distich of our grandmothers concerning the necessities of the trousseau:

"Something old and something new,
　Something borrowed and something blue."

CANCER.

WE HAVE become accustomed to the erudite discussion which has been going on among researches into the cause of cancer, and the claims and counterclaims of the metabolists and the infectionists no longer excite our hopeful etiologic minds. It is far too early probably, in fact, to trend toward either of these supposedly opposed theories of cancer. Indeed, some physiologists, knowing in the latest lore of protoplasmic structure and metabolism, can imagine a sort of infection or inoculation which might come within the scope of both theories and from its subtlety long escape the observation of the multitude of students of this dreadful scourge. Without discussing the failure (save in a negative and destructive sense) of the Harvard Cancer Commission or the vague and groping suppositions of the metabolists, we may well direct attention to work done by Gaylord, Clowes, and Baeslack, of Buffalo (a preliminary report of which appeared in the MEDICAL NEWS of January 14; as, perhaps, a gleam destined to brighten late or soon into the day of hope for millions of mankind. The results so far reported are meager, too meager and too far away from the deadly cancers of the human stomach and uterus and breast to be much more at present than a hopeful beginning; yet, on the other hand, perhaps not so far away despite their meagerness!

Gaylord and his coworkers, inoculating white mice with bits of mouse-tumor obtained from Jensen, of Copenhagen, and called by him adenocarcinoma, found that it could be readily communicated from mouse to mouse, twenty to seventy per cent. of the inoculations made being successful. About seven months after the inoculations of the tumors were begun they "noted, for the first time in a number of mice that the tumors, which had grown to a demonstrable size, ceased growing and underwent a form of spontaneous retrogression which terminated in the disappearance of the tumor without recurrence." Injecting the blood-serum of these mice which had recovered spontaneously, it was found that it possessed not only a strong immunizing power over recurrence in infected mice, but that it caused the disappearance of tumors not too far advanced and stopped the growth in all cases, with a diminution of the prominent general cachectic symptoms of the grave disease. Moreover, the serum of the mice so cured becomes in its turn an immune serum. The degree of the immunity conferred varied widely, but it was invariably immunizing in its action. In one case one-fifth of a cubic centimeter of the serum "caused the rapid retrogression and entire disappearance of two tumors in one animal and one in another, all of which were as large as peas, in the space of three days."

As to the nature of the curative serum these gentlemen incline to a present belief that it is not cytolytic in its action. The changes found in the epithelium of retrogressed tumors appear to be those suggestive of simple atrophy. The connective tissue stroma of the tumors was always largely overgrown, leaving only traces of epithelium—much the condition, in fact, described by Becker and Petersen as existing in the rare cases of marginal healing in cancers of man. These circumstances seem to be of especial significance, since they indicate a close correspondence of a very hopeful nature, between the conditions in the mice and in human individuals. Something more hopeful still, because pointing to a possibility of cure, these histologic similarities suggest that perhaps comparatively little of something or other is required in the infected blood-serum of man to make it too capable of tipping the balance favorably for the patient, since spontaneous cure in man is occasionally observed.

Thus the present case stands—rich in hopeful possibility, even on grounds so meager, yet as these summarized above. Few things so greatly important in medicine as the nature and curing of cancer burst forth complete at once. This looks like a glimmer of saving light. A year hence we shall be better able to say if it, indeed, be so, or only another *ignis fatuus* in this wretched desert all men would reclaim—as sad to humanity as another "city of dreadful night."

ECHOES AND NEWS.

NEW YORK.

American Journal of Surgery.—Dr. Joseph MacDonald announces that he has severed his connection as Manager and Managing Editor of the *International Journal of Surgery* with which he has been associated for the past fourteen years. This move was made for the purpose of enabling him to publish an independent practical surgical journal and he has purchased all rights in the *American Journal of Surgery and Gynecology*, and with the April number this journal, thoroughly modernized and largely increased in circulation, will be issued from New York as the *American Journal of Surgery*.

A New Training School for Nurses.—A training school for nurses has been started at the new French Hospital 450 West Thirty-fourth Street, New York. The course is to be two years including a two months probationary term, and will include experience in obstetrics and diseases of children, as well as all branches of general medicine, surgery and gynecology. Applicants are not required to speak French, but will receive instruction in the language as a part of their course. The hospital has a capacity of about 130 beds including private rooms, and both building and equipment are thoroughly up to date.

Extension of the Fight Against Tuberculosis to Brooklyn.—The committee for the prevention of tuberculosis of the Brooklyn Bureau of Charities, the formation of which has been under consideration by the board of directors of the bureau for some weeks, has been formally organized. The committee consists of the following persons: Dr. J. H. Raymond, chairman; William I. Nichols, secretary; Miss Margaret Dreier, treasurer; A. Abraham, Dr. H. Arrowsmith, Mrs. Andrew D. Baird, Mrs. Tunis G. Bergen, Dr. H. M. Briggs, Dr. Glenworth R. Butler, T. O. Callender, Dr. J. H. Darlington, Mrs. H. E. Dreier, Percy S. Dudley, Dr. H. A. Fairbairn, Dr. John F. Fitzgerald, Dr. J. W. Fleming, Mrs. R. W. Gage, Dr. Thomas L. Fogarty, Horace Greely, Mrs. James S. Hollinshead, Dr. T. M. Lloyd, Mrs. Willis L. Ogden, Edwin Reynolds, William Strauss, Benjamin Strauss, Mr. and Mrs. Alfred T. White, Dr. John S. Billings, the Rev. N. D. Hillis, Mrs. William Chandler Smith. The chairman will appoint an executive committee who will take actively in hand the work of the committee. The next meeting will be a public one, to be held in the hall of the Kings County Medical Society, on Bedford Avenue.

Meningitis Commission.—As a first step toward checking the great increase in the city's death rate, due to the inroads of cerebrospinal meningitis, Dr. Darlington, head of the Health Board, has appointed seven leading physicians a commission to thoroughly investigate the disease and, if unable to provide a cure, to find a preventative. The number of deaths last week from the disease were 76 as compared with 28 in the corresponding week of 1904. The total number of cases in the city from January 7 to March 11 was 386, of which 70 per cent. proved fatal. The number of cases of the disease in the corresponding period last year was 75. Four of the seven members of the commission have already agreed to serve and it is believed the other three will express their willingness to-day. The members are Dr. William M. Polk, chairman, dean of Cornell Medical College; Dr. Walter B. James, professor in the College of Physicians and Surgeons; Dr. William P. Northrup, professor of children's diseases in the University and Bellevue Hospital Medical College; Dr. Simon Flexner, of the Rockefeller Institute; Dr. Joshua M. Van Cott, pathologist at the Long Island Medical College; Dr. E. K. Dunham, pathologist of Carnegie Laboratory, and Dr. William K. Draper, visiting physician at Bellevue and Minturn Hospitals. "I have chosen these men for two reasons," said Dr. Darlington last week, "first, because every one of them is an authority in medicine and knows as much as is known to-day of cerebrospinal meningitis, and second, because, taken together, they represent all of the medical colleges of New York and will have the advantage of the laboratory work of those institutions." Dr. Darlington said that he expects the deaths from this disease will reach 1,200 before the season ends. Last week, he said, deaths from cerebrospinal meningitis raised the death record a full point, else it would have been the lowest in the city's history. The first meeting of the commission will be on next Tuesday. All of the members give their services free, while the $5,000 appropriated by the city will go toward defraying the expense of compiling data.

PHILADELPHIA.

A Mass Meeting.—In order to raise money for the Fred Douglass Memorial Hospital, a meeting was held in the Holy Trinity Church, where $1,000 were collected.

Bill Passes.—The legislature passed a bill regulating and licensing the practice of osteopaths; it also provides for the establishment of a State Board of Examiners.

Nurses' Home Dedicated.—The nurses of the Women's Hospital took possession of their new home after the exercises which took place last week. The new building is four stories high, and cost $20,000. The members of the board of managers were present at the dedication exercises.

Insane Patient Escapes.—Robert P. Kelly, who has been a patient at the Pennsylvania Hospital for Insane since January 3, 1905, because of melancholia due to business embarrassments, made his escape from that institution by climbing over the wall enclosure. The authorities are unable to locate him.

Hospital Reports.—During February there were admitted to the Hahnemann Hospital wards 155 patients and 249 were treated there, 195 of which were charity patients. In the same month 770 new patients were treated in the out-wards. The expenses of the Methodist Episcopal Hospital exceeded the income by $12,164 during the year just ended.

Enteric Fever on the Increase.—Last week 247 cases of typhoid fever were reported to the Board of Health; this number exceeds that of last week's figure by 69 cases. The increase is sectional, and these particular districts are supplied by water taken from the Delaware and Schuylkill rivers. The authorities are insisting upon the use of boiled water.

Work of the Visiting Nurse Society.—The nineteenth annual report of this society shows that 33,357 visits were made during the year just ended. It is the object of this organization to give to the poor the best possible home nursing, and to teach the head of the households to care and prepare food for the sick. The house, No. 1340 Lombard Street,

which the society has occupied for many years, was recently given to it by the will of J. Dundas Lippincott.

The Overcrowded Condition of Insane Hospitals to be Relieved.—At a conference, in which Governor Pennypacker, Speaker Walton and Chairman Plummer, of the appropriation committee, participated, it was decided to erect a one-story annex to each of the three insane hospitals, situated at Danville, Norristown and Warren. These structures are to be temporary, and when permanent buildings are erected the material of these structures is to be used in constructing consumptive camps.

The Crusade Against Tuberculosis.—This was the topic of D. L. F. Flick in an address before the Acorn Club. When asked his opinion of the danger of spitting on the sidewalks and in public places, and whether those people who expectorated in these places were not sufferers of tuberculosis, he replied to the question in the negative. He said " the poor consumptive is bearing more than his burden already and should not be made to share the responsibility of this evil." He informed the audience that a law should be passed prohibiting expectorating on the sidewalks and in public places.

Cerebrospinal Meningitis Prevalent.—Since the death of Dr. A. B. Craig, who contracted the disease while discharging his duty at the bedside of a patient, ill with the disease, many other cases have developed. This sad death, which must be placed in a parallel with the death of the soldier fighting for his country, has made the physicians of this city, at least, regard the disease as distinctly contagious instead of mildly contagious. The Board of Health has determined to placard the houses in which the disease occurs, and they have decided to fight it in a manner similar to that employed in rooting out smallpox. It has been suggested that the Council be asked to appropriate $5,000 or $10,000 to study the disease. Since the first of the year 26 cases have been reported; the last case that developed was first discovered while the boy was at school, so that the place had to be closed and fumigated.

Annual Meeting of the Directors of the White Haven Sanitarium.—In his annual address before the directors of this institution the president, Dr. L. F. Flick, suggested that it be put on a partial pay basis. He believes that it can be done in a manner which will avoid hardship to anyone. He recommends that $7 be charged patients for the first four weeks they are in the infirmary; $5 a week during the time they are in the sanatorium proper, and work from one to four hours a day; $3 a week during the time they are in the sanatorium proper, and work from four to eight hours a day; nothing to be charged for the month they are in the sanatorium proper, and work eight hours a day to harden. The institution would at all times have money in reserve to admit the very poor free he believes. Up to the present time the State has contributed $158,750, while the public has collected $156,422.89, so that the people have given nearly as much as the State. According to Dr. Flick's statement, 75 per cent. of the cases admitted have been restored to a condition of health, while 95 per cent. of the cases have left the institution improved. At the same meeting, General Wagner, president of the Third National Bank, offered a farm for convalescent patients. The tract of land is between Philadelphia and Bethlehem; if suited for a hospital, the farm, the General said, could be rented for a nominal amount.

Section of Otology and Laryngology of the College of Physicians of Philadelphia.—The meeting of this section was held March 15. Dr. Geo. M. Marshall read a paper on "A Case of Clonic Spasm of the Laryngeal and Pharyngeal Muscles Following a Cranial Injury." The case upon which the paper was based was exhibited. He was a man who claimed to have been sandbagged during the year 1901, and to have been operated upon because of a hemiplegia involving the arm and leg, of the right side, by Dr. Brewer, in New York, two days after the accident. The dura was slightly edematous but presented no other lesion. When the patient was seen at the Philadelphia Hospital he found it difficult to talk. Upon examination the muscles of the larynx and pharynx contracted from 154 to 165 times per minute. In discussing this case, Dr. Burr said there was some difficulty in obtaining a correct history, but from what he learned there was a cross paralysis, the left side of the face and the right arm and leg being involved. He believes there is a syphilitic basilar meningitis. Dr. F. B. Royer then read a paper on "The Complications and Sequelæ met in Laryngeal Diphtheria." He showed five cases. His paper was discussed by Drs. Griffith, Wharton, Jopson and Kyle.

Section of Medicine of the College of Physicians. —This section met March 13, where Dr. Stengel read a paper on "A Case of Tuberculous Meningitis Following Trauma in a Patient Having Tuberculosis of the Kidney, Giving a Positive Widal Reaction." The patient gave a history of trauma, the blow being received back of the ear. After the injury the patient began to vomit. Later he became stupid, although he could be aroused to answer questions; after replying he would again fall into the stupid condition. At times there were present involuntary urination. The pupils were unequal, and the movements of the eyes were incoordinate. Kernigs sign was present. The patient was in a typhoid state; the Widal reaction was positive on two occasions; nevertheless, Dr. Stengel believed the patient was suffering with tuberculous meningitis. The fluid obtained from lumbar puncture contained 60 per cent. mononuclear leucocytes, 12 per cent. transitional, 24 per cent. polymorphonuclear. The blood contained 21,800 leucocytes; blood cultures gave the staphylococcus. Later a slight facial palsy developed. The patient was now brought to operation with the idea of flushing the dura, in hopes that it might have the same effect that opening and flushing the peritoneum. At autopsy the left kidney was tuberculous, the left ureter contained many ulcers, there were many tubercules at the base of the brain. Dr. Francine, who was to read a paper on "Carbon Disulphide Poisoning," could not be present, but sent his paper and it was read by Dr. Krus. The substance is used extensively in manufacturing. Fifteen grains of the substance will prove fatal if taken. These patients, when at work, are exhilarated, but so soon as they leave the work they become depressed. When seen the patient was stupid, acting very much like a drunken man. The condition began with headache, mental depression, sometimes he became delirious during the night. Dr. Eshner exhibited the case of "Congenital Atrichia," which he reported at the last meeting.

Section on Gynecology of the College of Physicians of Philadelphia.—The meeting of this section was held March 16, where Dr. Geo. M. Boyd and Dr. A. G. Ellis read a paper on "Congenital Heart Disease." Owing to the absence of Dr. Boyd, Dr. Ellis read the paper. The article was based upon an infant upon which Dr. Ellis performed an autopsy at the Philadelphia Hospital, and found a transposition of the vessels of the heart. In looking up the clinical notes he found that the infant had lived 34 days, but during this time it had been cyanotic almost continuously, occasionally the blueness would disappear for a short time only. It suffered with dyspnea the greater part of the time. Although the child nursed fairly well it lost and gained weight alternately, so that at death it weighed a quarter of a pound less than at birth. At the autopsy Dr. Ellis found the heart globular in shape, the greater part of this organ was made up by the right side, especially the ventricle from which cavity the aorta arose. Beyond the origin of the vessel its course was normal; it gave off the usual three large branches from the arch, and beyond these it was joined by the ductus arteriosus, which was patulous. The coronary arteries arose from the aorta. The pulmonary artery took origin from the left ventricle, and then pursued its normal course. The foramen ovale was patulous. In discussing this paper, Dr. Coplin called attention to the operation that was performed by Anlog for ectopia cordis in 1888. This surgeon opened the chest by removing a piece of the sternum and then replaced the heart. Dr. John B. Deaver then read a paper on "Hysterectomy for Fibroids of the Uterus." He takes the ground that these growths should not be removed unless they give rise to symptoms, such as pressure, hemorrhage and pain. He is not so certain that many of these tumors undergo sarcomatous change. The treatment of fibroids of the uterus by electricity should, in his opinion, be condemned. Castration, for these neoplasms, he said, is irrational. Because of the frequency with which disease of the ovaries and tubes is associated with the fibroids he prefers to operate through the abdomen instead of through the vagina. He is very much opposed to the use of salt solution in the abdominal cavity. This paper was discussed by Drs. Noble, Clark, Shoemaker and Norris. Dr. A. P. Berg then read a paper on "Paraplegia Complicating Pregnancy." He is quite convinced that toxemia of pregnancy will give rise to disease of the nervous system. In the case which he reports, the woman developed a paraplegia, which he attributed to the toxemia affecting the spinal cord. His patient recovered completely some time after delivery. Drs. Rhein and Pickett discussed this paper. Dr. Theo. A. Erck read a paper on "Sarcomatous Degeneration of a Fibroid of the Uterus with Repeated Hemorrhages into the Tumor."

Philadelphia Pediatric Society.—This society met March 14. The scientific program was opened by Dr. E. C. Jones, who exhibited a family in whom five children have multiple exostoses but only three of the children could be brought. He said that the father, who is now dead, was similarly affected. The oldest child, now fifteen years old, has about fifty of these bone-like tumors scattered over his body. The growths made their first appearance at the age of four years. In the second child the tumors first appeared at the age of two years. He is now eight years and possesses about fifty of these tumors. Upon the other children the growths are less numerous. The doctor stated that there is no evidence of syphilis nor of gout, although there is a history of alcoholism in the family. Dr.

D. J. Milton Miller showed a case of chondrodystrophy fetalis. He called the society's attention to the fact that the height of a normal child at an age corresponding to the age of this child measures 45 inches, while the child exhibited measures but 36½ inches. It measures but 16 inches from the umbilicus to the sole of the feet. It has a very large head, the bridge of the nose is depressed, and in the lumbar region there is a well-marked lordosis. He maintained that the condition is due to some fault in the primary cartilage. The periosteum, he said, grows inward, and the development of the bone depended upon this structure. Dr. Chas. W. Burr then presented a case of Stuporous Insanity at Puberty. In giving a short sketch of the history, he said that the condition began after the boy had been constipated for three days. The first noticeable symptom was sleeplessness, and a tendency to wander around aimlessly. Then he became silent, did not ask for food, and finally refused to take food, stating his mother was trying to poison him. About four months ago (about three months after the onset of the disease) he stopped talking, and apparently paid no attention to anything, but if a limb were irritated he would merely draw it away. The patient passed urine and feces involuntarily. Occasionally he resisted movements; the reflexes were gone; about one month ago he began to talk, became observant, and can now be made to obey commands. His physical condition is improving, and Dr. Burr believes the prognosis is good. Dr. J. P. Crozer Griffith then read a paper on a "Fatal Case of Chorea." During the course of his paper he told the society that the movements of the patient became violent, and that the slightest excitement exaggerated them immensely. He noted the presence of a mitral systolic murmur. Toward the end of the disease the patient's speech became altered, and finally was unable to articulate, later the patient became delirious, and hyoscine was the only drug which succeeded in quieting him. He then became stuporous; finally coma set in and the patient died. Dr. Griffith believes death resulted from exhaustion. Dr. R. Max Goepp read a paper on a "Case of Necrotic Stomatitis Following Pneumonia and Measles." The *Bacillus diphtheriæ* and the *Staphylococcus pyogenes albus* were found in the slough. The condition cleared up after the application of the Paquelin cautery. He also reported a "Case of Malignant Scarlet Fever." The condition was diagnosed by the presence of scarlet fever in another child in the family and by the onset with convulsions. The child died in forty-eight hours.

CHICAGO.

Eastern Illinois Ophthalmological and Otological Society.—A society with this name was organized in Danville, Ill., March 7. Dr. Cassius M. Craig, of Champaign, was elected president; Dr. Charles P. Hoffman, of Danville, secretary, and the Committee ou Fee Bill consists of Drs. I. E. Huston and Elbert E. Clark, of Danville.

Ban on Soliciting Damage Suits.—A bill introduced by Mr. Burnett has passed the legislature prohibiting attorneys from soliciting personal or other damage cases. This measure was endorsed by the State Bar Association, and is directed against shyster lawyers, who make a business of drumming up this character of practice against members of the medical profession.

Bill to Limit Fees of Expert Witnesses.—A bill directed against physicians who make a business of appearing as expert witnesses in personal injury cases was recently introduced in the House, at Springfield, by Mr. Canady, limiting the fee to be paid an expert witness to $10. Physicians in Chicago now receive from $25 and upward for expert testimony, and it is asserted that a number of physicians make a livelihood by means of giving expert testimony.

Removal of Frank S. Betz Co.—This enterprising firm will leave their present building about May 1, and will move to their new plant at Hammond, Indiana. They leave a building a block long to go into a new building occupying over four acres of ground space. They have nearly twelve acres of land at Hammond, and over one thousand feet of switch track, which is connected with the Belt line, and can make shipments over this line much more promptly than in their old place; in fact, they can save from one to two days time in sending their goods to their customers.

Bill to Bar the Sale of Drugs.—A Mr. Clark, of Chicago, has introduced a sweeping bill regulating the sale of morphine and opium. Under the provisions of the proposed law these drugs may be sold only on prescription of a duly licensed physician. It is further stipulated that a druggist shall not refill a prescription unless certified to by the physician who gave the original prescription. The author of the bill asserts that close to 50 per cent. of the inmates in State insane asylums are suffering from the effects of these drugs. There is every indication that this bill will pass.

Care of the Insane.—According to a bill now pending in the State Legislature of Illinois, provision is made that after July 1, 1907, all insane patients who are a charge on the public shall be brought under the care of the State. This measure is clearly in line with the dictates of justice and humanity, and should tend to promote uniform and systematic action in dealing with the problem of the insane. There are at the present time outside of Cook County, in local poor-houses and other places not properly equipped for their care perhaps, one thousand insane patients. Cook County's Insane Hospital at Dunning, according to the Chicago *Daily News*, has an equal number. When any county has furnished the quota which it is permitted to contribute to the State institutions, any additional insane patients must accept such treatment as the County affords. It is obvious that every insane person in the State who is a charge on the public is entitled to treatment as good as the best accorded to others. It is also obvious that uniformity in this respect can be attained only by vesting the control of all the public institutions for the insane in a single body to be administered in conformity with the same general plan. At present the State insane hospitals lack the accommodations necessary to care for all the patients who might be transferred to them, but as the law, if passed, would not take effect for more than two years, there would be ample time in which to increase their capacity as far as might be necessary. Under the terms of the bill the Dunning institution would be turned over to the State without cost to the latter. The proposed law is a long step toward a wise and enlightened treatment of the problem for the insane. Humanity and justice require its immediate enactment.

CANADA.

Canadian Medical Journal Suspends Publication.—The *Canada Medical Record*, for many years conducted by Dr. F. W. Campbell, dean of the Medical Faculty of Bishop's College University, Montreal, has ceased publication, and has become amalgamated with the *Montreal Medical Journal.*

McGill Graduates in British Columbia.—The annual meeting of the Society of McGill graduates in British Columbia will be held in Vancouver on March 23, under the presidency of Dr. D. H. Harrison, of that city, who is at present in Southern California for the benefit of his health. The secretary is Dr. W. J. McGuigan, of Vancouver, and one of the principal items of business will be to arrange for a reunion in Montreal in 1906.

Winnipeg's Health Committee.—The City Council of Winnipeg, Manitoba, has appointed a brand new Health Committee, and they are getting down to work with great vigor. Its first work was to appoint a city bacteriologist in the person of Dr. Leeming, a native of India, but a graduate of the Manitoba Medical College, who has served as assistant to Dr. Gordon Bell, the provincial bacteriologist. The appointment of a competent staff of inspectors was the next item; and the aim of the Committee will be to put Winnipeg on a good sanitary basis early and systematically. That city does not desire to have any further epidemics of ₁typhoid fever to handle.

The New Alexandra Hospital, Montreal.—The erection of the new English contagious disease hospital, to be called the Alexandra Hospital, is progressing favorably. The buildings will be erected in a thorough fire-proof manner, and as the cost of this has exceeded expectations, the public will be again appealed to for financial support. The site comprises a block of land five hundred feet by three hundred feet and four hundred and fifty feet on another street. There are to be nine separate buildings in the group, while the seven pavilions constituting the hospital proper will be entirely separate. Each pavilion will have its own nursing staff and will be entirely isolated.

Amalgamation of Bishop's and McGill Medical Faculties.—The Medical Faculty of Bishop's College University, Montreal, will soon be amalgamated with the Medical Faculty of McGill University. A conference was held during the past week between the two faculties, and the Faculty of Bishop's, by an independent meeting has resolved to throw in its lot with McGill. Although the terms of amalgamation have not yet been definitely announced, it is understood that McGill has promised to grant the fullest and most generous terms both to the students and Faculty of Bishop's. Bishop's Faculty will be absorbed and the teaching staff will be granted associate positions on the McGill Faculty. The present term at Bishop's will be completed and the arrangements will go into effect for the next session in October.

The Canadian Association for the Prevention of Tuberculosis.—The fifth annual meeting of the Canadian Association for the Prevention of Tuberculosis was held at Ottawa on March 15, the gathering being attended by medical men from various parts of the Dominion of Canada. The annual report of the secretary, the Rev. Dr. Moore, of Ottawa, stated that a large deputation from all parts of the Dominion had waited on the Federal Government, with reference to the establishment of a sanitarium. The Premier had expressed his sympathy with the movement, and later on a resolution had been unanimously adopted by the House of Commons favoring governmental support in combating the disease. One result of this conference was that Dr. P. H. Bryce, chief medical officer for the Department of the Interior, was appointed the convener of a sub-committee, with the object of getting county councils and other public bodies to petition for the establishment of a sanatorium in each province, hoping, of course, for some help from the Dominion Government, and the response to this movement has been very gratifying. Twenty-four petitions have come from British Columbia alone. During the past year there were admitted to the association the British Columbia branch and the Association of Colchester, N. S. Literature was freely distributed to the extent of 785,000 leaves. In the evening, Prof. J. George Adami, of McGill University, delivered a lecture, at which His Excellency the Governor-General presided. The title of the lecture was "Adaptation and Consumption."

GENERAL.

Appointment of Dr. Dearborn.—George V. N. Dearborn, A.M. (Harvard), M.D., Ph.D. (Columbia), has been elected to the Professorship of Physiology in the Tufts College Medical and Dental Schools, Boston. More than six hundred students of both sexes are in attendance at these schools.

The Anti-Tuberculosis Movement in Youngstown and Grand Rapids.—The progress of a tuberculosis movement in Youngstown, Ohio, is described in a recent issue of *Charities*. Still another sign of the activity in this field comes from Grand Rapids, Michigan. After a quiet canvassing of the situation in that city, plans for the organization of an anti-tuberculosis society were laid, and on March 3, Dr. Victor C. Vaughan, of the University of Michigan, delivered by invitation a public address on the disease and the methods of combating it to a large and representative audience. Immediately following his lecture the formal movement was launched, a constitution and by-laws adopted, and about a hundred of the leading citizens of Grand Rapids handed in their names as members of the new society. The dues have been placed at one dollar a year, and new members are being added daily. A second meeting for the election of officers has been called, and the work is being pushed with enthusiasm.

The Dangers of Car Dust.—The popular interest displayed in the subject of car sanitation and car ventilation by the Boards of Health of the larger cities has evoked some criticism of the railroad companies for not giving more attention to a matter of such vital interest to their passengers. The laboratory of the Marine Hospital Service has been investigating this subject for some time. Dr. Walter Wyman, Surgeon-General of the Marine Hospital Service, says: "Just how much danger there is of contagion through vitiated air in the ordinary day coach now in use, or in the Pullman sleeping and palace cars, has not yet been definitely determined, and the matter is still being investigated. Information collected points to the State of Texas as having been the pioneer in this movement, due doubtless to its excellent railroad commission. It is held that there is much danger to the passengers of contracting contagious diseases from the fine dust arising from the carpets and upholstery while the cars are in motion, and which imperfect ventilation compels the passengers to inhale."

The Medical Corps of the United States Navy.—
A candidate for examination and appointment in the Medical Corps of the Navy must be between twenty-one and thirty years of age, and must apply to the Honorable Secretary of the Navy for permission to appear before a Naval Medical Examining Board. The application must be in the handwriting of the applicant, stating age and place of birth; also the place and State of which he is a permanent resident, and must be accompanied by letters or certificates from persons of repúte, testifying from personal knowledge to his good habits and moral character, and that he is a citizen of the United States. Such applications can be obtained by writing to Washington. When a candidate presents himself for examination on the date fixed by the president of the Board, he must bring with him testimonials as to character and professional fitness, diplomas, and a certificate that he is a citizen of the United States. While it is desirable that candidates should be graduates in medicine, such graduation is not essential. The examination usually occupies about nine days, and is conducted in the following order: 1. Physical. 2. Professional. 3. Collateral.

Physical Examination.—The physical examination is thorough, and the candidate is required to certify on oath that he is free from all mental, physical, and constitutional defects. Acuteness of vision, 12-20 for each eye, unaided by glasses, but capable of correction, by aid of lenses, to 20-20, is obligatory. Color perception must be normal and the teeth good. If the candidate is found to be physically disqualified his examination is concluded; if found to be physically qualified his examination is continued as follows: (1) Letter to the Board describing in detail his general and professional education. The professional examination will be in anatomy and physiology; surgery; medicine; pathology and microscopy; obstetrics and medical jurisprudence; materia medica and physiological action of drugs; chemistry and physics; hygiene and quarantine; general aptitude; literary and scientific branches. Seventy-five per cent. is required as a passing mark, 80 per cent. is required in most of the branches. Bandaging, tourniquets; four operations on cadaver; clinical cases (a written report being made in one case giving history, diagnosis, prognosis, treatment, one prescription, at least, being written out in full, in Latin) urinalysis (chemical and microscopical examination of one specimen of urine); practical microscopy, and recognition of five mounted specimens (histological, pathological, and bacteriological); recognition of surgical instruments. An oral examination follows the written work in each branch, and the required percentage is made up from the combined results of the written and oral examinations. The percentages given are not absolute, however, as losses in some branches may be made good in others, provided the standard is reached in the cardinal subjects of anatomy, physiology, medicine and surgery. The collateral examination embraces spelling, punctuation, the use of capital letters, grammar, arithmetic, geography (descriptive and physical), languages, history, general literature, elementary botany, geology and zoology. While due credit is given for a knowledge of languages and the sciences it is not essential except in the case of physics. A knowledge of the common school branches is essential, and deficiency in this respect will cause rejection even though passing marks may be gained in professional subjects. The Boards are required, under oath, to report on the physical, mental, moral, and professional qualifications of the candidate, so that the examinations are necessarily rigid and comprehensive, though simple and practical, and not beyond the attainments of any well educated physician. The oral and written questions are similar to those asked by the best medical colleges in examinations for graduation. A successful candidate, upon completion of his examination, will be notified by the president of the Board that he has been found qualified. With the consent of the Board, a candidate may withdraw at any period from further examination, and may at a future time present himself for reexamination. The Board may conclude the examination (written, oral and practical) at any time, and may deviate from this general plan as it may deem best for the interests of the naval service. The tenure of office in the Medical Corps of the Navy is for life, unless sooner terminated by removal, resignation, disability, or other casualty. No allowance will be made for the expenses of persons undergoing examination. All successful candidates will receive appointments as soon as qualified, and in the order of merit reported by the Board. The Officers of the Medical Corps of the Navy are as follows: Medical directors, medical inspectors, surgeons, passed assistant surgeons, and assistant surgeons. Vacancies in these grades (by death, or retirement at the age of 62 years) are filled in the order of seniority, and for each promotion a physical and a professional examination is required by law. Assistant surgeons are examined at the expiration of three years' service for promotion, and if successful become passed assistant surgeons. Through the provisions of a law enacted by the Fifty-seventh Congress, the Medical Corps of the Navy was increased 150 numbers; 25 to be appointed each calendar year for six years. The number of vacancies occurring through retirements, resignations, and casualties average about 10 a year. There are afforded, therefore, for candidates for the position of assistant surgeon about 35 appointments each year for the next six years.

The pay table is as follows:

	At Sea.	On Shore.	Allowances Per annum.
Assistant Surgeons, rank of Lieutenant (junior grade)............	$1,760.00	$1,496.00	$288.00
Passed Assistant Surgeons, rank of Lieutenant	2,200.00	1,870.00	432.00
After five years in the service...	2,400.00	2,040.00	432.00
After ten years in the service...	2,600.00	2,210.00	432.00
Surgeons, rank of Lieutenant Commander—			
After ten years in the service...	3,250.00	2,762.50	576.00
After fifteen years in the service.	3,500.00	2,975.00	576.00
Medical Inspectors, rank of Commander—			
After fifteen years in the service.	4,000.00	3,400.00	576.00
Medical Directors, rank of Captain—			
After fifteen years in the service.	4,500.00	3,825.00	720.00
Surgeon General, rank of Rear Admiral	5,500.00	5,500.00	720.00

Manuel Garcia Celebration.—Professor Manuel Garcia's hundredth birthday was celebrated in London last Friday by the presentation of a portrait and a banquet. The presentation took place at noon at the rooms of the London Laryngological Society, in the presence of representatives of kings and emperors, delegates of the world's greatest scientific and musical bodies, and some of the most notable personages of the age. Sir Felix Semon, C.V.O., chairman of the Garcia Committee, presided. Seated in a big arm chair on a platform the veteran musician and inventor of the laryngoscope, Professor Garcia, wearing his newly conferred orders, listened with evident pleasurable attention to the reading of addresses and telegrams from all parts of the globe. King Edward had made him Honorable Commander of the Royal Victorian Order. Emperor William had sent him by Professor Fraenkel the greatest distinction conferred in Germany, namely, a large gold medal for science, and his own sovereign, the King of Spain, had invested him with the Royal Order of Alfonso, at the same time congratulating him through his Charge d'Affaires, the Marquis de Villalobar, on behalf of himself and all his subjects. Professor Fraenkel, in a message from the Berlin Laryngological Society, congratulated the master on his entry into "the second century of his immortality." From noon until one o'clock messages and addresses were read in turn by representatives of the Royal Society of London, the Prussian Academy of Science, the Universities of Heidelberg, Königsberg and Manchester, numerous laryngological societies all over the world and the New York Academy of Medicine. In the address of the latter Dr. Harmon Smith, referring to Professor Garcia's invention of the laryngoscope, said that in New York alone fully thirty institutions relieved the suffering needs of countless thousands and that New York joined with all the world in testifying to the mighty debt which it owed to Professor Garcia, to whom it offered a tribute of its love, its gratitude and its praise. Sir Felix Semon, after reading out the telegrams of congratulation, made one remark which evoked immense applause. It was to the effect that, notwithstanding the disastrous war which was now raging between two countries, each of those said countries had taken good care to send messages of congratulation to Professor Garcia. The centenary committee then came forward and presented to Señor Garcia a portrait of himself by Mr. John S. Sargent, R. A., subscribed for by international contributions of numerous friends and admirers. Sir Felix Semon pulled aside a curtain and disclosed to view the Royal Academician's portrait, which represents Professor Garcia seated and half turned toward the right. At a banquet, which was held in the Hotel Cecil in the evening, Mr. Charters J. Symonds presided over a distinguished gathering of more than four hundred ladies and gentlemen. The menu was an elaborate and artistic production, bound with ribbons of the Spanish colors, a Spanish flag surmounting two photographs of Garcia, one of him taken a day or two ago, the other showing him as he was at the time of the invention of the laryngoscope. The chairman, in proposing the toast of the King, said that he had sitting on his right Lord Suffield, whom King Edward had sent to represent him on this occasion, a tribute from His Majesty which was greater than any of them had expected, for Lord Suffield was not one of the King's younger staff, but one with whom he had long had intimate acquaintance. The toast having been pledged, Mr. Symonds remained standing. He said his reason for doing so was that he wished to propose the health of two other sovereigns who had done honor to Professor Garcia, namely, the King of Spain and Emperor William of Germany.

He called upon the Marquis de Villalobar to read a telegram which had just been received from the King of Spain, which contained the heartiest con-

gratulations and best wishes to the "grand old Spaniard, who, by his invention, had glorified and exalted the Kingdom of Spain." Great cheering greeted the reading of this telegram, and the chairman then went on to say he believed the honor which the King of Spain had conferred on Señor Garcia carried with it the title of "His Excellency." Therefore, they would be able to address him in the future as "Your Excellency, Señor Garcia," a remark which again evoked enthusiastic cheering. Sir Felix Semon next rose and proposed the toast of the evening, that of the health of Señor Garcia, which he began by reverently addressing the centenarian as "My great and revered master." "It was," he said, "a solemn and most inspiring occasion upon which they were met to do honor to a many of eminence, a man who was born when the might of Napoleon was at its height, and who at the age of one hundred still retained all his mental and physical faculties, a blessing given to few. It was remarkable, also, that two professions, which had little or no points of contact, should be met to lay tribute at the feet of this great centenarian. He came of a family which would be indissolubly connected with music as long as there was any history of music, a family which had done inestimable work in the noble art of music, and Señor Garcia had, as a teacher of many distinguished singers, engraved his name forever on the roll of music teachers. He had created a school of singers who would ever cultivate the methods he had founded. But he had even greater claims upon the gratitude of mankind by his great invention of the laryngoscope, and that was why so many eminent members of the medical profession and of surgery were present on that occasion to lay a tribute of gratitude and congratulation at his feet." .

Señor Garcia, who was received with most enthusiastic cheers, was visibly moved, and after reading a few words of a speech in a trembling voice left the chairman to complete it, but the chairman apologized, saying that it was impossible for him to give these words such expression as had already come from the soul of the great centenarian. Sixteen societies, said Señor Garcia, called him "Father." "How," he asked, "could they expect him to find words to express his gratitude and to answer so many voices which called him 'Father.'" He asked those assembled "to try and think themselves one hundred years old—not the leaders, for they would never look it; they would never know it and no one would ever believe it—but the men might try, and he was sure that if they tried to answer these clamorous voices to which he had alluded they would say nought." Señor Garcia's little speech was greeted with prolonged cheering, which was renewed when he rose to leave. In fact, the scene of enthusiasm was almost indescribable. Professor Garcia, who was born in Madrid, Spain, March 17, 1805, was the son of Manuel Garcia, a famous Spanish tenor. His sister, Mme. Malibran, a celebrated opera singer, accompanied Señor Garcia to the United States in 1825, and later sang with great success in Paris, London and other cities. Mme. Viardot-Garcia, a younger sister of Professor Garcia, was also a celebrated singer. She married the late Louis Viardot, Director of the Paris Italian Opera, and retired from the stage in 1862.

Patent Medicine Advertisements Forbidden.—A new law forbids the publication in Norwegian newspapers of advertisements to further the sale of any and all foreign patent medicines.

Medicine in England.—Sir James Paget has followed up the lives of 1,000 medical students who had joined the medical school of St. Bartholomew's Hospital, with the following result: 23 met with distinguished success, 66 met with considerable success, 507 met with fair success, 124 met with very limited success, 56 failed, 96 discontinued medical studies while in pupilage, 41 died during pupilage, and 87 died within twelve years of commencing practice.

SPECIAL ARTICLE.

BYWAYS OF MEDICAL LITERATURE.—XXIV.

THE INCREASE OF QUACKERY.

From the information available gleaned from public and private sources, says an editorial writer in the February *Medical Magazine*, it would seem as though the practice of quackery was never so rife in England as at the present time. The country, and London in particular, is swarming with charlatans. There is hardly any disease, or class of diseases, which is left unexploited by this locust brood, and the cures range from faith healing and black magic to comparatively innocuous decoctions of "herbs." Of course the quacks could not flourish unless they were patronized by the public, and notwithstanding the advance of education and scientific education, the British public at the present day is quite as credulous in this respect as in the days of Queen Anne. To take an instance of the sort of stuff people will believe, one may turn to a recent number of the *Onlooker* in which a special article is devoted to the laudation of "a New Science." This new "Science" is called "Osteopathy." It is of American importation and gives the name and address of the practitioner who has come over from America because the American residents here "refused to be in London without him." Now what is this new "Science?" It is that "all pain and all disease come from pressure—pressure in the nerves or on the blood vessels by the dense tissues of the body, thereby obstructing the proper circulation of the blood and transmission of nerve force. Therefore the first thing an osteopathist does is to find out whether in the whole body there is the tiniest part dislocated or out of place, any muscle contracted, or blood-vessel pressed upon. To do this, he does not at first attend to the part of the body which is affected—he knows that the trouble will set up a corresponding irritation in the governing nerve centers of the spinal column. He therefore feels with educated fingers down the thirty-one nerve centers which are there, until he comes to the one which is functually deranged; and then, having localized the evil, he follows the course of the nerve till he comes to the place where the obstruction is, when he at once sets to work to remove it and set the blood freely circulating again. He treats successfully many of the dread complaints to which humanity is liable, some of which have been hitherto regarded as almost, if not quite, incurable, such as spinal curvature, incipient consumption, Bright's disease, diabetes, asthma, goiter, locomotor ataxia and paralysis." When one reads this paragraph one wonders how any man alive could pen such insane jargon; how the imagination of any one could run to such a grave excess of riot, so to speak. But underneath all this there is, to the lay individual, a ring of simplicity and effectiveness about the whole thing, and no doubt the particular exponent of this balderdash will attract numerous clients and extort handsome fees. London,

in particular, as has been said, is honeycombed to-day with these miscreants. In older days, before the dawn, of exact science, a large number of the so-called quacks were in reality honest men, who believed themselves possessed of special powers, and at that time nearly all practitioners dabbled in secret nostrums of their own, but at the present time the honest quack is practically non-existent, because, however small the smattering of science which he possesses, it is sufficient to enlighten him as to his ignorance.

SOME QUACKS OF BYGONE DAYS.

It may be of interest to quote some remarks from, a lecture delivered by Dr. Packard, of Philadelphia, to the Johns Hopkins Hospital Historical Club, on some of the most famous quacks of bygone times. He remarks that during the period of the Restoration especially, submission to the royal touch as a cure became very popular as a manifestation of loyalty. Another circumstance which contributed to maintain the royal touch in popular estimation was the fact that it was always accompanied by the gift of a gold piece to the patient from his sovereign. These were known as "touchpieces." It is interesting in this connection to recall that Dr. Samuel Johnson, the great lexicographer, was among those touched for this complaint by Queen Anne, the last of England's royalties to attempt the exercise of this healing faculty.

VALENTINE GREATRAKES.

In twenty-two years a careful list was kept of those of his subjects whom Charles II. touched for King's Evil, and their number amounted to over 92,000. There were, however, other claimants to the healing touch besides those of royal birth, among whom Valentine Greatrakes achieved a remarkable fame. He was born in County Waterford in the reign of Charles I., and, after an ordinary school education entered Trinity College, Dublin, from which place he did not graduate, as, owing to the Rebellion, his mother fled from Ireland, into England, where he lived in Devonshire and studied theology and philosophy under a German minister, the Reverend John Daniel Getsius. About the year 1624 he returned to Ireland. He was possessed of property, and was evidently held in some esteem for he became a justice of the peace and registrar for plantations.

How this quiet, contemplative, well-to-do country gentleman ever became possessed with the idea that he was gifted with the ability to heal disease by the touch of his hand will never be known. In 1662, however, he claimed to have discovered his supernatural gift, although for some time it appears he kept his virtue to himself, but at last, like the good man that he was, told his wife, who unkindly laughed at him. Nothing daunted, however, he began laying his hands upon various people in the neighborhood who suffered from scrofula or other diseases, and is said to have cured' very many of them. These doings made such a noise, however, that they came to the ears of the authorities, and the Bishop's Court at Lismore prohibited him from laying on hands in the future. He seems to have disobeyed the court's injunctions. As is the case with so, many quacks, he soon found titled victims. In January, 1665-66, the Earl of Orrery brought him over to England in order that he might lay his hands upon the wife of Lord Conway, who suffered from chronic headaches. Although he was unsuccessful with this patient, he, nevertheless, seems to have performed cures in a number of persons that lived in her neighborhood, so much so that an account of his cures in Warwickshire was. published by a Mr. Stubbe in which he stated "that

Mr. Greatrakes was possessed of some peculiar temperament, as his body was composed of some particular ferments, the effluvia whereof being introduced, sometimes by a light, sometimes by a violent friction, restore the temperament of the debilitated parts, regenerate the blood, and dissipate the heterogeneous ferments out of the bodies of the diseased, by the eyes, nose, mouth, hands and feet." Stubbe's account was written in the form of a letter to the famous Robert Boyle, Esq. The latter was extremely put out at being made party to what he was at first disposed to regard as the performances of a quack, but *mirabile dictu,* after witnessing some eight laying on of hands, even the great Boyle succumbed, and publicly announced that he could vouch for some of the wonderful results achieved by the healer. This English visit marked the climax of Greatrake's career. He made large sums of money, but within a few years his fame declined as rapidly as it had risen, and he died in obscurity. Queen Anne's poor eyesight rendered her a godsend to quack ophthalmologists. Two of these rascals the queen especially delighted to honor. One was a tailor named William Reade whom she knighted. The other was a shoemaker named Roger Grant. He was made oculist to the queen by special appointment. The champion quack ophthalmologist of the eighteenth century, however, was undoubtedly the Chevalier John Taylor. Dr. Brown Pusey, of Chicago, has recently published an account of his career founded upon his biography, which was published in London in 1761, with the following title: "The Life and Extraordinary History of the Chevalier, John Taylor, Ophthalmiator, Pontifical, Imperial and Royal; in two volumes; written from authentic materials and published by his son, John Taylor, Oculist; London, 1761." Dr. Pusey truly says, "in comparison with him the quacks of the present day are a cheap lot.' Dr. Pusey gives extracts from the hand-bills which it was his wont to distribute, and their glowing eloquence puts to shame all modern imitators. In the course of his book he narrated the tremendous distances he had traveled and the vast experience he had had. He was appointed Ophthalmiator Pontifical by Pope Benedict XIV., and was appointed oculist to George II., King of England; Augustus III., King of Poland; Frederick V., King of Denmark and Norway, and Frederick Adolphus, King of Sweden. As Dr. Pusey says, one of his important cases was in the person of a man who seems nearer to us than all these high personages, namely Händel, of whom he says, "I once thought to have had the same succes, having all circumstances in his favor, motions of the pupil, light, etc., but on drawing the curtain, we found the bottom defective."

AN EARLY SECRET REMEDY.

In a different category we must place Dr. Jonathan Goddard, the originator of "Goddard's Drops." We seldom realize nowadays when we prescribe aromatic spirits of ammonia that they were originally famous as a secret preparation known by the name of "Goddard's Drops." They were originated by Dr. Jonathan Goddard, a Fellow of the Royal Society, and Professor of Medicine in Gresham College. Dr. Goddard had a large practice, and was a professional adviser as well as an intimate friend of Oliver Cromwell. He had a laboratory in Gresham College, in which he manufactured various medicinal preparations, of which the drops became the most famous. He for some time kept their manufacture a secret, and sold them through apothecaries, but as this was contrary to his oath to the College of Physicians, he was obliged to reveal his secret to them, but only did so upon their promise that

the recipe should not be published until after his death. They were at first known as spiritus salis volatalis oleosus, or sal volatile drops. In "Doctors and Doctors," by Graham Everitt, there is a quotation from the Sloane MSS. 958, in which there is an entry, in a memorandum book, in the handwriting of John Coniers, an apothecary of Shoe Lane, which reads as follows:
"March 24, 1674-5. About ten o'clock that night my very good friend, Dr. Jonathan Goddard, reader of the physic lectures at Gresham College, suddenly fell down dead in the street, as he was entering a coach. He was a pretty corpulent and tall man, a bachelor between forty-five and fifty years of age; he was melancholy, inclined to be cynical, and used now and then to complain of giddiness in his head. He was an excellent mathematician, and some time physician to Oliver the Protector."

SPOT WARD.

Another substance which is now in general use, but of which the nature was at first kept secret by its inventor, is oil of vitriol or oil of sulphur. Joshua Ward, its discoverer, derived his nickname "Spot" Ward from a facial blemish. He was originally a chemist, and in the course of his work discovered a method of making oil of sulphur by the combustion of sulphur with saltpeter, the resulting compound being so cheap in its manufacture that it soon completely supplanted the real oil of vitriol in the market. Ward was a thoroughgoing quack, and employed every precaution to prevent the discovery of the nature of the substance which he used. He was a large, fat man, and used to drive around in a magnificent chariot drawn by four horses. He was high in the favor of George II., who provided him with a sort of dispensary and office in White Hall, at which he attended the poor and gave them his medicines for nothing at the expense of the king. Upon one occasion, when he had been paying a professional visit to his majesty, he turned his back on the king on leaving the room and started for the door. A court officer stepped forward and reminded him in a whisper that he should not turn his back on the king, to which he replied in a loud voice, "The king's seeing of my back is a matter of no consequence, but the breaking of my neck falling backwards is of consequence not only to him but to the poor."

Lady Mary W. Montague refers to Ward's preparation in a letter of 1748, and adds to it one of her usual keen reflections. "I find," she says, "that tar-water has succeeded to Ward's drops; and it is possible that some other form of quackery has by this time taken place of that. The English are, more than any other nation, infatuated with the prospect of universal medicine."

JOHN ST. JOHN LONG.

John St. John Long deserves to be ranked among the most successful quacks of all time. From his practice he is said to have derived an income of over £13,000 a year, and unfortunately for him, death terminated his career at a time when many victims cherished a belief that he was the greatest of healers. He was the son of a poor Irish peasant, and passed his youth in the village of Doneraile. He was possessed of a natural talent for drawing and painting, and after passing a short time in Dublin in the cultivation of these gifts, he established himself as an artist in Limerick. Here he painted portraits and gave instructions in painting and drawing to such pupils as he could procure. Finding the village of Limerick somewhat limited as a sphere for his activity, Long migrated to London where he worked for some time in the studio of Sir Thomas Lawrence. During this time he turned a few honest shillings by making anatomical drawings and paintings for the professors in the London medical schools. In the course of his work he picked up some crumbs of medical knowledge, and soon announced that he had discovered a wonderful liniment, by means of which he was not only able to cure most diseases, but also to discover the existence of latent disease in various organs. If, for example, this substance were applied over the chest of any person if they were healthy, and if there was no phthisical or other affection of the lungs, the application would be absolutely void of result. If, however, the lungs were in any way diseased, the substance would produce a counter-irritation resulting in the formation of a weeping sore. The acrid substance which flowed from this Long said was the essence of the disease. His enemies claimed that he used two distinct fluids to effect this wonderful result, one a bland and innoxious substance, the other a blistering liquid, which originally bore the name of St. John Long's liniment.

He also had a remedy in the form of vapor which was to be inhaled. For this purpose his patients would seat themselves around a large cabinet from which radiated a number of stems through which they inhaled the vapor. Long fitted up magnificent offices in a mansion in Harley street, and here the aristocracy flocked in swarms to inhale and to be rubbed. The list of Long's patients reads like a directory to the fashionable quarter of London.' But not only was he patronized by the citizens of the metropolis, but the sick and the foolish flocked from every quarter of the United Kingdom. The contemporary accounts of some of the scenes in Long's offices, whether written by his friends or his enemies, are most amusing. It was only possible for him to see patients for a few moments, and he would turn them over to one of his assistants, or else send them into the inhalation room to join the other patients sucking the miraculous vapor through Long's tubes.

One way in which he enormously increased his practice was to persuade healthy persons that he saw indications of latent disease within their systems, which could be demonstrated by an application of his wonderful liniment. As most of his patients were accompanied by various female relatives and friends on their visits to his office it was very easy for Long to cast his net about the healthy while bestowing his professioual attentions upon the sick. This trick, however, did not always pay as the sequel will show.

On Saturday, October 30, 1830, Long was brought to trial at the Old Bailey, charged with manslaughter in occasioning the death of Catherine Cashin. He pleaded not guilty to the indictment. The facts elicited at his trial were as follows:

"Miss Catherine Cashin was a young lady of good family in Ireland who had brought her younger sister up to London to be treated for phthisis. The elder sister, at the time of her arrival in London, was in perfect health. She had taken her sister a few times to Long's house, when the quack announced that he had discovered signs in her of latent consumption, and that if she did not put herself promptly under his care she would develop the disease within two months. This frightened the young woman to such an extent that she agreed to place herself in his hands. Accordingly, on August 3 she went to his offices and was rubbed with the famous liniment between her shoulders and on her back. Within a short time the parts began to ulcerate and become gangrenous and she died

on the 17th of the month. Before her death Mr., afterward Sir Benjamin Brodie, was called in, and at the trial he gave it as his opinion that her death was the result of the mortified sore upon her back. At the autopsy there was no evidence of any disease of the organs, save the large sloughing sore between the woman's shoulders. The woman employee of Long, who performed the actual rubbing on Miss Cashin's back, testified that she had rubbed the woman with the same lotion that had been used on a number of other persons, among them the Marchioness of Ormonde and Lady Harriet Butler. The wound was dressed with a cabbage leaf, and treated in a precisely similar manner to that of the other patients. A number of witnesses were called in behalf of the prisoner, among them some of the best known people and of the very highest social standing in London. The judge's charge was strongly in favor of the prisoner, though the jury found him guilty. His punishment, however, was not excessive, as he was fined only £250, which sum he pulled from his pocket in the courtroom." The account of the trial concludes, "having quitted the bar, he proceeded to the courtyard in company with his friends, where they got into a curricle of the Marquis of Sligo and rode off with his lordship amidst the clapping of his noble friends, and the hootings and hissing and laughter of the populace."

On November 10, 1830, Long was again brought before a coroner's jury, accused of manslaughter in having caused the death of Mrs. Colin Campbell Lloyd, the wife of a captain in the navy. Her medical attendant and surgeon, named George Vance, stated that he had been called in to see Mrs. Lloyd, and found her suffering from a large sloughing sore, covering practically the entire front of her thorax, and extending down so far that the sternum was found bare. She stated that she had been rubbed twice at St. John Long's house with his liniment. Mr. Brodie, who saw her, stated that the appearance of the sore was exactly similar to that which he had found on the back of Miss Cashin. Another surgeon, a Mr. Campbell, testified that he had seen Mrs. Lloyd some days before she had consulted Dr. Long, and that she had been in perfect health. She had visited the quack with a view to procuring relief from a slight throat affection. After examining her, Long had informed her that the throat trouble arose from extensive disease of the lungs, they being full of small ulcers, and recommended his inhalation treatment in addition to applications of his liniment to her chest. Her husband likewise testified that she had been in perfectly good health until after the rubbings at Long's. At the autopsy all Mrs. Lloyd's organs were perfectly normal, and the body showed no signs of disease, with the exception of the enormous sloughing sores over the chest and upper part of the abdomen. The jury found that the deceased had come to her death as the result of the application of a liniment to her chest by Dr. Long. When brought to the trial at the Old Bailey on the charge of having killed Mrs. Lloyd, the jury acquitted him.

In spite of all the expositions of Long's quackery, which were published not only in the medical but in the lay press, he continued to be upheld by a large and influential *clientèle*. His career was terminated at the early age of thirty-seven by phthisis pulmonalis, the very disease to which he had laid his most extravagant claims to cure. At his death it was found that, as a result of his nefarious practice, he had accumulated a snug fortune, which he left to his widow in Ireland. He was buried in Kensal Green Cemetery, and over his grave some of his admirers erected an elegant monument.

If in the twentieth century we are not blessed with quacks as simple as Valentine Greatrakes or as dangerous as St. John Long, it is solely due to the general advance of knowledge, for the quack in all ages accommodates himself to the prevailing tendencies of the time. Touching for king's evil would not pay nowadays, nor would the production of festering sores in order to extract the acrid humors' of the blood. The modern quack dabbles in electricity, massage, hypnotism, etc., all methods of cure which have been legitimately or honestly introduced as aids to the healing art. There is nothing in the law, as it stands, to prevent the practice of quackery in any form whatsoever; this is a "free" country, and people may practise without let or hindrance. A tremendous fraud and robbery are being perpetrated on the public. The Government approves of it, the medical profession is apathetic and perhaps powerless; so that at present there seems little chance of effective redress for many a long year to come.

EUGENE SUE AND MEDICINE.

Last December saw the centenary of Eugene Sue, known more particularly as the author of "The Mysteries of Paris" and "The Wandering Jew." The Sues, however, were doctors from father to son, and were all writers of many books. The first of the line published his "Human Anatomy, with Plates," in 1748. His elder son, Pierre, succeeded him as "surgeon of the city of Paris" in 1762, and stuck prudently to his medical last all through the Revolution, turning out dictionaries of surgery, whole books of anecdotes of medicine, post-mortem eulogies of physicians, until his death under the restored Bourbons in 1816. The younger son, Jean Joseph, who was to be father of Eugene, was an army surgeon, and served, like other men of his time, republic and empire and monarchy in turn. He went unharmed through the cruel Russian campaign of Napoleon, and, when the Bourbons came back, became physician of the king's military household. His books —for he, too, wrote many—all had a picturesque and impressionist quality; an example is his treatise on "the pain which follows (not accompanies) beheading by the guillotine!"

Coming from such a stock Eugene Sue properly became a romancer, but not until he had served a varied apprenticeship at the family trade. In his twentieth year, before his medical studies were completed, Eugene Sue was off as ambulance aid on the Spanish campaign of 1823, which was rather an expedition than a war. Then for six years he sailed as ship surgeon to the four quarters of the globe, with very wide-open eyes, as the reality of his descriptions in his outlandish tales show advantageously in comparison with other romancers. In 1827 he came in for sure-enough smells of gunpowder in the attack of the combined French, English and Russian fleets on Turks and Egyptians off the coast of Greece at Navarin.

Eugene Sue was barely twenty-six when he returned to Paris and quit the service of the State. The writing demon already possessed him, and the next year, 1830, he published his first sea novel, "Kenok, the Pirate." The same year his father died, and he came into a fortune which, at that time, was considered enormous, even by men of lofty ideas like Balzac; it was estimated as high as a million of francs! A new revolution came opportunely, and the rich young Sue had his social prominence enhanced by the fact that he had once been attached to the staff of the son of the expelled King Charles X. He drove English fashion along the Boulevard to the admiration of the young generation

of "dandies" like Alfred de Musset, who found their gospel of life in Byron. .

For five years Eugene Sue turned out his sea stories. They were rattling good so far as the telling went, though often better fitted in detail to the forecastle than to a lady's boudoir. Whatever may be said of his lack of syle, he had the talent of choosing proper names that strike and remain in the memory—" Plick and Plock," " Atar-Gull," " Coucaracha." The name of the house porter Pipelet in his " Mysteries of Paris" has passed into the French language as the nickname of concierge. This period of his writing he finished up with a five-volume octavo history of the French navy under Louis XIV.

As an interlude to this breathless existence of life and literature, such as it was, there is a medical story worth recalling, if only for the dubious light it throws on certain recent revivals. Eugene Sue's first cousin, the son of the musician Langlé, like himself, had begun the study of medicine. He caught a severe cold, which was followed by cough and hemorrhages and fits of suffocation. The other young doctors watched with him, and one set to work to bleed him—a sovereign remedy for congestion in those days. Relief followed, but after quarter of an hour the fits came back worse than ever. The young doctor bled the patient again and yet again, and like results to the eighth time! The results were satisfactory each time, but did not endure. The young men held a consultation, but could not agree. Finally, the same one who had previously operated established a record by a ninth bleeding, which fortunately was successful. It must be added that the young operator shortly abandoned the healing art. He says: "I saw that the nephew of Baron Sue was a vigorous subject!" This amazing doctor became the famous director of the Opera Veron, who. did so much for modern pre-Wagner music, from Cherubini, Auber, Halévy and Meyerbeer to Rossini. As to Langlé, he, too, gave up medicine after experiencing such heroic practice of it. With the devouring activity of the Sue family, he succeeded in three other professions—as playwright, singer and undertaker!

SOCIETY PROCEEDINGS.

PHILADELPHIA COUNTY MEDICAL SOCIETY.

Stated Meeting, held November 23, 1904.

The President, Roland G. Curtin, M.D., in the Chair.

Skiagraph of an Old Ununited Fracture of the Scaphoid Bone.—Dr. L. J. Hammond reported the following case: A young medical student had consulted him for a condition of pain in his right wrist, from which he had been suffering for more than two years. There was no tenderness to touch nor any visible signs of inflammation, and it was only when the wrist was abducted that the pain was intense. The condition had been variously diagnosed as rheumatism, sprain, tuberculous periostitis, and tenities. Treatment for these various conditions had given no relief. The X-ray revealed a fracture of the scaphoid bone, the fragments of which were united by a very loose fibrous connection. The interposed fibrous tissue was removed and the fragments of bone wired together. Perfect apposition of the fragments was secured, and they were held together by two small silver wire sutures. There was perfect restoration of all the wrist movements, with entire absence of pain.

An interesting point was the fact that, while the

patient recalled having fallen with the hand out-stretched and abducted, no immediate symptoms of pain, swelling or ecchymosis were sufficiently pronounced to demand surgical aid. Dr. Hammond said that experience in the surgical out-patients' department of city hospitals showed the frequency of fractures of the bones of the wrist and ankle-joints without recognition. The only treatment, he said, was to secure bony union, which could only be done by securing perfect apposition, either by wiring or any other of the mechanical means for this purpose. Dr. Hammond believed wiring to be by far the most reliable procedure.

Dr. Charles Lester Leonard referred to the obscure character of these fractures, which could be demonstrated in no other way than by the X-ray. This means of diagnosis was particularly valuable in the slight injuries occurring about the joint, the sprains, fractures and chipping of small fragments within the joint, which lead to incapacity of function so important to those depending upon their hands as a means of livelihood. He believes it the duty of the surgeon in injuries about the joints to have X-ray examinations made for the purpose of excluding these fractures, for a negative diagnosis is of much value to the patient in a saving of time and in the immediate institution of the proper treatment.

Typhoid Fever in Philadelphia.—Dr. Randolph Faries, in the consideration of this subject, said that typhoid fever does not exist in Philadelphia in such alarming numbers as the general public is given to believe. The apparently large proportion of the disease in this city he attributed to three conditions: Errors in diagnosis, cases contracted elsewhere, and duplicate cases. He enumerated sixteen diseases which may be mistaken for typhoid fever. No case should be reported to the Board of Health as typhoid fever unless a Widal reaction has been taken, and, in addition, the urine, feces, and catarrhal secretions examined. Especial care should be taken in examining the liver and spleen, in noting the course of the temperature, the nature of the pulse, the amount and kind of stupor, as well as the nervous symptoms present. Stress should be laid upon the blood spots and a blood count should be made. Dr. Faries believes that, with the municipal improvements of cleaner streets, better surface drainage and perfect under drainage, the abolition of cesspools, houses constructed with better scientific ventilation, careful disinfection of everything whereby typhoid may be transmitted, extreme vigilance on the part of the health authorities in reference to impure milk, adulterated foods, impure water, and a constant instruction to the general public in reference to those foods by which typhoid is often contracted, such as raw oysters, lettuce, overripe and unclean fruit, etc., it is reasonable to suppose there will come a time when a very few cases of typhoid fever, if any, will exist in Philadelphia.

Dr. Edward Martin observed that statistics showed a certain amount of transference of typhoid fever from one case to another, and that the reason for reporting the cases, so far as the public health is concerned, is to prevent this direct transference and to take precautions against a local epidemic. In most of the cases of typhoid in the well-to-do, the community is properly protected; but among the cases seen by the corps of assistants to the Bureau of Health, the importance of a report is very great. The Bureau would rather have a report of a case

which is not typhoid and look it up, than to have the case unreported and a possible spread of the contagion. The question of the disinfection of the dejecta he regards as a difficult one to overcome, and thinks we should not be indifferent to the people who get water below our pollutions. In the walking cases the urinary secretions may remain for a week a prolific source of infection. The Bureau of Health has made a statistical study of wells and cesspools and have been astonished to find upward of one hundred in such juxtaposition that the water must be infected. He regards the water supply as the main source of infection, and feels that Philadelphia will still be a typhoid-cursed city until it has a filtered water supply.

Dr. Faires, in closing the discussion, said that many of the cases were reported too quickly, but that the remedy was difficult, since the assistant inspectors of the health department were not allowed to interfere with the family physician. It was, therefore, manifestly the duty of the family physician to be especially careful in his diagnosis. While it is possible to ascertain the exact number of cases outside of the city, and the duplicate cases, it was not possible to estimate those cases of error in diagnosis.

Case of Trachoma Successfully Treated with the X-ray.—Drs. W. S. Newcomet and J. P. Krall reported this case and exhibited the patient, a girl of eighteen years. She had been subjected to all the operations for the cure of the condition, but without success. Treatment was begun in July, 1903, and continued until the first of the year. The inflammatory reaction was so intense that it was thought better to abandon the treatment. Later, however, it was found that she could count fingers at close range. The cornea of the eye was entirely clear and only with special illumination could there be seen fine blood vessels. The eye not treated with the X-ray showed all the symptoms that the treated eye formerly exhibited. The condition of the patient had been present since infancy, and she had been unable to see across the room. Treatment was given every other day for five minutes for about six weeks when the burn developed and treatment was withheld. The result, Dr. Newcomet believed, was due to the accidental burn produced in the course of treatment.

Dr. Jay F. Schamberg referred to a case of trachoma seen in the Polyclinic Hospital, less pronounced than the case exhibited, in the vascular injection of the cornea, but having a tremendous growth of vegetative excrescences uopn the conjunctivæ. The man had received about twenty treatments. The growths have almost entirely disappeared in both eyes and the conjunctivæ were fast approaching a normal condition. In technic, the eye was exposed by means of a clamp, the upper lid was everted and the clamps held by weights.

Dr. George E. Pfahler referred to the paper of Dr. Mayo, of London, and his results in treatment of trachoma by the X-ray, and especially to the value of the method in clearing up the cornea. He did not understand that any burns had been produced in the case of Dr. Mayo. The face at first was covered with a mask, but later no precautions were taken. The tube, a soft one, was placed at about nine inches from the patient, and the treatments were from three to five minutes in length. Personally, Dr. Pfahler had had no experience with the method.

Dr. Charles Lester Leonard regarded the case of much interest, both from the aspect of the ophthalmologist and from that of the X-ray worker. The condition still present in one eye, which had been symptomatically cured in the other, he thought showed a marked illustration of the possibilities of the X-ray in chronic conditions about the eye. The value of the method, he believes, depends not upon the production of a burn, but upon a specific action of the X-ray upon the autolytic ferments contained within the cells themselves. The X-ray, he stated, is not a cure-all, but an agency which assists nature by stimulating to action the self-contained elements within the cells.

Dr. M. K. Kassabian agreed with Dr. Leonard regarding the stimulating and irritating action of the X-rays upon the tissues, but believed further that there was a germicidal or inhibitory action upon the germ. In technic, he covers the Crookes' tubes with a dark cloth and darkens the room—preventing injury to the patient from the light because of the excessive photophobia. He attaches the everted eyelids by adhesive plaster to the forehead. He had four cases in the Philadelphia Hospital, two acute and two chronic. The acute cases had severe photophobia and lacrimation and were improved after four or five exposures.

Dr. Newcomet, in closing, said that he had been impressed, when in London, with what might be called the carelessness with which the cases there were treated; one-half of the men used little or no protection in the treatment, and one man used only wet gauze. In the treatment Dr. Newcomet uses a shield, and as much as possible avoids handling the cases.

Stated Meeting, held December 14, 1904.

The President, Roland G. Curtin, M.D., in the Chair.

Differential Diagnosis and Treatment of Acute Pelvic Peritonitis Associated with Gonorrheal Salpingitis.—Dr. Brooke M. Anspach in this paper drew attention to the fact that while acute pelvic peritonitis of gonorrheal origin is best treated expectantly during the acute stage, it occasionally bears a close resemblance to acute appendicitis in which the expectant plan of treatment would be dangerous. The diagnosis is based largely upon the mode of onset, the history of the patient, and the presence of gonorrhea. Bimanual palpation in an initial attack of acute pelvic peritonitis due to the gonococcus must be and is often negative. This obtains because of rigidity of the abdominal walls, and the slight structural change found early in these cases. After rest in bed, the use of salines and hot applications to the abdominal wall, the symptoms subside in from three to ten days. At this time examination is painless, the structural lesions are plainly evident, and operation should be performed. In case the expectant plan fails, and the patient becomes progressively worse, in view of the possibility of general peritonitis, no time should be lost in opening the abdomen. Several cases were given in detail.

Dr. Charles P. Noble, in the discussion, said that increased experience led him to expect less from conservatism in gonorrheal salpingitis than formerly. He agreed with Dr. Anspach in his views regarding operation in acute gonorrheal peritonitis. He recalled having operated twice in the acute stage. · In one case the peritonitis was quite diffuse; the patient recovered; In the other there was a large abscess to the left of the sigmoid. This also recovered. One of Dr. Noble's

cases, in which the result of conservatism was good, was the case of a young woman who had acquired gonorrhea, and in which peritonitis resulted in an extraperitoneal abscess. He had operated in the acute attack, drained her vaginam, and to his surprise the patient made an excellent recovery. The woman has since been married and has borne children. Unless the patient is a young woman, it is Dr. Noble's rule to take out both tubes, the uterus and ovaries. Dr. Noble stated that he had never seen a patient die of gonorrheal peritonitis.

Dr. John G. Clark said that the reason the gonococcus did not produce general peritonitis was because its chief habitat is the mucous membrane. As quickly as the gonococcus leaves the Fallopian tubes and enters Douglas's cul-de-sac the peritonitis is merely toxic, due to the toxins of the gonococcus. He believed it unwise to operate during an attack of gonorrheal peritonitis. Illustrative of this he cited a case in which the symptoms had increased in severity, and the question arose whether there was simply a gonorrheal peritonitis, or involvement of the tubes and ovaries. Operation was done, the tubes and uterus being removed and the ovaries left. Subsequently the woman developed a large abscess involving the ovary. Opening of the incision and further drainage were necessary. He emphasized the necessity of a close differential diagnosis and the importance of knowing when to wait until the acute attack had passed, and when not to wait but to operate for a more lethal type of infection. For the past few years it has been Dr. Clark's desire to conserve all tissues possible, because the usual individual who contracts gonorrhea is a young woman. He feels that the conservative policy in some instances works splendidly, but in the majority of cases badly.

Dr. Edward Martin said that his experience in this class of cases in recent years had been only as long as was requisite to transfer the patient to the hands of a competent gynecologist, but that in earlier days he had seen a good many of such cases, which had made prompt recovery under conservative treatment of the acute attack.

Dr. Anspach, in closing, called attention to the fact that in a good many of these cases of acute pelvic peritonitis, due to gonorrhea, not much is gained by bimanual dilatation. While all the cases were correctly diagnosed, had he not had the history and seen the associated signs of the gonorrheal infection, he could not have formed much of an opinion.

Significance of Abulic Symptoms in Cases of Mental Disease.—Dr. Robert H. Chase stated that besides hysteria, where it strongly prevails, abulia is common in all forms of nervous and mental disease in which the chief characteristic is a weakening or exhaustion of the mental processes. It is particularly conspicuous in melancholia, dementia præcox, and in the depressive types of general paresis; in some conditions of neurasthenia and psychasthenia; in the intoxication of opium and alcohol; and in the retardation of manic-depressive insanity. He divides it into systematized, localized and general abulia. Under the systematized he gives the abulia of sleep. Among the forms of general abulia was given the intellectual type, in which the trouble lies in a defect of the attention. He spoke of the rôle that attention played in the normal mechanism of the mind; and under the term aprosexia he gave its various defects in disease.

Dr. Charles K. Mills, in the discussion, said he believed papers of this kind of great use, even to those not particularly interested in mental and nervous affections, and that if there were presented to the profession more frequently the methods of studying the mental symptoms there would be given a better insight to the cases of insanity and cases not so regarded. He considered the subject a large one from the standpoint of the alienist.

On the Advisability of a National Department of Public Health and a Medical Cabinet Officer.—Dr. T. H. Evans said this was suggested by the late Dr. William Pepper. The writer favors it as a means to centralize and render more effective the many interests of the country that are medical. The supervision of education of children, so as to suit individual tastes, needs and abilities, is indicated. Physicians ought to control all matters which concern the physiological welfare of the citizen. The care of criminals, once apprehended by the law, belongs properly to medicine. Colonies for mental and moral degenerates, if established, would materially reduce crime. The physical defects of children should be understood as productive of later immorality, or conducive to it, if suitable education does not intervene. Education and licensing of practitioners of medicine and surgery in the opinion of the author alone belong to a central office, whose executive head should have a place in the cabinet of the President.

Dr. Edward Martin felt that in the main all were in accord with the views of Dr. Evans. The question of education, however, he thought should be a matter of State control. In regard to criminals he thought the matter of imprisonment not so much one of punishment as of protection for the rest of the community, and that too much leniency has been allowed on a basis of mental defect. The idea of centralization he thinks is applicable to the subjects of sanitation and prophylaxis, particularly against contagious diseases, and in regard to such general subjects as water pollution. The establishment of a National board, he thought, was hoped for by all physicians.

Dr. Charles K. Mills believed that much could be accomplished by the establishment of a central health department of some description. It is, however, a question more difficult of solution than would seem to physicians, who have only the physicians' side of the subject before them. Personally he would be very glad to see the medical profession represented in the Cabinet, and believed much good might come from such movement. It might, however, be better if a department of science were created with bureaus of different sort, including a National Bureau of Health, which would take cognizance of matter of this sort. The great advantage of such an office would be the unifying of methods of procedure concerning matters of health in all parts of the country. With such a national organization much might be accomplished in matters of quarantine, the pollution of rivers, the registration and examination of physicians, and such questions as physicians have the first right to consider. Those who have committed crime should, if their mental and physical health is a matter of question, receive that attention which is often not given to them both before and after trial and after conviction. Such questions as the care of the insane, the care of epileptics, the commission of crime by the young would receive the more humane attention, if there were some method of regulating their consideration, and if that method were, in part at least, national and centralized.

Dr. William S. Wadsworth thought it appropriate that the Philadelphia County Medical Society should recognize the needs of the community for a larger, broader and more intelligent handling of State medicine. He thought it not possible for men unversed in medical science to take care of the lives of human beings.

Various questions which should come under the head of such a national executive department, mentioned by Dr. Wadsworth, are the adulteration of foods, the study of sewage, the protection of life on railroads and in factories, child labor, the importation of hides and such materials, the quality of drugs, and patent medicines. He regards as highly desirable the presence of a medical man in the Cabinet.

Stated Meeting, held December 28, 1904.

Vice-President B. Franklin Stahl, M.D., in the Chair.

Food-Preservatives and Food Adulteration.—Dr. H. W. Wiley, Chief of the Bureau of Chemistry of the United States Department of Agriculture (by invitation) read a paper on this subject. He said that the necessity of preserving food in some way had been recognized since man emerged from his savage state. The development of the science of chemistry had placed in the hands of the manufacturer the means of preserving food before unknown and the means of matching foods in tints and colors. He believes that the education of the public in regard to artificial coloring of foods to be quite as effective as legislation. After the 2d of February he said the food law would require that all food products entering this country artificially colored should bear a label so stating. The material for coloring need not be declared, except in the one case of sulphate of copper. His advice to food makers is to cease using colors, and especially if the coloring is under suspicion of any kind. Concerning antiseptics in relation to foods, he thinks the rights of the consumer are paramount. He believes that there never should be an antiseptic admitted to foods, except when absolutely necessary, unless the consumer orders it for himself. There is, he thinks, a legitimate use of sulphurous acid, as employed in the fumigation of dried fruits, and the burning of the sulphur match in wine barrels which method has come down from antiquity, but when it is used as at the present time in enormous excess for preserving a poor wine and putting on the market a new wine before it is ripened, he declares its use to be unpardonable. He believes that the application of the principle of honesty would cover all the needs of a food law. Were Dr. Wiley to write a food law it would require that every food product be marked and be exactly what it was said to be.

Defects in Pennsylvania Food Legislation.—William W. Smithers, Esq. (by invitation) read a paper by this title. He said that the laws upon this subject now being enforced in Pennsylvania are not the expression of the wishes of the people, and that they result in unnecessary interference with manufacturers and merchants. He advocated the repeal of the Act of 1895 and the enactment of laws based upon the preservation of health and protection against fraud. He stated his belief that the office of Dairy and Food Commissioner was unconstitutional: that the existing food statutes are imperfect and open to many just complaints, and declared that every effort should be made to secure reasonable and adequate legislation upon this important subject.

Evaluation of Evidence as to the Pharmacologic Action of Food Preservatives.—Dr. Thomas L. Coley stated that as an economic principle it is apparent that a nation of eighty million people could not be fed from the farm to the table or from the local abattoir to the table, and there arises the complex problem of transportation of food in an edible condition. The use of chemical preservatives therefore becomes a necessity. Dr. Coley went over the grounds upon which these are used and reviewed the chief objections against their use. The dangers arising. from reputably prepared food to which preservatives have been added, he said, was as nothing in comparison to the dangers from foods having undergone putrefactive changes. A problem of such importance should be settled by medical men and not in courts of law with a lay jury. Legislative enactments should not be made in advance of scientific knowledge. There must be disabuse of the mind of the criminality of intent on the part of reputable manufacturers and a sharp line should be drawn between adulteration and food preservation. The question to be decided is the action of very minute doses of food preservatives over a protracted period. In order to illustrate the faulty interpretations from research work undertaken on a wrong basis, Dr. Coley cited the papers of Pfeiffer, Kionka and Harrington dealing with sulphite of soda. In all of these studies the amount of the drug used was higher than that employed for preservative purposes; too great quantities of meat were fed to the animals and no variety of diet was allowed. Further, the animals were confined, of questionable health in the beginning of the experiments, and the deductions of these authors were not warranted as far as the use of sulphite of soda as a food preservative is concerned.

BOOK REVIEWS.

DUALITY OF THOUGHT AND LANGUAGE. By EMIL SUTRO. The Physio-Psychic Society, New York and Berlin.

THIS volume is said to "show the supremacy of spirit over matter in man," and perhaps it does. At least, far be it from a humble reviewer to say that it does not do that—or anything else that might be mentioned—since any given page in the book is capable of reducing to a state of hopeless bewilderment the said reviewer's intellect. Possibly this is due to an excess of the material in this particular personality; but at any rate it becomes necessary to leave to those with a different mental equipment, whether that difference be spiritual or something else, the elucidation of Mr. Sutro's views on "the voice of the esophagus" and kindred topics.

CLINICAL HEMATOLOGY. A Practical Guide to the Examination of the Blood with Reference to Diagnosis. By JOHN C. DA COSTA, JR., M.D., Demonstrator of Clinical Medicine, Jefferson Medical College, etc., Second Edition, Revised and Enlarged. P. Blakiston's Son & Co., Philadelphia.

HEMATOLOGY, as a special branch of clinical diagnosis, has now developed to such proportions that no one who has not devoted years of time to its pursuit can venture to speak with any degree of authority upon its problems. Moreover, the technic of the various methods now in vogue is so complex and so delicate that only a specialist can master them. It is, therefore, a source of great gratification that Da Costa has prepared a new edition of his excellent book on Clinical Hematology. There are few treatises either in English or in any other language in which scientific precision and thoroughness are united with so notable a gift for exposition. The morphological characteristics of the corpuscles in the various anemias and leucemias are presented in a simple and convincing fashion. The recent advances in hematology, comprising the identi-

fication of new clinical entities such as trypanosomiasis, kala azar, Montana fever and chronic polycythemia; the correlation of blood pictures with a number of diseases hitherto unstudied, such as chloroma, syphilitic infection, variola, etc., and the proof of the septic nature of many of the septic infections, are all incorporated in a thoroughly critical and sane manner in the new edition. Among the improvements in technic described are Wright's stain, Milan's method of estimating coagulation time, Reudiger's serum test, cryoscopy, etc. The book is in every way a worthy addition to the scientific and to the practical library of the physician.

POVERTY. By ROBERT HUNTER. The Macmillan Company, New York.

MR. HUNTER himself says of his work: "The book as a whole has one aim, namely, to show the grievous need of certain social measures calculated to prevent the ruin and degradation of those working-people who are on the verge of poverty." Certainly, if it does not fulfil its purpose wherever it is read, the fault must lie with the reader. It is, above all, a book calculated to make people think—people who might easily, otherwise, never come in contact with the vital questions which it raises. These questions are set forth in a fashion that any one can comprehend. Mr. Hunter's conclusions are supported by statistics enough to be convincing, but not of the labyrinthine sort with which specialists are prone to bewilder the layman.

On the other hand, although he deals with things which might well be spoken with fire in the heart and tears in the eyes, he shows an admirable restraint and balance. His long and varied experience would furnish dramatic instances enough to fill his book from cover to cover, but he uses such sparingly, and all the more effectively.

He has done a distinct public service in separating clearly for the popular mind the problems of poverty and those of pauperism. For those who complacently affirm that the provisions of charity in the present day are so generous and varied that no one need suffer, it is very salutary to be told that "even if this were true, it would not materially lessen the sorrow of the poor."

Mr. Hunter does speak, in the chapters on "The Pauper" and "The Vagrant," of those who are dependent upon charity; but the greater part of his work is concerned with those who keep just above the line of pauperism, who do not habitually apply for assistance, but who are continuously ill clothed, ill housed and ill nourished, in spite of their best efforts. To select for quotation any one of the points he makes in demonstrating the magnitude and significance of this class would be an injustice to the others; and the reviewer can only refer his readers to the book itself where the problems of poverty, as they concern the poor in general, and the sick, the child, and the immigrant in particular, are treated with a psychological and economic insight which never lacks sympathy, and a sympathy which never lacks wisdom or degenerates into sentimentality.

A COMPOUND OF MEDICAL LATIN. By W. T. ST. CLAIR, A.M. Second Edition, Revised. P. Blakiston's Son & Co., Philadelphia.

THIS is a useful little volume. For the medical student whose knowledge of the Latin language is limited to the few etymological roots acquired during his adolescence the work will be found of value. Even to the college graduate, for many have no knowledge of Latin, it will prove of service.

Lightning Source UK Ltd.
Milton Keynes UK
UKHW021325100219
336936UK00006B/544/P